Cancer Metabolism

Historical Landmarks, New Concepts, and Opportunities

A subject collection from *Cold Spring Harbor Perspectives in Medicine*

Cancer Metabolism

Historical Landmarks, New Concepts, and Opportunities

A subject collection from *Cold Spring Harbor Perspectives in Medicine*

EDITED BY

Navdeep S. Chandel
Northwestern University

Karen H. Vousden
The Francis Crick Institute

Ralph J. DeBerardinis
University of Texas Southwestern Medical Center

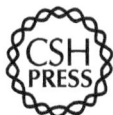

COLD SPRING HARBOR LABORATORY PRESS
Cold Spring Harbor, New York • www.cshlpress.org

Cancer Metabolism: Historical Landmarks, New Concepts, and Opportunities
A subject collection from *Cold Spring Harbor Perspectives in Medicine*
Articles online at www.cshperspectives.org

Executive Editor	Richard Sever
Project Supervisor	Barbara Acosta
Editorial Assistant	Danett Gil
Permissions Administrator	Carol Brown
Production Editor	Diane Schubach
Production Manager/Cover Designer	Denise Weiss
Publisher	John Inglis

Front cover artwork: Cover depicts cancer cells in the tumor microenvironment. Cover art created by Dr. Peter Jeffs (PeterJeffsArt.com).

Library of Congress Cataloging-in-Publication Data

Names: Chandel, Navdeep S. (Navdeep Singh), editor. | Vousden, Karen H., editor. | DeBerardinis, Ralph J., 1970- editor.
Title: Cancer metabolism : historical landmarks, new concepts, and opportunities / edited by Navdeep S. Chandel, Northwestern University, Karen H. Vousden, The Francis Crick Institute and Ralph J. DeBerardinis, University of Texas Southwestern Medical Center.
Description: Cold Spring Harbor, New York : Cold Spring Harbor Laboratory Press, [2025] | "A subject collection from Cold Spring Harbor Perspectives in Medicine." | Includes bibliographical references and index. | Summary: "Cancer cells display characteristic changes in metabolic pathways that may provide a growth advantage but also potentially make them vulnerable to therapies that target these pathways. This volume will discuss our knowledge of cancer cell metabolism and how this differs from processes in normal cells"-- Provided by publisher.
Identifiers: LCCN 2023048665 (print) | LCCN 2023048666 (ebook) | ISBN 9781621824701 (hardcover) | ISBN 9781621824718 (epub)
Subjects: LCSH: Cancer cells. | Cell metabolism. | Cancer cells--Growth. | Cancer cells--Growth--Regulation.
Classification: LCC RC269.7 .C366 2024 (print) | LCC RC269.7 (ebook) | DDC 616.99/4061--dc23/eng/20231201
LC record available at https://lccn.loc.gov/2023048665
LC ebook record available at https://lccn.loc.gov/2023048666

Contents

Contents

Preface

CANCER METABOLISM AS A DISCIPLINE predates the discovery that genetic mutations are causal drivers for tumor initiation and progression. In the 1920s, Otto Warburg, a pioneering biochemist, first noted that cancer cells preferentially consume glucose and produce lactate even in the presence of ample oxygen—a phenomenon now known as the Warburg effect. As genetics arrived and dominated our understanding of the molecular basis of cancer, interest in metabolism as a potential mechanistic driver of cancer waned. Even so, new diagnostic modalities like FDG-PET reinforced the basic premise of Warburg's work: that tumors display consistent metabolic differences from nonmalignant tissues, and that some of these differences could be exploited in the clinical arena.

Over the past 30 years or so, with the benefit of molecular tools and eventually new technologies in metabolic analysis, researchers have started to focus on why the Warburg effect is so pervasive in cancer cells and seems to provide a growth advantage to tumors. One prevailing theory is that high flow through glycolysis sustains the provision of glycolytic intermediates for anabolic pathways, supporting the synthesis of nucleotides, lipids, and amino acids essential for rapid cell proliferation. However, many recent studies have also positioned the mitochondria as central players in cancer metabolism. Traditionally seen as energy factories (the "powerhouse of the cell," in common parlance), mitochondria are now recognized for their roles in redox balance, in biosynthesis of macromolecules, and as signaling organelles controlling cell fate and function. They provide the necessary energy and building blocks for proliferating cancer cells while generating reactive oxygen species (ROS); these can function to promote oncogenic signaling while also inducing cell death, including ferroptosis.

Cancer cells, therefore, walk a metabolic tightrope, leveraging mitochondrial functions to their advantage while managing death-inducing ROS levels by increasing antioxidant levels to avoid self-destruction. Beyond their roles in biosynthesis and energy production, some metabolites promote tumor initiation and growth through signaling effects that influence gene expression and other activities beyond the traditional metabolic network. "Oncometabolites" like succinate, fumarate, and 2-hydroxyglutarate accumulate as a consequence of cancer-associated mutations in metabolic enzymes and inhibit α-ketoglutarate-dependent dioxygenases, leading to epigenetic changes that drive tumorigenesis.

Modern research has expanded on Warburg's findings, leading to the inescapable conclusion that "cancer metabolism" is far from uniform. Tumors exhibit an incredible degree of metabolic heterogeneity, not just between different types of cancer but sometimes even within different regions of the same tumor. This variability stems from a complex interplay of genetic mutations and environmental factors, producing distinct metabolic phenotypes that evolve as cancer progresses from localized disease that can often be cured by surgery to disseminated and therapeutically intractable metastatic disease. Understanding these shifting metabolic landscapes is crucial for developing targeted therapies.

The tumor microenvironment (TME) presents a unique set of challenges and opportunities for cancer cells. Nutrient availability in the TME is often limited, forcing cancer cells to adapt by activating nutrient-scavenging mechanisms such as autophagy and macropinocytosis. These pathways enable cancer cells to sustain growth under nutrient-deprived conditions and position metabolic adaptation as a mechanism of cancer progression. Interestingly, the metabolic demands and vulnerabilities of noncancerous cells within the TME, including immune cells, can also influence tumor progression.

Advances in our understanding of cancer metabolism have opened new avenues for therapy, particularly in targeting the selective metabolic dependencies of cancer cells. While early attempts at metabolic therapy faced challenges due to toxicity and metabolic plasticity, some modern approaches have been able to capitalize on tumor-specific liabilities. FDA-approved therapies in IDH-mutant leukemias capitalize on the fact that blocking mutant isoforms of these enzymes suppresses oncometabolite production. Moreover, combining metabolic therapies with standard treatments like chemotherapy, radiotherapy, and immunotherapy holds potential for more effective cancer treatment. Chemotherapy and radiotherapy target metabolic pathways and ROS biology, so identifying metabolic enzymes to enhance the efficacy of these therapies holds great promise. Moreover, a significant barrier to immunotherapy is overcoming the exhaustion of CD8 T cells, which have metabolic defects that could be strategically targeted.

The immense scope of metabolic heterogeneity in cancer means that a one-size-fits-all strategy is unlikely to succeed, however. A more personalized approach is necessary, where therapies are tailored to the specific metabolic vulnerabilities of a patient's tumor, particularly given the dynamic nature of cancer metabolism, which can change in response to treatment and disease progression. Diet plays a crucial role in influencing cancer metabolism, further complicating the relationship between nutrition and tumor growth. The future of cancer metabolism research lies in integrating advanced analytical techniques with patient stratification based on genetic mutations and other factors that govern metabolic dependencies. Using metabolomics, metabolic isotope tracers, and imaging technologies to map the metabolic landscape of tumors in real time could lead to the identification of predictive biomarkers and more effective therapeutic strategies.

In this book, a collection of chapters written by pioneers in the field of cancer metabolism highlight modern experiments that have revealed the many complexities of metabolic reprogramming during cancer initiation, progression, and metastasis, and identified opportunities to target these pathways for therapeutic benefit. An important legacy of research in cancer metabolism as highlighted in this book is that the ideas and techniques arising from this discipline have profoundly influenced numerous adjacent fields, including immunology, stem cell biology, and developmental biology. We are grateful to CSHL Press for allowing us to gather a collection of expert contributions and hope this book will be useful to new scientists entering the field. Maybe it will generate a small profit from CSHL Press for us to buy a glass of Bollinger champagne that the three of us can share.

NAVDEEP S. CHANDEL
KAREN H. VOUSDEN
RALPH J. DEBERARDINIS

Cancer Metabolism Historical Perspectives: A Chronicle of Controversies and Consensus

Chi V. Dang[1,2,3,4]

[1]Ludwig Institute for Cancer Research, New York, New York 10017, USA

[2]Department of Oncology, Johns Hopkins University School of Medicine, Baltimore, Maryland 21205, USA

[3]Department of Biochemistry and Molecular Biology, Johns Hopkins University Bloomberg School of Public Health, Baltimore, Maryland 21205, USA

[4]Bloomberg-Kimmel Institute for Cancer Immunotherapy, Sidney Kimmel Comprehensive Cancer Center, Johns Hopkins University, Baltimore, Maryland 21287, USA

Correspondence: cvdang@jhmi.edu; cdang@lcr.org

A century ago, Otto Warburg's work sparked the field of cancer metabolism, which has since taken a tortuous path. As evidence accumulated over the decades, consensus views of causes of cancer emerged, whereby genetic and epigenetic oncogenic drivers promoted immune evasion and induced new blood vessels and neoplastic metabolism to support tumor growth. Neoplastic cells abandon social cues of intercellular cooperation, escape tissue confinement, metastasize, and ultimately kill the host. Herein, key milestones in the study of cancer metabolism are chronicled with an emphasis on carbohydrate metabolism. The field began with a cancer cell–autonomous view that has been refined by a richer understanding of solid cancers as growing, immune-suppressive, complex organs comprising different cell types that are nourished by a variety of nutrients and variable amounts of oxygen through abnormal neovasculatures. Based on foundational historical studies, our current understanding of cancer metabolism offers a hopeful outlook for targeting metabolism to enhance cancer therapy.

The origin of life is thought to arise in part from a nascent nonenzymatic glycolytic pathway that is common to all self-sustaining life forms (Ralser 2018). In fact, the last hypothetical universal common ancestor (LUCA) of all cells is surmised to use nonoxidative sugar metabolism (Weiss et al. 2016). LUCA evolved long before the Great Oxidation Event resulting from the proliferation of photosynthetic organisms some 2.4 billion years ago (Holland 2006).

The availability of oxygen enabled the emergence of mitochondria as synthetic organelles to power eukaryotic metabolism and promote the evolution of metazoans. Oxygen availability also leads to reactive, toxic metabolic wastes. These byproducts, in addition to exogenous genotoxins, can corrupt the life-propagating encoded information, leading to cell growth arrest, death, or neoplastic cell transformation. In this way, the evolved metabolic processes of metazoans not only enable such complex life forms but also imperil them. In turn, deregulated neoplastic cell growth and proliferation also depend on these evolved metabolic pathways, but in ways that may distinguish neoplastic from physiologic metabolism.

EARLY CONCEPTS OF CANCER BIOLOGY

In 1885, Ernst Freund reported that blood glucose levels were elevated in individuals with cancer (Freund 1885) and proposed that glucose must sustain cancer. On this subject, the *New York Times* reported on December 23, 1887 that blood from the German Prince Frederick III, who married Queen Victoria's daughter, was to be analyzed for excess sugar to determine whether his laryngeal nodule was a cancer (Baron 1999). During this time, a small laryngeal biopsy by Morell Mackenzie, a leading head and neck surgeon sent by Queen Victoria, was rendered nonmalignant by Rudolph Virchow (Baron 1999). Based on the biopsy results, Mackenzie suggested that extensive surgical resection with high morbidity should not be undertaken. Unfortunately, for Prince Frederick, the nodule was not benign and progressive cancer was later diagnosed (Mackenzie 1888). The result of the Freund "diagnostic" blood test could not be found in the detailed Mackenzie report (Mackenzie 1888). In any event, the validity of Freund's test was questioned by a subsequent December 24, 1887 *New York Times* precis pointing to the possibility that the association of high blood sugar and cancer could be coincidental in patients with preexisting diabetes mellitus, and that one condition did not cause the other. Intriguingly, diabetes with hyperinsulinemia is now known to be a major risk factor for developing cancer (Gallagher and LeRoith 2020).

In parallel around the same time, some of the first information about cancer's interactions with the immune system and genomic alterations were uncovered. The surgeon William Coley noted that a patient with sarcoma underwent complete remission after a severe postsurgical wound infection with *Streptococcus pyogenes* and surmised that the infection was critical for the cure (Hoption Cann et al. 2003). In the 1890s, he developed a vaccine of killed bacteria (known as "Coley's toxins") to inoculate his patients and found complete remission of a sarcoma in his first patient. Arguably, this was the first cancer immunotherapy approach without the knowledge of the immediate cause of cancer or the role of tumor immunity. In 1902, Theodor Boveri speculated that malignant tumors could result from "certain abnormal chromosome constitution" based on his studies of chromosomes of fertilized urchin eggs and the appearance of tumor-like growths when chromosomes were present in imbalanced numbers (Boveri 2008), laying the groundwork for modern cancer genomics.

In the early 1900s, the cause of aneuploidy and the substance of heredity in chromosomes were unknown, but a clue for the cause of cancer was reported in a seminal 1911 paper (Rous 1911) by Peyton Rous, documenting that chicken tumor cell-free extracts can induce avian cancers. In this paper, Rous also noted spontaneous regression of these chicken tumors, which were found to have an "accumulation of lymphocytes," now known as tumor-infiltrating lymphocytes. Rous' observations were initially obscured but later led to the discovery of the Rous sarcoma virus, which proved to be foundational for the discovery of retroviral oncogenes.

The biochemistry of cancer was boosted by Otto Warburg who won the Nobel prize in 1931 for his discovery of cytochrome *c* oxidase (Warburg 1928). It was not his Nobel discovery, but a series of papers (Warburg 1930) in the 1920s underscoring the connection between altered glucose metabolism and cancer that brought Warburg into the limelight of cancer research. He provided evidence for what he believed to be the key cause of cancer—damaged cellular respiration.

In 1933, Hans Krebs found that among amino acids, glutamate-exposed guinea pig kidney consumed the most oxygen and noted an accompanying diminished ammonia level (Krebs 1935). In the same year, Dickens and Greville also noted that spleen, Jensen rat sarcoma, and rat or chick embryos produced large amounts of ammonia in the absence of sugar (Dickens and

Greville 1933). Krebs reported in 1935 the findings of an enzyme system for the synthesis of glutamine from glutamate and ammonia as well as the enzyme hydrolysis of glutamine, reversing the reaction (Krebs 1935). These observations documented the existence of glutamine synthetase and glutaminase, which are now known to play critical roles in tumor glutamine metabolism (Altman et al. 2016).

In 1945, Leuchtenberger and colleagues reported the striking finding of complete remissions of spontaneous murine mammary tumors treated with folic acid (Leuchtenberger et al. 1945). Based on these results, Sidney Farber treated 11 children with lethal acute lymphocytic leukemia (ALL) with folate and observed an "acceleration phenomenon" in the bone marrow of these patients (Farber 1949). This unexpected acceleration of the leukemia led Farber to the idea of using antifolates to treat leukemia. Farber reported clinical responses of childhood ALL to aminopterin in the landmark 1948 paper (Farber and Diamond 1948), underscoring the importance of inhibiting one-carbon metabolism in cancer and laying the foundation for modern chemotherapy (Stine et al. 2022). It should be noted that acute leukemias, which can proliferate in circulation, are distinctly different from solid tumors that have complex tumor microenvironments and grow slower. The rapid proliferation of leukemias requires heightened metabolism that renders them more responsive to cytotoxic therapies. A recent study using in vivo isotopic labeling and mass spectrometry (Fig. 1) underscores the difference between liquid and solid tumors, showing that tricarboxylic acid (TCA) cycling is higher in leukemia compared to solid tumors (Bartman et al. 2023).

Cancer neovascularization emerged in 1945 (Algire et al. 1945) as another key concept in cancer biology and one intimately connected to energy delivery and waste disposal. The work by Algire et al. recorded the appearance of new blood vessels in grafted normal tissues or tumor grafts. They observed that vascularization of normal transplanted tissues increased over a week and the emergence of arterioles and venules became visible. In contrast, tumors recruited new capillaries rapidly over 3 days evolving into large vessels that did not develop into arterioles or venules. The tumor neovasculature is disordered but the tumors continued to be able to recruit new vasculature as they grew (Folkman et al. 1971). Without neo-angiogenesis, solid tumors would be limited to sizes less than ∼200 μm in diameter, the limit of tissue oxygen diffusion (Carmeliet and Jain 2000).

In retrospect, synthesis of observations from the late 1800s into the 1950s provides a picture of solid cancer as a neoplastic mass, often with genomic changes, which can arise from a cell-free viral tumor extract, requires neovascularization, consumes glucose to produce lactate, consumes amino acids, converts glutamine to glutamate and ammonia, and is sensitive to one-carbon metabolism inhibition. The apparent conflicting observations that folate reduced the growth of mammary tumors but accelerated childhood leukemia suggest that fast-growing liquid tumors require folate for neoplastic growth and perhaps in the case of mammary tumors, folate may be required for the function of the antitumor arm of the immune system, although that was not appreciated at the time (Ron-Harel et al. 2016). More clearly, the observations of complete remissions induced by Coley's toxin underscored the importance of tumor immunity even before key concepts of innate and adaptive immunity were known.

OTTO WARBURG, CARL AND GERTY CORI, AND AEROBIC GLYCOLYSIS

Otto Warburg was a meticulous quantitative biochemist who innovated the "Warburg" manometric apparatus (Fig. 1A) that permitted precise measurements of glucose and oxygen consumption as well as carbon dioxide and lactate production by thin slices of normal or cancer tissues. His early studies of sea urchin eggs led to the finding that, upon fertilization, there was a rapid rise in oxygen consumption. Hence, he postulated that cancer tissue, being proliferative, would consume high amounts of oxygen relative to normal tissues. Instead of higher oxygen consumption, he reported in 1924 (Warburg 1930) that the Flexner–Jobling rat liver carcinoma tissue slices did not take up more oxygen than normal liver,

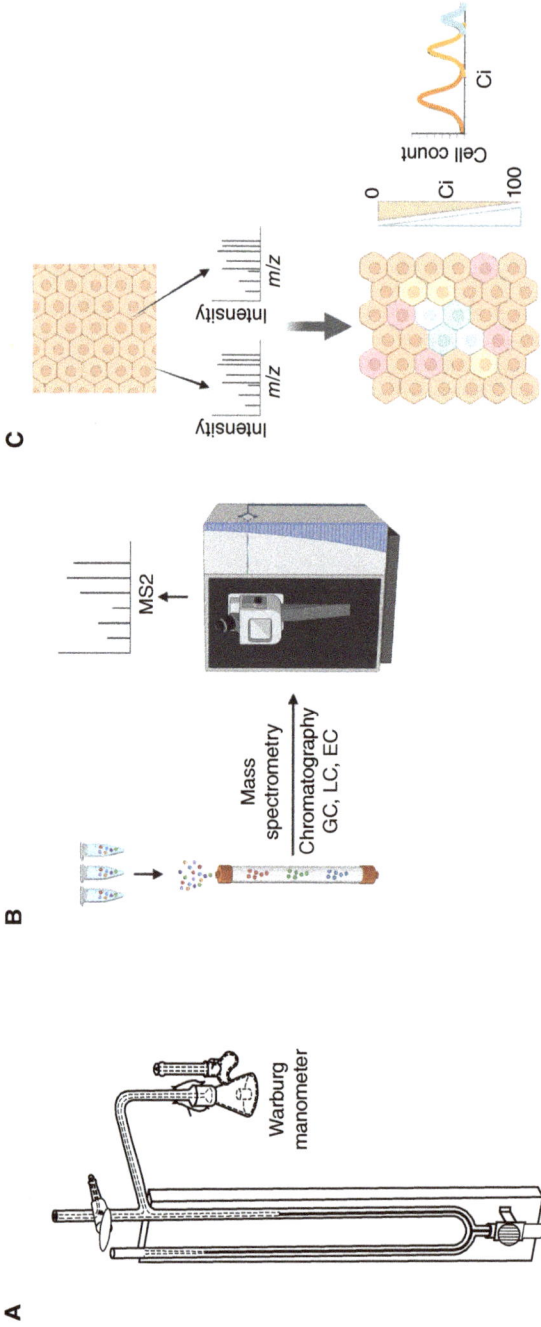

Figure 1. From Warburg manometer to mass spectrometry. Cancer metabolism research over the last century has been advanced by emerging technologies from the (*A*) Warburg manometer, to (*B*) mass spectrometry, and (*C*) illustration showing spatial mass spectrometry imaging of a tissue section that generates relative densities of metabolite signal intensity across the tissue section. The graph (*right*) depicts cell counts as a function of the distribution of signal intensities (Ci) of a metabolite. Each technological advance offers additional views of the complexity of cancer metabolism particularly in the context of the tumor immune microenvironment. (GC) Gas chromatography, (LC) liquid chromatography, (EC) electro-chemical. (Figure created with BioRender.com.)

Cite this article as *Cold Spring Harb Perspect Med* doi: 10.1101/cshperspect.a041530

but rather the carcinoma produced more lactate than normal liver under oxygenated conditions (Warburg 1925). Known as the Pasteur effect first described in 1861 (Racker 1974), oxygen was documented to suppress glycolysis in yeast. The converse whereby glucose suppresses respiration is known as the Crabtree effect (Crabtree 1929). As such, the heightened glycolytic feature in cancer tissues bypasses the Pasteur effect resulting in aerobic glycolysis, the ability to undergo glycolysis in the presence of oxygen that was coined the "Warburg effect" by Efraim Racker (Fig. 2; Racker 1972).

The propensity of cancers to take up glucose avidly and convert the vast majority to lactate, or the Warburg effect, became a paradigm for cancer research in the early and mid-1900s. This concept, generated largely from in vitro experiments, was studied in tumors by Carl and Gerty Cori and reported in 1925 (Cori and Cori 1925a, b). They found that glucose levels tend to be diminished in mouse and rat tumors compared to normal muscle. Likewise, tumor lactate levels were diminished compared to muscle in fasting animals. Hence, they reasoned that tumor lactate might be washed away by blood circulation and surmised that an increase in glucose by intraperitoneal injection could reveal the propensity of tumors to produce high lactate levels. Indeed, when glucose was administered, tumor glucose levels rose significantly and were accompanied by an elevation of tumor lactate, a phenomenon that was not seen with normal liver. Further, they found that blood lactate levels were more elevated in tumor-bearing animals than in non-tumor-bearing animals after glucose administration. Thus, they concluded that the in vivo experiments were not contradictory to the in vitro findings of Warburg, but rather the production of tumor lactate depends on the availability of circulating glucose. Their continued studies of glucose and lactate metabolism led to the 1947 Nobel prize discovery of the Cori cycle (Cori and Cori 1929), the conversion of glucose by muscle to lactate that in turn is converted to liver glycogen, which can be mobilized to produce circulating glucose (Fig. 3A).

Corroborating earlier studies of Rous sarcomas (Cori and Cori 1925b), Warburg and colleagues published in 1927 (Warburg et al. 1927) the study of tumor metabolism in vivo. The experimental approach was meticulous, requiring the dissection of normal or tumor arterial and venous vessels from the anesthetized animal for the collection of efferent and afferent blood (Fig. 3A). The major blood vessels were sampled, and a drop in glucose level was found in each case from the arterial to venous side. Compared to these normal differences in glucose levels, the drop across Jensen sarcomas were pronounced, suggesting that the consumption of glucose was higher in the tumor. When measuring arteriovenous differences in lactic acid level, they found that most organs consumed lactate, except for the brain (i.e., comparing levels in arterial vs. venous "Jugularis"). In contrast to evidence of lactate consumption by normal tissues, in all 10 Jensen tumors, venous lactate was much higher than arterial levels, indicating that Jensen tumors consumed glucose and produced lactate. These studies corroborated the findings by the Coris a few years earlier (Cori and Cori 1925b) and supported the notion of the Warburg effect in tumors (Fig. 3A). Intriguingly, these historical studies are now largely substantiated by more sophisticated mass spectrometry (Fig. 1B) with the use of isotopically labeled substrates such as glucose, lactate, or 2-deoxyglucose and modeling of metabolite distributions in vivo (Faubert et al. 2017; Liu et al. 2020; Bartman et al. 2023). Although lactate produced from glucose can be oxidized by tumors (Faubert et al. 2017), the Warburg effect has been documented in solid tumor models (Bartman et al. 2023), underscored by the utility of ^{18}F-2-deoxyglucose clinical imaging of human cancers (Fig. 3B; Som et al. 1980; Nolop et al. 1987).

CANCER METABOLISM CONTROVERSIES

The dogma of the Warburg effect providing an oversimplified view of cancer metabolism began to be challenged with controversies that crescendoed into the 1960s. Crabtree sought to determine whether Warburg metabolism is an "exclusive feature of malignant tissues" and whether anaerobic versus aerobic glycolysis have any relationships to the magnitude of respiration

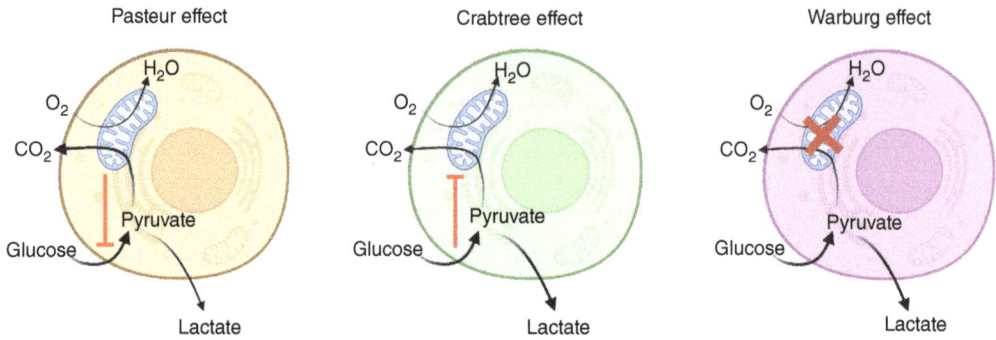

Figure 2. Pasteur, Crabtree, and Warburg effects. Generalized mammalian cells are depicted with the consumption of glucose through mitochondrial oxidation or glycolysis. Pasteur described the ability of oxygen to suppress yeast glycolysis that produces ethanol (not lactate as illustrated for mammalian cells), a phenomenon known as the Pasteur effect. Conversely, Crabtree found that some yeast strains demonstrated the ability of glucose to suppress respiration, known as the Crabtree effect. Warburg hypothesized that damaged mitochondria in cancer cells result in enhanced aerobic glycolysis, which bypasses the Pasteur effect, termed the Warburg effect. (Figure created with BioRender.com.)

(Crabtree 1928). Crabtree cited several publications documenting that nonmalignant tissues, such as the retina, placenta, and leukocytes, have high aerobic glycolysis, thereby questioning the validity of the Warburg hypothesis. Further, Crabtree used the Warburg manometer to study infectious nonmalignant lesions, such as pigeon pox, chicken vaccinia, or human warts or papillomas. He found that the excess glycolysis in pigeon pox slices was in the same order as those found by Warburg for tumor slices. Crabtree documented the elevation of glycolysis in Rous sarcoma tumors but surmised from his findings that changes accompanying the Warburg effect "… are not specific for malignant tissues but are a common feature of pathological overgrowths." Crabtree's historical findings presaged later studies that document virus-induced cellular glycolytic metabolism (Bissell et al. 1972; Thai et al. 2014).

The debate on the role of the Warburg effect in malignancies continued with camps on both sides digging into their positions. In studies of normal and tumor tissues, Elliott and Baker (1935) did not find differences in the Warburg effect between normal and tumor tissues (Elliott and Baker 1935) as compared to studies by Dickens (Dodds and Dickens 1940). Further, Boyland reported for the British Empire Cancer Campaign in 1940 and mentioned glycolysis, which

can be high in normal tissues, and hence is "… therefore impossible to consider this characteristic to be peculiar to tumours" (Boyland 1940a). This report resulted in a debate in *Nature* (March 30, 1940) between Dickens and Boyland about the merits of the Warburg effect in cancer (Boyland 1940b).

The ongoing debate on the Warburg effect was punctuated by Warburg's 1956 Science article that provided an overview titled "On the Origin of Cancer Cells" (Warburg 1956). He wrote with dogmatic authority, unshaken by contradictory data, that cancer cells have injured respiration (Fig. 2), and the resulting aerobic glycolysis causes cancer. He dismissed the roles of carcinogens and viruses in cancer, stating that "From this point of view, mutation and carcinogenic agent are not alternatives, but empty words, unless metabolically specified. Even more harmful in the struggle against cancer can be the continual discovery of miscellaneous cancer agents and cancer viruses, which, by obscuring the underlying phenomena, may hinder necessary preventive measures and thereby become responsible for cancer cases." Warburg's views on damaged respiration that drives glycolysis as a cause of cancer were challenged by Sidney Weinhouse (Weinhouse 1956) citing that isotope tracer studies revealed no difference between tumor and normal tissue in their conversion of glucose to

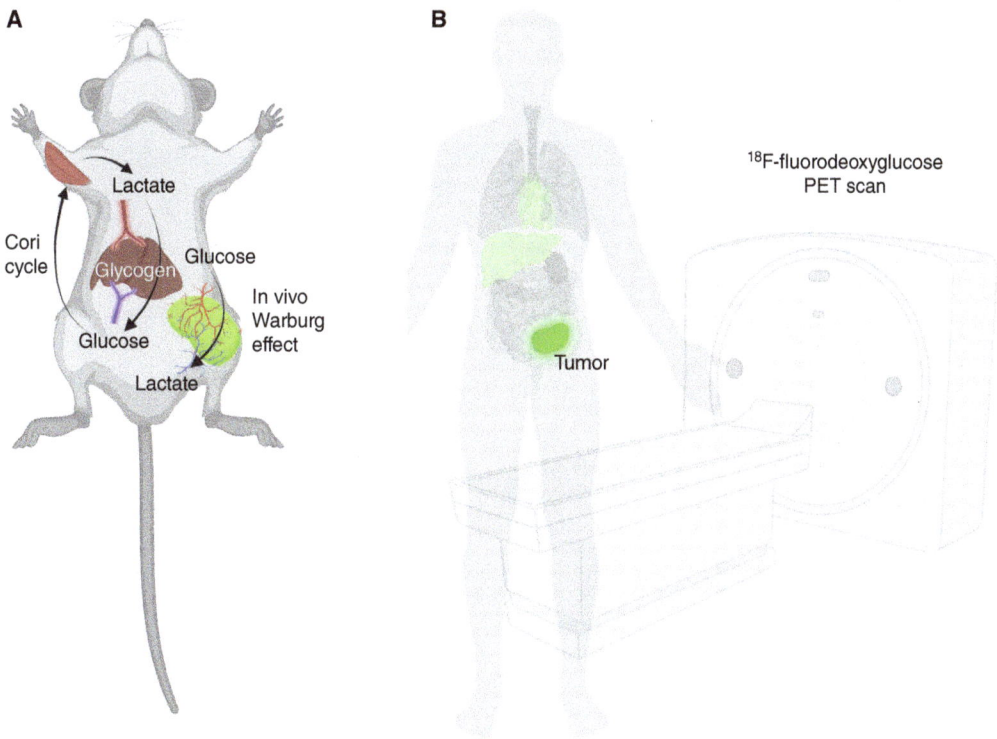

Figure 3. In vivo Warburg effect, the Cori cycle, and in vivo cancer positron emission tomography (PET) imaging. (A) By sampling arterial and venous blood across rodent normal organs, such as the liver, and tumors (green), Crabtree observed that increased glucose resulted in a higher lactate venous output from tumors than normal tissues, which tend to take up lactate from arterial blood. Warburg also documented that tumors have a propensity to convert high levels of glucose to lactate in vivo. In the case of liver, glycogen is produced through gluconeogenesis from muscle-generated lactate and in turn glucose released from glycogen can then be used by muscle in an interorgan circuit termed the Cori cycle. (B) The Warburg effect is exploited clinically to diagnose and monitor human cancers using an ^{18}F-fluorodeoxyglucose PET scan. Normal heart and liver also accumulate ^{18}F-labeled deoxyglucose, but tumors tend to have abnormally high uptake of the tracer (green). (Figure created with BioRender.com.)

carbon dioxide. Dean Burk (Burk and Schade 1956), another key figure, tipped the scale toward Warburg's aerobic glycolysis as a feature of cancer, but Burk acknowledged the validity of Weinhouse's objection to the concept of damaged mitochondria as a driver for malignancies. Warburg was wrong to dismiss an active role of mitochondria in tumorigenesis, in particular, since evidence shows the importance of mitochondrial function in cancer (Vasan et al. 2020).

Efraim Racker was a prolific biochemist who contributed fundamental insights into carbohydrate metabolism. His entry into cancer metabolism began with fundamental studies of glycolysis in the Ehrlich ascites tumor cells,

demonstrating that the conversion of glucose to lactate in cell extracts could be enhanced by the additional of purified phosphofructokinase and glyceraldehyde-3-phosphate dehydrogenase together with hexokinase, thereby defining the limiting glycolytic steps in ascites tumor extracts (Wu and Racker 1959). Skeptical of Warburg's damaged mitochondria hypothesis, Racker proposed that there are multiple causes of cancer, which share in common inefficient sodium-potassium ATPase pumps associated with aerobic glycolysis (Racker 1972). In 1981, Racker and Spector (1981) reported that the Src oncogenic kinase phosphorylates and suppresses the ATPase pump and thereby promotes aerobic glycolysis. This putative first link between an onco-gene and the Warburg effect further overshadows observations of aerobic glycolysis in normal cells, such as mitogen-activated lymphocytes (Hedeskov 1968) that in retrospect were perhaps the first reported glimpse of immunometabolism.

Racker's striking report of a link between an oncogene and tumor metabolism was, unfortunately, the result of scientific misconduct by his graduate student Spector (Racker 1989). The harbinger of misconduct was uncovered by the finding that [125]Iodine was spiked in his student's experiments to mimic the results of ^{32}P in the phosphorylation studies. The notion that Src drives the Warburg effect evaporated with this scandal. However, in 1983, Cooper in Hunter's laboratory and colleagues (Cooper et al. 1983) reported that enolase, phosphoglycerate kinase, and lactate dehydrogenase (LDH) were tyrosine phosphorylated in cells transformed by the Rous sarcoma virus bearing the v-Scr oncogene, but the functional significance was unclear. During this time, an early study of positron emission tomography (PET) using ^{18}F-fluoro-2-deoxy-glucose (FDG) showed enhanced glucose tumor uptake, assumed to be the Warburg effect, correlated with the degree of malignancy of cerebral gliomas (Di Chiro et al. 1982). The use of FDG PET (Fig. 3B) to detect altered cancer metabolism expanded (Hillner et al. 2008) and is now a standard of practice in clinical oncology.

The Warburg effect controversies distracted the literature from the key findings of Krebs (1935) and Dickens (Dodds and Dickens 1940) on the conversion of glutamine to glutamate and ammonia by normal tissues and the Jensen rat sarcoma. Glutamine was further shown by Eagle and coworkers in 1956 to be essential for mammalian cell growth in vitro (Eagle et al. 1956), providing the basis for Basal Medium Eagle. In 1983, consumption of glutamine was found to be increased in stimulated rat lymphocytes resulting in the production of glutamate, aspartate, and ammonia (Ardawi and Newsholme 1983). Brand reported (Brand et al. 1984) that concanavalin A–activated lymphocytes increased expression of glycolytic enzymes, enhancing glucose metabolism by 54-fold, whereby glucose was converted 90% to lactate and 1% was consumed for respi-

ration. This contrasts with resting lymphocytes that oxidize 27% of the glucose to CO_2. Glutamine use increased by eightfold in stimulated lymphocytes, producing glutamate, ammonia, aspartate, and CO_2. These foundational observations were largely forgotten in the current literature, but undoubtedly paved the way for recent studies on the use of glucose and glutamine for cancer metabolism (Cairns et al. 2011; DeBerardinis and Chandel 2016; Pavlova et al. 2022). In this respect, a recent tumor nutrient-partitioning study documents highest use of glutamine by tumor cells versus highest use of glucose by tumor myeloid cells in a mouse syngeneic MC38 colon tumor cell model (Reinfeld et al. 2021).

Warburg's controversial views on carbohydrate metabolism as the primary cause of cancer dominated the dialog on the biochemistry of cancer and ushered in an era of research on cancer metabolic pathways until the late 1970s when proto-oncogenes were discovered as precursors of viral oncogenes that drive neoplastic transformation. At the turn of the decade, in the 1980s, many oncogenes were discovered and documented to be altered in human cancers, opening a new chapter in cancer research focusing on the genetics of cancer (Varmus 1984). At this point, the interest in metabolism began to wane partly due to controversies over Warburg's dogmatic views and whether cancer metabolism is any different than normal metabolism. The field of cancer metabolism was further displaced by the view that oncogenes and tumor suppressors are the primary drivers of cancer with metabolism playing a subservient role to genetics.

ONCOGENES, TUMOR SUPPRESSORS, AND ALTERED TUMOR METABOLISM

The Src oncogene, fraudulently linked to the Warburg effect by Spector, appeared again with Ras in 1987, when Flier and coworkers (Flier et al. 1987) reported that rodent fibroblasts transfected with these oncogenes increased the mRNA expression of a glucose transporter and had increased uptake of 2-deoxyglucose. This connection between oncogenes and glucose uptake was further supported by the finding in 1989 that Ras and c-Mos-transformed NIH3T3 fibroblasts expressed more GADPH than control cells (Persons et al. 1989). Intriguingly, Myc expression did not result in increased glucose transporter expression or glucose uptake in the Flier study (Flier et al. 1987), but the levels of GAPDH in NIH3T3 appeared to correlate with Myc expression in the Persons study (Persons et al. 1989). However, the detailed mechanistic links between these oncogenes and elevation of the glucose transporter mRNA were missing. Within a decade of these findings, Myc-dependent genes in Myc-transformed Rat1a fibroblasts were identified based on the notion that the product of the MYC oncogene behaves as a transcription factor (Kato et al. 1990; Lewis et al. 1997).

To identify Myc-responsive genes, control or anchorage-independent Myc-transformed Rat1a fibroblasts were grown in suspension cultures. Through representational difference analysis, a form of PCR-assisted subtraction cloning, over 20 putative Myc-responsive genes were identified (Lewis et al. 1997). Among these, lactate dehydrogenase A (LDHA) was transcriptionally induced in Rat1a-Myc cells as evidenced by nuclear run-on assays and Myc-binding sites that are required for Myc transactivation of an LDHA promoter-luciferase reporter (Shim et al. 1997). Importantly, Myc transformation was dependent on LDHA. The finding of LDHA among putative Myc target genes functionally linked Myc to the Warburg effect, providing a firm mechanistic link between an oncogene and aerobic glycolysis. Semenza and coworkers (Wang et al. 1995) cloned the hypoxia-inducible factor (HIF) gene, which was shown to induce the expression of many glycolytic genes under hypoxic conditions (Firth et al. 1994; Semenza et al. 1994). The induction of these genes by HIF to mediate anaerobic glycolysis contrasts with the ability of Myc to induce glycolysis under aerobic conditions (Dang and Semenza 1999).

In addition to the hypoxic stabilization of HIF-1α and HIF-2α proteins, HIF-1 is also thought to be stabilized by upstream oncogenic signaling. In this regard, HIF-driven metabolic rewiring downstream of oncogenic drivers contributes to neoplastic glycolytic metabolism and angiogenesis. Activation of mTORC1 by amino acids and growth signaling through RHEB induces glucose metabolism through increasing Myc and HIF-1α activity and expression (Düvel et al. 2010). It is intriguing to note that MYC is central to PI3K inhibitor resistance (Muellner et al. 2011) and oncogenic alterations of metabolism downstream of PI3K-Akt (Hoxhaj and Manning 2020). Moreover, RAS induces pancreatic cancer glycolytic metabolism (Reinfeld et al. 2021) in a MYC-dependent manner (Ying et al. 2012). In this context, it should be noted that the RAS-ERK pathway has been shown to increase Myc expression and protein levels (Farrell and Sears 2014). As such, the potential collaboration between MYC and HIF signaling downstream of oncogenic pathways could be central to the Warburg effect seen in different cancers.

Subsequent to the observation on MYC-associated, glucose-deprivation-induced cell death (Shim et al. 1998), MYC overexpressing human cells were found to be addicted to glutamine (Yuneva et al. 2007), suggesting a role for MYC in regulating glutamine metabolism. In this respect, the Thompson (Wise et al. 2008) and Dang (Gao et al. 2009) laboratories independently reported the regulation of glutaminolysis by MYC, which activates glutaminase for the conversion of glutamine to glutamate and subsequent catabolism through the TCA cycle. Further, MYC is broadly involved in regulating many metabolic pathways including nucleotide and lipid metabolism (Dang 2012).

Based on their studies of the metabolism of activated T cells, Thompson and coworkers in 2002 reported that costimulation via CD28 triggered a PI3K-Akt-dependent activation of glycolysis (Frauwirth et al. 2002). While Akt was a known oncogene, first identified as the cellular homolog of v-Akt found in the rodent AKT8 retrovirus, activating mutations of PIK3Ca (PI3K) in human cancers were not reported until 2004 (Samuels et al. 2004). In this respect, activated Akt was documented to drive aerobic glycolysis (Elstrom et al. 2004) and subsequent studies underscore the ability of Akt to directly phosphorylate and activate HK2 and PFKBP2 (Hoxhaj and Manning 2020).

Loss-of-function of tumor suppressors also contributes to altered oncogenic metabolism

(Levine and Puzio-Kuter 2010; Humpton and Vousden 2016). For example, increased expression of the tumor suppressor PTEN, which opposes PI3K, resulted in heightened oxidative metabolism in vivo (Garcia-Cao et al. 2012), which is the phenotypic converse of the activation of glycolysis by PI3K (Hu et al. 2016). The tumor suppressor p53 tends to diminish glycolysis in favor of a more heightened oxidative metabolism (Humpton and Vousden 2016). This is in part driven by p53 activation of TIGAR as reported (Bensaad et al. 2006). Further, p53 induces synthesis of cytochrome c oxidase (SCO2) to drive mitochondrial respiration, such that loss of wild-type p53 decreased SCO2 expression, resulting in increased glycolysis (Matoba et al. 2006). Conversely, mitochondrial function affects p53 response. Inhibition of mitochondrial complex III or dihydroorotate dehydrogenase (DHODH) activity depletes pyrimidines and activates p53 (Ladds et al. 2018; Mick et al. 2020). In this respect, p53 is both downstream and upstream of metabolic perturbations. The tumor-suppressive effects of tuberous sclerosis complex TSC1 and TSC2 and alteration of metabolism are largely through their ability to inhibit mTOR activity (Manning and Cantley 2003). The tumor suppressor retinoblastoma (RB) has been implicated in glutamine metabolism, such that loss of Rb enhanced E2F-mediated expression of ASCT2- and E2F-independent increase in GLS (Reynolds et al. 2014).

Intriguingly, at the same time that canonical oncogenes were shown to impact metabolism, several core metabolic enzymes were shown to behave as tumor suppressors. Inherited mutations of several nuclear-encoded mitochondrial components, including succinate dehydrogenase subunits SDHB, SDHC, and SDHD and fumarate hydratase (FH), predispose to family syndromes of cancers such as pheochromocytoma, paraganglioma, leiomyosarcoma, and chromophobe renal cell carcinoma (Gottlieb and Tomlinson 2005). These findings suggest that these enzymes are tumor suppressive and the mechanism underlying their tumor-suppression function in part involves HIF stabilization (Selak et al. 2005) and epigenetic modification. For example, SDH mutation causes an accumulation

of succinate, which inhibits α-ketoglutarate-dependent prolyl hydroxylases and stabilizes HIF-1α (Selak et al. 2005), whereas FH mutations cause an accumulate of fumarate, which inhibits α-ketoglutarate-dependent demethylases and leads to epigenomic alterations that drive epithelial–mesenchymal transition (EMT) (Sciacovelli et al. 2016). These direct links between metabolic enzyme mutations and familial cancer underscore the importance of metabolic perturbation as a cancer driver.

EMERGING CANCER METABOLISM CONSENSUS

Considering general principles, it is apt to distinguish between maintenance and proliferative metabolism (Vander Heiden et al. 2009). Maintenance metabolism is required to sustain and renew cellular structures and functions by providing ATP to support membrane potentials and protein synthesis. These processes are diurnally dynamic, driven by the circadian clock core transcription factor Clock:Bmal1, whose oncogenic perturbation is documented (Sancar and Van Gelder 2021). As such, normal metabolic studies in vivo can be affected by this diurnal fluctuation that enables daily oscillation of cellular metabolism to synchronize with organismal feeding and fasting cycles.

Proliferative metabolism, on the other hand, can result from normal growth signaling such as activation of T cells, proliferation of bone marrow cells required to replace cellular blood components, or proliferation of the gut epithelium. Upon growth stimulation, signaling through Ras-MEK-ERK signaling cascade activates and stabilizes MYC to induce metabolic and growth-related mRNAs such as those for glucose or amino acid transporter to import nutrients for cell growth (Dang 2012). The influx of amino acids and growth signal transduction through PI3K-Akt-TSC2-RHEB activates mTOR to induce translation and protein synthesis (Cantor and Sabatini 2012). Together, MYC and mTOR can be envisioned to amplify transcription and translation (Hoxhaj and Manning 2020), respectively, of growth signaling and drive proliferative metabolism (Fig. 4). The hypoxia-independent

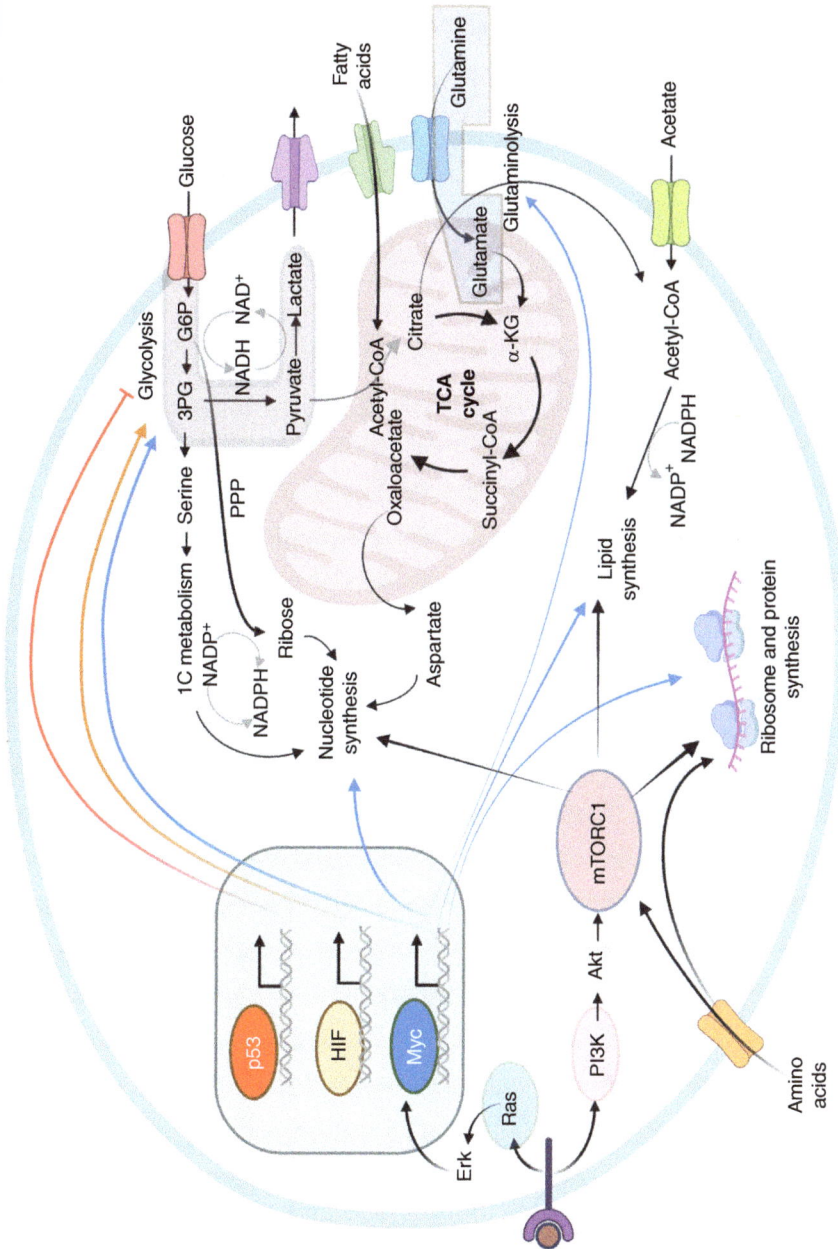

Figure 4. Oncogenic alterations of metabolism. The diagram shows a cell with an activated growth factor receptor (*left*) triggering signal transduction down the Ras-MEK-Erk pathway to activate Myc. Growth signal is also transmitted down the PI3K-Akt pathway to activate mTORC1, which senses amino acids for full activation. Myc, in turn, activates genes involved in anabolic metabolism, driving glycolysis, glutaminolysis, nucleotide, lipid, and protein synthesis. mTORC1 amplifies growth signaling by stimulating translation and protein synthesis for mass accumulation that includes its direct activation of nucleotide and lipid synthesis. The hypoxia-inducible factor (HIF) can be induced by mTORC1 and stabilized under hypoxia to induce anaerobic glycolysis. On the other hand, the tumor suppressor p53 suppresses glycolysis and induces mitochondrial respiration. Note that the prevalent human oncogenes Ras and PI3K are upstream of Myc and mTORC1, enabling transcriptional and translational amplification of oncogenic cell growth and proliferation. Fatty acids as an energy source through oxidation is depicted. (1C) One-carbon, (PPP) pentose phosphate pathway. (Figure created with BioRender.com.)

stabilization of HIF-1 is not necessary but can contribute to proliferative metabolism and induction of tumor neovascularization (Fig. 4). Tumor suppressors such as PTEN and TSC2 attenuate the growth signaling pathways driven by PI3K and mTORC1, respectively (Cantor and Sabatini 2012). Hence, loss of these tumor suppressors increased signaling through these oncogenic pathways and their effects on metabolism. P53 can attenuate Myc function by sensing an overactive Myc-Arf axis (Zindy et al. 1998) or suppress proliferation by sensing DNA replication or ribosomal stress (Lindström et al. 2022). p53 can sense ribosomal stress when MDM2 is bound to specific ribosomal subunits and release p53 from its grip. Increased p53 function, in turn, inhibits glycolysis and increases respiration (Fig. 4).

A key question is whether there are key differences between normal proliferative versus oncogenic metabolism (Vander Heiden et al. 2009). As discussed previously, the Warburg effect can be observed in cancers and normal tissues. For example, whereas resting T cells use less glycolysis and rely on oxidative metabolism, T-cell receptor (TCR) stimulation of murine T cells induces a proliferative metabolic program resembling that of malignant lymphocytes (Madden and Rathmell 2021). Specifically, stimulation of T cells with anti-CD3 and anti-CD28 drives glycolysis and glutaminolysis in a Myc-dependent fashion that enables proliferation, which does not depend on HIF-1α (Fig. 5A; Wang et al. 2011). Upon withdrawal of stimulation, T cells undergo apoptosis and some attain a resting memory oxidative metabolic state. In contrast to normal T cells, oncogenic NOTCH-driven T-cell lymphomas are dependent on constitutive MYC expression, which drives a constitutive proliferation metabolic profile that cannot return to a resting state (Zhou et al. 2022). In this regard, a difference in normal versus neoplastic proliferative metabolism is that the former can be turned off. In contrast, the latter is constitutively turned on, rendering the malignant state addicted to a constant supply of nutrients. Normal cells have mechanisms that sense nutrient deprivation such as AMPK, which can induce cell growth arrest. However, MYC-addicted cells are vulner-

able to glucose or glutamine deprivation–induced cell death as are AKT-addicted cells (Shim et al. 1998; Elstrom et al. 2004; Yuneva et al. 2007). Given these observations, are there sufficient therapeutic indices to exploit metabolism for cancer therapy?

METABOLIC THERAPY AND LESSONS LEARNED

When considering metabolic vulnerabilities of cancers, recent studies have highlighted the importance of tissue-specific metabolic effects of oncogenic drivers, metabolic plasticity, diet, as well as the impact of these features on the microbiome and antitumor immunity. Different oncogenes induce different metabolic profiles in the same organ. For example, in contrast to MYC, which drives glutamine and glucose metabolism in MYC-inducible liver cancer, MET oncogene-driven liver cancer expresses glutamine synthetase and hence appears less dependent on exogenous glutamine (Yuneva et al. 2012). On the other hand, the same oncogene can induce different metabolic effects in different tissues. Kras effects on branched chain amino metabolism are different in Kras, p53-loss-driven murine pancreatic adenocarcinoma versus non-small-cell lung cancer (NSCLC) (Mayers et al. 2016). In the former, branched chain amino acid (BCAA) uptake is diminished, whereas in NSCLC, the tumors incorporate BCAA into proteins. Hence, tissue-specific effects of oncogenes add to the complexity of tumor metabolism in vivo when considering the metabolic vulnerabilities of cancers.

Metabolic plasticity (Fendt et al. 2020) and metabolic stress such as activation of AMPK or the integrated stress-response pathways induce resistance to inhibition of cancer metabolism (Costa-Mattioli and Walter 2020). Metabolic plasticity was elegantly illustrated by Yuneva and coworkers using a MYC-inducible model of mouse HCC (Méndez-Lucas et al. 2020). They demonstrated that lost glutaminase (Gls) extended survival as seen with pharmacological Gls inhibition (Xiang et al. 2015). However, loss of hexokinase 2 (Hk2) did not extend survival. Intriguingly, loss of both Gls and Hk2 further

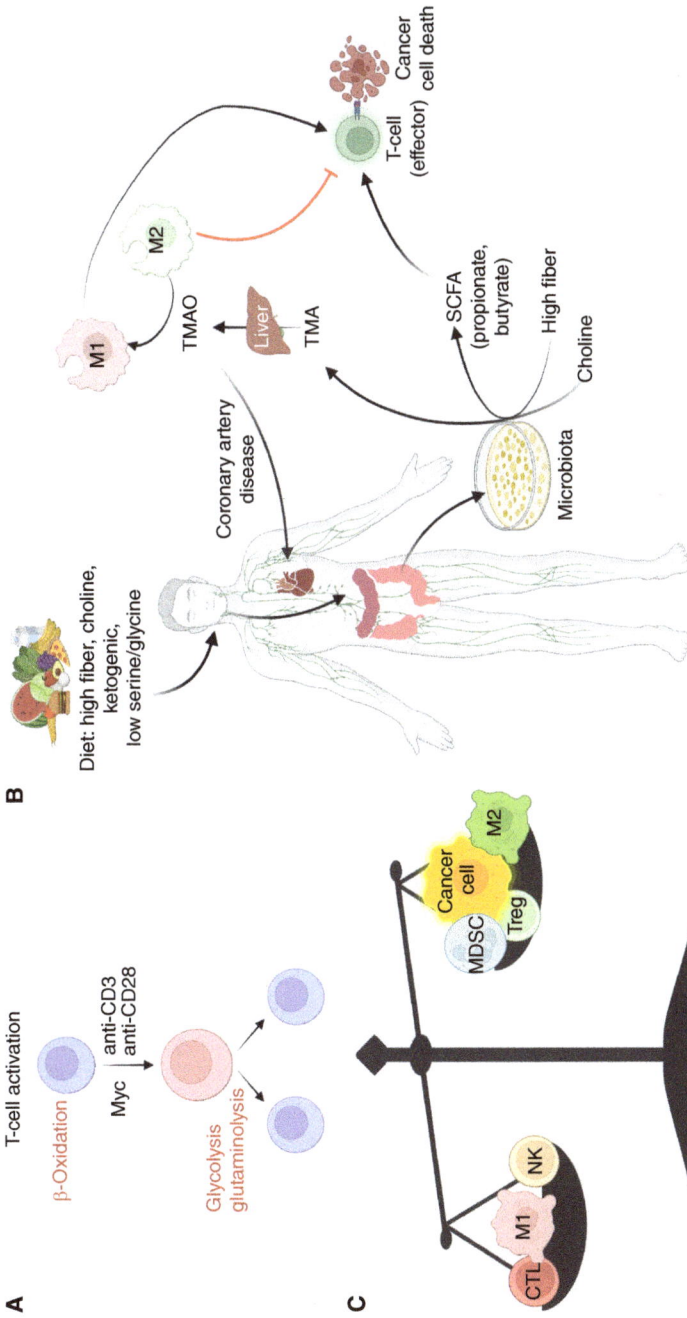

Figure 5. T-cell activation and the effect of diets on tumor and immune cell metabolism and fate. (*A*) Anti-CD3 plus anti-CD28 activation of resting primary murine T cells, which respires via β-oxidation, requires Myc, which activates glycolysis and glutaminolysis to drive biomass accumulation for cell proliferation. (*B*) Dietary high fiber or choline is shown to produce microbial short chain fatty acids (SCFAs) or trimethylamine (TMA) and liver-derived trimethylamine oxide (TMAO). SCFAs activate effector T cells, whereas TMAO polarizes macrophages toward inflammatory M1 states that increase coronary artery inflammation or enhance immune checkpoint blockade cancer therapy. Ketogenic diet affects the gut microbiota and tumor immunity; results from ongoing clinical studies are pending. Whether a serine/glycine deprivation diet proves to increase cancer therapy response in humans remains to be established. (*C*) The illustration depicts a scale balancing cells that have antitumor activity, such as cytotoxic CD8+ T cells (CD8), natural killer (NK) cells, or inflammatory M1 macrophages, versus cells, such as myeloid-derived suppressor cells (MDSCs), regulatory T (Treg) cells, or alternatively activated M2 macrophages that assist cancer cell growth. (CTL) Cytotoxic T-lymphocyte. (Figure created with BioRender.com.)

extended survival, but these double-knockout (KO) tumors eventually caused the demise of their hosts, indicating yet other ways that allow for neoplastic cells to circumvent metabolic blocks. This genetic evidence for metabolic plasticity is underscored by the cooperation between metabolic inhibitors, such as a combination of inhibitors of LDH and mitochondrial complex I, to slow tumor growth (Oshima et al. 2020).

Whereas loss of Hk2 did not extend survival of MYC-induced HCC, Hk2 is documented to be required for initiation and maintenance of murine KRas-driven lung cancer and ErbB2-driven breast cancer (Patra et al. 2013). Further, systemic deletion of Hk2 also reduced tumorigenesis in a diethylnitrosamine-induced murine model of HCC (DeWaal et al. 2018), and, importantly, loss of Hk2 did not affect T-cell proliferation or T-cell-mediated viral immunity (Mehta et al. 2018). Notably, some human multiple myelomas do not express hexokinase 1 and are highly sensitive to decreased HK2 (Xu et al. 2019). These observations suggest that HK2 is an example of an enzyme that appears to be cancer specific.

Under nutrient-depleted conditions, decreased mTOR activity and activation of AMPK induce ULK activity to drive autophagy, whereby autophagosomes are formed and destined for lysosomal degradation to recycle metabolites for survival (Onodera and Ohsumi 2005; Rabinowitz and White 2010). Further, mitophagy—a form of autophagy—is necessary to cull dysfunctional mitochondria. The maintenance of an $NAD^+/NADH$ ratio $\gg 1$ to drive oxidative anabolism is essential for cell function. As such, under nutrient deprivation, autophagy maintains NAD^+ levels (Kataura et al. 2022). When the conversion of NADH to NAD^+ is saturated via mitochondrial NADH malate-aspartate and glycerol-3-phosphate dehydrogenase shuttles, aerobic glycolysis is induced to regenerate cytosolic NAD^+ to drive GADPH-mediated catalysis (Wang et al. 2022). Hence, pathways that can regenerate cytosolic NAD^+ when NADH is in excess could increase in activity when other pathways are limited. Excessive NADH levels induce reductive stress (Mick et al. 2020) and activate as the transcriptional

corepressor CtBP to generate an adaptive transcriptome (Di et al. 2013).

In the study of MYC-driven murine liver cancer (Méndez-Lucas et al. 2020), the loss of Psat1, which drives one-carbon metabolism through serine and glycine, did not affect survival. However, withdrawal of serine and glycine from the diet as done previously by Vousden et al. (Maddocks et al. 2017) prolonged the survival of Psat KO but not wild-type tumor-bearing animals (Méndez-Lucas et al. 2020). These findings underscore that the effect of diet depends on the metabolic wiring of the tumor cells (Kalaany and Sabatini 2009; Lien and Vander Heiden 2019). What was not accounted for in these studies is the effect of diet on the host microbiome or immunity. Since the availability of dietary L-serine can affect the gut microbiota during inflammation (Kitamoto et al. 2020), whether a serine/glycine deprivation diet influences tumor immunity beyond a cancer cell–autonomous effect remains to be established. In this regard, the ketogenic diet can alter the host microbiome (Fig. 5B; Ang et al. 2020) and curb several models of mouse tumorigenesis. Ketogenic diet curbs tumor growth in a model of mouse pancreatic adenocarcinoma in combination with chemotherapy (Yang et al. 2022). Further, this combination also worked in immunocompromised mice, but sustained response was observed only in mice with an intact immune system. Intriguingly, a ketogenic diet alters gut and serum metabolome in dogs with implications on tumor immunity (Allenspach et al. 2022).

Dietary choline can induce inflammation through its conversion to trimethylamine (TMA) by the gut microbiota, and in turn oxidized by the liver to trimethylamine oxide (TMAO), which is well-implicated in provoking coronary artery disease (Wang et al. 2015). Dietary choline or administration of TMAO induces inflammatory M1 macrophages (Fig. 5B) that increase graft-versus-host response as well as response of tumors to immune checkpoint blockade (Wu et al. 2020; Mirji et al. 2022). As such, there is much more to learn about the effects of components of diet, such as high fiber content that generates microbial short chain fatty acids with immune modulatory activities (Fig. 5B), on

Cite this article as *Cold Spring Harb Perspect Med* doi: 10.1101/cshperspect.a041530

the microbiota that in turn increase cancer therapy responses (He et al. 2021; Spencer et al. 2021).

The idea of targeting metabolism for cancer treatment was championed by Sidney Farber who targeted nucleotide synthesis with the "anti-metabolite" aminopterin and subsequently methotrexate, which is still used clinically (Farber and Diamond 1948; Farber 1949). Together with asparaginase, an active therapy in lymphoblastic leukemias, this demonstrates that metabolic therapies can be active anticancer agents. However, other metabolic therapies have proven less efficacious. The fact that 2-deoxyglucose can inhibit glycolysis made it a candidate for studies in cancer patients, but studies from decades ago showed that it did not produce clear benefit, and patients had side effects such as diaphoresis (Landau et al. 1958). Likewise, the glutamine analog 6-diazo-5-oxo-1-norleucine (DON), which targets a multitude of glutamine using enzymes and hence is imprecise, was also tested in humans, but it appeared too toxic for clinical use (Magill et al. 1957). It is notable that a DON prodrug has significant preclinical efficacy against several tumor models in immunocompetent mice (Leone et al. 2019). Whether clinical trials on DON prodrug prove to be effective remains to be seen. Recent failures of metabolic inhibitors in the clinic result from either lack of activity or intolerable side effects. For example, CB-839, which is a highly specific glutaminase (GLS) inhibitor with little associated side effects, failed in a study of patients with renal cell carcinoma due to a lack of efficacy (Tannir et al. 2022). The use of the mitochondrial complex I inhibitor IACS-07549 failed in clinical studies because of neurotoxicity (Yap et al. 2023). However, an exception is the successful implementation of specific inhibitors for mutant isocitrate dehydrogenases, IDH1 and IDH2, for the treatment of cancers such as acute myelogenous leukemia (DiNardo et al. 2018). Here, the therapeutic index is widened by the specificity of the drugs for mutant versus wild-type enzymes.

CONCLUDING REMARKS

Over the past century, Warburg's studies on cancer metabolism and those reporting the use of Coley's toxin for cancer therapy lay the foundation for current studies that offer a hopeful outlook for new cancer therapeutic opportunities. Given the profound success of cancer immunotherapy, it should be noted that the use of metabolic inhibitors can interfere with or potentiate the antitumor arm of the immune system (Leone et al. 2019; Hermans et al. 2020). As such, the development of metabolic inhibitors to target cancer cells should also account for its potential adverse effect on antitumor immunity (Fig. 5C). Notably, a major challenge to effective immunotherapy is tumor acidity (Boedtkjer and Pedersen 2020; Tu et al. 2021; Gillies et al. 2022), whose mitigation in the clinical setting has not been sufficiently addressed by current research. The rapid improvement of mass spectrometry imaging (Ma and Fernández 2022) of tissues down to the single-cell level should provide the spatial resolution necessary to gain a richer understanding of the tumor immune microenvironment metabolic states (Fig. 1C) and potentially expose novel cancer metabolic vulnerabilities. The emerging field of immunometabolism (Buck et al. 2017; Leone and Powell 2020; Madden and Rathmell 2021; Stine et al. 2022) offers a richer understanding of metabolic vulnerabilities of immune versus cancer cells that is anticipated to provide novel druggable opportunities to enhance immunity while diminishing cancer cell viability.

ACKNOWLEDGMENTS

This historical perspective is from one viewpoint, and I realize that there may be alternative perspectives of the development of the field of cancer metabolism. In this respect, citations are limited and not meant to be comprehensive. I thank Adam Wolpaw, Rajeshkumar NV, and Zach Stine for comments. This work is supported in part by a Bloomberg Distinguished Professorship at Johns Hopkins, the Ludwig Institute for Cancer Research, and NCI grants R01 CA252225, CA051497, and CA053741.

REFERENCES

Algire GH, Chalkley HW, Legllais FY, Park HD. 1945. Vasculae reactions of normal and malignant tissues in vivo. I: Vascular reactions of mice to wounds and to normal and neoplastic transplants. *J Natl Cancer Inst* **6:** 73–85. doi:10 .1093/jnci/6.1.73

Allenspach K, Borcherding DC, Iennarella-Servantez CA, Mosichuk AP, Atherly T, Sahoo DK, Kathrani A, Suchodolski JS, Bourgois-Mochel A, Serao MR, et al. 2022. Ketogenic diets in healthy dogs induce gut and serum metabolome changes suggestive of anti-tumourigenic effects: a model for human ketotherapy trials. *Clin Transl Med* **12:** e1047. doi:10.1002/ctm2.1047

Altman BJ, Stine ZE, Dang CV. 2016. From Krebs to clinic: glutamine metabolism to cancer therapy. *Nat Rev Cancer* **16:** 619–634. doi:10.1038/nrc.2016.71

Ang QY, Alexander M, Newman JC, Tian Y, Cai J, Upadhyay V, Turnbaugh JA, Verdin E, Hall KD, Leibel RL, et al. 2020. Ketogenic diets alter the gut microbiome resulting in decreased intestinal Th17 cells. *Cell* **181:** 1263–1275. e16. doi:10.1016/j.cell.2020.04.027

Ardawi MS, Newsholme EA. 1983. Glutamine metabolism in lymphocytes of the rat. *Biochem J* **212:** 835–842. doi:10 .1042/bj2120835

Baron DN. 1999. A surgical mishap. *BMJ* **319:** 1360. doi:10 .1136/bmj.319.7221.1360

Bartman CR, Weilandt DR, Shen Y, Lee WD, Han Y, TeSlaa T, Jankowski CSR, Samarah L, Park NR, da Silva-Diz V, et al. 2023. Slow TCA flux and ATP production in primary solid tumours but not metastases. *Nature* **614:** 349–357. doi:10.1038/s41586-022-05661-6

Bensaad K, Tsuruta A, Selak MA, Vidal MN, Nakano K, Bartrons R, Gottlieb E, Vousden KH. 2006. TIGAR, a p53-inducible regulator of glycolysis and apoptosis. *Cell* **126:** 107–120. doi:10.1016/j.cell.2006.05.036

Bissell MJ, Hatie C, Rubin H. 1972. Patterns of glucose metabolism in normal and virus-transformed chick cells in tissue culture. *J Natl Cancer Inst* **49:** 555–565.

Boedtkjer E, Pedersen SF. 2020. The acidic tumor microenvironment as a driver of cancer. *Annu Rev Physiol* **82:** 103–126. doi:10.1146/annurev-physiol-021119-034627

Boveri T. 2008. Concerning the origin of malignant tumours by Theodor Boveri (translated and annotated by Henry Harris). *J Cell Sci* **121:** 1–84. doi:10.1242/jcs.025742

Boyland E. 1940a. The British Empire cancer campaign. *Nature* **145:** 246–248. doi:10.1038/145246a0

Boyland E. 1940b. Metabolism of tumours. *Nature* **145:** 513. doi:10.1038/145513a0

Brand K, Williams JF, Weidemann MJ. 1984. Glucose and glutamine metabolism in rat thymocytes. *Biochem J* **221:** 471–475. doi:10.1042/bj2210471

Buck MD, Sowell RT, Kaech SM, Pearce EL. 2017. Metabolic instruction of immunity. *Cell* **169:** 570–586. doi:10.1016/j .cell.2017.04.004

Burk D, Schade AL. 1956. On respiratory impairment in cancer cells. *Science* **124:** 270–272. doi:10.1126/science .124.3215.270

Cairns RA, Harris IS, Mak TW. 2011. Regulation of cancer cell metabolism. *Nat Rev Cancer* **11:** 85–95. doi:10.1038/ nrc2981

Cantor JR, Sabatini DM. 2012. Cancer cell metabolism: one hallmark, many faces. *Cancer Discov* **2:** 881–898. doi:10 .1158/2159-8290.CD-12-0345

Carmeliet P, Jain RK. 2000. Angiogenesis in cancer and other diseases. *Nature* **407:** 249–257. doi:10.1038/35025220

Cooper JA, Reiss NA, Schwartz RJ, Hunter T. 1983. Three glycolytic enzymes are phosphorylated at tyrosine in cells transformed by Rous sarcoma virus. *Nature* **302:** 218–223. doi:10.1038/302218a0

Cori CF, Cori GT. 1925a. The carbohydrate metabolism of tumors. I: The free sugar, lactic acid, and glycogen content of malignant tumors. *J Biol Chem* **64:** 11–22. doi:10.1016/ S0021-9258(18)84944-4

Cori CF, Cori GT. 1925b. The carbohydrate metabolism of tumors. II: Changes in the sugar, lactic acid, and CO_2 combining power of blood passing through a tumor. *J Biol Chem* **65:** 397–405. doi:10.1016/S0021-9258(18)84849-9

Cori CF, Cori GT. 1929. Glycogen formation in the liver from *d*- and *l*-lactic acid. *J Biol Chem* **81:** 389–403. doi:10.1016/ S0021-9258(18)83822-4

Costa-Mattioli M, Walter P. 2020. The integrated stress response: from mechanism to disease. *Science* **368:** eaat5314. doi:10.1126/science.aat5314

Crabtree HG. 1928. The carbohydrate metabolism of certain pathological overgrowths. *Biochem J* **22:** 1289–1298. doi:10.1042/bj0221289

Crabtree HG. 1929. Observations on the carbohydrate metabolism of tumours. *Biochem J* **23:** 536–545. doi:10.1042/ bj0230536

Dang CV. 2012. MYC on the path to cancer. *Cell* **149:** 22–35. doi:10.1016/j.cell.2012.03.003

Dang CV, Semenza GL. 1999. Oncogenic alterations of metabolism. *Trends Biochem Sci* **24:** 68–72. doi:10.1016/ S0968-0004(98)01344-9

DeBerardinis RJ, Chandel NS. 2016. Fundamentals of cancer metabolism. *Sci Adv* **2:** e1600200. doi:10.1126/sciadv .1600200

DeWaal D, Nogueira V, Terry AR, Patra KC, Jeon SM, Guzman G, Au J, Long CP, Antoniewicz MR, Hay N. 2018. Hexokinase-2 depletion inhibits glycolysis and induces oxidative phosphorylation in hepatocellular carcinoma and sensitizes to metformin. *Nat Commun* **9:** 446. doi:10.1038/s41467-017-02733-4

Di LJ, Byun JS, Wong MM, Wakano C, Taylor T, Bilke S, Baek S, Hunter K, Yang H, Lee M, et al. 2013. Genomewide profiles of CtBP link metabolism with genome stability and epithelial reprogramming in breast cancer. *Nat Commun* **4:** 1449. doi:10.1038/ncomms2438

Di Chiro G, DeLaPaz RL, Brooks RA, Sokoloff L, Kornblith PL, Smith BH, Patronas NJ, Kufta CV, Kessler RM, Johnston GS, et al. 1982. Glucose utilization of cerebral gliomas measured by ^{18}F-fluorodeoxyglucose and positron emission tomography. *Neurology* **32:** 1323–1323. doi:10 .1212/WNL.32.12.1323

Dickens F, Greville GD. 1933. Metabolism of normal and tumour tissue: ammonia and urea formation. *Biochem J* **27:** 1123–1133. doi:10.1042/bj0271123

DiNardo CD, Stein EM, de Botton S, Roboz GJ, Altman JK, Mims AS, Swords R, Collins RH, Mannis GN, Pollyea DA, et al. 2018. Durable remissions with ivosidenib in *IDH1*-mutated relapsed or refractory AML. *N Engl J Med* **378:** 2386–2398. doi:10.1056/NEJMoa1716984

Dodds EC, Dickens F. 1940. The biochemistry of malignant tissue. *Annu Rev Biochem* **9:** 423–458. doi:10.1146/an nurev.bi.09.070140.002231

Cite this article as *Cold Spring Harb Perspect Med* doi: 10.1101/cshperspect.a041530

Düvel K, Yecies JL, Menon S, Raman P, Lipovsky AI, Souza AL, Triantafellow E, Ma Q, Gorski R, Cleaver S, et al. 2010. Activation of a metabolic gene regulatory network downstream of mTOR complex 1. *Mol Cell* **39:** 171–183. doi:10.1016/j.molcel.2010.06.022

Eagle H, Oyama VI, Levy M, Horton CL, Fleischman R. 1956. The growth response of mammalian cells in tissue culture to L-glutamine and L-glutamic acid. *J Biol Chem* **218:** 607–616. doi:10.1016/S0021-9258(18)65826-0

Elliott KA, Baker Z. 1935. The respiratory quotients of normal and tumour tissue. *Biochem J* **29:** 2433–2441. doi:10.1042/bj0292433

Elstrom RL, Bauer DE, Buzzai M, Karnauskas R, Harris MH, Plas DR, Zhuang H, Cinalli RM, Alavi A, Rudin CM, et al. 2004. Akt stimulates aerobic glycolysis in cancer cells. *Cancer Res* **64:** 3892–3899. doi:10.1158/0008-5472.CAN-03-2904

Farber S. 1949. Some observations on the effect of folic acid antagonists on acute leukemia and other forms of incurable cancer. *Blood* **4:** 160–167. doi:10.1182/blood.V4.2.160.160

Farber S, Diamond LK. 1948. Temporary remissions in acute leukemia in children produced by folic acid antagonist, 4-aminopteroyl-glutamic acid. *N Engl J Med* **238:** 787–793. doi:10.1056/NEJM194806032382301

Farrell AS, Sears RC. 2014. MYC degradation. *Cold Spring Harb Perspect Med* **4:** a014365. doi:10.1101/cshperspect.a014365

Faubert B, Li KY, Cai L, Hensley CT, Kim J, Zacharias LG, Yang C, Do QN, Doucette S, Burguete D, et al. 2017. Lactate metabolism in human lung tumors. *Cell* **171:** 358–371.e9. doi:10.1016/j.cell.2017.09.019

Fendt SM, Frezza C, Erez A. 2020. Targeting metabolic plasticity and flexibility dynamics for cancer therapy. *Cancer Discov* **10:** 1797–1807. doi:10.1158/2159-8290.CD-20-0844

Firth JD, Ebert BL, Pugh CW, Ratcliffe PJ. 1994. Oxygen-regulated control elements in the phosphoglycerate kinase 1 and lactate dehydrogenase A genes: similarities with the erythropoietin 3′ enhancer. *Proc Natl Acad Sci* **91:** 6496–6500. doi:10.1073/pnas.91.14.6496

Flier JS, Mueckler MM, Usher P, Lodish HF. 1987. Elevated levels of glucose transport and transporter messenger RNA are induced by ras or src oncogenes. *Science* **235:** 1492–1495. doi:10.1126/science.3103217

Folkman J, Merler E, Abernathy C, Williams G. 1971. Isolation of a tumor factor responsible for angiogenesis. *J Exp Med* **133:** 275–288. doi:10.1084/jem.133.2.275

Frauwirth KA, Riley JL, Harris MH, Parry RV, Rathmell JC, Plas DR, Elstrom RL, June CH, Thompson CB. 2002. The CD28 signaling pathway regulates glucose metabolism. *Immunity* **16:** 769–777. doi:10.1016/S1074-7613(02)00323-0

Freund E. 1885. Zur diagnose des karzinoms [To diagnose carcinomas]. *Wiener Medizinische Blätter* **9:** 268–269.

Gallagher EJ, LeRoith D. 2020. Hyperinsulinaemia in cancer. *Nat Rev Cancer* **20:** 629–644. doi:10.1038/s41568-020-0295-5

Gao P, Tchernyshyov I, Chang TC, Lee YS, Kita K, Ochi T, Zeller KI, De Marzo AM, Van Eyk JE, Mendell JT, et al. 2009. c-Myc suppression of miR-23a/b enhances mitochondrial glutaminase expression and glutamine metabolism. *Nature* **458:** 762–765. doi:10.1038/nature07823

Garcia-Cao I, Song MS, Hobbs RM, Laurent G, Giorgi C, de Boer VC, Anastasiou D, Ito K, Sasaki AT, Rameh L, et al. 2012. Systemic elevation of PTEN induces a tumor-suppressive metabolic state. *Cell* **149:** 49–62. doi:10.1016/j.cell.2012.02.030

Gillies RJ, Ibrahim-Hashim A, Ordway B, Gatenby RA. 2022. Back to basic: trials and tribulations of alkalizing agents in cancer. *Front Oncol* **12:** 981718. doi:10.3389/fonc.2022.981718

Gottlieb E, Tomlinson IP. 2005. Mitochondrial tumour suppressors: a genetic and biochemical update. *Nat Rev Cancer* **5:** 857–866. doi:10.1038/nrc1737

He Y, Fu L, Li Y, Wang W, Gong M, Zhang J, Dong X, Huang J, Wang Q, Mackay CR, et al. 2021. Gut microbial metabolites facilitate anticancer therapy efficacy by modulating cytotoxic CD8+ T cell immunity. *Cell Metab* **33:** 988–1000.e7. doi:10.1016/j.cmet.2021.03.002

Hedeskov CJ. 1968. Early effects of phytohaemagglutinin on glucose metabolism of normal human lymphocytes. *Biochem J* **110:** 373–380. doi:10.1042/bj1100373

Hermans D, Gautam S, García-Cañaveras JC, Gromer D, Mitra S, Spolski R, Li P, Christensen S, Nguyen R, Lin JX, et al. 2020. Lactate dehydrogenase inhibition synergizes with IL-21 to promote CD8+ T cell stemness and antitumor immunity. *Proc Natl Acad Sci* **117:** 6047–6055. doi:10.1073/pnas.1920413117

Hillner BE, Siegel BA, Liu D, Shields AF, Gareen IF, Hanna L, Stine SH, Coleman RE. 2008. Impact of positron emission tomography/computed tomography and positron emission tomography (PET) alone on expected management of patients with cancer: initial results from the National Oncologic PET Registry. *J Clin Oncol* **26:** 2155–2161. doi:10.1200/JCO.2007.14.5631

Holland HD. 2006. The oxygenation of the atmosphere and oceans. *Philos Trans R Soc Lond B Biol Sci* **361:** 903–915. doi:10.1098/rstb.2006.1838

Hoption Cann SA, van Netten JP, van Netten C. 2003. Dr William Coley and tumour regression: a place in history or in the future. *Postgrad Med J* **79:** 672–680. doi:10.1093/postgradmedj/79.938.672

Hoxhaj G, Manning BD. 2020. The PI3K-AKT network at the interface of oncogenic signalling and cancer metabolism. *Nat Rev Cancer* **20:** 74–88. doi:10.1038/s41568-019-0216-7

Hu H, Juvekar A, Lyssiotis CA, Lien EC, Albeck JG, Oh D, Varma G, Hung YP, Ullas S, Lauring J, et al. 2016. Phosphoinositide 3-kinase regulates glycolysis through mobilization of aldolase from the actin cytoskeleton. *Cell* **164:** 433–446. doi:10.1016/j.cell.2015.12.042

Humpton TJ, Vousden KH. 2016. Regulation of cellular metabolism and hypoxia by p53. *Cold Spring Harb Perspect Med* **6:** a026146. doi:10.1101/cshperspect.a026146

Kalaany NY, Sabatini DM. 2009. Tumours with PI3K activation are resistant to dietary restriction. *Nature* **458:** 725–731. doi:10.1038/nature07782

Kataura T, Sedlackova L, Otten EG, Kumari R, Shapira D, Scialo F, Stefanatos R, Ishikawa KI, Kelly G, Seranova E, et al. 2022. Autophagy promotes cell survival by maintaining NAD levels. *Dev Cell* **57:** 2584–2598.e11. doi:10.1016/j.devcel.2022.10.008

Kato GJ, Barrett J, Villa-Garcia M, Dang CV. 1990. An amino-terminal c-myc domain required for neoplastic transformation activates transcription. *Mol Cell Biol* **10**: 5914–5920.

Kitamoto S, Alteri CJ, Rodrigues M, Nagao-Kitamoto H, Sugihara K, Himpsl SD, Bazzi M, Miyoshi M, Nishioka T, Hayashi A, et al. 2020. Dietary L-serine confers a competitive fitness advantage to Enterobacteriaceae in the inflamed gut. *Nat Microbiol* **5**: 116–125. doi:10.1038/s41564-019-0591-6

Krebs HA. 1935. Metabolism of amino acids: the synthesis of glutamine from glutamic acid and ammonia, and the enzymic hydrolysis of glutamine in animal tissues. *Biochem J* **29**: 1951–1969. doi:10.1042/bj0291951

Ladds M, van Leeuwen IMM, Drummond CJ, Chu S, Healy AR, Popova G, Pastor Fernández A, Mollick T, Darekar S, Sedimbi SK, et al. 2018. A DHODH inhibitor increases p53 synthesis and enhances tumor cell killing by p53 degradation blockage. *Nat Commun* **9**: 1107. doi:10.1038/s41467-018-03441-3

Landau BR, Laszlo J, Stengle J, Burk D. 1958. Certain metabolic and pharmacologic effects in cancer patients given infusions of 2-deoxy-D-glucose. *J Natl Cancer Inst* **21**: 485–494.

Leone RD, Powell JD. 2020. Metabolism of immune cells in cancer. *Nat Rev Cancer* **20**: 516–531. doi:10.1038/s41568-020-0273-y

Leone RD, Zhao L, Englert JM, Sun IM, Oh MH, Sun IH, Arwood ML, Bettencourt IA, Patel CH, Wen J, et al. 2019. Glutamine blockade induces divergent metabolic programs to overcome tumor immune evasion. *Science* **366**: 1013–1021. doi:10.1126/science.aav2588

Leuchtenberger R, Leuchtenberger C, Laszlo D, Lewisohn R. 1945. The influence of "folic acid" on spontaneous breast cancers in mice. *Science* **101**: 46. doi:10.1126/science.101.2611.46.a

Levine AJ, Puzio-Kuter AM. 2010. The control of the metabolic switch in cancers by oncogenes and tumor suppressor genes. *Science* **330**: 1340–1344. doi:10.1126/science.1193494

Lewis BC, Shim H, Li Q, Wu CS, Lee LA, Maity A, Dang CV. 1997. Identification of putative c-Myc-responsive genes: characterization of *rcl*, a novel growth-related gene. *Mol Cell Biol* **17**: 4967–4978. doi:10.1128/MCB.17.9.4967

Lien EC, Vander Heiden MG. 2019. A framework for examining how diet impacts tumour metabolism. *Nat Rev Cancer* **19**: 651–661. doi:10.1038/s41568-019-0198-5

Lindström MS, Bartek J, Maya-Mendoza A. 2022. P53 at the crossroad of DNA replication and ribosome biogenesis stress pathways. *Cell Death Differ* **29**: 972–982. doi:10.1038/s41418-022-00999-w

Liu S, Dai Z, Cooper DE, Kirsch DG, Locasale JW. 2020. Quantitative analysis of the physiological contributions of glucose to the TCA cycle. *Cell Metab* **32**: 619–628.e21. doi:10.1016/j.cmet.2020.09.005

Ma X, Fernández FM. 2022. Advances in mass spectrometry imaging for spatial cancer metabolomics. *Mass Spectrom Rev* e21804. doi:10.1002/mas.21804

Mackenzie M. 1888. *The fatal illness of Frederick the Noble.* Sampson Low, Marston, Searle & Rivington, London.

Madden MZ, Rathmell JC. 2021. The complex integration of T-cell metabolism and immunotherapy. *Cancer Discov* **11**: 1636–1643. doi:10.1158/2159-8290.CD-20-0569

Maddocks ODK, Athineos D, Cheung EC, Lee P, Zhang T, van den Broek NJF, Mackay GM, Labuschagne CF, Gay D, Kruiswijk F, et al. 2017. Modulating the therapeutic response of tumours to dietary serine and glycine starvation. *Nature* **544**: 372–376. doi:10.1038/nature22056

Magill GB, Myers WP, Reilly HC, Putnam RC, Magill JW, Sykes MP, Escher GC, Karnofsky DA, Burchenal JH. 1957. Pharmacological and initial therapeutic observations on 6-diazo-5-oxo-1-norleucine (DON) in human neoplastic disease. *Cancer* **10**: 1138–1150. doi:10.1002/1097-0142(195711/12)10:6<1138::AID-CNCR2820100608>3.0.CO;2-K

Manning BD, Cantley LC. 2003. Rheb fills a GAP between TSC and TOR. *Trends Biochem Sci* **28**: 573–576. doi:10.1016/j.tibs.2003.09.003

Matoba S, Kang JG, Patino WD, Wragg A, Boehm M, Gavrilova O, Hurley PJ, Bunz F, Hwang PM. 2006. P53 regulates mitochondrial respiration. *Science* **312**: 1650–1653. doi:10.1126/science.1126863

Mayers JR, Torrence ME, Danai LV, Papagiannakopoulos T, Davidson SM, Bauer MR, Lau AN, Ji BW, Dixit PD, Hosios AM, et al. 2016. Tissue of origin dictates branched-chain amino acid metabolism in mutant *Kras*-driven cancers. *Science* **353**: 1161–1165. doi:10.1126/science.aaf5171

Mehta MM, Weinberg SE, Steinert EM, Chhiba K, Martinez CA, Gao P, Perlman HR, Bryce P, Hay N, Chandel NS. 2018. Hexokinase 2 is dispensable for T cell-dependent immunity. *Cancer Metab* **6**: 10. doi:10.1186/s40170-018-0184-5

Méndez-Lucas A, Lin W, Driscoll PC, Legrave N, Novellas-demunt L, Xie C, Charles M, Wilson Z, Jones NP, Rayport S, et al. 2020. Identifying strategies to target the metabolic flexibility of tumours. *Nat Metab* **2**: 335–350. doi:10.1038/s42255-020-0195-8

Mick E, Titov DV, Skinner OS, Sharma R, Jourdain AA, Mootha VK. 2020. Distinct mitochondrial defects trigger the integrated stress response depending on the metabolic state of the cell. *eLife* **9**: e49178. doi:10.7554/eLife.49178

Mirji G, Worth A, Bhat SA, El Sayed M, Kannan T, Goldman AR, Tang HY, Liu Q, Auslander N, Dang CV, et al. 2022. The microbiome-derived metabolite TMAO drives immune activation and boosts responses to immune checkpoint blockade in pancreatic cancer. *Sci Immunol* **7**: eabn0704. doi:10.1126/sciimmunol.abn0704

Muellner MK, Uras IZ, Gapp BV, Kerzendorfer C, Smida M, Lechtermann H, Craig-Mueller N, Colinge J, Duernberger G, Nijman SM. 2011. A chemical-genetic screen reveals a mechanism of resistance to PI3K inhibitors in cancer. *Nat Chem Biol* **7**: 787–793. doi:10.1038/nchembio.695

Nolop KB, Rhodes CG, Brudin LH, Beaney RP, Krausz T, Jones T, Hughes JM. 1987. Glucose utilization in vivo by human pulmonary neoplasms. *Cancer* **60**: 2682–2689. doi:10.1002/1097-0142(19871201)60:11<2682::AID-CNCR2820601118>3.0.CO;2-H

Onodera J, Ohsumi Y. 2005. Autophagy is required for maintenance of amino acid levels and protein synthesis

Cite this article as *Cold Spring Harb Perspect Med* doi: 10.1101/cshperspect.a041530

under nitrogen starvation. *J Biol Chem* **280:** 31582–31586. doi:10.1074/jbc.M506736200

Oshima N, Ishida R, Kishimoto S, Beebe K, Brender JR, Yamamoto K, Urban D, Rai G, Johnson MS, Benavides G, et al. 2020. Dynamic imaging of LDH inhibition in tumors reveals rapid in vivo metabolic rewiring and vulnerability to combination therapy. *Cell Rep* **30:** 1798–1810.e4. doi:10.1016/j.celrep.2020.01.039

Patra KC, Wang Q, Bhaskar PT, Miller L, Wang Z, Wheaton W, Chandel N, Laakso M, Muller WJ, Allen EL, et al. 2013. Hexokinase 2 is required for tumor initiation and maintenance and its systemic deletion is therapeutic in mouse models of cancer. *Cancer Cell* **24:** 213–228. doi:10.1016/j.ccr.2013.06.014

Pavlova NN, Zhu J, Thompson CB. 2022. The hallmarks of cancer metabolism: still emerging. *Cell Metab* **34:** 355–377. doi:10.1016/j.cmet.2022.01.007

Persons DA, Schek N, Hall BL, Finn OJ. 1989. Increased expression of glycolysis-associated genes in oncogene-transformed and growth-accelerated states. *Mol Carcinog* **2:** 88–94. doi:10.1002/mc.2940020207

Rabinowitz JD, White E. 2010. Autophagy and metabolism. *Science* **330:** 1344–1348. doi:10.1126/science.1193497

Racker E. 1972. Bioenergetics and the problem of tumor growth. *Am Sci* **60:** 56–63.

Racker E. 1974. History of the Pasteur effect and its pathobiology. *Mol Cell Biochem* **5:** 17–23. doi:10.1007/BF01874168

Racker E. 1989. A view of misconduct in science. *Nature* **339:** 91–93. doi:10.1038/339091a0

Racker E, Spector M. 1981. Warburg effect revisited: merger of biochemistry and molecular biology. *Science* **213:** 303–307. doi:10.1126/science.6264596

Ralser M. 2018. An appeal to magic? The discovery of a non-enzymatic metabolism and its role in the origins of life. *Biochem J* **475:** 2577–2592. doi:10.1042/BCJ20160866

Reinfeld BI, Madden MZ, Wolf MM, Chytil A, Bader JE, Patterson AR, Sugiura A, Cohen AS, Ali A, Do BT, et al. 2021. Cell-programmed nutrient partitioning in the tumour microenvironment. *Nature* **593:** 282–288. doi:10.1038/s41586-021-03442-1

Reynolds MR, Lane AN, Robertson B, Kemp S, Liu Y, Hill BG, Dean DC, Clem BF. 2014. Control of glutamine metabolism by the tumor suppressor Rb. *Oncogene* **33:** 556–566. doi:10.1038/onc.2012.635

Ron-Harel N, Santos D, Ghergurovich JM, Sage PT, Reddy A, Lovitch SB, Dephoure N, Satterstrom FK, Sheffer M, Spinelli JB, et al. 2016. Mitochondrial biogenesis and proteome remodeling promote one-carbon metabolism for T cell activation. *Cell Metab* **24:** 104–117. doi:10.1016/j.cmet.2016.06.007

Rous P. 1911. A sarcoma of the fowl transmissible by an agent separable from the tumor cells. *J Exp Med* **13:** 397–411. doi:10.1084/jem.13.4.397

Samuels Y, Wang Z, Bardelli A, Silliman N, Ptak J, Szabo S, Yan H, Gazdar A, Powell SM, Riggins GJ, et al. 2004. High frequency of mutations of the *PIK3CA* gene in human cancers. *Science* **304:** 554. doi:10.1126/science.1096502

Sancar A, Van Gelder RN. 2021. Clocks, cancer, and chronochemotherapy. *Science* **371:** eabb0738. doi:10.1126/science.abb0738

Sciacovelli M, Gonçalves E, Johnson TI, Zecchini VR, da Costa AS, Gaude E, Drubbel AV, Theobald SJ, Abbo SR, Tran MG, et al. 2016. Fumarate is an epigenetic modifier that elicits epithelial-to-mesenchymal transition. *Nature* **537:** 544–547. doi:10.1038/nature19353

Selak MA, Armour SM, MacKenzie ED, Boulahbel H, Watson DG, Mansfield KD, Pan Y, Simon MC, Thompson CB, Gottlieb E. 2005. Succinate links TCA cycle dysfunction to oncogenesis by inhibiting HIF-α prolyl hydroxylase. *Cancer Cell* **7:** 77–85. doi:10.1016/j.ccr.2004.11.022

Semenza GL, Roth PH, Fang HM, Wang GL. 1994. Transcriptional regulation of genes encoding glycolytic enzymes by hypoxia-inducible factor 1. *J Biol Chem* **269:** 23757–23763. doi:10.1016/S0021-9258(17)31580-6

Shim H, Dolde C, Lewis BC, Wu CS, Dang G, Jungmann RA, Dalla-Favera R, Dang CV. 1997. c-Myc transactivation of *LDH-A*: implications for tumor metabolism and growth. *Proc Natl Acad Sci* **94:** 6658–6663. doi:10.1073/pnas.94.13.6658

Shim H, Chun YS, Lewis BC, Dang CV. 1998. A unique glucose-dependent apoptotic pathway induced by c-Myc. *Proc Natl Acad Sci* **95:** 1511–1516. doi:10.1073/pnas.95.4.1511

Som P, Atkins HL, Bandoypadhyay D, Fowler JS, MacGregor RR, Matsui K, Oster ZH, Sacker DF, Shiue CY, Turner H, et al. 1980. A fluorinated glucose analog, 2-fluoro-2-deoxy-D-glucose (F-18): nontoxic tracer for rapid tumor detection. *J Nucl Med* **21:** 670–675.

Spencer CN, McQuade JL, Gopalakrishnan V, McCulloch JA, Vetizou M, Cogdill AP, Khan MAW, Zhang X, White MG, Peterson CB, et al. 2021. Dietary fiber and probiotics influence the gut microbiome and melanoma immunotherapy response. *Science* **374:** 1632–1640. doi:10.1126/science.aaz7015

Stine ZE, Schug ZT, Salvino JM, Dang CV. 2022. Targeting cancer metabolism in the era of precision oncology. *Nat Rev Drug Discov* **21:** 141–162. doi:10.1038/s41573-021-00339-6

Tannir NM, Agarwal N, Porta C, Lawrence NJ, Motzer R, McGregor B, Lee RJ, Jain RK, Davis N, Appleman LJ, et al. 2022. Efficacy and safety of telaglenastat plus cabozantinib vs placebo plus cabozantinib in patients with advanced renal cell carcinoma: the CANTATA Randomized Clinical Trial. *JAMA Oncol* **8:** 1411–1418. doi:10.1001/jamaoncol.2022.3511

Thai M, Graham NA, Braas D, Nehil M, Komisopoulou E, Kurdistani SK, McCormick F, Graeber TG, Christofk HR. 2014. Adenovirus E4ORF1-induced MYC activation promotes host cell anabolic glucose metabolism and virus replication. *Cell Metab* **19:** 694–701. doi:10.1016/j.cmet.2014.03.009

Tu VY, Ayari A, O'Connor RS. 2021. Beyond the lactate paradox: how lactate and acidity impact T cell therapies against cancer. *Antibodies (Basel)* **10:** 25. doi:10.3390/antib10030025

Vander Heiden MG, Cantley LC, Thompson CB. 2009. Understanding the Warburg effect: the metabolic requirements of cell proliferation. *Science* **324:** 1029–1033. doi:10.1126/science.1160809

Varmus HE. 1984. The molecular genetics of cellular oncogenes. *Annu Rev Genet* **18:** 553–612. doi:10.1146/annurev.ge.18.120184.003005

Vasan K, Werner M, Chandel NS. 2020. Mitochondrial metabolism as a target for cancer therapy. *Cell Metab* **32:** 341–352. doi:10.1016/j.cmet.2020.06.019

Wang GL, Jiang BH, Rue EA, Semenza GL. 1995. Hypoxia-inducible factor 1 is a basic-helix-loop-helix-PAS heterodimer regulated by cellular O_2 tension. *Proc Natl Acad Sci* **92:** 5510–5514. doi:10.1073/pnas.92.12.5510

Wang R, Dillon CP, Shi LZ, Milasta S, Carter R, Finkelstein D, McCormick LL, Fitzgerald P, Chi H, Munger J, et al. 2011. The transcription factor Myc controls metabolic reprogramming upon T lymphocyte activation. *Immunity* **35:** 871–882. doi:10.1016/j.immuni.2011.09.021

Wang Z, Roberts AB, Buffa JA, Levison BS, Zhu W, Org E, Gu X, Huang Y, Zamanian-Daryoush M, Culley MK, et al. 2015. Non-lethal inhibition of gut microbial trimethylamine production for the treatment of atherosclerosis. *Cell* **163:** 1585–1595. doi:10.1016/j.cell.2015.11.055

Wang Y, Stancliffe E, Fowle-Grider R, Wang R, Wang C, Schwaiger-Haber M, Shriver LP, Patti GJ. 2022. Saturation of the mitochondrial NADH shuttles drives aerobic glycolysis in proliferating cells. *Mol Cell* **82:** 3270–3283. e9. doi:10.1016/j.molcel.2022.07.007

Warburg O. 1925. The metabolism of carcinoma cells. *J Cancer Res* **9:** 148–163. doi:10.1158/jcr.1925.148

Warburg O. 1928. The chemical constitution of respiration ferment. *Science* **68:** 437–443. doi:10.1126/science.68 .1767.437

Warburg OH. 1930. *The metabolism of tumors.* Constable, London.

Warburg O. 1956. On the origin of cancer cells. *Science* **123:** 309–314. doi:10.1126/science.123.3191.309

Warburg O, Wind F, Negelein E. 1927. The metabolism of tumors in the body. *J Gen Physiol* **8:** 519–530. doi:10 .1085/jgp.8.6.519

Weinhouse S. 1956. On respiratory impairment in cancer cells. *Science* **124:** 267–269. doi:10.1126/science.124 .3215.267

Weiss MC, Sousa FL, Mrnjavac N, Neukirchen S, Roettger M, Nelson-Sathi S, Martin WF. 2016. The physiology and habitat of the last universal common ancestor. *Nat Microbiol* **1:** 16116. doi:10.1038/nmicrobiol.2016.116

Wise DR, DeBerardinis RJ, Mancuso A, Sayed N, Zhang XY, Pfeiffer HK, Nissim I, Daikhin E, Yudkoff M, McMahon SB, et al. 2008. Myc regulates a transcriptional program that stimulates mitochondrial glutaminolysis and leads to glutamine addiction. *Proc Natl Acad Sci* **105:** 18782–18787. doi:10.1073/pnas.0810199105

Wu R, Racker E. 1959. Regulatory mechanisms in carbohydrate metabolism. III: Limiting factors in glycolysis of ascites tumor cells. *J Biol Chem* **234:** 1029–1035. doi:10 .1016/S0021-9258(18)98124-X

Wu K, Yuan Y, Yu H, Dai X, Wang S, Sun Z, Wang F, Fei H, Lin Q, Jiang H, et al. 2020. The gut microbial metabolite trimethylamine N-oxide aggravates GVHD by inducing M1 macrophage polarization in mice. *Blood* **136:** 501–515. doi:10.1182/blood.2019003990

Xiang Y, Stine ZE, Xia J, Lu Y, O'Connor RS, Altman BJ, Hsieh AL, Gouw AM, Thomas AG, Gao P, et al. 2015. Targeted inhibition of tumor-specific glutaminase diminishes cell-autonomous tumorigenesis. *J Clin Invest* **125:** 2293–2306. doi:10.1172/JCI75836

Xu S, Zhou T, Doh HM, Trinh KR, Catapang A, Lee JT, Braas D, Bayley NA, Yamada RE, Vasuthasawat A, et al. 2019. An HK2 antisense oligonucleotide induces synthetic lethality in HK1−HK2+ multiple myeloma. *Cancer Res* **79:** 2748–2760. doi:10.1158/0008-5472.CAN-18-2799

Yang L, TeSlaa T, Ng S, Nofal M, Wang L, Lan T, Zeng X, Cowan A, McBride M, Lu W, et al. 2022. Ketogenic diet and chemotherapy combine to disrupt pancreatic cancer metabolism and growth. *Med (N Y)* **3:** 119–136.

Yap TA, Daver N, Mahendra M, Zhang J, Kamiya-Matsuoka C, Meric-Bernstam F, Kantarjian HM, Ravandi F, Collins ME, Francesco MED, et al. 2023. Complex I inhibitor of oxidative phosphorylation in advanced solid tumors and acute myeloid leukemia: phase I trials. *Nat Med* **29:** 115–126. doi:10.1038/s41591-022-02103-8

Ying H, Kimmelman AC, Lyssiotis CA, Hua S, Chu GC, Fletcher-Sananikone E, Locasale JW, Son J, Zhang H, Coloff JL, et al. 2012. Oncogenic Kras maintains pancreatic tumors through regulation of anabolic glucose metabolism. *Cell* **149:** 656–670. doi:10.1016/j.cell.2012.01.058

Yuneva M, Zamboni N, Oefner P, Sachidanandam R, Lazebnik Y. 2007. Deficiency in glutamine but not glucose induces MYC-dependent apoptosis in human cells. *J Cell Biol* **178:** 93–105. doi:10.1083/jcb.200703099

Yuneva MO, Fan TW, Allen TD, Higashi RM, Ferraris DV, Tsukamoto T, Matés JM, Alonso FJ, Wang C, Seo Y, et al. 2012. The metabolic profile of tumors depends on both the responsible genetic lesion and tissue type. *Cell Metab* **15:** 157–170. doi:10.1016/j.cmet.2011.12.015

Zhou Y, Petrovic J, Zhao J, Zhang W, Bigdeli A, Zhang Z, Berger SL, Pear WS, Faryabi RB. 2022. EBF1 nuclear repositioning instructs chromatin refolding to promote therapy resistance in T leukemic cells. *Mol Cell* **82:** 1003–1020.e15. doi:10.1016/j.molcel.2022.01.015

Zindy F, Eischen CM, Randle DH, Kamijo T, Cleveland JL, Sherr CJ, Roussel MF. 1998. Myc signaling via the ARF tumor suppressor regulates p53-dependent apoptosis and immortalization. *Genes Dev* **12:** 2424–2433. doi:10.1101/ gad.12.15.2424

Imaging Tumor Metabolism

Thomas Ruan[1] and Kayvan R. Keshari[1,2,3]

[1]Department of Radiology, Memorial Sloan Kettering Cancer Center, New York, New York 10065, USA
[2]Molecular Pharmacology Program, Memorial Sloan Kettering Cancer Center, New York, New York 10065, USA
[3]Weill Cornell Graduate School, New York, New York 10065, USA

Correspondence: rahimikk@mskcc.org

Molecular imaging—the mapping of molecular and cellular processes in vivo—has the unique capability to interrogate cancer metabolism in its spatial contexts. This work describes the usage of the two most developed modalities for imaging metabolism in vivo: positron emission tomography (PET) and magnetic resonance (MR). These techniques can be used to probe glycolysis, glutamine metabolism, anabolic metabolism, redox state, hypoxia, and extracellular acidification. This review aims to provide an overview of the strengths and limitations of currently available molecular imaging strategies.

Cancer metabolism is spatially heterogeneous. The metabolic phenotypes involved in tumor progression evolve in response to local environmental drivers such as nutrient availability, perfusion, and hypoxia (Gatenby and Vincent 2003; Pavlova et al. 2022). Tumor metabolism must, therefore, be studied in its native contexts, and molecular imaging—the in vivo visualization of biochemical processes at molecular and cellular levels—is uniquely capable of shedding light on the spatial aspects of cancer metabolism (Rowe and Pomper 2022).

Molecular imaging methods detect metabolism-associated molecules, which are either endogenous or administered via perfusion. These in vivo methods yield insights into spatial heterogeneity, which are inaccessible by ex vivo or nonlocalized measurements. However, heterogeneity of signal can result from technical artifacts as well as the targeted biological processes

themselves. Proper interpretation of imaging data thus requires a clear understanding of signal generation, both in terms of the biochemical mechanisms of probe metabolism and the technical aspects of image formation.

When choosing an imaging method several factors must be considered, including spatial resolution, sensitivity, field of view, temporal resolution, and the potential for clinical translation. This review will describe applications of the two most common molecular imaging modalities: positron emission tomography (PET) and magnetic resonance spectroscopy or imaging (MRS/MRI).

POSITRON EMISSION TOMOGRAPHY (PET)

PET measures positron emission or β^+ decay, a process whereby an unstable radionuclide emits a positron that collides with an electron, creating γ rays measured by a closed ring of detectors (James and Gambhir 2012). PET does not produce reference images of the body and is typically paired with anatomic imaging by X-ray-computed tomography (CT) or an MRI. In the clinic, PET is typically paired with CT due to its fast scan acquisition and low cost. However, MRI provides superior soft-tissue contrast and reduced radiation exposure, making PET/MRI more appropriate for certain patients (Mayerhoefer et al. 2020). PET offers exceptional sensitivity due to negligible background signal; the lower detection limit is in the picomolar range and nano-to-milligram quantities of tracer molecules are typically delivered. PET also offers high spatial resolution (1–2 mm preclinical, 5–7 mm clinical) and can cover a large field of view, enabling whole-body imaging. Most PET probes, or tracers, are structural analogs of the metabolite they report on, differing only by an appended radioisotope moiety. The most commonly used isotope in PET tracer analogs is ^{18}F due to its long radioactive half-life of ~110 min and its structural similarity to a hydroxyl group. Even modest chemical modifications can alter interactions with transporters or enzymes in profound ways. Therefore, it is important to be aware that ^{18}F-functionalized probes do not undergo the same biochemistry as the metabolites they mimic. A different approach to PET probe design is to substitute an atom in the target metabolite with a radioisotope such as ^{11}C or [13]N. Substituted PET probes are attractive because they are biochemically identical to the metabolites they report on; however, the short half-lives of [11]C (20 min) and [13]N (10 min) make the application of these probes challenging (Neumann et al. 2007).

For a PET tracer to successfully inform on tumor metabolism, it must be differentially taken up by or retained within cancer cells over healthy tissue. The degree of differential uptake, or avidity, of a tracer is typically quantified in the clinic by the standardized uptake value (SUV), which is calculated by dividing measured radioactivity in a region of interest by the total activity of the injected dose per volume of the entire body (Thie 2004). Besides static SUV values, more sophisticated information can be obtained by kinetic modeling of dynamic PET data. The dynamic PET signal in a region of interest will depend on probe delivery through the blood, described by an input function, and irreversible retention of the probe in cells following a metabolic process (Carson 2003). A typical approach is compartmental modeling, where the PET probe is transported with linear first-order kinetics between compartments such as plasma, extracellular space, and intracellular space. In most cases, the final transfer step into intracellular space can be treated as unidirectional and irreversible. The relevant parameter derived from compartmental modeling is the net influx rate (K_i)—the linear rate of unidirectional probe uptake and trapping where all reversible compartments are in dynamic equilibrium.

Two major drawbacks limit the utility of PET imaging. First, PET tracers generate ionizing radiation, restricting the number of scans that can be safely performed on a single subject. Second, regardless of the radionuclide's chemical environment, positron emission always produces γ rays with identical energy. Thus, PET cannot distinguish between metabolites, and only indirectly measures metabolism as a function of probe uptake and retention.

MAGNETIC RESONANCE SPECTROSCOPY/IMAGING (MRS/MRI)

When atomic nuclei with a nonzero angular momentum quantum number (spin) are placed in a magnetic field, they align either with or against the field. The difference between these states of alignment—that is, their polarization—can be perturbed by radiofrequency excitation pulses, giving rise to a magnetic resonance (MR) signal. The frequency of a given nucleus's MR signal is specific to its local chemical environment. This phenomenon is known as chemical shift and allows the spectroscopic identification of different molecules. Spatially varying gradient magnetic fields allow for the localization of MR signals, producing an image showing signal intensity (magnetic resonance imaging; MRI) or a grid of localized MR spectra (magnetic resonance spectroscopy or spectroscopic imaging; MRS or MRSI). The most used isotopes in MR are ^{1}H and

^{13}C. Polarization levels for these nuclei at thermal equilibrium are quite low, resulting in poor MR sensitivity of $\sim 10^{-3}$–10^{-5} M. The most abundant and MR-sensitive nucleus is ^{1}H, so MRSI of endogenous ^{1}H is feasible for measuring metabolite pool sizes in vivo. However, ~99% of naturally occurring carbon is ^{12}C, which has zero spin and is undetectable by MR. MR detection of carbon thus requires the introduction of ^{13}C-enriched molecules in experiments that can be thought of as akin to isotope tracing by mass spectrometry. A conceptually similar experiment to ^{13}C MR tracing is an infusion of molecules labeled with ^{2}H, a technique called deuterium metabolic imaging (DMI).

The MR signal of ^{13}C-labeled probes can be dramatically magnified by a process termed hyperpolarization (HP) involving prepolarization of nuclei outside the detection magnet. The most common HP method is dissolution dynamic nuclear polarization (dDNP), whereby microwave radiation is used to transfer spin polarization from a free radical electron to ^{13}C nuclei at extremely low temperatures of ~1 K. After HP has been sufficiently built up, the frozen sample is rapidly dissolved by a heated buffer for injection (Ardenkjær-Larsen et al. 2003; Golman et al. 2003). More recently, methods coupling solution-state chemistry to separately polarized parahydrogen have been employed to achieve similar HP enhancements without the use of problematically low temperatures (Hövener et al. 2018; Gierse et al. 2023). In general, HP techniques increase the MR signal by several orders of magnitude, facilitating in vivo spatially resolved isotope tracing. It is important to note that the HP signal enhancement for a given nucleus has an effective lifetime—analogous to the half-life of radioactive nuclei—mediated by a process called T1 relaxation. Recent work has shown that the T1 time constant can be lengthened by the deuteration of the HP molecule or even the dissolution solvent (Keshari and Wilson 2014; Cho et al. 2018; Deh et al. 2024). However, the most effective strategy for mitigating T1 relaxation is the judicious selection of the ^{13}C enrichment position. Attached hydrogens undergo a dipolar cross-relaxation interaction with ^{13}C, making T1 relaxation efficient. For

this reason, most ^{13}C nuclei used for HP are in a carbonyl group (Keshari and Wilson 2014).

The key benefit of imaging metabolism with HP ^{13}C-enriched molecules is the use of chemical shift to separate signals coming from the injected molecule and its downstream metabolites (Brindle et al. 2011; Wang et al. 2019). For this to be possible, the chemical shifts of the probe molecule and its metabolic products must be sufficiently far apart for spectral resolution. MR experiments produce data in the form of signal intensities that are not inherently quantitative, so results are typically reported in ratios of metabolite-to-probe intensities. More sophisticated analyses fit HP MR data as a compartmental system, yielding kinetic rate constants with units of inverse seconds (Harrison et al. 2012; Bankson et al. 2015; Crane et al. 2021).

METABOLIC TARGETS

Glycolysis

The reprogramming of energy metabolism in cancer is an especially attractive target for molecular imaging due to its role as an integral requirement for cellular proliferation (Hanahan and Weinberg 2011). It should, therefore, come as no surprise that several of the most studied metabolic imaging strategies focus on the central feature of cancer energy metabolism: elevated glycolysis, also known as the Warburg effect (Fig. 1A; Warburg 1956).

Glucose

The paradigmatic success story of molecular imaging is perhaps [^{18}F]fluorodeoxyglucose (FDG) (Fig. 1Bi). PET of FDG is frequently used in the clinic to diagnose, stage, and monitor a range of cancers, with millions of scans performed in the United States every year (Alavi et al. 2004; Kelloff et al. 2005; Czernin et al. 2013; Rosenkrantz et al. 2016). FDG is an analog of glucose with ^{18}F substituted for the C2 hydroxyl group (Ido et al. 1978). FDG is readily imported into cells by the glucose transporters (GLUTs) and undergoes the reversible first step of glycolysis, phosphorylation of the C6 hydroxyl. However, fur-

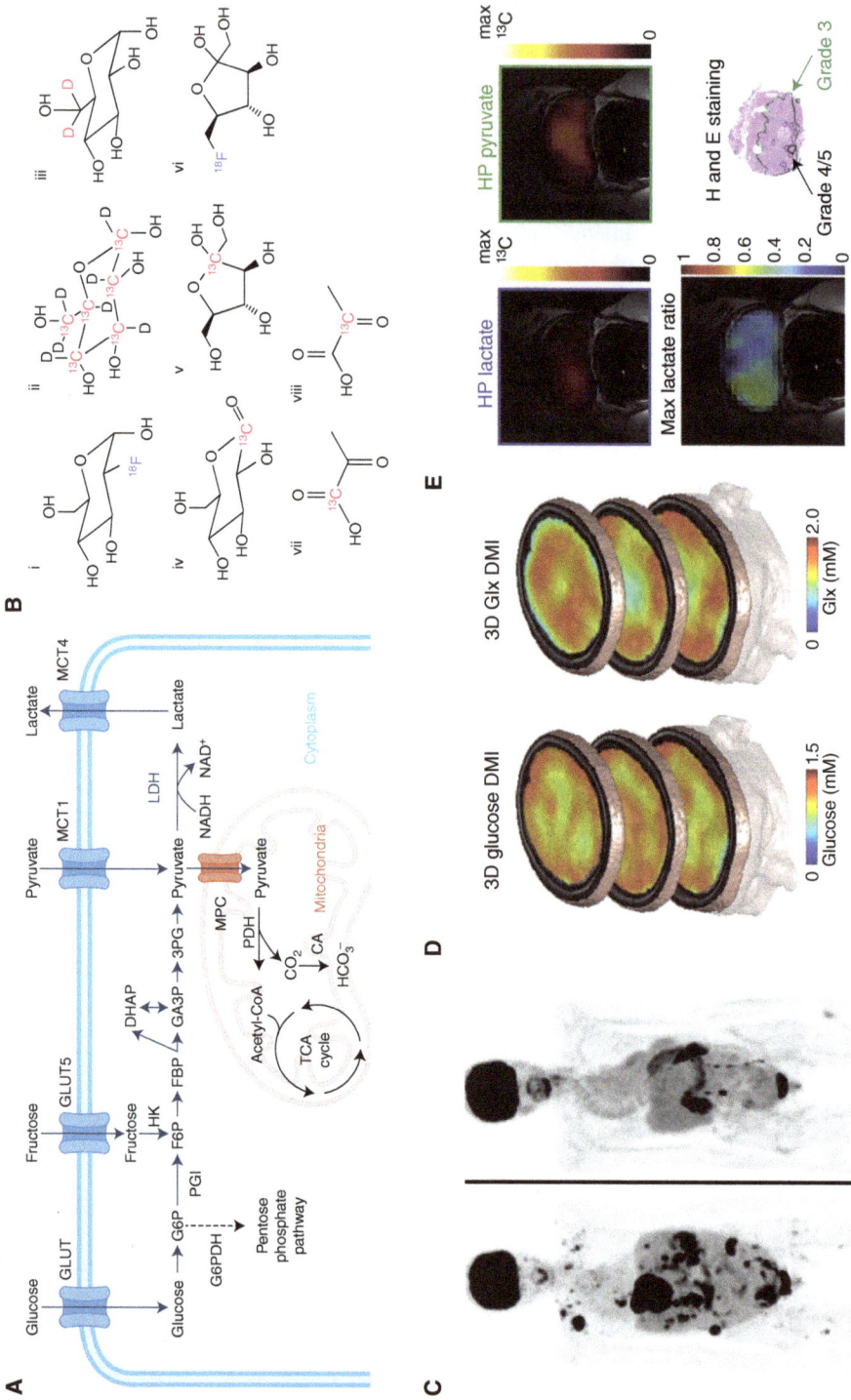

Figure 1. (*See following page for legend.*)

ther metabolism of FDG-6-phosphate through canonical glycolysis via phosphoglucose isomerase (PGI) is not possible due to the fluorine on C2. Since FDG-6-phosphate must be dephosphorylated before it can be effluxed, radioactivity in the cell is trapped in a dynamic equilibrium of uptake by GLUT, phosphorylation, and dephosphorylation (Gallagher et al. 1978). Thus, FDG-PET indirectly reports on the proximal aspects of glycolysis.

FDG is avidly taken up by any cells that consume large amounts of glucose, so FDG-PET is problematic for imaging tumors in the brain, which has high baseline levels of glycolysis (Fig. 1C). In other areas of the body, nonmalignant sources of accumulation can complicate FDG-PET imaging (Long and Smith 2011). Inflammation, for example, is a cause of nonspecific signals since activated inflammatory cells require high levels of glycolysis to function (Skoura et al. 2016). Knowledge of the underlying biochemical mechanism can help overcome this potential issue. Inflammatory cells also express high levels of glucose-6-phosphatase, the enzyme that dephosphorylates FDG-6-phos-

phate, and thus efflux radioactivity faster than tumor cells. As such, imaging at two time points can help differentiate between tumors and inflammation—while tumor and inflammatory cells will both show high SUV at an early time point, only tumor cells will retain the PET probe over a long time course (Alavi et al. 2004; Long and Smith 2011).

Historically, FDG-PET has not been used for imaging of prostate cancers, which tend to exhibit a modest Warburg effect. However, some evidence suggests that advanced prostate cancers that have become castration-resistant are amenable to FDG-PET as a result of dramatically increased glucose uptake (Jadvar 2016). Although FDG uptake is classically interpreted as a readout of glycolytic activity, there is some recent evidence suggesting that FDG uptake can also depend on flux through the pentose phosphate pathway (PPP) (Sambuceti et al. 2021). Silencing of hexose-6-phosphate dehydrogenase, the enzyme that catalyzes entry into the PPP in the endoplasmic reticulum, in mouse cell culture models of colon and breast cancer resulted in decreased FDG uptake despite in-

Figure 1. Molecular imaging of glycolysis. (A) Diagram of metabolites, enzymes, and transporters relevant to glycolysis. (G6P) Glucose-6-phosphate, (F6P) fructose-6-phosphate, (FBP) fructose-1,6-biphosphate, (GA3P) glyceraldehyde 3-phosphate, (DHAP) dihydroxyacetone phosphate, (3PG) 3-phosphoglycerate, (NAD$^+$/NADH) oxidized/reduced nicotinamide adenine dinucleotide, (CO$_2$) carbon dioxide, (HCO$_3^-$) bicarbonate, (acetyl-CoA) acetyl coenzyme A, (G6PDH) glucose-6-phosphate dehydrogenase, (PGI) phosphoglucose isomerase, (HK) hexokinase, (LDH) lactate dehydrogenase, (PDH) pyruvate dehydrogenase, (CA) carbonic anhydrase, (GLUT) glucose transporter, (MCT1/4) monocarboxylate transporter, (MPC) mitochondrial pyruvate carrier. (A created with BioRender.com.) (B) Chemical structures of probes for imaging glycolysis. (i) [^{18}F]fluorodeoxyglucose (FDG), (ii) [1,2,3,4,5,6,6'-^{2}H$_7$, U-^{13}C$_6$]-glucose, (iii) [6,6'-^{2}H$_2$]glucose, (iv) δ-[1-^{13}C]gluconolactone, (v) [2-^{13}C]fructose, (vi) 6-deoxy-6-[^{18}F]fluoro-D-fructose (6-[^{18}F]FDF), (vii) [1-^{13}C]pyruvate, (viii) [2-^{13}C]pyruvate. β-Emitting radioisotopes detected by positron emission tomograph (PET) are blue, and nuclei detected by magnetic resonance (MR) are red. (Structures created with ChemDraw). (C) PET-FDG maximum intensity projection images of patients with metastatic melanoma before (left) and after (right) BRAF inhibitor treatment. This image highlights the capability of PET to image metastasis over the whole body, and nonspecific FDG uptake in the brain and urinary system. (C reprinted from Czernin et al. 2013 under the terms of the Creative Commons Attribution License.) (D) Deuterium metabolic imaging (DMI) of orally administered [6,6'-^{2}H$_2$]glucose in brains of healthy humans. 3D maps of glucose (left) and glutamine/glutamate (Glx; right) show modestly heterogeneous delivery of deuterium-labeled substrate and conversion to Glx, with slightly lower Glx signal in the gray matter–rich ventricles. (D reprinted from De Feyter et al. 2018 under the terms of the Creative Commons Attribution-NonCommercial License.) (E) Hyperpolarization (HP) [1-^{13}C]pyruvate imaging of a prostate cancer patient. Data from an HP experiment can be represented in metabolite maps of lactate (top left), pyruvate (top right), or the ratio of product to substrate (bottom left). Color maps of signal intensity are overlaid on ^{1}H T2-weighted magnetic resonance imaging (MRI) images for anatomical reference. The lactate-to-pyruvate ratio is elevated in the left region of the prostate, corresponding to regions of higher Gleason grade in matched histology sections (bottom right). (E reprinted from Granlund et al. 2019, Elsevier © 2016.)

creases in glycolytic flux and lactate secretion (Marini et al. 2016). In this context, FDG-PET may report on NAPDH generation through the PPP, which is up-regulated in proliferative cancers. In all, although FDG-PET has become a workhorse clinical imaging modality, its lack of specificity has limited its effectiveness in basic research.

Other glucose-based PET probes have also been reported, although with limited application to imaging cancer metabolism. For example, PET of ^{11}C-labeled glucose has been used for PET imaging in brain cancer patients (Ericson et al. 1985; Spence et al. 1998). However, this probe is chemically identical to endogenous glucose and is not trapped in tumors like FDG. There have also been attempts to produce PET probes based on other sugars, such as 6-deoxy-6-[^{18}F]fluoro-D-fructose (6-[^{18}F]FDF), a radio analog of fructose (Fig. 1Bvi; Wuest et al. 2011). 6-[^{18}F]FDF is trapped in tumor cells by a similar mechanism to FDG, and has been used to image breast cancers that up-regulate the fructose transporter GLUT5 (Bouvet et al. 2014). In one comparative study, 6-[^{18}F]FDF uptake was shown to be more specific for breast cancers than FDG, indicating a potential clinical role for the imaging of sugars other than glucose (Wuest et al. 2017).

Elevated glucose uptake can be imaged directly with an MRI of HP uniformly ^{13}C-labeled glucose (Fig. 1Bii). The primary benefit of this approach is that it directly quantifies glucose metabolism in addition to uptake. An early demonstration of this technique on T47D cells in an NMR-compatible bioreactor system showed that lactate, and smaller amounts of dihydroxyacetone phosphate (DHAP) and 3-phosphoglyceric acid (3PG), can be detected from HP glucose (Harris et al. 2013). While imaging of mice implanted with EL4 and LL2 tumors detected HP glucose in tumors and organs such as the brain, heart, and kidney, only tumors produced HP lactate and, to a lesser extent, HP DHAP, bicarbonate, and 6-phosphogluconic acid (6PG) (Rodrigues et al. 2014). These latter two metabolites report on the shunting of glucose-6-phosphate to the PPP, demonstrating the ability of HP MR to simultaneously quantify multiple pathways. Another study linked the production of 6PG from HP glucose to the expression of telomerase reverse transcriptase, which up-regulates GLUT1 and glucose-6-phosphate dehydrogenase, in low-grade oligodendrogliomas (Viswanath et al. 2021a). MRS of HP glucose in glioblastoma models showed increased lactate production in a cell culture–based model, which produced a compact tumor, over a patient-derived model with an infiltrative phenotype (Mishkovsky et al. 2021). The biggest disadvantage of HP glucose is its short HP lifetime. Uniformly ^{13}C-labeled HP glucose has a T1 of only a few seconds, which is too short for in vivo detection of metabolism. Although synthetic strategies such as selective ^{13}C labeling or perdeuteration can help raise the T1 of glucose to ~10 sec (Mishkovsky et al. 2017), the fast HP decay of this probe still limits the achievable detection window.

A thermal (nonhyperpolarized) MR-based technique that targets glycolysis is glucose chemical exchange saturation transfer (glucoCEST). This method operates by saturating the MR signal of glucose hydroxyl hydrogens with a selective radiofrequency pulse. The exchange of the saturated nuclei with water hydrogens causes a decrease in the water ^{1}H MR signal. The extent of this attenuation correlates with the concentration of glucose, providing a method to sensitively measure local glucose concentrations. The median intensity and spatial distribution of the glucoCEST signal in xenograft tumors of two models of colorectal cancer (LS174T and SW1222) correlates with FDG-PET (Walker-Samuel et al. 2013). However, there was no significant correlation between glucoCEST uptake and perfusion, as measured by the common MRI contrast agent Gd-DTPA. These findings indicate that glucoCEST specifically reports on glucose uptake rather than perfusion of the delivered bolus. GlucoCEST is analogous to FDG-PET in that it measures glucose uptake, not subsequent metabolism. However, glucoCEST does not require the synthesis of a radiotracer, does not use ionizing radiation, and has a much higher spatial resolution than FDG-PET. Additionally, there may be contexts where glucoCEST is more sensitive to changes in glucose uptake than FDG-PET. For example, the metabolic response to doxorubicin treatment in mice implanted with 4T1 tumors was detected by glucoCEST but not FDG-PET (Capozza et al. 2022). The initial work of implementing glucoCEST in the clinic is underway (Xu et al. 2015; Bender et al. 2022), but this is still a nascent technology; for glucoCEST to supplant FDG-PET issues such as low sensitivity, susceptibility to subject motion, and full elucidation of signal compartmentalization must be addressed (Kim et al. 2022).

DMI is another MR-based technique for imaging glucose metabolism that has been gaining interest recently. The advantages of imaging deuterium-labeled molecules include experimental simplicity, high sensitivity, and low background noise (De Feyter and de Graaf 2021). A landmark study used DMI of $[6,6'-^2H_2]$glucose in rat and human brains to generate steady-state metabolic maps of glucose, lactate, and glutamine + glutamate (Glx; the signals from these similar metabolites overlap in the ^2H spectrum) (Fig. 1Biii; De Feyter et al. 2018). The ratio of lactate to Glx was higher in tumors, reflecting the Warburg phenotype of imbalance toward reductive metabolism of glucose (Fig. 1D). DMI has also been used to measure dynamic fluxes of glucose metabolism in mouse xenografts (Kreis et al. 2019; Markovic et al. 2021). While promising, this approach is hampered by long scan times and low spatial resolution associated with the poor MR sensitivity of deuterium. One promising solution to this problem measures decreases in the ^1H signals of glycolytic metabolites following administration of ^2H-labeled glucose to indirectly quantify ^2H enrichment (Rich et al. 2020). This method, described by its authors as "quantitative exchanged-label turnover MRS," may provide an easier path to clinical implementation for deuterium tracing experiments (Cember et al. 2022).

Besides imaging uptake and metabolism of glucose directly, other inputs and outputs of the glycolytic pathway have been investigated as molecular imaging targets. HP $[2-^{13}C]$fructose has been used to image the generation of fructose-6-phosphate in models of prostate cancer (Keshari et al. 2009) and fructose-1-phosphate

in hepatocellular carcinoma models (Fig. 1Bv; Tee et al. 2022). HP δ-$[1-^{13}C]$gluconolactone was developed as a probe of the oxidative portion of the PPP (Fig. 1Biv). In orthotopic models of glioblastoma in rats, the flux of HP δ-$[1-^{13}C]$ gluconolactone to HP $[^{13}C]$bicarbonate was higher in tumor tissue than contralateral or tumor-free control brains, and decreased in tumors upon silencing of TERT signaling (Batsios et al. 2021; Minami et al. 2023). There has also been some work on developing HP $[2-^{13}C]$dihydroxyacetone as a probe for gluconeogenesis, which enters glycolysis after phosphorylation to DHAP, although it has not yet been applied in the context of cancer metabolism (Moreno et al. 2017; Marco-Rius et al. 2021; Ragavan et al. 2021).

Lactate

Another popular target of molecular imaging is lactate, the predominant final product of glycolysis in tumors. This is due to its abundance and the ability to target it via a wide range of approaches. Historically, ^1H MRSI has been used in the clinic to measure lactate pool size, especially in brain cancers (Öz et al. 2014). Cross-validation studies show that higher-grade gliomas that exhibit high FDG-PET avidity also produce large amounts of lactate (Herholz et al. 1992). PET of $[3-^{11}C]$lactate has been used to measure lactate utilization in the healthy heart and brain (Herrero et al. 2007; Temma et al. 2018). This probe could be useful in studying cancers that have been shown to use lactate as a fuel source for the TCA cycle (Faubert et al. 2017).

HP pyruvate has been extensively investigated as a probe for lactate generation. $[1-^{13}C]$ pyruvate can build up high levels of polarization, has a long T1 (>60 sec), and is predominantly reduced to $[1-^{13}C]$lactate (chemical shift difference of ~12 ppm) via the lactate dehydrogenase complex (LDH) in tumor cells (Fig. 1Bvii; Albers et al. 2008; Keshari and Wilson 2014). HP pyruvate-to-lactate flux has been identified in a wide range of preclinical contexts as a biomarker of cancer metabolism, progression, and treatment response (Golman et al. 2006; Day et al. 2007; Albers et al. 2008; Hu et al. 2010, 2011; Park et al. 2010, 2012; Keshari et al. 2013; Serrao et al. 2016;

Dong et al. 2018; Grashei et al. 2022). $[1\text{-}^{13}C]$ Pyruvate is the first HP probe to be translated to the clinic (Kurhanewicz et al. 2019), with applications to patients with prostate cancer (Fig. 1E; Nelson et al. 2013; Aggarwal et al. 2017; Chen et al. 2020; Granlund et al. 2020; de Kouchkovsky et al. 2022), renal carcinomas (Tran et al. 2019; Tang et al. 2021; Ursprung et al. 2022), breast cancer (Gallagher et al. 2020; Woitek et al. 2020), brain cancer (Miloushev et al. 2018; Park et al. 2018; Zaccagna et al. 2022), and pancreatic cancer (Stødkilde-Jørgensen et al. 2020).

Elevated HP pyruvate-to-lactate flux is typically interpreted as a consequence of the Warburg effect. However, some evidence suggests that other factors also control the kinetics of HP pyruvate metabolism. Studies that correlate HP lactate generation with HP perfusion imaging (Lau et al. 2016) or mass spectrometry imaging of nonhyperpolarized ^{13}C-labeled pyruvate (Fala et al. 2021) indicate that one of the main determinants for increased HP pyruvate-to-lactate flux in tumors is the delivery of HP pyruvate. Additionally, pharmacological blockade of VEGF signaling, which decreases tumor vascularization, decreases HP pyruvate-to-lactate flux despite increases in LDH activity and lactate pool size (Bohndiek et al. 2012; Park et al. 2016). Elevated HP lactate formation also correlates with the expression of the pyruvate importer monocarboxylate transporter 1 (MCT1) in a variety of preclinical (Keshari et al. 2013; Xu et al. 2014; Sushentsev et al. 2022) and clinical contexts (Granlund et al. 2019; Gallagher et al. 2020). Overexpression of MCT1 in pancreatic carcinoma cells causes a marked increase in HP pyruvate-to-lactate flux, suggesting a possible rate-limiting role of membrane transport (Rao et al. 2020). Finally, pharmacological inhibition of LDH (Dutta et al. 2013; Varma et al. 2021) or indirect down-regulation of LDH through inhibition of upstream signaling (Dafni et al. 2010; Ward et al. 2010) dramatically ablates flux to lactate. Interestingly, there is some evidence that blocking off pyruvate reduction to lactate can result in compensatory increases in the utilization of other pathways, such as entry into the TCA cycle via pyruvate dehydrogenase (PDH) (Oshima et al. 2020). Overall, further work is required to clarify

the precise mechanisms influencing the kinetics of HP pyruvate metabolism.

HP $[1\text{-}^{13}C]$pyruvate readily reports on flux to lactate, but entry into the TCA cycle via PDH involves decarboxylation at the 1C position, forming $[^{13}C]$carbon dioxide that rapidly equilibrates to $[^{13}C]$bicarbonate via carbonic anhydrase (CA). Although $[^{13}C]$bicarbonate levels can be used as a proxy of pyruvate-derived carbon entry into the TCA cycle, the particulars of TCA cycle flux are functionally invisible to $[1\text{-}^{13}C]$pyruvate. To this end, HP $[2\text{-}^{13}C]$pyruvate (Fig. 1Bviii) has been investigated as a probe of TCA cycle flux in the production of glutamate, citrate, and acetylcarnitine (Schroeder et al. 2009; Marjańska et al. 2010; Park et al. 2013; Izquierdo-Garcia et al. 2015). Glutamate levels are responsive to pharmacological manipulation of pyruvate entry into the TCA cycle. Treatment with dichloroacetate, which indirectly activates PDH activity by inhibiting PDH kinase, increased HP glutamate formation in healthy rat brains (Park et al. 2013), whereas IDH1 mutant glioblastoma cells displayed a decrease in HP $[5\text{-}^{13}C]$glutamate generation concomitant with down-regulation of PDH expression (Izquierdo-Garcia et al. 2015). A pilot study on the clinical translation of HP $[2\text{-}^{13}C]$pyruvate in healthy brains of volunteers demonstrated that HP $[2\text{-}^{13}C]$pyruvate converted to lactate at a similar rate as $[1\text{-}^{13}C]$pyruvate (Chung et al. 2019). The full potential of $[2\text{-}^{13}C]$pyruvate has not yet been fully realized. Copolarization and injection of mixed $[1\text{-}^{13}C]$pyruvate and $[2\text{-}^{13}C]$pyruvate could allow simultaneous detection of the reductive and oxidative fates of pyruvate, expanding informational in a kind of multiplexing approach (Wilson et al. 2010; DeBerardinis and Keshari 2022). Another strategy is to use doubly labeled $[1,2\text{-}^{13}C_2]$pyruvate (Chen et al. 2012; Sriram et al. 2015), which can directly measure rates of key metabolic pathways in competition with each other.

In conclusion, glycolysis has presented ample targets for molecular imaging of cancer metabolism. FDG-PET and HP $[1\text{-}^{13}C]$pyruvate are the most used probes of their respective modalities, and several MR methods for the detection of glycolysis are in development.

Glutamine

Glutaminolysis

The second most attractive molecular imaging target for cancer after glucose is glutamine, which participates in several key tumor metabolic processes (Fig. 2A). Glutamine is involved in up-regulated proliferation through the biosynthesis of nucleotides or hexosamines and, via glutamate, can supply carbon to the TCA cycle for energy generation, amino acid synthesis, or reductive carboxylation (DeBerardinis and Cheng 2010; Altman et al. 2016). Early PET studies reported increased [13]N- or ^{11}C-labeled glutamine uptake in murine and canine tumor models, although the short half-lives of these radioisotopes (~10 and 20 min, respectively) limited detailed investigation (Gelbard et al. 1977; Qu et al. 2012).

Several fluorine-based analog probes have also been reported. [18]F-(2S,4R)4-fluoroglutamine (Fig. 2Biii) is the most used molecule because it resembles endogenous L-glutamine and shows differential uptake in xenograft models of glutamine-addicted gliomas and breast cancers (Lieberman et al. 2011; Qu et al. 2011; Liu et al. 2018). ^{18}F-glutamine has also been shown to accumulate in human patient tumors (Liu et al. 2018; Grkovski et al. 2020). A glutamine-based PET probe is especially useful for the clinical imaging of gliomas, where nonspecific uptake of glucose by the healthy brain makes conventional FDG-PET difficult (Fig. 2C; Venneti et al. 2015).

The mechanism by which tumor cells retain ^{18}F-glutamine has not been fully elucidated. Isolated rat kidney GLS1, the main isotype of glutaminase in tumors, can metabolize 4-fluoroglutamine to 4-fluoroglutamate in vitro (Cooper et al. 2012). However, a comparison of ^{18}F-glutamine and ^{18}F-glutamate showed uptake of both probes but long-term retention of ^{18}F-glutamine and rapid washout of ^{18}F-glutamate (Ploessl et al. 2012). This finding seems to suggest that although ^{18}F-glutamine is avidly taken up by tumor cells that up-regulate the neutral amino acid transporter ASCT2, the probe is not converted to glutamate. Inhibition of GLS in xenografts of triple-negative breast cancers that have high GLS expression results in increased ^{18}F-glutamine uptake, indicating that fluoroglutamine PET signal is sensitive to the intracellular pool size of glutamine (Zhou et al. 2017; Viswanath et al. 2021b).

Hyperpolarized glutamine has also been investigated as a probe for glutaminolysis. The C1 and C5 carbons of L-glutamine do not have directly bonded hydrogens and are ideal candidates for ^{13}C enrichment, with T1 values of 25 and 16 sec, respectively (Gallagher et al. 2008; Jensen et al. 2009). Unfortunately, the chemical shift difference between [1-^{13}C]glutamine and [1-^{13}C]glutamate is only 0.5 ppm, which is too small to feasibly separate. Conversely, HP [5-^{13}C]glutamine is a viable probe for glutaminolysis, with a favorable chemical shift difference between it and [5-^{13}C]glutamate of ~3.4 ppm. Early in vitro experiments with HP [5-^{13}C]glutamine in suspensions of glutamine-addicted tumor cells showed ready uptake and conversion to [5-^{13}C]glutamate (Gallagher et al. 2008b; Qu et al. 2011; Canapè et al. 2015). Experiments in rat liver tumor (Cabella et al. 2013) and mouse pancreatic ductal adenocarcinoma models (Eskandari et al. 2022) show that HP [5-^{13}C]glutamine is taken up and converted to [5-^{13}C]glutamate by tumors (Fig. 2D). Additionally, the T1 relaxation time of [5-^{13}C]glutamine can be extended by deuteration of the C4 carbon and replacement of the amide nitrogen with [15]N (Fig. 2Bi; Qu et al. 2011; Eskandari et al. 2022). While the comparatively shorter HP lifetime of HP [5-^{13}C]glutamine presents a challenge for clinical translation, isotope enrichment, and further modifications may make this probe useful for the in vivo characterization and development of next-generation glutaminase inhibitor drugs. Another avenue of exploration is HP-substituted ^{15}N-labeled glutamine analogs, which are well tolerated in vivo and show remarkably long T1s of 2.5–5 min (Chiavazza et al. 2013; Durst et al. 2016). However, the applicability of these probes to metabolic studies remains to be shown.

2-Hydroxyglutarate

Increased glutamine uptake is also seen in cancers with mutations in isocitrate dehydrogenase 1/2 (IDH1/2) that confer a gain-of-function phe-

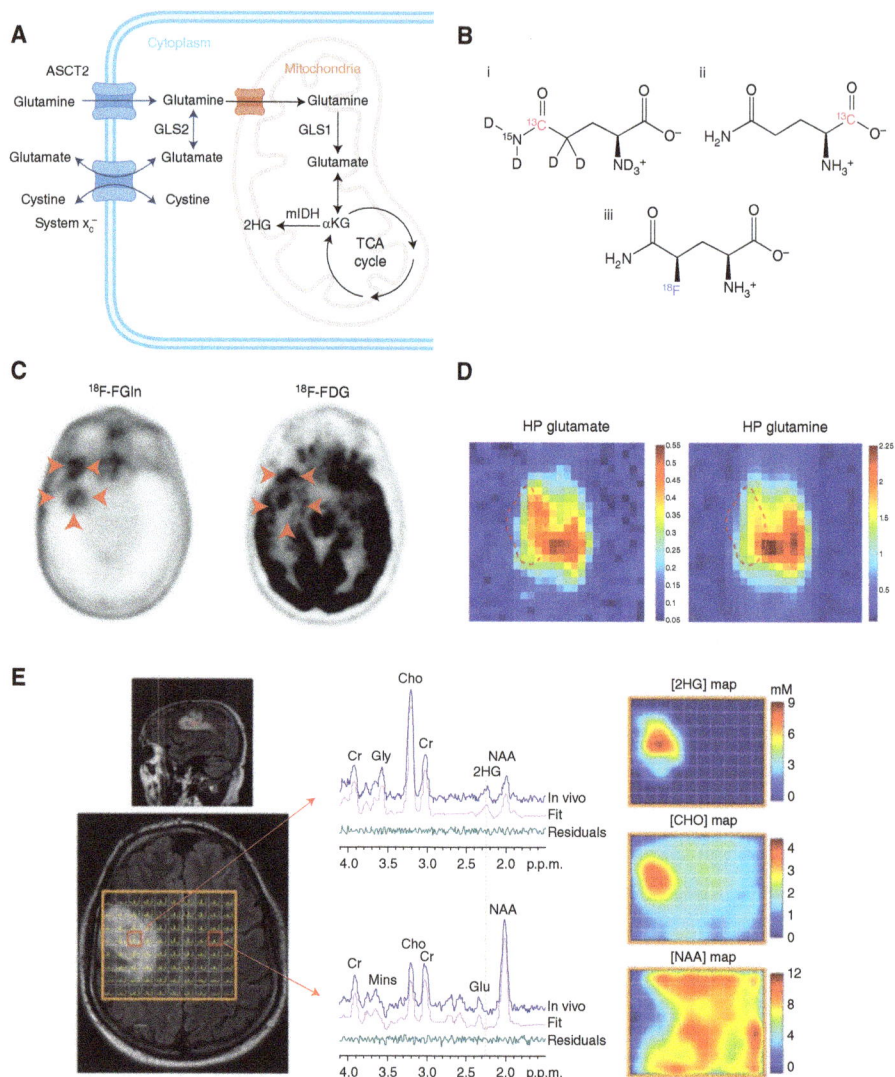

Figure 2. Molecular imaging of glutamine metabolism. (*A*) Diagram of metabolites, enzymes, and transporters relevant to glutamine metabolism. (αKG) α-ketoglutarate, (2HG) 2-hydroxyglutarate, (GLS1/2) glutaminase, (mIDH) mutant isocitrate dehydrogenase, (ASCT2) alanine–serine–cystine transporter 2. (*A* created with BioRender.com.) (*B*) Chemical structures of probes for imaging glutamine metabolism. (*i*) [5-^{13}C,4,4-^{2}H$_2$, 5-^{15}N]glutamine, (*ii*) [1-^{13}C]glutamine, (*iii*) ^{18}F-(2S,4R)4-fluoroglutamine. β-Emitting radioisotopes detected by positron emission tomography (PET) are blue, and nuclei detected by magnetic resonance (MR) are red. Structures created with ChemDraw. (*C*) ^{18}F-glutamine PET imaging of a glioblastoma patient (*left*) shows specific uptake in the tumor (red arrows) with minimal signal from the surrounding brain, whereas FDG-PET imaging of the same patient (*right*) shows indiscriminate uptake throughout the brain. (*C* reprinted from Venneti et al. 2015, The American Association for the Advancement of Science © 2015.) (*D*) Imaging of hyperpolarization (HP) [5-^{13}C]glutamine in a MIA PaCa-2 xenograft mouse model shows elevated glutaminolysis in tumor. Metabolic maps of HP glutamate (*left*) and HP glutamine (*right*) with tumor region indicated with red dotted line show decreased uptake of HP glutamine but similar HP glutamate production in tumor compared to surrounding tissue. (*D* reprinted from Eskandari et al. 2022 under the terms of Creative Commons Attribution-NonCommercial-NoDerivatives Licences 4.0 [CC BY-NC-ND].) (*E*) Clinical ^{1}H MRSI shows high 2HG production in mutant IDH2 glioma. 3D metabolic maps of 2HG (*left*), glutamine/glutamate (*center*), and lactate (*right*) show that regions of with high levels of 2HG correlate with high lactate production, but not glutamine/glutamate levels, which are relatively homogeneous throughout the imaging field of view. (*E* reprinted from Choi et al. 2012, Springer Link © 2012.)

Cite this article as *Cold Spring Harb Perspect Med* doi: 10.1101/cshperspect.a041551

notype where α-ketoglutarate (αKG) is converted to 2-hydroxyglutarate (2HG). Elevated 2HG production has been characterized as a central feature of metabolic reprogramming in a variety of cancers and is being investigated as a target for molecular imaging (Dang et al. 2009; Ježek 2020). ^{1}H MRSI measurement of 2HG pool size in glioma patients consistently shows that IDH mutant gliomas, but not healthy tissue or IDH wild-type tumors, produce large quantities of 2HG (Fig. 2E; Choi et al. 2012; Andronesi et al. 2016; An et al. 2017, 2018). In this way, 2HG can be thought of as an imaging biomarker of IDH mutation status.

In this vein, HP [1-^{13}C]glutamine (Fig. 2Bii) has been leveraged to image flux to 2HG in mouse xenografts of mutant IDH patient-derived chondrosarcoma cells (Salamanca-Cardona et al. 2017). Using ^{13}C mass spectrometry tracing experiments, this paper demonstrated that glutamine, not glucose, is the primary carbon source for 2HG. HP [1-^{13}C]αKG has also been used to measure 2HG formation in IDH mutant tumor cells and mouse models (Chaumeil et al. 2013; Miura et al. 2021). Targeting flux to 2HG may prove useful in the context of mutant IDH1 gliomas, which appear unsuitable for imaging with HP pyruvate (Chaumeil et al. 2016). Low cell permeability of αKG has hampered HP imaging capability, although chemical modifications such as esterification may help with this issue (Zacharias et al. 2012; AbuSalim et al. 2021; Singh et al. 2021).

Anabolism

Cancer cells also up-regulate pathways of anabolic metabolism to fuel unrestrained proliferation (Fig. 3A). This section presents examples of imaging probes that report on fatty acid, protein, and nucleoside salvage.

Fatty Acid Synthesis

Rapid tumor cell division is accompanied by high levels of de novo fatty acid biosynthesis, a pathway that produces the lipid bilayers that make up cell membranes. One of the building blocks of fatty acids is acetyl-CoA, which is synthesized from acetate. To that end, PET of

[^{11}C]acetate has been used as a strategy to image fatty acid synthesis in cancers (Fig. 3Bi). In the clinic, [^{11}C]acetate PET has been useful in imaging tumors that are not FDG avid such as prostate cancer, well-differentiated hepatocarcinoma, and multiple myelomas (Grassi et al. 2011; Chen et al. 2021). Uptake of [^{11}C]acetate is sensitive to inhibition of fatty acid synthase (FAS) in prostate cancer cells, indicating that [^{11}C]acetate could act as an imaging biomarker of fatty acid synthesis (Vāvere et al. 2008; Lewis et al. 2014). The first step of acetate metabolism is conversion to acetyl-CoA via acetyl-CoA synthetase (ACSS). ACSS1, the mitochondrial isoform of ACSS, is predominant in normal cells, and is used as an entry point for acetate into the TCA cycle. Tumor cells have low ACSS1 expression and instead up-regulate the cytosolic isoform ACSS2, diverting acetate incorporation into fatty acid synthesis (Yoshii et al. 2009). There has not been much success in developing ^{18}F-based acetate analogs as PET probes. Fluoroacetate is toxic at high doses and is used as a pesticide (Clarke 1991). Although ^{18}F-fluoroacetate is safe at low PET dosage concentration in nonhuman primates (Nishii et al. 2012), a study in healthy large animals showed that ^{18}F-fluoroacetate is mostly excreted through the blood and shows no specific uptake (Lindhe et al. 2009).

Acetate uptake has also been imaged with MR-based probes. DMI of infused ^{2}H-labeled acetate showed increased acetate uptake and reduced glutamate and glutamine labeling in tumors compared to healthy brain tissue in orthotopic models of glioma in rats, indicating reduced TCA cycle utilization by tumor cells (De Feyter et al. 2018). HP [1-^{13}C]acetate has also been used to measure TCA cycle flux in healthy rat hearts and kidneys, but this probe has yet to be applied to the context of cancer metabolism (Bastiaansen et al. 2015; Mikkelsen et al. 2017).

Amino Acid Uptake

Proliferative cancers display increased uptake of neutrally charged amino acids to fuel protein synthesis. The blood–brain barrier is permeable to neutrally charged amino acids, which are imported into cells by the L-type amino acid trans-

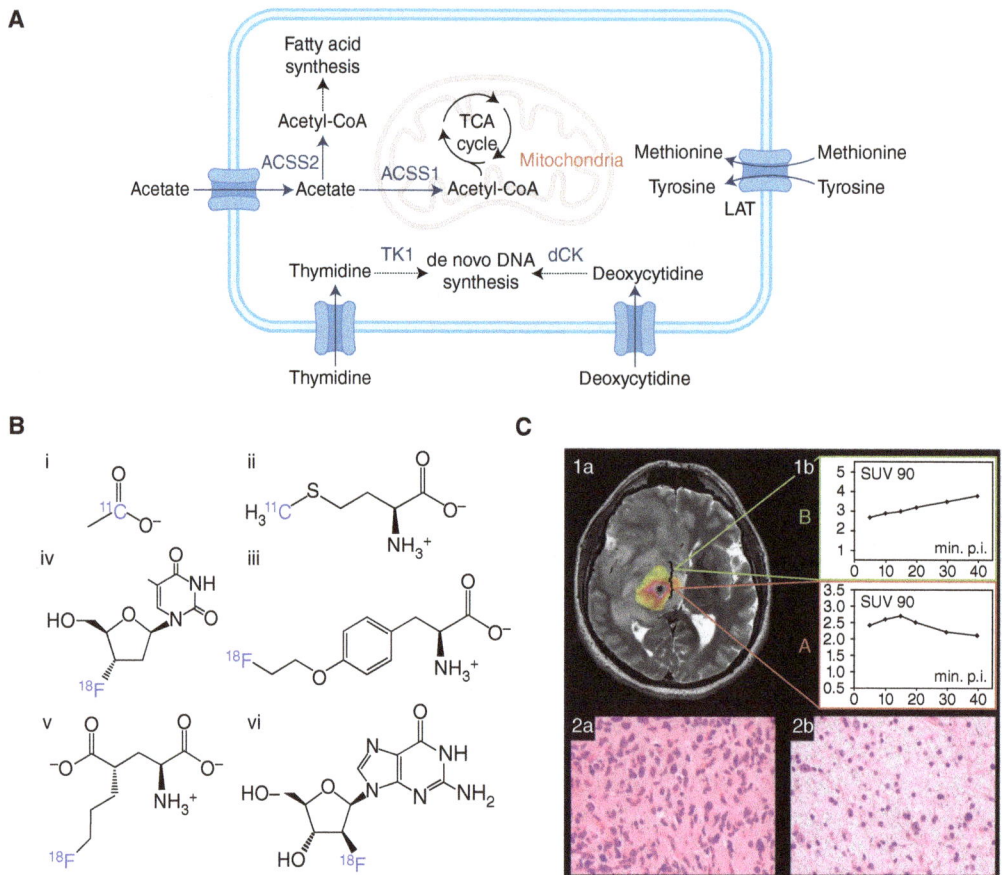

Figure 3. Molecular imaging of anabolic metabolism. (*A*) Diagram of metabolites, enzymes, and transporters relevant to anabolic metabolism. (ACSS1/2) acetyl-CoA synthase, (TK1) thymidine kinase, (dCK) deoxycytidine kinase, (LAT) large neutral amino acid transporter. (*A* created with BioRender.com.) (*B*) Chemical structures of probes for imaging glutamine metabolism. (*i*) [1-^{11}C]acetate, (*ii*) [^{11}C-methyl]L-methionine (^{11}C-MET), (*iii*) O-(2-[^{18}F]fluoroethyl)-L-tyrosine (^{18}FET), (*iv*) (S)-4-(3-[^{18}F]fluoropropyl)-L-glutamate ([^{18}F]FSPG), (*v*) [^{18}F]3′-deoxy-3′-fluorothymidine ([^{18}F]FLT), (*vi*) [^{18}F]clofarabine ([^{18}F]CFA). β-Emitting radioisotopes detected by positron emission tomography (PET) are blue, and nuclei detected by magnetic resonance (MR) are red. Structures created with ChemDraw. (*C*) Dynamic ^{18}FET imaging of a glioma patient reveals intratumoral heterogeneity. The single time point ^{18}FET image with anatomic magnetic resonance imaging (MRI) overlay (*left*) shows differential uptake of the probe. Kinetic data from specific regions (*right*) show the tumor periphery consistently accumulates ^{18}FET (*top*), whereas the interior has a quick initial uptake of tracer followed by a steady decline of PET signal (*bottom*). These time courses correspond to WHO grade III and II phenotypes, respectively, as identified by matched histopathology. (*C* reprinted, with permission, from Kunz et al. 2011, © The Author(s) 2011. Published by Oxford University Press on behalf of the Society for Neuro-Oncology.)

porters (LATs). Up-regulation of the LATs in many cancers has been interpreted as a mechanism for fueling proliferative protein synthesis (Okubo et al. 2010; Wang et al. 2015; Häfliger and Charles 2019).

The original and most implemented amino acid-based PET probe is [^{11}C-methyl]L-methi-

onine (^{11}C-MET) (Fig. 3Bii; Bustany et al. 1986). ^{11}C-MET has been successfully used to image gliomas in the clinic, outperforming FDG-PET, particularly in low-grade tumors (Singhal et al. 2008; Sharma et al. 2016; Xu et al. 2017; Ninatti et al. 2022). The high spatial resolution of PET can enable discrimination between intratumoral subcomponents; in one clinical study, low-grade astrocytomas showed increased ^{11}C-MET uptake in infiltrative exterior regions compared to interior regions with a solid tumor phenotype (Kracht et al. 2004).

As with all ^{11}C-based PET probes, the primary limitation of ^{11}C-MET is its short radioactive half-life. As such, there has been an effort to develop ^{18}F-labeled amino acid derivatives, the most notable example of which is O-(2-[^{18}F]fluoroethyl)-L-tyrosine ([18]FET) (Fig. 3Biii; Langen et al. 2017). [18]FET has found widespread success in the imaging of brain tumors. In particular, [18]FET has markedly high sensitivity in the disambiguation of high-grade gliomas from lesions that appear identically in standard MRI, such as brain metastases and primary lymphomas (Puranik et al. 2019). The long lifetime of [18]FET enables the measurement of probe uptake kinetics over the course of around an hour (Jansen et al. 2012, 2014; Lohmann et al. 2015). Dynamic information can be used to differentiate local phenotypes. For example, one kinetic study of [18]FET showed that low-grade gliomas constantly import and retain tracer, whereas high-grade tumors have an early peak of uptake followed by a steady decline of PET signal (Fig. 3C; Kunz et al. 2011). Heterogeneity within tumors was also observed in the form of "hot spots" of high-grade-like malignant regions. One factor that may play a part in differential probe dynamics is specific interactions with LAT1. One study used a model of purified LAT1 reconstituted in Xenopus oocytes to show that [18]FET is taken into cells by LAT1 but not effluxed (Habermeier et al. 2015). This asymmetry could help explain why [18]FET accumulates in high-LAT1 gliomas despite a lack of probe incorporation into cellular protein.

Another amino acid–based PET probe that has shown success is the glutamate analog (S)-4-(3-[^{18}F]fluoropropyl)-L-glutamate ([^{18}F]FSPG) (Fig. 3Biv; Koglin et al. 2011). [^{18}F]FSPG is imported into cells via system x_c^-, which exchanges glutamate for cystine. Up-regulation of system x_c^- has been observed in many cancers and has been linked to several factors promoting malignancy. Cystine imported by system x_c^- is reduced in the cell to cysteine, a precursor of glu-

tathione (GSH), the most abundant antioxidant molecule. Therefore, increased uptake of [^{18}F]FSPG by system x_c^- has been interpreted as an imaging biomarker of increased tumor cell resistance to oxidative stress (McCormick et al. 2018). In clinical trials spanning a variety of cancer types, [^{18}F]FSPG was shown to outperform FDG in distinguishing lesions (Baek et al. 2012; Kavanaugh et al. 2016; Park et al. 2020; Wardak et al. 2022).

Nucleoside Salvage

Another hallmark of the proliferating cancer cells is increased nucleoside metabolism. Uptake of [^{18}F]3'-deoxy-3'-fluorothymidine ([^{18}F]FLT), a PET analog of thymidine (Shields et al. 1998) has been shown to correlate to proliferation (Fig. 3Bv). [^{18}F]FLT is trapped in cells upon phosphorylation via thymidine kinase (TK), the first step in the de novo DNA biosynthesis pathway. [^{18}F]FLT has been used in the clinic as a sensitive probe of tumor proliferation in brain tumors (Chen et al. 2005; Choi et al. 2005). A limitation of [^{18}F]FLT is that it is specific to the thymidine salvage pathway. One study showed that [^{18}F]FLT is not avidly taken up by tumor subtypes that rely on de novo thymidine synthesis, a complementary and competitive pathway (McKinley et al. 2013). Therefore, care should be taken not to conflate [^{18}F]FLT uptake with more general proliferative markers, such as Ki67 staining.

Recent work has identified [^{18}F]clofarabine ([^{18}F]CFA) as a promising nucleoside analog PET probe for imaging of nucleoside salvage (Fig. 3Bvi; Kim et al. 2016). [^{18}F]CFA is a highly specific substrate for deoxycytidine kinase (dCK), and was shown to accumulate in leukemia cells. [^{18}F]CFA has also been investigated as a probe of immunotherapy response in preclinical models of glioma (Antonios et al. 2017). Activated T cells up-regulate dCK, so [^{18}F]CFA uptake can be interpreted as an imaging biomarker of activated T cell infiltration.

In conclusion, tumor cells power proliferative growth by up-regulating the biosynthesis of lipids, proteins, and DNA. These anabolic pathways can take up constituent carbon atoms from the extracellular space, allowing imaging of anabolism through the labeling of building block molecules such as acetate, amino acids, and nucleosides, respectively.

Phenotypic Consequences of Cancer Metabolism

This last section will focus on imaging probes that target phenotypic traits associated with cancer metabolism: altered redox balance, acidification of the tumor microenvironment (TME), and hypoxia.

Redox Status

Rapid proliferation generates high levels of reactive oxygen species, leading to an oxidative stress phenotype. Elevated levels of antioxidants, primarily GSH, have been identified as a mechanism for tumor resistance to radiation or chemotherapy. Infusion of ^{13}C-labeled glycine, a building block of GSH, allows direct measurement of GSH by ^{13}C MRS in tumors (Thelwall et al. 2005, 2012). However, the scan times for these experiments are prohibitively long for widespread application.

HP [1-^{13}C]dehydroascorbic acid (DHA) is a promising probe of redox status: it has a favorable T1 of 57 sec at 3 T, is preferentially taken up by tumor cells, and undergoes rapid reduction to [1-^{13}C]vitamin C with a chemical shift difference of 3.8 ppm (Fig. 4Ai; Bohndiek et al. 2011). There are two factors that influence the kinetics of DHA metabolism. First, DHA is reduced to vitamin C in the cell by enzymes that use GSH or NADPH as a cofactor, so the ratio of vitamin C to DHA functions as an indirect readout of the redox state of the cell. The ratio of HP DHA to vitamin C is elevated in lymphoma, prostate cancer, and colorectal cancer tumors, reflecting unbalanced redox phenotypes (Keshari et al. 2011; Timm et al. 2017). Another factor that influences the kinetics of DHA reduction is an expression of the GLUT transporters, which import DHA in addition to sugars. In a transgenic prostate cancer mouse model, increased vitamin C/DHA ratios in tumors correlated with avid FDG-PET uptake (Fig. 4B; Keshari et al. 2013). Immunohistochemistry confirmed that these tumors up-regulate GLUT3 and GLUT4, accounting for the increase of both PET and HP MR probe import. The path to clinical translation of HP DHA has been complicated by concerns with toxicity. In one study, formulations of DHA administered at 10 mg/kg dose to tumor-bearing mice induced respiratory arrest and cardiac depression (Timm et al. 2017). However, studies using large animals and nonhuman primates showed that doses of upward of 500 mg/kg can be well tolerated, suggesting differential pharmacology of DHA (Banerjee et al. 1953; Ducruet et al. 2011). More work on the mechanisms of DHA toxicity is required before clinical translation of this probe can progress.

^{11}C-labeled DHA and vitamin C have also been developed as PET probes for redox, although these molecules are less sensitive to changes in the chemotherapeutic depletion of GSH than HP DHA (Carroll et al. 2016, Qin et al. 2018). A recent alternative for imaging DHA/vitamin C redox is the PET probe ^{18}F-KS1, a modified radioanalog of vitamin C (Fig. 4Aii; Sai et al. 2019). ^{18}F-KS1 shows tumor specificity and favorable pharmacokinetics in rodent and nonhuman primate tumor models, making it attractive for clinical application (Damuka et al. 2022). The next step for ^{18}F-KS1 translation is a pilot study in humans. Another recently reported PET probe for redox is 4-[^{18}F]fluoro-1-naphthol ([^{18}F]4FN) (Pisaneschi et al. 2022). This probe is sensitive only to radical species with high redox potential, allowing specific imaging of innate immunity activation. Although [^{18}F]4FN has yet to be applied to the context of cancer metabolism, its mechanism provides the proof of concept of a tunable redox PET sensor, which may be leveraged for finer-grained quantification of intracellular redox states in cancer.

Extracellular pH

Acidification of the TME caused by excess lactate production is a widely observed cancer metabolic phenotype. Tumors evolve to thrive in this

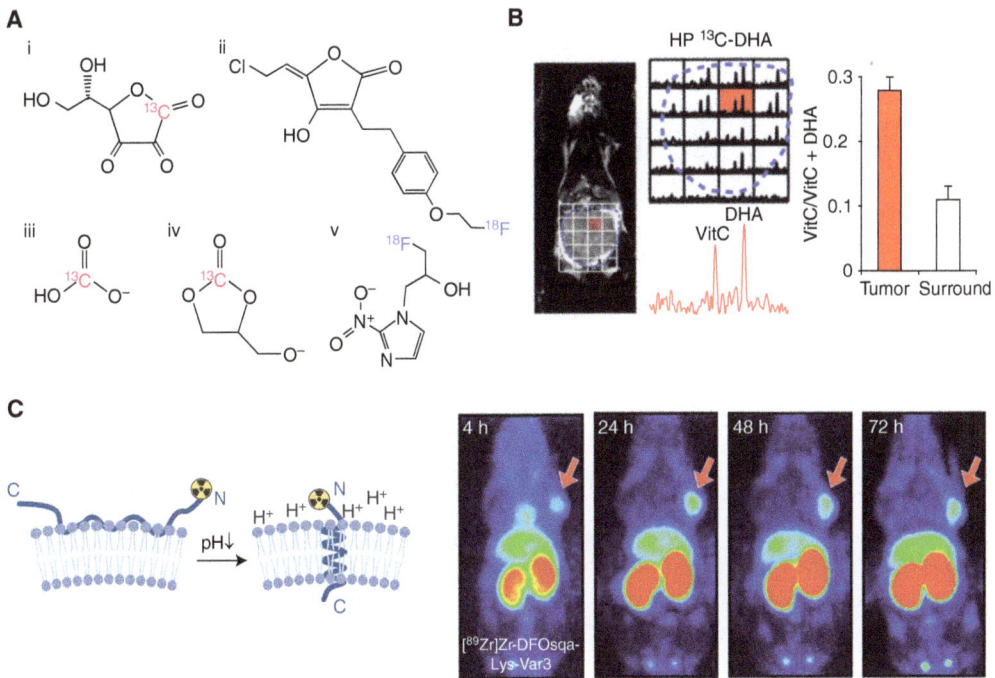

Figure 4. Molecular imaging of cancer metabolic phenotypes. (*A*) Chemical structures of probes for imaging redox, pH, and hypoxia. (*i*) [1-^{13}C]dehydroascorbic acid (DHA), (*ii*) (*E*)-5-(2-chloroethylidene)-3-((4-(2-[^{18}F] fluoroethoxy)benzyl)oxy)-4-hydroxyfuran-2(5H)-one (KS1), (*iii*) [^{13}C]bicarbonate, (*iv*) [1-^{13}C]1,2-glycerol car-bonate, (*v*) [^{18}F]fluoromisonidazole (^{18}F-FMISO). β-Emitting radioisotopes detected by positron emission to-mography (PET) are blue, and nuclei detected by magnetic resonance (MR) are red. Structures created with ChemDraw. (*B*) Measurement of intracellular redox states with magnetic resonance spectroscopic imaging (MRSI) of HP DHA. Anatomic coronal MR image of a transgenic model of prostate cancer mouse with tumor delineated with blue dashed line and overlaid spectra of HP DHA MRSI (*left*). Representative spectrum localized to the tumor (*bottom middle*) shows high uptake of DHA and conversion to vitamin C. Metabolite ratios summed over multiple spectra (*right*) show a 2.5-fold increase of flux of HP DHA to vitamin C in the tumor compared to surrounding healthy tissue, reflecting higher cellular concentrations of glutathione and increased transport of DHA via the glucose transporters GLUT1/3/4. (*B* reprinted, with permission, from Keshari et al. 2013, © SNMMI.) (*C*) Structure of pHLIP probe (*left*) shows DOTA chelator moiety, which can bind to copper radio-nuclides for PET imaging, bound to a 37-residue long peptide sequence. At neutral pH, the peptide has a random coil conformation, but in acidic environments can form an α-helical structure capable of stable transmembrane incorporation. Example whole-body coronal and axial PET images of ^{64}Cu-DOTA-pHLIP in prostate cancer xenograft mice (*right*) show higher probe uptake in LNCaP (*left*) over PC3 (*right*), corresponding with increased acidity in LNCaP (measured tumor pH_e = 6.78) compared to PC3 (measured tumor pH_e = 7.23). (*C*, created with BioRender, was adapted from Bauer et al. 2022 under the terms of the Creative Commons Attribution License (CC BY). Copyright © Bauer, Visca, Weerakkody, Cody, Samuels, Kaminsky, Andreev, Reshetnyak, and Lewis.).

acidic environment, with in vitro tumor cell pro-liferation maximized at a subphysiological pH of 6.8 (Gatenby and Gillies 2004; Zhang et al. 2010). Lowered extracellular pH (pH_e) has thus been investigated as an imaging biomarker of the Warburg effect. Imaging of pH_e is achieved with molecular probes that are sensitive to local changes in pH.

Historically, changes in pH were annotated using ^{31}P NMR spectroscopy and later spectro-scopic imaging by measuring chemical shift changes (Stubbs et al. 1992). While these could be enhanced through the use of an exogenous contrast agent (Gillies et al. 1994), these ap-proaches suffered from low sensitivity due to the nucleus chosen. pH imaging using ^{1}H MR approaches, including relaxivity or magnetization transfer, was more suited for spatially resolved pH maps given the sensitivity of ^1H MRI (Gillies et al. 2004). Relaxivity imaging involves the injection of a contrast agent, typically a gadolinium chelate, whose effect on the T1 relaxation of the water ^1H MR signal is pH-sensitive (Raghunand et al. 2002). Magnetization transfer experiments measure the exchange between labile hydrogens on an injected probe and bulk water. This exchange process is pH-dependent and can be measured with chemical exchange saturation transfer (CEST) techniques similar to those used in glucoCEST to indirectly infer pH (Ward and Balaban 2000; Sun and Sorensen 2008; Longo et al. 2014, 2016). One major drawback of both these methods is that the magnitude of the effect of pH on the signal is dependent on the local concentration of the contrast agents. These methods thus confound pH measurement with pharmacokinetic dynamics, requiring reproducible calibration curves. Since calibration of in vivo signals is often challenging, these methods have intrinsic issues with reproducibility and comparability across contexts.

Since PET signals are not inherently environmentally responsive, imaging pH_e with PET requires coupling probe retention to pH. One elegant strategy involves PET tracers conjugated to a pH (low) insertion peptide (pHLIP), a 36-amino acid-long peptide that only inserts into lipid bilayer membranes in an α-helical conformation at low pH (Reshetnyak et al. 2006). At physiological pH, pHLIP is in a random coil conformation and cannot insert into membranes. This means that a radioisotope-labeled pHLIP will only retain in membranes and give persistent PET signal in low pH regions. The first pHLIP-based PET probe was conjugated to ^{64}Cu, a radioisotope with an especially long half-life of ~12.8 h, and showed long-lasting uptake and retention in prostate cancer xenograft models (Fig. 4C; Văvere et al. 2009). Subsequent work has improved targeting specificity through structural modification of the peptide (Tapmeier et al. 2015; Wyatt et al. 2018) or substitution of ^{64}Cu with other radioisotopes such as ^{18}F (Daumar et al. 2012) or ^{89}Zr (Bauer et al. 2022). Cor-

relative histology of prostate cancer tumors showed that low pH_e regions detected by pHLIP-PET are associated with increased expression of carbonic anhydrase IX (CAIX), a tumor-associated acid-extruding protein (Viola-Villegas et al. 2014), linking imaging data to one molecular mechanism of TME acidification. So far there has been one phase I clinical trial of ^{18}F-labeled pHLIP (NCT04054986).

The most studied HP probe for acidification is [^{13}C]bicarbonate (Fig. 4Aiii; Gallagher et al. 2008). Bicarbonate is in pH-dependent equilibrium with carbon dioxide via CAIX, and up-regulation of CAIX is likely a predominant mechanism of tumor adaptation to hypoxia and TME acidification (Gallagher et al. 2015). The ratio of bicarbonate to carbon dioxide concentrations can be used to calculate pH using the Henderson–Hasselbach equation. Since carbon dioxide can freely diffuse across the cell membrane, the pH measured by HP bicarbonate does not distinguish between extracellular and intracellular compartments. However, some data suggest that this ratio is weighted to pH_e (Gallagher et al. 2011). One particular advantage of imaging injected bicarbonate is that it is an endogenous buffer molecule, making clinical translation possible. However, the solubility of sodium bicarbonate in suitable formulations for HP is poor R (Wilson et al. 2010). Recent work has addressed this limitation through the polarization of a carbonate precursor and rapid base-catalyzed hydrolysis to form HP bicarbonate (Korenchan et al. 2016). To this end, [1-^{13}C] 1,2-glycerol carbonate was used to measure grade-dependent acidification in transgenic mouse models of prostate cancer, where pH_e was markedly lower in higher-grade tumors (Fig. 4Aiv; Korenchan et al. 2019). Interestingly, in mice that had both low- and high-grade lesions, pH imaging allowed the separation of benign from aggressive tumor regions. This study also found a positive correlation between acidic TME regions and high expression of MCT4, the predominant exporter of lactate.

Besides HP bicarbonate, a number of molecules have been investigated for HP pH imaging: ^{13}C-enriched N-(2-acetamido-)2-aminoethanesulfonic acid (Flavell et al. 2015), [1,5-$^{13}C_2$]zy-

Cite this article as *Cold Spring Harb Perspect Med* doi: 10.1101/cshperspect.a041551

monic acid (Düwel et al. 2017), amino acid derivatives (Hundshammer et al. 2018), [2-^{13}C, D$_{10}$]diethylmalonic acid (Korenchan et al. 2017), ^{15}N-pyridine derivatives (Jiang et al. 2015), and ^{89}Y chelates (Jindal et al. 2010; Wang et al. 2020). Although these exotic probes all feature suitable in vitro HP probe characteristics such as favorable T1 times and chemical shift differences, it is unclear whether they have much translational utility due to issues with toxicity and in vivo uptake.

Hypoxia

Finally, a central feature of the TME that shapes tumor metabolic phenotypes is chronic and transient hypoxia. A reduction in oxygen limits the capacity for oxidative phosphorylation in tumor cells, driving the evolution of hypoxia-tolerant up-regulation of glycolysis. A number of methods have been developed to quantitatively image the partial pressure of oxygen, or concentration of oxygen dissolved in blood (pO$_2$).

The "gold standard" PET probe for hypoxia is [^{18}F]fluoromisonidazole (^{18}F-FMISO) (Fig. 4Av; Rasey et al. 1989; Koh et al. 1992). Upon entry into cells, the nitro group on ^{18}F-FMISO is rapidly reduced, primarily via xanthine oxide. In cells with physiological oxygen levels, reduced ^{18}F-FMISO is oxidized to its original form, which can then be exported out of the cell. However, oxidation is not possible in hypoxic cells and the reduced probe becomes trapped. Oxidation capacity is used as a proxy for oxygen concentration in the cell, making ^{18}F-FMISO an indirect reporter of hypoxia. ^{18}F-FMISO has been used to map hypoxic regions in a wide variety of cancers (Rajendran et al. 2006; Hendrickson et al. 2011; Hugonnet et al. 2011; Cheng et al. 2013; Tong et al. 2016). Widespread clinical translation of ^{18}F-FMISO as a diagnostic probe has proven difficult due to slow clearance of the probe from normoxic areas and consequently low tumor-to-background ratios. Therefore, other nitroimidazole-derived molecules are being explored for hypoxia imaging, the most promising of which is ^{18}F-FAZA, which shows favorable pharmacokinetics over ^{18}F-FMISO

and is currently under clinical investigation (Busk et al. 2013; Saga et al. 2015, 2016).

Oxygen levels can be directly imaged with electron paramagnetic resonance imaging (EPRI), a technique similar to MRI that instead detects unpaired electrons such as free radicals (Krishna et al. 2012). The high sensitivity and spatial resolution of EPRI have been used to map pO$_2$ in a variety of tumors (Yasui et al. 2017; Kishimoto et al. 2021; Virani et al. 2021). These studies tend to focus on the relationship between therapy resistance and hypoxia, a posited mechanism for tumor evasion to radiation. One comparative modality study in pancreatic cancer mouse xenograft models found that EPRI pO$_2$ measurements positively correlated with FDG-PET in the periphery of the tumor and negatively correlated in the center, indicating regional differences in response to hypoxia independent of glucose uptake (Yamamoto et al. 2020).

In conclusion, cancer metabolism can also be imaged from the perspective of the phenotypic features that both drive and arise in response to up-regulated proliferation. These characteristics include altered redox capacity in the cell, increased extracellular acidification, and transient or chronic hypoxia.

CONCLUDING REMARKS

This review has described various examples of PET and MR methods used to image cancer metabolism. We hope that this work provides a clear survey of the power of molecular imaging to investigate tumor metabolism in its native contexts. In the clinic, molecular imaging can delineate malignant regions based on their underlying metabolic phenotype, which might be invisible to anatomic imaging. In basic research, molecular imaging reveals aspects of spatial heterogeneity that guide the metabolism of cancers as they form, grow, and respond to treatment.

A molecular imaging research program is inherently interdisciplinary and recursive. Basic biology identifies suitable metabolic targets for molecular imaging. Chemists synthesize probes to target these metabolic processes, and nuclear physicists optimize methods for the detection of the probes in vivo. Biochemists characterize the metabolic mechanisms governing imaging signal formation, leveraging the findings of molecular imaging to suggest new avenues of investigation. Each of these phases relies upon and informs the others. Successful scientific discovery in metabolic imaging of cancer requires the perspectives from both the biology of metabolism and the development of molecular imaging techniques.

ACKNOWLEDGMENTS

We thank Garon Scott, Roxanne Morris, and Briana Turner for helpful comments.

REFERENCES

AbuSalim JE, Yamamoto K, Miura N, Blackman B, Brender JR, Mushti C, Seki T, Camphausen KA, Swenson RE, Krishna MC, et al. 2021. Simple esterification of $[1-^{13}C]$-α-ketoglutarate enhances membrane permeability and allows for noninvasive tracing of glutamate and glutamine production. *ACS Chem Biol* **16:** 2144–2150. doi:10.1021/acschembio.1c00561

Aggarwal R, Vigneron DB, Kurhanewicz J. 2017. Hyperpolarized $1-[^{13}C]$-pyruvate magnetic resonance imaging detects an early metabolic response to androgen ablation therapy in prostate cancer. *Eur Urol* **72:** 1028–1029. doi:10.1016/j.eururo.2017.07.022

Alavi A, Lakhani P, Mavi A, Kung JW, Zhuang H. 2004. PET: a revolution in medical imaging. *Radiol Clin North Am* **42:** 983–1001. doi:10.1016/j.rcl.2004.08.012

Albers MJ, Bok R, Chen AP, Cunningham CH, Zierhut ML, Zhang VY, Kohler SJ, Tropp J, Hurd RE, Yen Y-F, et al. 2008. Hyperpolarized ^{13}C lactate, pyruvate, and alanine: noninvasive biomarkers for prostate cancer detection and grading. *Cancer Res* **68:** 8607–8615. doi:10.1158/0008-5472.CAN-08-0749

Altman BJ, Stine ZE, Dang CV. 2016. From Krebs to clinic: glutamine metabolism to cancer therapy. *Nat Rev Cancer* **16:** 619–634. doi:10.1038/nrc.2016.71

An Z, Ganji SK, Tiwari V, Pinho MC, Patel T, Barnett S, Pan E, Mickey BE, Maher EA, Choi C. 2017. Detection of 2-hydroxyglutarate in brain tumors by triple-refocusing MR spectroscopy at 3T in vivo. *Magn Reson Med* **78:** 40–48. doi:10.1002/mrm.26347

An Z, Tiwari V, Ganji SK, Baxter J, Levy M, Pinho MC, Pan E, Maher EA, Patel TR, Mickey BE, et al. 2018. Echoplanar spectroscopic imaging with dual-readout alternated gradients (DRAG-EPSI) at 7 T: application for 2-hydroxyglutarate imaging in glioma patients. *Magn Reson Med* **79:** 1851–1861. doi:10.1002/mrm.26884

Andronesi OC, Loebel F, Bogner W, Marjańska M, Heiden MGV, Iafrate AJ, Dietrich J, Batchelor TT, Gerstner ER, Kaelin WG, et al. 2016. Treatment response assessment in IDH-mutant glioma patients by noninvasive 3D functional spectroscopic mapping of 2-hydroxyglutarate. *Clin Cancer Res* **22:** 1632–1641. doi:10.1158/1078-0432 .CCR-15-0656

Antonios JP, Soto H, Everson RG, Moughon DL, Wang AC, Orpilla J, Radu C, Ellingson BM, Lee JT, Cloughesy T, et al. 2017. Detection of immune responses after immunotherapy in glioblastoma using PET and MRI. *Proc Natl Acad Sci* **114:** 10220–10225. doi:10.1073/pnas.1706689114

Ardenkjær-Larsen JH, Fridlund B, Gram A, Hansson G, Hansson L, Lerche MH, Servin R, Thaning M, Golman K. 2003. Increase in signal-to-noise ratio of >10,000 times in liquid-state NMR. *Proc Natl Acad Sci* **100:** 10158–10163. doi:10.1073/pnas.1733835100

Baek S, Choi C-M, Ahn SH, Lee JW, Gong G, Ryu JS, Oh SJ, Bacher-Stier C, Fels L, Koglin N, et al. 2012. Exploratory clinical trial of (4S)-4-(3-[^{18}F]fluoropropyl)-L-glutamate for imaging x_C^- transporter using positron emission tomography in patients with non-small cell lung or breast cancer. *Clin Cancer Res* **18:** 5427–5437. doi:10.1158/ 1078-0432.CCR-12-0214

Banerjee S, Belavady B, Mukherjee AK. 1953. Effect of dehydroascorbic acid in rabbits. *Proc Soc Exp Biol Med* **83:** 133–135. doi:10.3181/00379727-83-20287

Bankson JA, Walker CM, Ramirez MS, Stefan W, Fuentes D, Merritt ME, Lee J, Sandulache VC, Chen Y, Phan L, et al. 2015. Kinetic modeling and constrained reconstruction of hyperpolarized $[1-^{13}C]$-pyruvate offers improved metabolic imaging of tumors. *Cancer Res* **75:** 4708–4717. doi:10.1158/0008-5472.CAN-15-0171

Bastiaansen JAM, Cheng T, Lei H, Gruetter R, Comment A. 2015. Direct noninvasive estimation of myocardial tricarboxylic acid cycle flux in vivo using hyperpolarized ^{13}C magnetic resonance. *J Mol Cell Cardiol* **87:** 129–137. doi:10.1016/j.yjmcc.2015.08.012

Batsios G, Taglang C, Cao P, Gillespie AM, Najac C, Subramani E, Wilson DM, Flavell RR, Larson PEZ, Ronen SM, et al. 2021. Imaging 6-phosphogluconolactonase activity in brain tumors in vivo using hyperpolarized δ-$[1-^{13}C]$gluconolactone. *Front Oncol* **11:** 589570. doi:10 .3389/fonc.2021.589570

Bauer D, Visca H, Weerakkody A, Carter LM, Samuels Z, Kaminsky S, Andreev OA, Reshetnyak YK, Lewis JS. 2022. PET imaging of acidic tumor environment with 89Zr-labeled pHLIP probes. *Front Oncol* **12:** 882541. doi:10 .3389/fonc.2022.882541

Bender B, Herz K, Deshmane A, Richter V, Tabatabai G, Schittenhelm J, Skardelly M, Scheffler K, Ernemann U, Kim M, et al. 2022. GLINT: GlucoCEST in neoplastic tumors at 3 T—clinical results of GlucoCEST in gliomas. *MAGMA* **35:** 77–85. doi:10.1007/s10334-021-00982-5

Bohndiek SE, Kettunen MI, Hu D, Kennedy BWC, Boren J, Gallagher FA, Brindle KM. 2011. Hyperpolarized $[1-^{13}C]$-ascorbic and dehydroascorbic acid: vitamin C as a probe for imaging redox status in vivo. *J Am Chem Soc* **133:** 11795–11801. doi:10.1021/ja2045925

Bohndiek SE, Kettunen MI, Hu D, Brindle KM. 2012. Hyperpolarized ^{13}C spectroscopy detects early changes in tumor vasculature and metabolism after VEGF neutralization. *Cancer Res* **72:** 854–864. doi:10.1158/0008-5472 .CAN-11-2795

Bouvet V, Jans HS, Wuest M, Soueidan O-M, Mercer J, McEwan AJ, West FG, Cheeseman CI, Wuest F. 2014.

Automated synthesis and dosimetry of 6-deoxy-6-[(18)F] fluoro-D-fructose (6-[(18)F]FDF): a radiotracer for imaging of GLUT5 in breast cancer. *Am J Nucl Med Mol Imaging* 4: 248–259.

Brindle KM, Bohndiek SE, Gallagher FA, Kettunen MI. 2011. Tumor imaging using hyperpolarized ^{13}C magnetic resonance spectroscopy. *Magn Reson Med* 66: 505–519. doi:10.1002/mrm.22999

Busk M, Mortensen LS, Nordsmark M, Overgaard J, Jakobsen S, Hansen KV, Theil J, Kallehauge JF, D'Andrea FP, Steiniche T, et al. 2013. PET hypoxia imaging with FAZA: reproducibility at baseline and during fractionated radiotherapy in tumour-bearing mice. *Eur J Nucl Med Mol Imaging* 40: 186–197. doi:10.1007/s00259-012-2258-x

Bustany P, Chatel M, Derlon JM, Darcel F, Sgouropoulos P, Soussaline F, Syrota A. 1986. Brain tumor protein synthesis and histological grades: a study by positron emission tomography (PET) with C11-L-methionine. *J Neurooncol* 3: 397–404. doi:10.1007/BF00165590

Cabella C, Karlsson M, Canapè C, Catanzaro G, Serra SC, Miragoli L, Poggi L, Uggeri F, Venturi L, Jensen PR, et al. 2013. In vivo and in vitro liver cancer metabolism observed with hyperpolarized [5-^{13}C]glutamine. *J Magn Reson* 232: 45–52. doi:10.1016/j.jmr.2013.04.010

Canapè C, Catanzaro G, Terreno E, Karlsson M, Lerche MH, Jensen PR. 2015. Probing treatment response of glutaminolytic prostate cancer cells to natural drugs with hyperpolarized [5-^{13}C]glutamine. *Magn Reson Med* 73: 2296–2305. doi:10.1002/mrm.25360

Capozza M, Anemone A, Dhakan C, Peruta MD, Bracesco M, Zullino S, Villano D, Terreno E, Longo DL, Aime S. 2022. GlucoCEST MRI for the evaluation response to chemotherapeutic and metabolic treatments in a murine triple-negative breast cancer: a comparison with [^{18}F]F-FDG-PET. *Mol Imaging Biol* 24: 126–134. doi:10.1007/s11307-021-01637-6

Carroll VN, Truillet C, Shen B, Flavell RR, Shao X, Evans MJ, VanBrocklin HF, Scott PJH, Chin FT, Wilson DM. 2016. [^{11}C]Ascorbic and [^{11}C]dehydroascorbic acid, an endogenous redox pair for sensing reactive oxygen species using positron emission tomography. *Chem Commun* 52: 4888–4890. doi:10.1039/C6CC00895J

Carson RE. 2003. Tracer kinetic modeling in PET. In *Positron emission tomography: basic science and clinical practice* (ed. Valk PE, et al.), pp. 147–179. Springer, Amsterdam.

Cember ATJ, Wilson NE, Rich LJ, Bagga P, Nanga RPR, Swago S, Swain A, Thakuri D, Elliot M, Schnall MD, et al. 2022. Integrating ^{1}H MRS and deuterium labeled glucose for mapping the dynamics of neural metabolism in humans. *Neuroimage* 251: 118977. doi:10.1016/j.neuroimage.2022.118977

Chaumeil MM, Larson PEZ, Yoshihara HAI, Danforth OM, Vigneron DB, Nelson SJ, Pieper RO, Phillips JJ, Ronen SM. 2013. Non-invasive in vivo assessment of IDH1 mutational status in glioma. *Nat Commun* 4: 2429. doi:10.1038/ncomms3429

Chaumeil MM, Radoul M, Najac C, Eriksson P, Viswanath P, Blough MD, Chesnelong C, Luchman HA, Cairncross JG, Ronen SM. 2016. Hyperpolarized ^{13}C MR imaging detects no lactate production in mutant IDH1 gliomas: implications for diagnosis and response monitoring. *Neuroimage Clin* 12: 180–189. doi:10.1016/j.nicl.2016.06.018

Chen W, Cloughesy T, Kamdar N, Satyamurthy N, Bergsneider M, Liau L, Mischel P, Czernin J, Phelps ME, Silverman DHS. 2005. Imaging proliferation in brain tumors with ^{18}F-FLT PET: comparison with ^{18}F-FDG. *J Nucl Med* 46: 945–952.

Chen AP, Hurd RE, Schroeder MA, Lau AZ, Gu Y, Lam WW, Barry J, Tropp J, Cunningham CH. 2012. Simultaneous investigation of cardiac pyruvate dehydrogenase flux, Krebs cycle metabolism and pH, using hyperpolarized [1,2-^{13}C$_2$]pyruvate in vivo. *NMR Biomed* 25: 305–311. doi:10.1002/nbm.1749

Chen H-Y, Aggarwal R, Bok RA, Ohliger MA, Zhu Z, Lee P, Gordon JW, Criekinge M van, Carvajal L, Slater JB, et al. 2020. Hyperpolarized ^{13}C-pyruvate MRI detects real-time metabolic flux in prostate cancer metastases to bone and liver: a clinical feasibility study. *Prostate Cancer P D* 23: 269–276. doi:10.1038/s41391-019-0180-z

Chen M, Zhu W, Du J, Yang C, Han B, Zhou D, Huo L, Zhuang J. 2021. 11C-acetate positron emission tomography is more precise than ^{18}F-fluorodeoxyglucose positron emission tomography in evaluating tumor burden and predicting disease risk of multiple myeloma. *Sci Rep* 11: 22188. doi:10.1038/s41598-021-01740-2

Cheng J, Lei L, Xu J, Sun Y, Zhang Y, Wang X, Pan L, Shao Z, Zhang Y, Liu G. 2013. ^{18}F-fluoromisonidazole PET/CT: a potential tool for predicting primary endocrine therapy resistance in breast cancer. *J Nucl Med* 54: 333–340. doi:10.2967/jnumed.112.111963

Chiavazza E, Viale A, Karlsson M, Aime S. 2013. ^{15}N-permethylated amino acids as efficient probes for MRI-DNP applications. *Contrast Media Mol Imaging* 8: 417–421. doi:10.1002/cmmi.1538

Cho A, Eskandari R, Miloushev VZ, Keshari KR. 2018. A non-synthetic approach to extending the lifetime of hyperpolarized molecules using D$_2$O solvation. *J Magn Reson* 295: 57–62. doi:10.1016/j.jmr.2018.08.001

Choi SJ, Kim JS, Kim JH, Oh SJ, Lee JG, Kim CJ, Ra YS, Yeo JS, Ryu JS, Moon DH. 2005. [^{18}f]3'-deoxy-3'-fluorothymidine PET for the diagnosis and grading of brain tumors. *Eur J Nucl Med Mol Imaging* 32: 653–659. doi:10.1007/s00259-004-1742-3

Choi C, Ganji SK, DeBerardinis RJ, Hatanpaa KJ, Rakheja D, Kovacs Z, Yang X-L, Mashimo T, Raisanen JM, Marin-Valencia I, et al. 2012. 2-Hydroxyglutarate detection by magnetic resonance spectroscopy in IDH-mutated patients with gliomas. *Nat Med* 18: 624–629. doi:10.1038/nm.2682

Chung BT, Chen H-Y, Gordon J, Mammoli D, Sriram R, Autry AW, Page LML, Chaumeil M, Shin P, Slater J, et al. 2019. First hyperpolarized [2-^{13}C]pyruvate MR studies of human brain metabolism. *J Magn Reson* 309: 106617. doi:10.1016/j.jmr.2019.106617

Clarke DD. 1991. Fluoroacetate and fluorocitrate: mechanism of action. *Neurochem Res* 16: 1055–1058.

Cooper AJL, Krasnikov BF, Pinto JT, Kung HF, Li J, Ploessl K. 2012. Comparative enzymology of (2S,4R)4-fluoroglutamine and (2S,4R)4-fluoroglutamate. *Comp Biochem Physiol B Biochem Mol Biol* 163: 108–120. doi:10.1016/j.cbpb.2012.05.010

Crane JC, Gordon JW, Chen H, Autry AW, Li Y, Olson MP, Kurhanewicz J, Vigneron DB, Larson PEZ, Xu D. 2021.

Hyperpolarized ^{13}C MRI data acquisition and analysis in prostate and brain at University of California, San Francisco. *NMR Biomed* **34**: e4280. doi:10.1002/nbm.4280

Czernin J, Allen-Auerbach M, Nathanson D, Herrmann K. 2013. PET/CT in oncology: current status and perspectives. *Curr Radiol Rep* **1**: 177–190. doi:10.1007/s40134-013-0016-x

Dafni H, Larson PEZ, Hu S, Yoshihara HAI, Ward CS, Venkatesh HS, Wang C, Zhang X, Vigneron DB, Ronen SM. 2010. Hyperpolarized ^{13}C spectroscopic imaging informs on hypoxia-inducible factor-1 and Myc activity downstream of platelet-derived growth factor receptor. *Cancer Res* **70**: 7400–7410. doi:10.1158/0008-5472.CAN-10-0883

Damuka N, Bashetti N, Mintz A, Bansode AH, Miller M, Krizan I, Furdui C, Bhoopal B, Gollapelli K, Kumar JS, et al. 2022. [^{18}f]KS1, a novel ascorbate-based ligand images ROS in tumor models of rodents and nonhuman primates. *Biomed Pharmacother* **156**: 113937. doi:10.1016/j.biopha.2022.113937

Dang L, White DW, Gross S, Bennett BD, Bittinger MA, Driggers EM, Fantin VR, Jang HG, Jin S, Keenan MC, et al. 2009. Cancer-associated IDH1 mutations produce 2-hydroxyglutarate. *Nature* **462**: 739–744. doi:10.1038/nature08617

Daumar P, Wanger-Baumann CA, Pillarsetty N, Fabrizio L, Carlin SD, Andreev OA, Reshetnyak YK, Lewis JS. 2012. Efficient ^{18}F-labeling of large 37-amino-acid pHLIP peptide analogues and their biological evaluation. *Bioconjug Chem* **23**: 1557–1566. doi:10.1021/bc3000222

Day SE, Kettunen MI, Gallagher FA, Hu DE, Lerche M, Wolber J, Golman K, Ardenkjaer-Larsen JH, Brindle KM. 2007. Detecting tumor response to treatment using hyperpolarized ^{13}C magnetic resonance imaging and spectroscopy. *Nat Med* **13**: 1382–1387. doi:10.1038/nm1650

DeBerardinis RJ, Cheng T. 2010. Q's next: the diverse functions of glutamine in metabolism, cell biology and cancer. *Oncogene* **29**: 313–324. doi:10.1038/onc.2009.358

DeBerardinis RJ, Keshari KR. 2022. Metabolic analysis as a driver for discovery, diagnosis, and therapy. *Cell* **185**: 2678–2689. doi:10.1016/j.cell.2022.06.029

De Feyter HMD, de Graaf RA. 2021. Deuterium metabolic imaging—back to the future. *J Magn Reson* **326**: 106932. doi:10.1016/j.jmr.2021.106932

De Feyter HMD, Behar KL, Corbin ZA, Fulbright RK, Brown PB, McIntyre S, Nixon TW, Rothman DL, de Graaf RA. 2018. Deuterium metabolic imaging (DMI) for MRI-based 3D mapping of metabolism in vivo. *Sci Adv* **4**: eaat7314. doi:10.1126/sciadv.aat7314

Deh K, Zhang G, Park AH, Cunningham CH, Bragagnolo ND, Lyashchenko S, Ahmmed S, Leftin A, Coffee E, Hricak H, et al. 2024. First in-human evaluation of [1-^{13}C] pyruvate in D$_2$O for hyperpolarized MRI of the brain: a safety and feasibility study. *Magn Reson Med* **11**: 10.1002/mrm.30002.

de Kouchkovsky I, Chen HY, Ohliger MA, Wang ZJ, Bok RA, Gordon JW, Larson PEZ, Frost M, Okamoto K, Cooperberg MR, et al. 2022. Hyperpolarized 1-[^{13}C]-pyruvate magnetic resonance imaging detects an early metabolic response to immune checkpoint inhibitor therapy in prostate cancer. *Eur Urol* **81**: 219–221. doi:10.1016/j.eururo.2021.10.015

Dong Y, Eskandari R, Ray C, Granlund KL, Santos-Cunha LD, Miloushev VZ, Tee SS, Jeong S, Aras O, Chen YB, et al. 2018. Hyperpolarized MRI visualizes Warburg effects and predicts treatment response to mTOR inhibitors in patient-derived ccRCC xenograft models. *Cancer Res* **79**: canres.2231.2018.

Ducruet AF, Mack WJ, Mocco J, Hoh DJ, Coon AL, D'Ambrosio AL, Winfree CJ, Pinsky DJ, Connolly ES. 2011. Preclinical evaluation of postischemic dehydroascorbic acid administration in a large-animal stroke model. *Transl Stroke Res* **2**: 399–403. doi:10.1007/s12975-011-0084-2

Durst M, Chiavazza E, Haase A, Aime S, Schwaiger M, Schulte RF. 2016. α-Trideuteromethyl[15N]glutamine: a long-lived hyperpolarized perfusion marker. *Magn Reson Med* **76**: 1900–1904. doi:10.1002/mrm.26104

Dutta P, Le A, Jagt DLV, Tsukamoto T, Martinez GV, Dang CV, Gillies RJ. 2013. Evaluation of LDH-A and glutaminase inhibition in vivo by hyperpolarized ^{13}C-pyruvate magnetic resonance spectroscopy of tumors. *Cancer Res* **73**: 4190–4195. doi:10.1158/0008-5472.CAN-13-0465

Düwel S, Hundshammer C, Gersch M, Feuerecker B, Steiger K, Buck A, Walch A, Haase A, Glaser SJ, Schwaiger M, et al. 2017. Imaging of pH in vivo using hyperpolarized ^{13}C-labelled zymonic acid. *Nat Commun* **8**: 15126. doi:10.1038/ncomms15126

Ericson K, Lilja A, Bergström M, Collins VP, Eriksson L, Ehrin E, von Hoist H, Lundqvist H, Längström B, Mosskin M. 1985. Positron emission tomography with ([11C] methyl)-L-methionine, [11C]D-glucose, and [68Ga] EDTA in supratentorial tumors. *J Comput Assist Tomogr* **9**: 683–689. doi:10.1097/00004728-198507010-00005

Eskandari R, Kim N, Mamakhanyan A, Saoi M, Zhang G, Berishaj M, Granlund KL, Poot AJ, Cross J, Thompson CB, et al. 2022. Hyperpolarized [5-^{13}C,4,4-^{2}H$_2$,5-^{15}N]-L-glutamine provides a means of annotating in vivo metabolic utilization of glutamine. *Proc Natl Acad Sci* **119**: e2120595119. doi:10.1073/pnas.2120595119

Fala M, Somai V, Dannhorn A, Hamm G, Gibson K, Couturier D, Hesketh R, Wright AJ, Takats Z, Bunch J, et al. 2021. Comparison of ^{13}C MRI of hyperpolarized [1-^{13}C] pyruvate and lactate with the corresponding mass spectrometry images in a murine lymphoma model. *Magn Reson Med* **85**: 3027–3035. doi:10.1002/mrm.28652

Faubert B, Li KY, Cai L, Hensley CT, Kim J, Zacharias LG, Yang C, Do QN, Doucette S, Burguete D, et al. 2017. Lactate metabolism in human lung tumors. *Cell* **171**: 358–371.e9. doi:10.1016/j.cell.2017.09.019

Flavell RR, von Morze C, Blecha JE, Korenchan DE, Criekinge MV, Sriram R, Gordon JW, Chen H-Y, Subramaniam S, Bok RA, et al. 2015. Application of Good's buffers to pH imaging using hyperpolarized ^{13}C MRI. *Chem Commun* **51**: 14119–14122. doi:10.1039/C5CC05348J

Gallagher BM, Fowler JS, Gutterson NI, MacGregor RR, Wan CN, Wolf AP. 1978. Metabolic trapping as a principle of radiopharmaceutical design: some factors resposible for the biodistribution of [^{18}F] 2-deoxy-2-fluoro-D-glucose. *J Nucl Med* **19**: 1154–1161.

Gallagher FA, Kettunen MI, Day SE, Hu DE, Ardenkjær-Larsen JH, Zandt RIT, Jensen PR, Karlsson M, Golman K,

Lerche MH, et al. 2008. Magnetic resonance imaging of pH in vivo using hyperpolarized ^{13}C-labelled bicarbonate. *Nature* **453**: 940–943. doi:10.1038/nature07017

Gallagher FA, Kettunen MI, Brindle KM. 2011. Imaging pH with hyperpolarized ^{13}C. *NMR Biomed* **24**: 1006–1015. doi:10.1002/nbm.1742

Gallagher FA, Sladen H, Kettunen MI, Serrao EM, Rodrigues TB, Wright A, Gill AB, McGuire S, Booth TC, Boren J, et al. 2015. Carbonic anhydrase activity monitored in vivo by hyperpolarized ^{13}C-magnetic resonance spectroscopy demonstrates its importance for pH regulation in tumors. *Cancer Res* **75**: 4109–4118. doi:10.1158/0008-5472.CAN-15-0857

Gallagher FA, Woitek R, McLean MA, Gill AB, Garcia RM, Provenzano E, Riemer F, Kaggie J, Chhabra A, Ursprung S, et al. 2020. Imaging breast cancer using hyperpolarized carbon-13 MRI. *Proc Natl Acad Sci* **117**: 2092–2098. doi:10.1073/pnas.1913841117

Gatenby RA, Gillies RJ. 2004. Why do cancers have high aerobic glycolysis? *Nat Rev Cancer* **4**: 891–899. doi:10.1038/nrc1478

Gatenby RA, Vincent TL. 2003. An evolutionary model of carcinogenesis. *Cancer Res* **63**: 6212–6220.

Gelbard AS, Christie TR, Clarke LP, Laughlin JS. 1977. Imaging of spontaneous canine tumours with ammonia and L-glutamine labeled with N-13. *J Nucl Med* **18**: 718–723.

Gierse M, Nagel L, Keim M, Lucas S, Speidel T, Lobmeyer T, Winter G, Josten F, Karaali S, Fellermann M, et al. 2023. Parahydrogen-polarized fumarate for preclinical in vivo metabolic magnetic resonance imaging. *J Am Chem Soc* **145**: 5960–5969. doi:10.1021/jacs.2c13830

Gillies RJ, Liu Z, Bhujwalla Z. 1994. 31P-MRS measurements of extracellular pH of tumors using 3-aminopropyl-phosphonate. *Am J Physiol* **267**: C195–C203. doi:10.1152/ajpcell.1994.267.1.C195

Gillies RJ, Raghunand N, Garcia-Martin ML, Gatenby RA. 2004. Ph imaging. A review of pH measurement methods and applications in cancers. *IEEE Eng Med Biol* **23**: 57–64. doi:10.1109/MEMB.2004.1360409

Golman K, Olsson LE, Axelsson O, Månsson S, Karlsson M, Petersson JS. 2003. Molecular imaging using hyperpolarized ^{13}C. *Br J Radiol* **76**: S118–S127. doi:10.1259/bjr/26631666

Golman K, Zandt RIT, Lerche M, Pehrson R, Ardenkjaer-Larsen JH. 2006. Metabolic imaging by hyperpolarized ^{13}C magnetic resonance imaging for in vivo tumor diagnosis. *Cancer Res* **66**: 10855–10860. doi:10.1158/0008-5472.CAN-06-2564

Granlund KL, Tee SS, Vargas HA, Lyashchenko SK, Reznik E, Fine S, Laudone V, Eastham JA, Touijer KA, Reuter VE, et al. 2020. Hyperpolarized MRI of human prostate cancer reveals increased lactate with tumor grade driven by monocarboxylate transporter 1. *Cell Metab* **31**: 105–114. e3. doi:10.1016/j.cmet.2019.08.024

Grashei M, Biechl P, Schilling F, Otto AM. 2022. Conversion of hyperpolarized [1-^{13}C]pyruvate in breast cancer cells depends on their malignancy, metabolic program and nutrient microenvironment. *Cancers (Basel)* **14**: 1845. doi:10.3390/cancers14071845

Grassi I, Nanni C, Allegri V, Morigi JJ, Montini GC, Castellucci P, Fanti S. 2011. The clinical use of PET with (11)C-acetate. *Am J Nucl Med Mol Imaging* **2**: 33–47.

Grkovski M, Goel R, Krebs S, Staton KD, Harding JJ, Mellinghoff IK, Humm JL, Dunphy MPS. 2020. Pharmacokinetic assessment of ^{18}F-(2S,4R)-4-fluoroglutamine in patients with cancer. *J Nucl Med* **61**: 357–366. doi:10.2967/jnumed.119.229740

Habermeier A, Graf J, Sandhöfer BF, Boissel J-P, Roesch F, Closs EI. 2015. System L amino acid transporter LAT1 accumulates O-(2-fluoroethyl)-L-tyrosine (FET). *Amino Acids* **47**: 335–344. doi:10.1007/s00726-014-1863-3

Häfliger P, Charles RP. 2019. The L-type amino acid transporter LAT1—an emerging target in cancer. *Int J Mol Sci* **20**: 2428. doi:10.3390/ijms20102428

Hanahan D, Weinberg RA. 2011. Hallmarks of cancer: the next generation. *Cell* **144**: 646–674. doi:10.1016/j.cell.2011.02.013

Harris T, Degani H, Frydman L. 2013. Hyperpolarized ^{13}C NMR studies of glucose metabolism in living breast cancer cell cultures. *NMR Biomed* **26**: 1831–1843. doi:10.1002/nbm.3024

Harrison C, Yang C, Jindal A, DeBerardinis RJ, Hooshyar MA, Merritt M, Sherry AD, Malloy CR. 2012. Comparison of kinetic models for analysis of pyruvate-to-lactate exchange by hyperpolarized ^{13}C NMR. *NMR Biomed* **25**: 1286–1294. doi:10.1002/nbm.2801

Hendrickson K, Phillips M, Smith W, Peterson L, Krohn K, Rajendran J. 2011. Hypoxia imaging with [F-18] FMISO-PET in head and neck cancer: potential for guiding intensity modulated radiation therapy in overcoming hypoxia-induced treatment resistance. *Radiother Oncol* **101**: 369–375. doi:10.1016/j.radonc.2011.07.029

Herholz K, Heindel W, Luyten PR, denHollander JA, Pietrzyk U, Voges J, Kugel H, Friedmann G, Heiss WD. 1992. In vivo imaging of glucose consumption and lactate concentration in human gliomas. *Ann Neurol* **31**: 319–327. doi:10.1002/ana.410310315

Herrero P, Dence CS, Coggan AR, Kisrieva-Ware Z, Eisenbeis P, Gropler RJ. 2007. L-3-11C-lactate as a PET tracer of myocardial lactate metabolism: a feasibility study. *J Nucl Med* **48**: 2046–2055. doi:10.2967/jnumed.107.044503

Hövener J, Pravdivtsev AN, Kidd B, Bowers CR, Glöggler S, Kovtunov KV, Plaumann M, Katz-Brull R, Buckenmaier K, Jerschow A, et al. 2018. Parahydrogen-based hyperpolarization for biomedicine. *Angew Chem Int Ed* **57**: 11140–11162. doi:10.1002/anie.201711842

Hu S, Lustig M, Balakrishnan A, Larson PEZ, Bok R, Kurhanewicz J, Nelson SJ, Goga A, Pauly JM, Vigneron DB. 2010. 3D compressed sensing for highly accelerated hyperpolarized ^{13}C MRSI with in vivo applications to transgenic mouse models of cancer. *Magn Reson Med* **63**: 312–321. doi:10.1002/mrm.22233

Hu S, Balakrishnan A, Bok RA, Anderton B, Larson PEZ, Nelson SJ, Kurhanewicz J, Vigneron DB, Goga A. 2011. ^{13}C-pyruvate imaging reveals alterations in glycolysis that precede c-Myc-induced tumor formation and regression. *Cell Metab* **14**: 131–142. doi:10.1016/j.cmet.2011.04.012

Hugonnet F, Fournier L, Medioni J, Smadja C, Hindié E, Huchet V, Itti E, Cuenod C-A, Chatellier G, Oudard S, et al. 2011. Metastatic renal cell carcinoma: relationship between initial metastasis hypoxia, change after 1 month's sunitinib, and therapeutic response: an ^{18}F-fluoromisonidazole PET/CT study. *J Nucl Med* **52**: 1048–1055. doi:10.2967/jnumed.110.084517

Hundshammer C, Düwel S, Ruseckas D, Topping G, Dzien P, Müller C, Feuerecker B, Hövener JB, Haase A, Schwaiger M, et al. 2018. Hyperpolarized amino acid derivatives as multivalent magnetic resonance pH sensor molecules. *Sensors* **18:** 600. doi:10.3390/s18020600

Ido T, Wan C, Casella V, Fowler JS, Wolf AP, Reivich M, Kuhl DE. 1978. Labeled 2-deoxy-D-glucose analogs. ^{18}F-labeled 2-deoxy-2-fluoro-D-glucose, 2-deoxy-2-fluoro-D-mannose and ^{14}C-2-deoxy-2-fluoro-D-glucose. *J Label Compd Radiopharm* **14:** 175–183. doi:10.1002/jlcr.2580140204

Izquierdo-Garcia JL, Viswanath P, Eriksson P, Cai L, Radoul M, Chaumeil MM, Blough M, Luchman HA, Weiss S, Cairncross JG, et al. 2015. *IDH1* mutation induces reprogramming of pyruvate metabolism. *Cancer Res* **75:** 2999–3009. doi:10.1158/0008-5472.CAN-15-0840

Jadvar H. 2016. Is there use for FDG-PET in prostate cancer? *Semin Nucl Med* **46:** 502–506. doi:10.1053/j.semnuclmed.2016.07.004

James ML, Gambhir SS. 2012. A molecular imaging primer: modalities, imaging agents, and applications. *Physiol Rev* **92:** 897–965. doi:10.1152/physrev.00049.2010

Jansen NL, Graute V, Armbruster L, Suchorska B, Lutz J, Eigenbrod S, Cumming P, Bartenstein P, Tonn JC, Kreth FW, et al. 2012. MRI-suspected low-grade glioma: is there a need to perform dynamic FET PET? *Eur J Nucl Med Mol Imaging* **39:** 1021–1029. doi:10.1007/s00259-012-2109-9

Jansen NL, Suchorska B, Wenter V, Eigenbrod S, Schmid-Tannwald C, Zwergal A, Niyazi M, Drexler M, Bartenstein P, Schnell O, et al. 2014. Dynamic ^{18}F-FET PET in newly diagnosed astrocytic low-grade glioma identifies high-risk patients. *J Nucl Med* **55:** 198–203. doi:10.2967/jnumed.113.122333

Jensen PR, Karlsson M, Meier S, Duus JØ, Lerche MH. 2009. Hyperpolarized amino acids for in vivo assays of transaminase activity. *Chemistry (Easton)* **15:** 10010–10012. doi:10.1002/chem.200901042

Ježek P. 2020. 2-Hydroxyglutarate in cancer cells. *Antioxid Redox Sign* **33:** 903–926. doi:10.1089/ars.2019.7902

Jiang W, Lumata L, Chen W, Zhang S, Kovacs Z, Sherry AD, Khemtong C. 2015. Hyperpolarized ^{15}N-pyridine derivatives as pH-sensitive MRI agents. *Sci Rep* **5:** 9104. doi:10.1038/srep09104

Jindal AK, Merritt ME, Suh EH, Malloy CR, Sherry AD, Kovács Z. 2010. Hyperpolarized [89]Y complexes as pH sensitive NMR probes. *J Am Chem Soc* **132:** 1784–1785. doi:10.1021/ja910278e

Kavanaugh G, Williams J, Morris AS, Nickels ML, Walker R, Koglin N, Stephens AW, Washington MK, Geevarghese SK, Liu Q, et al. 2016. Utility of [^{18}F]FSPG PET to image hepatocellular carcinoma: first clinical evaluation in a US population. *Mol Imaging Biol* **18:** 924–934. doi:10.1007/s11307-016-1007-0

Kelloff GJ, Hoffman JM, Johnson B, Scher HI, Siegel BA, Cheng EY, Cheson BD, O'Shaughnessy J, Guyton KZ, Mankoff DA, et al. 2005. Progress and promise of FDG-PET imaging for cancer patient management and oncologic drug development. *Clin Cancer Res* **11:** 2785–2808. doi:10.1158/1078-0432.CCR-04-2626

Keshari KR, Wilson DM. 2014. Chemistry and biochemistry of ^{13}C hyperpolarized magnetic resonance using dynamic nuclear polarization. *Chem Soc Rev* **43:** 1627–1659. doi:10.1039/C3CS60124B

Keshari KR, Wilson DM, Chen AP, Bok R, Larson PEZ, Hu S, Criekinge MV, Macdonald JM, Vigneron DB, Kurhanewicz J. 2009. Hyperpolarized [2-^{13}C]-fructose: a hemiketal DNP substrate for in vivo metabolic imaging. *J Am Chem Soc* **131:** 17591–17596. doi:10.1021/ja9049355

Keshari KR, Kurhanewicz J, Bok R, Larson PEZ, Vigneron DB, Wilson DM. 2011. Hyperpolarized ^{13}C dehydroascorbate as an endogenous redox sensor for in vivo metabolic imaging. *Proc Natl Acad Sci* **108:** 18606–18611. doi:10.1073/pnas.1106920108

Keshari KR, Sai V, Wang ZJ, VanBrocklin HF, Kurhanewicz J, Wilson DM. 2013. Hyperpolarized [1-^{13}C]dehydroascorbate MR spectroscopy in a murine model of prostate cancer: comparison with ^{18}F-FDG PET. *J Nucl Med* **54:** 922–928. doi:10.2967/jnumed.112.115402

Kim W, Le TM, Wei L, Poddar S, Bazzy J, Wang X, Uong NT, Abt ER, Capri JR, Austin WR, et al. 2016. [^{18}F]CFA as a clinically translatable probe for PET imaging of deoxycytidine kinase activity. *Proc Natl Acad Sci* **113:** 4027–4032. doi:10.1073/pnas.1524212113

Kim M, Eleftheriou A, Ravotto L, Weber B, Rivlin M, Navon G, Capozza M, Anemone A, Longo DL, Aime S, et al. 2022. What do we know about dynamic glucose-enhanced (DGE) MRI and how close is it to the clinics? Horizon 2020 GLINT consortium report. *MAGMA* **35:** 87–104. doi:10.1007/s10334-021-00994-1

Kishimoto S, Brender JR, Chandramouli GVR, Saida Y, Yamamoto K, Mitchell JB, Krishna MC. 2021. Hypoxia-activated prodrug evofosfamide treatment in pancreatic ductal adenocarcinoma xenografts alters the tumor redox status to potentiate radiotherapy. *Antioxid Redox Sign* **35:** 904–915. doi:10.1089/ars.2020.8131

Koglin N, Mueller A, Berndt M, Schmitt-Willich H, Toschi L, Stephens AW, Gekeler V, Friebe M, Dinkelborg LM. 2011. Specific PET imaging of x_C^- transporter activity using a ^{18}F-labeled glutamate derivative reveals a dominant pathway in tumor metabolism. *Clin Cancer Res* **17:** 6000–6011. doi:10.1158/1078-0432.CCR-11-0687

Koh W-J, Rasey JS, Evans ML, Grierson JR, Lewellen TK, Graham MM, Krohn KA, Griffin TW. 1992. Imaging of hypoxia in human tumors with [F-18]fluoromisonidazole. *Int J Radiat Oncol Biol Phys* **22:** 199–212. doi:10.1016/0360-3016(92)91001-4

Korenchan DE, Flavell RR, Baligand C, Sriram R, Neumann K, Sukumar S, VanBrocklin H, Vigneron DB, Wilson DM, Kurhanewicz J. 2016. Dynamic nuclear polarization of biocompatible ^{13}C-enriched carbonates for in vivo pH imaging. *Chem Commun* **52:** 3030–3033. doi:10.1039/C5CC09724J

Korenchan DE, Taglang C, von Morze C, Blecha JE, Gordon JW, Sriram R, Larson PEZ, Vigneron DB, VanBrocklin HF, Kurhanewicz J, et al. 2017. Dicarboxylic acids as pH sensors for hyperpolarized ^{13}C magnetic resonance spectroscopic imaging. *Analyst* **142:** 1429–1433. doi:10.1039/C7AN00076F

Korenchan DE, Bok R, Sriram R, Liu K, Santos RD, Qin H, Lobach I, Korn N, Wilson DM, Kurhanewicz J, et al. 2019. Hyperpolarized in vivo pH imaging reveals grade-dependent acidification in prostate cancer. *Oncotarget* **10:** 6096–6110. doi:10.18632/oncotarget.27225

Cite this article as *Cold Spring Harb Perspect Med* doi: 10.1101/cshperspect.a041551

Kracht LW, Miletic H, Busch S, Jacobs AH, Voges J, Hoevels M, Klein JC, Herholz K, Heiss WD. 2004. Delineation of brain tumor extent with [^{11}C]L-methionine positron emission tomography local comparison with stereotactic histopathology. *Clin Cancer Res* **10**: 7163–7170. doi:10.1158/1078-0432.CCR-04-0262

Kreis F, Wright AJ, Hesse F, Fala M, Hu D, Brindle KM. 2019. Measuring tumor glycolytic flux in vivo by using fast deuterium MRI. *Radiology* **294**: 191242.

Krishna MC, Matsumoto S, Yasui H, Saito K, Devasahayam N, Subramanian S, Mitchell JB. 2012. Electron paramagnetic resonance imaging of tumor pO$_2$. *Radiat Res* **177**: 376–386. doi:10.1667/RR2622.1

Kunz M, Thon N, Eigenbrod S, Hartmann C, Egensperger R, Herms J, Geisler J, la Fougere C, Lutz J, Linn J, et al. 2011. Hot spots in dynamic ^{18}FET-PET delineate malignant tumor parts within suspected WHO grade II gliomas. *Neuro Oncol* **13**: 307–316. doi:10.1093/neuonc/noq196

Kurhanewicz J, Vigneron DB, Ardenkjaer-Larsen JH, Bankson JA, Brindle K, Cunningham CH, Gallagher FA, Keshari KR, Kjaer A, Laustsen C, et al. 2019. Hyperpolarized ^{13}C MRI: path to clinical translation in oncology. *Neoplasia* **21**: 1–16. doi:10.1016/j.neo.2018.09.006

Langen KJ, Stoffels G, Filss C, Heinzel A, Stegmayr C, Lohmann P, Willuweit A, Neumaier B, Mottaghy FM, Galldiks N. 2017. Imaging of amino acid transport in brain tumours: positron emission tomography with O-(2-[^{18}F]fluoroethyl)-L-tyrosine (FET). *Methods* **130**: 124–134. doi:10.1016/j.ymeth.2017.05.019

Lau JYC, Chen AP, Gu Y, Cunningham CH. 2016. Voxel-by-voxel correlations of perfusion, substrate, and metabolite signals in dynamic hyperpolarized ^{13}C imaging. *NMR Biomed* **29**: 1038–1047. doi:10.1002/nbm.3564

Lewis DY, Boren J, Shaw GL, Bielik R, Ramos-Montoya A, Larkin TJ, Martins CP, Neal DE, Soloviev D, Brindle KM. 2014. Late imaging with [1-^{11}C]acetate improves detection of tumor fatty acid synthesis with PET. *J Nucl Med* **55**: 1144–1149. doi:10.2967/jnumed.113.134437

Lieberman BP, Ploessl K, Wang L, Qu W, Zha Z, Wise DR, Chodosh LA, Belka G, Thompson CB, Kung HF. 2011. PET imaging of glutaminolysis in tumors by ^{18}F-(2S,4R)4-fluoroglutamine. *J Nucl Med* **52**: 1947–1955. doi:10.2967/jnumed.111.093815

Lindhe Ö, Sun A, Ulin J, Rahman O, Långström B, Sörensen J. 2009. [^{18}F]Fluoroacetate is not a functional analogue of [11C]acetate in normal physiology. *Eur J Nucl Med Mol Imaging* **36**: 1453. doi:10.1007/s00259-009-1128-7

Liu F, Xu X, Zhu H, Zhang Y, Yang J, Zhang L, Li N, Zhu L, Kung HF, Yang Z. 2018. PET imaging of ^{18}F-(2S,4R)4-fluoroglutamine accumulation in breast cancer: from xenografts to patients. *Mol Pharm* **15**: 3448–3455. doi:10.1021/acs.molpharmaceut.8b00430

Lohmann P, Herzog H, Kops ER, Stoffels G, Judov N, Filss C, Galldiks N, Tellmann L, Weiss C, Sabel M, et al. 2015. Dual-time-point O-(2-[^{18}F]fluoroethyl)-L-tyrosine PET for grading of cerebral gliomas. *Eur Radiol* **25**: 3017–3024. doi:10.1007/s00330-015-3691-6

Long NM, Smith CS. 2011. Causes and imaging features of false positives and false negatives on ^{18}F-PET/CT in oncologic imaging. *Insights Imaging* **2**: 679–698. doi:10.1007/s13244-010-0062-3

Longo DL, Sun PZ, Consolino L, Michelotti FC, Uggeri F, Aime S. 2014. A general MRI-CEST ratiometric approach for pH imaging: demonstration of in vivo pH mapping with iobitridol. *J Am Chem Soc* **136**: 14333–14336. doi:10.1021/ja5059313

Longo DL, Bartoli A, Consolino L, Bardini P, Arena F, Schwaiger M, Aime S. 2016. In vivo imaging of tumor metabolism and acidosis by combining PET and MRI-CEST pH imaging. *Cancer Res* **76**: 6463–6470. doi:10.1158/0008-5472.CAN-16-0825

Marco-Rius I, Wright AJ, Hu D, Savic D, Miller JJ, Timm KN, Tyler D, Brindle KM, Comment A. 2021. Probing hepatic metabolism of [2-^{13}C]dihydroxyacetone in vivo with ^{1}H-decoupled hyperpolarized ^{13}C-MR. *Magnetic Reson Mater Phys Biol Med* **34**: 49–56. doi:10.1007/s10334-020-00884-y

Marini C, Ravera S, Buschiazzo A, Bianchi G, Orengo AM, Bruno S, Bottoni G, Emionite L, Pastorino F, Monteverde E, et al. 2016. Discovery of a novel glucose metabolism in cancer: the role of endoplasmic reticulum beyond glycolysis and pentose phosphate shunt. *Sci Rep* **6**: 25092. doi:10.1038/srep25092

Marjańska M, Iltis I, Shestov AA, Deelchand DK, Nelson C, Uğurbil K, Henry P-G. 2010. In vivo ^{13}C spectroscopy in the rat brain using hyperpolarized [1-^{13}C]pyruvate and [2-^{13}C]pyruvate. *J Magn Reson* **206**: 210–218. doi:10.1016/j.jmr.2010.07.006

Markovic S, Roussel T, Agemy L, Sasson K, Preise D, Scherz A, Frydman L. 2021. Deuterium MRSI characterizations of glucose metabolism in orthotopic pancreatic cancer mouse models. *NMR Biomed* **34**: e4569. doi:10.1002/nbm.4569

Mayerhoefer ME, Prosch H, Beer L, Tamandl D, Beyer T, Hoeller C, Berzaczy D, Raderer M, Preusser M, Hochmair M, et al. 2020. PET/MRI versus PET/CT in oncology: a prospective single-center study of 330 examinations focusing on implications for patient management and cost considerations. *Eur J Nucl Med Mol Imaging* **47**: 51–60. doi:10.1007/s00259-019-04452-y

McCormick PN, Greenwood HE, Glaser M, Maddocks ODK, Gendron T, Sander K, Gowrishankar G, Hoehne A, Zhang T, Shuhendler AJ, et al. 2018. Assessment of tumor redox status through (S)-4-(3-[^{18}F]fluoropropyl)-L-glutamic acid positron emission tomography imaging of system x$_c^-$ activity. *Cancer Res* **79**: canres.2634.2018.

McKinley ET, Ayers GD, Smith RA, Saleh SA, Zhao P, Washington MK, Coffey RJ, Manning HC. 2013. Limits of [^{18}F]-FLT PET as a biomarker of proliferation in oncology. *PLoS ONE* **8**: e58938. doi:10.1371/journal.pone.0058938

Mikkelsen EFR, Mariager CØ, Nørlinger T, Qi H, Schulte RF, Jakobsen S, Frøkiær J, Pedersen M, Stødkilde-Jørgensen H, Laustsen C. 2017. Hyperpolarized [1-^{13}C]-acetate renal metabolic clearance rate mapping. *Sci Rep* **7**: 16002. doi:10.1038/s41598-017-15929-x

Miloushev VZ, Granlund KL, Boltyanskiy R, Lyashchenko SK, DeAngelis LM, Mellinghoff IK, Brennan CW, Tabar V, Yang TJ, Holodny AI, et al. 2018. Metabolic imaging of the human brain with hyperpolarized ^{13}C pyruvate demonstrates ^{13}C lactate production in brain tumor patients. *Cancer Res* **78**: 3755–3760. doi:10.1158/0008-5472.CAN-18-0221

Minami N, Hong D, Taglang C, Batsios G, Gillespie AM, Viswanath P, Stevers N, Barger CJ, Costello JF, Ronen SM. 2023. Hyperpolarized δ-[1-^{13}C]gluconolactone imaging visualizes response to TERT or GABPB1 targeting therapy for glioblastoma. *Sci Rep* **13:** 5190. doi:10.1038/s41598-023-32463-1

Mishkovsky M, Anderson B, Karlsson M, Lerche MH, Sherry AD, Gruetter R, Kovacs Z, Comment A. 2017. Measuring glucose cerebral metabolism in the healthy mouse using hyperpolarized ^{13}C magnetic resonance. *Sci Rep* **7:** 11719. doi:10.1038/s41598-017-12086-z

Mishkovsky M, Gusyatiner O, Lanz B, Cudalbu C, Vassallo I, Hamou MF, Bloch J, Comment A, Gruetter R, Hegi ME. 2021. Hyperpolarized ^{13}C-glucose magnetic resonance highlights reduced aerobic glycolysis in vivo in infiltrative glioblastoma. *Sci Rep* **11:** 5771. doi:10.1038/s41598-021-85339-7

Miura N, Mushti C, Sail D, AbuSalim JE, Yamamoto K, Brender JR, Seki T, AbuSalim DI, Matsumoto S, Camphausen KA, et al. 2021. Synthesis of [1-^{13}C-5-^{12}C]-α-ketoglutarate enables noninvasive detection of 2-hydroxyglutarate. *NMR Biomed* **34:** e4588. doi:10.1002/nbm.4588

Moreno KX, Harrison CE, Merritt ME, Kovacs Z, Malloy CR, Sherry AD. 2017. Hyperpolarized δ-[1-^{13}C]gluconolactone as a probe of the pentose phosphate pathway. *NMR Biomed* **30:** e3713. doi:10.1002/nbm.3713

Nelson SJ, Kurhanewicz J, Vigneron DB, Larson PEZ, Harzstark AL, Ferrone M, van Criekinge M, Chang JW, Bok R, Park I, et al. 2013. Metabolic imaging of patients with prostate cancer using hyperpolarized [1-^{13}C]pyruvate. *Sci Transl Med* **5:** 198ra108. doi:10.1126/scitranslmed.3006070

Neumann K, Flavell R, Wilson DM. 2017. Exploring metabolism in vivo using endogenous ^{11}C metabolic tracers. *Semin Nucl Med* **47:** 461–473. doi:10.1053/j.semnuclmed.2017.05.003

Ninatti G, Sollini M, Bono B, Gozzi N, Fedorov D, Antunovic L, Gelardi F, Navarria P, Politi LS, Pessina F, et al. 2022. Preoperative [11C]methionine PET to personalize treatment decisions in patients with lower-grade gliomas. *Neuro Oncol* **24:** 1546–1556. doi:10.1093/neuonc/noac040

Nishii R, Tong W, Wendt R, Soghomonyan S, Mukhopadhyay U, Balatoni J, Mawlawi O, Bidaut L, Tinkey P, Borne A, et al. 2012. Pharmacokinetics, metabolism, biodistribution, radiation dosimetry, and toxicology of ^{18}F-fluoroacetate (^{18}F-FACE) in non-human primates. *Mol Imaging Biol* **14:** 213–224. doi:10.1007/s11307-011-0485-3

Okubo S, Zhen HN, Kawai N, Nishiyama Y, Haba R, Tamiya T. 2010. Correlation of L-methyl-11C-methionine (MET) uptake with L-type amino acid transporter 1 in human gliomas. *J Neuro Oncol* **99:** 217–225. doi:10.1007/s11060-010-0117-9

Oshima N, Ishida R, Kishimoto S, Beebe K, Brender JR, Yamamoto K, Urban D, Rai G, Johnson MS, Benavides G, et al. 2020. Dynamic imaging of LDH inhibition in tumors reveals rapid in vivo metabolic rewiring and vulnerability to combination therapy. *Cell Rep* **30:** 1798–1810.e4. doi:10.1016/j.celrep.2020.01.039

Öz G, Alger JR, Barker PB, Bartha R, Bizzi A, Boesch C, Bolan PJ, Brindle KM, Cudalbu C, Dinçer A, et al. 2014. Clinical proton MR spectroscopy in central nervous system disorders. *Radiology* **270:** 658–679. doi:10.1148/radiol.13130531

Park I, Larson PEZ, Zierhut ML, Hu S, Bok R, Ozawa T, Kurhanewicz J, Vigneron DB, VandenBerg SR, James CD, et al. 2010. Hyperpolarized ^{13}C magnetic resonance metabolic imaging: application to brain tumors. *Neuro Oncol* **12:** 133–144. doi:10.1093/neuonc/nop043

Park JM, Josan S, Jang T, Merchant M, Yen Y, Hurd RE, Recht L, Spielman DM, Mayer D. 2012. Metabolite kinetics in C6 rat glioma model using magnetic resonance spectroscopic imaging of hyperpolarized [1-^{13}C]pyruvate. *Magn Reson Med* **68:** 1886–1893. doi:10.1002/mrm.24181

Park JM, Josan S, Grafendorfer T, Yen Y, Hurd RE, Spielman DM, Mayer D. 2013. Measuring mitochondrial metabolism in rat brain in vivo using MR spectroscopy of hyperpolarized [2-^{13}C]pyruvate. *NMR Biomed* **26:** 1197–1203. doi:10.1002/nbm.2935

Park JM, Spielman DM, Josan S, Jang T, Merchant M, Hurd RE, Mayer D, Recht LD. 2016. Hyperpolarized ^{13}C-lactate to ^{13}C-bicarbonate ratio as a biomarker for monitoring the acute response of anti-vascular endothelial growth factor (anti-VEGF) treatment. *NMR Biomed* **29:** 650–659. doi:10.1002/nbm.3509

Park I, Larson PEZ, Gordon JW, Carvajal L, Chen H, Bok R, Criekinge MV, Ferrone M, Slater JB, Xu D, et al. 2018. Development of methods and feasibility of using hyperpolarized carbon-13 imaging data for evaluating brain metabolism in patient studies. *Magn Reson Med* **80:** 864–873. doi:10.1002/mrm.27077

Park SY, Mosci C, Kumar M, Wardak M, Koglin N, Bullich S, Mueller A, Berndt M, Stephens AW, Chin FT, et al. 2020. Initial evaluation of (4S)-4-(3-[^{18}F]fluoropropyl)-l-glutamate (FSPG) PET/CT imaging in patients with head and neck cancer, colorectal cancer, or non-Hodgkin lymphoma. *EJNMMI Res* **10:** 100. doi:10.1186/s13550-020-00678-2

Pavlova NN, Zhu J, Thompson CB. 2022. The hallmarks of cancer metabolism: still emerging. *Cell Metab* **34:** 355–377. doi:10.1016/j.cmet.2022.01.007

Pisaneschi F, Gammon ST, Paolillo V, Qureshy SA, Piwnica-Worms D. 2022. Imaging of innate immunity activation in vivo with a redox-tuned PET reporter. *Nat Biotechnol* **40:** 965–973. doi:10.1038/s41587-021-01169-y

Ploessl K, Wang L, Lieberman BP, Qu W, Kung HF. 2012. Comparative evaluation of ^{18}F-labeled glutamic acid and glutamine as tumor metabolic imaging agents. *J Nucl Med* **53:** 1616–1624. doi:10.2967/jnumed.111.101279

Puranik AD, Boon M, Purandare N, Rangarajan V, Gupta T, Moiyadi A, Shetty P, Sridhar E, Agrawal A, Dev I, et al. 2019. Utility of FET-PET in detecting high-grade gliomas presenting with equivocal MR imaging features. *World J Nucl Med* **18:** 266–272. doi:10.4103/wjnm.WJNM_89_18

Qin H, Carroll VN, Sriram R, Villanueva-Meyer JE, von Morze C, Wang ZJ, Mutch CA, Keshari KR, Flavell RR, Kurhanewicz J, et al. 2018. Imaging glutathione depletion in the rat brain using ascorbate-derived hyperpolarized MR and PET probes. *Sci Rep* **8:** 7928. doi:10.1038/s41598-018-26296-6

Qu W, Zha Z, Lieberman BP, Mancuso A, Stetz M, Rizzi R, Ploessl K, Wise D, Thompson C, Kung HF. 2011. Facile synthesis [5-^{13}C-4-^{2}H$_2$]-L-glutamine for hyperpolarized

MRS imaging of cancer cell metabolism. *Acad Radiol* **18:** 932–939. doi:10.1016/j.acra.2011.05.002

Qu W, Oya S, Lieberman BP, Ploessl K, Wang L, Wise DR, Divgi CR, Chodosh LA, Chodosh LP, Thompson CB, et al. 2012. Preparation and characterization of L-[5-^{11}C]-glutamine for metabolic imaging of tumors. *J Nucl Med* **53:** 98–105. doi:10.2967/jnumed.111.093831

Ragavan M, McLeod MA, Giacalone AG, Merritt ME. 2021. Hyperpolarized dihydroxyacetone is a sensitive probe of hepatic gluconeogenic state. *Metabolites* **11:** 441. doi:10.3390/metabo11070441

Raghunand N, Zhang S, Sherry AD, Gillies RJ. 2002. In vivo magnetic resonance imaging of tissue pH using a novel pH-sensitive contrast agent, GdDOTA-4AmP. *Acad Radiol* **9:** S481–S483. doi:10.1016/S1076-6332(03)80270-2

Rajendran JG, Schwartz DL, O'Sullivan J, Peterson LM, Ng P, Scharnhorst J, Grierson JR, Krohn KA. 2006. Tumor hypoxia imaging with [F-18] fluoromisonidazole positron emission tomography in head and neck cancer. *Clin Cancer Res* **12:** 5435–5441. doi:10.1158/1078-0432.CCR-05-1773

Rao Y, Gammon S, Zacharias NM, Liu T, Salzillo T, Xi Y, Wang J, Bhattacharya P, Piwnica-Worms D. 2020. Hyperpolarized [1-^{13}C]pyruvate-to-[1-^{13}C]lactate conversion is rate-limited by monocarboxylate transporter-1 in the plasma membrane. *Proc Natl Acad Sci* **117:** 22378–22389. doi:10.1073/pnas.2003537117

Rasey JS, Koh WJ, Grierson JR, Grunbaum Z, Krohn KA. 1989. Radiolabeled fluoromisonidazole as an imaging agent for tumor hypoxia. *Int J Radiat Oncol Biol Phys* **17:** 985–991. doi:10.1016/0360-3016(89)90146-6

Reshetnyak YK, Andreev OA, Lehnert U, Engelman DM. 2006. Translocation of molecules into cells by pH-dependent insertion of a transmembrane helix. *Proc Natl Acad Sci* **103:** 6460–6465. doi:10.1073/pnas.0601463103

Rich LJ, Bagga P, Wilson NE, Schnall MD, Detre JA, Haris M, Reddy R. 2020. ^{1}H magnetic resonance spectroscopy of ^{2}H-to-^{1}H exchange quantifies the dynamics of cellular metabolism in vivo. *Nat Biomed Eng* **4:** 335–342. doi:10.1038/s41551-019-0499-8

Rodrigues TB, Serrao EM, Kennedy BWC, Hu DE, Kettunen MI, Brindle KM. 2014. Magnetic resonance imaging of tumor glycolysis using hyperpolarized ^{13}C-labeled glucose. *Nat Med* **20:** 93–97. doi:10.1038/nm.3416

Rosenkrantz AB, Friedman K, Chandarana H, Melsaether A, Moy L, Ding YS, Jhaveri K, Beltran L, Jain R. 2016. Current status of hybrid PET/MRI in oncologic imaging. *Am J Roentgenol* **206:** 162–172. doi:10.2214/AJR.15.14968

Rowe SP, Pomper MG. 2022. Molecular imaging in oncology: current impact and future directions. *CA Cancer J Clin* **72:** 333–352. doi:10.3322/caac.21713

Saga T, Inubushi M, Koizumi M, Yoshikawa K, Zhang M, Tanimoto K, Horiike A, Yanagitani N, Ohyanagi F, Nishio M. 2015. Prognostic value of ^{18}F-fluoroazomycin arabinoside PET/CT in patients with advanced non-small-cell lung cancer. *Cancer Sci* **106:** 1554–1560. doi:10.1111/cas.12771

Saga T, Inubushi M, Koizumi M, Yoshikawa K, Zhang M-R, Obata T, Tanimoto K, Harada R, Uno T, Fujibayashi Y. 2016. Prognostic value of PET/CT with ^{18}F-fluoroazomycin arabinoside for patients with head and neck squamous

cell carcinomas receiving chemoradiotherapy. *Ann Nucl Med* **30:** 217–224. doi:10.1007/s12149-015-1048-5

Sai KKS, Bashetti N, Chen X, Norman S, Hines JW, Meka O, Kumar JVS, Devanathan S, Deep G, Furdui CM, et al. 2019. Initial biological evaluations of ^{18}F-KS1, a novel ascorbate derivative to image oxidative stress in cancer. *EJNMMI Res* **9:** 43. doi:10.1186/s13550-019-0513-x

Salamanca-Cardona L, Shah H, Poot AJ, Correa FM, Gialleonardo VD, Lui H, Miloushev VZ, Granlund KL, Tee SS, Cross JR, et al. 2017. In vivo imaging of glutamine metabolism to the oncometabolite 2-hydroxyglutarate in IDH1/2 mutant tumors. *Cell Metab* **26:** 830–841.e3. doi:10.1016/j.cmet.2017.10.001

Sambuceti G, Cossu V, Bauckneht M, Morbelli S, Orengo A, Carta S, Ravera S, Bruno S, Marini C. 2021. ^{18}F-fluoro-2-deoxy-D-glucose (FDG) uptake. What are we looking at? *Eur J Nucl Med Mol Imaging* **48:** 1278–1286. doi:10.1007/s00259-021-05368-2

Schroeder MA, Atherton HJ, Ball DR, Cole MA, Heather LC, Griffin JL, Clarke K, Radda GK, Tyler DJ. 2009. Real-time assessment of Krebs cycle metabolism using hyperpolarized C magnetic resonance spectroscopy. *FASEB J* **23:** 2529–2538. doi:10.1096/fj.09-129171

Serrao EM, Kettunen MI, Rodrigues TB, Dzien P, Wright AJ, Gopinathan A, Gallagher FA, Lewis DY, Frese KK, Almeida J, et al. 2016. MRI with hyperpolarised [1-^{13}C] pyruvate detects advanced pancreatic preneoplasia prior to invasive disease in a mouse model. *Gut* **65:** 465. doi:10.1136/gutjnl-2015-310114

Sharma R, D'Souza M, Jaimini A, Hazari PP, Saw S, Pandey S, Singh D, Solanki Y, Kumar N, Mishra AK, et al. 2016. A comparison study of ^{11}C-methionine and ^{18}F-fluorodeoxyglucose positron emission tomography-computed tomography scans in evaluation of patients with recurrent brain tumors. *Indian J Nucl Med* **31:** 93–102.

Shields AF, Grierson JR, Dohmen BM, Machulla HJ, Stayanoff JC, Lawhorn-Crews JM, Obradovich JE, Muzik O, Mangner TJ. 1998. Imaging proliferation in vivo with [F-18]FLT and positron emission tomography. *Nat Med* **4:** 1334–1336. doi:10.1038/3337

Singh J, Suh EH, Sharma G, Khen J, Hackett EP, Wen X, Sherry AD, Khemtong C, Malloy CR, Park JM, et al. 2021. ^{13}C-labeled diethyl ketoglutarate derivatives as hyperpolarized probes of 2-ketoglutarate dehydrogenase activity. *Anal Sens* **1:** 156–160. doi:10.1002/anse.202100021

Singhal T, Narayanan TK, Jain V, Mukherjee J, Mantil J. 2008. ^{11}C-L-methionine positron emission tomography in the clinical management of cerebral gliomas. *Mol Imaging Biol* **10:** 1–18. doi:10.1007/s11307-007-0115-2

Skoura E, Ardeshna K, Halsey R, Wan S, Kayani I. 2016. False-positive ^{18}F-FDG PET/CT imaging. *Clin Nucl Med* **41:** e171–e172. doi:10.1097/RLU.0000000000001083

Spence AM, Muzi M, Graham MM, O'Sullivan F, Krohn KA, Link JM, Lewellen TK, Lewellen B, Freeman SD, Berger MS, et al. 1998. Glucose metabolism in human malignant gliomas measured quantitatively with PET, 1-[C-11]glucose and FDG: analysis of the FDG lumped constant. *J Nucl Med* **39:** 440–448.

Sriram R, Criekinge MV, Hansen A, Wang ZJ, Vigneron DB, Wilson DM, Keshari KR, Kurhanewicz J. 2015. Real-time measurement of hyperpolarized lactate production and efflux as a biomarker of tumor aggressiveness in an MR compatible 3D cell culture bioreactor. *NMR Biomed* **28**: 1141–1149. doi:10.1002/nbm.3354

Stødkilde-Jørgensen H, Laustsen C, Hansen ESS, Schulte R, Ardenkjaer-Larsen JH, Comment A, Frøkiær J, Ringgaard S, Bertelsen LB, Ladekarl M, et al. 2020. Pilot study experiences with hyperpolarized [1-^{13}C]pyruvate MRI in pancreatic cancer patients. *J Magn Reson Imaging* **51**: 961–963. doi:10.1002/jmri.26888

Stubbs M, Bhujwalla ZM, Tozer GM, Rodrigues LM, Maxwell RJ, Morgan R, Howe FA, Griffiths JR. 1992. An assessment of ^{31}P MRS as a method of measuring pH in rat tumours. *NMR Biomed* **5**: 351–359. doi:10.1002/nbm.1940050606

Sun PZ, Sorensen AG. 2008. Imaging pH using the chemical exchange saturation transfer (CEST) MRI: correction of concomitant RF irradiation effects to quantify CEST MRI for chemical exchange rate and pH. *Magn Reson Med* **60**: 390–397. doi:10.1002/mrm.21653

Sushentsev N, McLean MA, Warren AY, Benjamin AJV, Brodie C, Frary A, Gill AB, Jones J, Kaggie JD, Lamb BW, et al. 2022. Hyperpolarised ^{13}C-MRI identifies the emergence of a glycolytic cell population within intermediate-risk human prostate cancer. *Nat Commun* **13**: 466. doi:10.1038/s41467-022-28069-2

Tang S, Meng MV, Slater JB, Gordon JW, Vigneron DB, Stohr BA, Larson PEZ, Wang ZJ. 2021. Metabolic imaging with hyperpolarized ^{13}C pyruvate magnetic resonance imaging in patients with renal tumors—initial experience. *Cancer* **127**: 2693–2704. doi:10.1002/cncr.33554

Tapmeier TT, Moshnikova A, Beech J, Allen D, Kinchesh P, Smart S, Harris A, McIntyre A, Engelman DM, Andreev OA, et al. 2015. The pH low insertion peptide pHLIP variant 3 as a novel marker of acidic malignant lesions. *Proc Natl Acad Sci* **112**: 9710–9715. doi:10.1073/pnas.1509488112

Tee SS, Kim N, Cullen Q, Eskandari R, Mamakhanyan A, Srouji RM, Chirayil R, Jeong S, Shakiba M, Kastenhuber ER, et al. 2022. Ketohexokinase-mediated fructose metabolism is lost in hepatocellular carcinoma and can be leveraged for metabolic imaging. *Sci Adv* **8**: eabm7985. doi:10.1126/sciadv.abm7985

Temma T, Kawashima H, Kondo N, Yamazaki M, Koshino K, Iida H. 2018. One-pot enzymatic synthesis of l-[3-^{11}C]lactate for pharmacokinetic analysis of lactate metabolism in rat brain. *Nucl Med Biol* **64–65**: 28–33. doi:10.1016/j.nucmedbio.2018.07.001

Thelwall PE, Yemin AY, Gillian TL, Simpson NE, Kasibhatla MS, Rabbani ZN, Macdonald JM, Blackband SJ, Gamcsik MP. 2005. Noninvasive in vivo detection of glutathione metabolism in tumors. *Cancer Res* **65**: 10149–10153. doi:10.1158/0008-5472.CAN-05-1781

Thelwall PE, Simpson NE, Rabbani ZN, Clark MD, Pourdeyhimi R, Macdonald JM, Blackband SJ, Gamcsik MP. 2012. In vivo MR studies of glycine and glutathione metabolism in a rat mammary tumor. *NMR Biomed* **25**: 271–278. doi:10.1002/nbm.1745

Thie JA. 2004. Understanding the standardized uptake value, its methods, and implications for usage. *J Nucl Med* **45**: 1431–1434.

Timm KN, Hu DE, Williams M, Wright AJ, Kettunen MI, Kennedy BWC, Larkin TJ, Dzien P, Marco-Rius I, Bohndiek SE, et al. 2017. Assessing oxidative stress in tumors by measuring the rate of hyperpolarized [1-^{13}C]dehydroascorbic acid reduction using ^{13}C magnetic resonance spectroscopy. *J Biol Chem* **292**: 1737–1748. doi:10.1074/jbc.M116.761536

Tong X, Srivatsan A, Jacobson O, Wang Y, Wang Z, Yang X, Niu G, Kiesewetter DO, Zheng H, Chen X. 2016. Monitoring tumor hypoxia using ^{18}F-FMISO PET and pharmacokinetics modeling after photodynamic therapy. *Sci Rep* **6**: 31551. doi:10.1038/srep31551

Tran M, Latifoltojar A, Neves JB, Papoutsaki M-V, Gong F, Comment A, Costa ASH, Glaser M, Tran-Dang MA, Sheikh SE, et al. 2019. First-in-human in vivo non-invasive assessment of intra-tumoral metabolic heterogeneity in renal cell carcinoma. *BJR Case Rep* **5**: 20190003.

Ursprung S, Woitek R, McLean MA, Priest AN, Crispin-Ortuzar M, Brodie CR, Gill AB, Gehrung M, Beer L, Riddick ACP, et al. 2022. Hyperpolarized ^{13}C-pyruvate metabolism as a surrogate for tumor grade and poor outcome in renal cell carcinoma—a proof of principle study. *Cancers (Basel)* **14**: 335. doi:10.3390/cancers14020335

Varma G, Seth P, de Souza PC, Callahan C, Pinto J, Vaidya M, Sonzogni O, Sukhatme V, Wulf GM, Grant AK. 2021. Visualizing the effects of lactate dehydrogenase (LDH) inhibition and *LDH-A* genetic ablation in breast and lung cancer with hyperpolarized pyruvate NMR. *NMR Biomed* **34**: e4560. doi:10.1002/nbm.4560

Vāvere AL, Kridel SJ, Wheeler FB, Lewis JS. 2008. 1-^{11}C-acetate as a PET radiopharmaceutical for imaging fatty acid synthase expression in prostate cancer. *J Nucl Med* **49**: 327–334. doi:10.2967/jnumed.107.046672

Vāvere AL, Biddlecombe GB, Spees WM, Garbow JR, Wijesinghe D, Andreev OA, Engelman DM, Reshetnyak YK, Lewis JS. 2009. A novel technology for the imaging of acidic prostate tumors by positron emission tomography. *Cancer Res* **69**: 4510–4516. doi:10.1158/0008-5472.CAN-08-3781

Venneti S, Dunphy MP, Zhang H, Pitter KL, Zanzonico P, Campos C, Carlin SD, Rocca GL, Lyashchenko S, Ploessl K, et al. 2015. Glutamine-based PET imaging facilitates enhanced metabolic evaluation of gliomas in vivo. *Sci Transl Med* **7**: 274ra17. doi:10.1126/scitranslmed.aaa1009

Viola-Villegas NT, Carlin SD, Ackerstaff E, Sevak KK, Divilov V, Serganova I, Kruchevsky N, Anderson M, Blasberg RG, Andreev OA, et al. 2014. Understanding the pharmacological properties of a metabolic PET tracer in prostate cancer. *Proc Natl Acad Sci* **111**: 7254–7259. doi:10.1073/pnas.1405240111

Virani N, Kwon J, Zhou H, Mason R, Berbeco R, Protti A. 2021. In vivo hypoxia characterization using blood oxygen level dependent magnetic resonance imaging in a preclinical glioblastoma mouse model. *Magn Reson Imaging* **76**: 52–60. doi:10.1016/j.mri.2020.11.003

Viswanath P, Batsios G, Ayyappan V, Taglang C, Gillespie AM, Larson PEZ, Luchman HA, Costello JF, Pieper RO, Ronen SM. 2021a. Metabolic imaging detects elevated glucose flux through the pentose phosphate pathway associated with TERT expression in low-grade gliomas. *Neuro Oncol* **23**: 1509–1522. doi:10.1093/neuonc/noab093

Viswanath V, Zhou R, Lee H, Li S, Cragin A, Doot RK, Mankoff DA, Pantel AR. 2021b. Kinetic modeling of ^{18}F-(2*S*,4*R*)4-fluoroglutamine in mouse models of breast cancer to estimate glutamine pool size as an indicator of tumor glutamine metabolism. *J Nucl Med* **62:** 1154–1162. doi:10.2967/jnumed.120.250977

Walker-Samuel S, Ramasawmy R, Torrealdea F, Rega M, Rajkumar V, Johnson SP, Richardson S, Gonçalves M, Parkes HG, Årstad E, et al. 2013. In vivo imaging of glucose uptake and metabolism in tumors. *Nat Med* **19:** 1067–1072. doi:10.1038/nm.3252

Wang P, Sun C, Zhu T, Xu Y. 2015. Structural insight into mechanisms for dynamic regulation of PKM2. *Protein Cell* **6:** 275–287. doi:10.1007/s13238-015-0132-x

Wang ZJ, Ohliger MA, Larson PEZ, Gordon JW, Bok RA, Slater J, Villanueva-Meyer JE, Hess CP, Kurhanewicz J, Vigneron DB. 2019. Hyperpolarized ¹³C MRI: state of the art and future directions. *Radiology* **291:** 182391.

Wang Q, Parish C, Niedbalski P, Ratnakar J, Kovacs Z, Lumata L. 2020. Hyperpolarized 89Y-EDTMP complex as a chemical shift-based NMR sensor for pH at the physiological range. *J Magn Reson* **320:** 106837. doi:10.1016/j.jmr.2020.106837

Warburg O. 1956. On the origin of cancer cells. *Science* **123:** 309–314. doi:10.1126/science.123.3191.309

Ward KM, Balaban RS. 2000. Determination of pH using water protons and chemical exchange dependent saturation transfer (CEST). *Magn Reson Med* **44:** 799–802. doi:10.1002/1522-2594(200011)44:5<799::AID-MRM18>3.0.CO;2-S

Ward CS, Venkatesh HS, Chaumeil MM, Brandes AH, VanCriekinge M, Dafni H, Sukumar S, Nelson SJ, Vigneron DB, Kurhanewicz J, et al. 2010. Noninvasive detection of target modulation following phosphatidylinositol 3-kinase inhibition using hyperpolarized ¹³C magnetic resonance spectroscopy. *Cancer Res* **70:** 1296–1305. doi:10.1158/0008-5472.CAN-09-2251

Wardak M, Sonni I, Fan AP, Minamimoto R, Jamali M, Hatami N, Zaharchuk G, Fischbein N, Nagpal S, Li G, et al. 2022. ¹⁸F-FSPG PET/CT imaging of system x_C^- transporter activity in patients with primary and metastatic brain tumors. *Radiology* **303:** 620–631. doi:10.1148/radiol.203296

Wilson DM, Keshari KR, Larson PEZ, Chen AP, Hu S, Criekinge MV, Bok R, Nelson SJ, Macdonald JM, Vigneron DB, et al. 2010. Multi-compound polarization by DNP allows simultaneous assessment of multiple enzymatic activities in vivo. *J Magn Reson* **205:** 141–147. doi:10.1016/j.jmr.2010.04.012

Woitek R, McLean MA, Gill AB, Grist JT, Provenzano E, Patterson AJ, Ursprung S, Torheim T, Zaccagna F, Locke M, et al. 2020. Hyperpolarized ¹³C MRI of tumor metabolism demonstrates early metabolic response to neoadjuvant chemotherapy in breast cancer. *Radiol Imaging Cancer* **2:** e200017. doi:10.1148/rycan.2020200017

Wuest M, Trayner BJ, Grant TN, Jans HS, Mercer JR, Murray D, West FG, McEwan AJB, Wuest F, Cheeseman CI. 2011. Radiopharmacological evaluation of 6-deoxy-6-[¹⁸F]fluoro-D-fructose as a radiotracer for PET imaging of GLUT5 in breast cancer. *Nucl Med Biol* **38:** 461–475. doi:10.1016/j.nucmedbio.2010.11.004

Wuest M, Hamann I, Bouvet V, Glubrecht D, Marshall A, Trayner B, Soueidan O, Krys D, Wagner M, Cheeseman C, et al. 2017. Molecular imaging of GLUT1 and GLUT5 in breast cancer: a multitracer PET imaging study in mice. *Mol Pharmacol* **93:** mol.117.110007.

Wyatt LC, Moshnikova A, Crawford T, Engelman DM, Andreev OA, Reshetnyak YK. 2018. Peptides of pHLIP family for targeted intracellular and extracellular delivery of cargo molecules to tumors. *Proc Natl Acad Sci* **115:** E2811–E2818. doi:10.1073/pnas.1715350115

Xu HN, Kadlececk S, Profka H, Glickson JD, Rizi R, Li LZ. 2014. Is higher lactate an indicator of tumor metastatic risk? A pilot MRS study using hyperpolarized ¹³C-pyruvate. *Acad Radiol* **21:** 223–231. doi:10.1016/j.acra.2013.11.014

Xu X, Chan KWY, Knutsson L, Artemov D, Xu J, Liu G, Kato Y, Lal B, Laterra J, McMahon MT, et al. 2015. Dynamic glucose enhanced (DGE) MRI for combined imaging of blood–brain barrier break down and increased blood volume in brain cancer. *Magnet Reson Med* **74:** 1556–1563. doi:10.1002/mrm.25995

Xu W, Gao L, Shao A, Zheng J, Zhang J. 2017. The performance of ¹¹C-methionine PET in the differential diagnosis of glioma recurrence. *Oncotarget* **8:** 91030–91039. doi:10.18632/oncotarget.19024

Yamamoto K, Brender JR, Seki T, Kishimoto S, Oshima N, Choudhuri R, Adler SS, Jagoda EM, Saito K, Devasahayam N, et al. 2020. Molecular imaging of the tumor microenvironment reveals the relationship between tumor oxygenation, glucose uptake, and glycolysis in pancreatic ductal adenocarcinoma. *Cancer Res* **80:** 2087–2093. doi:10.1158/0008-5472.CAN-19-0928

Yasui H, Kawai T, Matsumoto S, Saito K, Devasahayam N, Mitchell JB, Camphausen K, Inanami O, Krishna MC. 2017. Quantitative imaging of pO₂ in orthotopic murine gliomas: hypoxia correlates with resistance to radiation. *Free Radic Res* **51:** 861–871. doi:10.1080/10715762.2017.1388506

Yoshii Y, Waki A, Furukawa T, Kiyono Y, Mori T, Yoshii H, Kudo T, Okazawa H, Welch MJ, Fujibayashi Y. 2009. Tumor uptake of radiolabeled acetate reflects the expression of cytosolic acetyl-CoA synthetase: implications for the mechanism of acetate PET. *Nucl Med Biol* **36:** 771–777. doi:10.1016/j.nucmedbio.2009.05.006

Zaccagna F, McLean MA, Grist JT, Kaggie J, Mair R, Riemer F, Woitek R, Gill AB, Deen S, Daniels CJ, et al. 2022. Imaging glioblastoma metabolism by using hyperpolarized [1-¹³C]pyruvate demonstrates heterogeneity in lactate labeling: a proof of principle study. *Radiol Imaging Cancer* **4:** e210076. doi:10.1148/rycan.210076

Zacharias NM, Chan HR, Sailasuta N, Ross BD, Bhattacharya P. 2012. Real-time molecular imaging of tricarboxylic acid cycle metabolism in vivo by hyperpolarized 1-¹³C diethyl succinate. *J Am Chem Soc* **134:** 934–943. doi:10.1021/ja2040865

Zhang X, Lin Y, Gillies RJ. 2010. Tumor pH and its measurement. *J Nucl Med* **51:** 1167–1170. doi:10.2967/jnumed.109.068981

Zhou R, Pantel AR, Li S, Lieberman BP, Ploessl K, Choi H, Blankemeyer E, Lee H, Kung HF, Mach RH, et al. 2017. [¹⁸F](2S,4R)4-fluoroglutamine PET detects glutamine pool size changes in triple-negative breast cancer in response to glutaminase inhibition. *Cancer Res* **77:** 1476–1484. doi:10.1158/0008-5472.CAN-16-1945

Technologies for Decoding Cancer Metabolism with Spatial Resolution

Walter W. Chen,[1] **Michael E. Pacold,**[2] **David M. Sabatini,**[3] **and Naama Kanarek**[4,5]

[1]Division of Neonatal-Perinatal Medicine, Department of Pediatrics, Children's Medical Center Research Institute, University of Texas Southwestern Medical Center, Dallas, Texas 75390, USA

[2]Department of Radiation Oncology and Perlmutter Cancer Center, NYU Langone Health, New York, New York 10016, USA

[3]Institute of Organic Chemistry and Biochemistry of the Czech Academy of Sciences, 16610 Prague, Czech Republic

[4]Department of Pathology, Boston Children's Hospital, Harvard Medical School, Boston, Massachusetts 02115, USA

[5]Broad Institute of Harvard and Massachusetts Institute of Technology, Cambridge, Massachusetts 02142, USA

Correspondence: naama.kanarek@childrens.harvard.edu

It is increasingly appreciated that cancer cells adapt their metabolic pathways to support rapid growth and proliferation as well as survival, often even under the poor nutrient conditions that characterize some tumors. Cancer cells can also rewire their metabolism to circumvent chemotherapeutics that inhibit core metabolic pathways, such as nucleotide synthesis. A critical approach to the study of cancer metabolism is metabolite profiling (metabolomics), the set of technologies, usually based on mass spectrometry, that allow for the detection and quantification of metabolites in cancer cells and their environments. Metabolomics is a burgeoning field, driven by technological innovations in mass spectrometers, as well as novel approaches to isolate cells, subcellular compartments, and rare fluids, such as the interstitial fluid of tumors. Here, we discuss three emerging metabolomic technologies: spatial metabolomics, single-cell metabolomics, and organellar metabolomics. The use of these technologies along with more established profiling methods, like single-cell transcriptomics and proteomics, is likely to underlie new discoveries and questions in cancer research.

The study of cancer metabolism has been greatly enabled by the ability to define and measure the activity of metabolic pathways within cancer cells, often in the context of other large-scale data sets. Biological tools have improved to the point where it is routine to comprehensively measure the mRNA and protein levels of metabolic enzymes and transporters, their subcellular localizations, and the levels of precursor and product metabolites (DeBerardinis and Chandel 2016). While technological advancements in genomics, transcriptomics, and proteomics have propelled cancer metabolism research, the capacity to quantitate the cellular and extracellular concentrations of hundreds of metabolites (broadly defined as metabolomics) has made a unique contribution to our understanding of the metabolic adaptations that cancer cells use to drive tumor formation and metastasis (Olivares et al. 2015).

In the context of cancer metabolism research, most metabolomics approaches report the relative (on occasion absolute) quantification of metabolites in cells, culture media, biofluids, organs, and tumors. Labeled metabolites that include a stable isotope can be used to study the flux through a pathway, or decipher the metabolic fate of a metabolite that reveals metabolic decision-making in cancer cells (Faubert et al. 2021). New technologies that enable the measurement of metabolites with cellular and subcellular resolution are enabling the field to ask new biological questions. In this review, we discuss three examples of such technologies. Our goals are to motivate the application of these new technologies, and to emphasize the incentives for their further development.

SPATIAL METABOLOMICS

Nuclear magnetic resonance (NMR) and mass spectrometry-based metabolomics have yielded most of the data on which our modern understanding of metabolic pathways is built. Both techniques require the extraction of metabolites from the biological sample before analysis. Metabolite extraction, by definition, results in the loss of spatial information at the tissue, cellular, and subcellular levels. In contrast, technologies capable of identifying and quantifying metabolites directly in tissue sections enable us to ask questions about the compartmentalization of metabolism in situ at a wide variety of spatial scales (Fig. 1). Tissues compartmentalize metabolism at the millimeter scale: for example, liver zones that exhibit distinct dependences on oxidative phosphorylation (zone 1) versus glycolysis (zone 3) to produce ATP, which correlate with the relative abundances of oxygen and nutrients between these zones (Jungermann 1988). Similar differences are seen in the renal cortex, which is oxygen- and nutrient-rich relative to the medulla. Without careful dissection, these differences are near-impossible in the case of the liver; these

differences are obscured when extracting metabolites from bulk tissues.

The acquisition of metabolomics data requires the transfer of molecules from the solid phase to the gas phase (volatilization/desorption) with the concurrent charging of molecules (ionization), followed by the measurement of the mass-to-charge (m/z) ratio of the resulting ions. In contrast to electrospray (Cooks and Caprioli 2000), chemical, or electron impact ionization of bulk molecules emerging from gas or liquid chromatography, spatially resolved mass spectrometry requires spatially restricted volatilization and ionization. There are three primary methods for spatial volatilization and ionization: matrix-assisted laser desorption and ionization (MALDI), secondary ion mass spectrometry (SIMS), and desorption electrospray ionization (DESI). MALDI (Gilmore et al. 2019) requires the deposition of a crystalline chemical matrix above or below the tissue section, and diffusion of this matrix into the material to be analyzed. The matrix is excited by a high-energy laser that desorbs the matrix and analytes, followed by a charge transfer to the analytes in the gas phase. Scanning of the laser across the surface enables the spatial detection of analytes. MALDI is a soft ionization technique that, like electrospray, generates relatively fewer molecular fragments than hard ionization techniques, such as electron impact ionization. The resolution of MALDI is theoretically limited by the width of the laser beam, and in commercial instruments the minimum pixel size is often 10 µm × 10 µm.

SIMS requires a source of primary ions, usually generated in an ion gun. The primary ions can be individual atoms; clusters of atoms, as in gas cluster ion beam (GCIB) mass spectrometry; or ionized molecules. The ion beam is focused, steered, and fired at the sample, which is maintained under high vacuum, resulting in the transfer of charge to the molecules in the sample and the sputtering of ionized sample molecules off the surface. These ionized molecules are collected and analyzed by a directly coupled mass spectrometer. Scanning of the sample by steering magnets enables spatial volatilization and ionization of metabolites. SIMS instruments have high resolution, with a beam focus of 2 µm in diameter

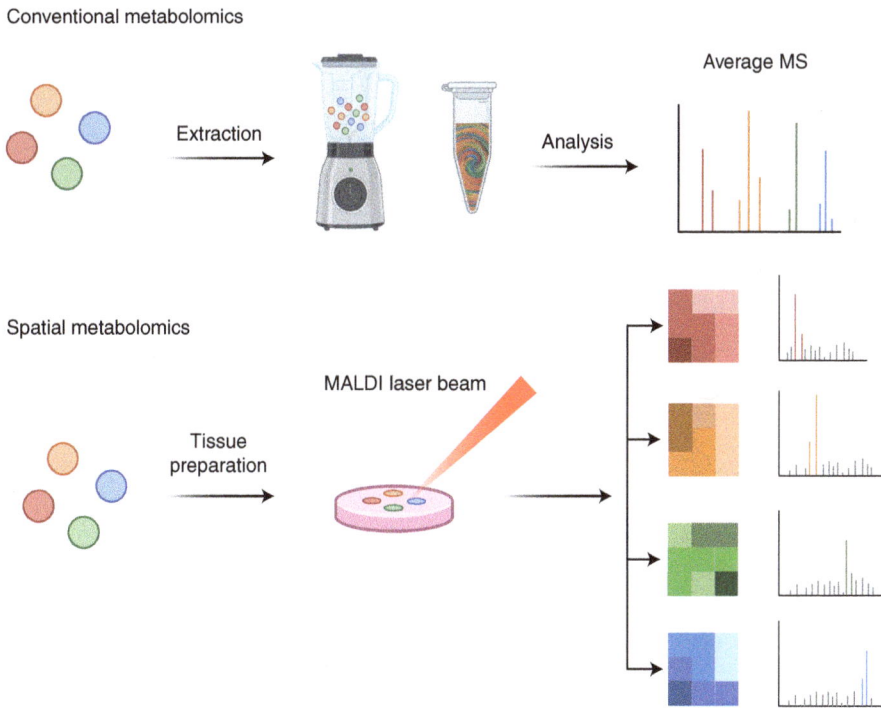

Figure 1. Fundamental differences between conventional metabolomics and spatial metabolomics. Conventional metabolomics approaches in heterogeneous tissues or tumors represent a weighted average of metabolites due to blending of metabolites during tissue processing. Spatial methods, such as matrix-assisted laser desorption and ionization (MALDI) or desorption electrospray ionization (DESI), enable spatial localization of metabolites, within the spatial and detection limits of current technologies. (MS) Mass spectrometry. (Figure created with BioRender.com.)

or less. Additionally, some SIMS research instruments, such as the 3D OrbiSIMS, readily detect polar metabolites (Passarelli et al. 2017), which are typically more difficult to detect with the MALDI approach.

In DESI, an electrospray source generates ionized droplets that strike the surface of the sample at an angle, and thus simultaneously extract and ionize metabolites from the sample. The metabolites enter the inlet of the mass spectrometer, which is placed nearby. Scanning the electrospray source over the material enables spatial ionization of metabolites. The resolution of DESI (maximum 8–10 μm; more commonly 100–350 μm) is limited by the spread of the droplet beam, and efficient ionization and detection are best achieved when the spray and mass spectrometry inlet are both extremely close to the sample (Campbell et al. 2012; Li et al. 2023).

Separation of ions is a necessary step before mass spectrometry as mass spectrometers cannot distinguish structural isomers without fragmentation analysis. Commercially available spatial metabolomics instruments use ion mobility spectrometry (IMS) (Gabelica and Marklund 2018), in which molecules are pulled through a drift gas by electrical fields and separated by collisional cross section, to separate molecules before analysis by mass spectrometry. IMS is analogous to chromatographic separation of molecules by their bulk properties in GC-MS or liquid chromatography-mass spectrometry (LC-MS), but requires much shorter times for separation, and is compatible with the acquisition times of spatial metabolomics data collection.

Ions generated by MALDI are frequently detected and quantitated by a time-of-flight (TOF) mass spectrometer, which has a wide m/z detection range, high resolution, and rapid acquisition times. Orbitrap mass spectrometers, which have comparable resolutions, do not have sufficiently short cycle times to acquire spatial metabolomic data rapidly, but higher resolution orbitrap instruments, which have shorter cycle times, should be suitable for this purpose in the future.

As discussed in the next section, efficient single-cell metabolomics will ultimately require improvements in the sensitivity of the detection methods for metabolites, because they are present at low absolute quantities in individual cells even when at high intracellular concentrations. For example, a eukaryotic cell with a volume ~2 picoliters that contains glutathione at a concentration of 10 mM (Phillips and Milo 2009) has an absolute amount of 20 femtomoles or 12×10^9 molecules of glutathione. Glutathione is one of the most abundant metabolites in the cell. The same cell would contain ~1×10^9 or fewer molecules of each of the amino acids, which are present at 10–100 µM concentrations. A typical mass spectrometer has a detection limit of ~30 fg of material (Russ et al. 2011), which corresponds to 200 attomoles or 1.64×10^8 amino acid molecules. In theory, this sensitivity should allow the detection and quantitation of amino acids and glutathione in a single cell if all those metabolites can be volatilized and ionized. However, volatilization and ionization of metabolites, as well as ion transfer within the mass spectrometer, are not completely efficient processes, making it unlikely that current mass spectrometry technology will allow detection of all metabolites at the single-cell level unless perfectly efficient desorption and ionization techniques are developed.

In general, nonpolar metabolites such as lipids are more easily volatilized and ionized by MALDI, the most widely available spatial metabolomics technique. Consequently, detection of polar metabolites is frequently worse than detection and quantitation of nonpolar metabolites. Standard tissue fixation, embedding, and staining techniques also increase the risk of loss of polar and nonpolar metabolites due to the extensive use of solvents that extract both polar and nonpolar metabolites.

Volatilization and ionization take place at a 10 µm × 10 µm or 20 µm × 20 µm scale, which

requires tens of hours of acquisition time for a 1 cm × 1 cm tissue slice. Because mass spectrometry cannot always distinguish between molecules that have identical masses, but different structures (structural isomers, including molecules of different handedness, or enantiomers), mass spectrometry analysis should ideally be preceded by an analytical technique capable of doing so at a timescale that will not unduly prolong data acquisition. As mentioned above, most MALDI spatial MS instruments use a variant of IMS, which has the speed to resolve structural isomers in the gas phase that makes it compatible with spatial metabolomics. However, current IMS has limited separation power, in part due to the short length of the flight tubes used for separating molecules. Longer tracks, such as those used in technologies such as structures for lossless ion manipulations (SLIM) (Tolmachev et al. 2014), could improve small molecule separations before detection by mass spectrometry.

Current spatial metabolomics methods also can detect a wider array of metabolites from frozen tissue rather than formalin-fixed, paraffin-embedded (FFPE) tissue, which constitutes the majority of pathology specimens. Nevertheless, a limited number of metabolites, particularly lipids, can be detected in FFPE sections (Denti et al. 2022). Finally, even under optimal conditions, spatial metabolomics methods detect a more limited set of metabolites than conventional LC-MS-based metabolomics techniques.

Each pixel from a spatial metabolomics data acquisition or analysis contains, at a minimum, thousands of features. Each feature has an ion mobility retention time, precursor ion (intact ion), and product ion (fragmentation) data from mass spectrometry. These features must be annotated with known metabolites or classified as unknown features (which may or may not correspond to endogenous metabolites; see the Metabolomics Standard Initiative [Sumner et al. 2007]). Most LC-MS analyses generate hundreds of megabytes of data, but data files for imaging MS runs start in the terabyte range and increase in size. The development of software packages that can analyze and detect spatial distributions in these metabolites in an automated manner will enable more widespread use of spatial metabolomics.

Cite this article as *Cold Spring Harb Perspect Med* doi: 10.1101/cshperspect.a041553

The ultimate spatial metabolomics instrument would detect any metabolite at tissue to subcellular concentrations quantitatively and in real time. The latter may be possible with advances in magnetic resonance imaging and MR spectroscopy, while the former will be enabled by improvements in tissue processing and mass spectrometer sensitivity and specificity. The development of improved spatial metabolomics instruments will enable researchers to ask fundamental questions about metabolite sharing and compartmentalization, such as the identities and concentrations of metabolites in the extracellular or extratumoral space. The use of spatial metabolomics with labeled metabolites, particularly when model organisms or patients are administered stable isotope-labeled metabolites before analyses, also will allow us to answer fundamental questions about metabolite physiology in whole organisms, such as demonstrating the regions of the brain that differentially use ketones and glutamate when glucose is restricted or gluconeogenesis in the renal cortex and glycolysis in the renal medulla (Wang et al. 2022).

SINGLE-CELL METABOLOMICS

Heterogeneity is an intrinsic feature of cell populations, organs, and tumors. Cell-to-cell variation is evident in the heterogeneous transcriptional (Aldridge and Teichmann 2020), metabolic (Kim and DeBerardinis 2019; Kondo et al. 2021), epigenetic (Easwaran et al. 2014), and proteomic (Maier et al. 2009) profiles that emerge whenever single-cell approaches are used. Techniques with single-cell resolution have been transformative for several fields, including cancer biology (Baslan and Hicks 2017; Vitale et al. 2021), immunology (Chen et al. 2019), and for understanding the differences between the normal and pathological states of diverse tissues (Haber et al. 2017; Halpern et al. 2017; Montoro et al. 2018; Solé-Boldo et al. 2020).

The vast majority of single-cell results emanate from single-cell transcriptomics, while other omics studies provide orthogonal information at a single-cell resolution: single-cell transcriptomics studies are sometimes enhanced by other analyses of the cellular function and state, includ-

ing cell mass (Kimmerling et al. 2018) and growth (Godin et al. 2010), as well as proteomic (Genshaft et al. 2016), genomic (Dey et al. 2015), epigenetic (Angermueller et al. 2016), and metabolomic profiles (Vandereyken et al. 2023). These additional measurements provide comprehensive profiling of the cell state and identify cellular changes that do not manifest transcriptionally. Each of these modules informs a complimentary aspect of cell state and function. Specifically, metabolomics provides a unique data set of metabolite levels that reflect changes that result from fluctuations in the environment of the cell and intracellular signaling, and inform the functional activity of the cell. Furthermore, cell metabolism can regulate the function (Shyh-Chang et al. 2013; Palmer et al. 2015), differentiation, and proliferation of individual cells within a population (Vander Heiden et al. 2009).

Metabolic heterogeneity within cell populations is common and influences disease outcome and treatment responses (Robertson-Tessi et al. 2015). Moreover, critical individual cells can shift the behavior of a whole population, such as in tumor progression (DeBerardinis and Chandel 2016; Vander Heiden and DeBerardinis 2017), inflammation (Kominsky et al. 2010), and the response to treatment—especially metabolic-based therapy for cancer (Luengo et al. 2017), and autoimmune diseases (Piranavan et al. 2020). We increasingly appreciate that metabolic heterogeneity has a major impact on life and health spans (Vander Heiden and DeBerardinis 2017; Condon and Sabatini 2019).

Single-cell transcriptomics (Xiao et al. 2019; Rohlenova et al. 2020) or proteomics (Hartmann and Bendall 2020; Hartmann et al. 2021) allow for high throughput analysis, and are often used to profile metabolic pathways in lieu of more direct measurements of single-cell metabolites, and can serve as a proxy of the metabolic state of single cells. An advantage of this approach over the measurements of metabolites is that it relies on single-cell technologies that are more advanced and accessible, but an obvious disadvantage is that these measurements fall short of reflecting the actual metabolic state of the cell. It goes without saying that mRNA and protein abundance report on the general state of the cell, but not necessarily on the fast-changing metabolic state. Fast changes in and outside the cell, such as an acute nutritional shortage, oxidative and reductive distress, the allosteric regulation of enzymes, and rapid response to cell signaling, will often not be detected by transcriptomic and proteomic methods.

Single-cell metabolomics has been of interest to the metabolism and general life sciences community for more than a decade (Boggio et al. 2011; Svatoš 2011), and the field has witnessed constant progress in performance driven by technological advancements (Tajik et al. 2022). Technological approaches to perform single-cell metabolomics mostly rely on mass spectrometry, and although they vary, they can be generally grouped into two types: sample ionization using a high-energy beam, which is usually assisted by a stabilizing matrix; and direct injection of the sample to the mass spectrometer, sometimes after an ion separation step such as chromatography (Zhang et al. 2023).

As discussed in the Spatial Metabolomics section, single-cell metabolomics can be achieved by spatial metabolomics (Shrestha 2020b; Taylor et al. 2021) using MALDI mass spectrometry (Dueñas and Lee 2021), SIMS (Kurczy et al. 2010; Senyo et al. 2013), or DESI (Saunders et al. 2023). These are highly precise methods that can achieve single-cell or near single-cell resolution with high numbers of cells (Rappez et al. 2021) across tissues (Boggio et al. 2011; Qi et al. 2018; Saunders et al. 2023), with good examples from various mouse tissues, such as the kidney (Zhao et al. 2018) and tumors (Dilillo et al. 2017), and in primary human epithelial cells (from cheek swabs) (Bergman and Lanekoff 2017). There are even reports of using a <2 μm pixel size to detect a few select ions at the organelle level in cultured mamalian cells (Bien et al. 2022), and in primary sea slug cells (Castro et al. 2021). Furthermore, isotope tracing has been integrated into spatial metabolomics, as was shown for the mouse kidney and brain (Wang et al. 2022), and as the resolution of this method improves, it will enable more accurate assessment of the relative flux of assessed metabolic pathways.

Recent advances have improved the application of laser ionization-based technology to single-cell metabolomics. Cao et al. (2024) applied an innovative single-cell metabolomics method they named high-throughput single-cell metabolomics (hi-scMet) to study hematopoietic stem cell (HSC) differentiation. The method incorporates a fluorescence-activated cell sorting (FACS)-sorted HSC population loaded onto ferric oxide nanoparticles as the matrix, and then analyzed by MALDI. The use of nanoparticles allowed for much higher throughput in comparison to micropipette methods and the method enables consistent detection of 100 metabolites. Of note, single-cell resolution is essential for the study of this rare population in its natural environment given the presence of fully differentiated hematpoietic cells that are orders of magnitude more abundant and will otherwise mask the metabolic features of HSCs in any population-based study. However, a limitation of this method is the FACS sorting step that introduces metabolic shifts in the cells.

A limitation of spatial metabolomics is the necessity to use a matrix that is essentially premixed with the sample to enable sample fixation. This is a limitation for two main reasons. One is the technical noise introduced by the matrix, which is discussed in the section Spatial Metabolomics, but this is an even bigger problem when trying to analyze single cells in which the abundances of metabolites is very low to begin with (Fig. 2A). A second limitation of having to fix the sample is that it excludes fresh, live cells from analyses. For example, lymphocytes freshly isolated from blood must be first smeared on a slide and fixed and only then analyzed, as are cultured cells grown in suspension. This limitation is a serious hurdle because the cellular metabolic state is extremely dynamic and transient, with changes happening on the order of seconds and continuing even when samples are placed on ice. Therefore, single-cell metabolomics will have greater value if it can be performed routinely on live cells.

Indeed, techniques for single-cell metabolomics of live cells are currently available, but are limited because the extreme technical challenges of most approaches leads to low throughput (Hiyama et al. 2015; Onjiko et al. 2015; Zhang and Vertes 2015; Chen et al. 2016a; Lee et al. 2016; Pan et al. 2016; Zhang et al. 2016; Bergman

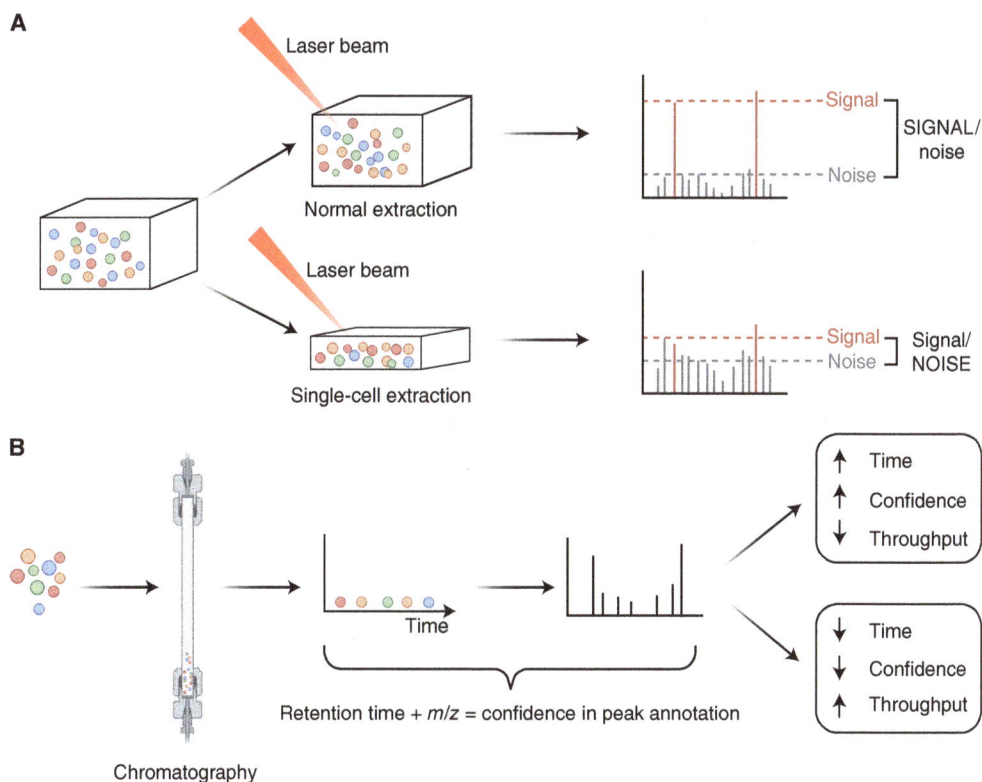

Figure 2. Two major single-cell metabolomics approaches. (*A*) Spatial single-cell metabolomics that is based on matrix-assisted methods is limited by the matrix itself that introduces noise. The higher the resolution, the smaller is the signal-to-noise ratio. However, spatial single-cell metabolomics can be performed in relatively high throughput. (*B*) Single-cell metabolomics that is based on direct injection of the cell—with or without analytical separation methods such as chromatography (as depicted in the figure) or other ion separation methods—is often very low throughput, with time-based ion separation introducing an internal time-consuming step to the analysis. (Figure created with BioRender.com.)

and Lanekoff 2017; Zhu et al. 2017, 2018; Sun et al. 2018; Artyomov and Van den Bossche 2020; Shrestha 2020a,b). For example, a published report on single-cell metabolomics of human hepatocytes included five or six cells in each analysis (Fukano et al. 2012), and a study that profiled the metabolome of individual neurons included 18 cells in each cohort (Zhu et al. 2018). However, progress is being made, and some studies report improved throughput, with numbers per group that can reach 120 cultured cells (Qin et al. 2024). This might be still too few to achieve satisfactory statistical power given the variation between individual cells.

An important aspect of single-cell metabolomics is its application alongside another 'omics analyses, such as proteomics, transcriptomics, or genomics, which can report on cell type and state that are often hard (or impossible) to decipher from the metabolome alone.

Spatial analysis can include metabolomics with either proteomics (Hu et al. 2023), transcriptomics, or epigenomics (Nikopoulou et al. 2023) from the same cell. Paired omics studies that included live single-cell metabolomics have been paired with single-cell proteomics (Baysoy et al. 2023; Wu et al. 2024), but other analyses such as transcriptomics or epigenomics can better inform cell type and differentiation states. Furthermore, single-cell transcriptomics is a very developed field, with excellent, extremely advanced data analysis tools and well-studied gene-expression signatures that can be highly informative regarding metabolic pathways.

The challenges that hinder single-cell metabolomics of live cells are significant. Metabolites are highly labile (even at low temperatures), metabolites do not share any unifying chemistry, and the metabolome cannot be amplified (unlike DNA or RNA) or tagged and barcoded (unlike proteins or nucleic acids) to analyze multiple cells in parallel (Specht et al. 2021). Therefore, it is not surprising that the methods for single-cell metabolomics that have been used to date are low throughput, require specific instrumentation and skills, and are unsuited for large-scale cell state assessments (Zenobi 2013). Additionally, the abundance of metabolites in a single cell is very low, and achieving a reliable separation between background noise and true signal is difficult. However, it is encouraging that the sensitivity of many mass spectrometers is sufficient to detect metabolites from a single cell, as demonstrated in real-world examples (Fukano et al. 2012; Hiyama et al. 2015; Onjiko et al. 2015; Zhang and Vertes 2015; Chen et al. 2016a; Lee et al. 2016; Pan et al. 2016; Zhang et al. 2016; Bergman and Lanekoff 2017; Zhu et al. 2017, 2018; Sun et al. 2018; Artyomov and Van den Bossche 2020; Shrestha 2020a,b), and this sensitivity will only continue to improve as new mass spectrometers are developed specifically for single-cell analyses.

Yet, there are several practical limitations to live single-cell metabolomics that will be hard to overcome. Sample preparation is complicated; it is essential to handle the single cell in a way that maintains its viability, and, critically, its metabolome, which is far more labile than its transcriptome and proteome. Additionally, dilution of the single-cell metabolome by adding extraction buffer must be minimized to maintain, as much as possible, the metabolites extracted from individual cells within a detectable range. Data normalization is another challenge; to compare the abundance of a metabolite of interest between cells, the cell volume should be accounted for. This parameter is better addressed in spatial metabolomics, where often at least one dimension of the cell can be directly measured.

A forward-looking perspective of live single-cell metabolomics will include several key leaps in this important developing technology (Fig. 2B). First, to achieve biologically and statistically significant single-cell metabolomics data, the number of analyzed cells per experiment must be high to account for stochasticity. As such, single-cell metabolomics approaches must be high throughput and considerably faster interrogative workflows will be needed. Unlike most of the methods discussed here, current metabolite profiling approaches usually use LC-MS, which is highly time-consuming (~30 min per sample), limiting the number of cells that can be analyzed in a reasonable period of time. Second, metabolomics data on its own, without paired multiomics, lack information regarding cell type and state. Other paired omics are important for the correct interpretation of metabolomics data, and the field will benefit tremendously when metabolomics of live cells are added as a paired technology to the world of multiomics. With these advancements, single-cell metabolomics of live cells will surely contribute significantly to discovery and innovation in biology and medicine.

ORGANELLAR METABOLOMICS

Metabolic organelles, such as mitochondria and lysosomes, play crucial roles in the metabolism of cancer cells. As a result of their compartmentalized nature, organelles contain unique repertoires of proteins, lipids, and metabolites that enable diverse biochemical processes and the generation of distinct metabolic landscapes. To fully understand how these organelles contribute to cancer metabolism, it is thus important to be able to assess the changes in metabolism occurring within the organelles themselves. While whole-cell metabolomic studies have provided important insights into various aspects of cancer metabolism pertaining to organelles, interrogation of metabolites at a whole-cell level can miss various changes in organellar metabolism as the amount of a metabolite in a given subcellular location can be just a small fraction of the total whole-cell pool.

A straightforward approach to comprehensively profile organellar metabolomes is to homogenize cells, directly isolate the organelle of interest, and interrogate the metabolic contents via mass spectrometry. Historically though, this has been challenging for several reasons. Metabolites, unlike proteins and nucleic acids, are considerably more labile and metabolite pools can begin to change from the native state by either residual enzymatic or transporter activity during the course of organellar isolation even when the workflow is done at 4°C (Bowsher and Tobin 2001; Ross-Inta et al. 2008; Matuszczyk et al. 2015); thus, methods for studying organellar metabolites require very rapid isolation. In addition, it is also essential that the isolation strategy have sufficient specificity such that the organelle of interest is adequately purified away from contaminants (e.g., other organelles) so that one is truly interrogating the desired subcellular compartment. Finally, traditional buffers for isolating organelles often contain large amounts of solutes, such as sucrose and mannitol, which can carry over into the extracted metabolite sample and consequently interfere with interrogation of metabolites by the popular method of LC/MS (Roede et al. 2012; Chen et al. 2016b).

To address these technical barriers for the study of organellar metabolites, a methodology using an epitope-tagged protein localized to an organellar membrane (i.e., an "organellar tag") and rapid immunoisolation of the cognate organelles in an LC/MS-compatible format has been developed, with the first instance of the technique applied to the fast immunopurification of mitochondria (MITO-IP) (Chen et al. 2016b, 2017). In the MITO-IP, expression of a 3XHA-tagged protein localized to the outer mitochondrial membrane (i.e., the "MITO-Tag") allows for the rapid and specific anti-hemagglutinin (HA) immunocapture of mitochondria from cultured human cells in a workflow that is compatible with LC/MS-based metabolomics and other downstream assays (Fig. 3A). Potassium-phosphate-buffered saline (KPBS), a simplified organellar isolation buffer comprised of only KCl and KH_2PO_4, maintains mitochondrial integrity and eliminates the introduction of small-molecule contaminants (e.g., sucrose, mannitol) into the LC/MS workflow that occurs when using tra-

ditional mitochondrial isolation buffers. In addition, by leveraging the high affinity, highly specific interaction between the MITO-Tag and the cognate anti-HA antibody, the presence of multiple copies of the MITO-Tag per mitochondrion, and the speed of a magnet-based isolation workflow, the MITO-IP technique allows for the purification of mitochondria within 10 min of cellular homogenization. In contrast to previous mitochondrial isolation methods that would compromise speed for specificity or vice versa, the MITO-IP technique offers both, thereby enabling robust metabolomic interrogation of mitochondria from cultured human cells.

Given the utility of the technique, the MITO-IP methodology has now been adapted for the interrogation of other organelles and for the study of organelles in complex biological systems, resulting in a family of useful rapid organellar immunopurification approaches using organellar tags (Fig. 3B). There are now methods in cultured cells for the isolation of lysosomes (LYSO-IP) (Abu-Remaileh et al. 2017), peroxisomes (PEROXO-IP) (Ray et al. 2020), endosomes (ENDO-IP) (Park et al. 2022), melanosomes (MELANO-IP) (Adelmann et al. 2020), Golgi (GOLGI-IP) (Fasimoye et al. 2023), and synaptic vesicles (SV-IP) (Chantranupong et al. 2020). Transgenic mice, such as "MITO-Tag Mice" (The Jackson Laboratory strain #032290) (Bayraktar et al. 2019) and "LysoTag Mice" (The Jackson Laboratory strain #035401) (Laqtom et al. 2022), in which expression of the corresponding organellar tag can be activated via Cre recombinase, have also been generated to allow for rapid isolation and metabolic profiling of mitochondria and lysosomes, respectively, from specific cell types in complex tissues in vivo without the need for cell sorting, which can improve the speed of the workflow and reduce distortion of the organellar metabolic profile. Transgenic mice designed with a similar strategy as the MITO-Tag Mice but with a different organellar tag have also been developed (The Jackson Laboratory strain #032675) and enable cell-type-specific isolation of mitochondria in vivo as well (Fecher et al. 2019).

Evidenced by hundreds of requests on Addgene for the plasmids harboring different organellar tags, this family of rapid organellar

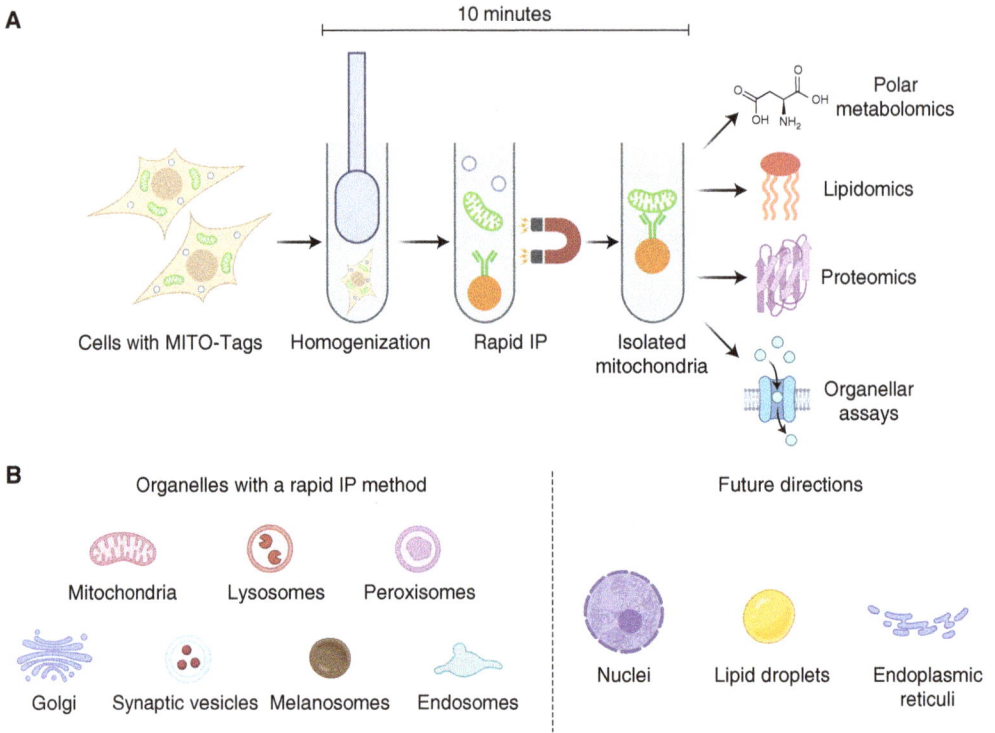

Figure 3. Rapid organellar immunopurification. (*A*) Immunopurification of mitochondria (MITO-IP) workflow. Cells expressing the MITO-Tag (i.e., 3XHA-tagged outer mitochondrial membrane protein) are harvested and homogenized, thereby liberating mitochondria (green), which can subsequently be rapidly immunopurified away from other cellular material using magnetic beads conjugated to anti-hemagglutinin (HA) antibodies. The resulting mitochondrial isolate can then be used for a variety of purposes, such as polar metabolomics, lipidomics, proteomics, and organellar assays (e.g., metabolite uptake assays). Of note, purified mitochondria can be obtained within 10 min of cellular homogenization. (*B*) Rapid organellar immunopurification landscape. Mammalian organelles with and without a rapid immunopurification method akin to the MITO-IP are shown. Organelles with a developed method include mitochondria, lysosomes, peroxisomes, Golgi, synaptic vesicles, melanosomes, and endosomes. Organelles that could be pursued in the future include nuclei, lipid droplets, and endoplasmic reticuli. (Figure created with BioRender.com.)

immunopurification methods has become a popular way to study organellar metabolism and biology. Indeed, the techniques have been used with various metabolomic pipelines (targeted and untargeted polar metabolomics, stable isotope tracing, and lipidomics) (Chen et al. 2016b; Abu-Remaileh et al. 2017; Bayraktar et al. 2019; Adelmann et al. 2020; Chantranupong et al. 2020; Kory et al. 2020; Soula et al. 2020; Sun et al. 2021; Wang et al. 2021; Laqtom et al. 2022; Trefely et al. 2022; Xiao et al. 2022; Fasimoye et al. 2023; Scharenberg et al. 2023), absolute-quantification metabolomics for measurements of organellar metabolite concentrations (Chen et al. 2016b; Abu-Remaileh et al. 2017; Wyant et al. 2017), proteomics (Wyant et al. 2018; Bayraktar et al. 2019; Chantranupong et al. 2020; Ray et al. 2020; Wang et al. 2021; Laqtom et al. 2022; Park et al. 2022; Fasimoye et al. 2023), and metabolite transport assays of purified organelles (Abu-Remaileh et al. 2017; Wyant et al. 2017; Wang et al. 2021). Of note, the metabolomic studies that have been undertaken underscore the importance of directly interrogating metabolites at the organellar level as the corresponding whole-cell/whole-tissue analyses do not fully capture the dynamics of the organellar metabolic landscape.

Looking ahead, there are several areas that are relatively unexplored with regards to the aforementioned rapid organellar immunopurification methods and cancer metabolism. Firstly, the nucleus, while now felt to be a site of localized metabolic processes, represents a challenge because of nuclear pores, which generally allow molecules <40 kDa (e.g., metabolites) to passively move across the nuclear membrane (Lin and Hoelz 2019). Future attempts to rapidly isolate nuclei for metabolomics will thus need to address this problem of metabolites leaking out of nuclei during isolation. The endoplasmic reticulum and lipid droplets represent other organelles intimately connected to cellular metabolism that lack rapid-isolation approaches akin to the MITO-IP, although both organelles should be amenable to such pursuits (Fig. 3B). Other interesting applications of these epitope tag-based immunopurification techniques will take full advantage of the ability to rapidly isolate organelles with cell-type specificity in complex systems without the need for cell sorting, which improves the speed of the workflow and reduces distortion of the organellar metabolic profile. For example, generating cells in which expression of the organellar tag is under the control of a promoter only active in a certain cell type would have utility in studying cancer metabolism in both coculture and organoid systems in vitro. Furthermore, xenograft mouse models using implanted cancer cells expressing an organellar tag would allow for more accurate interrogation of organellar metabolites originating from the cancer cells and not the accompanying stroma when processing the bulk tumor. Using MITO-Tag and LysoTag mice in established cancer models and various Cre recombinase drivers could also allow for selective assessment of organellar metabolites within not just cancer cells but also noncancerous cells in the tumor microenvironment, such as nervous tissue (Winkler et al. 2023) and different immune cells (Makowski et al. 2020), both of which are now appreciated to play a significant role in cancer dynamics. Taken together, given the importance of organelles in cancer metabolism and what has already been achieved using rapid organellar immunopurification methods, we thus believe that there is much future potential for these techniques in the study of cancer metabolism.

SUMMARY

Metabolomics data add a key layer of information that we increasingly recognize is necessary for understanding cancer at the cell and organismal levels. New technologies enabling the measurement of metabolites at cellular and subcellular resolutions should drive exciting new discoveries, likely in combination with other high-resolution approaches to measure proteins and RNAs. Day-to-day metabolite profiling of cells in bulk and in biofluids will continue to serve as the most robust and broadly used application of metabolomics. However, precedence with transcriptomics and proteomics has shown that as technologies move to increasing resolutions, unexpected discoveries are made that lead to new biological questions. There is no reason to think that metabolomics will not follow this same path.

ACKNOWLEDGMENTS

We thank these funding sources for supporting our work: W.W.C is supported by AAP Marshall Klaus Neonatal-Perinatal Research Award, Thrasher Research Fund Early Career Award, and Children's Health Fellow Research Scholar Award—the content of this manuscript does not necessarily represent the official views of Children's Health. D.M.S. received support from the US NIH (R01 CA103866, R01 CA129105, and R01 AI47389) and funding from the Institute of Organic Chemistry and Biochemistry of the Czech Academy of Sciences and Pershing Square Philanthropies; M.E.P. is supported by a Damon Runyon-Rachleff Innovation Award (DRR 63-20), a Pershing Square Sohn Prize for Young Investigators in Cancer Research, the Tara Miller Melanoma Foundation—MRA Young Investigator Award (668365), a Basic Research Grant from the Harry J. Lloyd Charitable Trust, an ACS Research Scholar Award (RSG-21-115-01-MM), an NIGMS R35 MIRA from the NIH (1R35GM147119), an Irma T. Hirschl Career Scientist Award, a Concern Foundation

Conquer Cancer Now Grant, and a Scholar-Innovator Award from the Harrington Discovery Institute; N.K. is supported by the NIH/NCI (1R01CA282477-01A1, 1R01CA279550-01), the STARR Cancer Consortium, Boston Children's Hospital Research Executive Council, Richard and Susan Smith Family Foundation, Binational Science Foundation, N.K. is a Pew Scholar. We acknowledge Sophie Tanenbaum and BioRender.com for assistance with the generation of figures.

REFERENCES

Abu-Remaileh M, Wyant GA, Kim C, Laqtom NN, Abbasi M, Chan SH, Freinkman E, Sabatini DM. 2017. Lysosomal metabolomics reveals V-ATPase- and mTOR-dependent regulation of amino acid efflux from lysosomes. *Science* 358: 807–813. doi:10.1126/science.aan6298

Adelmann CH, Traunbauer AK, Chen B, Condon KJ, Chan SH, Kunchok T, Lewis CA, Sabatini DM. 2020. MFSD12 mediates the import of cysteine into melanosomes and lysosomes. *Nature* 588: 699–704. doi:10.1038/s41586-020-2937-x

Aldridge S, Teichmann SA. 2020. Single cell transcriptomics comes of age. *Nat Commun* 11: 4307. doi:10.1038/s41467-020-18158-5

Angermueller C, Clark SJ, Lee HJ, Macaulay IC, Teng MJ, Hu TX, Krueger F, Smallwood S, Ponting CP, Voet T, et al. 2016. Parallel single-cell sequencing links transcriptional and epigenetic heterogeneity. *Nat Methods* 13: 229–232. doi:10.1038/nmeth.3728

Artyomov MN, Van den Bossche J. 2020. Immunometabolism in the single-cell era. *Cell Metab* 32: 710–725. doi:10.1016/j.cmet.2020.09.013

Baslan T, Hicks J. 2017. Unravelling biology and shifting paradigms in cancer with single-cell sequencing. *Nat Rev Cancer* 17: 557–569. doi:10.1038/nrc.2017.58

Bayraktar EC, Baudrier L, Özerdem C, Lewis CA, Chan SH, Kunchok T, Abu-Remaileh M, Cangelosi AL, Sabatini DM, Birsoy K, et al. 2019. MITO-Tag mice enable rapid isolation and multimodal profiling of mitochondria from specific cell types in vivo. *Proc Natl Acad Sci* 116: 303–312. doi:10.1073/pnas.1816656115

Baysoy A, Bai Z, Satija R, Fan R. 2023. The technological landscape and applications of single-cell multi-omics. *Nat Rev Mol Cell Biol* 24: 695–713. doi:10.1038/s41580-023-00615-w

Bergman HM, Lanekoff I. 2017. Profiling and quantifying endogenous molecules in single cells using nano-DESI MS. *Analyst* 142: 3639–3647. doi:10.1039/C7AN00885F

Bien T, Koerfer K, Schwenzfeier J, Dreisewerd K, Soltwisch J. 2022. Mass spectrometry imaging to explore molecular heterogeneity in cell culture. *Proc Natl Acad Sci* 119: e2114365119. doi:10.1073/pnas.2114365119

Boggio KJ, Obasuyi E, Sugino K, Nelson SB, Agar NYR, Agar JN. 2011. Recent advances in single-cell MALDI mass spectrometry imaging and potential clinical impact. *Exp Rev Proteomics* 8: 591–604. doi:10.1586/epr.11.53

Bowsher CG, Tobin AK. 2001. Compartmentation of metabolism within mitochondria and plastids. *J Exp Bot* 52: 513–527. doi:10.1093/jexbot/52.356.513

Campbell DI, Ferreira CR, Eberlin LS, Cooks RG. 2012. Improved spatial resolution in the imaging of biological tissue using desorption electrospray ionization. *Anal Bioanal Chem* 404: 389–398. doi:10.1007/s00216-012-6173-6

Cao J, Yao QJ, Wu J, Chen X, Huang L, Liu W, Qian K, Wan JJ, Zhou BO. 2024. Deciphering the metabolic heterogeneity of hematopoietic stem cells with single-cell resolution. *Cell Metab* 36: 209–221.e6. doi:10.1016/j.cmet.2023.12.005

Castro DC, Xie YR, Rubakhin SS, Romanova EV, Sweedler JV. 2021. Image-guided MALDI mass spectrometry for high-throughput single-organelle characterization. *Nat Methods* 18: 1233–1238. doi:10.1038/s41592-021-01277-2

Chantranupong L, Saulnier JL, Wang W, Jones DR, Pacold ME, Sabatini BL. 2020. Rapid purification and metabolomic profiling of synaptic vesicles from mammalian brain. *eLife* 9: e59699. doi:10.7554/eLife.59699

Chen F, Lin L, Zhang J, He Z, Uchiyama K, Lin JM. 2016a. Single-cell analysis using drop-on-demand inkjet printing and probe electrospray ionization mass spectrometry. *Anal Chem* 88: 4354–4360. doi:10.1021/acs.analchem.5b04749

Chen WW, Freinkman E, Wang T, Birsoy K, Sabatini DM. 2016b. Absolute quantification of matrix metabolites reveals the dynamics of mitochondrial metabolism. *Cell* 166: 1324–1337.e11. doi:10.1016/j.cell.2016.07.040

Chen WW, Freinkman E, Sabatini DM. 2017. Rapid immunopurification of mitochondria for metabolite profiling and absolute quantification of matrix metabolites. *Nat Protoc* 12: 2215–2231. doi:10.1038/nprot.2017.104

Chen H, Ye F, Guo G. 2019. Revolutionizing immunology with single-cell RNA sequencing. *Cell Mol Immunol* 16: 242–249. doi:10.1038/s41423-019-0214-4

Condon KJ, Sabatini DM. 2019. Nutrient regulation of mTORC1 at a glance. *J Cell Sci* 132: jcs222570. doi:10.1242/jcs.222570

Cooks G, Caprioli R. 2000. Special feature on electrospray ionization. *J Mass Spectrom* 35: 761. doi:10.1002/1096-9888(200007)35:7<761::AID-JMS38>3.0.CO;2-U

DeBerardinis RJ, Chandel NS. 2016. Fundamentals of cancer metabolism. *Sci Adv* 2: e1600200. doi:10.1126/sciadv.1600200

Denti V, Capitoli G, Piga I, Clerici F, Pagani L, Criscuolo L, Bindi G, Principi L, Chinello C, Paglia G, et al. 2022. Spatial multiomics of lipids, N-glycans, and tryptic peptides on a single FFPE tissue section. *J Proteome Res* 21: 2798–2809.

Dey SS, Kester L, Spanjaard B, Bienko M, van Oudenaarden A. 2015. Integrated genome and transcriptome sequencing of the same cell. *Nat Biotechnol* 33: 285–289. doi:10.1038/nbt.3129

Dilillo M, Ait-Belkacem R, Esteve C, Pellegrini D, Nicolardi S, Costa M, Vannini E, Graaf EL, Caleo M, McDonnell LA. 2017. Ultra-high mass resolution MALDI imaging mass spectrometry of proteins and metabolites in a mouse model of glioblastoma. *Sci Rep* 7: 603. doi:10.1038/s41598-017-00703-w

Dueñas ME, Lee YJ. 2021. Single-cell metabolomics by mass spectrometry imaging. *Adv Exp Med Biol* **1280:** 69–82. doi:10.1007/978-3-030-51652-9_5

Easwaran H, Tsai HC, Baylin SB. 2014. Cancer epigenetics: tumor heterogeneity, plasticity of stem-like states, and drug resistance. *Mol Cell* **54:** 716–727. doi:10.1016/j.molcel.2014.05.015

Fasimoye R, Dong W, Nirujogi RS, Rawat ES, Iguchi M, Nyame K, Phung TK, Bagnoli E, Prescott AR, Alessi DR, et al. 2023. Golgi-IP, a tool for multimodal analysis of Golgi molecular content. *Proc Natl Acad Sci* **120:** e2219953120. doi:10.1073/pnas.2219953120

Faubert B, Tasdogan A, Morrison SJ, Mathews TP, DeBerardinis RJ. 2021. Stable isotope tracing to assess tumor metabolism in vivo. *Nat Protoc* **16:** 5123–5145. doi:10.1038/s41596-021-00605-2

Fecher C, Trovò L, Müller SA, Snaidero N, Wettmarshausen J, Heink S, Ortiz O, Wagner I, Kühn R, Hartmann J, et al. 2019. Cell-type-specific profiling of brain mitochondria reveals functional and molecular diversity. *Nat Neurosci* **22:** 1731–1742. doi:10.1038/s41593-019-0479-z

Fukano Y, Tsuyama N, Mizuno H, Date S, Takano M, Masujima T. 2012. Drug metabolite heterogeneity in cultured single cells profiled by pico-trapping direct mass spectrometry. *Nanomedicine (Lond)* **7:** 1365–1374. doi:10.2217/nnm.12.34

Gabelica V, Marklund E. 2018. Fundamentals of ion mobility spectrometry. *Curr Opin Chem Biol* **42:** 51–59. doi:10.1016/j.cbpa.2017.10.022

Genshaft AS, Li S, Gallant CJ, Darmanis S, Prakadan SM, Ziegler CG, Lundberg M, Fredriksson S, Hong J, Regev A, et al. 2016. Multiplexed, targeted profiling of single-cell proteomes and transcriptomes in a single reaction. *Genome Biol* **17:** 188. doi:10.1186/s13059-016-1045-6

Gilmore IS, Heiles S, Pieterse CL. 2019. Metabolic imaging at the single-cell scale: recent advances in mass spectrometry imaging. *Annu Rev Anal Chem (Palo Alto Calif)* **12:** 201–224. doi:10.1146/annurev-anchem-061318-115516

Godin M, Delgado FF, Son S, Grover WH, Bryan AK, Tzur A, Jorgensen P, Payer K, Grossman AD, Kirschner MW, et al. 2010. Using buoyant mass to measure the growth of single cells. *Nat Methods* **7:** 387–390. doi:10.1038/nmeth.1452

Haber AL, Biton M, Rogel N, Herbst RH, Shekhar K, Smillie C, Burgin G, Delorey TM, Howitt MR, Katz Y, et al. 2017. A single-cell survey of the small intestinal epithelium. *Nature* **551:** 333–339. doi:10.1038/nature24489

Halpern KB, Shenhav R, Matcovitch-Natan O, Tóth B, Lemze D, Golan M, Massasa EE, Baydatch S, Landen S, Moor AE, et al. 2017. Single-cell spatial reconstruction reveals global division of labor in the mammalian liver. *Nature* **542:** 352–356. doi:10.1038/nature21065

Hartmann FJ, Bendall SC. 2020. Immune monitoring using mass cytometry and related high-dimensional imaging approaches. *Nat Rev Rheumatol* **16:** 87–99. doi:10.1038/s41584-019-0338-z

Hartmann FJ, Mrdjen D, McCaffrey E, Glass DR, Greenwald NF, Bharadwaj A, Khair Z, Verberk SGS, Baranski A, Baskar R, et al. 2021. Single-cell metabolic profiling of human cytotoxic T cells. *Nat Biotechnol* **39:** 186–197. doi:10.1038/s41587-020-0651-8

Hiyama E, Ali A, Amer S, Harada T, Shimamoto K, Furushima R, Abouleila Y, Emara S, Masujima T. 2015. Direct lipido-metabolomics of single floating cells for analysis of circulating tumor cells by live single-cell mass spectrometry. *Anal Sci* **31:** 1215–1217. doi:10.2116/analsci.31.1215

Hu T, Allam M, Cai S, Henderson W, Yueh B, Garipcan A, Ievlev AV, Afkarian M, Beyaz S, Coskun AF. 2023. Single-cell spatial metabolomics with cell-type specific protein profiling for tissue systems biology. *Nat Commun* **14:** 8260. doi:10.1038/s41467-023-43917-5

Jungermann K. 1988. Metabolic zonation of liver parenchyma. *Semin Liver Dis* **8:** 329–341. doi:10.1055/s-2008-1040554

Kim J, DeBerardinis RJ. 2019. Mechanisms and implications of metabolic heterogeneity in cancer. *Cell Metab* **30:** 434–446. doi:10.1016/j.cmet.2019.08.013

Kimmerling RJ, Prakadan SM, Gupta AJ, Calistri NL, Stevens MM, Olcum S, Cermak N, Drake RS, Pelton K, De Smet F, et al. 2018. Linking single-cell measurements of mass, growth rate, and gene expression. *Genome Biol* **19:** 207. doi:10.1186/s13059-018-1576-0

Kominsky DJ, Campbell EL, Colgan SP. 2010. Metabolic shifts in immunity and inflammation. *J Immunol* **184:** 4062–4068. doi:10.4049/jimmunol.0903002

Kondo H, Ratcliffe CDH, Hooper S, Ellis J, MacRae JI, Hennequart M, Dunsby CW, Anderson KI, Sahai E. 2021. Single-cell resolved imaging reveals intra-tumor heterogeneity in glycolysis, transitions between metabolic states, and their regulatory mechanisms. *Cell Rep* **34:** 108750. doi:10.1016/j.celrep.2021.108750

Kory N, uit de Bos J, van der Rijt S, Jankovic N, Güra M, Arp N, Pena IA, Prakash G, Chan SH, Kunchok T, et al. 2020. MCART1/SLC25A51 is required for mitochondrial NAD transport. *Sci Adv* **6:** eabe5310. doi:10.1126/sciadv.abe5310

Kurczy ME, Piehowski PD, Van Bell CT, Heien ML, Winograd N, Ewing AG. 2010. Mass spectrometry imaging of mating *Tetrahymena* show that changes in cell morphology regulate lipid domain formation. *Proc Natl Acad Sci* **107:** 2751–2756. doi:10.1073/pnas.0908101107

Laqtom NN, Dong W, Medoh UN, Cangelosi AL, Dharamdasani V, Chan SH, Kunchok T, Lewis CA, Heinze I, Tang R, et al. 2022. CLN3 is required for the clearance of glycerophosphodiesters from lysosomes. *Nature* **609:** 1005–1011. doi:10.1038/s41586-022-05221-y

Lee JK, Jansson ET, Nam HG, Zare RN. 2016. High-resolution live-cell imaging and analysis by laser desorption/ionization droplet delivery mass spectrometry. *Anal Chem* **88:** 5453–5461. doi:10.1021/acs.analchem.6b00881

Li X, Hu H, Laskin J. 2023. High-resolution integrated microfluidic probe for mass spectrometry imaging of biological tissues. *Anal Chim Acta* **1279:** 341830. doi:10.1016/j.aca.2023.341830

Lin DH, Hoelz A. 2019. The structure of the nuclear pore complex (an update). *Annu Rev Biochem* **88:** 725–783. doi:10.1146/annurev-biochem-062917-011901

Luengo A, Gui DY, Vander Heiden MG. 2017. Targeting metabolism for cancer therapy. *Cell Chem Biol* **24:** 1161–1180. doi:10.1016/j.chembiol.2017.08.028

Maier T, Güell M, Serrano L. 2009. Correlation of mRNA and protein in complex biological samples. *FEBS Lett* **583:** 3966–3973. doi:10.1016/j.febslet.2009.10.036

Makowski L, Chaib M, Rathmell JC. 2020. Immunometabolism: from basic mechanisms to translation. *Immunol Rev* **295:** 5–14. doi:10.1111/imr.12858

Matuszczyk J-C, Teleki A, Pfizenmaier J, Takors R. 2015. Compartment-specific metabolomics for CHO reveals that ATP pools in mitochondria are much lower than in cytosol. *Biotechnol J* **10:** 1639–1650. doi:10.1002/biot.201500060

Montoro DT, Haber AL, Biton M, Vinarsky V, Lin B, Birket SE, Yuan F, Chen S, Leung HM, Villoria J, et al. 2018. A revised airway epithelial hierarchy includes CFTR-expressing ionocytes. *Nature* **560:** 319–324. doi:10.1038/s41586-018-0393-7

Nikopoulou C, Kleinenkuhnen N, Parekh S, Sandoval T, Ziegenhain C, Schneider F, Giavalisco P, Donahue K-F, Vesting AJ, Kirchner M, et al. 2023. Spatial and single-cell profiling of the metabolome, transcriptome and epigenome of the aging mouse liver. *Nat Aging* **3:** 1430–1445. doi:10.1038/s43587-023-00513-y

Olivares O, Däbritz JHM, King A, Gottlieb E, Halsey C. 2015. Research into cancer metabolomics: towards a clinical metamorphosis. *Semin Cell Dev Biol* **43:** 52–64. doi:10.1016/j.semcdb.2015.09.008

Onjiko RM, Moody SA, Nemes P. 2015. Single-cell mass spectrometry reveals small molecules that affect cell fates in the 16-cell embryo. *Proc Natl Acad Sci* **112:** 6545–6550. doi:10.1073/pnas.1423682112

Palmer CS, Ostrowski M, Balderson B, Christian N, Crowe SM. 2015. Glucose metabolism regulates T cell activation, differentiation, and functions. *Front Immunol* **6:** 1. doi:10.3389/fimmu.2015.00001

Pan N, Rao W, Standke SJ, Yang Z. 2016. Using dicationic ion-pairing compounds to enhance the single cell mass spectrometry analysis using the single-probe: a microscale sampling and ionization device. *Anal Chem* **88:** 6812–6819. doi:10.1021/acs.analchem.6b01284

Park H, Hundley FV, Yu Q, Overmyer KA, Brademan DR, Serrano L, Paulo JA, Paoli JC, Swarup S, Coon JJ, et al. 2022. Spatial snapshots of amyloid precursor protein intramembrane processing via early endosome proteomics. *Nat Commun* **13:** 6112. doi:10.1038/s41467-022-33881-x

Passarelli MK, Pirkl A, Moellers R, Grinfeld D, Kollmer F, Havelund R, Newman CF, Marshall PS, Arlinghaus H, Alexander MR, et al. 2017. The 3D OrbiSIMS-label-free metabolic imaging with subcellular lateral resolution and high mass-resolving power. *Nat Methods* **14:** 1175–1183. doi:10.1038/nmeth.4504

Phillips R, Milo R. 2009. A feeling for the numbers in biology. *Proc Natl Acad Sci* **106:** 21465–21471. doi:10.1073/pnas.0907732106

Piranavan P, Bhamra M, Perl A. 2020. Metabolic targets for treatment of autoimmune diseases. *ImmunoMetabolism* **2:** e200012. doi:10.20900/immunometab20200012

Qi M, Philip MC, Yang N, Sweedler JV. 2018. Single cell neurometabolomics. *ACS Chem Neurosci* **9:** 40–50. doi:10.1021/acschemneuro.7b00304

Qin S, Zhang Y, Shi M, Miao D, Lu J, Wen L, Bai Y. 2024. In-depth organic mass cytometry reveals differential contents of 3-hydroxybutanoic acid at the single-cell level. *Nat Commun* **15:** 4387. doi:10.1038/s41467-024-48865-2

Rappez L, Stadler M, Triana S, Gathungu RM, Ovchinnikova K, Phapale P, Heikenwalder M, Alexandrov T. 2021. SpaceM reveals metabolic states of single cells. *Nat Methods* **18:** 799–805. doi:10.1038/s41592-021-01198-0

Ray GJ, Boydston EA, Shortt E, Wyant GA, Lourido S, Chen WW, Sabatini DM. 2020. A PEROXO-tag enables rapid isolation of peroxisomes from human cells. *iScience* **23:** 101109. doi:10.1016/j.isci.2020.101109

Robertson-Tessi M, Gillies RJ, Gatenby RA, Anderson AR. 2015. Impact of metabolic heterogeneity on tumor growth, invasion, and treatment outcomes. *Cancer Res* **75:** 1567–1579. doi:10.1158/0008-5472.CAN-14-1428

Roede JR, Park Y, Li S, Strobel FH, Jones DP. 2012. Detailed mitochondrial phenotyping by high resolution metabolomics. *PLoS ONE* **7:** e33020. doi:10.1371/journal.pone.0033020

Rohlenova K, Goveia J, García-Caballero M, Subramanian A, Kalucka J, Treps L, Falkenberg KD, de Rooij L, Zheng Y, Lin L, et al. 2020. Single-cell RNA sequencing maps endothelial metabolic plasticity in pathological angiogenesis. *Cell Metab* **31:** 862–877.e14. doi:10.1016/j.cmet.2020.03.009

Ross-Inta C, Tsai C-Y, Giulivi C. 2008. The mitochondrial pool of free amino acids reflects the composition of mitochondrial DNA-encoded proteins: indication of a post-translational quality control for protein synthesis. *Biosci Rep* **28:** 239–249. doi:10.1042/BSR20080090

Russ CW IV, Prest H, Wells G. 2011. Why use signal-to-noise as a measure of MS performance when it is often meaningless? Agilent Technologies, Wilmington, DE. https://www.agilent.com/cs/library/technicaloverviews/public/5990-8341EN.pdf?srsltid=AfmBOopfL3G46N6qDZJLXjYYWM4kSiGbsfoTvZxU0KbyQY08Zjv-skcT

Saunders KDG, Lewis HM, Beste DJ, Cexus O, Bailey MJ. 2023. Spatial single cell metabolomics: current challenges and future developments. *Curr Opin Chem Biol* **75:** 102327. doi:10.1016/j.cbpa.2023.102327

Scharenberg SG, Dong W, Ghoochani A, Nyame K, Levin-Konigsberg R, Krishnan AR, Rawat ES, Spees K, Bassik MC, Abu-Remaileh M. 2023. An SPNS1-dependent lysosomal lipid transport pathway that enables cell survival under choline limitation. *Sci Adv* **9:** eadf8966. doi:10.1126/sciadv.adf8966

Senyo SE, Steinhauser ML, Pizzimenti CL, Yang VK, Cai L, Wang M, Wu TD, Guerquin-Kern JL, Lechene CP, Lee RT. 2013. Mammalian heart renewal by pre-existing cardiomyocytes. *Nature* **493:** 433–436. doi:10.1038/nature11682

Shrestha B. 2020a. *Single cell metabolism.* Humana, New York.

Shrestha B. 2020b. Single-cell metabolomics by mass spectrometry. *Methods Mol Biol* **2064:** 1–8. doi:10.1007/978-1-4939-9831-9_1

Shyh-Chang N, Daley GQ, Cantley LC. 2013. Stem cell metabolism in tissue development and aging. *Development* **140:** 2535–2547. doi:10.1242/dev.091777

Solé-Boldo L, Raddatz G, Schütz S, Mallm JP, Rippe K, Lonsdorf AS, Rodríguez-Paredes M, Lyko F. 2020. Single-cell transcriptomes of the human skin reveal age-related loss of fibroblast priming. *Commun Biol* **3:** 188. doi:10.1038/s42003-020-0922-4

Soula M, Weber RA, Zilka O, Alwaseem H, La K, Yen F, Molina H, Garcia-Bermudez J, Pratt DA, Birsoy K. 2020. Metabolic determinants of cancer cell sensitivity to canonical ferroptosis inducers. *Nat Chem Biol* **16:** 1351–1360. doi:10.1038/s41589-020-0613-y

Cite this article as *Cold Spring Harb Perspect Med* doi: 10.1101/cshperspect.a041553

Specht H, Emmott E, Petelski AA, Huffman RG, Perlman DH, Serra M, Kharchenko P, Koller A, Slavov N. 2021. Single-cell proteomic and transcriptomic analysis of macrophage heterogeneity using SCoPE2. *Genome Biol* **22:** 50. doi:10.1186/s13059-021-02267-5

Sumner LW, Amberg A, Barrett D, Beale MH, Beger R, Daykin CA, Fan TW, Fiehn O, Goodacre R, Griffin JL, et al. 2007. Proposed minimum reporting standards for chemical analysis Chemical Analysis Working Group (CAWG) Metabolomics Standards Initiative (MSI). *Metabolomics* **3:** 211–221. doi:10.1007/s11306-007-0082-2

Sun M, Yang Z, Wawrik B. 2018. Metabolomic fingerprints of individual algal cells using the single-probe mass spectrometry technique. *Front Plant Sci* **9:** 571. doi:10.3389/fpls.2018.00571

Sun Y, Rahbani JF, Jedrychowski MP, Riley CL, Vidoni S, Bogoslavski D, Hu B, Dumesic PA, Zeng X, Wang AB, et al. 2021. Mitochondrial TNAP controls thermogenesis by hydrolysis of phosphocreatine. *Nature* **593:** 580–585. doi:10.1038/s41586-021-03533-z

Svatoš A. 2011. Single-cell metabolomics comes of age: new developments in mass spectrometry profiling and imaging. *Anal Chem* **83:** 5037–5044. doi:10.1021/ac2003592

Tajik M, Baharfar M, Donald WA. 2022. Single-cell mass spectrometry. *Trends Biotechnol* **40:** 1374–1392. doi:10.1016/j.tibtech.2022.04.004

Taylor MJ, Lukowski JK, Anderton CR. 2021. Spatially resolved mass spectrometry at the single cell: recent innovations in proteomics and metabolomics. *J Am Soc Mass Spectrom* **32:** 872–894. doi:10.1021/jasms.0c00439

Tolmachev AV, Webb IK, Ibrahim YM, Garimella SV, Zhang X, Anderson GA, Smith RD. 2014. Characterization of ion dynamics in structures for lossless ion manipulations. *Anal Chem* **86:** 9162–9168. doi:10.1021/ac502054p

Trefely S, Huber K, Liu J, Noji M, Stransky S, Singh J, Doan MT, Lovell CD, von Krusenstiern E, Jiang H, et al. 2022. Quantitative subcellular acyl-CoA analysis reveals distinct nuclear metabolism and isoleucine-dependent histone propionylation. *Mol Cell* **82:** 447–462.e6. doi:10.1016/j.molcel.2021.11.006

Vandereyken K, Sifrim A, Thienpont B, Voet T. 2023. Methods and applications for single-cell and spatial multiomics. *Nat Rev Genet* **24:** 494–515. doi:10.1038/s41576-023-00580-2

Vander Heiden MG, DeBerardinis RJ. 2017. Understanding the intersections between metabolism and cancer biology. *Cell* **168:** 657–669. doi:10.1016/j.cell.2016.12.039

Vander Heiden MG, Cantley LC, Thompson CB. 2009. Understanding the Warburg effect: the metabolic requirements of cell proliferation. *Science* **324:** 1029–1033. doi:10.1126/science.1160809

Vitale I, Shema E, Loi S, Galluzzi L. 2021. Intratumoral heterogeneity in cancer progression and response to immunotherapy. *Nat Med* **27:** 212–224. doi:10.1038/s41591-021-01233-9

Wang Y, Yen FS, Zhu XG, Timson RC, Weber R, Xing C, Liu Y, Allwein B, Luo H, Yeh H-W, et al. 2021. SLC25A39 is necessary for mitochondrial glutathione import in mammalian cells. *Nature* **599:** 136–140. doi:10.1038/s41586-021-04025-w

Wang L, Xing X, Zeng X, Jackson SR, TeSlaa T, Al-Dalahmah O, Samarah LZ, Goodwin K, Yang L, McReynolds MR, et al. 2022. Spatially resolved isotope tracing reveals tissue

metabolic activity. *Nat Methods* **19:** 223–230. doi:10.1038/s41592-021-01378-y

Winkler F, Venkatesh HS, Amit M, Batchelor T, Demir IE, Deneen B, Gutmann DH, Hervey-Jumper S, Kuner T, Mabbott D, et al. 2023. Cancer neuroscience: state of the field, emerging directions. *Cell* **186:** 1689–1707. doi:10.1016/j.cell.2023.02.002

Wu J, Xu Q-Q, Jiang Y-R, Chen J-B, Ying W-X, Fan Q-X, Wang H-F, Wang Y, Shi S-W, Pan J-Z, et al. 2024. One-shot single-cell proteome and metabolome analysis strategy for the same single cell. *Anal Chem* **96:** 5499–5508. doi:10.1021/acs.analchem.3c05659

Wyant GA, Abu-Remaileh M, Wolfson RL, Chen WW, Freinkman E, Danai LV, Vander Heiden MG, Sabatini DM. 2017. mTORC1 activator SLC38A9 is required to efflux essential amino acids from lysosomes and use protein as a nutrient. *Cell* **171:** 642–654.e12. doi:10.1016/j.cell.2017.09.046

Wyant GA, Abu-Remaileh M, Frenkel EM, Laqtom NN, Dharamdasani V, Lewis CA, Chan SH, Heinze I, Ori A, Sabatini DM. 2018. NUFIP1 is a ribosome receptor for starvation-induced ribophagy. *Science* **360:** 751–758. doi:10.1126/science.aar2663

Xiao Z, Dai Z, Locasale JW. 2019. Metabolic landscape of the tumor microenvironment at single cell resolution. *Nat Commun* **10:** 3763. doi:10.1038/s41467-019-11738-0

Xiao H, Bozi LHM, Sun Y, Riley CL, Philip VM, Chen M, Li J, Zhang T, Mills EL, Emont MP, et al. 2022. Architecture of the outbred brown fat proteome defines regulators of metabolic physiology. *Cell* **185:** 4654–4673.e28. doi:10.1016/j.cell.2022.10.003

Zenobi R. 2013. Single-cell metabolomics: analytical and biological perspectives. *Science* **342:** 1243259. doi:10.1126/science.1243259

Zhang L, Vertes A. 2015. Energy charge, redox state, and metabolite turnover in single human hepatocytes revealed by capillary microsampling mass spectrometry. *Anal Chem* **87:** 10397–10405. doi:10.1021/acs.analchem.5b02502

Zhang XC, Wei ZW, Gong XY, Si XY, Zhao YY, Yang CD, Zhang SC, Zhang XR. 2016. Integrated droplet-based microextraction with ESI-MS for removal of matrix interference in single-cell analysis. *Sci Rep* **6:** 24730. doi:10.1038/srep24730

Zhang C, Le Dévédec SE, Ali A, Hankemeier T. 2023. Single-cell metabolomics by mass spectrometry: ready for primetime? *Curr Opin Biotechnol* **82:** 102963. doi:10.1016/j.copbio.2023.102963

Zhao C, Xie P, Yong T, Wang H, Chung ACK, Cai Z. 2018. MALDI-MS imaging reveals asymmetric spatial distribution of lipid metabolites from bisphenol S-induced nephrotoxicity. *Anal Chem* **90:** 3196–3204. doi:10.1021/acs.analchem.7b04540

Zhu H, Zou G, Wang N, Zhuang M, Xiong W, Huang G. 2017. Single-neuron identification of chemical constituents, physiological changes, and metabolism using mass spectrometry. *Proc Natl Acad Sci* **114:** 2586–2591. doi:10.1073/pnas.1615557114

Zhu H, Wang N, Yao L, Chen Q, Zhang R, Qian J, Hou Y, Guo W, Fan S, Liu S, et al. 2018. Moderate UV exposure enhances learning and memory by promoting a novel glutamate biosynthetic pathway in the brain. *Cell* **173:** 1716–1727.e17. doi:10.1016/j.cell.2018.04.014

Oncogenic Control of Metabolism

Natalya N. Pavlova[1] and Craig B. Thompson[2]

[1]Oncological Sciences, Huntsman Cancer Institute, University of Utah, Salt Lake City, Utah 84112, USA

[2]Cancer Biology and Genetics Program, Memorial Sloan Kettering Cancer Center, New York, New York 10065, USA

Correspondence: natasha.pavlova@hci.utah.edu

A cell committed to proliferation must reshape its metabolism to enable robust yet balanced production of building blocks for the assembly of proteins, lipids, nucleic acids, and other macromolecules, from which two functional daughter cells can be produced. The metabolic remodeling associated with proliferation is orchestrated by a number of pro-proliferative signaling nodes, which include phosphatidylinositol-3 kinase (PI3K), the RAS family of small GTPases, and transcription factor *c-myc*. In metazoan cells, these signals are activated in a paracrine manner via growth factor–mediated activation of receptor (or receptor-associated) tyrosine kinases. Such stimuli are limited in duration and therefore allow the metabolism of target cells to return to the resting state once the proliferation demands have been satisfied. Cancer cells acquire activating genetic alterations within common pro-proliferative signaling nodes. These alterations lock cellular nutrient uptake and utilization into a perpetual progrowth state, leading to the aberrant accumulation and spread of cancer cells.

A century ago, German physiologist Otto Warburg made a discovery that tumors—regardless of their type—consumed high quantities of glucose. Furthermore, Warburg found that tumors handled the glucose they acquired differently from that of normal tissues (Warburg et al. 1927). Even with ample oxygen available, tumors preferred to ferment glucose into a three-carbon molecule of lactate rather than oxidize it to completion (that is, to CO_2) through respiration.

This seminal discovery—later termed aerobic glycolysis—gave rise to a compelling notion that altered cell metabolism constitutes the very foundation of tumorigenesis. But why do tumors catabolize glucose in a manner so distinct from normal tissues (such as, for instance, muscle or liver)? Warburg's initial explanation of this phenomenon was undoubtedly influenced by the discovery by Pauly and Rajewsky (1956), who demonstrated that X-rays—already known to be carcinogenic—were directly damaging to tissue respiration. Accordingly, Warburg interpreted the aerobic glycolysis he had observed in tumors as a manifestation of the "irreversible injury to respiration," which leaves cells with the fermentative route as the sole option of deriving energy from glucose (Warburg 1956).

In the decades that followed, numerous studies have refuted Warburg's own explanation of this phenomenon, revealing that tumors do retain—and rely on—the capacity for oxidative phosphorylation (Cavalli et al. 1997; Weinberg et al. 2010; Martínez-Reyes et al. 2020). Today, the tumor's ravenous appetite for glucose is being exploited in standard-of-care tumor-imaging approaches, wherein the accumulation of the radiolabeled glucose analog ^{18}F-deoxyglucose allows an oncologist to pinpoint the location of a tumor in one's body (Ben-Haim and Ell 2009). However, the mechanism and the utility of such profligate use of glucose by tumors has remained unclear for decades after Warburg's original discovery. As the field of cancer metabolism underwent a renaissance at the dawn of the twenty-first century, a new crop of discoveries exposed this seemingly aberrant handling of glucose as but one aspect of a grander scheme of tumor-associated metabolic remodeling (Ward and Thompson 2012; DeBerardinis and Chandel 2016). Furthermore, aerobic glycolysis has revealed itself as not being the consequence of something that cancer cells have lost—but on the contrary, driven by something they have gained.

UPSTANDING CITIZENS AND RULE-BREAKERS

Cancer is a disease of progressive accumulation of cells that have evaded the control mechanisms that hold proliferation of cells in a multicellular organism in check. In contrast to unicellular organisms, which make their proliferative decisions based on the favorability of the surrounding environment, metazoan cells have essentially relinquished autonomous decision-making on issues of not only proliferation, but even survival itself (Hanahan and Weinberg 2000). Proliferation and survival of metazoan cells is controlled by highly specific paracrine instructions—including signals carried by soluble growth factors (for example, EGF or HGF), which bind and activate corresponding plasma membrane–localized receptor tyrosine kinases (RTKs) such as EGFR or c-Met (Aaronson 1991). A complementary set of instructions comes from integrin-mediated attachments of cells to the specific components of the extracellular matrix (Giancotti and Ruoslahti 1999). Acting together, these signals transmit prosurvival and pro-proliferative messages to the recipient cell.

Cancer cells circumvent the need for external instructions that their normal counterparts live via acquiring somatic genetic·alterations—gain-of-function alterations in proto-oncogenes, and loss-of-function alterations in tumor suppressors (Weinberg 1994; Hunter 1997; Sherr 2004). The scale of these alterations ranges from point mutations and small indels to larger-scale gene deletions, amplifications, translocations, and whole-chromosome aneuploidies (Vogelstein et al. 2013). The first oncogenes discovered were derivatives of host genes hijacked by a peculiar class of viruses that gives rise to transmissible cancers in birds—such as Rous sarcoma virus—which harbors a truncated form of the non-RTK c-Src (Stehelin et al. 1976), and avian myelocytomatosis virus MC29, which contains a variant of the transcription factor *c-myc* (Vennstrom et al. 1982). These discoveries were followed by the realization that the very same genes—termed proto-oncogenes—that become hijacked by viruses are, in fact, common targets of somatic genetic alteration in tumors in general (Vogt 2012). With the advent of genome sequencing technologies, the collaborative initiatives aimed at sequencing tens of thousands of tumors yielded a comprehensive view of human genes subject to recurrent genomic alteration in cancer (Ding et al. 2018; ICGC/TCGA Pan-Cancer Analysis of Whole Genomes Consortium 2020). However, the work of functional characterization of these alterations and their causal involvement in cancer continues to the present day.

Functionally, the predominant class of causative tumor-associated genetic alterations targets major signaling hubs that transmit growth factor–delivered instructions on issues of cell growth, proliferation, and eventual attrition via programmed cell death mechanisms (Hunter 1997; Hanahan and Weinberg 2000). Among commonly identified oncogenic alterations are point mutations within KRAS, PIK3CA, and EGFR genes, as well as amplifications of *c-myc*, Erbb2/HER2, and c-Met. Conversely, tumor suppressor genes such as p53, PTEN, and Rb suffer the opposite fate in tumors, wherein the loss-of-function alterations in this class of genes deregulate growth and survival of cancer cells (Vogelstein and Kinzler 2004).

Cite this article as *Cold Spring Harb Perspect Med* doi: 10.1101/cshperspect.a041531

Collectively, these alterations lock the proproliferative, prosurvival signaling machinery of a healthy cell into a perpetual "on" state, which, in turn, drives uncontrolled cell accumulation. Importantly, as the explosion of discoveries in the first decade of the twenty-first century revealed, the signaling pathways that are targeted with genetic alteration in cancer do not merely transmit commands to the cell to grow and divide. Rather, these signals can exert direct and immediate control over the cell's metabolic networks, promptly expanding and reorienting them to ensure that the task of replicative cell division—in essence, a monumental construction project—is a success.

THE DINNER BELL FOR THE CELL

In unicellular organisms, a signal that initiates proliferation is nutrient availability itself (Fig. 1A). Linking the commitment to proliferation directly to nutrient availability allows unicellular organisms to make the most out of their changing environments. Nutrient sensing in yeast is carried out by a set of dedicated receptors, among which are G-protein-coupled receptors (GPCRs), which sense sources of fermentable carbon, as well as receptors for reduced nitrogen and phosphate (Thevelein and de Winde 1999; Giots et al. 2003; Georis et al. 2011). When activated, these sensors directly stimulate the cell's decision-making ma-

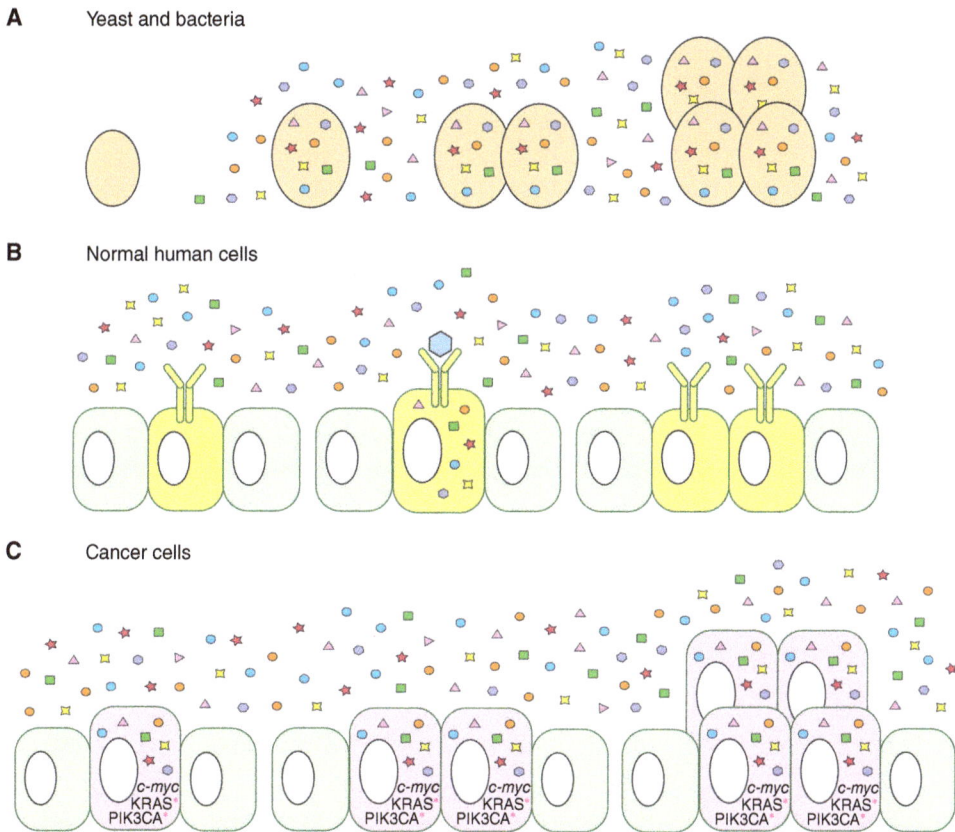

Figure 1. Autonomous and nonautonomous decision-making strategies in nutrient acquisition. (A) Unicellular organisms import nutrients at will and use nutrient availability as a cue for proliferation. (B) Normal metazoan cells import nutrients and engage in proliferation in response to cell-type-specific paracrine stimuli (i.e., growth factors), which are limited in duration. (C) Cancer cells harbor oncogenes (such as mutant alleles of KRAS, PIK3CA, or amplification of c-myc), which result in constitutive activation of the major nutrient import and utilization signals, leading to disordered cell accumulation. Asterisks indicate genes that are frequently altered in cancer.

chinery, instructing the yeast cell to build biomass and proliferate.

In contrast to the unicellular organisms, metazoan cells are surrounded by plentiful nutrients, delivered to them via plasma and interstitial fluid (Kratz and Lewandrowski 1998). The supply of nutrients is maintained via a combination of feeding behavior, nutrient release from internal stores, and their de novo synthesis. Accordingly, GPCR-based glucose sensing in metazoans has been demoted to serving a handful of specialized functions—for instance, as taste receptors (Ahmad and Dalziel 2020). Yet despite the cornucopia of nutrients around them, metazoan cells have relinquished the autonomy to access those nutrients to a remarkable extent (Fig. 1B). Indeed, neurons and lymphocytes deprived of growth factors were found to be unable to import glucose in the quantities needed to even maintain their mitochondrial potential and ATP production (Rathmell et al. 2000; Lindsten et al. 2003).

As follow-up studies have shown, the metazoan cells' ability to import glucose is controlled by growth factor–associated phosphoinositide-3 kinase (PI3K)/Akt signaling. The PI3K/Akt module integrates paracrine progrowth/prosurvival inputs transmitted via both RTKs and cellular attachments to the extracellular matrix. Importantly, alterations that lead to an aberrantly activated PI3K/Akt signaling represent a dominant class of genetic alterations in human cancer (Fig. 1C; Yuan and Cantley 2008). Such alterations include amplifications and mutations in various RTKs and activating mutations in the catalytic and regulatory subunits of PI3K. Loss-of-function alterations within PTEN and INPP4B tumor suppressors, which normally serve to counterbalance the PI3K activity, are also frequently found in tumors. Underscoring its key role in enabling glucose uptake, ectopic expression of a constitutively active form of Akt was found to be sufficient for cells to access glucose around them, bypassing the need for both growth factor– and attachment-mediated instructions for doing so (Rathmell et al. 2003; Schafer et al. 2009).

Why is glucose unable to enter the cell in the absence of growth factors? Mechanistically, acti-

vation of Akt downstream of PI3K allows the glucose transporter GLUT1, which, in resting cells, is sequestered within endocytic vesicles in the cell's interior, to be translocated to the plasma membrane (Wieman et al. 2007). To this end, Akt phosphorylates and inhibits thioredoxin-interacting protein (TXNIP), an α-arrestin that interacts with GLUT1 and facilitates its clathrin-mediated endocytosis, thereby sequestering GLUT1 away from the plasma membrane (Waldhart et al. 2017). In addition, tumor suppressor PTEN can direct GLUT1 to the endosomal compartment directly via sequestering sorting nexin 27 (SNX27), such that tumor-associated loss of PTEN further facilitates GLUT1 translocation to the cell surface (Fig. 2; Shinde and Maddika 2017).

Signaling via Akt also promotes the activity of the enzyme hexokinase 2 (HK2)—the first enzyme in the glycolysis cascade—which, in turn, phosphorylates and thereby traps glucose molecules within the cell. To this end, phosphorylation by Akt promotes the localization of HK2 at the outer mitochondrial membrane, where its proximity to mitochondria-generated ATP enhances the rate of phosphorylation-mediated glucose capture (Miyamoto et al. 2008). The pivotal role of GLUT1 and HK2 in mediating the cell's ability to access glucose is shown by the discovery that cellular bioenergetics and survival in the absence of growth factors can be restored by merely expressing a combination of recombinant GLUT1 and HK2 (Rathmell et al. 2003).

Activating mutations in the small GTPase KRAS also facilitate autonomous glucose uptake by up-regulating GLUT1 and HK2 at the transcriptional level (Ying et al. 2012). Amplification of another key oncogene, c-myc, also facilitates the uptake of glucose by simultaneously transactivating GLUT1, while also repressing the expression of TXNIP (Osthus et al. 2000; Shen et al. 2015).

Besides soluble growth factor deprivation, detachment of epithelial cells from the extracellular matrix also compromises glucose uptake, cellular mitochondrial potential, and ATP generation, all of which can be restored via ectopic expression of constitutively active Akt or PI3K alleles, or the HER2/erbb2 oncogene (Schafer et al. 2009). Collectively, these studies indicate

Cite this article as *Cold Spring Harb Perspect Med* doi: 10.1101/cshperspect.a041531

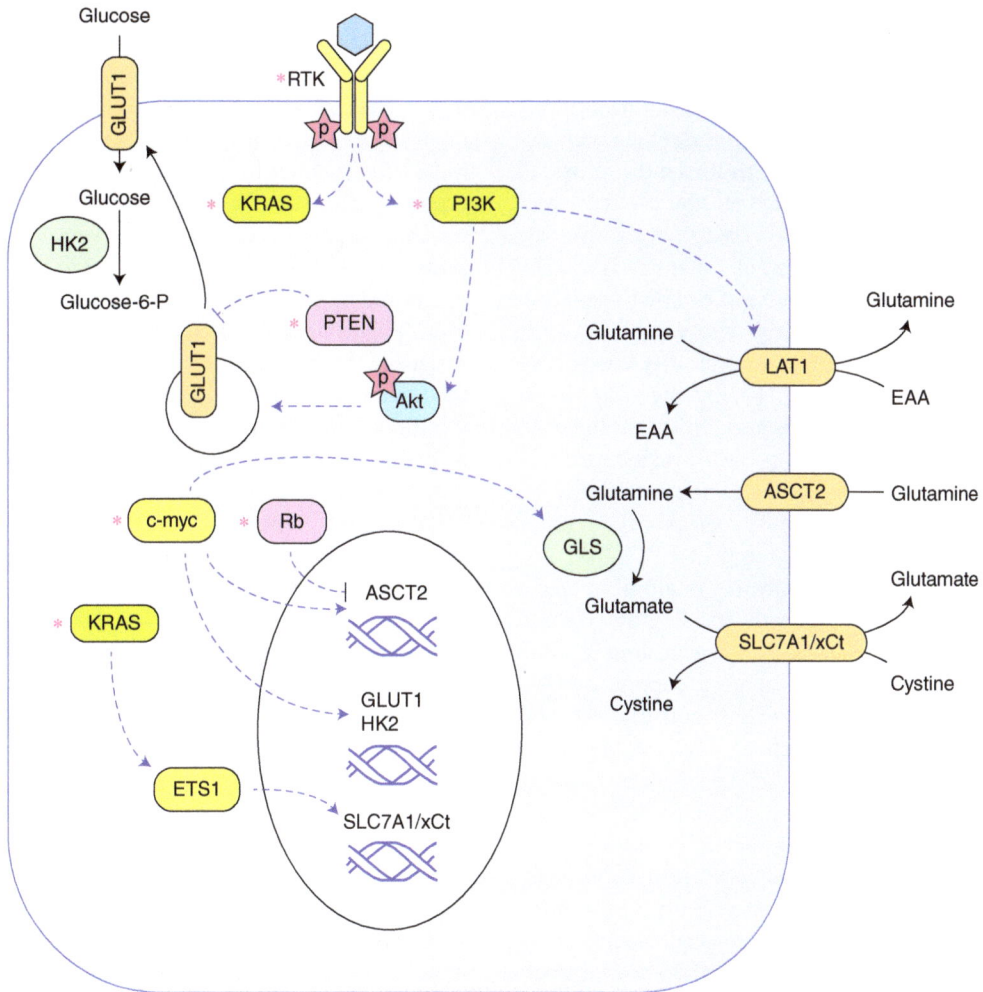

Figure 2. Growth signal–associated regulation of nutrient uptake. Remodeling of nutrient uptake by the major progrowth signaling effectors. (GLUT1) Glucose transporter 1, (RTK) receptor tyrosine kinase, (HK2) hexokinase 2, (GLS) glutaminase. Asterisks indicate genes that are frequently altered in cancer.

that the flow of glucose into the cell is not a passive process to merely replenish what has already been consumed. On the contrary, it exists under direct and immediate control of a set of paracrine signals delivered to cells via growth factors and substratum attachments.

Growth and proliferation of cells also requires a supply of amino acids, the uptake of which is similarly controlled by progrowth signals. Thus, aberrant activation of PI3K and Akt, as well as loss of PTEN all up-regulate the expression of the components of system L/LAT1, a plasma membrane–localized transporter in charge

of importing most essential amino acids into the cell (Edinger and Thompson 2002; Palm et al. 2017). Furthermore, the uptake of cysteine (in its oxidized dimeric form, cystine) is facilitated by the transporter xCt, the plasma membrane localization of which can be promoted by activating mutations of the RTK EGFR (Tsuchihashi et al. 2016). KRAS-driven activation of the ETS1 transcription factor also promotes xCt expression on the transcriptional level (Fig. 2; Lim et al. 2019).

While some amino acids are primarily used in protein synthesis, others fulfill additional pro-anabolic roles in a proliferating cell. Thus, a non-essential amino acid glutamine serves as an obligate donor of reduced nitrogen for the synthesis of purine and pyrimidine nucleotides, hexosamine units, and several nonessential amino acids—especially those insufficiently provided through circulation, such as aspartate and asparagine (Zhang et al. 2017). Further, the five-carbon molecular skeleton of glutamine is used by cells as a preferred source of carbon to replenish the pools of the tricarboxylic acid (TCA) cycle intermediates in a process of anaplerosis (DeBerardinis et al. 2007). Finally, the ability to accumulate glutamine is also critical for the cell's import of essential amino acids via the system L/LAT1 transporter, as their entry into the cell is coupled to glutamine export (Nicklin et al. 2009).

The cellular capacity for glutamine uptake is governed by progrowth transcription factors *c-myc* and E2F3. Thus, oncogenic amplification of *c-myc* gene and loss of tumor suppressor Rb (a negative regulator of E2F3) constitutively upregulates transcription of a major glutamine transporter ASCT2/SLC1A5 (Wise et al. 2008; Reynolds et al. 2014). In summary, multiple signaling hubs work together to ensure the cell's access to an array of necessary nutrients needed for proliferation, and this dependency becomes subverted by cancer cells through acquisition of oncogenic alterations and loss of tumor suppressors.

CENTRAL CARBON METABOLISM RISES TO THE TASK

Non-proliferative cells are primarily concerned with maintaining their ATP generation; thus, the predominant fate of glucose in such cells is its stepwise oxidation in a series of biochemical reactions of central carbon metabolism. Glucose catabolism is composed of two parts: cytosol-localized glycolysis and mitochondria-localized TCA. Oxidation of glucose-derived carbon in these reactions yields a crop of electrons, which are then loaded onto specialized electron carrier molecules, nicotinamide adenine dinucleotide (NAD^+) and flavin adenine dinucleotide (FAD), to generate NADH and $FADH_2$. The electrons

are fed into the mitochondria-localized electron transport chain (ETC), restoring the carriers back to NAD^+ and FAD. The pumping of H^+ into the intermembrane space and the movement of the electrons through the sequence of the ETC complexes to the terminal electron acceptor O_2 produces the inner membrane's electrostatic potential, which, in turn, powers ATP synthesis. The total energy yield from oxidizing one molecule of glucose to CO_2 is equivalent to 36 ATP molecules—two from the electrons harvested during the glycolysis stage and 34 from the those harvested in the TCA cycle.

In contrast, the metabolic needs of a cell committed to proliferation change dramatically due to a steep rise in demand for building blocks to generate new biomass (Vander Heiden et al. 2009; Lunt and Vander Heiden 2011; Chandel 2021). To fulfill the demand for building blocks required for proliferation, the same progrowth signals that facilitate nutrient uptake also orchestrate expansion and remodeling of the entire central carbon metabolism toward serving this monumental task. The nature of this realignment is tripartite: (1) expansion of the flow of glucose-derived carbon through glycolysis, (2) establishment of a number of off-ramps in which select glycolytic and TCA cycle intermediates can leave central carbon metabolism to be used as building blocks for anabolic reactions, and (3) increase the availability of the NADPH, a donor of reducing equivalents for several pivotal anabolic processes—including synthesis of fatty acids, cholesterol, deoxyribonucleotides, and proline.

At the transcriptional level, expansion of glucose-derived carbon flux through glycolysis is orchestrated by *c-myc*, which promotes expression of virtually every glycolytic enzyme (Dang et al. 2006). KRAS activation can further enhance the expression of HK2 and phophofructokinase-1 (PFK1) (Ying et al. 2012). In addition, PI3K/Akt signaling potentiates the activity of PFK1 by phosphorylating and activating PFKFB2 (Novellasdemunt et al. 2013), an enzyme in charge of producing fructose-2,6-bisphosphate, which acts as an allosteric activator of PFK1. Furthermore, PI3K-driven cytoskeletal remodeling helps liberate glycolytic enzyme aldolase, facili-

 Cite this article as *Cold Spring Harb Perspect Med* doi: 10.1101/cshperspect.a041531

tating its activation (Hu et al. 2016). Finally, loss of tumor suppressor p53 expands the glycolytic flow by down-regulating the Tp53-induced glycolysis and apoptosis regulator (TIGAR), which acts by lowering fructose-2,6-bisphosphate levels, causing PFK1 inhibition (Fig. 3; Bensaad et al. 2006).

Establishment of off-ramps that shunt glucose carbons into branching pathways that sustain biosynthesis is also coordinated by growth-associated signals (Fig. 3). For instance, the entry of glucose-6-phosphate into the pentose phosphate pathway, where it can be oxidized to generate NADPH as well as fuel the production of ribose-5-phosphate

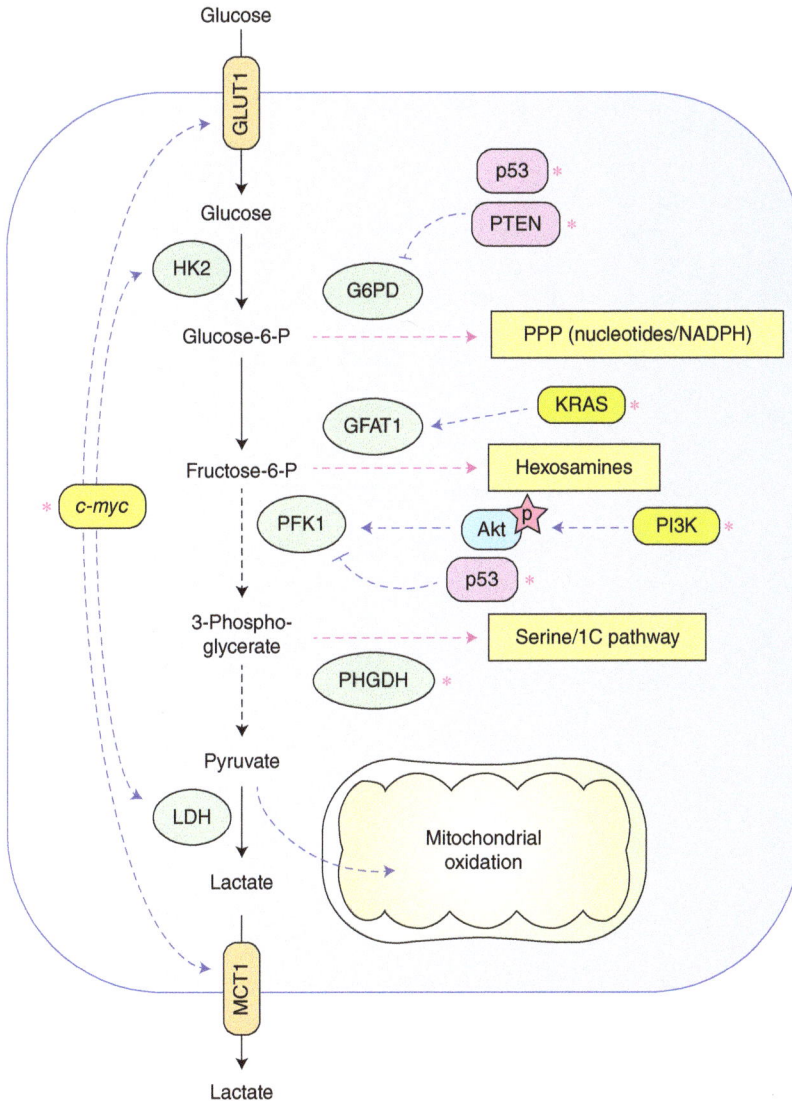

Figure 3. Growth signal–associated remodeling of glycolysis. Remodeling of the glycolytic pathway by the major progrowth signaling effectors. (G6PD) Glucose-6-phosphate dehydrogenase, (GFAT1) glutamine-fructose-6-phosphate transaminase 1, (PFK1) phosphofructokinase 1, (PHGDH) phosphoglycerate dehydrogenase, (LDH) lactate dehydrogenase, (MCT1) monocarboxylate transporter 1, (PPP) pentose phosphate pathway, (1C pathway) one-carbon pathway. Asterisks indicate genes that are frequently altered in cancer.

to build new nucleotides, is controlled by the enzyme glucose-6-phosphate dehydrogenase (G6PD). While *G6PD* mRNA expression is promoted by PI3K signaling (Wagle et al. 1998), both p53 and PTEN tumor suppressors can directly bind G6PD, preventing its dimerization and activation (Jiang et al. 2011; Hong et al. 2014). One rung of the glycolysis ladder lower, fructose-6-phosphate serves as the proximal substrate for the hexosamine pathway, which produces UDP-GlcNAc to drive protein glycosylation. Expression of the gatekeeping enzyme in this pathway, glutamine-fructose-6-phosphate transaminase 1 (GFAT1) is positively regulated by KRAS-mediated signaling (Fig. 3; Ying et al. 2012).

The use of the three-carbon glycolytic intermediate 3-phosphoglycerate to fuel serine biosynthesis can be facilitated in select types of solid tumors directly via genomic amplification of the enzyme phosphoglycerate dehydrogenase (PHGDH) (Mullarky et al. 2011; Possemato et al. 2011). Expanding the access to serine not only helps fulfill the demands for protein synthesis but also fuels the expansive one-carbon metabolism network, in which the distal carbon of the serine molecule goes on to serve a wide range of metabolic roles. These include provisions of methyl groups for cellular methylation reactions in a form of *S*-adenosylmethionine (SAM), biosynthesis of nucleotides, and generation of NADPH from $NADP^+$ (Ducker and Rabinowitz 2017).

The TCA cycle, too, becomes reconfigured from being predominantly an electron-harvesting machine into a production line for diverse building blocks to build new biomass. Thus, TCA-derived citrate leaves the mitochondria to be cleaved in the cytosol by the enzyme ATP citrate lyase (ACLY) into oxaloacetate and acetyl-CoA (Bauer et al. 2005). The ACLY-catalyzed reaction is facilitated by Akt signaling—both via Akt directly phosphorylating the Ser455 residue of ACLY, as well as through Akt-mediated relief of GSK3β-mediated inhibitory phosphorylation (Hughes et al. 1992; Berwick et al. 2002). ACLY-driven production of cytosolic acetyl-CoA is a key limiting step for the synthesis of fatty acids and cholesterol, which are required by proliferating cells to build new membranes (Fig. 4).

Oxaloacetate transamination into aspartate is another key probiosynthetic function of the TCA cycle. Aspartate is not only used for protein synthesis but also to generate nucleotides and asparagine; interestingly, aspartate levels are among the lowest of all amino acids and most cells lack transporters that would allow them to import sufficient quantities of aspartate to maintain growth (Sullivan et al. 2018).

Given the sheer volume of the anabolic reactions that require reducing equivalents in a form of NADPH, the demand for NADPH rises steeply with proliferation. To help meet this demand, activated Akt directly phosphorylates and activates the NAD kinase 1 (NADK1), which converts NAD^+ into $NADP^+$, thereby expanding the pool of this important electron carrier (Hoxhaj et al. 2019). A mirror reaction, catalyzed by NADK2, increases the pool of NADPH in the mitochondrial compartment, where it serves to facilitate proline biosynthesis (Schwörer et al. 2020; Zhu et al. 2021). Working in tandem, NADK1 and NADK2 build up the total cellular NADPH capacity to meet the demands of proliferation (Fig. 4).

Despite the dramatic expansion of the glycolytic flux under direction of growth-associated signals, a relatively minor fraction of this extra glucose carbon ends up entering mitochondria for oxidation. Strikingly, the entry of pyruvate into mitochondria was shown to be not only dispensable, but, in fact, to restrain tumorigenesis in at least some cancer contexts. Indeed, genetic inactivation of mitochondrial pyruvate carrier (MPC1) in a mouse model of colorectal cancer model was found to facilitate tumor initiation and aggressiveness (Bensard et al. 2020).

Diversion of glucose-derived carbon away from mitochondria is also controlled by the pro-growth signals. Thus, both *c-myc* and mutant KRAS act by up-regulating the expression of the lactate dehydrogenase (LDH) enzyme as well as of the monocarboxylate transporter (MCT1) (Ying et al. 2012; Wahlström and Henriksson 2015). LDH can convert pyruvate to lactate in a reaction that also regenerates one NAD^+ equivalent from NADH. This reaction is followed by the expulsion of the resultant lactate out of the cell via the MCT1 transporter. Thus,

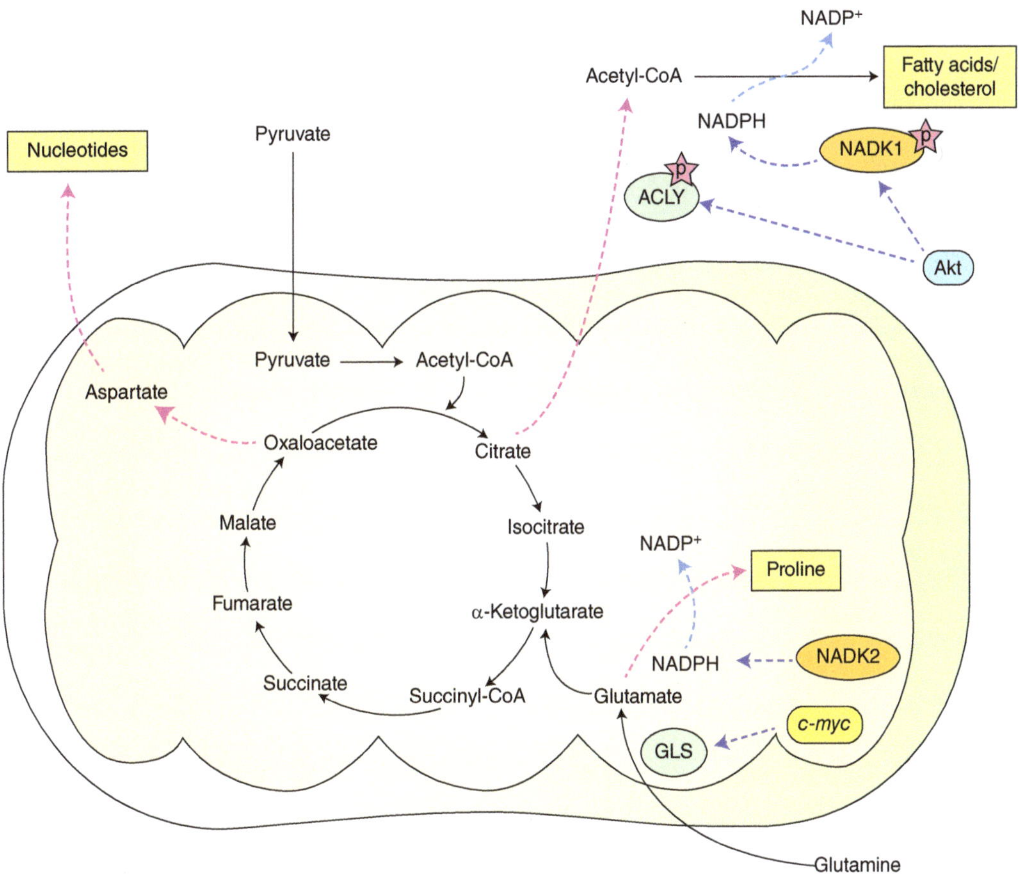

Figure 4. Growth signal–associated remodeling of the tricarboxylic acid (TCA) cycle to support the synthesis of macromolecular precursors. Facilitation of the TCA cycle outflows to support anabolic growth by the major progrowth signaling effectors. (ACLY) ATP-citrate lyase, (NADK1/2) nicotinamide adenine dinucleotide kinase 1/2.

oncogenic lesions harbored by cancer cells promote glycolysis through NAD^+ regeneration and the diversion of glucose carbon into lactate production regardless of the availability of oxygen. This phenomenon is termed aerobic glycolysis—or, in honor of its discoverer—the Warburg effect.

The logic behind this, at first glance, paradoxical way of handling glucose has been made clearer by the discoveries of the past two decades (Vander Heiden et al. 2009; DeBerardinis and Chandel 2020; Luengo et al. 2021). Thus, diverting glycolysis-derived pyruvate away from mitochondria and into lactate allows a cell to maintain high levels of glycolytic flux in support of the

various biosynthetic off-ramps, while safely disposing with the excess of glucose-derived carbon the cell has amassed following activation of progrowth signaling. Preventing mass entry of pyruvate into mitochondria for its oxidation allows a cell to (1) avoid overloading the ETC, which could otherwise lead to the spontaneous discharge of electrons into the surrounding aqueous milieu, generating reactive oxygen species, (2) prevent accumulation of ATP and citrate, which allosterically inhibit the glycolytic cascade at the level of PFK1, and (3) maintain the availability of NAD^+ carriers to help the TCA cycle moving forward and facilitate biosynthetic reactions that require NAD^+ as a cofactor.

Viewed in this way, the propensity of cancer cells for aerobic glycolysis (i.e., the Warburg effect) is not a cancer-specific metabolic aberration, but rather, an adaptation central to the establishment of the pro-proliferative state, shared by cancer and normal proliferating cells alike (Frauwirth et al. 2002; Fitzgerald et al. 2018). The crucial difference between the two contexts is that while in normal cells the commitment to proliferation and the attendant changes in carbon metabolism are limited in duration, metabolism of cancer cells becomes locked in this state by oncogene activation and/or tumor suppressor loss.

NITROGEN ON A BUDGET

Commitment to proliferation imposes high demand for sources of reduced nitrogen for building nucleotides, hexosamines, nonessential amino acids, polyamines, and other nitrogen-containing molecules. As discussed earlier, glutamine is a principal donor of reduced nitrogen in anabolic metabolism (Zhang et al. 2017). Like glucose, the anabolic use of glutamine is orchestrated by the same progrowth pathways that become commonly hijacked in cancer. For instance, KRAS-transformed cells markedly elevate the flux through the hexosamine biosynthesis pathway (Kim et al. 2020). In addition, the use of glutamine for nucleotide biosynthesis is coordinated by *c-myc*-driven up-regulation of numerous nucleotide biosynthetic enzymes, among which are thymidylate synthase (TS), inosine monophosphate dehydrogenase 2 (IMPDH2), and phosphoribosyl pyrophosphate synthetase 2 (PRPS2) (Mannava et al. 2008). Alongside *c-myc*, activation of mTORC1 downstream of PI3K/Akt signaling further facilitates production of both purines—via transcriptional up-regulation of ATF4—and pyrimidines —via the activating phosphorylation of the multienzyme complex CAD (Ben-Sahra et al. 2013, 2016). The latter is also subject to positive regulation via Erk-mediated phosphorylation (Graves et al. 2000).

The five-carbon skeleton of the glutamine molecule plays a crucial role in central carbon metabolism. Specifically, glutamine is first deamidated by the mitochondria-localized enzyme

glutaminase (GLS) to produce glutamate, which is consequently deaminated into α-ketoglutarate. Consequently, glutamine-derived α-ketoglutarate helps replenish the stocks of TCA cycle intermediates, such that the outflows of the TCA carbon into anabolic processes such as lipid biosynthesis and generation of aspartate and asparagine can be sustained to promote cell growth and proliferation. Of note, the first step of glutaminolysis is also facilitated by *c-myc*, which acts by suppressing miR-23a/b expression, which, in turn, releases GLS transcript from the inhibitory action of miRNAs (Gao et al. 2009).

Other oncogenes can further elevate the cellular demand for glutamine. Thus, activating mutations in the catalytic subunit of PI3K promotes expression of glutamate-pyruvate transaminase 2 (GPT2), further enhancing α-ketoglutarate production (Hao et al. 2016). In addition, non-small-cell lung carcinoma–associated activating mutations in EGFR were found to promote the reductive flux of glutamine-derived carbon into citrate even in the presence of oxygen, which elevates the demand for glutamine even further (Chen et al. 2019). Finally, import of cystine through the xCt transporter depletes cellular glutamate, imposing yet more demand on the glutaminolysis flux, which further increases cellular glutamine usage (Romero et al. 2017).

The large demand of transformed cells for glutamine is underscored by the findings from metabolomic studies, which reveal that glutamine is profoundly depleted in tumors (Roberts et al. 1956; Márquez et al. 1989; Kamphorst et al. 2015; Pan et al. 2016). To counter the deficit of glutamine, cells have developed diverse ways to sense and respond to glutamine depletion. Thus, glutamine depletion prevents E3 ligase CRBN-mediated proteasomal degradation of the GLUL enzyme, leading to GLUL accumulation (Nguyen et al. 2016). Interestingly, while hyperactive *c-myc* increases the cellular demand for glutamine, it also balances these demands via transcriptionally up-regulating the enzyme glutamine synthetase (GLUL), which allows cells to produce glutamine from glutamate and ammonium de novo (Fig. 5; Bott et al. 2015).

Second, availability of glutamine is sensed by mTORC1 via a noncanonical, ARF1 GTPase-

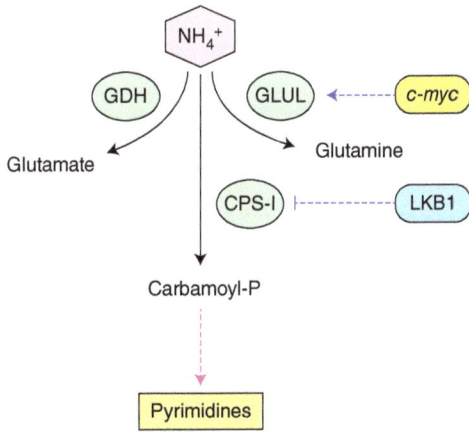

Figure 5. Cancer cells can reincorporate ammonium to support growth. Repurposing of inorganic ammonium (NH_4^+) for biosynthesis in cancer cells. (GDH) Glutamate dehydrogenase, (CPS-I) carbamoyl phosphate synthetase I, (GLUL) glutamate-ammonia ligase (glutamine synthetase).

mediated mechanism, which allows a cell to adjust its translation rate upon encountering glutamine deficit (Jewell et al. 2015; Meng et al. 2020). Third, glutamine deficit leads to depletion of glutamine-loaded tRNAs, which selectively compromise translation of proteins that contain polyglutamine (polyQ) tracts, causing their mistranslation via translational frameshifting. Of note, polyQ tracts are frequently found in proteins involved in transcription, which may help link the cell's transcriptional output directly to the nutrient status of a cell (Pavlova et al. 2020).

An additional consequence of the high flux through the GLS enzyme in proliferating cells is the accumulation of ammonium (NH_4^+). Although originally regarded as merely metabolic waste, ammonium can play an important role in allowing oncogene-transformed cells to supplement their limited pools of nutrients. First, ammonium accumulation facilitates autophagy, allowing cells to digest intracellular proteins and organelles as a stop-gap measure in critically low nutrient conditions (Eng et al. 2010; Cheong et al. 2011). In addition, high concentrations of ammonium detected in tumors allow regenerating glutamate via direct amination of the TCA cycle–derived α-ketoglutarate (Spinelli et al.

2017). Finally, loss of the tumor suppressor LKB1 allows lung cancer cells to use NH_4^+ as a substrate for pyrimidine synthesis by switching from glutamine-utilizing enzyme carbamoyl phosphate synthetase II (CPS-II) to the ammonium-utilizing isoform, CPS-I, which is normally only expressed in liver (Kim et al. 2017). The switch to CPS-I allows cells to fuel pyrimidine synthesis with ammonium, while reserving the limited glutamine for those biosynthetic reactions in which it cannot be substituted (Fig. 5).

While glutamine can be limiting in many tumor contexts, the interstitial fluid of select tumor types—for instance, $KRas^{G12D}$; $p53^{fl/fl}$; *Pdx1-Cre*-driven murine pancreatic tumors—has been reported to be deficient in arginine (Sullivan et al. 2019). Arginine deficiency may arise from the combination of tumor-residing myeloid cell metabolism as well as consumption of arginine by cancer cells themselves (Apiz Saab et al. 2023). The need for arginine in proliferating cells is not limited to protein synthesis; rather, arginine also fuels production of polycationic molecules called polyamines. Abundant in proliferating cells, polyamines avidly bind to nucleic acids owing to their positive electrostatic charge. Polyamines regulate DNA replication, gene transcription, and translation through not yet fully understood mechanisms (Gallo et al. 1986; Miller-Fleming et al. 2015). In a manner analogous to other proliferation-associated anabolic processes, production of polyamines is directly coordinated by oncogenes: thus, the initiating enzyme in polyamine biosynthesis, ornithine decarboxylase (ODC), is up-regulated by *c-myc* at the transcriptional level, while its translation is facilitated by RAS/ERK/eIF4E signaling cascade (Bello-Fernandez et al. 1993; Graff et al. 1997).

Taken together, oncogene-associated signaling facilitates uptake and utilization of nitrogen sources in numerous biosynthetic processes, which can eventually lead to the depletion of high-demand substrates in established tumors. Cancer cells meet this challenge by rewiring their metabolic pathways to facilitate de novo synthesis and frugal use of nitrogen sources available to them, thereby maintaining cell accumulation even when preferred sources of reduced nitrogen are limiting.

DINNER OF OPPORTUNISTS

Transformed cells eventually outgrow the nutrient supplies around them, leading to the depletion of high-demand nutrients and emergence of nutrient gradients within established tumors

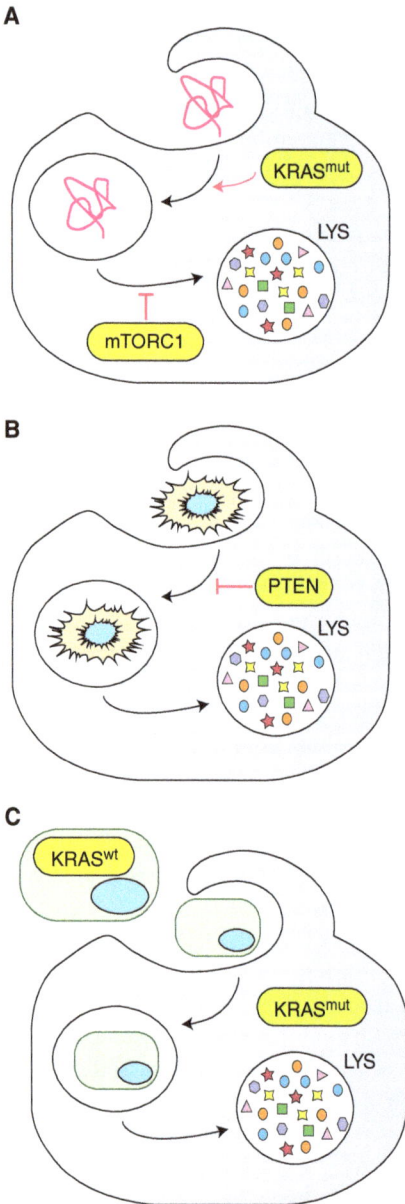

Figure 6. Opportunistic nutrient acquisition strategies in cancer cells. Capture and lysosome-mediated degradation of (*A*) extracellular proteins, (*B*) dead cells, and (*C*) living cells. (LYS) Lysosome.

(Kamphorst et al. 2015; Pan et al. 2016). Autophagy can provide a starved cell with a source of bioenergetic substrates to sustain the energy charge, as well as help maintain pools of TCA cycle metabolites and nucleotides (Guo et al. 2011, 2016; Yang et al. 2011). However, autophagy cannot yield a net positive flux of nutrients needed to build new biomass. To solve this problem, some oncogenes allow cells to engage in opportunistic modes of nutrient acquisition, which involves nonspecific engulfment and lysosome-based digestion of extracellular proteins and even entire cells as a source of low-molecular weight nutrients (Palm and Thompson 2017; Finicle et al. 2018).

Thus, KRAS oncogene can promote the nonspecific, fluid-phase uptake, termed macropinocytosis, to supplement the dwindling stores of amino acids via digesting captured proteins as well as scavenging unsaturated fatty acids from extracellular lysophospholipids (Commisso et al. 2013; Kamphorst et al. 2013). Notably, lysosome-based degradation of captured proteins is inhibited by active mTORC1, the principal sensor of free amino acid supply in the cell (Fig. 6A; Palm et al. 2015; Nofal et al. 2017). In this way, mTORC1 helps cells to optimize their mode of amino acid acquisition to the nutrient status of the surrounding microenvironment. Furthermore, loss of PTEN can also unlock the cell's ability to obtain missing nutrients from captured proteins and even entire dead cells (Fig. 6B; Kim et al. 2018). Even live cells can be engulfed and utilized as a nutrient source by cancer cells via the process of entosis (Hamann et al. 2017). Of note, altered cytoskeletal dynamics of KRAS-transformed cells increase their entotic capacity, making KRAS-transformed cells more likely to capture and digest their nontransformed neighbors than to be consumed as food themselves (Fig. 6C; Sun et al. 2014).

CONCLUDING REMARKS

For many years, anabolic metabolism of a proliferating cell has been viewed as a passive consequence of the progrowth state, in which biosynthetic enzymes draw the necessary substrates from the existing metabolite pools, while the latter become replenished in a homeostatic manner. However, the studies of the past two decades have revealed that growth-associated signals act in concert to promptly remodel and expand the metabolic repertoire of the cell so that it can fulfill the task of proliferation through the enhanced expression and activity of key metabolic enzymes and nutrient transporters. Acquisition of oncogenic lesions and loss of tumor suppressors lock the transformed cell in a progrowth metabolic state in perpetuity, enabling improper accumulation of cancer cells within the target tissue and eventually beyond its confines.

COMPETING INTEREST STATEMENT

C.B.T. is a founder of Agios Pharmaceuticals and is on the Board of Directors of Regeneron and Charles River Laboratories.

REFERENCES

Aaronson SA. 1991. Growth factors and cancer. *Science* **254:** 1146–1153. doi:10.1126/science.1659742

Ahmad R, Dalziel JE. 2020. G protein-coupled receptors in taste physiology and pharmacology. *Front Pharmacol* **11:** 587664. doi:10.3389/fphar.2020.587664

Apiz Saab JJ, Dzierozynski LN, Jonker PB, AminiTabrizi R, Shah H, Menjivar RE, Scott AJ, Nwosu ZC, Zhu Z, Chen RN, et al. 2023. Pancreatic tumors exhibit myeloid-driven amino acid stress and upregulate arginine biosynthesis. *eLife* **12:** e81289. doi:10.7554/eLife.81289

Bauer DE, Hatzivassiliou G, Zhao F, Andreadis C, Thompson CB. 2005. ATP citrate lyase is an important component of cell growth and transformation. *Oncogene* **24:** 6314–6322. doi:10.1038/sj.onc.1208773

Bello-Fernandez C, Packham G, Cleveland JL. 1993. The ornithine decarboxylase gene is a transcriptional target of c-Myc. *Proc Natl Acad Sci* **90:** 7804–7808. doi:10.1073/pnas.90.16.7804

Ben-Haim S, Ell P. 2009. ^{18}F-FDG PET and PET/CT in the evaluation of cancer treatment response. *J Nucl Med* **50:** 88–99. doi:10.2967/jnumed.108.054205

Bensaad K, Tsuruta A, Selak MA, Vidal MN, Nakano K, Bartrons R, Gottlieb E, Vousden KH. 2006. TIGAR, a p53-inducible regulator of glycolysis and apoptosis. *Cell* **126:** 107–120. doi:10.1016/j.cell.2006.05.036

Ben-Sahra I, Howell JJ, Asara JM, Manning BD. 2013. Stimulation of de novo pyrimidine synthesis by growth signaling through mTOR and S6K1. *Science* **339:** 1323–1328. doi:10.1126/science.1228792

Ben-Sahra I, Hoxhaj G, Ricoult SJH, Asara JM, Manning BD. 2016. mTORC1 induces purine synthesis through control of the mitochondrial tetrahydrofolate cycle. *Science* **351:** 728–733. doi:10.1126/science.aad0489

Bensard CL, Wisidagama DR, Olson KA, Berg JA, Krah NM, Schell JC, Nowinski SM, Fogarty S, Bott AJ, Wei P, et al. 2020. Regulation of tumor initiation by the mitochondrial pyruvate carrier. *Cell Metab* **31:** 284–300.e7. doi:10.1016/j.cmet.2019.11.002

Berwick DC, Hers I, Heesom KJ, Moule SK, Tavaré JM. 2002. The identification of ATP-citrate lyase as a protein kinase B (Akt) substrate in primary adipocytes. *J Biol Chem* **277:** 33895–33900. doi:10.1074/jbc.M204681200

Bott AJ, Peng IC, Fan Y, Faubert B, Zhao L, Li J, Neidler S, Sun Y, Jaber N, Krokowski D, et al. 2015. Oncogenic Myc induces expression of glutamine synthetase through promoter demethylation. *Cell Metab* **22:** 1068–1077. doi:10.1016/j.cmet.2015.09.025

Cavalli LR, Varella-Garcia M, Liang BC. 1997. Diminished tumorigenic phenotype after depletion of mitochondrial DNA. *Cell Growth Differ* **8:** 1189–1198.

Chandel NS. 2021. Metabolism of proliferating cells. *Cold Spring Harb Perspect Biol* **13:** a040618. doi:10.1101/cshperspect.a040618

Chen PH, Cai L, Huffman K, Yang C, Kim J, Faubert B, Boroughs L, Ko B, Sudderth J, McMillan EA, et al. 2019. Metabolic diversity in human non-small cell lung cancer cells. *Mol Cell* **76:** 838–851.e5. doi:10.1016/j.molcel.2019.08.028

Cheong H, Lindsten T, Wu J, Lu C, Thompson CB. 2011. Ammonia-induced autophagy is independent of ULK1/ULK2 kinases. *Proc Natl Acad Sci* **108:** 11121–11126. doi:10.1073/pnas.1107969108

Commisso C, Davidson SM, Soydaner-Azeloglu RG, Parker SJ, Kamphorst JJ, Hackett S, Grabocka E, Nofal M, Drebin JA, Thompson CB, et al. 2013. Macropinocytosis of protein is an amino acid supply route in Ras-transformed cells. *Nature* **497:** 633–637. doi:10.1038/nature12138

Dang CV, O'Donnell KA, Zeller KI, Nguyen T, Osthus RC, Li F. 2006. The c-Myc target gene network. *Semin Cancer Biol* **16:** 253–264. doi:10.1016/j.semcancer.2006.07.014

DeBerardinis RJ, Chandel NS. 2016. Fundamentals of cancer metabolism. *Sci Adv* **2:** e1600200. doi:10.1126/sciadv.1600200

DeBerardinis RJ, Chandel NS. 2020. We need to talk about the Warburg effect. *Nat Metab* **2:** 127–129. doi:10.1038/s42255-020-0172-2

DeBerardinis RJ, Mancuso A, Daikhin E, Nissim I, Yudkoff M, Wehrli S, Thompson CB. 2007. Beyond aerobic glycolysis: transformed cells can engage in glutamine metabolism that exceeds the requirement for protein and nucleotide synthesis. *Proc Natl Acad Sci* **104:** 19345–19350. doi:10.1073/pnas.0709747104

Ding L, Bailey MH, Porta-Pardo E, Thorsson V, Colaprico A, Bertrand D, Gibbs DL, Weerasinghe A, Huang KL, Tokheim C, et al. 2018. Perspective on oncogenic processes at the end of the beginning of cancer genomics. *Cell* **173:** 305–320.e10. doi:10.1016/j.cell.2018.03.033

Ducker GS, Rabinowitz JD. 2017. One-carbon metabolism in health and disease. *Cell Metab* **25:** 27–42. doi:10.1016/j.cmet.2016.08.009

Edinger AL, Thompson CB. 2002. Akt maintains cell size and survival by increasing mTOR-dependent nutrient uptake. *Mol Biol Cell* **13:** 2276–2288. doi:10.1091/mbc.01-12-0584

Eng CH, Yu K, Lucas J, White E, Abraham RT. 2010. Ammonia derived from glutaminolysis is a diffusible regulator of autophagy. *Sci Signal* **3:** ra31. doi:10.1126/scisignal.2000911

Finicle BT, Jayashankar V, Edinger AL. 2018. Nutrient scavenging in cancer. *Nat Rev Cancer* **18:** 619–633. doi:10.1038/s41568-018-0048-x

Fitzgerald G, Soro-Arnaiz I, De Bock K. 2018. The Warburg effect in endothelial cells and its potential as an anti-angiogenic target in cancer. *Front Cell Dev Biol* **6:** 100. doi:10.3389/fcell.2018.00100

Frauwirth KA, Riley JL, Harris MH, Parry RV, Rathmell JC, Plas DR, Elstrom RL, June CH, Thompson CB. 2002. The CD28 signaling pathway regulates glucose metabolism. *Immunity* **16:** 769–777. doi:10.1016/S1074-7613(02)00323-0

Gallo CJ, Koza RA, Herbst EJ. 1986. Polyamines and HeLa-cell DNA replication. *Biochem J* **238:** 37–42. doi:10.1042/bj2380037

Gao P, Tchernyshyov I, Chang TC, Lee YS, Kita K, Ochi T, Zeller KI, De Marzo AM, Van Eyk JE, Mendell JT, et al. 2009. c-Myc suppression of miR-23a/b enhances mitochondrial glutaminase expression and glutamine metabolism. *Nature* **458:** 762–765. doi:10.1038/nature07823

Georis I, Tate JJ, Cooper TG, Dubois E. 2011. Nitrogen-responsive regulation of GATA protein family activators Gln3 and Gat1 occurs by two distinct pathways, one inhibited by rapamycin and the other by methionine sulfoximine. *J Biol Chem* **286:** 44897–44912. doi:10.1074/jbc.M111.290577

Giancotti FG, Ruoslahti E. 1999. Integrin signaling. *Science* **285:** 1028–1032. doi:10.1126/science.285.5430.1028

Giots F, Donaton MC, Thevelein JM. 2003. Inorganic phosphate is sensed by specific phosphate carriers and acts in concert with glucose as a nutrient signal for activation of the protein kinase A pathway in the yeast *Saccharomyces cerevisiae*. *Mol Microbiol* **47:** 1163–1181. doi:10.1046/j.1365-2958.2003.03365.x

Graff JR, De Benedetti A, Olson JW, Tamez P, Casero RA Jr, Zimmer SG. 1997. Translation of ODC mRNA and polyamine transport are suppressed in *ras*-transformed CREF cells by depleting translation initiation factor 4E. *Biochem Biophys Res Commun* **240:** 15–20. doi:10.1006/bbrc.1997.7592

Graves LM, Guy HI, Kozlowski P, Huang M, Lazarowski E, Pope RM, Collins MA, Dahlstrand EN, Earp HS III, Evans DR. 2000. Regulation of carbamoyl phosphate synthetase by MAP kinase. *Nature* **403:** 328–332. doi:10.1038/35002111

Guo JY, Chen HY, Mathew R, Fan J, Strohecker AM, Karsli-Uzunbas G, Kamphorst JJ, Chen G, Lemons JM, Karantza V, et al. 2011. Activated Ras requires autophagy to maintain oxidative metabolism and tumorigenesis. *Genes Dev* **25:** 460–470. doi:10.1101/gad.2016311

Guo JY, Teng X, Laddha SV, Ma S, Van Nostrand SC, Yang Y, Khor S, Chan CS, Rabinowitz JD, White E. 2016. Autophagy provides metabolic substrates to maintain energy charge and nucleotide pools in Ras-driven lung cancer cells. *Genes Dev* **30:** 1704–1717. doi:10.1101/gad.283416.116

Hamann JC, Surcel A, Chen R, Teragawa C, Albeck JG, Robinson DN, Overholtzer M. 2017. Entosis is induced by glucose starvation. *Cell Rep* **20:** 201–210. doi:10.1016/j.celrep.2017.06.037

Hanahan D, Weinberg RA. 2000. The hallmarks of cancer. *Cell* **100:** 57–70. doi:10.1016/S0092-8674(00)81683-9

Hao Y, Samuels Y, Li Q, Krokowski D, Guan BJ, Wang C, Jin Z, Dong B, Cao B, Feng X, et al. 2016. Oncogenic PIK3CA mutations reprogram glutamine metabolism in colorectal cancer. *Nat Commun* **7:** 11971. doi:10.1038/ncomms11971

Hong X, Song R, Song H, Zheng T, Wang J, Liang Y, Qi S, Lu Z, Song X, Jiang H, et al. 2014. PTEN antagonises Tcl1/hnRNPK-mediated G6PD pre-mRNA splicing which contributes to hepatocarcinogenesis. *Gut* **63:** 1635–1647. doi:10.1136/gutjnl-2013-305302

Hoxhaj G, Ben-Sahra I, Lockwood SE, Timson RC, Byles V, Henning GT, Gao P, Selfors LM, Asara JM, Manning BD. 2019. Direct stimulation of NADP$^+$ synthesis through Akt-mediated phosphorylation of NAD kinase. *Science* **363:** 1088–1092. doi:10.1126/science.aau3903

Hu H, Juvekar A, Lyssiotis CA, Lien EC, Albeck JG, Oh D, Varma G, Hung YP, Ullas S, Lauring J, et al. 2016. Phosphoinositide 3-kinase regulates glycolysis through mobilization of aldolase from the actin cytoskeleton. *Cell* **164:** 433–446. doi:10.1016/j.cell.2015.12.042

Hughes K, Ramakrishna S, Benjamin WB, Woodgett JR. 1992. Identification of multifunctional ATP-citrate lyase kinase as the α-isoform of glycogen synthase kinase-3. *Biochem J* **288:** 309–314. doi:10.1042/bj2880309

Hunter T. 1997. Oncoprotein networks. *Cell* **88:** 333–346. doi:10.1016/S0092-8674(00)81872-3

ICGC/TCGA Pan-Cancer Analysis of Whole Genomes Consortium. 2020. Pan-cancer analysis of whole genomes. *Nature* **578:** 82–93. doi:10.1038/s41586-020-1969-6

Jewell JL, Kim YC, Russell RC, Yu FX, Park HW, Plouffe SW, Tagliabracci VS, Guan KL. 2015. Metabolism. Differential regulation of mTORC1 by leucine and glutamine. *Science* **347:** 194–198. doi:10.1126/science.1259472

Jiang P, Du W, Wang X, Mancuso A, Gao X, Wu M, Yang X. 2011. P53 regulates biosynthesis through direct inactivation of glucose-6-phosphate dehydrogenase. *Nat Cell Biol* **13:** 310–316. doi:10.1038/ncb2172

Kamphorst JJ, Cross JR, Fan J, de Stanchina E, Mathew R, White EP, Thompson CB, Rabinowitz JD. 2013. Hypoxic and Ras-transformed cells support growth by scavenging unsaturated fatty acids from lysophospholipids. *Proc Natl Acad Sci* **110:** 8882–8887. doi:10.1073/pnas.1307237110

Kamphorst JJ, Nofal M, Commisso C, Hackett SR, Lu W, Grabocka E, Vander Heiden MG, Miller G, Drebin JA, Bar-Sagi D, et al. 2015. Human pancreatic cancer tumors are nutrient poor and tumor cells actively scavenge extracellular protein. *Cancer Res* **75:** 544–553. doi:10.1158/0008-5472.CAN-14-2211

Kim J, Hu Z, Cai L, Li K, Choi E, Faubert B, Bezwada D, Rodriguez-Canales J, Villalobos P, Lin YF, et al. 2017. CPS1 maintains pyrimidine pools and DNA synthesis in KRAS/LKB1-mutant lung cancer cells. *Nature* **546:** 168–172. doi:10.1038/nature22359

Kim SM, Nguyen TT, Ravi A, Kubiniok P, Finicle BT, Jayashankar V, Malacrida L, Hou J, Robertson J, Gao D, et al. 2018. PTEN deficiency and AMPK activation promote nutrient scavenging and anabolism in prostate cancer

Cite this article as *Cold Spring Harb Perspect Med* doi: 10.1101/cshperspect.a041531

cells. *Cancer Discov* **8**: 866–883. doi:10.1158/2159-8290 .CD-17-1215

Kim J, Lee HM, Cai F, Ko B, Yang C, Lieu EL, Muhammad N, Rhyne S, Li K, Haloul M, et al. 2020. The hexosamine biosynthesis pathway is a targetable liability in KRAS/ LKB1 mutant lung cancer. *Nat Metab* **2**: 1401–1412. doi:10.1038/s42255-020-00316-0

Kratz A, Lewandrowski KB. 1998. Case records of the Massachusetts General Hospital. Weekly clinicopathological exercises. Normal reference laboratory values. *N Engl J Med* **339**: 1063–1072. doi:10.1056/NEJM19981008 3391508

Lim JKM, Delaidelli A, Minaker SW, Zhang HF, Colovic M, Yang H, Negri GL, von Karstedt S, Lockwood WW, Schaffer P, et al. 2019. Cystine/glutamate antiporter xCT (SLC7A11) facilitates oncogenic RAS transformation by preserving intracellular redox balance. *Proc Natl Acad Sci* **116**: 9433–9442. doi:10.1073/pnas.1821323116

Lindsten T, Golden JA, Zong WX, Minarcik J, Harris MH, Thompson CB. 2003. The proapoptotic activities of Bax and Bak limit the size of the neural stem cell pool. *J Neurosci* **23**: 11112–11119. doi:10.1523/JNEUROSCI.23-35-11112.2003

Luengo A, Li Z, Gui DY, Sullivan LB, Zagorulya M, Do BT, Ferreira R, Naamati A, Ali A, Lewis CA, et al. 2021. Increased demand for NAD$^+$ relative to ATP drives aerobic glycolysis. *Mol Cell* **81**: 691–707.e6. doi:10.1016/j.molcel .2020.12.012

Lunt SY, Vander Heiden MG. 2011. Aerobic glycolysis: meeting the metabolic requirements of cell proliferation. *Annu Rev Cell Dev Biol* **27**: 441–464. doi:10.1146/annurev-cell bio-092910-154237

Mannava S, Grachtchouk V, Wheeler LJ, Im M, Zhuang D, Slavina EG, Mathews CK, Shewach DS, Nikiforov MA. 2008. Direct role of nucleotide metabolism in C-MYC-dependent proliferation of melanoma cells. *Cell Cycle* **7**: 2392–2400. doi:10.4161/cc.6390

Márquez J, Sánchez-Jiménez F, Medina MA, Quesada AR, Nunez de Castro I. 1989. Nitrogen metabolism in tumor bearing mice. *Arch Biochem Biophys* **268**: 667–675. doi:10 .1016/0003-9861(89)90335-4

Martínez-Reyes I, Cardona LR, Kong H, Vasan K, McElroy GS, Werner M, Kihshen H, Reczek CR, Weinberg SE, Gao P, et al. 2020. Mitochondrial ubiquinol oxidation is necessary for tumour growth. *Nature* **585**: 288–292. doi:10 .1038/s41586-020-2475-6

Meng D, Yang Q, Wang H, Melick CH, Navlani R, Frank AR, Jewell JL. 2020. Glutamine and asparagine activate mTORC1 independently of Rag GTPases. *J Biol Chem* **295**: 2890–2899. doi:10.1074/jbc.AC119.011578

Miller-Fleming L, Olin-Sandoval V, Campbell K, Ralser M. 2015. Remaining mysteries of molecular biology: the role of polyamines in the cell. *J Mol Biol* **427**: 3389–3406. doi:10 .1016/j.jmb.2015.06.020

Miyamoto S, Murphy AN, Brown JH. 2008. Akt mediates mitochondrial protection in cardiomyocytes through phosphorylation of mitochondrial hexokinase-II. *Cell Death Differ* **15**: 521–529. doi:10.1038/sj.cdd.4402285

Mullarky E, Mattaini KR, Vander Heiden MG, Cantley LC, Locasale JW. 2011. *PHGDH* amplification and altered glucose metabolism in human melanoma. *Pigment Cell Mel-*

anoma Res **24**: 1112–1115. doi:10.1111/j.1755-148X.2011 .00919.x

Nguyen TV, Lee JE, Sweredoski MJ, Yang SJ, Jeon SJ, Harrison JS, Yim JH, Lee SG, Handa H, Kuhlman B, et al. 2016. Glutamine triggers acetylation-dependent degradation of glutamine synthetase via the thalidomide receptor cereblon. *Mol Cell* **61**: 809–820. doi:10.1016/j.molcel.2016.02 .032

Nicklin P, Bergman P, Zhang B, Triantafellow E, Wang H, Nyfeler B, Yang H, Hild M, Kung C, Wilson C, et al. 2009. Bidirectional transport of amino acids regulates mTOR and autophagy. *Cell* **136**: 521–534. doi:10.1016/j.cell .2008.11.044

Nofal M, Zhang K, Han S, Rabinowitz JD. 2017. mTOR inhibition restores amino acid balance in cells dependent on catabolism of extracellular protein. *Mol Cell* **67**: 936–946. e5. doi:10.1016/j.molcel.2017.08.011

Novellasdemunt L, Tato I, Navarro-Sabate A, Ruiz-Meana M, Mendez-Lucas A, Perales JC, Garcia-Dorado D, Ventura F, Bartrons R, Rosa JL. 2013. Akt-dependent activation of the heart 6-phosphofructo-2-kinase/fructose-2,6-bisphosphatase (PFKFB2) isoenzyme by amino acids. *J Biol Chem* **288**: 10640–10651. doi:10.1074/jbc.M113.455998

Osthus RC, Shim H, Kim S, Li Q, Reddy R, Mukherjee M, Xu Y, Wonsey D, Lee LA, Dang CV. 2000. Deregulation of glucose transporter 1 and glycolytic gene expression by c-Myc. *J Biol Chem* **275**: 21797–21800. doi:10.1074/jbc .C000023200

Palm W, Thompson CB. 2017. Nutrient acquisition strategies of mammalian cells. *Nature* **546**: 234–242. doi:10.1038/ nature22379

Palm W, Park Y, Wright K, Pavlova NN, Tuveson DA, Thompson CB. 2015. The utilization of extracellular proteins as nutrients is suppressed by mTORC1. *Cell* **162**: 259–270. doi:10.1016/j.cell.2015.06.017

Palm W, Araki J, King B, DeMatteo RG, Thompson CB. 2017. Critical role for PI3-kinase in regulating the use of proteins as an amino acid source. *Proc Natl Acad Sci* **114**: E8628–E8636. doi:10.1073/pnas.1712726114

Pan M, Reid MA, Lowman XH, Kulkarni RP, Tran TQ, Liu X, Yang Y, Hernandez-Davies JE, Rosales KK, Li H, et al. 2016. Regional glutamine deficiency in tumours promotes dedifferentiation through inhibition of histone demethylation. *Nat Cell Biol* **18**: 1090–1101. doi:10.1038/ncb3410

Pauly H, Rajewsky B. 1956. The effect of roentgen rays on tissue respiration. *Strahlentherapie* **99**: 383–386.

Pavlova NN, King B, Josselsohn RH, Violante S, Macera VL, Vardhana SA, Cross JR, Thompson CB. 2020. Translation in amino-acid-poor environments is limited by tRNA (Gln) charging. *eLife* **9**: e62307. doi:10.7554/eLife.62307

Possemato R, Marks KM, Shaul YD, Pacold ME, Kim D, Birsoy K, Sethumadhavan S, Woo HK, Jang HG, Jha AK, et al. 2011. Functional genomics reveal that the serine synthesis pathway is essential in breast cancer. *Nature* **476**: 346–350. doi:10.1038/nature10350

Rathmell JC, Vander Heiden MG, Harris MH, Frauwirth KA, Thompson CB. 2000. In the absence of extrinsic signals, nutrient utilization by lymphocytes is insufficient to maintain either cell size or viability. *Mol Cell* **6**: 683–692. doi:10 .1016/S1097-2765(00)00066-6

Rathmell JC, Fox CJ, Plas DR, Hammerman PS, Cinalli RM, Thompson CB. 2003. Akt-directed glucose metabolism can prevent Bax conformation change and promote growth factor-independent survival. *Mol Cell Biol* **23:** 7315–7328. doi:10.1128/MCB.23.20.7315-7328.2003

Reynolds MR, Lane AN, Robertson B, Kemp S, Liu Y, Hill BG, Dean DC, Clem BF. 2014. Control of glutamine metabolism by the tumor suppressor Rb. *Oncogene* **33:** 556–566. doi:10.1038/onc.2012.635

Roberts E, Simonsen DG, Tanaka KK, Tanaka T. 1956. Free amino acids in growing and regressing ascites cell tumors: host resistance and chemical agents. *Cancer Res* **16:** 970–978.

Romero R, Sayin VI, Davidson SM, Bauer MR, Singh SX, LeBoeuf SE, Karakousi TR, Ellis DC, Bhutkar A, Sánchez-Rivera FJ, et al. 2017. Keap1 loss promotes Kras-driven lung cancer and results in dependence on glutaminolysis. *Nat Med* **23:** 1362–1368. doi:10.1038/nm.4407

Schafer ZT, Grassian AR, Song L, Jiang Z, Gerhart-Hines Z, Irie HY, Gao S, Puigserver P, Brugge JS. 2009. Antioxidant and oncogene rescue of metabolic defects caused by loss of matrix attachment. *Nature* **461:** 109–113. doi:10.1038/nature08268

Schwörer S, Berisa M, Violante S, Qin W, Zhu J, Hendrickson RC, Cross JR, Thompson CB. 2020. Proline biosynthesis is a vent for TGFβ-induced mitochondrial redox stress. *EMBO J* **39:** e103334. doi:10.15252/embj.2019103334

Shen L, O'Shea JM, Kaadige MR, Cunha A, Wilde BR, Cohen AL, Welm AL, Ayer DE. 2015. Metabolic reprogramming in triple-negative breast cancer through Myc suppression of TXNIP. *Proc Natl Acad Sci* **112:** 5425–5430. doi:10.1073/pnas.1501555112

Sherr CJ. 2004. Principles of tumor suppression. *Cell* **116:** 235–246. doi:10.1016/S0092-8674(03)01075-4

Shinde SR, Maddika S. 2017. PTEN regulates glucose transporter recycling by impairing SNX27 retromer assembly. *Cell Rep* **21:** 1655–1666. doi:10.1016/j.celrep.2017.10.053

Spinelli JB, Yoon H, Ringel AE, Jeanfavre S, Clish CB, Haigis MC. 2017. Metabolic recycling of ammonia via glutamate dehydrogenase supports breast cancer biomass. *Science* **358:** 941–946. doi:10.1126/science.aam9305

Stehelin D, Varmus HE, Bishop JM, Vogt PK. 1976. DNA related to the transforming gene(s) of avian sarcoma viruses is present in normal avian DNA. *Nature* **260:** 170–173. doi:10.1038/260170a0

Sullivan LB, Luengo A, Danai LV, Bush LN, Diehl FF, Hosios AM, Lau AN, Elmiligy S, Malstrom S, Lewis CA, et al. 2018. Aspartate is an endogenous metabolic limitation for tumour growth. *Nat Cell Biol* **20:** 782–788. doi:10.1038/s41556-018-0125-0

Sullivan MR, Danai LV, Lewis CA, Chan SH, Gui DY, Kunchok T, Dennstedt EA, Vander Heiden MG, Muir A. 2019. Quantification of microenvironmental metabolites in murine cancers reveals determinants of tumor nutrient availability. *eLife* **8:** e44235. doi:10.7554/eLife.44235

Sun Q, Luo T, Ren Y, Florey O, Shirasawa S, Sasazuki T, Robinson DN, Overholtzer M. 2014. Competition between human cells by entosis. *Cell Res* **24:** 1299–1310. doi:10.1038/cr.2014.138

Thevelein JM, De Winde JH. 1999. Novel sensing mechanisms and targets for the cAMP-protein kinase A pathway in the yeast *Saccharomyces cerevisiae*. *Mol Microbiol* **33:** 904–918. doi:10.1046/j.1365-2958.1999.01538.x

Tsuchihashi K, Okazaki S, Ohmura M, Ishikawa M, Sampetrean O, Onishi N, Wakimoto H, Yoshikawa M, Seishima R, Iwasaki Y, et al. 2016. The EGF receptor promotes the malignant potential of glioma by regulating amino acid transport system xc(–). *Cancer Res* **76:** 2954–2963. doi:10.1158/0008-5472.CAN-15-2121

Vander Heiden MG, Cantley LC, Thompson CB. 2009. Understanding the Warburg effect: the metabolic requirements of cell proliferation. *Science* **324:** 1029–1033. doi:10.1126/science.1160809

Vennstrom B, Sheiness D, Zabielski J, Bishop JM. 1982. Isolation and characterization of c-myc, a cellular homolog of the oncogene (v-myc) of avian myelocytomatosis virus strain 29. *J Virol* **42:** 773–779. doi:10.1128/jvi.42.3.773-779.1982

Vogelstein B, Kinzler KW. 2004. Cancer genes and the pathways they control. *Nat Med* **10:** 789–799. doi:10.1038/nm1087

Vogelstein B, Papadopoulos N, Velculescu VE, Zhou S, Diaz LA Jr, Kinzler KW. 2013. Cancer genome landscapes. *Science* **339:** 1546–1558. doi:10.1126/science.1235122

Vogt PK. 2012. Retroviral oncogenes: a historical primer. *Nat Rev Cancer* **12:** 639–648. doi:10.1038/nrc3320

Wagle A, Jivraj S, Garlock GL, Stapleton SR. 1998. Insulin regulation of glucose-6-phosphate dehydrogenase gene expression is rapamycin-sensitive and requires phosphatidylinositol 3-kinase. *J Biol Chem* **273:** 14968–14974. doi:10.1074/jbc.273.24.14968

Wahlström T, Henriksson MA. 2015. Impact of MYC in regulation of tumor cell metabolism. *Biochim Biophys Acta* **1849:** 563–569. doi:10.1016/j.bbagrm.2014.07.004

Waldhart AN, Dykstra H, Peck AS, Boguslawski EA, Madaj ZB, Wen J, Veldkamp K, Hollowell M, Zheng B, Cantley LC, et al. 2017. Phosphorylation of TXNIP by AKT mediates acute influx of glucose in response to insulin. *Cell Rep* **19:** 2005–2013. doi:10.1016/j.celrep.2017.05.041

Warburg O. 1956. On respiratory impairment in cancer cells. *Science* **124:** 269–270. doi:10.1126/science.124.3215.269

Warburg O, Wind F, Negelein E. 1927. The metabolism of tumors in the body. *J Gen Physiol* **8:** 519–530. doi:10.1085/jgp.8.6.519

Ward PS, Thompson CB. 2012. Metabolic reprogramming: a cancer hallmark even Warburg did not anticipate. *Cancer Cell* **21:** 297–308. doi:10.1016/j.ccr.2012.02.014

Weinberg RA. 1994. Oncogenes and tumor suppressor genes. *CA Cancer J Clin* **44:** 160–170. doi:10.3322/canjclin.44.3.160

Weinberg F, Hamanaka R, Wheaton WW, Weinberg S, Joseph J, Lopez M, Kalyanaraman B, Mutlu GM, Budinger GR, Chandel NS. 2010. Mitochondrial metabolism and ROS generation are essential for Kras-mediated tumorigenicity. *Proc Natl Acad Sci* **107:** 8788–8793. doi:10.1073/pnas.1003428107

Wieman HL, Wofford JA, Rathmell JC. 2007. Cytokine stimulation promotes glucose uptake via phosphatidylinositol-3 kinase/Akt regulation of Glut1 activity and trafficking. *Mol Biol Cell* **18:** 1437–1446. doi:10.1091/mbc.e06-07-0593

Wise DR, DeBerardinis RJ, Mancuso A, Sayed N, Zhang XY, Pfeiffer HK, Nissim I, Daikhin E, Yudkoff M, McMahon SB, et al. 2008. Myc regulates a transcriptional program that stimulates mitochondrial glutaminolysis and leads to glutamine addiction. *Proc Natl Acad Sci* **105:** 18782–18787. doi:10.1073/pnas.0810199105

Yang S, Wang X, Contino G, Liesa M, Sahin E, Ying H, Bause A, Li Y, Stommel JM, Dell'antonio G, et al. 2011. Pancreatic cancers require autophagy for tumor growth. *Genes Dev* **25:** 717–729. doi:10.1101/gad.2016111

Ying H, Kimmelman AC, Lyssiotis CA, Hua S, Chu GC, Fletcher-Sananikone E, Locasale JW, Son J, Zhang H, Coloff JL, et al. 2012. Oncogenic Kras maintains pancreatic tumors through regulation of anabolic glucose metabolism. *Cell* **149:** 656–670. doi:10.1016/j.cell.2012.01.058

Yuan TL, Cantley LC. 2008. PI3K pathway alterations in cancer: variations on a theme. *Oncogene* **27:** 5497–5510. doi:10.1038/onc.2008.245

Zhang J, Pavlova NN, Thompson CB. 2017. Cancer cell metabolism: the essential role of the nonessential amino acid, glutamine. *EMBO J* **36:** 1302–1315. doi:10.15252/embj .201696151

Zhu J, Schwörer S, Berisa M, Kyung YJ, Ryu KW, Yi J, Jiang X, Cross JR, Thompson CB. 2021. Mitochondrial NADP(H) generation is essential for proline biosynthesis. *Science* **372:** 968–972. doi:10.1126/science .abd5491

Lessons Learned from Cancer Metabolism for Physiology and Disease

Sydney L. Campbell and Heather R. Christofk

Department of Biological Chemistry, University of California, Los Angeles, Los Angeles, California 90095, USA

Correspondence: hchristofk@mednet.ucla.edu

Tumor cells divide rapidly and dramatically alter their metabolism to meet biosynthetic and bioenergetic needs. Through studying the aberrant metabolism of cancer cells, other contexts in which metabolism drives cell state transitions become apparent. In this work, we will discuss how principles established by the field of cancer metabolism have led to discoveries in the contexts of physiology and tissue injury, mammalian embryonic development, and virus infection. We present specific examples of findings from each of these fields that have been shaped by the study of cancer metabolism. We also discuss the next important scientific questions facing these subject areas collectively. Altogether, these examples demonstrate that the study of "cancer metabolism" is indeed the study of cell metabolism in the context of a tumor, and undoubtedly discoveries from each of the fields discussed here will continue to build on each other in the future.

As described elsewhere, the observations documented by Otto Warburg in the 1920s that cancer cells up-regulate glycolysis in the presence of oxygen laid the foundation for the field of cancer metabolism as we know it today. Although it is now clear that Warburg's conclusions painted an oversimplified picture of tumor cell metabolism, a valuable understanding borne out of Warburg's observations is that highly proliferative cells, like cancer cells, have different metabolic needs than cells that are not dividing, such as the majority of cells in healthy tissues. Importantly, cancer is not the only context in which cells need to proliferate, nor is proliferation the only cell activity in which altered metabolism should be considered.

In this work, we discuss how the lessons learned from studying cancer metabolism have led to important findings in three key areas: tissue homeostasis, in physiological and injury contexts; mammalian embryonic development, which requires massive cell proliferation and controlled differentiation; and virus infection. Our objective is not to provide a comprehensive review of each of these broad subject areas, but instead to highlight specific examples of discoveries in these fields that were informed by previous or parallel discoveries in the cancer metabolism field. We will also outline the key scientific challenges facing cell metabolism research and discuss ways that all of these fields, including cancer metabolism, can move forward together.

Tumor cells and cells in the contexts described in this work share several defining features that can be controlled by or lead to major changes in cell metabolism; we refer to these unifying themes throughout (Fig. 1). The first unifying theme is that cellular proliferation requires increased nutrient consumption and macromolecule biosynthesis to support biomass generation. Although this unifying theme has been exemplified by studies in cancer cells, cells in a developing embryo or in tissues undergoing renewal or repair must also be metabolically programmed to divide rapidly, albeit in a more highly controlled manner. Although viral replication does not necessarily require cell division, it does require up-regulation of metabolic pathways associated with proliferation that generate biomass. Included in this theme is flexibility to utilize different carbon sources to meet energetic and biosynthetic needs in these settings. The second unifying theme is the bidirectional relationship between metabolism and cell identity transitions. Tumor cells frequently exhibit aberrant differentiation that can be linked to altered metabolism. Similarly, successful embryonic development is dependent on defined differentiation steps that require precise

metabolic regulation. Tissue repair often involves the dedifferentiation and redifferentiation of epithelial cells to replace the damaged tissue, and metabolism is emerging as a potential level of regulation for these processes. The last unifying theme is diet as a means to control cell metabolism in vivo. Tumor cells have specific metabolic dependencies that can be exploited by dietary restriction of the nutrients they require. This discovery has led to the study of diet and systemic metabolism in regulating tissue homeostasis, promoting proper embryonic development, and limiting virus infection. The examples we discuss highlight these unifying themes as the common threads linking tumor cells to cells in physiology, development, and infection.

TISSUE HOMEOSTASIS

It is now well understood that there is a bidirectional relationship between metabolism and cell state (Fig. 1, Theme 2), which has implications for cell metabolism in systemic disease and tissue injury. Differentiated cells in healthy tissues typically proliferate only to maintain cell number and homeostasis, and thus are usually quite sta-

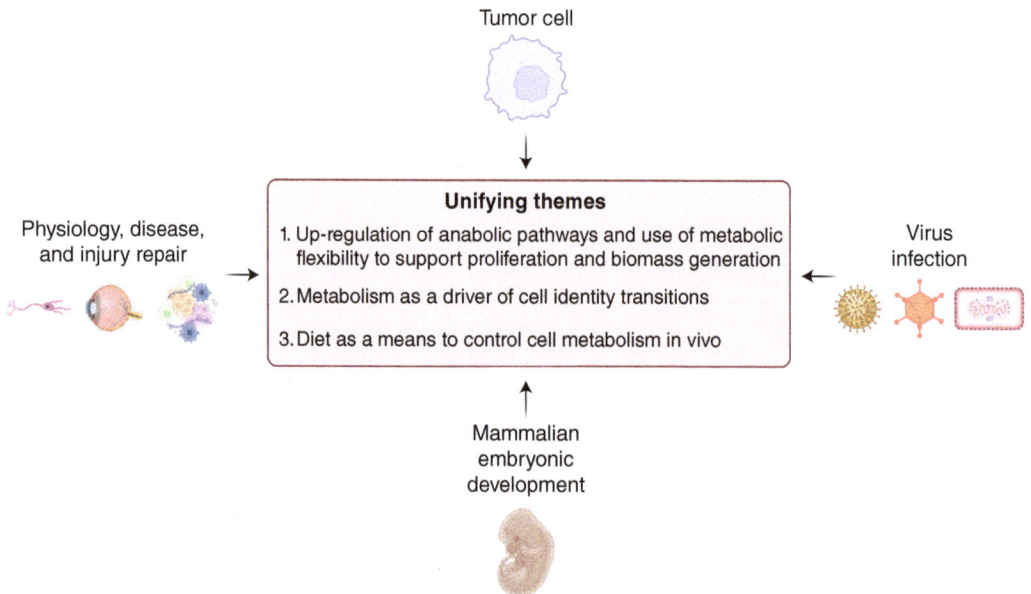

Figure 1. Unifying themes in cellular metabolism research inspired by cancer metabolism discoveries. An outline of topics discussed in this paper. (Figure created with BioRender.com.)

Cite this article as *Cold Spring Harb Perspect Med* doi: 10.1101/cshperspect.a041554

ble metabolically. In the context of systemic disease or tissue injury, on the other hand, cells can alter their metabolism considerably and in ways that contribute to disease or tissue repair. In this section, we discuss how understanding cancer metabolism has shaped the studies of cell metabolism in two biological contexts: physiology and disease, and tissue repair. The latter subsection will include a discussion of adult tissue stem cell metabolism, and how principles from cancer metabolism might be applied to future study of these cells.

Physiology and Disease

Although the field of cancer metabolism started with the idea that tumor cells have generally common dysfunctional metabolism, by comparing cancer cell lines derived from different tissues it has become clear that not only do cancer cells have different metabolic phenotypes based on their oncogenic drivers, but they also differ in metabolism at baseline according to tissue type. Consistently, tumor interstitial fluid samples from varied cancer types have different metabolic profiles linked to their tissues of origin (Sullivan et al. 2019). The evidence of tissue specificity, combined with advances in metabolic measurement and tracing techniques, has led to the comprehensive profiling of nutrient utilization in different tissues in healthy animals (Hui et al. 2017; Jang et al. 2019; Neinast et al. 2019). These methods for whole-organism metabolic profiling and tracing enable a more meaningful interpretation of how tissue-specific metabolic disruptions contribute to disease. For example, leptin-deficient *db/db* mice display increased serine utilization by the liver compared to wild-type mice. Ultimately, a serine-supplemented diet can ameliorate neuropathy progression in this mouse model of type II diabetes (Fig. 1, Theme 3; Handzlik et al. 2023).

Studies of cancer metabolism and the nutritional dependencies of tumor cells have led to the design of diet-based strategies to either directly limit tumor growth or improve the efficacy of existing cancer drugs. For instance, a serine- and glycine-deficient diet can limit cancer growth in autochthonous mouse models of lymphoma and intestinal cancer (Maddocks et al. 2017). Subsequent studies have shown that deprivation of serine and glycine can sensitize other cancer cell types to radiation in vitro and can be an effective therapy when combined with PHGDH inhibitors in vivo to limit the growth of HCT116 xenografts (Tajan et al. 2021; Falcone et al. 2022).

These discoveries have promoted the examination of metabolic vulnerabilities in other diseases; an example of serine metabolism is macular telangiectasia type 2 (MacTel). MacTel patients experience gradual loss of central vision due to swelling of macular blood vessels. Although it was known that MacTel patients had low serine levels in their serum, it was unknown whether or how this nutritional imbalance contributed to this progressive disease. Through metabolomics analysis, it was found that MacTel patients also have elevated serum levels of deoxysphinganine. Interestingly, mice fed a serine- and glycine-deficient diet for 2 weeks also showed the same increase in deoxysphinganine not only in the serum but also in the retina and sciatic nerve (Fig. 1, Theme 3). Further, these mice displayed reduced eye responsiveness similar to that observed in MacTel patients, indicating that the low serine levels and corresponding increased deoxysphinganine levels in the serum are likely causative of some MacTel pathology. Indeed, treating human retinal organoids with fenofibrate, which drives degradation of deoxysphinganine, protects the organoids from the toxic effects of deoxysphinganine (Gantner et al. 2019).

Tissue Stem Cells and Injury Repair

One reason for metabolic differences between tumor cells and normal differentiated tissue cells is that tumor cells proliferate in a rapid and uncontrolled manner (Vander Heiden et al. 2009). However, many postnatal tissues also have resident stem cell compartments with proliferative capacity that are crucial to injury recovery and overall tissue homeostasis (Fig. 1, Theme 1; Shapira and Christofk 2020). Some of these populations, such as stem cells in the crypt regions of the small intestine, are constantly proliferating to maintain continual cell turnover in that tissue.

Other adult stem cells, such as hematopoietic stem cells, remain mostly dormant and do not proliferate until activated by a stimulus. There is growing evidence that the metabolism of adult stem cells contributes to their unique biology and role in tissue homeostasis.

Just as metabolism changes significantly during oncogenic transformation, changes in metabolism are now known to regulate adult stem cell activation and differentiation. For example, hair follicle stem cells undergo metabolic rewiring as they transition from their typical dormant state to an activated state of hair growth; this transition is particularly marked by an increase in lactate dehydrogenase A (LDHA) activity (Fig. 1, Theme 2). LDHA deletion blocks hair follicle activation, whereas inhibition of the mitochondrial pyruvate carrier promotes hair growth, indicating that this population can be controlled metabolically (Flores et al. 2017). In addition to the metabolic transitions occurring during stem cell activation, diet-derived nutrients can also regulate stemness phenotypes. A high-fat diet, for instance, increases the renewal capacity of intestinal stem cells through up-regulation of PPAR-δ and Wnt signaling. Sustained PPAR-δ signaling in turn increases the ability of intestinal stem and progenitor cells to form adenomas ex vivo (Beyaz et al. 2016). Caloric restriction can similarly promote the renewal and proliferation capacities of intestinal stem cells and progenitors via a CPT1-dependent increase in fatty acid oxidation (Fig. 1, Theme 3); treatment with a fatty acid oxidation agonist can restore the renewal capacity of intestinal stem cells isolated from aged mice (Mihaylova et al. 2018). Finally, decreases in systemic vitamin C levels due to reduced dietary intake can limit the number and regenerative capacity of hematopoietic stem cells in mice through reducing TET2 activity (Agathocleous et al. 2017). Interestingly, these data are corroborated by human data showing that patients with hematological malignancies typically have lower vitamin C levels than those who do not (Huijskens et al. 2016; Liu et al. 2016).

In contrast to stem cell populations that are always present, some tissues exhibit facultative stem cell–like populations that arise and prolif-erate only as needed. These latter cells typically derive from differentiated cells that start to express typical stemness markers and sometimes markers of other cell types in that tissue (Shapira and Christofk 2020). These dedifferentiated cells can proliferate during injury repair and then differentiate back to a normal epithelial cell type of that tissue. An example of this cell type is hepatic progenitor cells (HPCs) in the liver. Upon liver damage, especially in chronic damage, normal hepatocytes or cholangiocytes can give rise to *Axin2*-expressing bipotent HPCs (Huch et al. 2013). Because such facultative "stem cells" appear only in response to an injury stimulus, comprise a small percentage of the tissue, and are not always well defined in terms of markers, the metabolism of cells like HPCs has not been well studied. However, they most likely undergo metabolic changes as they dedifferentiate, increase proliferation, and redifferentiate like the adult stem cells described above.

Proper activity of facultative adult stem cells requires precise regulation of the dedifferentiation and redifferentiation of a normal tissue cell; metabolic abnormalities can disrupt these processes (Fig. 1, Theme 2). For example, gain-of-function *IDH2* mutation, which has been thoroughly discussed in Gunn and Losman (2024), can negatively impact liver repair. Expression of gain-of-function mutant IDH2^{R172K} in hepatocytes drives production of the oncometabolite 2-hydroxyglutarate but does not cause abnormal phenotypes in adult mouse liver. Upon 3,5-diethoxycarbonyl-1,4-dihydrocollidin-induced liver injury, however, IDH2^{R172K}-expressing mice exhibit strong depletion of mature hepatocytes as evidenced by reduced *HNF-4α* gene expression. Although the cells that proliferate in response to injury are not HPCs by the current definition, as they do not express the HPC marker *Sox9*, their lack of expression of mature hepatocyte markers indicates that *IDH2* mutation impairs proper restoration of hepatocyte differentiation required for healing after acute injury (Saha et al. 2014). Expression of KRAS^{G12D} in mouse hepatocytes in vivo alongside IDH2^{R172K} acts synergistically to promote development of intrahepatic cholangiocarcinoma (Saha et al. 2014). Indeed, these are two bona fide oncogenic hits, but an implication is that the metabolic phenotype caused by IDH2^{R172K} sets the stage for KRAS^{G12D} to form a tumor.

The role of cell plasticity, like that observed in adult stem cells in tumorigenesis, is a topic of active research. A term introduced in pediatric cancers is "developmental pliancy," meaning the innate capability of a cell at a specific developmental stage to adapt to its environment or context. As initially defined, this adaptability is achieved through epigenetic modifications that promote open chromatin, but there are likely other ways pliability can be established. A more pliable cell is, in turn, more susceptible to transformation by oncogenic insult or mutation (Chen et al. 2015). More recently, it has been proposed that this term be applied to adult cells as well in terms of oncogenic transformation, but instead of a specific developmental stage, the pliability corresponds to a specific state of differentiation, thus termed "cellular pliancy" (Puisieux et al. 2018). Given that metabolism can direct stem cell fate, it is likely that the metabolic context of the cell can in turn impact the pliability of a cell, as in the IDH2^{R172K} mechanism described here. Whether dietary nutrients can control not only adult tissue stem cell homeostasis but also their propensity for oncogenic transformation is an exciting area for further study.

MAMMALIAN EMBRYONIC DEVELOPMENT

As a mammalian embryo develops, it grows from a single fertilized oocyte to a multicellular blastocyst and placenta. This cell division must be highly controlled for a healthy organism to develop, which is in stark contrast to the uncontrolled proliferation of cancer cells. However, in both cases, the cells need to leverage the materials available in their microenvironment to meet their biosynthetic needs (Fig. 1, Theme 1).

The connection between cell metabolism and epigenetic modifications is well established in cancer and in mammalian cells generally, but this link is especially critical in a developing organism as metabolic enzymes are tied to the initial activation of transcription. A fertilized oocyte does not begin transcription until it has grown from the one-cell stage to the two-cell stage in mice, or the four-cell stage to the eight-cell stage in humans, and under-

goes a process called zygotic genome activation. In both murine and human embryos at these analogous stages, TCA cycle enzymes citrate synthase (CS), aconitase 2 (ACO2), isocitrate dehydrogenase (IDH), pyruvate dehydrogenase (PDH), and pyruvate carboxylase (PC) translocate from the mitochondria to the nucleus (Nagaraj et al. 2017). This localization is required for the establishment of H3K27 acetylation, which promotes transcription. Although enzymatic assays and metabolomic measurements in isolated nuclei do indicate that these enzymes are metabolically active (Nagaraj et al. 2017), it is unclear how exactly generation of TCA cycle metabolites such as α-ketoglutarate is driving the generation of these chromatin marks, although such metabolites have been shown to regulate chromatin modifiers (Campbell and Wellen 2018). Notably, unexpected nuclear localization of PDH, as well as other metabolic enzymes like acetyl-CoA synthetase 2 (ACSS2) and ATP-citrate lyase (ACLY), occurs in different cancer cell types (Sutendra et al. 2014; Schug et al. 2015; Sivanand et al. 2018). Further studies of these translocations could continue to reveal parallels between cancer and embryonic development in terms of linking metabolic enzyme localization with dramatic changes in gene expression and cell state (Fig. 1, Theme 2).

Just like cancer cells, the cells in the developing embryo shift their usage of available glucose, pyruvate, and lactate to meet their biosynthetic and bioenergetic needs (Fig. 1, Theme 1). During the earliest stages of embryonic development, the fertilized oocyte only has access to the nutrients available in its direct microenvironment, most importantly maternal pyruvate and lactate, which alone are enough to sustain the developing embryo up to the eight-cell stage in the human embryo. After this point, embryonic glucose uptake increases substantially between the eight-cell and blastocyst stages (Leese and Barton 1984). Although initially thought that glucose uptake increases mainly to meet energy demands in the developing embryo (Johnson et al. 2003), in fact, this increase primarily fuels biomass synthesis. The eight- to 16-cell transition is critical because it marks the earliest lineage division; the compacted cells in the inner cell mass become totipotent blastocysts, whereas the polar cells on the outer edge become the trophecto-derm, which is a crucial layer in implantation and placenta development. Metabolomics tracing at this stage in preimplanted embryos reveals that glucose actually is not at all incorporated into TCA cycle intermediates, and instead it is used in the pentose phosphate and hexosamine biosynthesis pathways to generate biomass (Chi et al. 2020). Remarkably, exogenous pyruvate and lactate provide sufficient carbons to sustain the TCA cycle in the 16-cell embryo.

A key feature of cancer metabolism is the ability of tumor cells to rapidly switch between metabolic substrates, like glucose and glutamine, in the face of potentially nutrient-deprived microenvironmental conditions. These observations have inspired studies to address whether developing embryos are similarly metabolically flexible (Fig. 1, Theme 1). In murine embryos, genes encoding glycolytic enzymes are expressed at very low levels until the morula stage, which explains in part why glucose cannot be substituted for maternal pyruvate and lactate before the inner cell mass forms. However, following zygotic gene activation, development can be rescued under pyruvate deprivation if glucose and other α-ketoacids are supplemented. α-ketobutyrate, for example, can be reduced by LDHB to generate NAD^+ (Sharpley et al. 2021). The observation that two-cell embryos could continue to develop when other α-ketoacids are substituted for pyruvate brought to light the importance of maintaining a high NAD^+:NADH ratio during development; the total NAD^+ and NADH pool becomes more oxidized over progression from oocyte to blastocyst. If pyruvate is absent but the NAD^+:NADH ratio is maintained, the developing embryo can up-regulate glucose metabolism to fuel the TCA cycle in a MYC-dependent manner. This metabolic plasticity increases even further at the morula stage, wherein the cells can adjust to total nutrient deprivation by up-regulating fatty acid oxidation (Sharpley et al. 2021). Thus, although the early stages of preimplantation embryo development are metabolically rigid, over the course of development the embryo acquires the ability to utilize a wider range of metabolic substrates (Fig. 1, Theme 1).

Studying cancer metabolism has taught us to examine spatial variations in metabolism, because cells within the same tumor mass can exhibit differences in metabolism depending on vascularization, ECM deposition, and stromal cell composition. Likewise, recent studies have found changes in glucose utilization within different embryonic compartments. Rapid proliferation of cells continues throughout embryo development and, in addition, the placenta starts to form at the start of midgestation, around E10 in mice. Thus, unlike preimplantation development in which the blastocyst is directly exposed to whatever nutrients are available in the surrounding uterus, after E10 the placenta regulates passage of nutrients from the mother to the embryo. Reflective of this unique role of the placenta, infusing pregnant mice with ^{13}C-glucose reveals distinct metabolite labeling patterns in the placenta and embryo. For example, although a significant fraction of ribose is labeled from maternal glucose in both the placenta and embryo within 4 h of infusion, the embryo displays an increased contribution of maternal glucose to nucleotide bases of purines, indicating higher de novo purine synthesis in the embryo (Solmonson et al. 2022). Further proliferation and compartmental specialization must occur as the embryo starts to develop organs. Interestingly, at E9.5, labeling from ^{13}C-glucose in TCA cycle intermediates is higher in the placenta than in the embryo, but this is reversed by E12.5, at which point labeling of TCA cycle metabolites is equal to or higher than that observed in the placenta. Interestingly, this time point coincides with very early development of the heart, liver, and brain, all of which rely on oxidative metabolism (Fig. 1, Theme 2; Solmonson et al. 2022). This increase in TCA cycle usage is important not only for organ development, but also for embryo viability. Mouse embryos homozygous for a pathogenic mutant of lipoyltransferase-1 (LIPT1), which transfers a required cofactor to key TCA cycle enzymes, are lost around E11.5, which is in the range of when this TCA cycle transition occurs. Indeed, again through infusion experiments, it was found that these embryos do not display the increased TCA cycle usage by E11, although placental function is normal (Solmonson et al. 2022).

Because the early embryo is entirely reliant on exogenous maternal nutrients, the microenvironmental conditions play a critical role in the health of a developing organism. The importance of maternal health has been understood for centuries and has led to the common use of prenatal vitamins and supplements. However, in the face of globally increasing rates of obesity and diabetes, it is vital to understand how excess dietary fat and sugar and changes in maternal blood glucose levels affect development. Indeed, ^{13}C-glucose tracing studies in pregnant Akita mice, an established mouse model of diabetes and hyperglycemia, demonstrate that the toxic metabolite sorbitol accumulates in fetal tissues of hyperglycemic dams during mid-to-late gestation, although the impact of sorbitol on fetal development remains to be explored (Perez-Ramirez et al. 2024). Additionally, although tracing experiments in this data set were conducted at a time when the fetus was developing its own circulatory system independent from the mother, fetuses from Akita dams continued to incorporate ^{13}C-glucose from maternal serum into the carbon backbones of metabolites (Perez-Ramirez et al. 2024). This adjustment to a specific maternal nutritional context is in line with the evidence for increased metabolic plasticity over the course of embryo development. Further understanding of fetal nutrient utilization will enable the design of strategies, including diet optimization, to promote the metabolic health of both mothers and infants (Fig. 1, Theme 3).

Finally, it is important to note that mammalian development is not limited to the proliferation and cell fate changes that occur in the embryo. Metabolic transitions are undoubtedly occurring in tissues between pre- and postweaning, during adolescence, and over the course of aging. Defining changes in metabolism throughout these states and how they might be affected by diet or metabolic syndrome are areas for future discovery.

VIRUS INFECTION

Cancer cell metabolism is altered in part according to the tumor cell's changing biosynthetic needs. This is mirrored in viral infection; viruses must replicate to survive, and as obligate intracellular parasites, they are completely reliant on materials available in the host cell for replication.

Thus, viruses also manipulate cell metabolism to meet their replication needs (Fig. 1, Theme 1). Notably, there are myriad types of viruses with diverse structures and modes of replication. In this section, rather than outline the specifics of viral diversity and how each type can alter metabolism as has been previously described (Thaker et al. 2019), we will discuss virus infection broadly and highlight key metabolic pathways applicable to multiple virus types.

All viruses contain either RNA or DNA and a protein capsid that protects the nucleic acid, so at a minimum these structures must be synthesized with each replication. Beyond those components, some viruses have specialized structures; for example, certain viruses require fatty acids to synthesize lipid envelopes. Just as cancer cells can switch between carbon sources depending on what is available and what is required to meet their specific biosynthetic needs, viruses can also change the primary nutrients utilized by the host cell (Fig. 1, Theme 1). For example, SARS-CoV-2 infection leads to reduced oxidation of glutamine and increased incorporation of glucose into the TCA cycle via PC, although the precise mechanisms by which this occurs are unclear (Mullen et al. 2021). Epstein–Barr virus (EBV) infects B cells and drives increased expression of the serine transporter ASCT2 while also increasing de novo serine synthesis via viral protein EBNA2 and MYC. Increased serine levels achieved through these metabolic changes support increased nucleotide synthesis required by the replicating virus (Wang et al. 2019). In this way, EBV maximizes the use of available extracellular serine while also protecting against serine deprivation; however, growing cells in serine-free media does limit the growth of EBV-infected cells in vitro (Wang et al. 2019).

Not only does virus infection lead to changes in cell metabolism that resemble those seen in tumor cells, viruses also hijack signaling pathways that are frequently dysregulated in cancer. For example, adenoviral infection of MCF10A breast epithelial cells leads to increased glucose uptake and lactate production. Specifically, the viral gene product E4ORF1 was found to be responsible for causing this increase in a MYC-dependent manner. E4ORF1 interacts with

MYC in the nucleus to promote expression of MYC targets like *PFKM* and *HK2* (Thai et al. 2014). The increased MYC transcriptional activity also drives glutamine uptake and increased use of reductive carboxylation to fuel the TCA cycle. Inhibiting reductive carboxylation via treatment with glutaminase inhibitors significantly limits adenovirus replication (Thai et al. 2014). Interestingly, GLS inhibition can also limit replication of herpes simplex virus 1 (HSV-1) in human foreskin fibroblasts and of influenza virus in normal human bronchial epithelial cells, indicating that the use of glutamine for TCA cycle flux could be leveraged by multiple virus types to meet their replication needs (Thai et al. 2015).

As observed in cancer cells, multiple types of viruses can disrupt proper cellular nutrient sensing via mTORC1. Adenovirus, for instance, activates mTORC1 signaling downstream from PI3K in a manner dependent on viral gene products E4ORF1 and E4ORF4 (O'Shea et al. 2005). Interestingly, these proteins can activate mTORC1 signaling in kidney epithelial cells even when the cells are grown in phosphate-buffered saline entirely without nutrients or growth factor signaling. Through add-back experiments, it was found that E4ORF1 and E4ORF4 work in the same pathways as growth factors and glucose, respectively, in terms of mTORC1 activation (O'Shea et al. 2005). Because mTORC1 can signal nutrient abundance and thus promote anabolic biosynthesis pathways, it makes sense that viruses would take advantage of this pathway to support their own synthesis needs; for example, the pox virus vaccinia activates mTORC1 signaling to promote massive viral protein synthesis, although the extent to which the virus can achieve this is cell-type dependent (Meade et al. 2019). Promisingly, mTOR inhibitors have been shown to limit viral reproduction of adenovirus, vaccinia virus, and SARS-CoV-2, among others (O'Shea et al. 2005; Meade et al. 2019; Mullen et al. 2021).

Methionine has emerged as a key nutrient in tumor cell metabolism because of its requirement for generating *S*-adenosyl methionine (SAM), the donor for histone and DNA methylation, and because of its key roles in nucleotide generation and redox balance. Viruses can also leverage methionine metabolism to support virion replication. A recent study showed that methionine can regulate the complex gene expression of the replication cycle of EBV. After EBV infection, the virus remains in the latent phase in B cells, replicating at low levels until the more immunogenic lytic phase is activated. Tenfold methionine restriction in vitro leads to the derepression of latency-promoting genes and lytic cycle antigen genes in multiple cell lines, likely because of the loss of DNA and histone methylation at the promoter regions of these genes (Guo et al. 2022). Dietary methionine restriction led to the expression of lytic cycle antigen genes in vivo in an EBV model (Fig. 1, Theme 3; Guo et al. 2022). Although these experiments were performed in an immunocompromised model, promoting expression of these antigen genes via methionine restriction could make the infected cells more vulnerable to healthy immune cells and thus could be leveraged therapeutically.

So far, the characterization of the changes in cell metabolism that occur with virus infection is limited, both in the sense that only a handful of types of viruses have been studied and that these studies have been conducted either in vitro or in immunocompromised mice. Importantly, it can be challenging to successfully generate immunocompetent in vivo models for human viruses in mice because of differences in genetics, surface protein expression, and innate immune response between species (Sarkar and Heise 2019). Further, as described in Hathaway et al. (2024), metabolism is an important regulator of immune cell differentiation and function. The development of immunocompetent models of virus infection will be essential to fully understand the effects of virus infection on immune cell metabolism.

KEY NEXT QUESTIONS AND SCIENTIFIC CHALLENGES

As stated in a recent review of cancer metabolism, what separates tumor cell metabolism from other cell metabolism is that the tumor cells exist in a cancer patient (Finley 2023), meaning that "cancer metabolism" is simply the study of cell metabolism in a cancer cell. A major concept that has emerged from examining cancer metabolism is that cell metabolism is highly context dependent, whether that context is a response to injury, a developing embryo, a virus-infected cell, or, of course, a tumor cell. Given that we have come to appreciate the metabolic commonalities between these settings, the key next questions and challenges described in this section apply to not only studying cancer metabolism but to investigating cell metabolism altogether.

Related to the point of context dependence, tumor metabolism studies and cancer research in general have greatly highlighted the need for studying cellular processes in vivo. Conditions historically used for cell culture do not mimic physiological nutrient concentrations, and cell metabolism can change dramatically in response to different culture methods, such as two-dimensional versus organoid culture. In vivo tracing and measurement strategies have seen dramatic improvement in recent years, and going forward it would be prudent to identify phenotypes in vivo to follow up on in vitro molecular studies, as opposed to the reverse order, which is how studies have been typically designed up to this point.

A further challenge with in vivo molecular studies is cellular heterogeneity within tissues. Most strategies for isolation of specific cells from a tissue rely on expression of some type of fluorescent marker that enables the enrichment of those cells via FACS. However, cell metabolism is highly responsive to environmental changes, and such sorting techniques are far too slow to permit accurate metabolite measurements. Advances in isolating subcellular organelles via magnetic bead pulldowns, for example, may have the potential to be adapted for use with tissue. Overall, moving toward primarily using in vivo models and developing strategies to study cell-type-specific metabolism within those models will improve the translational potential of discoveries.

Another key challenge facing researchers of cell metabolism is establishing precise causative links between laboratory observations and specific nutrients that mediate specific downstream cellular processes. Public health diet studies, for example, frequently correlate intake of a particular nutrient or vitamin with a certain positive or negative health outcome. Dietary intervention is a tractable therapeutic strategy, but to maximize the therapeutic potential of dietary changes we must understand at the molecular level how different cell types in tissues of interest respond to specific nutrients and how these systems might interact with one another in the body.

In line with this, it is important to understand the contribution of biological variability to metabolic profiles and responses. Only recently have studies begun to include both male and female mice in experiments or to focus on recruitment of diverse patients for clinical trials. Undoubtedly, sex and ancestry can underlie metabolic phenotypes and responses in cancer and in the contexts described in this article. Although perhaps the most difficult challenge of the ones described here, accounting for biological variability in metabolism research will dramatically increase the potential clinical applications of molecular studies.

CONCLUDING REMARKS

The expansion of principles developed from studying tumor cell metabolism into other important scientific areas highlights how, at its core, the study of cancer metabolism is the study of cell metabolism. In this work, we have highlighted specific examples of ways tumor metabolism has informed or paralleled discoveries in tissue homeostasis, mammalian development, and viral infection. Going forward, these fields will undoubtedly continue to impact and build on one another, which will strengthen our understanding of cell metabolism and hopefully move toward highly effective treatment and prevention strategies for all cancer types. Warburg was convinced that he had made a discovery relevant specifically to cancer cells, when in fact the identification of aberrant tumor cell metabolism has led to important discoveries that extend far beyond cancer. With this in mind, it will be exciting to see what lessons we continue to learn from cancer metabolism in the future.

ACKNOWLEDGMENTS

The authors thank A. Krall and B. Wilde for their helpful suggestions and editing of this paper.

REFERENCES

Reference is also in this subject collection.

Agathocleous M, Meacham CE, Burgess RJ, Piskounova E, Zhao Z, Crane GM, Cowin BL, Bruner E, Murphy MM, Chen W, et al. 2017. Ascorbate regulates haematopoietic stem cell function and leukaemogenesis. *Nature* 549: 476–481. doi:10.1038/nature23876

Beyaz S, Mana MD, Roper J, Kedrin D, Saadatpour A, Hong SJ, Bauer-Rowe KE, Xifaras ME, Akkad A, Arias E, et al. 2016. High-fat diet enhances stemness and tumorigenicity of intestinal progenitors. *Nature* 531: 53–58. doi:10.1038/nature17173

Campbell SL, Wellen KE. 2018. Metabolic signaling to the nucleus in cancer. *Mol Cell* 71: 398–408. doi:10.1016/j.molcel.2018.07.015

Chen X, Pappo A, Dyer MA. 2015. Pediatric solid tumor genomics and developmental pliancy. *Oncogene* 34: 5207–5215. doi:10.1038/onc.2014.474

Chi F, Sharpley MS, Nagaraj R, Roy SS, Banerjee U. 2020. Glycolysis-independent glucose metabolism distinguishes TE from ICM fate during mammalian embryogenesis. *Dev Cell* 53: 9–26.e4. doi:10.1016/j.devcel.2020.02.015

Falcone M, Uribe AH, Papalazarou V, Newman AC, Athineos D, Stevenson K, Sauvé CEG, Gao Y, Kim JK, Del Latto M, et al. 2022. Sensitisation of cancer cells to radiotherapy by serine and glycine starvation. *Br J Cancer* 127: 1773–1786. doi:10.1038/s41416-022-01965-6

Finley LWS. 2023. What is cancer metabolism? *Cell* 186: 1670–1688. doi:10.1016/j.cell.2023.01.038

Flores A, Schell J, Krall AS, Jelinek D, Miranda M, Grigorian M, Braas D, White AC, Zhou JL, Graham NA, et al. 2017. Lactate dehydrogenase activity drives hair follicle stem cell activation. *Nat Cell Biol* 19: 1017–1026. doi:10.1038/ncb3575

Gantner ML, Eade K, Wallace M, Handzlik MK, Fallon R, Trombley J, Bonelli R, Giles S, Harkins-Perry S, Heeren TFC, et al. 2019. Serine and lipid metabolism in macular disease and peripheral neuropathy. *N Engl J Med* 381: 1422–1433. doi:10.1056/NEJMoa1815111

* Gunn K, Losman JA. 2024. Isocitrate dehydrogenase mutations in cancer: mechanisms of transformation and metabolic liability. *Cold Spring Harb Perspect Med* doi:10.1101/cshperspect.a041537

Guo R, Liang JH, Zhang Y, Lutchenkov M, Li Z, Wang Y, Trujillo-Alonso V, Puri R, Giulino-Roth L, Gewurz BE. 2022. Methionine metabolism controls the B cell EBV epigenome and viral latency. *Cell Metab* 34: 1280–1297.e9. doi:10.1016/j.cmet.2022.08.008

Handzlik MK, Gengatharan JM, Frizzi KE, McGregor GH, Martino C, Rahman G, Gonzalez A, Moreno AM, Green CR, Guernsey LS, et al. 2023. Insulin-regulated serine and lipid metabolism drive peripheral neuropathy. *Nature* 614: 118–124. doi:10.1038/s41586-022-05637-6

* Hathaway ES, Jennings EQ, Rathmell JC. 2024. Immunometabolic maladaptations to the tumor microenvironment. *Cold Spring Harb Perspect Med* doi:10.1101/cshperspect.a041547

Huch M, Dorrell C, Boj SF, Van Es JH, Li VSW, Van De Wetering M, Sato T, Hamer K, Sasaki N, Finegold MJ, et al. 2013. In vitro expansion of single Lgr5+ liver stem cells induced by Wnt-driven regeneration. *Nature* 494: 247–250. doi:10.1038/nature11826

Hui S, Ghergurovich JM, Morscher RJ, Jang C, Teng X, Lu W, Esparza LA, Reya T, Zhan L, Yanxiang Guo J, et al. 2017. Glucose feeds the TCA cycle via circulating lactate. *Nature* 551: 115–118. doi:10.1038/nature24057

Huijskens MJAJ, Wodzig WKWH, Walczak M, Germeraad WTV, Bos GMJ. 2016. Ascorbic acid serum levels are reduced in patients with hematological malignancies. *Results Immunol* 6: 8–10. doi:10.1016/j.rinim.2016.01.001

Jang C, Hui S, Zeng X, Cowan AJ, Wang L, Chen L, Morscher RJ, Reyes J, Frezza C, Hwang HY, et al. 2019. Metabolite exchange between mammalian organs quantified in pigs. *Cell Metab* 30: 594–606.e3. doi:10.1016/j.cmet.2019.06.002

Johnson MT, Mahmood S, Patel MS. 2003. Intermediary metabolism and energetics during murine early embryogenesis. *J Biol Chem* 278: 31457–31460. doi:10.1074/jbc.R300002200

Leese H, Barton A. 1984. Pyruvate and glucose uptake by mouse ova and preimplantation embryos. *J Reprod Fertil* 72: 9–13. doi:10.1530/jrf.0.0720009

Liu M, Ohtani H, Zhou W, Ørskov AD, Charlet J, Zhang YW, Shen H, Baylin SB, Liang G, Grønbæk K, et al. 2016. Vitamin C increases viral mimicry induced by 5-aza-2′-deoxycytidine. *Proc Natl Acad Sci* 113: 10238–10244. doi:10.1073/pnas.1612262113

Maddocks ODK, Athineos D, Cheung EC, Lee P, Zhang T, Van Den Broek NJF, Mackay GM, Labuschagne CF, Gay D, Kruiswijk F, et al. 2017. Modulating the therapeutic response of tumours to dietary serine and glycine starvation. *Nature* 544: 372–376. doi:10.1038/nature22056

Meade N, King M, Munger J, Walsh D. 2019. mTOR dysregulation by vaccinia virus F17 controls multiple processes with varying roles in infection. *J Virol* 93: e00784-19. doi:10.1128/JVI.00784-19

Mihaylova MM, Cheng CW, Cao AQ, Tripathi S, Mana MD, Bauer-Rowe KE, Abu-Remaileh M, Clavain L, Erdemir A, Lewis CA, et al. 2018. Fasting activates fatty acid oxidation to enhance intestinal stem cell function during homeostasis and aging. *Cell Stem Cell* 22: 769–778.e4. doi:10.1016/j.stem.2018.04.001

Mullen PJ, Garcia G, Purkayastha A, Matulionis N, Schmid EW, Momcilovic M, Sen C, Langerman J, Ramaiah A, Shackelford DB, et al. 2021. SARS-CoV-2 infection rewires host cell metabolism and is potentially susceptible to mTORC1 inhibition. *Nat Commun* 12: 1–10. doi:10.1038/s41467-021-22166-4

Nagaraj R, Sharpley MS, Chi F, Braas D, Zhou Y, Kim R, Clark AT, Banerjee U. 2017. Nuclear localization of mitochondrial TCA cycle enzymes as a critical step in mammalian zygotic genome activation. *Cell* 168: 210–223.e11. doi:10.1016/j.cell.2016.12.026

Neinast MD, Jang C, Hui S, Murashige DS, Chu Q, Morscher RJ, Li X, Zhan L, White E, Anthony TG, et al. 2019. Quantitative analysis of the whole-body metabolic fate of branched-chain amino acids. *Cell Metab* 29: 417–429.e4. doi:10.1016/j.cmet.2018.10.013

O'Shea C, Klupsch K, Choi S, Bagus B, Soria C, Shen J, McCormick F, Stokoe D. 2005. Adenoviral proteins mimic nutrient/growth signals to activate the mTOR pathway for viral replication. *EMBO J* **24:** 1211–1221. doi:10.1038/sj.emboj.7600597

Perez-Ramirez CA, Nakano H, Law RC, Matulionis N, Thompson J, Pfeiffer A, Park JO, Nakano A, Christofk HR. 2024. Atlas of fetal metabolism during mid-to-late gestation and diabetic pregnancy. *Cell* **187:** 204–215.e14. doi:10.1016/j.cell.2023.11.011

Puisieux A, Pommier RM, Morel A, Lavial F. 2018. Cellular pliancy and the multistep process of tumorigenesis. *Cancer Cell* **33:** 164–172. doi:10.1016/j.ccell.2018.01.007

Saha SK, Parachoniak CA, Ghanta KS, Fitamant J, Ross KN, Najem MS, Gurumurthy S, Akbay EA, Sia D, Cornella H, et al. 2014. Mutant IDH inhibits HNF-4α to block hepatocyte differentiation and promote biliary cancer. *Nature* **513:** 110–114. doi:10.1038/nature13441

Sarkar S, Heise MT. 2019. Mouse models as resources for studying infectious diseases. *Clin Ther* **41:** 1912–1922. doi:10.1016/j.clinthera.2019.08.010

Schug ZT, Peck B, Jones DT, Zhang Q, Grosskurth S, Alam IS, Goodwin LM, Smethurst E, Mason S, Blyth K, et al. 2015. Acetyl-CoA synthetase 2 promotes acetate utilization and maintains cancer cell growth under metabolic stress. *Cancer Cell* **27:** 57–71. doi:10.1016/j.ccell.2014.12.002

Shapira SN, Christofk HR. 2020. Metabolic regulation of tissue stem cells. *Trends Cell Biol* **30:** 566–576. doi:10.1016/j.tcb.2020.04.004

Sharpley MS, Chi F, Hoeve JT, Banerjee U. 2021. Metabolic plasticity drives development during mammalian embryogenesis. *Dev Cell* **56:** 2329–2347.e6. doi:10.1016/j.devcel.2021.07.020

Sivanand S, Viney I, Wellen KE. 2018. Spatiotemporal control of acetyl-CoA metabolism in chromatin regulation. *Trends Biochem Sci* **43:** 61–74. doi:10.1016/j.tibs.2017.11.004

Solmonson A, Faubert B, Gu W, Rao A, Cowdin MA, Menendez-Montes I, Kelekar S, Rogers TJ, Pan C, Guevara G, et al. 2022. Compartmentalized metabolism supports midgestation mammalian development. *Nature* **604:** 349–353. doi:10.1038/s41586-022-04557-9

Sullivan MR, Danai LV, Lewis CA, Chan SH, Gui DY, Kunchok T, Dennstedt EA, Vander Heiden MG, Muir A. 2019. Quantification of microenvironmental metabolites in murine cancers reveals determinants of tumor nutrient availability. *eLife* **8:** 1–27. doi:10.7554/eLife.44235

Sutendra G, Kinnaird A, Dromparis P, Paulin R, Stenson TH, Haromy A, Hashimoto K, Zhang N, Flaim E, Michelakis ED. 2014. A nuclear pyruvate dehydrogenase complex is important for the generation of acetyl-CoA and histone acetylation. *Cell* **158:** 84–97. doi:10.1016/j.cell.2014.04.046

Tajan M, Hennequart M, Cheung EC, Zani F, Hock AK, Legrave N, Maddocks ODK, Ridgway RA, Athineos D, Suárez-Bonnet A, et al. 2021. Serine synthesis pathway inhibition cooperates with dietary serine and glycine limitation for cancer therapy. *Nat Commun* **12:** 1–16. doi:10.1038/s41467-020-20223-y

Thai M, Graham NA, Braas D, Nehil M, Komisopoulou E, Kurdistani SK, Mccormick F, Graeber TG, Christofk HR. 2014. Adenovirus E4ORF1-induced MYC activation promotes host cell anabolic glucose metabolism and virus replication. *Cell Metab* **19:** 694–701. doi:10.1016/j.cmet.2014.03.009

Thai M, Thaker SK, Feng J, Du Y, Hu H, Ting Wu T, Graeber TG, Braas D, Christofk HR. 2015. MYC-induced reprogramming of glutamine catabolism supports optimal virus replication. *Nat Commun* **6:** 8873. doi:10.1038/ncomms9873

Thaker SK, Ch'ng J, Christofk HR. 2019. Viral hijacking of cellular metabolism. *BMC Biol* **17:** 59. doi:10.1186/s12915-019-0678-9

Vander Heiden MG, Cantley LC, Thompson CB. 2009. Understanding the Warburg effect: the metabolic requirements of cell proliferation. *Science* **324:** 1029–1033. doi:10.1126/science.1160809

Wang LW, Shen H, Nobre L, Ersing I, Paulo JA, Trudeau S, Wang Z, Smith NA, Ma Y, Reinstadler B, et al. 2019. Epstein–Barr-virus-induced one-carbon metabolism drives B cell transformation. *Cell Metab* **30:** 539–555.e11. doi:10.1016/j.cmet.2019.06.003

Growth Signaling Networks Orchestrate Cancer Metabolic Networks

Brendan D. Manning[1,2] and Christian C. Dibble[3]

[1]Department of Molecular Metabolism, Harvard T.H. Chan School of Public Health, Boston, Massachusetts 02115, USA

[2]Department of Cell Biology, Harvard Medical School, Boston, Massachusetts 02115, USA

[3]Department of Pathology, Cancer Research Institute, Beth Israel Deaconess Medical Center, Harvard Medical School, Boston, Massachusetts 02115, USA

Correspondence: bmanning@hsph.harvard.edu

Normal cells grow and divide only when instructed to by signaling pathways stimulated by exogenous growth factors. A nearly ubiquitous feature of cancer cells is their capacity to grow independent of such signals, in an uncontrolled, cell-intrinsic manner. This property arises due to the frequent oncogenic activation of core growth factor signaling pathway components, including receptor tyrosine kinases, PI3K-AKT, RAS-RAF, mTORC1, and MYC, leading to the aberrant propagation of pro-growth signals independent of exogenous growth factors. The growth of both normal and cancer cells requires the acquisition of nutrients and their anabolic conversion to the primary macromolecules underlying biomass production (protein, nucleic acids, and lipids). The core growth factor signaling pathways exert tight regulation of these metabolic processes and the oncogenic activation of these pathways drive the key metabolic properties of cancer cells and tumors. Here, we review the molecular mechanisms through which these growth signaling pathways control and coordinate cancer metabolism.

At its essence, cancer is a disease of uncontrolled cell growth, proliferation, and survival. In an otherwise favorable nutrient environment, normal metazoan cells with capacity to proliferate (i.e., nonterminally differentiated cells) do so only when instructed to by growth factor signaling pathways (Fig. 1A). Growth factors, collectively referring to exogenous hormones, morphogens, cytokines, and chemokines, derived from the same cell (autocrine), cells and cell types sharing a given niche (para-crine), or cells comprising distant organs (endocrine) are the molecular means through which cells communicate with one another to coordinate developmental and homeostatic processes across tissues and the whole organism. Cells receive these signals upon growth factor engagement of cognate receptors on the surface of responsive cells, the most common of which are G-protein-coupled receptors (GPCRs) and receptor tyrosine kinases (RTKs), which propagate the signal through the stimulation of signal transduction pathways trig-

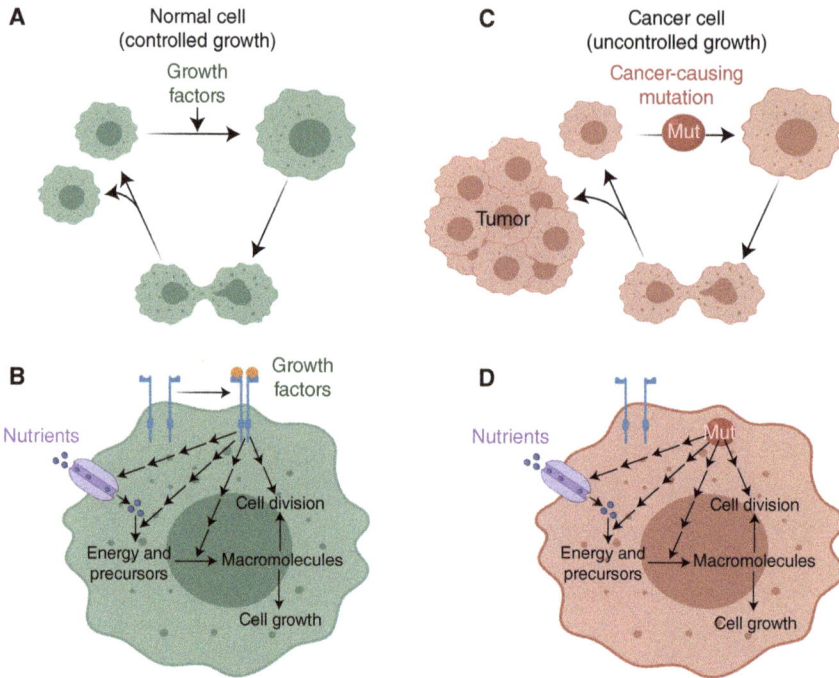

Figure 1. Cancer cells acquire growth factor-independent growth that involves uncontrolled signaling-mediated changes in cell metabolism. (*A*) Normal cells proliferate only when they are instructed to by exogenous growth factors (e.g., mitogens, cytokines, hormones, etc.), which stimulate their growth and division. (*B*) Growth factor signaling pathways stimulate nutrient uptake, the use of nutrients to produce anabolic precursors and cofactors (ATP, NADPH, NEAAs, nucleotides, and cytosolic acetyl-coenzyme A [CoA]), and the anabolic synthesis of macromolecules essential for cell growth and division (proteins, nucleic acids, and lipids). (*C*) Cancer cells acquire mutations that disconnect their growth and division from the need for exogenous growth factors, thus leading to uncontrolled growth. (*D*) The mutations leading to uncontrolled growth chronically activate the signaling pathways that drive the metabolic processes underlying growth and division. (Figure generated with BioRender; biorender.com.)

gered by receptor-proximal events on the cytosolic face of the plasma membrane. The molecular nature, strength, duration, and combination of signals received, together with the recipient cell type, dictate the downstream cellular response, which include growth, cell division, survival, death, migration, differentiation, or other specialized functions. Importantly, a nearly ubiquitous feature of cancer cells is their capacity to grow, proliferate, and survive in a cell-intrinsic manner independent of growth factor–initiated signals (Fig. 1C). This property stems from the fact that many of the most common oncogenes and tumor suppressors in human cancer are key components of growth factor signaling pathways, with their cancer-causing mutations leading to constitutive, growth factor–independent activation of the core signaling

mechanisms that promote cell growth, proliferation, and survival (Sanchez-Vega et al. 2018).

The metabolism of a cancer cell often resembles that of normal cells induced to proliferate by growth factor signaling pathways. Thus, it is no surprise that growth factor signaling controls proliferative metabolism to coordinate its regulation with other cellular processes, such as organellar biogenesis and cell-cycle progression (Fig. 1B). Constitutive activation of these signaling pathways is a major driver of the metabolic program of cancer cells (Fig. 1D). Nutrient availability is fundamental to cellular metabolism, as nutrients dictate intracellular substrate accessible for flux into metabolic pathways. Likewise, the accumulation of metabolic products can influence metabolic flux via feedback regulation of

Cite this article as *Cold Spring Harb Perspect Med* doi: 10.1101/cshperspect.a041543

metabolic enzymes. Cell signaling pathways add a critical additional layer of control over metabolic networks as they can sense and regulate nutrient uptake into cells, while also controlling processes that consume metabolic products, via biosynthesis for instance, thus affecting their rate of clearance to sustain metabolic flux.

Here, we discuss the core growth factor signaling pathways driving cell growth, proliferation, and survival in both normal and cancer cells, with a focus on how they exert both direct and indirect control over nutrient uptake and cellular metabolism. In doing so, we review findings on acute regulation of metabolic activity via growth factor–regulated protein kinases and their direct phosphorylation of metabolic enzymes, as well as more delayed control of metabolic pathways through downstream transcriptional regulation of nutrient transporters and metabolic enzymes. Perturbations in adaptive stress signaling pathways also play a critical role in cancer metabolism, including those influencing p53, LKB1-AMPK, and KEAP1-NRF2 (Kruiswijk et al. 2015; Harris and DeNicola 2020; Trefts and Shaw 2021), but we focus our attention here on the major growth factor signaling pathways underlying oncogenesis (Fig. 2). This is not meant to be an exhaustive review of the many mechanisms through which signaling pathways control cellular metabolism but rather focuses on connectivity between the most common signaling and metabolic pathways driving the aberrant growth properties of cancer cells.

CORE ONCOGENIC SIGNALING PATHWAYS DRIVE CELL-INTRINSIC GROWTH AND SURVIVAL

The nearly ubiquitous independence of cancer cells from exogenous growth factors for their growth and survival can arise through numerous non-mutually exclusive genetic alterations acquired as normal cells transform into cancer cells. While tumor suppressors that regulate genome integrity (e.g., p53) or the cell cycle (e.g., CDKN2A) are commonly lost in human cancers, large cancer genome studies, such as The Cancer Genome Atlas (TCGA, www.cancer.gov/ccg/research/genome-sequencing/tcga), have revealed

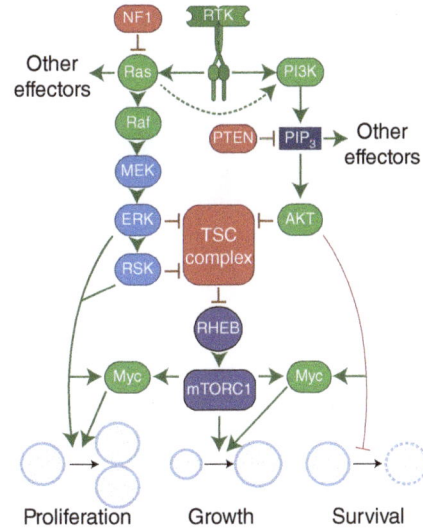

Figure 2. Core growth factor–stimulated pathways that most frequently acquire mutations leading to their aberrant growth factor–independent activation in cancer. RTKs activate the PI3K and RAS signaling pathways, which can be negatively regulated by PTEN and NF1, respectively. Activated PI3K generates the lipid second messenger PIP3, which regulates multiple downstream effectors, a major one being the Ser/Thr kinase AKT. AKT has many downstream substrates influencing cell growth and survival. Activated (GTP-bound) RAS binds to and activates many downstream effectors, including PI3K (dashed line), a major one being the Ser/Thr kinase RAF. RAF activation stimulates a protein kinase cascade leading to activation of ERK and RSK, which have many downstream substrates influencing cell growth and proliferation. The TSC protein complex inhibits RHEB, which when active (GTP-bound) directly binds to and stimulates the Ser/Thr kinase complex mTORC1, a major promoter of cell growth. The growth factor stimulated kinases, AKT, ERK, and RSK, all phosphorylate TSC2 within the TSC complex and relieve its inhibition of Rheb, thereby activating mTORC1 in response to these signals. These protein kinases, as well as mTORC1, also promote the accumulation and activation of MYC, a transcription factor that drives the expression of gene targets required for cell growth and proliferation. Oncogenes in this signaling network are depicted in green, whereas tumor suppressors are red. (Figure generated with BioRender; biorender.com.)

that genes encoding components of growth factor–regulated signaling pathways, collectively, constitute the most common class of oncogenes and tumor suppressors (Sanchez-Vega et al. 2018).

Atop key cancer signaling pathways sit a large number of plasma-membrane resident RTKs that initiate intracellular signaling upon binding growth factors. Oncogenic mutations or genomic amplification of these RTKs constitutively increase their protein kinase activity independent of growth factor ligand stimulation, with oncogenic alterations of EGFR and FGFR family members being the most common. Activated receptors propagate signals through *trans*-autophosphorylation of specific tyrosine residues on both their own cytosolic domains and on Src homology 2 (SH2) domain-containing proteins that dock onto specific phosphorylated tyrosines. These tyrosine-phosphorylation events lead to plasma membrane recruitment and activation of key downstream signaling proteins, including the class Ia phosphoinositide 3-kinases (PI3Ks) and regulators of the RAS family of small GTPases (Fig. 2). Two of the most common oncogenes across human cancer lineages are those encoding the p110α catalytic subunit of PI3K (*PIK3CA*) and K-Ras (*KRAS*) (Sanchez-Vega et al. 2018).

PIK3CA is the most common single oncogene in human cancer, which is oncogenically activated through a combination of hotspot somatic mutations (most often affecting the PI3K-p110α residues H1047, E545, or E542) and gene amplification (Zhang et al. 2017). Growth factor or oncogenic activation brings PI3K to the plasma membrane where its lipid kinase activity is stimulated and it phosphorylates its phospholipid substrate phosphatidylinositol 4,5-bisphosphate (PIP_2) to produce the lipid second messenger phosphatidylinositol 3,4,5-trisphosphate (PIP_3) (Fruman et al. 2017). Importantly, one of the most commonly lost tumor suppressors in human cancers is PTEN (Zhang et al. 2017; Sanchez-Vega et al. 2018), a lipid phosphatase that counters PI3K activity by converting PIP_3 back to PIP_2. Thus, growth-factor-independent accumulation of PIP_3 at the plasma membrane is common in cancer cells, with PIP_3 serving to recruit and activate effector proteins to further propagate downstream signaling events. The best characterized of these PIP_3-binding effectors is the serine/threonine protein kinase AKT (also known as protein kinase B [PKB]), which has three isoforms (AKT1/PKBα, AKT2/PKβ,

and AKT3/PKBγ) that exhibit partial functional redundancy but variable expression patterns (Manning and Toker 2017). Although far less frequent than PI3K activation or PTEN loss, AKT activation also occurs in cancer due to point mutations (e.g., AKT1-E17K) and amplifications that promote increased plasma membrane recruitment and activation that is at least partially independent of PIP_3 accumulation. Activated AKT subsequently phosphorylates and regulates dozens of downstream targets to promote cell growth and survival and, as discussed further below, alter cellular metabolism (Manning and Toker 2017; Hoxhaj and Manning 2020).

As another core transducer of growth factor and RTK signaling, isoforms of the RAS GTPase, particularly K-RAS and to a lesser extent H-RAS and N-RAS, are commonly mutated and potent oncogenes (Li et al. 2018; Sanchez-Vega et al. 2018). Like other small GTPases, RAS family members function as signaling switches by cycling between two distinct conformations dictated by the guanine nucleotide, GTP or GDP, to which they are bound. Generally, downstream signaling effectors are specifically engaged and activated by RAS in its GTP-bound form. The active GTP-bound form of RAS is promoted by RTK-mediated recruitment of guanine nucleotide exchange factors (GEFs), such as "son of sevenless" (SOS), which facilitate the release of GDP from RAS and thus permit GTP binding (Karnoub and Weinberg 2008). Conversion of RAS to its inactive GDP-bound state is facilitated by RAS-specific GTPase-activating proteins (GAPs), such as neurofibromatosis 1 (NF1), which stimulate the intrinsic GTPase activity of RAS to hydrolyze GTP to GDP (Maertens and Cichowski 2014). Oncogenic RAS proteins accumulate in their GTP-bound active form independent of RTK signaling due to a variety of genetic events, the most common of which impair their GTPase activity (e.g., K-RAS G12 mutations) (Haigis 2017). Of the many RAS-GAPs, the NF1 tumor suppressor is the most frequently inactivated in cancer, a genetic event that also leads to increased RAS-GTP accumulation and downstream signaling (Maertens and Cichowski 2014; Li et al. 2018; Sanchez-Vega et al. 2018). RAS-GTP has several direct effectors, including PI3K and the RAF family of protein kinases, with the B-RAF isoform itself being a potent oncogene very frequently activated in certain cancers. RAF activation downstream of RAS-GTP stimulates the canonical extracellular signal-regulated kinase (ERK) (also known as mitogen-activated protein kinase [MAPK]) signaling cascade leading to activation of the protein kinase ERK, which phosphorylates and regulates many downstream targets (Lavoie et al. 2020). Oncogenic RAS signaling has profound effects on cancer cell metabolism (Kerk et al. 2021; Mukhopadhyay et al. 2021).

The PI3K and RAS pathways converge on the regulation of a number of shared downstream targets that influence cell growth and survival, and we focus on two global regulators of cellular metabolism and growth here, mTORC1 and MYC (Fig. 2). The protein kinase mechanistic target of rapamycin (mTOR) complex 1 (mTORC1) is widely known as a downstream effector of PI3K-AKT signaling, but can be independently activated by the RAS-ERK pathway. Growth factor–stimulated activation of mTORC1 is largely controlled by convergent regulation of the tuberous sclerosis complex (TSC) protein complex, comprised of the tumor suppressors TSC1 and TSC2, together with the protein TBC1D7. In the absence of growth factors, the TSC complex suppresses mTORC1 activation by acting as a GAP for the small GTPase RHEB, which in its GTP-bound state directly engages and simulates the kinase activity of mTORC1 (Valvezan and Manning 2019). Upon growth factor stimulation, several protein kinases activated downstream of PI3K and RAS, including AKT, ERK, and RSK, directly phosphorylate TSC2 and relieve the ability of the TSC complex to inhibit RHEB's activation of mTORC1 (Inoki et al. 2002; Manning et al. 2002; Roux et al. 2004; Ma et al. 2005; Menon et al. 2014). While TSC1, TSC2, Rheb, and components of mTORC1 more rarely acquire functional mutations in sporadic cancers, there are a large number of tumor suppressors and proto-oncogenes within the signaling network that converges on regulation of the TSC complex. Hence, aberrant inactivation of the TSC complex and growth factor–independent activation of mTORC1 signaling occurs in the majority of cancers (Ilagan and Manning 2016;

Zhang et al. 2017; Sanchez-Vega et al. 2018). mTORC1 regulates numerous downstream targets involved in cell growth control, largely by promoting anabolic processes while inhibiting catabolic processes, as detailed below (Torrence and Manning 2018; Valvezan and Manning 2019). In addition to targets acutely phosphorylated downstream of mTORC1, pro-growth signaling through mTORC1 has been found to activate specific transcription factors, including HIF1α, SREBP1/2, and ATF4, and stimulate expression of their metabolic gene targets (Zhong et al. 2000; Hudson et al. 2002; Adams 2007; Porstmann et al. 2008; Düvel et al. 2010; Ben-Sahra et al. 2016; Park et al. 2017; Torrence et al. 2021). Canonically, each of these transcription factors are activated separately upon depletion of specific nutrients, including oxygen (HIF1α), lipids (SREBP1/2), and amino acids (ATF4) in an mTORC1-independent manner; such nutrient-deprived conditions inhibit mTORC1 signaling (Torrence and Manning 2018). However, under nutrient-rich conditions, these global regulators of specific metabolic pathways are activated together downstream of mTORC1 signaling to promote anabolic growth rather than their canonical roles in adaptation to nutrient depletion.

MYC (or c-MYC) is a ubiquitous growth-promoting basic helix–loop–helix (bHLH) transcription factor with a relatively rapid turnover rate, whose abundance is regulated by multiple signaling pathways (Stine et al. 2015). Notably, both the RAS-ERK and PI3K-AKT pathways direct phosphorylation events on the MYC protein that block its ubiquitination and degradation (Sears et al. 2000; Farrell and Sears 2014). In addition, mTORC1 can promote MYC accumulation by enhancing the translation of its mRNA, while also increasing the transactivating function of MYC at its downstream target genes (Gera et al. 2004; Wall et al. 2008; Csibi et al. 2014; Cho et al. 2021). In addition to being a downstream effector of growth signaling pathways, MYC (and to a lesser extent, its paralogs N-MYC and L-MYC) is itself a potent oncogenic protein that is pathologically activated in more than 20% of human cancers due typically to gene amplification or chromosomal translocations (Schaub et al. 2018; Dhanasekaran et al. 2022).

MYC drives transcription from DNA-binding elements called E-boxes, which are shared targets for bHLH transcription factors found in the promoters of thousands of genes, including those encoding key metabolic enzymes activated in proliferating cells (Stine et al. 2015). It has been proposed that under controlled physiological conditions MYC engages a canonical set of gene promoters through E-boxes for which it has a high affinity, whereas the oncogenic overexpression and dysregulation of MYC leads to its promiscuous regulation of genes with lower affinity E-boxes that are normally targets of other bHLH transcription factors (e.g., HIF1, SREBP). Thus, when considering the contributions of MYC to cancer development and progression, including the metabolic program of cancer cells, it is important to understand the mechanism(s) of its activation and the degree to which its abundance is elevated.

GROWTH SIGNALING PATHWAYS IMPACT THE METABOLIC HALLMARKS OF A CANCER CELL

Nearly all cancer cell–intrinsic metabolic properties, many of which are detailed in this collection, can be influenced by core oncogenic signaling pathways. Here, we discuss the transcriptional and posttranslational regulatory mechanisms through which the most commonly activated signaling pathways in human cancer (PI3K, RAS, mTORC1, and MYC) influence metabolic hallmarks of cancer cells, including enhanced nutrient uptake, production of energy and anabolic precursors, and synthesis of macromolecules (Fig. 1D).

Nutrient Acquisition

Most fundamental to cancer cell propagation and tumor growth is the need to acquire readily usable sources of carbon (e.g., glucose), nitrogen (e.g., glutamine), and any other essential nutrient that cells cannot make on their own (e.g., vitamins and essential amino acids). The nutrient content of a cancer cell's anatomic niche can vary widely, and hence the strategies employed to acquire essential nutrients from the microenvironment can be distinct between different cancer types, whether it be in nutrient-rich environments, such as in blood-borne cancers, or environments where nutrients are believed to be relatively scarce, such as in stroma-dominated cancers like pancreatic ductal adenocarcinoma (PDAC). In general, the various mechanisms of nutrient acquisition are under the control of the core oncogenic signaling pathways that drive tumorigenesis (Fig. 3).

The controlled uptake of glucose into cells and tissues is critical for both systemic and cellular metabolic homeostasis. As a primary downstream effector of insulin signaling, the PI3K-AKT pathway plays a critical role in stimulating postprandial glucose uptake into insulin-responsive tissues such as skeletal muscle and adipose, which is predominantly driven by translocation of the glucose transporter GLUT4 to the plasma membrane (Manning and Toker 2017). AKT signaling has also been found to be both necessary and sufficient for promoting plasma membrane accumulation and glucose uptake via GLUT1 (SLC2A1), which is the dominant glucose transporter expressed in many cancer cells (Rathmell et al. 2003; Wieman et al. 2007; Makinoshima et al. 2015; Siska et al. 2016). One molecular mechanism contributing to this posttranslational induction of GLUT1-driven glucose uptake is likely the AKT-mediated inhibitory phosphorylation of thioredoxin-interacting protein (TXNIP), which directs GLUT1 internalization and decreased glucose uptake (Hong et al. 2016; Waldhart et al. 2017). In addition, GLUT1 and other glucose transporters are under the transcriptional control of MYC and HIF1α (Gordan et al. 2007), the latter of which is canonically stabilized under conditions of hypoxia but can be up-regulated under normoxic conditions through an mTORC1-dependent increase in its translation (Zhong et al. 2000; Laughner et al. 2001; Hudson et al. 2002; Thomas et al. 2006; Düvel et al. 2010). Indeed, treatment of cell and tumor models with mTORC1 inhibitors, such as rapamycin or its analogs (collectively referred to as rapalogs), can lead to down-regulation of GLUT1 expression and glucose uptake via decreased HIF1α levels (Majumder et al. 2004; Düvel et al. 2010). Ultimately, the sustained uptake, cellular retention, and further metabolism

Cite this article as *Cold Spring Harb Perspect Med* doi: 10.1101/cshperspect.a041543

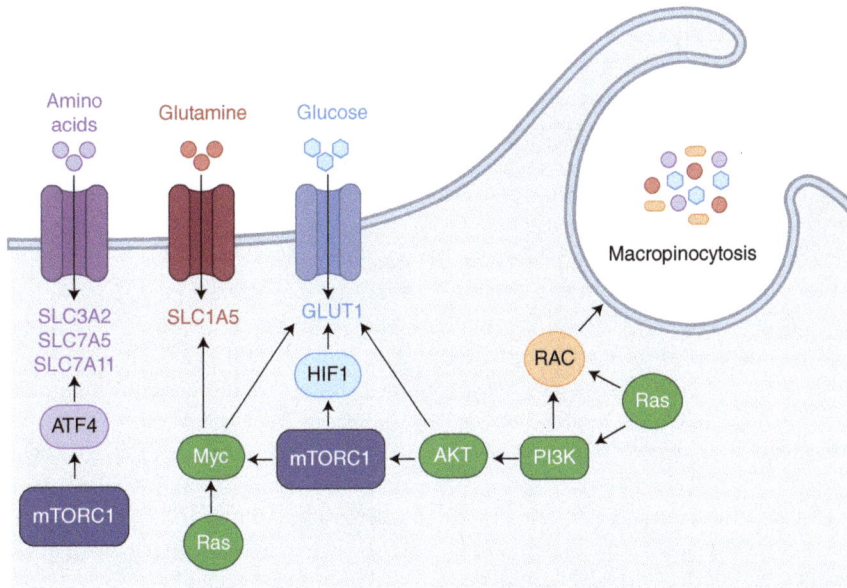

Figure 3. Oncogenic signaling pathways drive nutrient uptake. Oncogenes (green) and their downstream effectors, including the MYC, ATF4, and HIF1 transcription factors, promote the expression and/or cell surface residency of major transporters of glucose, glutamine, and a variety of amino acids. In addition, both PI3K and RAS can enhance RAC-mediated macropinocytosis, a form of bulk fluid phase uptake of extracellular materials. (Figure generated with BioRender; biorender.com.)

of glucose requires its phosphorylation and conversion to glucose 6-phosphate, which is also promoted by PI3K-AKT signaling (see below).

Amino acid uptake is also key to cell growth and is often enhanced in cancer cells. Glutamine provides a nitrogen source for the synthesis of nonessential amino acids (NEAAs) and nucleotides and can also serve as a carbon source for replenishing TCA cycle intermediates depleted in biosynthetic reactions (i.e., anaplerosis). In addition, glutamine and its deamidated product glutamate are also required as efflux substrates for specific amino acid antiporters that take up essential amino acids. While the uptake of glutamine and other amino acids can be mediated by several different transporters, which vary between cell types and tissues, much attention has been paid to a subset of amino acid antiporters that are frequently up-regulated in cancer. These include the neutral amino acid transporter SLC1A5, which is a major glutamine transporter in cancer cells, and two heterodimeric antiporters in SLC7A5-SLC3A2 (LAT1), which transport

large neutral amino acids such as leucine, and SLC7A11-SLC3A2 (xCT), which transports cystine, an oxidized dimer of cysteine and the primary form in serum (Bhutia et al. 2015; Kandasamy et al. 2018). MYC is a major driver of glutamine uptake and metabolism, and MYC-transformed cells have been found to be dependent on glutamine for their survival (Yuneva et al. 2007; Wise et al. 2008). Importantly, SLC1A5 is a canonical MYC target gene, making MYC activation in cancer a major determinant of SLC1A5 overexpression and enhanced glutamine uptake. Both MYC and HIF2α have also been found to stimulate the expression of SLC7A5, and the glutamine taken up through SLC1A5 can facilitate SLC7A5-mediated transport of essential amino acids (e.g., leucine) by acting as an efflux substrate (Gao et al. 2009; Nicklin et al. 2009; Elorza et al. 2012). Finally, the expression of SLC1A5, SLC7A5, SLC7A11, and SLC3A2, among other transporters, has been found to be increased downstream of mTORC1 signaling in an ATF4-dependent manner (Park et al. 2017; Torrence et al. 2021). Thus, these amino acid transporters commonly overexpressed in human cancers are likely induced by common oncogenic signaling pathways through the convergent regulation of these transcription factors.

While proliferating cells, including cancer cells, often exhibit enhanced capacity to synthesize both nucleotides and lipids de novo (discussed below), these key macromolecules for growth and proliferation can also be acquired from the tumor microenvironment via nucleotide salvage pathways, involving cell-surface transporters for nucleobases or nucleosides, or a variety of established transporters for fatty acids and cholesterol. However, relatively little is known about direct mechanisms through which core oncogenic signaling pathways control these transporters, especially those involved in nucleobase and nucleoside uptake. Much attention has been paid to the role of the long chain fatty acid transporter CD36, which is expressed in many cancer cells, as well as tumor stromal cells, and has been found to enhance tumor growth and metastasis (Guerrero-Rodríguez et al. 2022). Putative mechanisms through which oncogenic signaling pathways promote CD36 expression or overexpression in distinct cancer subtypes are unknown. However, a study in cardiomyocytes found that CD36 recruitment to the plasma membrane is controlled through a mechanism similar to that of GLUT4 in insulin-responsive skeletal muscle and adipose tissue (Samovski et al. 2012). This study indicated that, like GLUT4, CD36 resides on intracellular vesicles that are stimulated to translocate to the plasma membrane in response to AKT-dependent phosphorylation and inhibition of the Rab-GAP AS160/TBC1D4. If this mechanism is at play in cancer cells, then those with oncogenic PI3K-AKT signaling could have increased cell-surface CD36 and enhanced uptake of free fatty acids. CD36 has also been shown to stimulate intracellular signaling in response to a variety of extracellular ligands, including fatty acids, which may contribute to its role in promoting tumorigenesis (Guerrero-Rodríguez et al. 2022). In addition, fatty acid transport proteins (FATPs) of the SLC27A family, which also possess acyl-coenzyme A (CoA) synthetase activity, appear to play an important role in fatty acid uptake into cancer cells, but how oncogenic signaling events impact the abundance, localization, or function of these proteins in cancer is poorly understood (Acharya et al. 2023).

In addition to nutrient-specific plasma membrane transporters, fluid-phase endocytic processes such as macropinocytosis have also emerged as important mechanisms used by cancer cells to acquire key nutrients from the tumor microenvironment (Puccini et al. 2022). The interstitial environment immediately surrounding cancer cells can sometimes be nutrient-sparse but macromolecule-rich, with a prime example being pancreatic adenocarcinoma (PDAC). Abundant extracellular macromolecules, such as albumin, apolipoproteins, extracellular matrix proteins, cell debris, and necrotic cells, can be nonselectively engulfed into intracellular vesicles (macropinosomes) and trafficked to the lysosome for hydrolysis into their nutrient components. The resulting amino acids, fatty acids, nucleosides, and carbohydrates can then be released into the cytosol for use by the cancer cell (Puccini et al. 2022). There is much evidence that oncogenic signaling pathways can promote macropinocytosis in certain types of cancer. This cellular process was first described to be induced by oncogenic RAS (Bar-Sagi and Feramisco 1986), which is a major oncogenic driver of PDAC, and macropinocytosis-mediated scavenging of extracellular protein has been found to serve as an important alternative route of amino acid uptake into RAS-transformed cancer cells (Commisso et al. 2013; Kamphorst et al. 2015; Palm et al. 2015; Davidson et al. 2017). Oncogenic PI3K signaling, via direct activating mutations or loss of PTEN, have also been found to promote macropinocytosis (Kim et al. 2018; Jayashankar and Edinger 2020), and PI3K has been suggested to be both necessary and sufficient for the induction of macropinocytosis downstream of oncogenic RAS (Rodriguez-Viciana et al. 1997). Mechanistically, the initiation of macropinocytosis requires activation of the small GTPase RAC1 (Fig. 3), which induces reorganization of the actin cytoskeleton to promote membrane ruffling and engulfment of extracellular material into macropinosomes (Puccini et al. 2022). Several distinct

Cite this article as *Cold Spring Harb Perspect Med* doi: 10.1101/cshperspect.a041543

mechanisms have been uncovered by which oncogenic RAS and PI3K signaling activate RAC1, one of which is the plasma membrane recruitment of RAC1 GEFs via binding directly to the PI3K lipid product PIP_3. A recent study also found a new role for the enzyme ATP citrate lyase (ACLY), which catalyzes the cytosolic conversion of citrate to acetyl-CoA, a substrate for both de novo lipid synthesis and protein acetylation, in promoting macropinocytosis in cancer cells (Puccini et al. 2023). ACLY was found to interact with the cortical actin cytoskeleton and provide substrate for acetylation of an actin capping protein that controls the actin remodeling underlying macropinocytosis. Interestingly, AKT directly phosphorylates and promotes the activity of ACLY (Berwick et al. 2002; Lee et al. 2014; Martinez Calejman et al. 2020), raising the untested possibility that AKT signaling might influence macropinocytosis via its regulation of ACLY.

Bioenergetics and Redox Homeostasis

To proliferate, both normal and cancer cells must sustain catabolic pathways to provide a source of energy, in the form of ATP. However, the demand for ATP in a proliferating cell is believed to be only modestly higher than in a quiescent or terminally differentiated cell maintaining its homeostatic state (Lunt and Vander Heiden 2011). Proliferating cells exhibit a larger demand for anabolic processes to support the synthesis of macromolecules needed to produce more cells. Importantly, catabolic and anabolic metabolism must be carefully coordinated in proliferating cells to maintain balance between reduction and oxidation (redox) states. Thus, the signaling pathways driving cancer development and progression must promote anabolic growth within this framework (Fig. 4).

Most tumors take up a lot more glucose than normal tissues, and this glucose is trapped within the cell and activated for further metabolism by its conversion to glucose 6-phosphate through the action of hexokinases (HKs). This nearly universal property underlies the widespread use of fluorodeoxyglucose-positron emission tomography (FDG-PET) for detecting and monitoring tumors. There is evidence that oncogenic signaling

pathways drive this behavior, as pathway inhibitors can decrease the tumor FDG-PET signal, an effect that might predict subsequent treatment response in some settings (e.g., Engelman et al. 2008; Ben-Haim and Ell 2009; Day et al. 2019). The PI3K-AKT-mTORC1 pathway promotes glucose uptake and its glycolytic conversion to lactate (e.g., aerobic glycolysis) through multiple mechanisms (Fig. 4; Elstrom et al. 2004; Majumder et al. 2004; Düvel et al. 2010; Hoxhaj and Manning 2020; Hosios and Manning 2021). HK2 appears to be the primary hexokinase expressed in many cancers and has been found to be essential for tumor formation and progression in mouse tumor models, including those driven by the PI3K-AKT pathway (Patra et al. 2013; Nogueira et al. 2018). AKT signaling has been found to promote HK2 subcellular localization to the surface of the mitochondria, where its activity is believed to be highest and it has the capacity to suppress apoptosis (Robey and Hay 2006). AKT appears to directly phosphorylate HK2 and stimulate its mitochondrial localization in cardiomyocytes (Roberts et al. 2013), and a separate study found that HK2 phosphorylation influences its activity, glucose uptake, and lactate production (Yang et al. 2018). Interestingly, a specific splice variant of activated K-RAS (K-RAS4A) was found to directly bind to HK1 at the mitochondria and promote its enzymatic activity, suggesting an additional direct mechanism through which oncogenic signaling can promote glucose metabolism in cancer cells (Amendola et al. 2019). The PI3K-AKT pathway may exert additional direct stimulatory effects on glycolytic enzymes that function downstream of hexokinase to enhance the glycolytic catabolism of glucose-6-phosphate (Deprez et al. 1997; Hu et al. 2016; Lee et al. 2017; Hoxhaj and Manning 2020). However, like glucose transporters, HK isoforms and glycolytic enzymes are highly expressed in cancer cells, and this is mediated, in large part, through a combination of transcription factors downstream of the core oncogenic pathways, including MYC and HIF1 (Semenza 2003; Stine et al. 2015).

In many cancer cells, as well as normal cells induced to proliferate, the excess glucose taken up is glycolytically converted to lactate, thus yielding just two molecules of ATP, in contrast

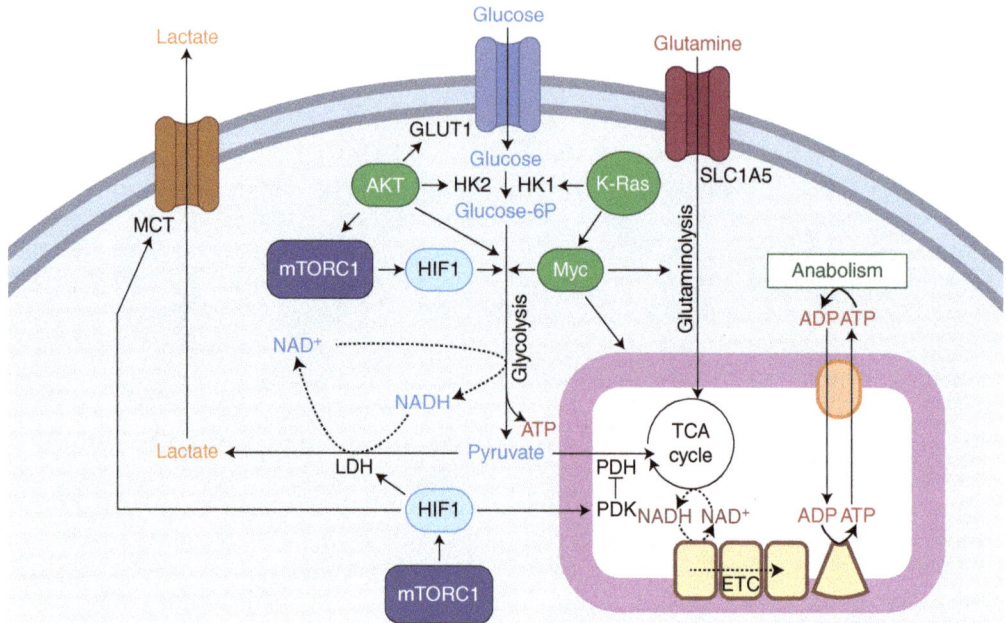

Figure 4. Oncogenic signaling pathways drive aerobic glycolysis, while maintaining mitochondrial function. AKT stimulates an increase in glycolysis by directly phosphorylating and regulating the activity of a subset of glycolytic enzymes, while also increasing the expression of nearly all the enzymes of glycolysis, as well as lactate dehydrogenase (LDH), pyruvate dehydrogenase (PDH) kinase (PDK), and the monocarboxylate transporters (MCTs), via a mechanistic target of rapamycin (mTOR) complex 1 (mTORC1)-mediated increase in the HIF1 transcription factor. RAS4A binds to and stimulates the activity of HK1. MYC also stimulates expression of glycolytic enzymes, as well as those of glutamine uptake and catabolism (glutaminolysis) and mitochondrial function. Finally, oncogenic signaling can influence the electron transport chain (ETC) and tricarboxylic acid (TCA) cycle indirectly by promoting ATP turnover through anabolic processes. (Figure generated with BioRender; biorender.com.)

to its full oxidation in the mitochondria yielding more than 30 ATPs (Lunt and Vander Heiden 2011). The advantages of aerobic glycolysis to rapidly proliferating cells remains a point of debate (DeBerardinis and Chandel 2020). However, a key metabolic property of aerobic glycolysis is that it is self-sustaining with respect to redox homeostasis, as the cytosolic NAD^+ essential for glycolysis can be rapidly restored through the NADH-oxidizing conversion of pyruvate to lactate via lactate dehydrogenase (LDH). Subsequent secretion of lactate through monocarboxylate transporters (MCTs) is then essential to maintain the directionality of the reversible LDH reaction (Fig. 4). This preferential directing of glycolytic pyruvate toward conversion to lactate and away from mitochondrial metabolism

appears to be reinforced in cancer cells via the common transcriptional up-regulation of isoforms of LDH and MCT, as well as pyruvate dehydrogenase (PDH) kinase (PDK), which attenuates PDH activity and the entry of pyruvate carbon into the TCA cycle. This transcriptional control is likely driven, in part, by oncogenic signaling events leading to activation of MYC and HIF1 (Semenza 2003; Stine et al. 2015), although FOXM1 has been implicated in the increased expression of LDH in *PIK3CA*-mutant breast cancers (Ros et al. 2020).

Mitochondria play an important role in the proliferative metabolism of cancer cells, contributing to both their bioenergetic and anabolic demands. Like normal cells, cancer cell mitochondria are able to oxidize various substrates,

 Cite this article as *Cold Spring Harb Perspect Med* doi: 10.1101/cshperspect.a041543

including glucose-derived pyruvate, amino acids, and lipids to generate ATP. While MYC has gene targets that can enhance mitochondrial function (Stine et al. 2015), there is relatively little known about direct control mechanisms through which oncogenic signaling stimulates mitochondrial metabolism in cancer cells. As alluded to above, a driving force behind aerobic glycolysis in cancer cells is the need to regenerate NAD^+, which can also occur through various mitochondrial redox shuttles. These shuttles, which can become saturated in highly glycolytic cells, ultimately require the donation of electrons from NADH in the mitochondrial matrix to complex I of the electron transport chain (ETC). The continued flow of electrons through the ETC is dictated by the rate of intracellular ATP turnover to sustain ample concentrations of ADP as a substrate in the mitochondrial matrix for ATP synthase (complex V) (Luengo et al. 2021; Wang et al. 2022). Therefore, the cellular rate of ATP consumption influences both mitochondrial respiration and aerobic glycolysis (Fig. 4). As described below, oncogenic signaling pathways drive ATP-consuming anabolic processes to promote cell growth, the most energetically demanding of which is protein synthesis. Thus, these pathways likely influence compartment-specific redox balance indirectly. Finally, the tricarboxylic acid (TCA) cycle is an important source of intermediates that serve as precursors for the synthesis of nonessential amino acids, nucleotides, and lipids. Replenishment of these intermediates through anaplerotic reactions is required to maintain TCA cycle function. One mechanism promoting anaplerosis is the MYC-induced expression of SLC1A5, which imports glutamine, and the glutaminolysis enzymes glutaminase (GLS) and glutamate dehydrogenase (GDH), which convert glutamine to the TCA-cycle intermediate α-ketoglutarate (Fig. 4; Wise et al. 2008).

Anabolic Cofactor and Precursor Synthesis

The cofactors and precursors required for the synthesis of key macromolecules essential for cell growth and division, including proteins, nucleic acids, and lipids, are not inherently abundant in cells. Growth factor signaling pathways, especially those that are oncogenically activated in cancer, can promote the exogenous uptake of certain precursor nutrients (see above) and stimulate the de novo synthesis of certain cofactors and macromolecular building blocks.

An abundance of reducing power in the form of NADPH is required for the synthesis of all dNTPs and lipids plus some nonessential amino acids and is critical for the protection of cells from oxidative stress. There are many metabolic pathways in the cell that can reduce $NADP^+$ to generate NADPH, the most prominent of which is the oxidative pentose phosphate pathway (oxPPP) in the cytosol and one-carbon metabolism pathway in the mitochondria. Through the action of two dehydrogenases, the oxPPP produces two molecules of NADPH while converting glucose-6-phosphate into the ribose-5-phosphate required for nucleotide synthesis (Fig. 5A). A major metabolic determinant of glucose-6-phosphate flux into the oxPPP, rather than into glycolysis, is the availability of $NADP^+$, the rate-limiting substrate for the first enzyme in the oxPPP, glucose-6-phosphate dehydrogenase (G6PD). Therefore, sustained flux into the oxPPP requires the continuous turnover of NADPH to $NADP^+$ during reductive biosynthesis (e.g., lipid synthesis) or neutralization of reactive oxygen species (ROS), which likely contribute to the frequent up-regulation of this pathway in cancer (Patra and Hay 2014). However, the intracellular pool of $NADP^+$ available for NADPH-producing dehydrogenases such as G6PD can also be increased through the action of NAD kinase (NADK), which through its metabolite kinase activity can convert a portion of the much more abundant cytosolic pool of NAD^+ to $NADP^+$. AKT can directly phosphorylate NADK and stimulate an increase in its catalytic activity, thus linking both normal and oncogenic PI3K-AKT signaling to the regulated expansion of intracellular $NADP^+$ and NADPH pools (Hoxhaj et al. 2019). In addition, the expression of NADPH-producing enzymes is often elevated in cancer cells via the action of transcription factors that can be activated downstream of oncogenic signaling pathways, including SREBP, ATF4, and NRF2 (Düvel et al. 2010; DeNicola et al. 2011; Mitsuishi et al. 2012; Torrence et al. 2021).

ATF4, for instance, drives expression of key one-carbon metabolism enzymes that can promote NADPH generation in the mitochondrial matrix (Fan et al. 2014; Ben-Sahra et al. 2016; Yang and Vousden 2016; Torrence et al. 2021).

While quiescent cells predominantly acquire the nucleotides they need for RNA synthesis and genome maintenance through salvage pathways requiring uptake of nucleosides or nucleobases, proliferating cells, such as cancer cells or activated immune cells, stimulate an increase in de novo nucleotide synthesis pathways to meet the extra demands for growth and proliferation (Fig. 5B; Ali and Ben-Sahra 2023). Proliferating cells achieve this by increasing metabolic flux through both the nucleotide synthesis pathways themselves and the metabolic pathways that produce essential precursors for nucleotide synthesis. A key example of the latter is the PPP, which provides the ribose sugar moiety for all nucleotides. In addition to the oxPPP (discussed above), growth factor and oncogenic signaling pathways can also enhance the nonoxidative PPP, which is a series of reversible reactions that convert intermediates of glycolysis into ribose-5-phosphate without generating NADPH. An isoform of the enzyme required to make ribose-5-phosphate from both the oxidative and nonoxidative PPPs, ribose-5-phosphate isomerase (RPIA), can be transcriptionally up-regulated by MYC downstream of KRAS, as observed in mouse models of PDAC (Ying et al. 2012; Santana-Codina et al. 2018). Bicarbonate (HCO_3^-) is a carbon source required for catalytic assembly of both pyrimidine and purine bases. A specific bicarbonate transporter, SLC4A7, is translated in response to growth factor signaling through mTORC1 to provide the excess intracellular bicarbonate required for de novo nucleotide synthesis in growing cells and tumors, beyond the homeostatic role of bicarbonate in maintaining cellular pH balance (Ali et al. 2022). In addition to promoting the uptake of glutamine, a major nitrogen source for both pyrimidine and purine base synthesis, MYC drives expression of several genes encoding the core metabolic enzymes of the de novo pyrimidine and purine synthesis pathways, contributing to the common up-regulation of both pathways in cancer (Stine et al.

2015). mTORC1 signaling has been found to promote an increase in de novo purine synthesis in a manner dependent on the transcription factors MYC, SREBP, and ATF4, the latter of which promotes expression of genes encoding mitochondrial one-carbon metabolism enzymes required to produce the formyl units essential for two reactions in the catalytic assembly of the purine base (Ben-Sahra et al. 2016). Purine synthesis is also under acute regulation by growth factor and oncogenic RAS stimulated signaling pathways, with ERK2 directly phosphorylating and activating the de novo purine synthesis enzyme phosphoribosylformylglycinamidine synthase (PFAS) (Ali et al. 2020). Both the RAS-ERK and mTORC1-S6K1 pathways can also acutely stimulate de novo pyrimidine synthesis via distinct phosphorylation sites on CAD (carbamoyl-phosphate synthetase, aspartate transcarbamoylase, dihydroorotase). This large multifunctional enzyme catalyzes the first three steps in this pathway, and its phosphorylation stimulates its activity and metabolic flux through pyrimidine synthesis (Graves et al. 2000; Ben-Sahra et al. 2013; Robitaille et al. 2013). Thus, the core signaling pathways activated in human cancers promote, at multiple levels, the de novo synthesis of both purine and pyrimidine nucleotides, ensuring ample supplies for the enhanced RNA and DNA synthesis required for cell growth and division.

Human cells can produce 11 out of the 20 proteinogenic amino acids required, and the metabolic pathways that produce most of these NEAAs are often up-regulated in cancer (Fig. 5C; Choi and Coloff 2019). The NEAA glutamate, generally produced via GLS from exogenously acquired glutamine, a process promoted by MYC, serves as the essential nitrogen source for converting α-keto acids to α-amino acids through transaminase reactions. Oncogenic MYC has also been found to promote the synthesis of proline from glutamate (Liu et al. 2012). Importantly, the metabolic pathways producing the specific α-keto acid substrates, the transaminases themselves, and other enzymes of NEAA synthesis are often elevated in human cancers, with much of this originating at the level of gene expression. While this is likely the product

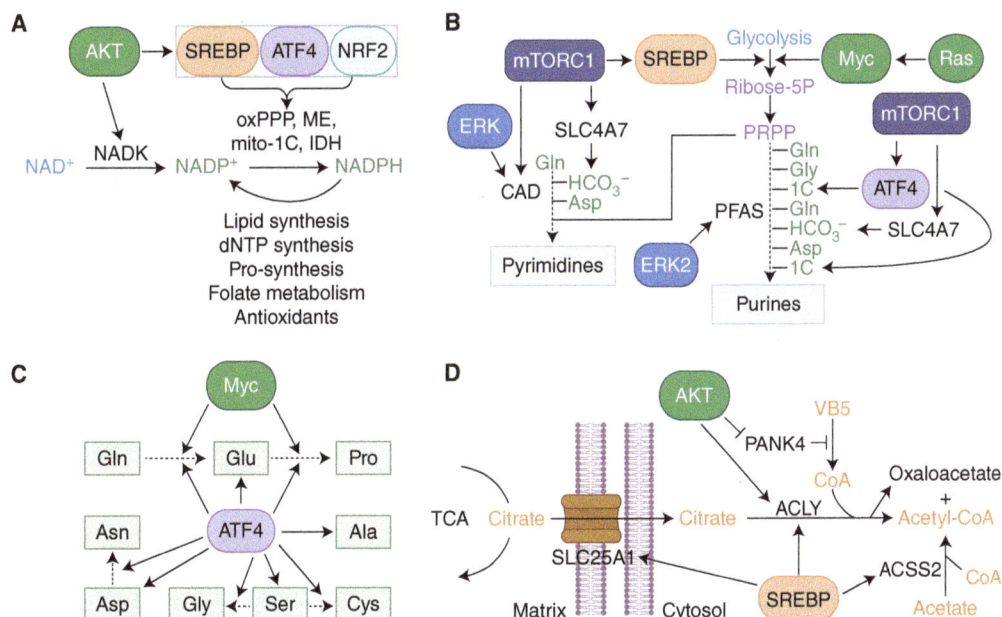

Figure 5. Oncogenic signaling pathways enhance the production of anabolic precursors and cofactors. (*A*) Components of oncogenic signaling pathways can increase the availability of cellular reducing power. NADPH is produced by enzymes that reduce $NADP^+$, which can be transcriptionally up-regulated by growth factor–regulated transcription factors. $NADP^+$ is regenerated through a variety of reducing cellular processes and can be produced through the NAD kinase (NADK)-dependent phosphorylation of NAD^+, an activity enhanced by AKT-mediated phosphorylation of NADK. (*B*) Oncogenic signaling pathways increase de novo nucleotide synthesis through a variety of mechanisms. SREBP and MYC increase the oxidative and nonoxidative pentose phosphate pathway (PPP), respectively, to increase ribose-5-phosphate, which upon conversion to PRPP provides the ribose moiety to both pyrimidines and purines. Other moieties comprising the pyrimidine and purine bases are assembled in a series of metabolic reactions, with specific oncogenic signaling components influencing either the nucleotide synthesis enzymes themselves (e.g., CAD, PFAS) or the availability of substrates of the enzymes (e.g., 1C units, HCO_3^-), as depicted. (*C*) The enzymes of nonessential amino acid (NEAA) synthesis are transcriptionally induced by MYC and ATF4, which can be activated downstream of oncogenic signaling pathways. (*D*) Oncogenic signaling pathways can enhance the production of cytosolic acetyl-CoA. AKT directly phosphorylates PANK4 and ACLY to respectively increase CoA synthesis and the conversion of cytosolic citrate to acetyl-CoA and oxaloacetate. The SREBP transcription factors can increase expression of SLC25A1, ACLY, and ACSS2 to increase cytosolic acetyl-CoA production. (Figure generated with BioRender; biorender.com.)

of several different transcription factors active in cancer cells, nearly all enzymes involved in NEAA synthesis are gene targets of the ATF4 transcription factor, which, as stated above, can be activated under pro-growth conditions by mTORC1 signaling (Ben-Sahra et al. 2016; Park et al. 2017; Torrence et al. 2021). Interestingly, while these NEAAs are required for protein synthesis, they vary from essential amino acids in that they are also utilized for a variety of other metabolic processes necessary for cell growth and survival, such as nucleotide and glutathione synthesis, perhaps explaining why human cells have maintained the capacity to synthesize these particular amino acids (Choi and Coloff 2019).

In addition to being an essential TCA-cycle carbon source in the mitochondria and the substrate for protein acetylation in all cellular compartments, acetyl-CoA is the building block from which all intracellular fatty acids and sterols are synthesized de novo in the cytosol (Fig. 5D; Guertin and Wellen 2023). The cofactor CoA is the major carrier of activated acyl groups in the cell, including acetate and the long chain fatty acids that comprise phospholipids. CoA is synthesized de novo from the essential vitamin pantothenate (vitamin B5), and this biosynthetic pathway has been found to be acutely and directly stimulated by PI3K-AKT signaling. This regulation is mediated in part by the AKT-mediated inhibitory phosphorylation of pantothenate kinase 4 (PANK4), a rate-limiting suppressor of CoA synthesis (Dibble et al. 2022). As mentioned above, AKT also directly phosphorylates and stimulates ACLY, the enzyme that produces cytosolic acetyl-CoA from TCA cycle–derived citrate (Berwick et al. 2002; Lee et al. 2014; Martinez Calejman et al. 2020). Therefore, PI3K-Akt signaling acutely and concomitantly stimulates the carbon acquisition (via glucose uptake), cofactor synthesis, and enzyme activity required to produce cytosolic acetyl-CoA pools. In addition, the proteins required for the synthesis of cytosolic acetyl-CoA, including the mitochondrial citrate carrier (CIC/SLC25A1), ACLY, and acyl-CoA synthetase short-chain family member 2 (ACSS2), which can generate acetyl-CoA from acetate and CoA, are all encoded by gene targets of the SREBP family of transcription factors and are therefore elevated in their expression downstream of the PI3K-mTOR pathway (Fig. 5D; Porstmann et al. 2008; Düvel et al. 2010).

Macromolecular Synthesis

Ultimately, the growth of both normal and cancer cells requires the conversion of nutrients, energy, and reducing equivalents into the macromolecules that comprise cells, which must double their content prior to cell division. While macromolecular composition can vary widely between cell types, generally cellular dry mass is comprised of >50% protein, followed by nucleic acids and lipids, with smaller proportions of complex carbohydrates (Lunt and Vander Heiden 2011). While the core signaling pathways driving cell growth and division promote precursor acquisition and synthesis (as described above), they also stimulate macromolecular synthesis from these precursors.

The amino acid components of protein are the biggest contributor to biomass in proliferating cells (Hosios et al. 2016), and the stimulation of protein synthesis is a fundamental function of growth factor and oncogenic signaling pathways (Fig. 6A). Oncogenic RTK, RAS, and PI3K signaling can all activate mTORC1 in a growth factor–independent manner, and mTORC1 enhances protein synthesis at multiple levels, from acute induction of mRNA translation initiation to the promotion of ribosome biogenesis leading to a global increase in cellular protein synthesis. While the molecular mechanisms have been reviewed elsewhere (Valvezan and Manning 2019; Liu and Sabatini 2020), mTORC1 acutely stimulates cap-dependent translation from mRNAs containing a $5'$-terminal oligopyrimidine (TOP) cis-regulatory element, which include those encoding nearly all protein subunits of the ribosome (rProteins) and the majority of translation factors. This mTORC1-dependent regulation is achieved, in part, by controlling access to the major mRNA $5'$-cap-binding protein eukaryotic translation initiation factor 4E (eIF4E), which recruits the translation initiation complex. Parallel to mTORC1, oncogenic signaling through the RAS-ERK pathway can independently promote translation initiation through phosphorylation and activation of eIF4E by MAPK-interacting Ser/Thr kinase 1 (MNK1), which is activated directly downstream of ERK (Kovalski et al. 2022). Importantly, eIF4E has been found to be genetically limiting for RAS-driven cellular transformation and tumorigenesis (Truitt et al. 2015). While mTORC1 stimulates the mRNA translation of ribosomal proteins and translation factors, MYC can induce their gene transcription, thereby further enhancing global protein synthesis downstream of oncogenic signaling pathways in cancer (Fig. 6A; van Riggelen et al. 2010; Stine et al. 2015).

Proliferating cells, whether normal or cancerous, boost nucleotide synthesis to meet the increased demand for nucleic acids, the most abundant of which are ribosomal RNA (rRNA) and genomic DNA. As described above, both mTORC1 and MYC coinduce nucleotide synthesis and ribosome biogenesis. A likely reason that these processes are coupled in their regulation is the fact that ribosomes are comprised of >50% rRNA, and ribosome biogenesis substantially increases the demand for nucleotides to support rRNA synthesis. To reinforce this coupling, both mTORC1 and MYC exert downstream control of rRNA synthesis via the RNA Pol I– and III–mediated transcription of the genes encoding the four major rRNAs, as well as their splicing, maturation, and assembly into ribosomes (Fig. 6A; van Riggelen et al. 2010; Valvezan and Manning 2019). Outside of supplying more nucleotides, mechanisms of direct control of DNA synthesis by oncogenic signaling pathways are less well defined. Proliferating cells do not appear to maintain substantial pools of dNTPs to facilitate DNA synthesis, rather, they draw from a larger pool of NTPs that ribonucleotide reductase (RNR) converts to dNTPs for

DNA replication as cells enter S phase of the cell cycle, when dNTP concentrations are at their highest (Aye et al. 2015). Oncogenic signaling pathways can indirectly influence this conversion through their promotion of the G_1 to S phase transition, which the RAS-ERK pathway does through multiple downstream mechanisms (Lavoie et al. 2020), some of which can also increase RNR subunit expression, stability, and function in S phase (Fig. 6B; Aye et al. 2015). Among other cell-cycle-regulating transcription factors, MYC also likely induces expression of RNR subunits (Liu et al. 2008).

Like nucleotide synthesis, de novo lipid synthesis might be limited outside of specialized cell

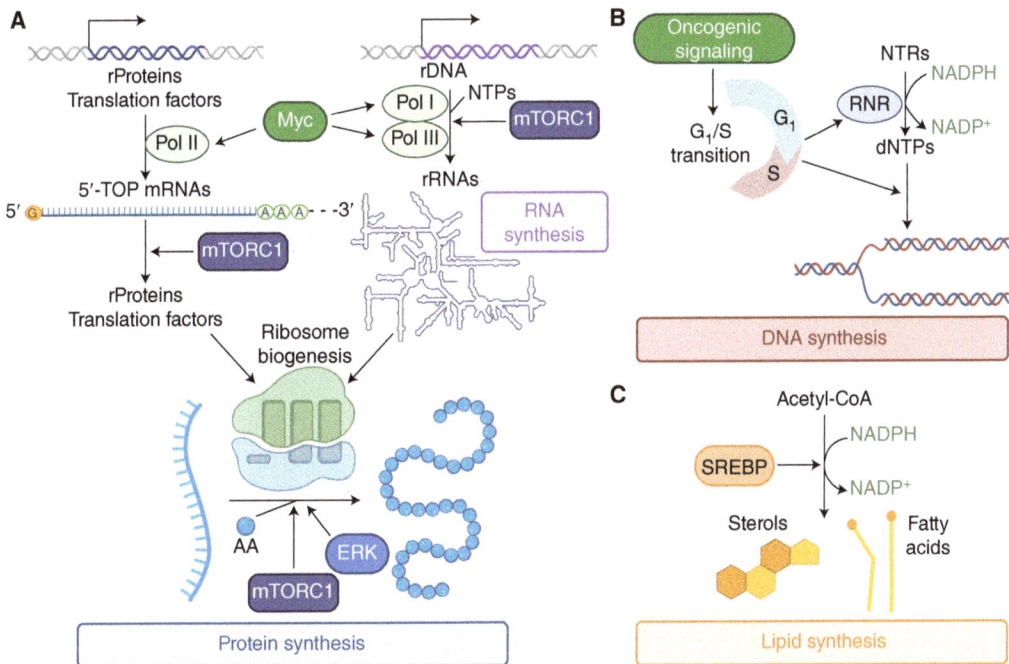

Figure 6. Oncogenic signaling pathways stimulate the synthesis of macromolecules required for cell growth and proliferation. (A) Components of oncogenic signaling pathways promote ribosome biogenesis and protein synthesis. MYC drives the pol II–mediated transcription of genes for rProteins and translation factors, which are encoded by mRNAs with 5′TOP sequences that are selectively translated in response to mechanistic target of rapamycin (mTOR) complex 1 (mTORC1) signaling. Both MYC and mTORC1 promote the pol I– and III–mediated expression of ribosomal RNA (rRNAs), the most abundant RNA species in cells, which complex with the newly synthesized rProteins to produce ribosomes. In addition, both mTORC1 and ERK signaling promote cap-dependent translation initiation. (B) Oncogenic signaling events promote cell-cycle entry at the G_1/S transition, at which point ribonucleotide reductase (RNR) converts NTPs into the dNTPs needed for DNA replication during S phase. (C) Oncogenic signaling promotes de novo lipid synthesis via the SREBP transcription factors, which induce the expression of nearly all enzymes required for sterol and fatty acid synthesis. (Figure generated with BioRender; biorender.com.)

types and tissues but is stimulated in proliferating cells, including cancer cells (Menendez and Lupu 2007; Snaebjornsson et al. 2020). In addition to the mechanisms increasing cytosolic NADPH and acetyl-CoA discussed above, both of which are needed in high abundance for de novo lipid synthesis, the enzymes of fatty acid and sterol synthesis are transcriptionally induced downstream of growth factor and oncogenic signaling pathways, at least in part, through mTORC1-mediated induction of SREBP1 and SREBP2 (Fig. 6C; Porstmann et al. 2008; Düvel et al. 2010). Expression of oncogenic RAS and PI3K is sufficient to stimulate de novo lipid synthesis in cells, and this induction is dependent on mTORC1 and its regulation SREBP1/2 (Ricoult et al. 2016). The fatty acids produced in response to mTORC1-SREBP regulation may be particularly important for membrane phospholipid production, and mTORC1 has been found to prevent the lysosome-mediated turnover of membrane phospholipids (Hosios et al. 2022). Thus, oncogenic signaling likely drives de novo lipid synthesis to support the expansion of both organellar and plasma membranes in growing cells.

Other Pathways in Cancer Metabolism

There is evidence that several additional metabolic enzymes and pathways are also controlled by growth factor signaling pathways, at least in part through mTORC1 activation, and are up-regulated in cancer cells. While the proposed mechanisms and molecular consequences vary between studies, mTORC1 signaling has been shown to enhance the S-adenosylmethionine (SAM)-dependent N^6-methyadenosine (m^6A) methylation of mRNAs to enhance cell and tumor growth (Cho et al. 2021; Villa et al. 2021). Polyamines (putrescine, spermidine, and spermine) have been found to play multiple functions in promoting cell growth and survival, and their synthesis and accumulation are frequently elevated in cancer through the action of oncogenic signaling pathways (Casero et al. 2018). For instance, MYC has been found to promote expression of ornithine decarboxylase (ODC), the rate-limiting enzyme of polyamine

synthesis that yields putrescine, and oncogenic RAS has been proposed to promote the stabilization of ODC mRNA through mTORC1 signaling (Bello-Fernandez et al. 1993; Origanti et al. 2012). In addition, oncogenic KRAS has been shown to drive polyamine synthesis in PDAC models through a MEK-dependent transcriptional mechanism affecting ODC and the enzyme ornithine aminotransferase (OAT), which mediates synthesis of the polyamine precursor ornithine from glutamine (Lee et al. 2023). The synthesis of longer chain polyamines, spermidine and spermine, from putrescine requires the production of decarboxy-SAM from SAM via the enzyme SAM decarboxylase (AMD1), the stability and activity of which has been found to be promoted by mTORC1 signaling in PTEN-deficient prostate cancer (Zabala-Letona et al. 2017). Through its induction of ATF4, mTORC1 signaling also increases synthesis of the Glu-Cys-Gly tripeptide glutathione, the most abundant antioxidant molecule in cells, via transcriptional up-regulation of the major cystine transporter SLC7A11 (Torrence et al. 2021). PI3K-AKT signaling also enhances glutathione production by up-regulating the expression of glutathione biosynthesis genes through mechanisms that stabilize the transcription factor NRF2 (Lien et al. 2016). While additional molecular mechanisms await discovery, the core oncogenic signaling pathways likely influence nearly all aspects of the metabolic program of cancer cells.

THERAPEUTIC PERSPECTIVES AND CONCLUSIONS

With the knowledge that oncogenic signaling pathways control key metabolic processes in tumors, one must consider these effects when predicting and evaluating the response or resistance to therapeutics targeting specific oncogenic alterations. Pharmacological inhibitors of RTKs, PI3K, B-RAF, and mTOR have all been approved for clinical use in different cancer settings. It is possible that the most effective use of these inhibitors would take advantage of specific metabolic dependencies that might arise from their

 Cite this article as *Cold Spring Harb Perspect Med* doi: 10.1101/cshperspect.a041543

use, by combining them with inhibitors of specific metabolic pathways for instance. However, an important feature of metabolic control by cancer-driving signaling pathways that should be evident from the discussion above is that multiple layers of redundancy have evolved in the control of critical metabolic pathways in cancer cells. Furthermore, the most common oncogenic events in human cancer activate RTKs, RAS, or PI3K signaling, which all converge on a shared set of downstream effectors, such as mTORC1 and MYC, to drive the key features of cancer metabolism that promote uncontrolled cell growth. This redundancy in growth signaling appears to underlie both innate and acquired resistance to oncogene-targeted therapeutics. For instance, while allosteric mTORC1 inhibitors, such as rapalogs, have shown limited clinical effectiveness as single-agent cancer treatments, sustained activation (or reactivation) of mTORC1 following treatment with an oncogene-targeted therapy has been found in multiple independent studies to drive resistance to that therapy (for review, see Ilagan and Manning 2016). Relatedly, sustained activation of SREBP1 and de novo lipid synthesis has been found to underlie the resistance of BRAF-mutant melanoma to BRAF inhibitors (Talebi et al. 2018). Specific metabolic vulnerabilities might also arise from the uncontrolled nature of growth signaling pathways in tumors. An example of this has been revealed in studies of cell and tumor models of small cell lung cancer and TSC, which are respectively driven by aberrant activation of MYC and mTORC1, two signaling effectors that drive both nucleotide synthesis and ribosome biogenesis. These cells and tumors with enhanced ribosome biogenesis are highly susceptible to clinically used compounds that inhibit the synthesis of guanine nucleotides, which are the most abundant class of nucleotide comprising the rRNA that must be produced in abundance in such settings (Valvezan et al. 2017, 2020; Huang et al. 2018, 2021). Finally, it is also possible that the use of specific signaling pathway inhibitors, such as rapalogs, might simply slow the growth of tumors while increasing tumor cell fitness, in part by relieving the anabolic burden on such cells. These are all important considerations for

ongoing studies to unravel the complex relationship between cancer signaling networks and metabolic networks and how best to treat cancers with the growing arsenal of pharmacological compounds that target these networks.

ACKNOWLEDGMENTS

The authors apologize to colleagues whose work they were unable to discuss due to space constraints. Research in the Manning and Dibble laboratories related to the subject of this review was supported by grants to B.D.M. from the NIH (R35-CA197459 and P01-CA120964) and C.C.D. from the V Foundation for Cancer Research (V Scholar Grant V2019-009). The authors declare no competing interests.

REFERENCES

Acharya R, Shetty SS, Kumari NS. 2023. Fatty acid transport proteins (FATPs) in cancer. *Chem Phys Lipids* **250:** 105269. doi:10.1016/j.chemphyslip.2022.105269

Adams CM. 2007. Role of the transcription factor ATF4 in the anabolic actions of insulin and the anti-anabolic actions of glucocorticoids. *J Biol Chem* **282:** 16744–16753. doi:10.1074/jbc.M610510200

Ali ES, Ben-Sahra I. 2023. Regulation of nucleotide metabolism in cancers and immune disorders. *Trends Cell Biol* S0962-8924(23)00044-2. doi:10.1016/j.tcb.2023.03.003

Ali ES, Sahu U, Villa E, O'Hara BP, Gao P, Beaudet C, Wood AW, Asara JM, Ben-Sahra I. 2020. ERK2 phosphorylates PFAS to mediate posttranslational control of de novo purine synthesis. *Mol Cell* **78:** 1178–1191.e6. doi:10.1016/j.molcel.2020.05.001

Ali ES, Lipońska A, O'Hara BP, Amici DR, Torno MD, Gao P, Asara JM, Yap MF, Mendillo ML, Ben-Sahra I. 2022. The mTORC1-SLC4A7 axis stimulates bicarbonate import to enhance de novo nucleotide synthesis. *Mol Cell* **82:** 3284–3298.e7. doi:10.1016/j.molcel.2022.06.008

Amendola CR, Mahaffey JP, Parker SJ, Ahearn IM, Chen WC, Zhou M, Court H, Shi J, Mendoza SL, Morten MJ, et al. 2019. KRAS4A directly regulates hexokinase 1. *Nature* **576:** 482–486. doi:10.1038/s41586-019-1832-9

Aye Y, Li M, Long MJ, Weiss RS. 2015. Ribonucleotide reductase and cancer: biological mechanisms and targeted therapies. *Oncogene* **34:** 2011–2021. doi:10.1038/onc.2014.155

Bar-Sagi D, Feramisco JR. 1986. Induction of membrane ruffling and fluid-phase pinocytosis in quiescent fibroblasts by ras proteins. *Science* **233:** 1061–1068. doi:10.1126/science.3090687

Bello-Fernandez C, Packham G, Cleveland JL. 1993. The ornithine decarboxylase gene is a transcriptional target of c-Myc. *Proc Natl Acad Sci* **90:** 7804–7808. doi:10.1073/pnas.90.16.7804

Ben-Haim S, Ell P. 2009. 18F-FDG PET and PET/CT in the evaluation of cancer treatment response. *J Nucl Med* **50:** 88–99. doi:10.2967/jnumed.108.054205

Ben-Sahra I, Howell JJ, Asara JM, Manning BD. 2013. Stimulation of de novo pyrimidine synthesis by growth signaling through mTOR and S6K1. *Science* **339:** 1323–1328. doi:10.1126/science.1228792

Ben-Sahra I, Hoxhaj G, Ricoult SJ, Asara JM, Manning BD. 2016. mTORC1 induces purine synthesis through control of the mitochondrial tetrahydrofolate cycle. *Science* **351:** 728–733. doi:10.1126/science.aad0489

Berwick DC, Hers I, Heesom KJ, Moule SK, Tavará JM. 2002. The identification of ATP-citrate lyase as a protein kinase B (Akt) substrate in primary adipocytes. *J Biol Chem* **277:** 33895–33900. doi:10.1074/jbc.M204681200

Bhutia YD, Babu E, Ramachandran S, Ganapathy V. 2015. Amino acid transporters in cancer and their relevance to "glutamine addiction": novel targets for the design of a new class of anticancer drugs. *Cancer Res* **75:** 1782–1788. doi:10.1158/0008-5472.CAN-14-3745

Casero RA Jr, Murray Stewart T, Pegg AE. 2018. Polyamine metabolism and cancer: treatments, challenges and opportunities. *Nat Rev Cancer* **18:** 681–695. doi:10.1038/s41568-018-0050-3

Cho S, Lee G, Pickering BF, Jang C, Park JH, He L, Mathur L, Kim SS, Jung S, Tang HW, et al. 2021. mTORC1 promotes cell growth via m⁶A-dependent mRNA degradation. *Mol Cell* **81:** 2064–2075.e8. doi:10.1016/j.molcel.2021.03.010

Choi BH, Coloff JL. 2019. The diverse functions of non-essential amino acids in cancer. *Cancers (Basel)* **11:** 675. doi:10.3390/cancers11050675

Commisso C, Davidson SM, Soydaner-Azeloglu RG, Parker SJ, Kamphorst JJ, Hackett S, Grabocka E, Nofal M, Drebin JA, Thompson CB, et al. 2013. Macropinocytosis of protein is an amino acid supply route in ras-transformed cells. *Nature* **497:** 633–637. doi:10.1038/nature12138

Csibi A, Lee G, Yoon SO, Tong H, Ilter D, Elia I, Fendt SM, Roberts TM, Blenis J. 2014. The mTORC1/S6K1 pathway regulates glutamine metabolism through the eIF4B-dependent control of c-Myc translation. *Curr Biol* **24:** 2274–2280. doi:10.1016/j.cub.2014.08.007

Davidson SM, Jonas O, Keibler MA, Hou HW, Luengo A, Mayers JR, Wyckoff J, Del Rosario AM, Whitman M, Chin CR, et al. 2017. Direct evidence for cancer-cell-autonomous extracellular protein catabolism in pancreatic tumors. *Nat Med* **23:** 235–241. doi:10.1038/nm.4256

Day TA, Shirai K, O'Brien PE, Matheus MG, Godwin K, Sood AJ, Kompelli A, Vick JA, Martin D, Vitale-Cross L, et al. 2019. Inhibition of mTOR signaling and clinical activity of rapamycin in head and neck cancer in a window of opportunity trial. *Clin Cancer Res* **25:** 1156–1164. doi:10.1158/1078-0432.CCR-18-2024

DeBerardinis RJ, Chandel NS. 2020. We need to talk about the Warburg effect. *Nat Metab* **2:** 127–129. doi:10.1038/s42255-020-0172-2

DeNicola GM, Karreth FA, Humpton TJ, Gopinathan A, Wei C, Frese K, Mangal D, Yu KH, Yeo CJ, Calhoun ES, et al. 2011. Oncogene-induced Nrf2 transcription promotes ROS detoxification and tumorigenesis. *Nature* **475:** 106–109. doi:10.1038/nature10189

Deprez J, Vertommen D, Alessi DR, Hue L, Rider MH. 1997. Phosphorylation and activation of heart 6-phospho-

fructo-2-kinase by protein kinase B and other protein kinases of the insulin signaling cascades. *J Biol Chem* **272:** 17269–17275. doi:10.1074/jbc.272.28.17269

Dhanasekaran R, Deutzmann A, Mahauad-Fernandez WD, Hansen AS, Gouw AM, Felsher DW. 2022. The MYC oncogene—the grand orchestrator of cancer growth and immune evasion. *Nat Rev Clin Oncol* **19:** 23–36. doi:10.1038/s41571-021-00549-2

Dibble CC, Barritt SA, Perry GE, Lien EC, Geck RC, DuBois-Coyne SE, Bartee D, Zengeya TT, Cohen EB, Yuan M, et al. 2022. PI3K drives the de novo synthesis of coenzyme A from vitamin B5. *Nature* **608:** 192–198. doi:10.1038/s41586-022-04984-8

Düvel K, Yecies JL, Menon S, Raman P, Lipovsky AI, Souza AL, Triantafellow E, Ma Q, Gorski R, Cleaver S, et al. 2010. Activation of a metabolic gene regulatory network downstream of mTOR complex 1. *Mol Cell* **39:** 171–183. doi:10.1016/j.molcel.2010.06.022

Elorza A, Soro-Arnáiz I, Meléndez-Rodríguez F, Rodríguez-Vaello V, Marsboom G, de Cárcer G, Acosta-Iborra B, Albacete-Albacete L, Ordóñez A, Serrano-Oviedo L, et al. 2012. HIF2α acts as an mTORC1 activator through the amino acid carrier SLC7A5. *Mol Cell* **48:** 681–691. doi:10.1016/j.molcel.2012.09.017

Elstrom RL, Bauer DE, Buzzai M, Karnauskas R, Harris MH, Plas DR, Zhuang H, Cinalli RM, Alavi A, Rudin CM, et al. 2004. Akt stimulates aerobic glycolysis in cancer cells. *Cancer Res* **64:** 3892–3899. doi:10.1158/0008-5472.CAN-03-2904

Engelman JA, Chen L, Tan X, Crosby K, Guimaraes AR, Upadhyay R, Maira M, McNamara K, Perera SA, Song Y, et al. 2008. Effective use of PI3K and MEK inhibitors to treat mutant kras G12D and PIK3CA H1047R murine lung cancers. *Nat Med* **14:** 1351–1356. doi:10.1038/nm.1890

Fan J, Ye J, Kamphorst JJ, Shlomi T, Thompson CB, Rabinowitz JD. 2014. Quantitative flux analysis reveals folate-dependent NADPH production. *Nature* **510:** 298–302. doi:10.1038/nature13236

Farrell AS, Sears RC. 2014. MYC degradation. *Cold Spring Harb Perspect Med* **4:** a014365. doi:10.1101/cshperspect.a014365

Fruman DA, Chiu H, Hopkins BD, Bagrodia S, Cantley LC, Abraham RT. 2017. The PI3K pathway in human disease. *Cell* **170:** 605–635. doi:10.1016/j.cell.2017.07.029

Gao P, Tchernyshyov I, Chang TC, Lee YS, Kita K, Ochi T, Zeller KI, De Marzo AM, Van Eyk JE, Mendell JT, et al. 2009. c-Myc suppression of miR-23a/b enhances mitochondrial glutaminase expression and glutamine metabolism. *Nature* **458:** 762–765. doi:10.1038/nature07823

Gera JF, Mellinghoff IK, Shi Y, Rettig MB, Tran C, Hsu JH, Sawyers CL, Lichtenstein AK. 2004. AKT activity determines sensitivity to mammalian target of rapamycin (mTOR) inhibitors by regulating cyclin D1 and c-myc expression. *J Biol Chem* **279:** 2737–2746. doi:10.1074/jbc.M309999200

Gordan JD, Thompson CB, Simon MC. 2007. HIF and c-Myc: sibling rivals for control of cancer cell metabolism and proliferation. *Cancer Cell* **12:** 108–113. doi:10.1016/j.ccr.2007.07.006

Graves LM, Guy HI, Kozlowski P, Huang M, Lazarowski E, Pope RM, Collins MA, Dahlstrand EN, Earp HS III, Evans

DR. 2000. Regulation of carbamoyl phosphate synthetase by MAP kinase. *Nature* **403**: 328–332. doi:10.1038/35002111

Guerrero-Rodríguez SL, Mata-Cruz C, Pérez-Tapia SM, Velasco-Velázquez MA. 2022. Role of CD36 in cancer progression, stemness, and targeting. *Front Cell Dev Biol* **10**: 1079076. doi:10.3389/fcell.2022.1079076

Guertin DA, Wellen KE. 2023. Acetyl-CoA metabolism in cancer. *Nat Rev Cancer* **23**: 156–172. doi:10.1038/s41568-022-00543-5

Haigis KM. 2017. KRAS alleles: the devil is in the detail. *Trends Cancer* **3**: 686–697. doi:10.1016/j.trecan.2017.08.006

Harris IS, DeNicola GM. 2020. The complex interplay between antioxidants and ROS in cancer. *Trends Cell Biol* **30**: 440–451. doi:10.1016/j.tcb.2020.03.002

Hong SY, Yu FX, Luo Y, Hagen T. 2016. Oncogenic activation of the PI3K/Akt pathway promotes cellular glucose uptake by downregulating the expression of thioredoxin-interacting protein. *Cell Signal* **28**: 377–383. doi:10.1016/j.cellsig.2016.01.011

Hosios AM, Manning BD. 2021. Cancer signaling drives cancer metabolism: AKT and the Warburg effect. *Cancer Res* **81**: 4896–4898. doi:10.1158/0008-5472.CAN-21-2647

Hosios AM, Hecht VC, Danai LV, Johnson MO, Rathmell JC, Steinhauser ML, Manalis SR, Vander Heiden MG. 2016. Amino acids rather than glucose account for the majority of cell mass in proliferating mammalian cells. *Dev Cell* **36**: 540–549. doi:10.1016/j.devcel.2016.02.012

Hosios AM, Wilkinson ME, McNamara MC, Kalafut KC, Torrence ME, Asara JM, Manning BD. 2022. mTORC1 regulates a lysosome-dependent adaptive shift in intracellular lipid species. *Nat Metab* **4**: 1792–1811. doi:10.1038/s42255-022-00706-6

Hoxhaj G, Manning BD. 2020. The PI3K–AKT network at the interface of oncogenic signalling and cancer metabolism. *Nat Rev Cancer* **20**: 74–88. doi:10.1038/s41568-019-0216-7

Hoxhaj G, Ben-Sahra I, Lockwood SE, Timson RC, Byles V, Henning GT, Gao P, Selfors LM, Asara JM, Manning BD. 2019. Direct stimulation of $NADP^+$ synthesis through Akt-mediated phosphorylation of NAD kinase. *Science* **363**: 1088–1092. doi:10.1126/science.aau3903

Hu H, Juvekar A, Lyssiotis CA, Lien EC, Albeck JG, Oh D, Varma G, Hung YP, Ullas S, Lauring J, et al. 2016. Phosphoinositide 3-kinase regulates glycolysis through mobilization of aldolase from the actin cytoskeleton. *Cell* **164**: 433–446. doi:10.1016/j.cell.2015.12.042

Huang F, Ni M, Chalishazar MD, Huffman KE, Kim J, Cai L, Shi X, Cai F, Zacharias LG, Ireland AS, et al. 2018. Inosine monophosphate dehydrogenase dependence in a subset of small cell lung cancers. *Cell Metab* **28**: 369–382.e5. doi:10.1016/j.cmet.2018.06.005

Huang F, Huffman KE, Wang Z, Wang X, Li K, Cai F, Yang C, Cai L, Shih TS, Zacharias LG, et al. 2021. Guanosine triphosphate links MYC-dependent metabolic and ribosome programs in small-cell lung cancer. *J Clin Invest* **131**: e139929. doi:10.1172/JCI139929

Hudson CC, Liu M, Chiang GG, Otterness DM, Loomis DC, Kaper F, Giaccia AJ, Abraham RT. 2002. Regulation of hypoxia-inducible factor 1α expression and function by the mammalian target of rapamycin. *Mol Cell Biol* **22**: 7004–7014. doi:10.1128/MCB.22.20.7004-7014.2002

Ilagan E, Manning BD. 2016. Emerging role of mTOR in the response to cancer therapeutics. *Trends Cancer* **2**: 241–251. doi:10.1016/j.trecan.2016.03.008

Inoki K, Li Y, Zhu T, Wu J, Guan KL. 2002. TSC2 is phosphorylated and inhibited by Akt and suppresses mTOR signalling. *Nat Cell Biol* **4**: 648–657. doi:10.1038/ncb839

Jayashankar V, Edinger AL. 2020. Macropinocytosis confers resistance to therapies targeting cancer anabolism. *Nat Commun* **11**: 1121. doi:10.1038/s41467-020-14928-3

Kamphorst JJ, Nofal M, Commisso C, Hackett SR, Lu W, Grabocka E, Vander Heiden MG, Miller G, Drebin JA, Bar-Sagi D, et al. 2015. Human pancreatic cancer tumors are nutrient poor and tumor cells actively scavenge extracellular protein. *Cancer Res* **75**: 544–553. doi:10.1158/0008-5472.CAN-14-2211

Kandasamy P, Gyimesi G, Kanai Y, Hediger MA. 2018. Amino acid transporters revisited: new views in health and disease. *Trends Biochem Sci* **43**: 752–789. doi:10.1016/j.tibs.2018.05.003

Karnoub AE, Weinberg RA. 2008. Ras oncogenes: split personalities. *Nat Rev Mol Cell Biol* **9**: 517–531. doi:10.1038/nrm2438

Kerk SA, Papagiannakopoulos T, Shah YM, Lyssiotis CA. 2021. Metabolic networks in mutant KRAS-driven tumours: tissue specificities and the microenvironment. *Nat Rev* **21**: 510–525. doi:10.1038/s41568-021-00375-9

Kim SM, Nguyen TT, Ravi A, Kubiniok P, Finicle BT, Jayashankar V, Malacrida L, Hou J, Robertson J, Gao D, et al. 2018. PTEN deficiency and AMPK activation promote nutrient scavenging and anabolism in prostate cancer cells. *Cancer Discov* **8**: 866–883. doi:10.1158/2159-8290.CD-17-1215

Kovalski JR, Kuzuoglu-Ozturk D, Ruggero D. 2022. Protein synthesis control in cancer: selectivity and therapeutic targeting. *EMBO J* **41**: e109823. doi:10.15252/embj.2021109823

Kruiswijk F, Labuschagne CF, Vousden KH. 2015. P53 in survival, death and metabolic health: a lifeguard with a license to kill. *Nat Rev Mol Cell Biol* **16**: 393–405. doi:10.1038/nrm4007

Laughner E, Taghavi P, Chiles K, Mahon PC, Semenza GL. 2001. HER2 (neu) signaling increases the rate of hypoxia-inducible factor 1α (HIF-1α) synthesis: novel mechanism for HIF-1-mediated vascular endothelial growth factor expression. *Mol Cell Biol* **21**: 3995–4004. doi:10.1128/MCB.21.12.3995-4004.2001

Lavoie H, Gagnon J, Therrien M. 2020. ERK signalling: a master regulator of cell behaviour, life and fate. *Nat Rev Mol Cell Biol* **21**: 607–632. doi:10.1038/s41580-020-0255-7

Lee JV, Carrer A, Shah S, Snyder NW, Wei S, Venneti S, Worth AJ, Yuan ZF, Lim HW, Liu S, et al. 2014. Akt-dependent metabolic reprogramming regulates tumor cell histone acetylation. *Cell Metab* **20**: 306–319. doi:10.1016/j.cmet.2014.06.004

Lee JH, Liu R, Li J, Zhang C, Wang Y, Cai Q, Qian X, Xia Y, Zheng Y, Piao Y, et al. 2017. Stabilization of phosphofructokinase 1 platelet isoform by AKT promotes tumorigenesis. *Nat Commun* **8**: 949. doi:10.1038/s41467-017-00906-9

Lee MS, Dennis C, Naqvi I, Dailey L, Lorzadeh A, Ye G, Zaytouni T, Adler A, Hitchcock DS, Lin L, et al. 2023. Ornithine aminotransferase supports polyamine synthesis in pancreatic cancer. *Nature* **616:** 339–347. doi:10.1038/s41586-023-05891-2

Li S, Balmain A, Counter CM. 2018. A model for RAS mutation patterns in cancers: finding the sweet spot. *Nat Rev Cancer* **18:** 767–777. doi:10.1038/s41568-018-0076-6

Lien EC, Lyssiotis CA, Juvekar A, Hu H, Asara JM, Cantley LC, Toker A. 2016. Glutathione biosynthesis is a metabolic vulnerability in PI(3)K/Akt-driven breast cancer. *Nat Cell Biol* **18:** 572–578. doi:10.1038/ncb3341

Liu GY, Sabatini DM. 2020. mTOR at the nexus of nutrition, growth, ageing and disease. *Nat Rev Mol Cell Biol* **21:** 183–203. doi:10.1038/s41580-019-0199-y

Liu YC, Li F, Handler J, Huang CR, Xiang Y, Neretti N, Sedivy JM, Zeller KI, Dang CV. 2008. Global regulation of nucleotide biosynthetic genes by c-Myc. *PLoS ONE* **3:** e2722. doi:10.1371/journal.pone.0002722

Liu W, Le A, Hancock C, Lane AN, Dang CV, Fan TW, Phang JM. 2012. Reprogramming of proline and glutamine metabolism contributes to the proliferative and metabolic responses regulated by oncogenic transcription factor c-MYC. *Proc Natl Acad Sci* **109:** 8983–8988. doi:10.1073/pnas.1203244109

Luengo A, Li Z, Gui DY, Sullivan LB, Zagorulya M, Do BT, Ferreira R, Naamati A, Ali A, Lewis CA, et al. 2021. Increased demand for NAD$^+$ relative to ATP drives aerobic glycolysis. *Mol Cell* **81:** 691–707.e6. doi:10.1016/j.molcel.2020.12.012

Lunt SY, Vander Heiden MG. 2011. Aerobic glycolysis: meeting the metabolic requirements of cell proliferation. *Annu Rev Cell Dev Biol* **27:** 441–464. doi:10.1146/annurev-cellbio-092910-154237

Ma L, Chen Z, Erdjument-Bromage H, Tempst P, Pandolfi PP. 2005. Phosphorylation and functional inactivation of TSC2 by Erk implications for tuberous sclerosis and cancer pathogenesis. *Cell* **121:** 179–193. doi:10.1016/j.cell.2005.02.031

Maertens O, Cichowski K. 2014. An expanding role for RAS GTPase activating proteins (RAS GAPs) in cancer. *Adv Biol Regul* **55:** 1–14. doi:10.1016/j.jbior.2014.04.002

Majumder PK, Febbo PG, Bikoff R, Berger R, Xue Q, McMahon LM, Manola J, Brugarolas J, McDonnell TJ, Golub TR, et al. 2004. mTOR inhibition reverses Akt-dependent prostate intraepithelial neoplasia through regulation of apoptotic and HIF-1-dependent pathways. *Nat Med* **10:** 594–601. doi:10.1038/nm1052

Makinoshima H, Takita M, Saruwatari K, Umemura S, Obata Y, Ishii J, Matsumoto S, Sugiyama E, Ochiai A, Abe R, et al. 2015. Signaling through the phosphatidylinositol 3-kinase (PI3K)/mammalian target of rapamycin (mTOR) axis is responsible for aerobic glycolysis mediated by glucose transporter in epidermal growth factor receptor (EGFR)-mutated lung adenocarcinoma. *J Biol Chem* **290:** 17495–17504. doi:10.1074/jbc.M115.660498

Manning BD, Toker A. 2017. AKT/PKB signaling: navigating the network. *Cell* **169:** 381–405. doi:10.1016/j.cell.2017.04.001

Manning BD, Tee AR, Logsdon MN, Blenis J, Cantley LC. 2002. Identification of the tuberous sclerosis complex-2 tumor suppressor gene product tuberin as a target of the phosphoinositide 3-kinase/Akt pathway. *Mol Cell* **10:** 151–162. doi:10.1016/S1097-2765(02)00568-3

Martinez Calejman C, Trefely S, Entwisle SW, Luciano A, Jung SM, Hsiao W, Torres A, Hung CM, Li H, Snyder NW, et al. 2020. mTORC2-AKT signaling to ATP-citrate lyase drives brown adipogenesis and de novo lipogenesis. *Nat Commun* **11:** 575. doi:10.1038/s41467-020-14430-w

Menendez JA, Lupu R. 2007. Fatty acid synthase and the lipogenic phenotype in cancer pathogenesis. *Nat Rev Cancer* **7:** 763–777. doi:10.1038/nrc2222

Menon S, Dibble CC, Talbott G, Hoxhaj G, Valvezan AJ, Takahashi H, Cantley LC, Manning BD. 2014. Spatial control of the TSC complex integrates insulin and nutrient regulation of mTORC1 at the lysosome. *Cell* **156:** 771–785. doi:10.1016/j.cell.2013.11.049

Mitsuishi Y, Taguchi K, Kawatani Y, Shibata T, Nukiwa T, Aburatani H, Yamamoto M, Motohashi H. 2012. Nrf2 redirects glucose and glutamine into anabolic pathways in metabolic reprogramming. *Cancer Cell* **22:** 66–79. doi:10.1016/j.ccr.2012.05.016

Mukhopadhyay S, Vander Heiden MG, McCormick F. 2021. The metabolic landscape of RAS-driven cancers from biology to therapy. *Nat Cancer* **2:** 271–283. doi:10.1038/s43018-021-00184-x

Nicklin P, Bergman P, Zhang B, Triantafellow E, Wang H, Nyfeler B, Yang H, Hild M, Kung C, Wilson C, et al. 2009. Bidirectional transport of amino acids regulates mTOR and autophagy. *Cell* **136:** 521–534. doi:10.1016/j.cell.2008.11.044

Nogueira V, Patra KC, Hay N. 2018. Selective eradication of cancer displaying hyperactive Akt by exploiting the metabolic consequences of Akt activation. *eLife* **7:** e32213. doi:10.7554/eLife.32213

Origanti S, Nowotarski SL, Carr TD, Sass-Kuhn S, Xiao L, Wang JY, Shantz LM. 2012. Ornithine decarboxylase mRNA is stabilized in an mTORC1-dependent manner in Ras-transformed cells. *Biochem J* **442:** 199–207. doi:10.1042/BJ20111464

Palm W, Park Y, Wright K, Pavlova NN, Tuveson DA, Thompson CB. 2015. The utilization of extracellular proteins as nutrients is suppressed by mTORC1. *Cell* **162:** 259–270. doi:10.1016/j.cell.2015.06.017

Park Y, Reyna-Neyra A, Philippe L, Thoreen CC. 2017. mTORC1 balances cellular amino acid supply with demand for protein synthesis through post-transcriptional control of ATF4. *Cell Rep* **19:** 1083–1090. doi:10.1016/j.celrep.2017.04.042

Patra KC, Hay N. 2014. The pentose phosphate pathway and cancer. *Trends Biochem Sci* **39:** 347–354. doi:10.1016/j.tibs.2014.06.005

Patra KC, Wang Q, Bhaskar PT, Miller L, Wang Z, Wheaton W, Chandel N, Laakso M, Muller WJ, Allen EL, et al. 2013. Hexokinase 2 is required for tumor initiation and maintenance and its systemic deletion is therapeutic in mouse models of cancer. *Cancer Cell* **24:** 213–228. doi:10.1016/j.ccr.2013.06.014

Porstmann T, Santos CR, Griffiths B, Cully M, Wu M, Leevers S, Griffiths JR, Chung YL, Schulze A. 2008. SREBP activity is regulated by mTORC1 and contributes to Akt-dependent cell growth. *Cell Metab* **8:** 224–236. doi:10.1016/j.cmet.2008.07.007

Cite this article as *Cold Spring Harb Perspect Med* doi: 10.1101/cshperspect.a041543

Puccini J, Badgley MA, Bar-Sagi D. 2022. Exploiting cancer's drinking problem: regulation and therapeutic potential of macropinocytosis. *Trends Cancer* **8:** 54–64. doi:10.1016/j.trecan.2021.09.004

Puccini J, Wei J, Tong L, Bar-Sagi D. 2023. Cytoskeletal association of ATP citrate lyase controls the mechanodynamics of macropinocytosis. *Proc Natl Acad Sci* **120:** e2213272120. doi:10.1073/pnas.2213272120

Rathmell JC, Fox CJ, Plas DR, Hammerman PS, Cinalli RM, Thompson CB. 2003. Akt-directed glucose metabolism can prevent bax conformation change and promote growth factor-independent survival. *Mol Cell Biol* **23:** 7315–7328. doi:10.1128/MCB.23.20.7315-7328.2003

Ricoult SJ, Yecies JL, Ben-Sahra I, Manning BD. 2016. Oncogenic PI3K and K-Ras stimulate de novo lipid synthesis through mTORC1 and SREBP. *Oncogene* **35:** 1250–1260. doi:10.1038/onc.2015.179

Roberts DJ, Tan-Sah VP, Smith JM, Miyamoto S. 2013. Akt phosphorylates HK-II at Thr-473 and increases mitochondrial HK-II association to protect cardiomyocytes. *J Biol Chem* **288:** 23798–23806. doi:10.1074/jbc.M113.482026

Robey RB, Hay N. 2006. Mitochondrial hexokinases, novel mediators of the antiapoptotic effects of growth factors and Akt. *Oncogene* **25:** 4683–4696. doi:10.1038/sj.onc.1209595

Robitaille AM, Christen S, Shimobayashi M, Cornu M, Fava LL, Moes S, Prescianotto-Baschong C, Sauer U, Jenoe P, Hall MN. 2013. Quantitative phosphoproteomics reveal mTORC1 activates de novo pyrimidine synthesis. *Science* **339:** 1320–1323. doi:10.1126/science.1228771

Rodriguez-Viciana P, Warne PH, Khwaja A, Marte BM, Pappin D, Das P, Waterfield MD, Ridley A, Downward J. 1997. Role of phosphoinositide 3-OH kinase in cell transformation and control of the actin cytoskeleton by Ras. *Cell* **89:** 457–467. doi:10.1016/S0092-8674(00)80226-3

Ros S, Wright AJ, D'Santos P, Hu DE, Hesketh RL, Lubling Y, Georgopoulou D, Lerda G, Couturier DL, Razavi P, et al. 2020. Metabolic imaging detects resistance to PI3Kα inhibition mediated by persistent FOXM1 expression in ER[+] breast cancer. *Cancer Cell* **38:** 516–533.e9. doi:10.1016/j.ccell.2020.08.016

Roux PP, Ballif BA, Anjum R, Gygi SP, Blenis J. 2004. Tumor-promoting phorbol esters and activated Ras inactivate the tuberous sclerosis tumor suppressor complex via p90 ribosomal S6 kinase. *Proc Natl Acad Sci* **101:** 13489–13494. doi:10.1073/pnas.0405659101

Samovski D, Su X, Xu Y, Abumrad NA, Stahl PD. 2012. Insulin and AMPK regulate FA translocase/CD36 plasma membrane recruitment in cardiomyocytes via Rab GAP AS160 and Rab8a Rab GTPase. *J Lipid Res* **53:** 709–717. doi:10.1194/jlr.M023424

Sanchez-Vega F, Mina M, Armenia J, Chatila WK, Luna A, La KC, Dimitriadoy S, Liu DL, Kantheti HS, Saghafinia S, et al. 2018. Oncogenic signaling pathways in the cancer genome atlas. *Cell* **173:** 321–337.e10. doi:10.1016/j.cell.2018.03.035

Santana-Codina N, Roeth AA, Zhang Y, Yang A, Mashadova O, Asara JM, Wang X, Bronson RT, Lyssiotis CA, Ying H, et al. 2018. Oncogenic KRAS supports pancreatic cancer through regulation of nucleotide synthesis. *Nat Commun* **9:** 4945. doi:10.1038/s41467-018-07472-8

Schaub FX, Dhankani V, Berger AC, Trivedi M, Richardson AB, Shaw R, Zhao W, Zhang X, Ventura A, Liu Y, et al. 2018. Pan-cancer alterations of the MYC oncogene and its proximal network across the cancer genome atlas. *Cell Syst* **6:** 282–300.e2. doi:10.1016/j.cels.2018.03.003

Sears R, Nuckolls F, Haura E, Taya Y, Tamai K, Nevins JR. 2000. Multiple Ras-dependent phosphorylation pathways regulate Myc protein stability. *Genes Dev* **14:** 2501–2514. doi:10.1101/gad.836800

Semenza GL. 2003. Targeting HIF-1 for cancer therapy. *Nat Rev Cancer* **3:** 721–732. doi:10.1038/nrc1187

Siska PJ, van der Windt GJ, Kishton RJ, Cohen S, Eisner W, MacIver NJ, Kater AP, Weinberg JB, Rathmell JC. 2016. Suppression of Glut1 and glucose metabolism by decreased Akt/mTORC1 signaling drives T cell impairment in B cell leukemia. *J Immunol* **197:** 2532–2540. doi:10.4049/jimmunol.1502464

Snaebjornsson MT, Janaki-Raman S, Schulze A. 2020. Greasing the wheels of the cancer machine: the role of lipid metabolism in cancer. *Cell Metab* **31:** 62–76. doi:10.1016/j.cmet.2019.11.010

Stine ZE, Walton ZE, Altman BJ, Hsieh AL, Dang CV. 2015. MYC, metabolism, and cancer. *Cancer Discov* **5:** 1024–1039. doi:10.1158/2159-8290.CD-15-0507

Talebi A, Dehairs J, Rambow F, Rogiers A, Nittner D, Derua R, Vanderhoydonc F, Duarte JAG, Bosisio F, Van den Eynde K, et al. 2018. Sustained SREBP-1-dependent lipogenesis as a key mediator of resistance to BRAF-targeted therapy. *Nat Commun* **9:** 2500. doi:10.1038/s41467-018-04664-0

Thomas GV, Tran C, Mellinghoff IK, Welsbie DS, Chan E, Fueger B, Czernin J, Sawyers CL. 2006. Hypoxia-inducible factor determines sensitivity to inhibitors of mTOR in kidney cancer. *Nat Med* **12:** 122–127. doi:10.1038/nm1337

Torrence ME, Manning BD. 2018. Nutrient sensing in cancer. *Annu Rev Cancer Biol* **2:** 251–269. doi:10.1146/annurev-cancerbio-030617-050329

Torrence ME, MacArthur MR, Hosios AM, Valvezan AJ, Asara JM, Mitchell JR, Manning BD. 2021. The mTORC1-mediated activation of ATF4 promotes protein and glutathione synthesis downstream of growth signals. *eLife* **10:** e63326. doi:10.7554/eLife.63326

Trefts E, Shaw RJ. 2021. AMPK: restoring metabolic homeostasis over space and time. *Mol Cell* **81:** 3677–3690. doi:10.1016/j.molcel.2021.08.015

Truitt ML, Conn CS, Shi Z, Pang X, Tokuyasu T, Coady AM, Seo Y, Barna M, Ruggero D. 2015. Differential requirements for eIF4E dose in normal development and cancer. *Cell* **162:** 59–71. doi:10.1016/j.cell.2015.05.049

Valvezan AJ, Manning BD. 2019. Molecular logic of mTORC1 signalling as a metabolic rheostat. *Nat Metab* **1:** 321–333. doi:10.1038/s42255-019-0038-7

Valvezan AJ, Turner M, Belaid A, Lam HC, Miller SK, McNamara MC, Baglini C, Housden BE, Perrimon N, Kwiatkowski DJ, et al. 2017. mTORC1 couples nucleotide synthesis to nucleotide demand resulting in a targetable metabolic vulnerability. *Cancer Cell* **32:** 624–638.e5. doi:10.1016/j.ccell.2017.09.013

Valvezan AJ, McNamara MC, Miller SK, Torrence ME, Asara JM, Henske EP, Manning BD. 2020. IMPDH inhibitors for antitumor therapy in tuberous sclerosis complex. *JCI Insight* **5:** e135071. doi:10.1172/jci.insight.135071

van Riggelen J, Yetil A, Felsher DW. 2010. MYC as a regulator of ribosome biogenesis and protein synthesis. *Nat Rev Cancer* **10:** 301–309. doi:10.1038/nrc2819

Villa E, Sahu U, O'Hara BP, Ali ES, Helmin KA, Asara JM, Gao P, Singer BD, Ben-Sahra I. 2021. mTORC1 stimulates cell growth through SAM synthesis and m^{6}A mRNA-dependent control of protein synthesis. *Mol Cell* **81:** 2076–2093.e9. doi:10.1016/j.molcel.2021.03.009

Waldhart AN, Dykstra H, Peck AS, Boguslawski EA, Madaj ZB, Wen J, Veldkamp K, Hollowell M, Zheng B, Cantley LC, et al. 2017. Phosphorylation of TXNIP by AKT mediates acute influx of glucose in response to insulin. *Cell Rep* **19:** 2005–2013. doi:10.1016/j.celrep.2017.05.041

Wall M, Poortinga G, Hannan KM, Pearson RB, Hannan RD, McArthur GA. 2008. Translational control of c-MYC by rapamycin promotes terminal myeloid differentiation. *Blood* **112:** 2305–2317. doi:10.1182/blood-2007-09-111856

Wang Y, Stancliffe E, Fowle-Grider R, Wang R, Wang C, Schwaiger-Haber M, Shriver LP, Patti GJ. 2022. Saturation of the mitochondrial NADH shuttles drives aerobic glycolysis in proliferating cells. *Mol Cell* **82:** 3270–3283.e9. doi:10.1016/j.molcel.2022.07.007

Wieman HL, Wofford JA, Rathmell JC. 2007. Cytokine stimulation promotes glucose uptake via phosphatidylinositol-3 kinase/Akt regulation of Glut1 activity and trafficking. *Mol Biol Cell* **18:** 1437–1446. doi:10.1091/mbc.e06-07-0593

Wise DR, DeBerardinis RJ, Mancuso A, Sayed N, Zhang XY, Pfeiffer HK, Nissim I, Daikhin E, Yudkoff M, McMahon SB, et al. 2008. Myc regulates a transcriptional program that stimulates mitochondrial glutaminolysis and leads to glutamine addiction. *Proc Natl Acad Sci* **105:** 18782–18787. doi:10.1073/pnas.0810199105

Yang M, Vousden KH. 2016. Serine and one-carbon metabolism in cancer. *Nat Rev Cancer* **16:** 650–652. doi:10.1038/nrc.2016.81

Yang T, Ren C, Qiao P, Han X, Wang L, Lv S, Sun Y, Liu Z, Du Y, Yu Z. 2018. PIM2-mediated phosphorylation of hexokinase 2 is critical for tumor growth and paclitaxel resistance in breast cancer. *Oncogene* **37:** 5997–6009. doi:10.1038/s41388-018-0386-x

Ying H, Kimmelman AC, Lyssiotis CA, Hua S, Chu GC, Fletcher-Sananikone E, Locasale JW, Son J, Zhang H, Coloff JL, et al. 2012. Oncogenic kras maintains pancreatic tumors through regulation of anabolic glucose metabolism. *Cell* **149:** 656–670. doi:10.1016/j.cell.2012.01.058

Yuneva M, Zamboni N, Oefner P, Sachidanandam R, Lazebnik Y. 2007. Deficiency in glutamine but not glucose induces MYC-dependent apoptosis in human cells. *J Cell Biol* **178:** 93–105. doi:10.1083/jcb.200703099

Zabala-Letona A, Arruabarrena-Aristorena A, Martín-Martín N, Fernandez-Ruiz S, Sutherland JD, Clasquin M, Tomas-Cortazar J, Jimenez J, Torres I, Quang P, et al. 2017. mTORC1-dependent AMD1 regulation sustains polyamine metabolism in prostate cancer. *Nature* **547:** 109–113. doi:10.1038/nature22964

Zhang Y, Kwok-Shing Ng P, Kucherlapati M, Chen F, Liu Y, Tsang YH, de Velasco G, Jeong KJ, Akbani R, Hadjipanayis A, et al. 2017. A pan-cancer proteogenomic atlas of PI3K/AKT/mTOR pathway alterations. *Cancer Cell* **31:** 820–832.e3. doi:10.1016/j.ccell.2017.04.013

Zhong H, Chiles K, Feldser D, Laughner E, Hanrahan C, Georgescu MM, Simons JW, Semenza GL. 2000. Modulation of hypoxia-inducible factor 1α expression by the epidermal growth factor/phosphatidylinositol 3-kinase/PTEN/AKT/FRAP pathway in human prostate cancer cells: implications for tumor angiogenesis and therapeutics. *Cancer Res* **60:** 1541–1545.

Metabolic Signaling in Cancer

Laura V. Pinheiro,[1,2,3,4] Pedro Costa-Pinheiro,[1,3,4] and Kathryn E. Wellen[1,3]

[1]Department of Cancer Biology, Perelman School of Medicine; [2]Biochemistry and Molecular Biophysics Graduate Group, Perelman School of Medicine; [3]Abramson Family Cancer Research Institute, University of Pennsylvania, Philadelphia, Pennsylvania 19104-6160, USA

Correspondence: wellenk@upenn.edu

Metabolic reprogramming in cancer allows cells to survive in harsh environments and sustain macromolecular biosynthesis to support proliferation. In addition, metabolites play crucial roles as signaling molecules. Metabolite fluctuations are detected by various sensors in the cell to regulate gene expression, metabolism, and signal transduction. Metabolic signaling mechanisms contribute to tumorigenesis by altering the physiology of cancer cells themselves, as well as that of neighboring cells in the tumor microenvironment. In this review, we discuss principles of metabolic signaling and provide examples of how cancer cells take advantage of metabolic signals to promote cell proliferation and evade the immune system, thereby contributing to tumor growth and progression.

Metabolism comprises the chemical reactions carried out by cells that result in the breakdown of nutrients (catabolism) and the synthesis of macromolecules (anabolism), including lipids, carbohydrates, proteins, and nucleic acids. Metabolites generated by these processes play additional signaling roles as substrates for posttranslational modifications (PTMs) of proteins, as cofactors for enzymatic reactions, and as allosteric regulators of enzymes (Campbell and Wellen 2018; Figlia et al. 2020; Baker and Rutter 2023). Through these functions, metabolites can modulate metabolism, gene expression, and signal transduction, thereby playing crucial roles in cellular communication. These nutrient sensing and signaling mechanisms enable tuning of cellular processes to fluctuations in nutrient uptake and metabolism. Cancer cells can disrupt or co-opt the normal control of metabolic signaling pathways to promote survival, proliferation, and immune evasion.

In this review, we first discuss principles of metabolic signaling and then provide examples of metabolic signaling in cancer, considering both intracellular and cell–cell cross-talk mechanisms. We close with a discussion of emerging aspects of metabolic signaling and technologies.

PRINCIPLES OF METABOLITE SENSING AND SIGNALING

Properties of Metabolic Signals

Three essential properties of a metabolic signaling mechanism are (1) a metabolite whose abun-

[4]These authors contributed equally to this work.

dance changes in response to nutrient availability or metabolic reprogramming; (2) a sensor that can detect the changes in the abundance of the metabolite; and (3) the ability to implement or tune a biological response or set of responses as metabolite abundance changes. Metabolic signaling can occur through mechanisms that involve either covalent modifications or noncovalent interactions of the metabolite with proteins or other macromolecules (Fig. 1).

Covalent Metabolite Signaling

Histones and nonhistone proteins can acquire PTMs, such as phosphorylation, acetylation, and methylation. These covalent modifications can affect the structural and biochemical properties of the protein, thus impacting function (Figlia et al. 2020). Although some modifications can occur nonenzymatically, most PTMs are added and removed through enzymatic reactions, many of which use metabolites as substrates (Reid et al. 2017; Figlia et al. 2020).

The biochemical properties of the enzymes that catalyze these reactions are key determinants of whether metabolic fluctuations will impact protein PTMs. One of these properties is the Michaelis constant (K_m), the substrate concentration at which an enzyme is working at half of its maximal rate. If a substrate concentration is near the K_m that defines that particular enzyme–substrate relationship, then small alterations in substrate concentration can have significant effects on the reaction rate (Reid et al. 2017). As a result,

changes in cellular metabolism can directly impact the rate at which some PTMs are added or removed from proteins, thereby modulating protein functions in a metabolically responsive manner (Reid et al. 2017; Campbell and Wellen 2018; Figlia et al. 2020). Acetylation, for example, is often metabolically responsive because acetyl-CoA concentrations in the cell fluctuate near the K_m values for some acetyltransferases (Fig. 2). Conversely, phosphorylation is typically not metabolically responsive because cellular ATP concentrations are orders of magnitude higher than most kinase K_m values for ATP; thus, changes in ATP abundance do not impact kinase reaction rates (Fig. 2). Although there is a growing list of metabolically sensitive PTMs (Trefely et al. 2020), we will focus on acetylation and methylation as the most abundant and well-studied marks.

Acetylation

Histone lysine acetylation modulates gene expression in part by increasing chromatin accessibility. Specifically, acetylation neutralizes the positive charge on histone lysines, which loosens the interaction with the negatively charged DNA backbone. Designated readers can then bind to acetylated lysine residues, where they function as protein effectors of these modifications to regulate transcriptional programs and biological outcomes. Acetyl-CoA, a key intermediate in cellular metabolism, is the substrate used for protein acetylation. Acetyl-CoA is generated during nu-

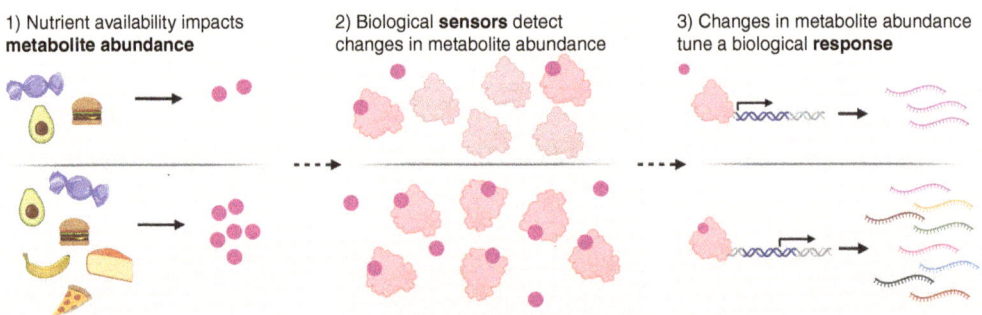

1) Nutrient availability impacts **metabolite abundance**

2) Biological **sensors** detect changes in metabolite abundance

3) Changes in metabolite abundance tune a biological **response**

Figure 1. Key properties of metabolic signaling mechanisms. (Figure created with BioRender.com.)

Cite this article as *Cold Spring Harb Perspect Med* doi: 10.1101/cshperspect.a041544

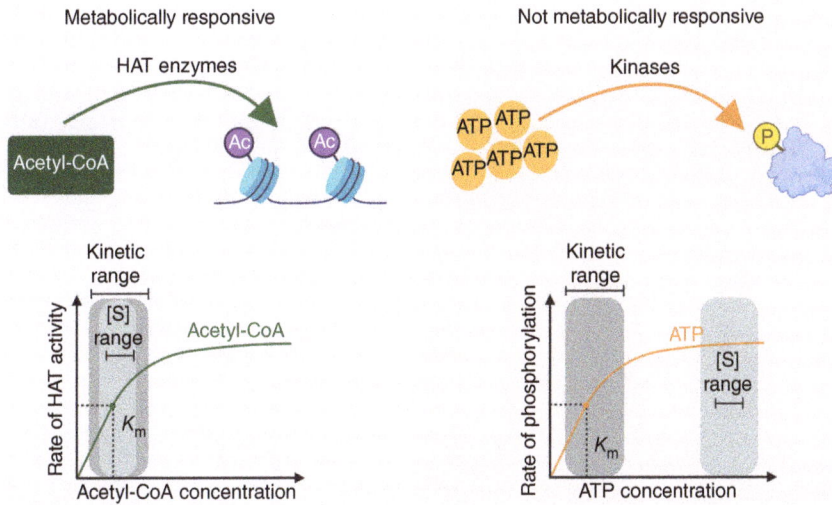

Figure 2. Metabolic regulation of posttranslational modifications (PTMs). PTMs are metabolically sensitive when substrate concentrations fluctuate in response to nutrient availability near the K_m for the substrate of the relevant enzymes (in the example in the *left* panel, acetyl-CoA abundance impacts acetylation in this manner). Conversely, when physiological substrate concentrations always exceed the relevant enzyme's K_m for the substrate, the modification is not responsive to metabolism (e.g., in the *right* panel, fluctuations in ATP in cells do not impact the rate of phosphorylation). (Figure created with BioRender.com.)

trient catabolism, and its abundance is sensitive to the availability of extracellular nutrients (Guertin and Wellen 2023). Correspondingly, histone acetylation is highly sensitive to the abundance of acetyl-CoA, and some other proteins can also be acetylated in a nutrient-responsive manner, impacting their functions (Fig. 3). In addition to lysine acetylation, emerging evidence indicates that acetylation of RNA and generation of acetylated derivatives of metabolites may also be metabolically responsive (Levy et al. 2020; Guertin and Wellen 2023).

Although acetylation reactions can occur nonenzymatically, most lysine acetylation outside of the mitochondria is carried out by lysine acetyltransferase (KAT) enzymes (Reid et al. 2017; Figlia et al. 2020). At the whole-cell level, acetyl-CoA abundance ranges between ~3 and 20 µM in mammalian cells (Lee et al. 2014; Chen et al. 2016); however, the precise concentration range of acetyl-CoA within the nucleus has not been established and might be different from that in whole cells. Nevertheless, many KATs have K_m values near to physiological acetyl-CoA concen-

trations (Wiktorowicz et al. 1981; Lee et al. 2014; Reid et al. 2017), likely enabling the regulation of histone and nonhistone protein acetylation in accordance with nutrient availability (Cai et al. 2011; Lee et al. 2014; Mariño et al. 2014). Moreover, the free CoA produced by KATs upon the transfer of the acetyl moiety to a lysine acts as a feedback inhibitor of the enzymes; therefore, the local acetyl-CoA:CoA ratio, which is affected by the cell's metabolic activity, is also likely important for control of acetylation (Fig. 3; Lee et al. 2014; Montgomery et al. 2016).

Removal of acetyl groups is catalyzed by Zn^{2+}-dependent class I and II histone deacetylases (HDACs) and by NAD^+-dependent sirtuins (class III HDACs) (Menzies et al. 2016). SIRT1 and SIRT3, in particular, are sensitive to the levels of NAD^+, because their corresponding K_m values for NAD^+ are near the physiological NAD^+ abundance in cells (Xie et al. 2020). Although SIRT1 and SIRT3 are sensitive to fluctuations in NAD^+ levels, class I and II HDACs can be inhibited by specific metabolites, including the short-chain fatty acid (SCFA) butyrate, a ma-

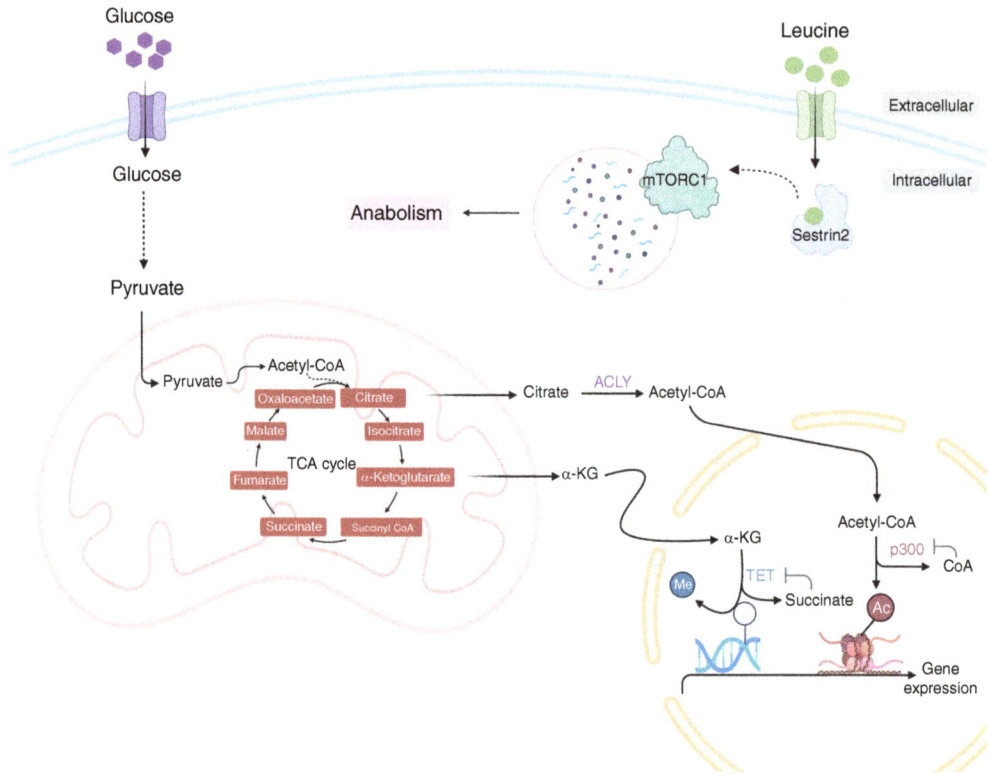

Figure 3. Metabolites can control signaling by both covalent and noncovalent mechanisms, depicted by examples in this figure. Metabolites such as α-ketoglutarate and acetyl-CoA are used by chromatin-modifying enzymes such as histone acetyltransferases (HATs) and ten–eleven translocation (TET) enzymes, which catalyze multistep DNA demethylation, to regulate gene expression. The amino acid leucine plays a role in the noncovalent regulation of signaling by binding to Sestrin2, which disrupts its interaction with GATOR2, allowing activation of mTORC1. (Figure created with BioRender.com.)

jor product of the microbiota, and the ketone body β-hydroxybutyrate (Candido et al. 1978; Shimazu et al. 2013).

Methylation

Proteins, DNA, and RNA can become methylated (Fig. 3). Histone methylation can occur on lysine or arginine residues and can repress or activate gene transcription, depending on the site and the number of methyl groups added. Methylation of DNA on cytosine nucleobases generally represses gene transcription, and both histone and DNA methylation reactions are catalyzed by methyltransferases that use S-adenosylmethionine (SAM) as a methyl donor (Locasale 2013). SAM is a metabolite generated through the coupled methionine and folate cycles, which comprise a metabolic network known as one-carbon metabolism, and it supplies methyl (or one-carbon) units for numerous processes, including DNA and histone methylation (Locasale 2013; Campbell and Wellen 2018). For a detailed discussion of one-carbon metabolism, please refer to the review by Lim and Metallo (2024).

Like acetylation, methylation is sensitive to changes in methionine and SAM abundance, as the K_m values of various methyltransferases are near physiological concentrations of SAM, which have been measured at ~3–60 µM in cells (Reid et al. 2017). S-adenosyl homocysteine (SAH), a product of methyltransferase reactions, can also inhibit methyltransferases (Reid et al.

2017). Methionine restriction of cells in culture decreases SAM abundance with a consequent drop in histone methylation; this is similarly observed in liver tissue during dietary methionine restriction in mice (Mentch et al. 2015). Notably, consuming a diet low in methionine has also been shown to reduce plasma levels of methionine metabolites in humans (Gao et al. 2019; Olsen et al. 2020), although a correlation of this diet with decreased histone methylation has not been established.

Removal of methyl groups from histones is achieved by histone demethylase enzymes, and removal from DNA is carried out in a multistep process by ten–eleven translocation (TET) methylcytosine dioxygenases. Histone demethylases and TET enzymes belong to a broad class of 2-oxoglutarate-dependent dioxygenases (2-OGDD), which require 2-oxoglutarate (also known as α-ketoglutarate; α-KG) as an obligatory cofactor (Fig. 3; Martínez-Reyes and Chandel 2020). 2-OGDD enzymes are competitively inhibited by other metabolites with structures that are similar to that of α-KG, including succinate, fumarate, (D)-2-hydroxyglutarate (2-HG), and (L)-2-HG (Fig. 3). Notably, D-2-HG is the product of mutant isocitrate dehydrogenase (IDH1 and IDH2) enzymes, which occur in some cancers and drive a hypermethylation phenotype through the regulation of 2-OGDD enzymes. Gunn and Losman (2024) discuss such regulation in greater depth.

Noncovalent Mechanisms of Nutrient-Dependent Sensing and Signaling

Metabolites also participate in metabolic regulation and signaling via noncovalent interactions between metabolites and proteins. Such regulation is well known for its roles in tuning metabolic flux (Baker and Rutter 2023). For example, the glycolytic enzyme phosphofructokinase (PFK1) is allosterically activated or inhibited by different upstream or downstream metabolites (e.g., fructose 2,6-bisphosphate, which is produced from PFK1's substrate fructose-6-phosphate, activates the enzyme, whereas downstream products citrate and ATP exert inhibitory effects), allowing glycolysis to be regulated according to the metabolic needs of the cell. Similarly, noncovalent interactions between metabolites and signaling proteins can tether metabolic state to signal transduction pathways regulating growth and metabolism. Major examples include nutrient sensing through the mTORC1 and AMPK pathways, which are briefly described below and covered in greater depth in Manning and Dibble (2024).

mTOR: Nutrient Sensor and Regulator of Anabolism

In eukaryotic cells, mechanistic target of rapamycin (mTOR) forms two distinct complexes, mTORC1 (which contains the partner protein RAPTOR) and mTORC2 (which contains RICTOR) (Liu and Sabatini 2020). mTORC1 is a master regulator of growth and metabolism that integrates growth factor signals with nutrient availability (Blommaart et al. 1995; Wolfson et al. 2016). The mTORC1 network contains multiple nutrient sensors that detect and respond to the availability of amino acids, glucose, SAM, and cholesterol. For example, Sestrin2 is a leucine sensor. Under low amino acid conditions, Sestrin2 sequesters GATOR2, a positive regulator of mTORC1 (Saxton et al. 2016; Wolfson et al. 2016). However, when leucine is abundant, it binds to Sestrin2, releasing GATOR2 to activate mTORC1 (Saxton et al. 2016; Wolfson et al. 2016). Importantly, leucine binds to Sestrin2 with a K_d of 20 µM, which is approximately the half-maximal concentration at which leucine activates mTORC1 signaling (Wolfson et al. 2016). Active mTORC1 regulates downstream signaling pathways to promote biosynthesis and cell growth (Liu and Sabatini 2020).

AMPK: Energy Sensor and Regulator of Catabolism

AMP-activated protein kinase (AMPK) is a key metabolic node, sensing the energy status of a eukaryotic cell by measuring fluctuations in the levels of adenine nucleotides (Hardie et al. 2016). Canonically, AMPK is activated by binding of AMP, and to a lesser extent ADP, to the enzyme's γ subunit (Gowans et al. 2013; Li et al. 2015; Hardie et al. 2016). ATP binds competitively with AMP and ADP at this site; when ATP replaces AMP in the γ subunit of AMPK, it promotes the separation between the nucleotide-binding pocket of AMPK and its catalytic domain, exposing phosphorylation sites to the activity of phosphatases and subsequent inactivation. Thus, the levels of AMP, ADP, and ATP constitute an important metric for the energy status of a cell, called the "energy charge" calculated by ([ATP] + ½ [ADP])/([AMP] + [ADP] + [ATP]) (Atkinson and Walton 1967). Nutrient deprivation reduces ATP levels, with a corresponding increase in AMP and ADP and subsequent activation of AMPK (Gowans et al. 2013). This initiates a cascade of reactions that culminate in the activation of catabolic pathways to increase levels of ATP, including increased autophagy and enhanced mitochondrial biogenesis and metabolism. On the other hand, when ATP levels are high (i.e., when nutrients are abundant), AMPK is inactivated, enabling progrowth pathways to drive anabolism (Quirós et al. 2016). Indeed, AMPK is a key negative regulator of mTORC1. Whereas in normal cells AMPK and mTOR work together to balance energy generation and biosynthesis in accordance with cellular needs and in response to exogenous growth factor signals, oncogenic signaling can drive aberrant hyperactivation of proproliferative pathways, promoting tumor growth.

METABOLIC SIGNALING IN CANCER

Metabolic reprogramming is a hallmark of cancer. In this section, we will illustrate examples of how metabolic signals are altered in cancer, discussing both intracellular and cell–cell signaling cross-talk mechanisms, and how these pathways are impacted by environmental nutrient availability and cancer cell metabolic reprogramming.

Metabolic Signaling Mechanisms in Cancer Cells

Tumor cells frequently reside in harsh environments where they must contend with nutrient scarcity, oxygen deprivation, and the resulting competition for resources. As such, nutrient sensing and adaptive mechanisms contribute to cancer cell plasticity and ability to survive

and proliferate. Moreover, cell-intrinsic signals, such as metabolic reprogramming driven by oncogenic signaling, can also co-opt metabolic signaling mechanisms to promote growth. As highlighted earlier, one of the most notable instances of co-opting metabolic signaling in cancer is mediated by mutant IDH1 and IDH2 enzymes, which produce the oncometabolite D-2-HG, leading to inhibition of 2-OGDD enzymes and, as a result, DNA and histone hypermethylation and inhibition of cell differentiation. Here, we discuss additional roles of metabolic signaling mechanisms in tumorigenesis.

Acetyl-CoA Metabolism

The availability of nutrients, including glucose, acetate, and palmitate, impacts acetyl-CoA abundance in cells, leading to changes in the acetylation of histones and other proteins, including transcription factors. Such regulation has been shown to be important for the implementation of specific gene expression programs in cancer cells, including those enabling cell migration, metastasis, and lipogenesis (Gao et al. 2016; Lee et al. 2018; Altea-Manzano et al. 2023).

In addition to nutrient availability, oncogenic and growth factor–driven metabolic reprogramming events, such as those mediated by the PI3K–AKT pathway, modulate acetyl-CoA production and histone acetylation. In particular, activated AKT phosphorylates ATP citrate lyase (ACLY), promoting sustained acetyl-CoA production and histone acetylation even under nutrient restriction; accordingly, phosphorylation of AKT at Ser473 correlates with global histone acetylation in human gliomas and prostate tumors (Lee et al. 2014). Insulin and other growth factors can also exogenously activate the AKT–ACLY–histone acetylation axis (Carrer et al. 2019; Senapati et al. 2019). Another example is the adipocyte-secreted factor leptin, which was shown to promote AMPK activation in breast cancer cells, leading to inhibition of acetyl-CoA carboxylase 1 (ACC1), thereby increasing acetyl-CoA abundance and acetylation of Smad2 to promote the expression of genes involved in epithelial–mesenchymal transition (EMT) (Rios Garcia et al. 2017). Regulation of expression of

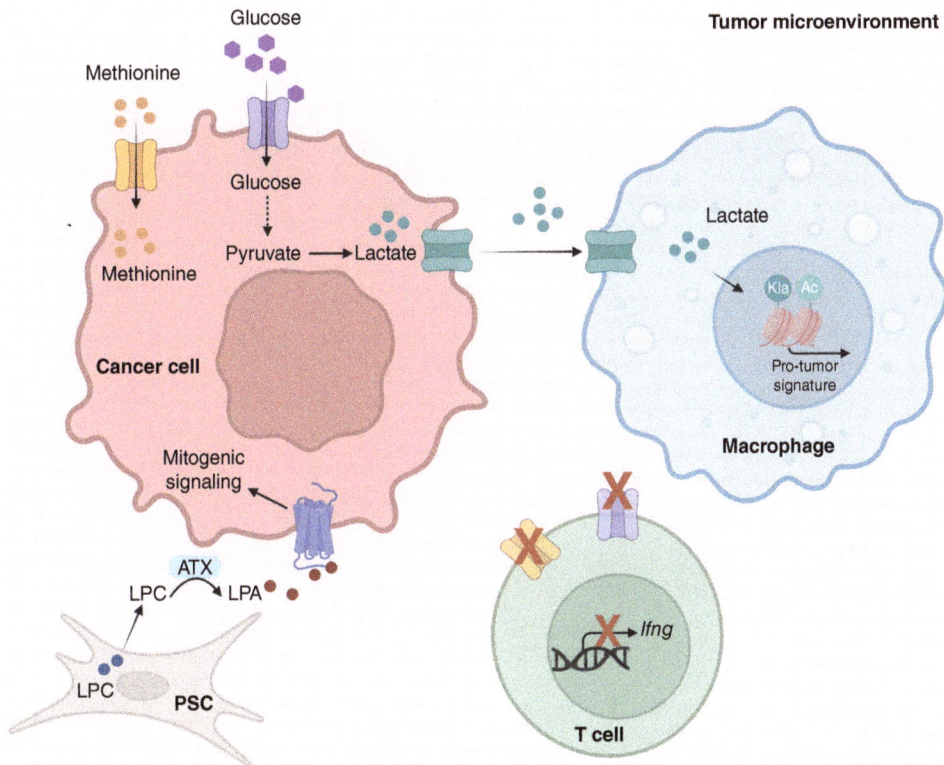

Figure 4. Metabolic cross talk in the tumor microenvironment (TME). The TME is characterized by harsh nutrient conditions where different cells compete for, but also share, resources. A few examples are depicted in this figure. Tumor cells consume high amounts of glucose (purple, glucose transporter) resulting in excessive lactate production and secretion. This exogenous lactate is taken up by macrophages, and subsequently impacts gene expression leading to a protumor macrophage signature, in part through regulation of chromatin modifications. High consumption of glucose and methionine (yellow, methionine transporter) by tumor cells has been implicated in the reduction of T-cell activity, promoting evasion of anticancer immunity. Finally, pancreatic stellate cells (PSCs) have been shown to secret lysophosphatidylcholines (LPCs), which are then converted to lysophosphatidic acid (LPA) by the extracellular enzyme autotaxin (ATX); LPA supports cancer cell mitogenic signaling and growth through interaction with cell surface receptors. (Figure created with BioRender.com.)

enzymes involved in acetyl-CoA metabolism in tumors can also impact histone acetylation and gene expression. In hepatocellular carcinoma (HCC), for example, reduced expression of the acetyl-CoA hydrolase ACOT12 promotes preservation of acetyl-CoA levels to boost histone acetylation and EMT gene expression (Lu et al. 2019).

One-Carbon Metabolism

Similar to acetyl-CoA metabolism, metabolic reprogramming in cancer cells can also impact SAM pools and methylation. For example, in a

mouse model of pancreatic cancer, *Kras* mutation concomitant with loss of the tumor-suppressor *Lkb1* (KL) was found to drive glucose uptake and its use for the biosynthesis of the one-carbon-unit donor serine. Methyl groups from serine are transferred to tetrahydrofolate and used in the methionine cycle to regenerate methionine from homocysteine for SAM synthesis. The increased serine and SAM synthesis thus allows KL tumors to sustain higher levels of DNA methylation and renders them susceptible to inhibition of DNA methyltransferases (Kottakis et al. 2016). On the other hand, nicotinamide *N*-methyltransferase (NNMT) is overexpressed in several cancers and can suppress methylation potential by depleting SAM pools, because NNMT methylates nicotinamide utilizing SAM as the methyl donor (Ulanovskaya et al. 2013; Gao et al. 2021). NNMT overexpression is associated with a poor prognosis in several cancer types, leading to interest in inhibiting NNMT for cancer treatment (Gao et al. 2021).

Overall, both nutrient availability and cancer cell metabolic reprogramming impact acetyl-CoA and SAM abundance, consequently regulating acetylation and methylation and contributing to cancerous phenotypes.

Cross-Talk Mechanisms in the Tumor Microenvironment

Tumors are made up of a heterogeneous mixture composed of a variety of cell types including cancer cells, immune cells, fibroblasts, endothelial cells, and adipocytes, among others (Lyssiotis and Kimmelman 2017; Elia and Haigis 2021; Martínez-Reyes and Chandel 2021). This multicellular milieu is termed the tumor microenvironment (TME). Cells in the TME often exchange or compete for available metabolites to sustain growth, proliferation, and function (Lyssiotis and Kimmelman 2017). These metabolites can serve in signaling roles at the cell surface or be taken up and metabolized intracellularly. We will discuss some examples of cellular cross talk below, with a focus on metabolites as signaling molecules.

Glucose, Lactate, and Acetate

Cancer cells have long been characterized for their ability to uptake copious amounts of glucose for lactate production even when oxygen is present, a phenomenon termed aerobic glycolysis or the Warburg effect (Koppenol et al. 2011). This glycolytic phenotype and resulting depletion of glucose in the TME can affect the function of nearby immune cells and antitumor immunity. T-cell activation and function have been described to be regulated by glucose through at least two mechanisms (Elia and Haigis 2021). First, the glycolytic intermediate phosphoenolpyruvate (PEP) acts as a signaling metabolite that

indirectly increases cytoplasmic calcium in T cells (Ho et al. 2015). PEP availability is sensed by sarco/endoplasmic reticulum Ca^{2+}-ATPase (SERCA), which transports calcium from the cytosol into the endoplasmic reticulum (ER); mechanistically, PEP promotes oxidation of cysteine residues on SERCA, thus inhibiting calcium uptake. Cytoplasmic calcium availability and signaling to the calcium-responsive transcription factor nuclear factor of activated T cells (NFAT) then drives T cells to an effector function phenotype. Lack of glycolysis in T cells due to competition for glucose with highly glycolytic tumors results in low abundance of intracellular PEP in T cells and consequent suppression of T-cell function (Ho et al. 2015; Baker and Rutter 2023). Second, the pool of acetyl-CoA that exists outside of the mitochondria (i.e., the nuclear-cytosolic pool) is sensitive to the rate of glycolysis and required for histone acetylation. Reduced glycolysis can thus suppress histone acetylation and subsequently reduce the expression of the interferon γ gene (*IFNG*), a cytokine used by T cells for their cytotoxic functions (Fig. 4; Peng et al. 2016). Acetate, an alternative carbon source that can be used for the synthesis of acetyl-CoA, can rescue cytokine production in the absence of glucose-derived acetyl-CoA by maintaining histone acetylation and chromatin accessibility (Qiu et al. 2019).

A key product of glycolysis, lactate, itself functions as a signaling metabolite involved in cell–cell cross talk. Evidence has emerged that lactate plays a key role in modulating the phenotype of tumor-associated macrophages (TAMs). Macrophages are cells of the innate immune system and can either have antitumor functions or functions that support tumor growth. Interestingly, lactate induces a gene expression program in macrophages that is supportive of tumor growth (Colegio et al. 2014; Noe et al. 2021). This may occur through several possible mechanisms (Fig. 4). One proposed mechanism is through the regulation of acetyl-CoA production and histone acetylation (Noe et al. 2021); extracellular lactate is imported into macrophages and converted to pyruvate and subsequently citrate via the TCA cycle, enabling acetyl-CoA generation through ACLY. ACLY-dependent histone acetylation has been implicated in the acquisition of an anti-inflammatory macrophage phenotype (Covarrubias et al. 2016). Lactate can also be used as a precursor for another chemical modification called lactylation (Zhang et al. 2019). Histone lactylation is associated with the acquisition of a wound-healing, anti-inflammatory, protumor phenotype in macrophages that had been previously polarized toward a proinflammatory phenotype (Zhang et al. 2019). Of note, the metabolic route from lactate to lysine lactylation remains to be defined, and the modification can also derive from the reactive glycolytic by-product methylglyoxal (Gaffney et al. 2020). Lactate may also be sensed by the α-KG-dependent proline hydroxylase, PHD2, which hydroxylates HIF1α and targets it for degradation; specifically, lactate inhibits PHD2 by competing with the cosubstrate α-KG for binding (Feng et al. 2022). Although implicated in promoting an inflammatory phenotype in adipose tissue macrophages (Feng et al. 2022), lactate-dependent HIF1α stabilization is implicated in polarizing TAMs toward a homeostatic, protumor phenotype (Colegio et al. 2014). Finally, lactate is also sensed extracellularly by G-protein coupled receptors (GPCRs) in macrophages (Elia and Haigis 2021). In breast cancer, this signaling event supports tumor cell–macrophage cross talk and promotes metastasis (Elia and Haigis 2021); similarly, lactate-induced GPCR signaling in endothelial cells supports angiogenesis (Morland et al. 2017; Bader et al. 2020).

Thus, cancer cell glycolysis, leading to glucose limitation and elevated lactate in the TME, impacts the function of nearby macrophages and T cells in part through metabolic signaling functions, facilitating the evasion of immune defenses.

Methionine

In addition to its roles in cancer cells, methionine metabolism modulates the biology of T cells and fibroblasts in the TME. Some cancer cells have elevated expression of the methionine transporter SLC43A2, exhausting methionine available in the TME (Fig. 4). This results in diminished CD8[+] T-cell methionine metabolism and subsequent loss of methylation at specific loci important for CD8[+] T-cell viability and function (Bian et al. 2020).

Metabolic regulation of histone methylation has also been implicated in the tumor-supporting functions of cancer-associated fibroblasts (CAFs). In particular, high expression of NNMT was detected in the stroma of metastatic ovarian tumors. NNMT depletes SAM pools, reducing histone methylation in CAFs, and thereby modulating the expression of genes associated with cytokine secretion and extracellular matrix production (Eckert et al. 2019).

Fatty Acids and Other Lipids

The availability of lipids in the TME can be impacted by various factors including diet and production or consumption by different types of cells (Beyaz et al. 2016; Michelet et al. 2018; Auciello et al. 2019; Ringel et al. 2020; Lien et al. 2021; Altea-Manzano et al. 2023). Lipids function as key components of membranes, and fatty acids can be catabolized as fuel, but different classes of lipids can also exert diverse signaling functions.

SCFAs are a class of fatty acids that are largely produced by microbiota through the fermentation of dietary fibers; key SCFAs include acetate, propionate, and butyrate (Carretta et al. 2021; Mirzaei et al. 2021). Because of their local production in the gastrointestinal (GI) tract, butyrate and other SCFAs have been heavily studied in the context of GI cancers (Carretta et al. 2021; Mirzaei et al. 2021). Notably, although butyrate is a major fuel source in healthy colonocytes, in colon cancer cells it accumulates and inhibits HDACs, boosting histone acetylation and promoting an antiproliferative gene expression profile (Donohoe et al. 2012). Accordingly, butyrate production by gut microbes has been shown to be at the root of dietary fiber's protective action against colon cancer (Donohoe et al. 2014). SCFAs can also exert their effects by signaling through GPCRs. The expression of most GPCRs that respond to SCFAs is lost in malignancy, suggesting that SCFA-induced GPCR signaling has antitumor functions (Thangaraju et al. 2009; Tang et al. 2011; Carretta et al. 2021; Mirzaei et al. 2021).

Fatty acids also modulate peroxisome proliferator-activated receptor (PPAR) signaling.

PPARs are transcription factors that respond to different classes of lipids via ligand binding to subsequently regulate gene expression. Diets that are high in fat sustain tumor growth in certain types of cancer, and one mechanism by which this occurs is through dietary fatty acids and their effect on PPARs. In particular, a high-fat diet (HFD), and fatty acids like palmitic acid, which are abundant in HFD, activate PPARδ signaling in intestinal stem cells and progenitor cells to enhance their ability to initiate tumors (Beyaz et al. 2016). Similarly, obesity induces a PPAR-driven accumulation of lipids in natural killer (NK) cells, which are immune cells with cytotoxic antitumor functions. In the context of obesity, with active PPAR signaling and a high intracellular lipid load, NK cells become dysfunctional and allow for sustained tumor growth (Michelet et al. 2018).

Specific lipids, notably lysophosphatidic acid (LPA), exert protumorigenic signaling roles. LPA signals through several GPCRs, promoting cell proliferation and migration (Mills and Moolenaar 2003; Dorsam and Gutkind 2007). In pancreatic cancer, pancreatic stellate cells (PSCs) present in the microenvironment secrete lysophosphatidylcholines, which are converted to LPA extracellularly by the enzyme autotaxin to support tumor growth (Fig. 4; Auciello et al. 2019; Snaebjornsson et al. 2020). Lipid metabolism thus exerts diverse signaling functions in cancer biology.

Ketone Bodies

Diets low in carbohydrates but with high amounts of fat (i.e., ketogenic diets) drive increased hepatic production of the ketone bodies β-hydroxybutyrate (BHB), acetoacetate, and acetone. Ketone bodies can be used as metabolic fuel for extrahepatic tissues, but they also serve in signaling roles, including through inhibiting HDACs and binding to GPCRs (Puchalska and Crawford 2021). For example, ketogenic diets were found to potently inhibit tumor growth in a mouse model of colorectal cancer. This was tied to BHB-dependent signaling through a GPCR, HCAR2 (Dmitrieva-Posocco et al. 2022). The ketogenic enzyme 3-hydroxy-3-methylglutaryl-CoA synthase (HMGCS2) has also been found to be enriched in intestinal stem cells, where it functions to preserve stemness. Mechanistically, BHB inhibits HDACs, which in turn enhances Notch signaling to promote self-renewal, functions that are boosted in mice fed a ketogenic diet (Cheng et al. 2019). Additionally, studies have connected the ketone body, acetoacetate, with oncogenic BRAF signaling in melanoma (Kang et al. 2015; Xia et al. 2017). $BRAF^{V600E}$ was shown to promote the intracellular accumulation of acetoacetate via up-regulation of the ketogenic enzyme HMG-CoA lyase (HMGCL), which led to increased binding of mutant BRAF to MEK1 with subsequent activation of MEK–ERK signaling (Kang et al. 2015). Notably, dietary manipulation of acetoacetate availability impacted $BRAF^{V600E}$ mutant tumors, with a ketogenic diet enhancing and lipid-lowering agents decreasing tumor growth (Xia et al. 2017).

CONCLUDING REMARKS: EMERGING ASPECTS OF METABOLIC SIGNALING IN CANCER

As we have discussed throughout this review, signaling functions of metabolites play crucial roles in cancer in supporting proliferation and tumor growth and in evading immune destruction. This can occur through both nutrient-sensitive chemical modifications and through protein–metabolite interactions that impact protein function without the formation of covalent bonds. Understanding the roles of metabolites as signaling molecules remains a highly active area of research. Key areas of exploration to advance our understanding of metabolic signaling mechanisms in cancer include improving the measurement of metabolism spatially across tumors and in subcellular compartments and identifying metabolite–protein interactions.

It is intuitive that a key aspect of metabolic signaling is compartmentalization, in that metabolites may be present within multiple compartments of the cell, and metabolite sensing depends on local concentrations in the vicinity of the sensor. Yet, despite the recognition that compartmentalization is a key component of metabolic regulation, the detection, tracking, and quantification of metabolites in subcellular compartments remains a challenge. General strategies for assessing subcellular metabolite abundance involve either the use of fluorescent or bioluminescent metabolite biosensors or biochemical fractionation followed by metabolite quantification by mass spectrometry (Liu et al. 2015; Wellen and Snyder 2019). Biosensors enable the assessment of metabolites in intact cells but are currently available for a limited number of metabolites. Fractionation strategies are disruptive and can alter metabolism from that in the intact cell, although recent technologies enabling rapid cell fractionation and strategies to account for metabolic perturbations that occur during fractionation are facilitating new insights into compartmentalized metabolism (Abu-Remaileh et al. 2017; Chen et al. 2017; Trefely et al. 2022). Recently, studies have provided evidence that the nucleus is a site of active metabolism that is at least in part distinct from that of the cytosol (Ryu et al. 2018; Trefely et al. 2022). Further development and use of sensitive experimental strategies will aid in defining the abundance and regulation of metabolites in compartments of interest, including the nucleus. In terms of metabolic compartmentalization within different cell types in a tumor, mass spectrometry imaging has become a key technology for resolving spatial differences in metabolism in tissues and will undoubtedly play a key role in resolving metabolic signaling mechanisms, particularly pertaining to cell–cell communication, in tumors in the coming years (Planque et al. 2023).

Many metabolic enzymes have been known for decades to be regulated allosterically by their products or related metabolites; yet the broader roles of metabolites in interacting with and impacting the function of other proteins in the cell remains minimally explored. Recent technological advancements are beginning to shed light into this area of biology. MIDAS (mass spectrometry integrated with equilibrium dialysis for the discovery of allostery systematically) combines equilibrium dialysis with metabolome analysis by mass spectrometry to identify metabolites interacting with a protein of interest (Hicks et al. 2023). Initial work describing this approach identified numerous novel protein–metabolite

interactions, including inhibition of lactate dehydrogenase A by long-chain fatty acyl-CoA binding (Hicks et al. 2023). Reciprocally, thermal proteome profiling allows the identification of proteins that interact with a given metabolite, based on the principle that most protein–ligand binding interactions will stabilize the tertiary structure of the protein. The thermal stability of proteins in complex samples in the presence or absence of metabolites can be interrogated rapidly using multiplexed quantitative mass spectrometry (MS)-based proteomics (Franken et al. 2015; Reinhard et al. 2015). Such an approach was recently used to discover that intracellular lactate binds to and inhibits sentrin-specific protease 1 (SENP1). SENP1 is responsible for the SUMOylation of the anaphase-promoting complex (APC) 4 leading to its inactivation and disruption of the APC (Liu et al. 2023). By inhibiting SENP1, lactate contributes to the stabilization of the APC, promoting sustained high proliferation rates (Liu et al. 2023). With an expanding experimental toolbox and the vast potential for metabolites to exert signaling functions, we predict that rapid progress in understanding how metabolites regulate cell biology in normal and pathological states will continue to drive fundamental advances in cancer biology.

ACKNOWLEDGMENTS

L.V.P. was supported by T32DK007314. P.C.-P. was supported by K00CA245802. Work in the laboratory of K.E.W. has been supported by R01CA174761, R01CA248315, R01CA262055, R01CA228339, and Ludwig Cancer Research. Figures were made using Biorender.com.

REFERENCES

*Reference is also in this subject collection.

Abu-Remaileh M, Wyant GA, Kim C, Laqtom NN, Abbasi M, Chan SH, Freinkman E, Sabatini DM. 2017. Lysosomal metabolomics reveals V-ATPase- and mTOR-dependent regulation of amino acid efflux from lysosomes. *Science* **358:** 807–813. doi:10.1126/science.aan6298

Altea-Manzano P, Doglioni G, Liu Y, Cuadros AM, Nolan E, Fernández-García J, Wu Q, Planque M, Laue KJ, Cidre-Aranaz F, et al. 2023. A palmitate-rich metastatic niche enables metastasis growth via p65 acetylation resulting in pro-metastatic NF-κB signaling. *Nat Cancer* **4:** 344–364. doi:10.1038/s43018-023-00513-2

Atkinson DE, Walton GM. 1967. Adenosine triphosphate conservation in metabolic regulation. Rat liver citrate cleavage enzyme. *J Biol Chem* **242:** 3239–3241. doi:10.1016/S0021-9258(18)95956-9

Auciello FR, Bulusu V, Oon C, Tait-Mulder J, Berry M, Bhattacharyya S, Tumanov S, Allen-Petersen BL, Link J, Kendsersky ND, et al. 2019. A stromal lysolipid-autotaxin signaling axis promotes pancreatic tumor progression. *Cancer Discov* **9:** 617–627. doi:10.1158/2159-8290.CD-18-1212

Bader JE, Voss K, Rathmell JC. 2020. Targeting metabolism to improve the tumor microenvironment for cancer immunotherapy. *Mol Cell* **78:** 1019–1033. doi:10.1016/j.molcel.2020.05.034

Baker SA, Rutter J. 2023. Metabolites as signalling molecules. *Nat Rev Mol Cell Biol* **24:** 355–374. doi:10.1038/s41580-022-00572-w

Beyaz S, Mana MD, Roper J, Kedrin D, Saadatpour A, Hong SJ, Bauer-Rowe KE, Xifaras ME, Akkad A, Arias E, et al. 2016. High-fat diet enhances stemness and tumorigenicity of intestinal progenitors. *Nature* **531:** 53–58. doi:10.1038/nature17173

Bian Y, Li W, Kremer DM, Sajjakulnukit P, Li S, Crespo J, Nwosu ZC, Zhang L, Czerwonka A, Pawlowska A, et al. 2020. Cancer SLC43A2 alters T cell methionine metabolism and histone methylation. *Nature* **585:** 277–282. doi:10.1038/s41586-020-2682-1

Blommaart EF, Luiken JJ, Blommaart PJ, van Woerkom GM, Meijer AJ. 1995. Phosphorylation of ribosomal protein S6 is inhibitory for autophagy in isolated rat hepatocytes. *J Biol Chem* **270:** 2320–2326. doi:10.1074/jbc.270.5.2320

Cai L, Sutter BM, Li B, Tu BP. 2011. Acetyl-CoA induces cell growth and proliferation by promoting the acetylation of histones at growth genes. *Mol Cell* **42:** 426–437. doi:10.1016/j.molcel.2011.05.004

Campbell SL, Wellen KE. 2018. Metabolic signaling to the nucleus in cancer. *Mol Cell* **71:** 398–408. doi:10.1016/j.molcel.2018.07.015

Candido EP, Reeves R, Davie JR. 1978. Sodium butyrate inhibits histone deacetylation in cultured cells. *Cell* **14:** 105–113. doi:10.1016/0092-8674(78)90305-7

Carrer A, Trefely S, Zhao S, Campbell SL, Norgard RJ, Schultz KC, Sidoli S, Parris JLD, Affronti HC, Sivanand S, et al. 2019. Acetyl-CoA metabolism supports multistep pancreatic tumorigenesis. *Cancer Discov* **9:** 416–435. doi:10.1158/2159-8290.CD-18-0567

Carretta MD, Quiroga J, López R, Hidalgo MA, Burgos RA. 2021. Participation of short-chain fatty acids and their receptors in gut inflammation and colon cancer. *Front Physiol* **12:** 662739. doi:10.3389/fphys.2021.662739

Chen WW, Freinkman E, Wang T, Birsoy K, Sabatini DM. 2016. Absolute quantification of matrix metabolites reveals the dynamics of mitochondrial metabolism. *Cell* **166:** 1324–1337.e11. doi:10.1016/j.cell.2016.07.040

Chen WW, Freinkman E, Sabatini DM. 2017. Rapid immunopurification of mitochondria for metabolite profiling and absolute quantification of matrix metabolites. *Nat Protoc* **12:** 2215–2231. doi:10.1038/nprot.2017.104

Cheng CW, Biton M, Haber AL, Gunduz N, Eng G, Gaynor LT, Tripathi S, Calibasi-Kocal G, Rickett S, Butty VL, et al. 2019. Ketone body signaling mediates intestinal stem cell homeostasis and adaptation to diet. *Cell* **178:** 1115–1131.e15. doi:10.1016/j.cell.2019.07.048

Colegio OR, Chu NQ, Szabo AL, Chu T, Rhebergen AM, Jairam V, Cyrus N, Brokowski CE, Eisenbarth SC, Phillips GM, et al. 2014. Functional polarization of tumour-associated macrophages by tumour-derived lactic acid. *Nature* **513:** 559–563. doi:10.1038/nature13490

Covarrubias AJ, Aksoylar HI, Yu J, Snyder NW, Worth AJ, Iyer SS, Wang J, Ben-Sahra I, Byles V, Polynne-Stapornkul T, et al. 2016. Akt-mTORC1 signaling regulates Acly to integrate metabolic input to control of macrophage activation. *eLife* **5:** e11612. doi:10.7554/eLife.11612

Dmitrieva-Posocco O, Wong AC, Lundgren P, Golos AM, Descamps HC, Dohnalová L, Cramer Z, Tian Y, Yueh B, Eskiocak O, et al. 2022. β-hydroxybutyrate suppresses colorectal cancer. *Nature* **605:** 160–165. doi:10.1038/s41586-022-04649-6

Donohoe DR, Collins LB, Wali A, Bigler R, Sun W, Bultman SJ. 2012. The Warburg effect dictates the mechanism of butyrate-mediated histone acetylation and cell proliferation. *Mol Cell* **48:** 612–626. doi:10.1016/j.molcel.2012.08.033

Donohoe DR, Holley D, Collins LB, Montgomery SA, Whitmore AC, Hillhouse A, Curry KP, Renner SW, Greenwalt A, Ryan EP, et al. 2014. A gnotobiotic mouse model demonstrates that dietary fiber protects against colorectal tumorigenesis in a microbiota- and butyrate-dependent manner. *Cancer Discov* **4:** 1387–1397. doi:10.1158/2159-8290.CD-14-0501

Dorsam RT, Gutkind JS. 2007. G-protein-coupled receptors and cancer. *Nat Rev Cancer* **7:** 79–94. doi:10.1038/nrc2069

Eckert MA, Coscia F, Chryplewicz A, Chang JW, Hernandez KM, Pan S, Tienda SM, Nahotko DA, Li G, Blaženović I, et al. 2019. Proteomics reveals NNMT as a master metabolic regulator of cancer-associated fibroblasts. *Nature* **569:** 723–728. doi:10.1038/s41586-019-1173-8

Elia I, Haigis MC. 2021. Metabolites and the tumour microenvironment: from cellular mechanisms to systemic metabolism. *Nat Metab* **3:** 21–32. doi:10.1038/s42255-020-00317-z

Feng T, Zhao X, Gu P, Yang W, Wang C, Guo Q, Long Q, Liu Q, Cheng Y, Li J, et al. 2022. Adipocyte-derived lactate is a signalling metabolite that potentiates adipose macrophage inflammation via targeting PHD2. *Nat Commun* **13:** 5208. doi:10.1038/s41467-022-32871-3

Figlia G, Willnow P, Teleman AA. 2020. Metabolites regulate cell signaling and growth via covalent modification of proteins. *Dev Cell* **54:** 156–170. doi:10.1016/j.devcel.2020.06.036

Franken H, Mathieson T, Childs D, Sweetman GM, Werner T, Tögel I, Doce C, Gade S, Bantscheff M, Drewes G, et al. 2015. Thermal proteome profiling for unbiased identification of direct and indirect drug targets using multiplexed quantitative mass spectrometry. *Nat Protoc* **10:** 1567–1593. doi:10.1038/nprot.2015.101

Gaffney DO, Jennings EQ, Anderson CC, Marentette JO, Shi T, Schou Oxvig AM, Streeter MD, Johannsen M, Spiegel DA, Chapman E, et al. 2020. Non-enzymatic lysine lactoylation of glycolytic enzymes. *Cell Chem Biol* 27: 206–213. e6. doi:10.1016/j.chembiol.2019.11.005

Gao X, Lin SH, Ren F, Li JT, Chen JJ, Yao CB, Yang HB, Jiang SX, Yan GQ, Wang D, et al. 2016. Acetate functions as an epigenetic metabolite to promote lipid synthesis under hypoxia. *Nat Commun* 7: 11960. doi:10.1038/ncomms11960

Gao X, Sanderson SM, Dai Z, Reid MA, Cooper DE, Lu M, Richie JP, Ciccarella A, Calcagnotto A, Mikhael PG, et al. 2019. Dietary methionine influences therapy in mouse cancer models and alters human metabolism. *Nature* 572: 397–401. doi:10.1038/s41586-019-1437-3

Gao Y, Martin NI, van Haren MJ. 2021. Nicotinamide *N*-methyl transferase (NNMT): an emerging therapeutic target. *Drug Discov Today* 26: 2699–2706. doi:10.1016/j.drudis.2021.05.011

Gowans GJ, Hawley SA, Ross FA, Hardie DG. 2013. AMP is a true physiological regulator of AMP-activated protein kinase by both allosteric activation and enhancing net phosphorylation. *Cell Metab* 18: 556–566. doi:10.1016/j.cmet.2013.08.019

Guertin DA, Wellen KE. 2023. Acetyl-CoA metabolism in cancer. *Nat Rev Cancer* 23: 156–172. doi:10.1038/s41568-022-00543-5

* Gunn K, Losman JA. 2024. Isocitrate dehydrogenase mutations in cancer: mechanisms of transformation and metabolic liability. *Cold Spring Harb Perspect Med* doi:10.1101/cshperspect.a041537

Hardie DG, Schaffer BE, Brunet A. 2016. AMPK: an energy-sensing pathway with multiple inputs and outputs. *Trends Cell Biol* 26: 190–201. doi:10.1016/j.tcb.2015.10.013

Hicks KG, Cluntun AA, Schubert HL, Hackett SR, Berg JA, Leonard PG, Ajalla Aleixo MA, Zhou Y, Bott AJ, Salvatore SR, et al. 2023. Protein-metabolite interactomics of carbohydrate metabolism reveal regulation of lactate dehydrogenase. *Science* 379: 996–1003. doi:10.1126/science.abm3452

Ho PC, Bihuniak JD, Macintyre AN, Staron M, Liu X, Amezquita R, Tsui YC, Cui G, Micevic G, Perales JC, et al. 2015. Phosphoenolpyruvate is a metabolic checkpoint of antitumor T cell responses. *Cell* 162: 1217–1228. doi:10.1016/j.cell.2015.08.012

Kang HB, Fan J, Lin R, Elf S, Ji Q, Zhao L, Jin L, Seo JH, Shan C, Arbiser JL, et al. 2015. Metabolic rewiring by oncogenic BRAF V600E links ketogenesis pathway to BRAF-MEK1 signaling. *Mol Cell* 59: 345–358. doi:10.1016/j.molcel.2015.05.037

Koppenol WH, Bounds PL, Dang CV. 2011. Otto Warburg's contributions to current concepts of cancer metabolism. *Nat Rev Cancer* 11: 325–337. doi:10.1038/nrc3038

Kottakis F, Nicolay BN, Roumane A, Karnik R, Gu H, Nagle JM, Boukhali M, Hayward MC, Li YY, Chen T, et al. 2016. LKB1 loss links serine metabolism to DNA methylation and tumorigenesis. *Nature* 539: 390–395. doi:10.1038/nature20132

Lee JV, Carrer A, Shah S, Snyder NW, Wei S, Venneti S, Worth AJ, Yuan ZF, Lim HW, Liu S, et al. 2014. Akt-dependent metabolic reprogramming regulates tumor cell histone acetylation. *Cell Metab* 20: 306–319. doi:10.1016/j.cmet.2014.06.004

Lee JV, Berry CT, Kim K, Sen P, Kim T, Carrer A, Trefely S, Zhao S, Fernandez S, Barney LE, et al. 2018. Acetyl-CoA

promotes glioblastoma cell adhesion and migration through Ca^{2+}-NFAT signaling. *Genes Dev* 32: 497–511. doi:10.1101/gad.311027.117

Levy MJ, Montgomery DC, Sardiu ME, Montano JL, Bergholtz SE, Nance KD, Thorpe AL, Fox SD, Lin Q, Andresson T, et al. 2020. A systems chemoproteomic analysis of Acyl-CoA/protein interaction networks. *Cell Chem Biol* 27: 322–333.e5. doi:10.1016/j.chembiol.2019.11.011

Li X, Wang L, Zhou XE, Ke J, de Waal PW, Gu X, Tan MH, Wang D, Wu D, Xu HE, et al. 2015. Structural basis of AMPK regulation by adenine nucleotides and glycogen. *Cell Res* 25: 50–66. doi:10.1038/cr.2014.150

Lien EC, Westermark AM, Zhang Y, Yuan C, Li Z, Lau AN, Sapp KM, Wolpin BM, Vander Heiden MG. 2021. Low glycaemic diets alter lipid metabolism to influence tumour growth. *Nature* 599: 302–307. doi:10.1038/s41586-021-04049-2

* Lim EW, Metallo CM. 2024. Tracing the diverse paths of one-carbon metabolism in cancer and beyond. *Cold Spring Harb Perspect Med* doi:10.1101/cshperspect.a041533

Liu GY, Sabatini DM. 2020. mTOR at the nexus of nutrition, growth, ageing and disease. *Nat Rev Mol Cell Biol* 21: 183–203. doi:10.1038/s41580-019-0199-y

Liu D, Evans T, Zhang F. 2015. Applications and advances of metabolite biosensors for metabolic engineering. *Metab Eng* 31: 35–43. doi:10.1016/j.ymben.2015.06.008

Liu W, Wang Y, Bozi LHM, Fischer PD, Jedrychowski MP, Xiao H, Wu T, Darabedian N, He X, Mills EL, et al. 2023. Lactate regulates cell cycle by remodelling the anaphase promoting complex. *Nature* 616: 790–797. doi:10.1038/s41586-023-05939-3

Locasale JW. 2013. Serine, glycine and one-carbon units: cancer metabolism in full circle. *Nat Rev Cancer* 13: 572–583. doi:10.1038/nrc3557

Lu M, Zhu WW, Wang X, Tang JJ, Zhang KL, Yu GY, Shao WQ, Lin ZF, Wang SH, Lu L, et al. 2019. ACOT12-dependent alteration of acetyl-CoA drives hepatocellular carcinoma metastasis by epigenetic induction of epithelial-mesenchymal transition. *Cell Metab* 29: 886–900.e5. doi:10.1016/j.cmet.2018.12.019

Lyssiotis CA, Kimmelman AC. 2017. Metabolic interactions in the tumor microenvironment. *Trends Cell Biol* 27: 863–875. doi:10.1016/j.tcb.2017.06.003

* Manning BD, Dibble CC. 2024. Growth signalling networks orchestrate cancer metabolic networks. *Cold Spring Harb Perspect Med* doi:10.1101/cshperspect.a041543

Mariño G, Pietrocola F, Eisenberg T, Kong Y, Malik SA, Andryushkova A, Schroeder S, Pendl T, Harger A, Niso-Santano M, et al. 2014. Regulation of autophagy by cytosolic acetyl-coenzyme A. *Mol Cell* 53: 710–725. doi:10.1016/j.molcel.2014.01.016

Martínez-Reyes I, Chandel NS. 2020. Mitochondrial TCA cycle metabolites control physiology and disease. *Nat Commun* 11: 102. doi:10.1038/s41467-019-13668-3

Martínez-Reyes I, Chandel NS. 2021. Cancer metabolism: looking forward. *Nat Rev Cancer* 21: 669–680. doi:10.1038/s41568-021-00378-6

Mentch SJ, Mehrmohamadi M, Huang L, Liu X, Gupta D, Mattocks D, Gómez Padilla P, Ables G, Bamman MM, Thalacker-Mercer AE, et al. 2015. Histone methylation dynamics and gene regulation occur through the sensing

of one-carbon metabolism. *Cell Metab* **22:** 861–873. doi:10
.1016/j.cmet.2015.08.024

Menzies KJ, Zhang H, Katsyuba E, Auwerx J. 2016. Protein
acetylation in metabolism—metabolites and cofactors.
Nat Rev Endocrinol **12:** 43–60. doi:10.1038/nrendo.2015
.181

Michelet X, Dyck L, Hogan A, Loftus RM, Duquette D, Wei K,
Beyaz S, Tavakkoli A, Foley C, Donnelly R, et al. 2018.
Metabolic reprogramming of natural killer cells in obesity
limits antitumor responses. *Nat Immunol* **19:** 1330–1340.
doi:10.1038/s41590-018-0251-7

Mills GB, Moolenaar WH. 2003. The emerging role of lysophosphatidic acid in cancer. *Nat Rev Cancer* **3:** 582–591.
doi:10.1038/nrc1143

Mirzaei R, Afaghi A, Babakhani S, Sohrabi MR, Hosseini-
Fard SR, Babolhavaeji K, Khani Ali Akbari S, Yousefima-
shouf R, Karampoor S. 2021. Role of microbiota-derived
short-chain fatty acids in cancer development and prevention. *Biomed Pharmacother* **139:** 111619. doi:10.1016/j
.biopha.2021.111619

Montgomery DC, Garlick JM, Kulkarni RA, Kennedy S, Al-
lali-Hassani A, Kuo YM, Andrews AJ, Wu H, Vedadi M,
Meier JL. 2016. Global profiling of acetyltransferase feedback regulation. *J Am Chem Soc* **138:** 6388–6391. doi:10
.1021/jacs.6b03036

Morland C, Andersson KA, Haugen OP, Hadzic A, Kleppa L,
Gille A, Rinholm JE, Palibrk V, Diget EH, Kennedy LH, et
al. 2017. Exercise induces cerebral VEGF and angiogenesis
via the lactate receptor HCAR1. *Nat Commun* **8:** 15557.
doi:10.1038/ncomms15557

Noe JT, Rendon BE, Geller AE, Conroy LR, Morrissey SM,
Young LEA, Bruntz RC, Kim EJ, Wise-Mitchell A, Barbosa
de Souza Rizzo M, et al. 2021. Lactate supports a metabolic-
epigenetic link in macrophage polarization. *Sci Adv* **7:**
eabi8602. doi:10.1126/sciadv.abi8602

Olsen T, Øvrebø B, Haj-Yasein N, Lee S, Svendsen K, Hjorth
M, Bastani NE, Norheim F, Drevon CA, Refsum H, et al.
2020. Effects of dietary methionine and cysteine restriction
on plasma biomarkers, serum fibroblast growth factor 21,
and adipose tissue gene expression in women with overweight or obesity: a double-blind randomized controlled
pilot study. *J Transl Med* **18:** 122. doi:10.1186/s12967-020-
02288-x

Peng M, Yin N, Chhangawala S, Xu K, Leslie CS, Li MO. 2016.
Aerobic glycolysis promotes T helper 1 cell differentiation
through an epigenetic mechanism. *Science* **354:** 481–484.
doi:10.1126/science.aaf6284

Planque M, Igelmann S, Ferreira Campos AM, Fendt SM.
2023. Spatial metabolomics principles and application to
cancer research. *Curr Opin Chem Biol* **76:** 102362. doi:10
.1016/j.cbpa.2023.102362

Puchalska P, Crawford PA. 2021. Metabolic and signaling
roles of ketone bodies in health and disease. *Annu
Rev Nutr* **41:** 49–77. doi:10.1146/annurev-nutr-111120-
111518

Qiu J, Villa M, Sanin DE, Buck MD, O'Sullivan D, Ching R,
Matsushita M, Grzes KM, Winkler F, Chang CH, et al.
2019. Acetate promotes T cell effector function during
glucose restriction. *Cell Rep* **27:** 2063–2074.e5. doi:10
.1016/j.celrep.2019.04.022

Quirós PM, Mottis A, Auwerx J. 2016. Mitonuclear communication in homeostasis and stress. *Nat Rev Mol Cell Biol*
17: 213–226. doi:10.1038/nrm.2016.23

Reid MA, Dai Z, Locasale JW. 2017. The impact of cellular
metabolism on chromatin dynamics and epigenetics. *Nat
Cell Biol* **19:** 1298–1306. doi:10.1038/ncb3629

Reinhard FB, Eberhard D, Werner T, Franken H, Childs D,
Doce C, Savitski MF, Huber W, Bantscheff M, Savitski
MM, et al. 2015. Thermal proteome profiling monitors
ligand interactions with cellular membrane proteins. *Nat
Methods* **12:** 1129–1131. doi:10.1038/nmeth.3652

Ringel AE, Drijvers JM, Baker GJ, Catozzi A, García-Cañaveras JC, Gassaway BM, Miller BC, Juneja VR, Nguyen
TH, Joshi S, et al. 2020. Obesity shapes metabolism in
the tumor microenvironment to suppress anti-tumor immunity. *Cell* **183:** 1848–1866.e26. doi:10.1016/j.cell.2020
.11.009

Rios Garcia M, Steinbauer B, Srivastava K, Singhal M, Mat-
tijssen F, Maida A, Christian S, Hess-Stumpp H, Augustin
HG, Müller-Decker K, et al. 2017. Acetyl-CoA carboxylase
1-dependent protein acetylation controls breast cancer
metastasis and recurrence. *Cell Metab* **26:** 842–855.e5.
doi:10.1016/j.cmet.2017.09.018

Ryu KW, Nandu T, Kim J, Challa S, DeBerardinis RJ, Kraus
WL. 2018. Metabolic regulation of transcription through
compartmentalized NAD$^+$ biosynthesis. *Science* **360:**
eaan5780. doi:10.1126/science.aan5780

Saxton RA, Knockenhauer KE, Wolfson RL, Chantranupong
L, Pacold ME, Wang T, Schwartz TU, Sabatini DM. 2016.
Structural basis for leucine sensing by the Sestrin2-
mTORC1 pathway. *Science* **351:** 53–58. doi:10.1126/sci
ence.aad2087

Senapati P, Kato H, Lee M, Leung A, Thai C, Sanchez A,
Gallagher EJ, LeRoith D, Seewaldt VL, Ann DK, et al.
2019. Hyperinsulinemia promotes aberrant histone acetylation in triple-negative breast cancer. *Epigenetics Chromatin* **12:** 44. doi:10.1186/s13072-019-0290-9

Shimazu T, Hirschey MD, Newman J, He W, Shirakawa K, Le
Moan N, Grueter CA, Lim H, Saunders LR, Stevens RD, et
al. 2013. Suppression of oxidative stress by β-hydroxybutyrate, an endogenous histone deacetylase inhibitor. *Science* **339:** 211–214. doi:10.1126/science.1227166

Snaebjornsson MT, Janaki-Raman S, Schulze A. 2020. Greasing the wheels of the cancer machine: the role of lipid
metabolism in cancer. *Cell Metab* **31:** 62–76. doi:10
.1016/j.cmet.2019.11.010

Tang Y, Chen Y, Jiang H, Robbins GT, Nie D. 2011. G-protein-
coupled receptor for short-chain fatty acids suppresses
colon cancer. *Int J Cancer* **128:** 847–856. doi:10.1002/ijc
.25638

Thangaraju M, Cresci GA, Liu K, Ananth S, Gnanaprakasam
JP, Browning DD, Mellinger JD, Smith SB, Digby GJ,
Lambert NA, et al. 2009. GPR109A is a G-protein-
coupled receptor for the bacterial fermentation product
butyrate and functions as a tumor suppressor in colon.
Cancer Res **69:** 2826–2832. doi:10.1158/0008-5472
.CAN-08-4466

Trefely S, Lovell CD, Snyder NW, Wellen KE. 2020. Compart-
mentalised acyl-CoA metabolism and roles in chromatin
regulation. *Mol Metab* **38:** 100941. doi:10.1016/j.molmet
.2020.01.005

Trefely S, Huber K, Liu J, Noji M, Stransky S, Singh J, Doan MT, Lovell CD, von Krusenstiern E, Jiang H, et al. 2022. Quantitative subcellular acyl-CoA analysis reveals distinct nuclear metabolism and isoleucine-dependent histone propionylation. *Mol Cell* **82:** 447–462.e6. doi:10.1016/j.molcel.2021.11.006

Ulanovskaya OA, Zuhl AM, Cravatt BF. 2013. NNMT promotes epigenetic remodeling in cancer by creating a metabolic methylation sink. *Nat Chem Biol* **9:** 300–306. doi:10.1038/nchembio.1204

Wellen KE, Snyder NW. 2019. Should we consider subcellular compartmentalization of metabolites, and if so, how do we measure them? *Curr Opin Clin Nutr Metab Care* **22:** 347–354. doi:10.1097/MCO.0000000000000580

Wiktorowicz JE, Campos KL, Bonner J. 1981. Substrate and product inhibition initial rate kinetics of histone acetyltransferase. *Biochemistry* **20:** 1464–1467. doi:10.1021/bi00509a009

Wolfson RL, Chantranupong L, Saxton RA, Shen K, Scaria SM, Cantor JR, Sabatini DM. 2016. Sestrin2 is a leucine sensor for the mTORC1 pathway. *Science* **351:** 43–48. doi:10.1126/science.aab2674

Xia S, Lin R, Jin L, Zhao L, Kang HB, Pan Y, Liu S, Qian G, Qian Z, Konstantakou E, et al. 2017. Prevention of dietary-fat-fueled ketogenesis attenuates BRAF V600E tumor growth. *Cell Metab* **25:** 358–373. doi:10.1016/j.cmet.2016.12.010

Xie N, Zhang L, Gao W, Huang C, Huber PE, Zhou X, Li C, Shen G, Zou B. 2020. NAD^+ metabolism: pathophysiologic mechanisms and therapeutic potential. *Signal Transduct Target Ther* **5:** 227. doi:10.1038/s41392-020-00311-7

Zhang D, Tang Z, Huang H, Zhou G, Cui C, Weng Y, Liu W, Kim S, Lee S, Perez-Neut M, et al. 2019. Metabolic regulation of gene expression by histone lactylation. *Nature* **574:** 575–580. doi:10.1038/s41586-019-1678-1

Understanding the Warburg Effect in Cancer

Zhaoqi Li,[1,2] Muhammad Bin Munim,[1,2] Daniel A. Sharygin,[1,2] Brooke J. Bevis,[1] and Matthew G. Vander Heiden[1,2,3]

[1]Koch Institute for Integrative Cancer Research, Massachusetts Institute of Technology, Cambridge, Massachusetts 02139, USA

[2]Department of Biology, Massachusetts Institute of Technology, Cambridge, Massachusetts 02139, USA

[3]Dana-Farber Cancer Institute, Boston, Massachusetts 02115, USA

Correspondence: mvh@mit.edu

Rapidly proliferating cells, including cancer cells, adapt metabolism to meet the increased energetic and biosynthetic demands of cell growth and division. Many rapidly proliferating cells exhibit increased glucose consumption and fermentation regardless of oxygen availability, a phenotype termed aerobic glycolysis or the Warburg effect in cancer. Several explanations for why cells engage in aerobic glycolysis and how it supports proliferation have been proposed, but none can fully explain all conditions and data where aerobic glycolysis is observed. Nevertheless, there is convincing evidence that the Warburg effect is important for the proliferation of many cancers, and that inhibiting either glucose uptake or fermentation can impair tumor growth. Here, we discuss what is known about metabolism associated with aerobic glycolysis and the evidence supporting various explanations for why aerobic glycolysis may be important in cancer and other contexts.

Cell growth and proliferation necessitate the transformation of extracellular nutrients into biomass. Life uses diverse strategies to support biomass accumulation that range from carbon fixation by photosynthetic organisms to direct biomass incorporation of consumed nutrients by heterotrophic organisms. Glucose is a primary and preferred nutrient source for many animal cells, including many cancer cells, and pathways involving glucose catabolism are conserved across all domains of life. Generally speaking, in nonproliferating cells, the complete oxidation of glucose to CO_2 enables maximum ATP production via oxidative phosphorylation, a process that requires consumption of oxygen (Fig. 1).

Fermentation of glucose-derived pyruvate can produce ATP in glycolysis without using oxidative phosphorylation, and thus can work in the absence of oxygen, but because glucose is not fully oxidized, far less ATP can be produced. Thus, fermentation is the major route of ATP generation in anaerobic conditions. However, regardless of oxygen availability, many rapidly proliferating cells, including most cancer cells, also increase glucose uptake and ferment much of that glucose. This phenomenon, known as aerobic glycolysis or the Warburg effect in cancer, has been the topic of extensive research for more than a century (Vander Heiden et al. 2009; Koppenol et al. 2011).

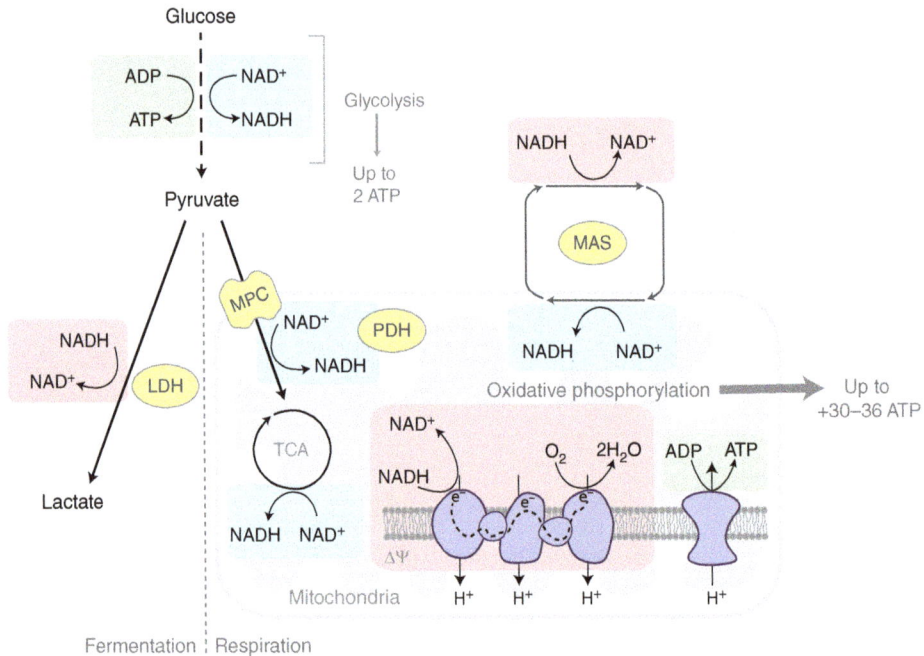

Figure 1. Role of glycolysis, fermentation, and oxidative phosphorylation in redox metabolism and ATP generation. Schematic showing the metabolism of glucose to pyruvate by glycolysis, with the subsequent metabolism of pyruvate to make lactate (fermentation in mammalian cells) versus the further oxidation of pyruvate in the mitochondria, which can support ATP production via oxidative phosphorylation. Metabolism of glucose to lactate to make ATP does not require oxygen, while metabolism of glucose-derived pyruvate in the mitochondria to support oxidative phosphorylation can produce more ATP, but requires consumption of oxygen (respiration) to regenerate NAD$^+$. The proteins involved in the differential metabolism of pyruvate (LDH [lactate dehydrogenase], MPC [mitochondrial pyruvate carrier], PDH [pyruvate dehydrogenase complex]) as well as the malate–aspartate shuttle (MAS) as a route to transfer electrons from cytosolic NADH to the mitochondria are also shown.

An association between aerobic glycolysis and rapid proliferation is not universal, but is generally conserved from bacteria to humans (De Deken 1966; Wolfe 2005; Liberti and Locasale 2016). The signal transduction pathways that promote this phenotype in cancer and immune cells have been extensively studied (Frauwirth et al. 2002; Elstrom et al. 2004; Krawczyk et al. 2010; Sun et al. 2011; Kaplon et al. 2013; Xu et al. 2021); however, a metabolic rationale for how aerobic glycolysis supports proliferation remains controversial. Nevertheless, the widespread utilization of aerobic glycolysis during rapid proliferation suggests there are strong selective pressures to maintain this phenotype over evolutionary timescales. This also argues that the underlying explanation for why cancer cells exhibit the Warburg effect cannot be specific to cancer. Rather, aerobic gly-

colysis must reflect some aspect of proliferative metabolism that is found in many different species and contexts even if the propensity of cancers to exhibit this phenotype provides additional benefits for cancers in some settings. Nevertheless, the increased glucose uptake associated with the Warburg effect is leveraged for cancer staging and imaging of therapeutic responses via the use of ^{18}F-fluorodeoxyglucose-positron emission tomography (FDG-PET) scan (Vander Heiden et al. 2009), and targeting aspects of aerobic glycolysis have been proposed as potential ways to treat cancer (Luengo et al. 2017).

ROLE OF GLUCOSE IN METABOLISM

All life must harness energy from the environment and use that energy to maintain homeo-

Cite this article as *Cold Spring Harb Perspect Med* doi: 10.1101/cshperspect.a041532

stasis as well as support any increase in biomass. This includes maintaining an ATP/ADP ratio where favorable hydrolysis of ATP to ADP can be coupled to otherwise unfavorable reactions. This necessitates that cells constantly phosphorylate ADP to produce ATP, which occurs through two major pathways in mammalian cells: glycolysis and mitochondrial oxidative phosphorylation (Fig. 1). Both routes of ATP production can be supported via the oxidation of glucose, although oxidative phosphorylation can be driven by oxidation of other nutrients including fatty acids and amino acids.

Glucose is an important nutrient for many cells and tissues in mammals, as well as other organisms, and mammalian cells use ATP to trap passively transported glucose in cells via phosphorylation to glucose-6-phosphate, which serves as the initial substrate for glucose oxidation by glycolysis (Fig. 2). Metabolism of glucose-6-phosphate into pyruvate net generates two molecules of ATP and two molecules of NADH in the Embden–Meyerhoff–Parnas pathway of glycolysis used by most organisms, including mammals. Apart from ATP and NADH, the end product of glycolysis is two molecules of pyruvate. The partial oxidation of glucose to pyruvate requires a constant source of NAD^+ to act as an electron acceptor and support carbon oxidation, accounting for NADH generation by this pathway (Fig. 1). Importantly, NAD^+ must be regenerated from NADH to enable continued glycolysis. This must occur by the subsequent transfer of electrons to a final electron acceptor, such as oxygen or glucose-derived pyruvate. In the absence of oxygen or another suitable acceptor, the pyruvate can be fermented to a more reduced molecule, such as lactate or ethanol, to regenerate NAD^+. Thus, fermentation enables glycolysis to proceed even when oxygen is absent (Harris 2002). If oxygen is available, pyruvate can be further oxidized

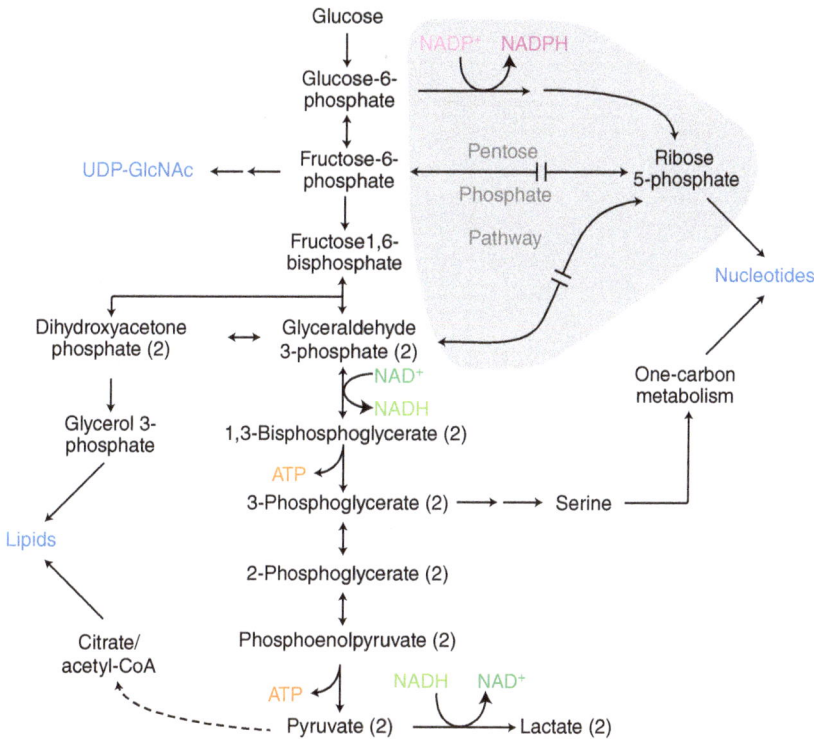

Figure 2. Relationship between glycolysis and biomass production. Schematic showing glycolysis and the pentose phosphate pathway, and how to select glycolytic intermediates are related to the indicated biomass components. Pyruvate kinase catalyzes the conversion of phosphoenolpyruvate to pyruvate.

in the mitochondria to support additional ATP production via oxidative phosphorylation, or provide a source of carbon for biomass components derived from further metabolism of pyruvate. Electron disposal is necessary to support both the oxidation of pyruvate via the pyruvate dehydrogenase complex (PDH) and the TCA cycle, with the transfer of electrons to oxygen being coupled to the generation of an electrochemical proton gradient that supports oxidative phosphorylation.

By generating its own electron acceptor, fermentation provides a clear advantage to cells to allow continued ATP production in the absence of oxygen (Harris 2002), but the product of fermentation differs across organisms. Mammalian cells ferment pyruvate into lactate, while yeast and bacteria use pathways that convert pyruvate into a variety of molecules such as ethanol, hydrogen, acetic acid, and/or formic acid (Smid and Lacroix 2013). In all cases, fermentation can sustain redox balance and glycolytic flux, but comes at the cost of a diminished ATP yield per molecule of glucose metabolized. Oxidative phosphorylation produces around 15 times more ATP per molecule of glucose oxidized than fermentation (Fig. 1). Thus, provided oxygen is available, oxidative phosphorylation enables efficient ATP synthesis when nutrients are limited. However, this raises the question of why many rapidly proliferating cells from all kingdoms of life favor high rates of fermentation even when oxygen is available. That is, why is aerobic glycolysis associated with rapid proliferation in many different cells and contexts, including cancers?

USE OF AEROBIC GLYCOLYSIS IN CANCER

The propensity for cells to engage in aerobic glycolysis during rapid growth has been broadly observed across life, including in cancer, where Warburg first observed approximately a century ago that tumor cells have high glucose uptake and lactate excretion (Warburg et al. 1924; Vander Heiden et al. 2009; Koppenol et al. 2011). Knowing that fermentation can be induced in respiration-deficient cells, Warburg hypothesized that an "irreversible injury to respiration"

may be a prerequisite for oncogenic transformation (Warburg 1956). While this hypothesis has since been disproven (Weinhouse 1976; Vander Heiden et al. 2009), it is still argued that an inability to do oxidative phosphorylation to drive fermentation is potentially beneficial to cancer even though there is clear evidence that most cancers continue to consume oxygen, and that mitochondrial respiration is required for tumor growth (Gatenby and Gillies 2004; Weinberg et al. 2010; Tan et al. 2015; Vander Heiden and DeBerardinis 2017; Bajzikova et al. 2019; Martínez-Reyes et al. 2020). That respiration is required for tumor growth is supported by the reality of aerobic glycolysis and the Warburg effect, which involves increased glucose uptake and a relative increase in fermentation, with continued and sometimes increased rates of respiration (Vander Heiden et al. 2009).

Several molecular events that favor aerobic glycolysis have been described, including increased expression of lactate dehydrogenase (LDH), down-regulation of the mitochondrial pyruvate carrier (MPC), and negative regulation of PDH activity (Fig. 1; Shim et al. 1997; Fantin et al. 2006; Kim et al. 2006; Papandreou et al. 2006; Kaplon et al. 2013; Schell et al. 2014; Vacanti et al. 2014; Yang et al. 2014; Ždralević et al. 2018; Luengo et al. 2021). Pharmacological inhibition or genetic disruption of these metabolic nodes disrupts aerobic glycolysis and slows cancer cell proliferation and tumor growth across many different models and cancer types, arguing that many cancers are indeed functionally dependent on aerobic glycolysis (Shim et al. 1997; Fantin et al. 2006; Kaplon et al. 2013; Schell et al. 2014; Vander Heiden and DeBerardinis 2017; Luengo et al. 2021). This dependence on aerobic glycolysis also argues that some aspect of this phenotype must be beneficial for the proliferation in cancer.

POSSIBLE EXPLANATIONS FOR WHY AEROBIC GLYCOLYSIS BENEFITS CANCER

A role for aerobic glycolysis in rapidly proliferating cancer cells has been extensively studied, and many explanations for this metabolic phenotype have been proposed. The appreciation

Cite this article as *Cold Spring Harb Perspect Med* doi: 10.1101/cshperspect.a041532

that angiogenesis can be limiting for tumor growth led to the hypothesis that tumor hypoxia may select for a metabolic phenotype that favors aerobic glycolysis. That is, a need to survive conditions with low oxygen due to insufficient vasculature selects for cells that rely more on an anaerobic metabolism and they persist even when cells gain access to oxygen (Gatenby and Gillies 2004). While the propensity of cancers to rely on aerobic glycolysis may prove beneficial for enduring periods of hypoxia that cancer cells encounter, this is an unsatisfying explanation for why aerobic glycolysis is broadly associated with cancer (Vander Heiden et al. 2009). Aerobic glycolysis is prevalent in cancers that are exposed to the highest oxygen tensions among human cancers, such as lung cancers and leukemia, and the phenotype is particularly prominent in cultured cancer cells that are persistently exposed to hyperoxia in culture. Aerobic glycolysis is also associated with increased glucose uptake, and thus vascularization is also needed to deliver the glucose that supports high rates of glucose consumption. Finally, aerobic glycolysis is a phenotype associated with proliferation across many cell types and contexts, including rapidly proliferating immune cells (Wang et al. 1976), and thus in many contexts, it cannot be a product of hypoxia selection, but rather must reflect some property also found in many other cells ranging from microbes to metazoans.

The fermentation of glucose to ethanol provides an advantage to some microbes as a strategy to suppress the growth of other organisms, allowing them to better compete for carbon resources. This has led some to hypothesize that cancer cells may derive analogous advantages, with high rates of lactate secretion leading to immune suppression or other phenotypes that benefit the cancer at the expense of the host (Chang et al. 2015; Apostolova and Pearce 2022). Again, while the use of the fermentative waste product as a toxic byproduct that benefits either microbes or cancer cells has been shown to occur in some contexts, it is far more likely that this is a secondary gain from a process that is already happening rather than the primary explanation for why aerobic glycolysis occurs in the first place. Apart from the prevalence of

aerobic glycolysis across many different examples of proliferation, there is also evidence that aerobic glycolysis occurs in some nonproliferative normal contexts, such as the mammalian retina (Agathocleous et al. 2012; Hurley 2021), where it is hard to reconcile toxic metabolite production as being beneficial.

One explanation based on theory is that aerobic glycolysis provides advantages for ATP generation over oxidative phosphorylation, and thus energetic reasons drive selection of this phenotype for reasons that are not apparent from consideration of ATP yield alone. For example, it has been argued that ATP production by glycolysis is faster than ATP production by oxidative phosphorylation, and thus the use of glycolysis may enable cells to proliferate faster than cells that use slower oxidative phosphorylation when nutrients are not limiting (Pfeiffer et al. 2001; Lunt and Vander Heiden 2011). Although up to 15 times, more ATP is produced per molecule of glucose when utilizing oxidative phosphorylation over glycolytic fermentation, the flux observed for aerobic glycolysis relative to aerobic respiration is ~10–50 times greater, raising a question about whether there really is a difference in energy production over a given period of time between these two pathways (Shestov et al. 2014). Nevertheless, it has been shown that cancer cells in tumors compete for glucose with other cell types in the tumors, including immune cells (Chang et al. 2015) and evolutionary game theory suggests pathways with a low yield, but high rates of ATP production, are favored when cells compete for resources (Pfeiffer et al. 2001). However, studies have identified macrophages as being the most glucose-avid cell type in at least some tumors (Reinfeld et al. 2021). Additionally, uncoupling mitochondria, which reduces the rate of ATP production, or increases the rate of ATP consumption, can increase the proliferation rate of some cancer cells (Fang et al. 2010; Luengo et al. 2021). Furthermore, both theoretical and experimental data have suggested that many cancers have excess ATP (Racker 1983; Fang et al. 2010; Vander Heiden et al. 2010; Vander Heiden and DeBerardinis 2017; Luengo et al. 2021), with ATP demand of cancers being less than that of normal tissue (Bartman et al. 2023). This suggests that ATP may not be limiting for proliferation of many cancers and argues against a faster rate of ATP production being a general explanation for why the Warburg effect is beneficial in cancer.

Modeling efforts have claimed that ATP production by aerobic glycolysis is more proteome efficient than oxidative phosphorylation, and have proposed this as an explanation for why aerobic glycolysis is beneficial for proliferation (Vazquez et al. 2010; Basan et al. 2015). Indeed, far fewer enzymes are needed to support ATP production by fermentation than are needed to support ATP production by oxidative phosphorylation. However, an argument for proteome efficiency to make ATP only works if cells are ATP limited, and as discussed above, this is not the case for many cancers. A more recent study also argued against glycolysis being more proteome efficient in some contexts, showing that producing ATP by oxidative phosphorylation is more proteome efficient in both lymphocytes and some yeast, yet these organisms engage in aerobic glycolysis when proliferating (Shen et al. 2024). Also arguing against this explanation, most cancers require mitochondrial respiration (Weinberg et al. 2010; Tan et al. 2015; Vander Heiden and DeBerardinis 2017; Bajzikova et al. 2019; Martínez-Reyes et al. 2020), meaning resources must be allocated to generate the protein machinery to support this metabolism in addition to the enzymes needed for fermentation. Cells with the most access to vasculature in human lung tumors also paradoxically exhibit the highest rates of glucose metabolism (Hensley et al. 2016), consistent with a concurrent use of oxidative metabolism in cancer cells with high glucose uptake.

Another proposed benefit of the Warburg effect is limiting the production of reactive oxygen species (ROS) (Anastasiou et al. 2011; Ghanbari Movahed et al. 2019). ROS are byproducts of mitochondrial respiration and, at sufficiently high levels, can cause oxidative damage to DNA, proteins, and lipids, contributing to cellular dysfunction and death. A high rate of glycolysis will shift some of the burden of ATP production away from oxidative phosphoryla-

tion and also has been proposed to promote NADPH generation via the pentose phosphate pathway that branches from glycolysis (Fig. 2; Anastasiou et al. 2011). NADPH is important to keep glutathione reduced and limit damage from ROS. Yeast can engage in cycles of oxidative and fermentative metabolism, with fermentation used to limit ROS production during genome duplications (Tu et al. 2005). High levels of ROS can also modulate signaling pathways that promote the Warburg effect. For instance, ROS activates hypoxia-inducible factor 1α (HIF-1α)-mediated transcription of glycolytic enzymes and pyruvate dehydrogenase kinase (PDK) (Semba et al. 2016; Tafani et al. 2016). PDK inhibits the oxidation of pyruvate via phosphorylating PDH, reducing the flux of pyruvate into the mitochondria and promoting lactate production (Kim et al. 2006; Papandreou et al. 2006). However, at least some rapidly proliferating cells engaged in aerobic glycolysis also exhibit a very low (reduced) $NAD^+/NADH$ ratio with saturated mitochondrial electron transport (Luengo et al. 2021; Wang et al. 2022), a context that will promote ROS production (Vander Heiden and DeBerardinis 2017).

Aerobic glycolysis has been proposed to occur as a consequence of cell signaling downstream from growth-promoting pathways. The phosphoinositide 3-kinase (PI3K)/AKT signaling axis is commonly activated in cancer cells, and this enhances both glucose uptake and glycolysis (Vander Heiden et al. 2009; Hoxhaj and Manning 2020). This increased glycolytic flux, typically observed under proliferative conditions, can exceed the V_{max} of PDH, resulting in pyruvate accumulation and lactate production (Curi et al. 1988). A role for PI3K in driving LDH expression and aerobic glycolysis in immune cells has also been reported (Xu et al. 2021). Other oncogenic proteins, such as the MYC transcription factor, can also promote the expression of LDH to support increased production of lactate (Shim et al. 1997). The fact that these growth-promoting pathways also promote aerobic glycolysis further argues that this pathway is beneficial, but by themselves do not explain why they are supportive of cell proliferation.

AEROBIC GLYCOLYSIS AND BIOMASS SYNTHESIS

It has been argued that aerobic glycolysis must be beneficial for biomass production, as this would fit with why its promotion is linked to progrowth signaling pathways and its association with proliferation (Vander Heiden et al. 2009). Indeed, studies in proliferating lymphocytes and fibroblasts have linked the use of aerobic glycolysis to nucleotide synthesis (Wang et al. 1976; Pouysségur et al. 1980). In further support of a link between biomass accumulation and aerobic glycolysis, proliferating cells, including most cancer cells, express the M2 isoform of the glycolytic enzyme pyruvate kinase (PKM2), which catalyzes the conversion of phosphoenolpyruvate to pyruvate (Fig. 2; Dayton et al. 2016). PKM2 is the less active, regulatable isoform of pyruvate kinase, and decreased PKM2 activity has been associated with aerobic glycolysis (Christofk et al. 2008). Reduced PKM2 activity has been proposed to enable the accumulation of glycolytic intermediates to support carbon shunting into the pentose phosphate and serine synthesis pathways for biomass synthesis (Anastasiou et al. 2011; Chaneton et al. 2012; Ye et al. 2012; Dayton et al. 2016). While a role for aerobic glycolysis in supporting biomass accumulation is plausible, less active PKM2 does not necessarily lead to the accumulation of glycolytic intermediates, although does favor nucleotide synthesis (Lunt et al. 2015; Davidson et al. 2022). It is unlikely that any benefit of aerobic glycolysis is to produce only one biomass component, even though some biomass precursors such as ribose-phosphate or UDP-GlcNAc are necessarily generated from intermediates in glycolysis. Rather it is more likely aerobic glycolysis is part of a metabolic program that enables the production of many biomass components.

Insight into understanding a potential role for aerobic glycolysis in supporting proliferation came from the observation that suppressing aerobic glycolysis, either through LDH inhibition, suppression of lactate export, or PDH activation, results in a decreased (reduced) cellular NAD^+/NADH ratio (Benjamin et al. 2018; Luengo et al. 2021; Wang et al. 2022). These results suggest that blocking fermentation through multiple independent methods suppresses NADH to NAD^+ conversion, and thus limits oxidized biomass production (Fig. 3). Maintenance of a functional respiratory chain is also required for most cancer cells to proliferate and for tumors to grow (Weinberg et al. 2010; Wheaton et al. 2014; Zhang et al. 2014; Tan et al. 2015; Bajzikova et al. 2019). Beyond a role in ATP production via oxidative phosphorylation, respiration also enables NAD^+ regeneration, and orthogonal methods of NAD^+ production can restore proliferation in respiration-deficient

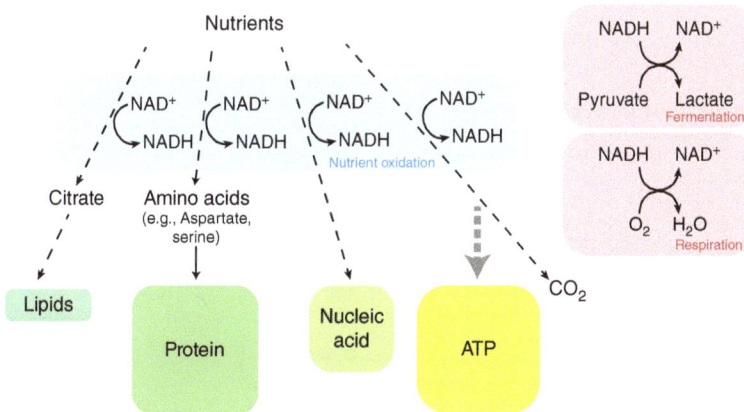

Figure 3. The role of oxidation reactions in biomass production. Schematic showing that regeneration of NAD^+ via either pyruvate to lactate conversion or oxygen consumption is important to support the oxidation reactions necessary to produce ATP as well as many biomass components.

cells (Birsoy et al. 2015; Sullivan et al. 2015; Titov et al. 2016). The surprising insight from these studies was the demonstration that an essential role of mitochondrial respiration in proliferating cells may not be for ATP production, but rather for NAD^+ regeneration.

NAD^+ is required for the biosynthesis of oxidized biomass components (Fig. 3), such as the amino acids aspartate and serine, purine and pyrimidine nucleotides, and precursors for fatty acid and lipid synthesis (Birsoy et al. 2015; Sullivan et al. 2015, 2018; Bao et al. 2016; Vander Heiden and DeBerardinis 2017; Garcia-Bermudez et al. 2018; Murphy et al. 2018; Diehl et al. 2019; Li et al. 2022). In other words, to transform environmental nutrients into biomass, a cell must continually engage in the consumption of NAD^+ and production of NADH, necessitating access to electron acceptors to regenerate the NAD^+ needed to sustain growth. Thus, in rapidly proliferating cells, the production of oxidized biomass is an important donor to the respiratory chain in addition to any pyruvate oxidation for ATP. These insights in understanding proliferative metabolism in cancer have reshaped our understanding of which metabolic requirements are most limiting for proliferation and better contextualized the reality of aerobic glycolysis as a metabolic phenotype. In light of our modern understanding, aerobic glycolysis should be best considered as the fermentation of glucose concurrent with respiration, not the fermentation of glucose in lieu of respiration.

TOWARD A UNIFYING EXPLANATION FOR AEROBIC GLYCOLYSIS IN DIFFERENT CONTEXTS

An explanation for the Warburg effect must take into account the use of aerobic glycolysis in other contexts. The preferential fermentation of pyruvate into lactate has been observed in nontransformed mammalian cells, including lymphocytes and stem cells (Wang et al. 1976; Frauwirth et al. 2002; Intlekofer and Finley 2019). Microorganisms, such as the yeast *Saccharomyces cerevisiae*, also perform aerobic glycolysis during instances of rapid growth, despite the

fact that these organisms ferment pyruvate into ethanol instead of lactate (De Deken 1966). Recent insights into the metabolism of photosynthetic organisms, such as the green algae *Chlamydomonas reinhardtii*, have led to the observation that fermentation, rather than oxidation, is the preferred fate of pyruvate during nonphotosynthetic growth (Strenkert et al. 2019). The striking conservation of aerobic glycolysis in cells, tissues, and organisms across these diverse metabolic niches and lifestyles suggests that the engagement of fermentation during proliferation is an ancient metabolic trait. Moreover, the divergence of the terminal fermentation end products in these organisms argues that it is the redox consequences of this pathway, not the carbon fate of pyruvate, that has prevailed over evolutionary timescales, even if some organisms select a particular carbon fate for secondary gain. Supporting this notion, endowing yeast with the ability to generate NAD^+ independent of respiration is sufficient to suppress aerobic glycolysis without altering proliferation rates (Vemuri et al. 2007; Luengo et al. 2021).

A clue toward what drives aerobic glycolysis can be found from studies where mitochondrial NADH oxidation is pharmacologically uncoupled from ATP production. In this context, aerobic glycolysis is inhibited and the oxygen consumption rate is increased, indicating that electron transport is not limited for substrate in many cells doing aerobic glycolysis (Luengo et al. 2021; Wang et al. 2022). Rather, the extent of respiration is determined by the ability to dispose of a product of oxidative phosphorylation, ATP, because excess ATP saturates the malate–aspartate shuttle (Fig. 1), limiting NADH regeneration by mitochondria (Luengo et al. 2021; Wang et al. 2022). Either uncoupling respiration from ATP production or increasing ATP consumption is sufficient to elevate the rate of electron transport in fermentation-defective cells, elevating the rate of NAD^+ regeneration and increasing proliferation without increasing fermentation (Luengo et al. 2021; Wang et al. 2022). Thus, when aerobic glycolysis is inhibited, proliferating cells have increased reliance on respiration to provide the NAD^+ required to sustain biomass production. However, since the electron transport chain is coupled to ATP production, an inability to remove ATP from the system constrains NAD^+ regeneration despite excess oxygen (Fig. 4). Indeed, several studies examining the role of fermentation in proliferation all point to a model where excess ATP limits NAD^+ regeneration (Birsoy et al. 2015; Sullivan et al. 2015; Titov et al. 2016; Hanse et al. 2017; Benjamin et al. 2018; Luengo et al. 2021; Wang et al. 2022; Broeks et al. 2023). Together, this argues that the stoichiometric production of NAD^+ and ATP by the electron transport chain becomes an issue in contexts where cells have biochemical processes that require more NAD^+ than ATP and suggests that in many contexts aerobic glycolysis may be a consequence of demand for NAD^+ exceeding demand for ATP (Luengo et al. 2021).

CONCLUDING REMARKS AND OPEN QUESTIONS

While a link to $NAD^+/NADH$ metabolism is likely part of why aerobic glycolysis is associated with proliferation, when taken in isolation, the proposition that fermentation in proliferating cells serves to regenerate NAD^+ cannot be the

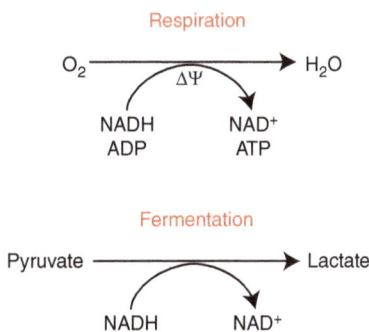

Figure 4. Increased demand for NAD^+ relative to ATP can promote aerobic glycolysis. Because NAD^+ regeneration by mitochondrial respiration is coupled to the generation of a proton gradient/mitochondrial membrane potential ($\Delta\Psi$), which is consumed to make ATP (see Fig. 1), if demand for NAD^+ regeneration exceeds the demand for ATP production, the $NAD^+/NADH$ ratio in cells will decrease (become more reduced) and promote fermentation.

full explanation for the Warburg effect. The conversion of glucose into lactate is redox-neutral and thus is incapable of net-producing NAD^+ (Fig. 1). The catabolism of glucose through glycolysis consumes NAD^+, and in the context of high glucose consumption, elevated fermentation only serves to regenerate, rather than yield, NAD^+. The fact that the majority of pyruvate in the cell is derived from glucose means that the only metabolic output of the conversion of glucose to lactate is ATP. Thus, it remains an open question as to why rapidly proliferating cells perform aerobic glycolysis while simultaneously increasing glucose uptake when the evidence in most cases argues against ATP being limited.

There are many mechanisms that could function to suppress aerobic glycolysis as a way to regenerate NAD^+. For example, beyond the microbial solutions for increasing NAD^+ regeneration at the expense of ATP production, the mammalian genome encodes a family of uncoupling proteins (UCPs) whose activity could bypass the need for NAD^+ regeneration through fermentation. UCP expression has been associated with cancer in rare instances (Valle et al. 2010; Robbins and Zhao 2011; Kawashima et al. 2020), but does not appear to be generally selected for in cancer. Moreover, futile ATP-burning processes have been observed in human tissues and cancers (Fang et al. 2010; Kazak et al. 2015; Yao et al. 2016), but how common these processes are in cancer has not been studied. Beyond mammalian systems, yeast and some bacteria contain NADH dehydrogenases that are able to regenerate NAD^+ with diminished ATP-generating capacity or that are independent of ATP production altogether. The yeast NADH dehydrogenase (Ndi1) regenerates NAD^+ without coupling electron transfer to a proton motive force, and many different organisms contain water-forming NAD(P)H oxidases that directly consume oxygen to regenerate NAD^+ (Higuchi et al. 2000; Iwata et al. 2012; Wheaton et al. 2014; Titov et al. 2016; Martínez-Reyes et al. 2020). The existence of these mechanisms of fermentation-independent NAD^+ regeneration raises the question as to why these pathways are not engaged in instances where aerobic glycolysis is used, including cancers.

The prevalence of alternative forms of glycolysis and fermentation in prokaryotes such as the Entner–Doudoroff pathway and mixed acid fermentation further complicates the notion of finding a truly unified mechanism underlying aerobic glycolysis. Understanding prokaryotic metabolism with respect to proteome efficiency and ATP yield is much more plausible, and some metabolic phenotypes have been shown to provide the flexibility to respond to large shifts in nutrient conditions that are never experienced by cells in metazoans (Flamholz et al. 2013; Law et al. 2024). Nevertheless, the existence of pathways that enable NAD^+ regeneration at the expense of maximal ATP production to support the proliferation of some microbes (Higuchi et al. 2000; Iwata et al. 2012) highlights that cells need solutions for meeting the redox constraints of biomass production in addition to meeting the demand for ATP.

Since the first description of aerobic glycolysis in cancer by Warburg et al. (1924), we have made substantial leaps in understanding both the biochemical and genetic mechanisms underlying this phenomenon. Interpretations on the origins and teleology of this metabolic phenotype have evolved over time. The link between proliferation and aerobic glycolysis is widespread across life, and a unifying mechanism that links aerobic glycolysis to every particular instance in which it is observed may not be possible. However, the fact that this phenotype is evident in many contexts spanning all kingdoms of life argues against it being driven by factors unique to cancer. Rather, like many phenotypes in cancer, the association between the Warburg effect and cancer is likely yet another example of how cancer co-opts otherwise normal cellular processes to support inappropriate proliferation and survival in abnormal tissue contexts.

COMPETING INTEREST STATEMENT

Z.L. is a current employee and shareholder of Sesame Therapeutics. M.G.V.H. is a scientific advisor for Agios Pharmaceuticals, iTeos Therapeutics, Faeth Therapeutics, Sage Therapeutics, Lime Therapeutics, Pretzel Therapeutic

DROIA Ventures, MPM Capital, and Auron Therapeutics.

ACKNOWLEDGMENTS

The authors apologize for undoubtedly missing many important references. M.G.V.H acknowledges past and present support from the Lustgarten Foundation, the MIT Center for Precision Cancer Medicine, the Ludwig Center at MIT, and the NCI (R35CA242379, R01CA201276, R01CA259253, P30CA14051).

REFERENCES

Agathocleous M, Love NK, Randlett O, Harris JJ, Liu J, Murray AJ, Harris WA. 2012. Metabolic differentiation in the embryonic retina. *Nat Cell Biol* **14:** 859–864. doi:10.1038/ncb2531

Anastasiou D, Poulogiannis G, Asara JM, Boxer MB, Jiang JK, Shen M, Bellinger G, Sasaki AT, Locasale JW, Auld DS, et al. 2011. Inhibition of pyruvate kinase M2 by reactive oxygen species contributes to cellular antioxidant responses. *Science* **334:** 1278–1283. doi:10.1126/science.1211485

Apostolova P, Pearce EL. 2022. Lactic acid and lactate: revisiting the physiological roles in the tumor microenvironment. *Trends Immunol* **43:** 969–977. doi:10.1016/j.it.2022.10.005

Bajzikova M, Kovarova J, Coelho AR, Boukalova S, Oh S, Rohlenova K, Svec D, Hubackova S, Endaya B, Judasova K, et al. 2019. Reactivation of dihydroorotate dehydrogenase-driven pyrimidine biosynthesis restores tumor growth of respiration-deficient cancer cells. *Cell Metab* **29:** 399–416.e10. doi:10.1016/j.cmet.2018.10.014

Bao XR, Ong SE, Goldberger O, Peng J, Sharma R, Thompson DA, Vafai SB, Cox AG, Marutani E, Ichinose F, et al. 2016. Mitochondrial dysfunction remodels one-carbon metabolism in human cells. *eLife* **5:** e10575. doi:10.7554/eLife.10575

Bartman CR, Weilandt DR, Shen Y, Lee WD, Han Y, TeSlaa T, Jankowski CSR, Samarah L, Park NR, da Silva-Diz V, et al. 2023. Slow TCA flux and ATP production in primary solid tumours but not metastases. *Nature* **614:** 349–357. doi:10.1038/s41586-022-05661-6

Basan M, Hui S, Okano H, Zhang Z, Shen Y, Williamson JR, Hwa T. 2015. Overflow metabolism in *Escherichia coli* results from efficient proteome allocation. *Nature* **528:** 99–104. doi:10.1038/nature15765

Benjamin D, Robay D, Hindupur SK, Pohlmann J, Colombi M, El-Shemerly MY, Maira SM, Moroni C, Lane HA, Hall MN. 2018. Dual inhibition of the lactate transporters MCT1 and MCT4 is synthetic lethal with metformin due to NAD^+ depletion in cancer cells. *Cell Rep* **25:** 3047–3058.e4. doi:10.1016/j.celrep.2018.11.043

Birsoy K, Wang T, Chen WW, Freinkman E, Abu-Remaileh M, Sabatini DM. 2015. An essential role of the mitochondrial electron transport chain in cell proliferation is to

Cite this article as *Cold Spring Harb Perspect Med* doi: 10.1101/cshperspect.a041532

enable aspartate synthesis. *Cell* **162:** 540–551. doi:10 .1016/j.cell.2015.07.016

Broeks MH, Meijer NWF, Westland D, Bosma M, Gerrits J, German HM, Ciapaite J, van Karnebeek CDM, Wanders RJA, Zwartkruis FJT, et al. 2023. The malate-aspartate shuttle is important for de novo serine biosynthesis. *Cell Rep* **42:** 113043. doi:10.1016/j.celrep.2023.113043

Chaneton B, Hillmann P, Zheng L, Martin AC, Maddocks OD, Chokkathukalam A, Coyle JE, Jankevics A, Holding FP, Vousden KH, et al. 2012. Serine is a natural ligand and allosteric activator of pyruvate kinase M2. *Nature* **491:** 458–462. doi:10.1038/nature11540

Chang CH, Qiu J, O'Sullivan D, Buck MD, Noguchi T, Curtis JD, Chen Q, Gindin M, Gubin MM, van der Windt GJ, et al. 2015. Metabolic competition in the tumor microenvironment is a driver of cancer progression. *Cell* **162:** 1229–1241. doi:10.1016/j.cell.2015.08.016

Christofk HR, Vander Heiden MG, Harris MH, Ramanathan A, Gerszten RE, Wei R, Fleming MD, Schreiber SL, Cantley LC. 2008. The M2 splice isoform of pyruvate kinase is important for cancer metabolism and tumour growth. *Nature* **452:** 230–233. doi:10.1038/nature06734

Curi R, Newsholme P, Newsholme EA. 1988. Metabolism of pyruvate by isolated rat mesenteric lymphocytes, lymphocyte mitochondria and isolated mouse macrophages. *Biochem J* **250:** 383–388. doi:10.1042/bj2500383

Davidson SM, Schmidt DR, Heyman JE, O'Brien JP, Liu AC, Israelsen WJ, Dayton TL, Sehgal R, Bronson RT, Freinkman E, et al. 2022. Pyruvate kinase M1 suppresses development and progression of prostate adenocarcinoma. *Cancer Res* **82:** 2403–2416. doi:10.1158/0008-5472 .CAN-21-2352

Dayton TL, Jacks T, Vander Heiden MG. 2016. PKM2, cancer metabolism, and the road ahead. *EMBO Rep* **17:** 1721–1730. doi:10.15252/embr.201643300

De Deken RH. 1966. The Crabtree effect: a regulatory system in yeast. *J Gen Microbiol* **44:** 149–156. doi:10.1099/ 00221287-44-2-149

Diehl FF, Lewis CA, Fiske BP, Vander Heiden MG. 2019. Cellular redox state constrains serine synthesis and nucleotide production to impact cell proliferation. *Nat Metab* **1:** 861–867. doi:10.1038/s42255-019-0108-x

Elstrom RL, Bauer DE, Buzzai M, Karnauskas R, Harris MH, Plas DR, Zhuang H, Cinalli RM, Alavi A, Rudin CM, et al. 2004. Akt stimulates aerobic glycolysis in cancer cells. *Cancer Res* **64:** 3892–3899. doi:10.1158/0008-5472 .CAN-03-2904

Fang M, Shen Z, Huang S, Zhao L, Chen S, Mak TW, Wang X. 2010. The ER UDPase ENTPD5 promotes protein N-glycosylation, the Warburg effect, and proliferation in the PTEN pathway. *Cell* **143:** 711–724. doi:10.1016/j.cell .2010.10.010

Fantin VR, St-Pierre J, Leder P. 2006. Attenuation of LDH-A expression uncovers a link between glycolysis, mitochondrial physiology, and tumor maintenance. *Cancer Cell* **9:** 425–434. doi:10.1016/j.ccr.2006.04.023

Flamholz A, Noor E, Bar-Even A, Liebermeister W, Milo R. 2013. Glycolytic strategy as a tradeoff between energy yield and protein cost. *Proc Natl Acad Sci* **110:** 10039–10044. doi:10.1073/pnas.1215283110

Frauwirth KA, Riley JL, Harris MH, Parry RV, Rathmell JC, Plas DR, Elstrom RL, June CH, Thompson CB. 2002.

The CD28 signaling pathway regulates glucose metabolism. *Immunity* **16:** 769–777. doi:10.1016/S1074-7613 (02)00323-0

Garcia-Bermudez J, Baudrier L, La K, Zhu XG, Fidelin J, Sviderskiy VO, Papagiannakopoulos T, Molina H, Snuderl M, Lewis CA, et al. 2018. Aspartate is a limiting metabolite for cancer cell proliferation under hypoxia and in tumours. *Nat Cell Biol* **20:** 775–781. doi:10.1038/ s41556-018-0118-z

Gatenby RA, Gillies RJ. 2004. Why do cancers have high aerobic glycolysis? *Nat Rev Cancer* **4:** 891–899. doi:10 .1038/nrc1478

Ghanbari Movahed Z, Rastegari-Pouyani M, Mohammadi MH, Mansouri K. 2019. Cancer cells change their glucose metabolism to overcome increased ROS: one step from cancer cell to cancer stem cell? *Biomed Pharmacother* **112:** 108690. doi:10.1016/j.biopha.2019.108690

Hanse EA, Ruan C, Kachman M, Wang D, Lowman XH, Kelekar A. 2017. Cytosolic malate dehydrogenase activity helps support glycolysis in actively proliferating cells and cancer. *Oncogene* **36:** 3915–3924. doi:10.1038/onc.2017 .36

Harris AL. 2002. Hypoxia—a key regulatory factor in tumour growth. *Nat Rev Cancer* **2:** 38–47. doi:10.1038/ nrc704

Hensley CT, Faubert B, Yuan Q, Lev-Cohain N, Jin E, Kim J, Jiang L, Ko B, Skelton R, Loudat L, et al. 2016. Metabolic heterogeneity in human lung tumors. *Cell* **164:** 681–694. doi:10.1016/j.cell.2015.12.034

Higuchi M, Yamamoto Y, Kamio Y. 2000. Molecular biology of oxygen tolerance in lactic acid bacteria: functions of NADH oxidases and Dpr in oxidative stress. *J Biosci Bioeng* **90:** 484–493. doi:10.1016/S1389-1723(01)80028-1

Hoxhaj G, Manning BD. 2020. The PI3K-AKT network at the interface of oncogenic signalling and cancer metabolism. *Nat Rev Cancer* **20:** 74–88. doi:10.1038/s41568-019-0216-7

Hurley JB. 2021. Retina metabolism and metabolism in the pigmented epithelium: a busy intersection. *Annu Rev Vis Sci* **7:** 665–692. doi:10.1146/annurev-vision-100419-115156

Intlekofer AM, Finley LWS. 2019. Metabolic signatures of cancer cells and stem cells. *Nat Metab* **1:** 177–188. doi:10 .1038/s42255-019-0032-0

Iwata M, Lee Y, Yamashita T, Yagi T, Iwata S, Cameron AD, Maher MJ. 2012. The structure of the yeast NADH dehydrogenase (Ndi1) reveals overlapping binding sites for water- and lipid-soluble substrates. *Proc Natl Acad Sci* **109:** 15247–15252. doi:10.1073/pnas.1210059109

Kaplon J, Zheng L, Meissl K, Chaneton B, Selivanov VA, Mackay G, van der Burg SH, Verdegaal EM, Cascante M, Shlomi T, et al. 2013. A key role for mitochondrial gatekeeper pyruvate dehydrogenase in oncogene-induced senescence. *Nature* **498:** 109–112. doi:10.1038/nature 12154

Kawashima M, Bensaad K, Zois CE, Barberis A, Bridges E, Wigfield S, Lagerholm C, Dmitriev RI, Tokiwa M, Toi M, et al. 2020. Disruption of hypoxia-inducible fatty acid binding protein 7 induces beige fat-like differentiation and thermogenesis in breast cancer cells. *Cancer Metab* **8:** 13. doi:10.1186/s40170-020-00219-4

Kazak L, Chouchani ET, Jedrychowski MP, Erickson BK, Shinoda K, Cohen P, Vetrivelan R, Lu GZ, Laznik-Bogoslavski D, Hasenfuss SC, et al. 2015. A creatine-driven substrate cycle enhances energy expenditure and thermogenesis in beige fat. *Cell* **163:** 643–655. doi:10.1016/j.cell.2015.09.035

Kim JW, Tchernyshyov I, Semenza GL, Dang CV. 2006. HIF-1-mediated expression of pyruvate dehydrogenase kinase: a metabolic switch required for cellular adaptation to hypoxia. *Cell Metab* **3:** 177–185. doi:10.1016/j.cmet.2006.02.002

Koppenol WH, Bounds PL, Dang CV. 2011. Otto Warburg's contributions to current concepts of cancer metabolism. *Nat Rev Cancer* **11:** 325–337. doi:10.1038/nrc3038

Krawczyk CM, Holowka T, Sun J, Blagih J, Amiel E, DeBerardinis RJ, Cross JR, Jung E, Thompson CB, Jones RG, et al. 2010. Toll-like receptor-induced changes in glycolytic metabolism regulate dendritic cell activation. *Blood* **115:** 4742–4749. doi:10.1182/blood-2009-10-249540

Law RC, Nurwono G, Park JO. 2024. A parallel glycolysis provides a selective advantage through rapid growth acceleration. *Nat Chem Biol* **20:** 314–322. doi:10.1038/s41589-023-01395-2

Li Z, Ji BW, Dixit PD, Tchourine K, Lien EC, Hosios AM, Abbott KL, Rutter JC, Westermark AM, Gorodetsky EF, et al. 2022. Cancer cells depend on environmental lipids for proliferation when electron acceptors are limited. *Nat Metab* **4:** 711–723. doi:10.1038/s42255-022-00588-8

Liberti MV, Locasale JW. 2016. The Warburg effect: how does it benefit cancer cells? *Trends Biochem Sci* **41:** 211–218. doi:10.1016/j.tibs.2015.12.001

Luengo A, Gui DY, Vander Heiden MG. 2017. Targeting metabolism for cancer therapy. *Cell Chem Biol* **24:** 1161–1180. doi:10.1016/j.chembiol.2017.08.028

Luengo A, Li Z, Gui DY, Sullivan LB, Zagorulya M, Do BT, Ferreira R, Naamati A, Ali A, Lewis CA, et al. 2021. Increased demand for NAD$^+$ relative to ATP drives aerobic glycolysis. *Mol Cell* **81:** 691–707.e6. doi:10.1016/j.molcel.2020.12.012

Lunt SY, Vander Heiden MG. 2011. Aerobic glycolysis: meeting the metabolic requirements of cell proliferation. *Annu Rev Cell Dev Biol* **27:** 441–464. doi:10.1146/annurev-cellbio-092910-154237

Lunt SY, Muralidhar V, Hosios AM, Israelsen WJ, Gui DY, Newhouse L, Ogrodzinski M, Hecht V, Xu K, Acevedo PN, et al. 2015. Pyruvate kinase isoform expression alters nucleotide synthesis to impact cell proliferation. *Mol Cell* **57:** 95–107. doi:10.1016/j.molcel.2014.10.027

Martínez-Reyes I, Cardona LR, Kong H, Vasan K, McElroy GS, Werner M, Kihshen H, Reczek CR, Weinberg SE, Gao P, et al. 2020. Mitochondrial ubiquinol oxidation is necessary for tumour growth. *Nature* **585:** 288–292. doi:10.1038/s41586-020-2475-6

Murphy JP, Giacomantonio MA, Paulo JA, Everley RA, Kennedy BE, Pathak GP, Clements DR, Kim Y, Dai C, Sharif T, et al. 2018. The NAD$^+$ salvage pathway supports PHGDH-driven serine biosynthesis. *Cell Rep* **24:** 2381–2391.e5. doi:10.1016/j.celrep.2018.07.086

Papandreou I, Cairns RA, Fontana L, Lim AL, Denko NC. 2006. HIF-1 mediates adaptation to hypoxia by actively downregulating mitochondrial oxygen consumption. *Cell Metab* **3:** 187–197. doi:10.1016/j.cmet.2006.01.012

Pfeiffer T, Schuster S, Bonhoeffer S. 2001. Cooperation and competition in the evolution of ATP-producing pathways. *Science* **292:** 504–507. doi:10.1126/science.1058079

Pouysségur J, Franchi A, Silvestre P. 1980. Relationship between increased aerobic glycolysis and DNA synthesis initiation studied using glycolytic mutant fibroblasts. *Nature* **287:** 445–447. doi:10.1038/287445a0

Racker E. 1983. The Warburg effect: two years later. *Science* **222:** 232. doi:10.1126/science.6312561

Reinfeld BI, Madden MZ, Wolf MM, Chytil A, Bader JE, Patterson AR, Sugiura A, Cohen AS, Ali A, Do BT, et al. 2021. Cell-programmed nutrient partitioning in the tumour microenvironment. *Nature* **593:** 282–288. doi:10.1038/s41586-021-03442-1

Robbins D, Zhao Y. 2011. New aspects of mitochondrial uncoupling proteins (UCPs) and their roles in tumorigenesis. *Int J Mol Sci* **12:** 5285–5293. doi:10.3390/ijms12085285

Schell JC, Olson KA, Jiang L, Hawkins AJ, Van Vranken JG, Xie J, Egnatchik RA, Earl EG, DeBerardinis RJ, Rutter J. 2014. A role for the mitochondrial pyruvate carrier as a repressor of the Warburg effect and colon cancer cell growth. *Mol Cell* **56:** 400–413. doi:10.1016/j.molcel.2014.09.026

Semba H, Takeda N, Isagawa T, Sugiura Y, Honda K, Wake M, Miyazawa H, Yamaguchi Y, Miura M, Jenkins DM, et al. 2016. HIF-1α-PDK1 axis-induced active glycolysis plays an essential role in macrophage migratory capacity. *Nat Commun* **7:** 11635. doi:10.1038/ncomms11635

Shen Y, Dinh HV, Cruz ER, Chen Z, Bartman CR, Xiao T, Call CM, Ryseck RP, Pratas J, Weilandt D, et al. 2024. Mitochondrial ATP generation is more proteome efficient than glycolysis. *Nat Chem Biol* doi:10.1038/s41589-024-01571-y

Shestov AA, Liu X, Ser Z, Cluntun AA, Hung YP, Huang L, Kim D, Le A, Yellen G, Albeck JG, et al. 2014. Quantitative determinants of aerobic glycolysis identify flux through the enzyme GAPDH as a limiting step. *eLife* **3:** e03342. doi:10.7554/eLife.03342

Shim H, Dolde C, Lewis BC, Wu CS, Dang G, Jungmann RA, Dalla-Favera R, Dang CV. 1997. c-Myc transactivation of *LDH-A*: implications for tumor metabolism and growth. *Proc Natl Acad Sci* **94:** 6658–6663. doi:10.1073/pnas.94.13.6658

Smid EJ, Lacroix C. 2013. Microbe-microbe interactions in mixed culture food fermentations. *Curr Opin Biotechnol* **24:** 148–154. doi:10.1016/j.copbio.2012.11.007

Strenkert D, Schmollinger S, Gallaher SD, Salomé PA, Purvine SO, Nicora CD, Mettler-Altmann T, Soubeyrand E, Weber APM, Lipton MS, et al. 2019. Multiomics resolution of molecular events during a day in the life of Chlamydomonas. *Proc Natl Acad Sci* **116:** 2374–2383. doi:10.1073/pnas.1815238116

Sullivan LB, Gui DY, Hosios AM, Bush LN, Freinkman E, Vander Heiden MG. 2015. Supporting aspartate biosynthesis is an essential function of respiration in proliferating cells. *Cell* **162:** 552–563. doi:10.1016/j.cell.2015.07.017

Sullivan LB, Luengo A, Danai LV, Bush LN, Diehl FF, Hosios AM, Lau AN, Elmiligy S, Malstrom S, Lewis CA, et al. 2018. Aspartate is an endogenous metabolic limitation for tumour growth. *Nat Cell Biol* **20:** 782–788. doi:10.1038/s41556-018-0125-0

Sun Q, Chen X, Ma J, Peng H, Wang F, Zha X, Wang Y, Jing Y, Yang H, Chen R, et al. 2011. Mammalian target of rapamycin up-regulation of pyruvate kinase isoenzyme type M2 is critical for aerobic glycolysis and tumor growth. *Proc Natl Acad Sci* **108:** 4129–4134. doi:10.1073/pnas.1014769108

Tafani M, Sansone L, Limana F, Arcangeli T, De Santis E, Polese M, Fini M, Russo MA. 2016. The interplay of reactive oxygen species, hypoxia, inflammation, and sirtuins in cancer initiation and progression. *Oxid Med Cell Longev* **2016:** 3907147. doi:10.1155/2016/3907147

Tan AS, Baty JW, Dong LF, Bezawork-Geleta A, Endaya B, Goodwin J, Bajzikova M, Kovarova J, Peterka M, Yan B, et al. 2015. Mitochondrial genome acquisition restores respiratory function and tumorigenic potential of cancer cells without mitochondrial DNA. *Cell Metab* **21:** 81–94. doi:10.1016/j.cmet.2014.12.003

Titov DV, Cracan V, Goodman RP, Peng J, Grabarek Z, Mootha VK. 2016. Complementation of mitochondrial electron transport chain by manipulation of the NAD$^+$/NADH ratio. *Science* **352:** 231–235. doi:10.1126/science.aad4017

Tu BP, Kudlicki A, Rowicka M, McKnight SL. 2005. Logic of the yeast metabolic cycle: temporal compartmentalization of cellular processes. *Science* **310:** 1152–1158. doi:10.1126/science.1120499

Vacanti NM, Divakaruni AS, Green CR, Parker SJ, Henry RR, Ciaraldi TP, Murphy AN, Metallo CM. 2014. Regulation of substrate utilization by the mitochondrial pyruvate carrier. *Mol Cell* **56:** 425–435. doi:10.1016/j.molcel.2014.09.024

Valle A, Oliver J, Roca P. 2010. Role of uncoupling proteins in cancer. *Cancers (Basel)* **2:** 567–591. doi:10.3390/cancers2020567

Vander Heiden MG, DeBerardinis RJ. 2017. Understanding the intersections between metabolism and cancer biology. *Cell* **168:** 657–669. doi:10.1016/j.cell.2016.12.039

Vander Heiden MG, Cantley LC, Thompson CB. 2009. Understanding the Warburg effect: the metabolic requirements of cell proliferation. *Science* **324:** 1029–1033. doi:10.1126/science.1160809

Vander Heiden MG, Locasale JW, Swanson KD, Sharfi H, Heffron GJ, Amador-Noguez D, Christofk HR, Wagner G, Rabinowitz JD, Asara JM, et al. 2010. Evidence for an alternative glycolytic pathway in rapidly proliferating cells. *Science* **329:** 1492–1499. doi:10.1126/science.1188015

Vazquez A, Liu J, Zhou Y, Oltvai ZN. 2010. Catabolic efficiency of aerobic glycolysis: the Warburg effect revisited. *BMC Syst Biol* **4:** 58. doi:10.1186/1752-0509-4-58

Vemuri GN, Eiteman MA, McEwen JE, Olsson L, Nielsen J. 2007. Increasing NADH oxidation reduces overflow metabolism in *Saccharomyces cerevisiae*. *Proc Natl Acad Sci* **104:** 2402–2407. doi:10.1073/pnas.0607469104

Wang T, Marquardt C, Foker J. 1976. Aerobic glycolysis during lymphocyte proliferation. *Nature* **261:** 702–705. doi:10.1038/261702a0

Wang Y, Stancliffe E, Fowle-Grider R, Wang R, Wang C, Schwaiger-Haber M, Shriver LP, Patti GJ. 2022. Saturation of the mitochondrial NADH shuttles drives aerobic glycolysis in proliferating cells. *Mol Cell* **82:** 3270–3283. e9. doi:10.1016/j.molcel.2022.07.007

Warburg O. 1956. On the origin of cancer cells. *Science* **123:** 309–314. doi:10.1126/science.123.3191.309

Warburg O, Posener K, Negelein E. 1924. Ueber den Stoffwechsel der Tumoren. *Biochem Z* **152:** 319–344.

Weinberg F, Hamanaka R, Wheaton WW, Weinberg S, Joseph J, Lopez M, Kalyanaraman B, Mutlu GM, Budinger GR, Chandel NS. 2010. Mitochondrial metabolism and ROS generation are essential for Kras-mediated tumorigenicity. *Proc Natl Acad Sci* **107:** 8788–8793. doi:10.1073/pnas.1003428107

Weinhouse S. 1976. The Warburg hypothesis fifty years later. *Z Krebsforsch Klin Onkol Cancer Res Clin Oncol* **87:** 115–126. doi:10.1007/BF00284370

Wheaton WW, Weinberg SE, Hamanaka RB, Soberanes S, Sullivan LB, Anso E, Glasauer A, Dufour E, Mutlu GM, Budigner GS, et al. 2014. Metformin inhibits mitochondrial complex I of cancer cells to reduce tumorigenesis. *eLife* **3:** e02242. doi:10.7554/eLife.02242

Wolfe AJ. 2005. The acetate switch. *Microbiol Mol Biol Rev* **69:** 12–50. doi:10.1128/MMBR.69.1.12-50.2005

Xu K, Yin N, Peng M, Stamatiades EG, Shyu A, Li P, Zhang X, Do MH, Wang Z, Capistrano KJ, et al. 2021. Glycolysis fuels phosphoinositide 3-kinase signaling to bolster T cell immunity. *Science* **371:** 405–410. doi:10.1126/science.abb2683

Yang C, Ko B, Hensley CT, Jiang L, Wasti AT, Kim J, Sudderth J, Calvaruso MA, Lumata L, Mitsche M, et al. 2014. Glutamine oxidation maintains the TCA cycle and cell survival during impaired mitochondrial pyruvate transport. *Mol Cell* **56:** 414–424. doi:10.1016/j.molcel.2014.09.025

Yao CH, Fowle-Grider R, Mahieu NG, Liu GY, Chen YJ, Wang R, Singh M, Potter GS, Gross RW, Schaefer J, et al. 2016. Exogenous fatty acids are the preferred source of membrane lipids in proliferating fibroblasts. *Cell Chem Biol* **23:** 483–493. doi:10.1016/j.chembiol.2016.03.007

Ye J, Mancuso A, Tong X, Ward PS, Fan J, Rabinowitz JD, Thompson CB. 2012. Pyruvate kinase M2 promotes de novo serine synthesis to sustain mTORC1 activity and cell proliferation. *Proc Natl Acad Sci* **109:** 6904–6909. doi:10.1073/pnas.1204176109

Ždralević M, Brand A, Di Ianni L, Dettmer K, Reinders J, Singer K, Peter K, Schnell A, Bruss C, Decking SM, et al. 2018. Double genetic disruption of lactate dehydrogenases A and B is required to ablate the "Warburg effect" restricting tumor growth to oxidative metabolism. *J Biol Chem* **293:** 15947–15961. doi:10.1074/jbc.RA118.004180

Zhang X, Fryknäs M, Hernlund E, Fayad W, De Milito A, Olofsson MH, Gogvadze V, Dang L, Påhlman S, Schughart LA, et al. 2014. Induction of mitochondrial dysfunction as a strategy for targeting tumour cells in metabolically compromised microenvironments. *Nat Commun* **5:** 3295. doi:10.1038/ncomms4295

Mitochondria and Cancer

Timothy C. Kenny and Kıvanç Birsoy

Laboratory of Metabolic Regulation and Genetics, The Rockefeller University, New York, New York 10065, USA

Correspondence: kbirsoy@rockefeller.edu

Mitochondria are semiautonomous organelles with diverse metabolic and cellular functions including anabolism and energy production through oxidative phosphorylation. Following the pioneering observations of Otto Warburg nearly a century ago, an immense body of work has examined the role of mitochondria in cancer pathogenesis and progression. Here, we summarize the current state of the field, which has coalesced around the position that functional mitochondria are required for cancer cell proliferation. In this review, we discuss how mitochondria influence tumorigenesis by impacting anabolism, intracellular signaling, and the tumor microenvironment. Consistent with their critical functions in tumor formation, mitochondria have become an attractive target for cancer therapy. We provide a comprehensive update on the numerous therapeutic modalities targeting the mitochondria of cancer cells making their way through clinical trials.

Mitochondria are dynamic organelles that originated through the endosymbiosis with α-proteobacteria within protoeukaryotic cells (Archibald 2015). While their primary function lies in energy production through oxidative phosphorylation (OXPHOS), mitochondria also play critical roles in iron–sulfur cluster biogenesis, macromolecule synthesis, calcium homeostasis, redox balance, cell death, and cellular signaling (Tan and Finkel 2020; Chakrabarty and Chandel 2021). Given these extensive arrays of functions performed by mitochondria, mitochondrial dysfunction is observed in numerous human pathologies, including neurodegeneration and cancer.

The connection between mitochondria and cancer has been recognized for more than a century, since Warburg's (1956) seminal observation that tumor cells exhibit enhanced glucose uptake and lactate production regardless of oxygen presence. This phenomenon, also known as aerobic glycolysis, is a prominent feature observed in most, but not all, cancers and forms the basis for the clinical imaging of tumors in patients using fluorodeoxyglucose positron emission tomography (FDG-PET) (Fletcher et al. 2008). During that period, Warburg believed that this phenomenon that now bears his name—the "Warburg effect" indicates a deficiency in mitochondrial respiration and proposed that the "irreversible injury of respiration" is a universal underlying factor in cancer development (Warburg 1956). For a long time, this has led to the misconception that mitochondrial metabolism is dispensable for tumor growth (DeBerardinis and Chandel 2020). However, research in the cancer metabolism field over the last two decades has highlighted a more nuanced role of mitochondrial metabolism in cancer. Contrary to earlier assumptions, it is now evident that while some tumors exhibit deficiencies in mitochondrial metabolism, the majority of cancer cells rely on functional mitochondria for their growth and progression.

What then causes the Warburg effect? It is now widely believed that aerobic glycolysis of cancer cells supports the biosynthetic needs rather than the energetic demands of rapidly dividing cells (DeBerardinis and Chandel 2020). Indeed, enhanced glycolytic activity leads to the accumulation of glycolytic intermediates, which can be used by biosynthetic pathways, driving anabolic metabolism. Supporting this notion, in vivo studies have shown that cancer cells exhibit higher glycolytic flux and lower tricarboxylic acid (TCA) cycle activity compared to normal tissues (Bartman et al. 2023). Recent studies suggest that aerobic glycolysis is a consequence of cellular demand for NAD^+ in excess of that for ATP or saturation of mitochondrial NADH shuttles (Luengo et al. 2021; Wang et al. 2022). In their study using the NCI-60 panel of cell lines, the Patti group demonstrated a correlation between the rate of aerobic glycolysis, as indicated by lactate secretion and mitochondrial NADH shuttle activity, rather than the cellular proliferation rate (Wang et al. 2022). In this model, the rate of glycolysis outpaces the ability of the malate–aspartate shuttle (MAS) and the glycerol 3-phosphate shuttle (G3PS) to transport NADH to the mitochondria. In turn, this bottleneck drives the fermentation of glucose to lactate as a compensatory mechanism (Wang et al. 2022).

Advancements in our understanding of mitochondria and cancer have evolved since Warburg's initial observations in the 1920s, but many aspects remain to be explored. In this review, we aim to provide an overview of the current understanding of the essential role of mitochondria in cancer, their impact on cancer pathogenesis and progression, and explore potential strategies for targeting mitochondria in cancer therapy.

THE RELIANCE OF CANCER CELLS ON FUNCTIONAL MITOCHONDRIA

Most metazoan cells rely on mitochondria for their survival and proliferation. However, there are exceptional cases where cells have deviated from this norm. For example, red blood cells undergo a unique process of maturation where they eliminate their mitochondria during the terminal stages of differentiation, allowing them to stop proliferating and specialize in their primary function of oxygen transport (Dzierzak and Philipsen 2013). In experimental systems, human cells deprived of mitochondria can survive for a limited period in culture but are unable to proliferate (Correia-Melo et al. 2017). These results indicate an essential role for mitochondria in supporting cell division and growth, but their precise role in eukaryotic cell fitness is still not fully understood. However, insights can be gained from rare organisms that lack mitochondria, such as the eukaryotic microorganism oxymonad *Monoceromonoides* sp. (Karnkowska et al. 2016). To compensate for the absence of mitochondria, this organism has developed an alternative system that replaced the mitochondrial iron–sulfur cluster assembly pathway with a bacterial sulfur mobilization system in the cytosol, enabling it to perform essential functions typically carried out by mitochondria. These observations strongly point to iron–sulfur cluster synthesis as the critical role of mitochondria in cell proliferation. Consistently, iron–sulfur clusters play essential roles in numerous cellular processes, including energy production, DNA replication, and redox homeostasis (Rouault 2015).

Among the metabolic pathways in mitochondria, electron transport chain (ETC) activity is particularly relevant for cell proliferation. ETC comprises four enzyme complexes that facilitate the transfer of electrons from donors, such as NADH, to oxygen, the final electron acceptor. This process involves the pumping of protons into the intermembrane space, establishing a gradient across the inner mitochondrial membrane. The F_0F_1 ATPase uses this gradient to drive ATP synthesis (Mitchell 1961). The ETC is fueled by electron donors produced through metabolic pathways, such as glycolysis, the TCA cycle, and β-oxidation (Fig. 1). Consequently, ETC activity impacts a range of processes beyond energy balance, such as reactive oxygen species (ROS) production and mitochondrial membrane potential. In addition to ATP production, the ETC is also involved in maintaining cellular

Cite this article as *Cold Spring Harb Perspect Med* doi: 10.1101/cshperspect.a041534

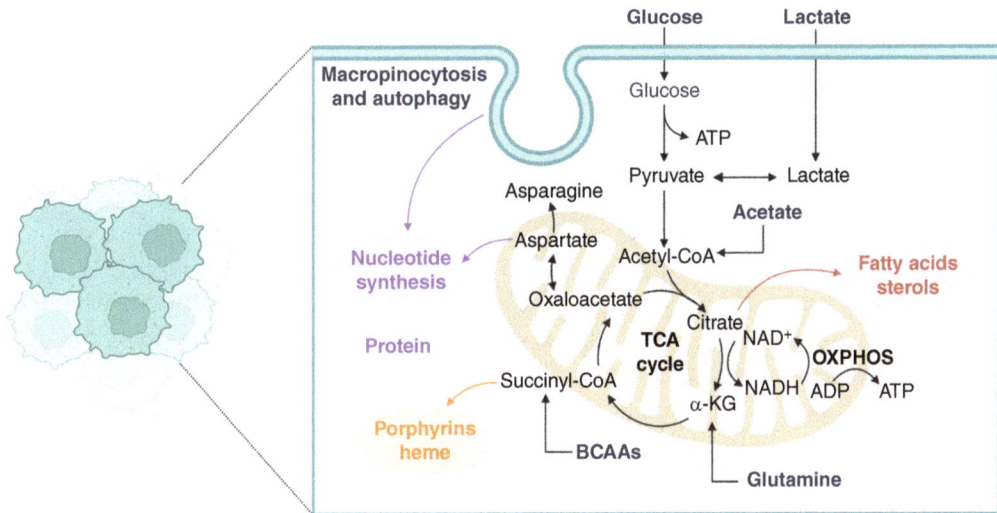

Figure 1. The tricarboxylic acid (TCA) cycle fuels cancer metabolism. Mitochondrial TCA cycle intermediates serve as precursors for the biosynthesis needed for cancer cell growth. Cancer cells display unique metabolic strategies to fuel the TCA cycle with multiple fuel inputs. (Figure created with Biorender.com.)

redox balance, regulating the ratio of reduced to oxidized molecules (NADH and NAD$^+$), which is crucial for maintaining the appropriate cellular environment for proliferation.

Disruptions or dysfunctions in the ETC can have significant consequences for tumor growth. One of the first definitive evidence for the essential function of ETC has been generated by the Chandel laboratory in 2010. In an in vivo mouse model of K-Ras-driven lung cancer, the loss of mitochondrial transcription factor A (TFAM), a crucial factor for mitochondrial DNA (mtDNA) replication, resulted in the inhibition of tumor formation (Fig. 2; Weinberg et al. 2010; Guo et al. 2011). Remarkably, most human tumors select against truncating mutations in complexes III and V, and cancer cell lines with homoplasmic truncating mutations in complex I are unable to form xenografts (Iommarini et al. 2014; Martínez-Reyes et al. 2020). Unbiased genetic screens conducted in vivo provide further evidence for the crucial role of ETC function in cancer (Fig. 3; Biancur et al. 2021; Zhu et al. 2021). These genetic screens identified components of ETC and heme synthesis as essential genes for the growth of Kras mutant tumors. Similar studies have consistently identified mitochondrial and OXPHOS genes as essential for the growth of cancer cells,

especially under conditions matching the tumor microenvironment such as hypoxia (Arroyo et al. 2016; Jain et al. 2020; Rossiter et al. 2021; Thomas et al. 2021; Michl et al. 2022).

Additional compelling evidence to support the essential role of ETC comes from observations of the horizontal transfer of mitochondria and/or mtDNA between cells. One of the first examples of this phenomenon used murine breast cancer 4T1 and melanoma B16 cells depleted of mtDNA (ρ^0) by extended culture in low-dose ethidium bromide (Tan et al. 2015). When these cells were injected into mice, there was significant latency in tumor growth compared to the parental cell lines. Strikingly, all tumors that formed from ρ^0 cells had acquired the mitochondrial genome from the host, indicating the strong selective pressure to retain mtDNA and ETC during tumor formation. In a follow-up study, the same group used mice with fluorescently tagged mitochondria to demonstrate that ρ^0 cells acquired whole mitochondria from host cells to restore ETC and mitochondrial activity (Dong et al. 2017). Notably, the precise mechanism by which mitochondria and/or mtDNA are horizontally transferred between cells is unclear, but such modes of transfer may include tunneling nanotubes, gap junctions, cell fusion, or extracellular vesicles (Dong et al.

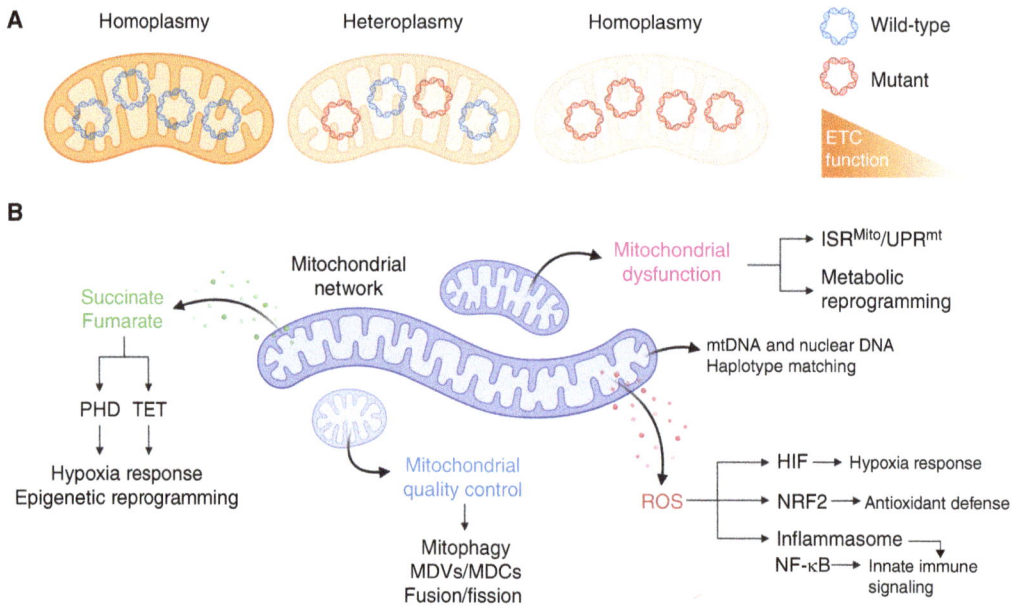

Figure 2. Mitochondrial DNA (mtDNA) mutations and genetics influence cancer cell biology. (*A*) Accumulation of loss-of-function mtDNA mutations affects electron transport chain (ETC) function. Homoplasmic loss-of-function mtDNA mutations are rarely found in human tumors. (*B*) The myriad ways in which mitochondria and the metabolites they produce impact cellular biology. (Figure created with Biorender.com.)

2023). More recently, positron emission tomography (PET) radiotracers have been used to measure mitochondrial membrane potential in vivo highlighting that mitochondria are, in fact, functional in cancer (Momcilovic et al. 2019). Interestingly, the extent of the mitochondrial membrane potential of in vivo non-small-cell lung cancer is associated with spatial and structural features of the mitochondrial network (Han et al. 2023). Further, highlighting the importance of mitochondria in cancer, in vivo isotope tracing in mice and humans with ^{13}C-glucose demonstrated that ETC function is required for TCA cycle metabolism (Pachnis et al. 2022). In totality, these observations speak to the essential role for mitochondrial metabolism in tumor growth leading to the next logical question—why?

THE ESSENTIAL ROLE OF MITOCHONDRIAL RESPIRATION IN TUMOR GROWTH

Why do cancer cells require ETC to grow? While early studies primarily focused on the role of energy production, recent investigations have suggested that the synthesis of amino acids may provide the answer. These findings build upon earlier observations by Guiseppe Attardi and colleagues, who demonstrated that human cells lacking mtDNA are unable to proliferate unless supraphysiological levels of pyruvate are supplied (King and Attardi 1989). However, the specific reason why pyruvate rescues the proliferation of highly glycolytic cancer cells remained unclear until recently (Van Vranken and Rutter 2015). Two studies published back-to-back in 2015 addressed this question and reached the same conclusion as to why the ETC is essential for proliferation (Birsoy et al. 2015; Sullivan et al. 2015).

Given that pyruvate has many potential metabolic fates when supplemented to respiration-deficient cells, Sullivan et al. (2015) sought to identify alternative metabolic substrates that could support the growth of respiration-deficient cells to uncover its essential function. They found that α-ketobutyrate, which can serve as a substrate for lactate dehydrogenase to regenerate NAD$^+$, could also rescue the proliferation defects

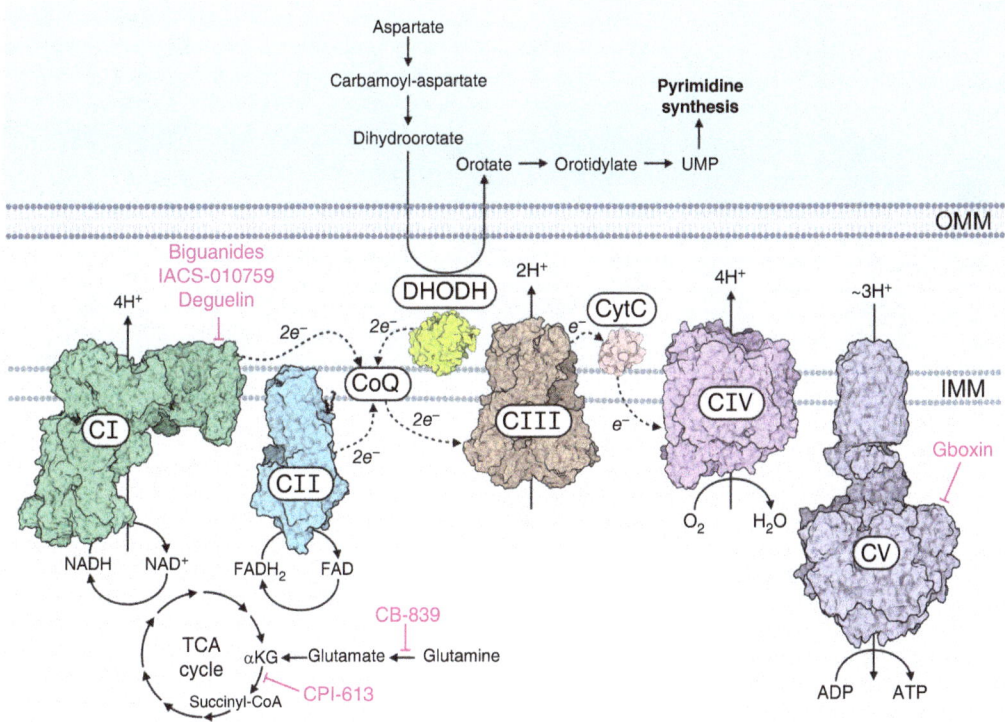

Figure 3. Essential functions of the electron transport chain (ETC) and targets for cancer therapy. The five complexes of the ETC embedded in the mitochondrial inner membrane produce the majority of ATP used by cancer cells. Complexes I and II oxidize electron carriers NADH and FADH$_2$ to NAD$^+$ and FAD, respectively. This oxidation is critical for the continued activity of the tricarboxylic acid (TCA) cycle to support the biosynthetic needs of cancer cells. During the conversion of dihydroorotate to orotate, a key step in de novo pyrimidine synthesis, DHODH donates electrons to mitochondrial ubiquinone (CoQ). Inhibitors of the ETC and mitochondrial metabolism, which show therapeutic promise in treating cancer, are highlighted in pink. Atomic structures: complex I (PDB: 6RFR), complex II (PDB: 1ZOY), DHODH (PDB: 4LS1), complex III (PDB: 6QPE), cytochrome *c* (PDB: 2B4Z), complex IV (PDB: 5Z62), complex V/ATP synthase (PDB: 5FL7). (Figure created with Biorender.com.)

of respiration-deficient cells. These results suggested that restoration of the NAD$^+$/NADH ratio was required for the proliferation of cells with compromised ETC. Further metabolomics experiments hinted that reduced aspartate levels could underlie these observations (Sullivan et al. 2015). In a complementary approach, Birsoy et al. (2015) used a CRISPR screen with sgRNAs targeting ∼3000 metabolic genes to identify synthetic lethal interactions with ETC inhibition. This approach identified aspartate production by GOT1, a cytosolic aspartate aminotransferase, as essential under complex I inhibition by phenformin but not in normal growth conditions. Importantly, both studies demon-

strated that increasing aspartate availability could largely rescue the proliferation of defects of ETC mutant cells, highlighting the essential role for the ETC to enable aspartate synthesis. Indeed, it was later demonstrated that aspartate availability was a determining factor in sensitivity to ETC inhibition (Garcia-Bermudez et al. 2018).

In addition to its essential role under ETC inhibition, aspartate is also a limiting metabolite for cancer cells to grow under hypoxia or as tumors in vivo (Garcia-Bermudez et al. 2018; Sullivan et al. 2018). Indeed, to compensate for the loss of aspartate production under hypoxic conditions, pancreatic ductal adenocarcinoma

(PDAC) cells up-regulate the uptake of extracellular proteins through macropinocytosis in vivo (Garcia-Bermudez et al. 2022). Similarly, liver cancers engage in hypoxia-induced macropinocytosis to enable growth under nutrient limitation (Zhang et al. 2022). Finally, when depleted of glutamine, cancer cells depend on p53-mediated up-regulation of SLC1A3, an aspartate transporter, to maintain the ETC and TCA cycle activity to promote de novo glutamate, glutamine, and nucleotide synthesis (Tajan et al. 2018).

Why do cells need aspartate? In addition to its proteinogenic role, aspartate is a metabolite precursor for nucleotides. Indeed, upon ETC inhibition, cancer cells display severe deficiencies for nucleotides, which are required for RNA and DNA synthesis. More recent work on the essential function of the ETC has converged on the same theme. Temporal analysis of ρ^0 4T1 breast cancer cells after host mtDNA acquisition revealed that respiratory recovery coincided with the reactivation of DHODH (Bajzikova et al. 2019). DHODH, which converts dihydroorotate to orotate in the de novo pyrimidine synthesis pathway, donates two electrons to the ETC in the course of the reaction. Indeed, using cancer cells lacking a functional complex III, another group demonstrated that the ETC was required for the oxidation of ubiquinol back to ubiquinone so that it could accept electrons from DHODH and enable pyrimidine synthesis (Martínez-Reyes et al. 2020). Using elegant genetic complementation experiments, they demonstrated that the oxidation of ubiquinol to ubiquinone and not NAD^+ regeneration or ATP synthesis was the essential ETC function for tumor growth (Martínez-Reyes et al. 2020). Taken together, these results suggest that cancer cells require a functional ETC for the oxidation of ubiquinol, which in turn is necessary for DHODH activity and the maintenance of the oxidative TCA cycle for macromolecule biosynthesis. Yet another metabolic fate of aspartate is the production of asparagine through asparagine synthase (ASNS) activity. The reduced synthesis of asparagine from aspartate may underlie the proliferation defects of cancer cells with ETC dysfunction (Krall et al. 2021). Indeed, the combination of ETC inhibitors and asparagine depletion via L-asparaginase, a clinical drug that depletes serum asparagine, effectively limits the growth of some tumors. The decrease in asparagine levels may be the critical link leading to the activation of integrated stress response during chronic ETC inhibition (Mick et al. 2020).

NUTRIENTS THAT FUEL TCA CYCLE

Cancer cells use diverse metabolic substrates to fuel their TCA cycle. This metabolic plasticity is a defining feature of cancer cells and a prominent means of resistance to metabolic intervention by tumors. The classic textbook fuel of the TCA cycle is pyruvate generated from glucose by glycolysis. Work in the past decade, however, has shed light on the many metabolic inputs cancer cells can use to drive the TCA cycle. The flow of carbons through the TCA cycle itself has recently been demonstrated to be less fixed and immutable as previously thought (Arnold et al. 2022).

As elaborated above, cancer cells engage in aerobic glycolysis and secrete lactate. However, lactate itself can be used as a metabolic substrate to fuel the TCA cycle and the metabolism of cancer cells. In culture, cancer cells use exogenous lactate to generate pyruvate and drive lipid synthesis (Chen et al. 2016). In vivo, human non-small-cell lung carcinoma (NSCLC) tumors also use lactate as a carbon source for the TCA cycle. Remarkably, TCA cycle intermediates derived from lactate exceed those produced from glucose, suggesting that human tumors prefer lactate as a TCA cycle fuel (Faubert et al. 2017). Indeed, quantitative flux analysis in mice revealed that tumors and most tissues use lactate as a primary source of carbon for the TCA cycle (Hui et al. 2017). Similarly, ammonia, another byproduct of cancer cell metabolism, can be assimilated into the central carbon metabolism of breast cancer cells by reverse glutamate dehydrogenase (GDH) flux to recycle nitrogen for amino acid synthesis and proliferation (Spinelli et al. 2017). Kras/LKB1 mutant NSCLC cells use CPS1 to condense ammonia and bicarbonate to generate carbamoyl phosphate for de novo pyrimidine synthesis (Kim et al. 2017).

Under hypoxia or ETC inhibition, cancer cells can use alternative fuel sources to drive

TCA cycle progression thereby enabling the biosynthesis of macromolecules needed for cell proliferation. One such mechanism is through glutamine-dependent reductive carboxylation to generate citrate thereby enabling de novo lipid synthesis (Wise et al. 2011; Metallo et al. 2012; Mullen et al. 2012). This pathway relies on the activities of cytosolic and mitochondrial localized $NADP^+$/NADHPH-dependent isocitrate dehydrogenases, Interestingly, this reductive carboxylation is essential for survival during anchorage-independent growth—a key step in the metastatic cascade (Jiang et al. 2016) Acetate can also be used by cancer cells as a fuel source for the TCA cycle and macromolecule biosynthesis. Acetate is readily taken up by multiple cancer types and incorporated into the acetyl-CoA pool by ACSS2 (Comerford et al. 2014; Mashimo et al. 2014). Acetate-derived acetyl-CoA, in turn, can be used for the TCA cycle, thereby enabling the de novo synthesis of amino acids and nucleotides. Acetyl-CoA also serves as a building block for fatty acid and sterol biosynthesis as well as a substrate for histone and protein acetylation. Interestingly, the contribution of acetate-derived carbons to the TCA cycle rivals that of glucose despite significantly lower levels of glucose than acetate in the tumor microenvironment. Acetate-derived TCA cycle intermediates are unique to tumor cells as surrounding normal tissue shows little fractional enrichment from acetate (Comerford et al. 2014; Mashimo et al. 2014). Branched-chain amino acids, such as leucine, can also be used as a substrate to generate TCA cycle intermediates and support nucleotide synthesis (Tönjes et al. 2013; Mayers et al. 2016; Carrer et al. 2019; Neinast et al. 2019; Sivanand and Vander Heiden 2020).

Highlighting the metabolic flexibility of cancer cells, tumors can also bypass their need for de novo lipogenesis through the scavenging of unsaturated fatty acids from lysophospholipids (Kamphorst et al. 2013; Gharpure et al. 2018). Scavenging of tumor cells for alternative substrates to meet metabolic demands upon nutrient limitation is a common theme in cancer biology. Upon glucose limitation, ribose derived from extracellular uridine or RNA can be used to fuel the central carbon metabolism of PDAC

cells (Nwosu et al. 2023; Skinner et al. 2023). Glutamine deprivation in PDAC cells also triggers the hexosamine salvage pathway to generate glucosamine from hyaluronic acid in the extracellular matrix (Campbell et al. 2021; Kim et al. 2021). Breast cancer cells that have metastasized to the lung use extracellular pyruvate to generate αKG through pyruvate transamination. These metastatic breast cancer cells, in turn, use this αKG to drive prolyl hydroxylase activity and reshape their extracellular matrix for colonization (Elia et al. 2019). These few examples highlight a growing body of literature showing the myriad substrates cancer cells can use to drive central carbon metabolism and thereby satisfy their need for energy and macromolecule synthesis.

The remarkable metabolic plasticity of cancer has recently been corroborated in human patients using sophisticated metabolic tracing studies that use intraoperative intravenous infusions. In a cohort of NSCLC patients, intraoperative ^{13}C-glucose infusion revealed intra- and intertumoral metabolic heterogeneity in vivo (Hensley et al. 2016). 1,2-^{13}C-glucose tracing in patients with triple-negative breast cancer (TNBC) showed that TNBC tumors preferentially break down glucose by glycolysis rather than the oxidative pentose phosphate pathway (oxPPP); although some metabolites, such as ribose phosphate, are predominately produced by oxPPP (Ghergurovich et al. 2021). ^{13}C-glucose tracing in a cohort of pediatric cancer patients with tumors of diverse histologies showed that neuroblastomas preferentially obtained labeled lactate from the blood rather than generating it from glucose via glycolysis on their own (Johnston et al. 2021). These observations gleaned from labeling ratios suggest that neuroblastomas engage in lactate transport, likely through MCT1. Interestingly, melanoma cells with higher expression of MCT1 are more efficient at forming distant metastases than their counterparts with low MCT1 expression, suggesting that obtaining lactate from the microenvironment is a critical metabolic bottleneck in the metastatic cascade (Tasdogan et al. 2020). Taken together, these studies highlight the influence of tumor etiology and the microenvironment on the metabolic fuel choices of cancer cells. Although some cancers display preferred routes to satisfy their metabolic needs, cancer cells are incredibly resourceful and drastically reprogram their metabolism to support continued proliferation and disease progression.

mtDNA MUTATIONS IN CANCER INITIATION AND PROGRESSION

Almost half of all tumors carry somatic mutations in their mtDNA (Ju et al. 2014). Among these, some tumor types such as thyroid, kidney, and colorectal cancer have significantly higher rates of mtDNA mutations (Ju et al. 2014; Yuan et al. 2020; Gorelick et al. 2021). Among these, truncating mtDNA deletions preferentially target complex I (Gorelick et al. 2021) and have been proposed to be causal to some tumor types such as benign renal oncocytoma (Gopal et al. 2018).

Multiple copies of mtDNA are present within a single mitochondrion resulting in hundreds to thousands of copies of mtDNA per eukaryotic cell. Mitochondrial genetics, therefore, uses specialized nomenclature when discussing mtDNA mutations or variants. While homoplasmy is used to describe a state in which all mtDNA strains are identical in sequence at a given locus, heteroplasmy refers to a state in which differences exist in the mitochondrial genome at a specific locus. Consistent with an essential role of mitochondrial metabolism in cancer cell growth, the vast majority of mtDNA mutations in cancer are heteroplasmic with frequencies not approaching 100% (Ju et al. 2014; Yuan et al. 2020). These observations suggest there is a strong selective pressure to maintain some nonmutated mtDNA copies so that the ETC function is not entirely lost. Despite this, there are clear phenotypic effects of mtDNA mutations in cancer that affect disease susceptibility, progression, and response to therapy. One of the most poignant examples of how mtDNA influences cancer progression makes use of transmitochondrial cytoplasmic hybrid (cybrid) technology in which ρ^0 cells devoid of mtDNA are fused to enucleated cells with a mitochondrial genome of non- and highly metastatic murine cancer cells (Ishikawa et al. 2008). Using tail vein injections and spontaneous metastasis assays, the authors described the striking ability of metastatic mtDNA with missense complex I mutations to impart a metastatic phenotype to cells with nonmetastatic nuclei. Similarly, nonmetastatic mtDNA blunted the metastatic potential of cells with metastatic nuclei. Since this seminal observation nearly 15 years ago, many reports have used similar or complementary approaches to show that mtDNA could influence cancer cell biology (for review, see Kenny et al. 2019; Kopinski et al. 2021; Kim et al. 2022; Welch et al. 2022). Of note, using mice in which the same nuclear genome is paired with nonpathogenic mtDNA from different strains, it has been shown that tumor incidence and progression are phenotypically influenced by mtDNA (Latorre-Pellicer et al. 2016; Brinker et al. 2017; Chattopadhyay et al. 2022).

It has proved difficult to efficiently edit the mitochondrial genome to generate specific mutations, athough substantial progress has recently been made (Bacman et al. 2020; Nissanka and Moraes 2020; Mok et al. 2022; Lee et al. 2023). These approaches have made it possible to dissect the influence of a specific mtDNA mutation in a truly isogenic system. In such an approach, mtDNA base editing was used to generate murine melanoma cells with 40% or 60% heteroplasmy of a truncating mutation in mt-ND5 of complex I (Mahmood et al. 2024). Cells with higher heteroplasmy relied more heavily on aerobic glycolysis but did not show any difference in tumor growth in vivo. Surprisingly, cancer from high heteroplasmy cells were more sensitive to immune checkpoint blockade, suggesting a connection between cancer mtDNA and immune recognition. Consistently, melanoma patients with mtDNA mutations of high heteroplasmy (>50%) were more responsive to immunotherapy than patients with no or low heteroplasmy mtDNA mutations (Mahmood et al. 2024). Interestingly, the rejection of autologous iPSC-derived cells has been linked to the acquisition of de novo mtDNA mutations during reprogramming, which are recognized by the immune system as neoantigens (Deuse et al. 2019). Taken together, mtDNA has the ability to influence cancer biology at all stages of the disease—from susceptibility and tumor formation to metastasis and therapy response. The mechanisms by which mtDNA variations and mutations impart these effects are not fully clear, but work in recent years has centered on retrograde—mitochondria to the nucleus—signaling as a key player. These signaling pathways and their role in cancer have been reviewed elsewhere (Mottis et al. 2019; Anderson and Haynes 2020; Inigo and Chandra 2022). Consistent with their role in cancer biology, mtDNA mutations can be exploited for cancer therapy (Birsoy et al. 2014).

In addition to mtDNA-encoded mutations, nuclear-encoded mitochondrial genes are also mutated in cancer. In particular, mutations in nuclear-encoded TCA cycle genes generate oncometabolites, which drive tumor formation and growth. Notably, loss-of-function mutations in succinate dehydrogenase (SDH), which characterize patients with hereditary paragangliomas and pheochromocytomas result in succinate accumulation. Similarly, loss-of-function mutations in fumarate hydratase (FH) observed in patients with hereditary leiomyomatosis and renal cell cancer cause fumarate accumulation. Renal cell carcinoma tumors have also been shown to accumulate L-2-hydroxyglutarate (L-2HG) through reduced expression of L-2HG dehydrogenase (L2HGDH) (Shim et al. 2014). These oncometabolites—succinate, fumarate, and L-2HG—inhibit α-ketoglutarate dependent dioxygenases thereby increasing histone and DNA methylation. At the same time, these oncometabolites can mimic hypoxia by inhibiting prolyl hydroxylases thereby stabilizing hypoxia-inducible factor 1α (HIF1α). The resulting epigenetic and transcriptional changes are thought to contribute to the etiology of these unique cancers (Vasan et al. 2020). For example, fumarate accumulation in FH-deficient cancers modifies the epigenome to induce an epithelial-to-mesenchymal (EMT) transcriptional state, thereby increasing the invasiveness and aggressivity of these tumors (Sciacovelli et al. 2016). SDH-deficient tumors use pyruvate carboxylase activity for oxaloacetate generation (Cardaci et al. 2015; Lussey-Lepoutre et al. 2015), while FH-deficient tumors engage in glutamine-dependent reductive carboxylation to generate citrate for macromolecule biosynthesis (Wise et al. 2011; Metallo et al. 2012; Mullen et al. 2012). These studies highlight the plasticity of metabolic strategies used by cancer cells to enable proliferation.

The rewired metabolism of oncometabolite-driven tumors can be exploited for diagnostic purposes. For example, the presence of succinyl-adenosine or succinic-cysteine in plasma has been identified as a reliable biomarker of FH-deficient tumors (Zheng et al. 2023). Oncometabolite-driven tumors also exhibit unique metabolic vulnerabilities. For example, heme oxygenase activity is synthetic lethal in cells lacking FH (Frezza et al. 2011). While SDH and FH-deficient tumors lack a fully functional TCA cycle and thereby rely solely on glycolysis for ATP production, they still depend on mitochondrial metabolism for TCA cycle anaplerosis to feed biosynthetic pathways essential for proliferation and growth.

TARGETING MITOCHONDRIA FOR CANCER THERAPY

A consequence of their essential role in cancer, mitochondria represent an attractive target for cancer therapy. Targeting mitochondria has emerged as an attractive anticancer therapy with approaches ranging from targeting mitochondrial metabolism to mitochondrial proteostasis. One such therapeutic compound is metformin, most well-known as a first-line therapy for patients with type 2 diabetes. Evidence for metformin's antineoplastic activity first came from retrospective studies of patients on the drug for blood glucose control (Evans et al. 2005). Following these clinical observations, multiple groups confirmed the anticancer activity of metformin in preclinical models (Buzzai et al. 2007; Hirsch et al. 2009; Memmott et al. 2010; Algire et al. 2011). Importantly, the effective metformin doses used in preclinical models are easily achievable in the clinic (Chandel et al. 2016). Accordingly, there are hundreds of clinical trials assessing the efficacy of metformin as an anticancer agent with mixed outcomes thus far (Vasan et al. 2020). Metformin is dependent on OCT3 for transport into the cell (Madera et al. 2015; Cai et al. 2019; Vasan et al. 2020), which may explain the variability in clinical responses and suggest biomarkers may be needed to identify patients who will maximally respond to the drug. Metformin's cellular mechanism of action is likely due to its ability to bind and partially inhibit mitochondrial complex I. Indeed, recent work resolved the structure of biguanides, such as metformin, bound to complex I (Bridges et al. 2023). In addition to OCT transporters, metformin is dependent on mitochondrial membrane potential for import into the mitochondrial matrix (Bridges et al. 2014; Wheaton et al. 2014). A recently developed PET radiotracer capable of measuring mitochondrial membrane potential in vivo may provide another effective means to nominate patients who will benefit from metformin treatment (Momcilovic et al. 2019; Han et al. 2023). Other biguanides, such as phenformin, have also shown efficacy in preclinical tumor models (Shackelford et al. 2013; Birsoy et al. 2014). Additionally, other complex I inhibitors (IACS-100759, deguelin) or inhibitors of other ETC complexes (Gboxin) have displayed impressive antitumor effects in preclinical models (Molina et al. 2018; Naguib et al. 2018; Shi et al. 2019; Zhang et al. 2019). Similarly, OXPHOS has been targeted for cancer therapy by inhibiting mitochondrial transcription and translation, thereby blocking production of the key ETC subunits encoded in mtDNA (Škrtić et al. 2011; Kuntz et al. 2017; Bonekamp et al. 2020). As elaborated above, ETC function is required for de novo pyrimidine synthesis by sustaining DHODH activity. Consistent with this, DHODH inhibition has been shown to be efficacious in preclinical work across multiple tumor types (Sykes et al. 2016; Brown et al. 2017; Mathur et al. 2017; Koundinya et al. 2018; Ladds et al. 2018; Li et al. 2019). Similarly, the TCA cycle is integral to produce intermediate metabolites for growth and has been targeted for cancer therapy, most notably with CPI-613, which inhibits α-ketoglutarate dehydrogenase and pyruvate dehydrogenase (Pardee et al. 2014; Stuart et al. 2014; Alistar et al. 2016). Glutamine represents a major carbon source for the generation of TCA cycle intermediates necessary for macromolecule biosynthesis. This is accomplished by the activity of glutaminase, which converts glutamine to glutamate, which can then feed into the TCA as α-ketoglutarate through dehydrogenase or transaminase reactions. Naturally, GLS1 has proven an attractive therapeutic target for cancer with the inhibitor CB-839 currently in clinical trials (Le et al. 2012; Shroff et al. 2015; Xiang et al. 2015; Romero et al. 2017). In addition to targeting mitochondrial metabolism, targeting mitochondrial homeostasis has also emerged as a therapeutic modality. G-TPP, an inhibitor of mitochondrial HSP90/TRAP1, causes proteotoxic stress in the mitochondria, to which cancer cells are more sensitive (Kang et al. 2010; Siegelin et al. 2011; Zhang et al. 2016). Recent reviews have cataloged the many mitochondrial targets for cancer therapy and highlighted their progression through clinical trials (Missiroli et al. 2020; Vasan et al. 2020; Tan et al. 2021; de Beauchamp et al. 2022).

One of the most exciting compounds to target the ETC of cancer cell mitochondria has been IACS-010759, a highly selective complex I inhibitor with very high favorable pharmacology, prompting clinical trials. The preclinical work of IACS-010759 displayed impressive antitumor effects in vitro and in vivo using syngeneic transplant and xenograft models with no observed toxicity to noncancerous tissue (Molina et al. 2018). The results of two dose-escalation phase I clinical trials with IACS-010759 in patients with relapsed/refractory acute myeloid leukemia and advanced solid tumors were recently released, prompting the discontinuation of both trials (Yap et al. 2023). Unexpectedly, both studies identified emergent dose-limiting toxicities including elevated blood lactate and neurotoxicity (Yap et al. 2023). The adverse effects of these clinical trials give pause to the idea of moving ahead with this therapeutic modality. Indeed, some have called for a suspension of mitochondria-targeting cancer therapies (Zhang and Dang 2023). It is clear that the preclinical models used to assess the efficacy and toxicity of these inhibitors fail to capture the nuanced effect of ETC inhibition on organismal physiology. The advancement of these inhibitors to the clinic should be done with great caution and the potential side effects of ETC inhibition, such as peripheral toxicity, should be reassessed. Another area of concern with ETC inhibitors for cancer treatment is their effect on the immune system. Immunotherapy and adoptive cellular therapy are increasingly important treatment modalities for cancer. Their efficacy, in large part, relies on the cytotoxic function of T cells, a key immune effector cell population for cancer treatment. Especially in the activated state, T cells depend on many of the same metabolic pathways used by cancer cells (Andrejeva and Rathmell 2017). Given the similar metabolic strategies used by cancer cells and T cells, it is likely that any interventions to target the mitochondrial metabolism of cancer cells would also affect T cells. Indeed, mitochondrial metabolism and the ETC is essential for the function of regulatory T cells and the proliferation of effector T cells (Sena et al. 2013; Tarasenko et al. 2017; Chapman et al. 2018; Bailis et al. 2019; Fu et al. 2019; Weinberg et al. 2019; Field et al. 2020). Similarly, increased flux through glycolysis and the TCA cycle is a defining feature of naive T cells upon activation (Frauwirth et al. 2002; Menk et al. 2018; Ma et al. 2019). Cancer therapies targeting the ETC and the TCA cycle, therefore, will impede tumor immune responses. Future efforts will undoubtedly focus on mitigating the side effects of these inhibitors on noncancer cells to unlock their full therapeutic potential. The field will be waiting with bated breath as the results of ongoing clinical trials are released. Until then, we may need to rethink how to target mitochondrial metabolism for cancer therapy. Perhaps combinatorial approaches of these compounds with other treatment modalities will enhance therapeutic response and minimize adverse events.

CONCLUSION

Observations made by Otto Warburg nearly 100 years ago have shaped the field of cancer metabolism and influenced the views of generations of scientists as to the essentiality of mitochondria in cancer. Work in the last 20–30 years has dispelled the myth that mitochondria are unnecessary for cancer cell growth. Mitochondria and their metabolism are, in fact, essential to the growth and proliferation of cancer cells. Work in the last 10 years, especially, has demonstrated that functional mitochondria are required for anabolism, specifically the de novo generation of nucleotides. While their role in anabolism is necessary for tumor growth, mitochondria significantly impact tumorigenesis and progression

through signaling, intracellular communication, and interactions of tumor cells with their environment. Consistent with such a prominent influence on all aspects of cancer biology, mitochondria have become an attractive target for therapy. Preclinical work has been extremely promising showing that targeting various aspects of mitochondrial metabolism are potent anticancer strategies. Recent clinical trials, however, have highlighted the risk of targeting these essential pathways in humans as severe toxicities were seen in cancer patients, specifically in the nervous system. The jury is out on the fate of these therapeutic modalities in the clinic. Rational design of combination therapies and more precise identification of patients who would benefit from cancer metabolism therapies may unlock the enormous potential of this anticancer approach.

REFERENCES

Algire C, Amrein L, Bazile M, David S, Zakikhani M, Pollak M. 2011. Diet and tumor LKB1 expression interact to determine sensitivity to anti-neoplastic effects of metformin in vivo. *Oncogene* **30:** 1174–1182. doi:10.1038/onc.2010.483

Alistar AT, Desnoyers R, D'Agostino RJ, Pasche B. 2016. CPI-613 enhances FOLFIRINOX response rate in stage IV pancreatic cancer. *Ann Oncol* **27:** vi228. doi:10.1093/annonc/mdw371.67

Anderson NS, Haynes CM. 2020. Folding the mitochondrial UPR into the integrated stress response. *Trends Cell Biol* **30:** 428–439. doi:10.1016/j.tcb.2020.03.001

Andrejeva G, Rathmell JC. 2017. Similarities and distinctions of cancer and immune metabolism in inflammation and tumors. *Cell Metab* **26:** 49–70. doi:10.1016/j.cmet.2017.06.004

Archibald JM. 2015. Endosymbiosis and eukaryotic cell evolution. *Curr Biol* **25:** R911–R921. doi:10.1016/j.cub.2015.07.055

Arnold PK, Jackson BT, Paras KI, Brunner JS, Hart ML, Newsom OJ, Alibekoff SP, Endress J, Drill E, Sullivan LB, et al. 2022. A non-canonical tricarboxylic acid cycle underlies cellular identity. *Nature* **603:** 477–481. doi:10.1038/s41586-022-04475-w

Arroyo JD, Jourdain AA, Calvo SE, Ballarano CA, Doench JG, Root DE, Mootha VK. 2016. A genome-wide CRISPR death screen identifies genes essential for oxidative phosphorylation. *Cell Metab* **24:** 875–885. doi:10.1016/j.cmet.2016.08.017

Bacman SR, Gammage PA, Minczuk M, Moraes CT. 2020. Manipulation of mitochondrial genes and mtDNA heteroplasmy. *Methods Cell Biol* **155:** 441–487. doi:10.1016/bs.mcb.2019.12.004

Bailis W, Shyer JA, Zhao J, Canaveras JCG, Al Khazal FJ, Qu R, Steach HR, Bielecki P, Khan O, Jackson R, et al. 2019. Distinct modes of mitochondrial metabolism uncouple T cell differentiation and function. *Nature* **571**: 403–407. doi:10.1038/s41586-019-1311-3

Bajzikova M, Kovarova J, Coelho AR, Boukalova S, Oh S, Rohlenova K, Svec D, Hubackova S, Endaya B, Judasova K, et al. 2019. Reactivation of dihydroorotate dehydrogenase-driven pyrimidine biosynthesis restores tumor growth of respiration-deficient cancer cells. *Cell Metab* **29**: 399–416.e10. doi:10.1016/j.cmet.2018.10.014

Bartman CR, Weilandt DR, Shen Y, Lee WD, Han Y, TeSlaa T, Jankowski CSR, Samarah L, Park NR, da Silva-Diz V, et al. 2023. Slow TCA flux and ATP production in primary solid tumours but not metastases. *Nature* **614**: 349–357.

Biancur DE, Kapner KS, Yamamoto K, Banh RS, Neggers JE, Sohn ASW, Wu W, Manguso RT, Brown A, Root DE, et al. 2021. Functional genomics identifies metabolic vulnerabilities in pancreatic cancer. *Cell Metab* **33**: 199–210.e8. doi:10.1016/j.cmet.2020.10.018

Birsoy K, Possemato R, Lorbeer FK, Bayraktar EC, Thiru P, Yucel B, Wang T, Chen WW, Clish CB, Sabatini DM. 2014. Metabolic determinants of cancer cell sensitivity to glucose limitation and biguanides. *Nature* **508**: 108–112. doi:10.1038/nature13110

Birsoy K, Wang T, Chen WW, Freinkman E, Abu-Remaileh M, Sabatini DM. 2015. An essential role of the mitochondrial electron transport chain in cell proliferation is to enable aspartate synthesis. *Cell* **162**: 540–551. doi:10.1016/j.cell.2015.07.016

Bonekamp NA, Peter B, Hillen HS, Felser A, Bergbrede T, Choidas A, Horn M, Unger A, Di Lucrezia R, Atanassov I, et al. 2020. Small-molecule inhibitors of human mitochondrial DNA transcription. *Nature* **588**: 712–716. doi:10.1038/s41586-020-03048-z

Bridges HR, Jones AJY, Pollak MN, Hirst J. 2014. Effects of metformin and other biguanides on oxidative phosphorylation in mitochondria. *Biochem J* **462**: 475–487. doi:10.1042/BJ20140620

Bridges HR, Blaza JN, Yin Z, Chung I, Pollak MN, Hirst J. 2023. Structural basis of mammalian respiratory complex I inhibition by medicinal biguanides. *Science* **379**: 351–357. doi:10.1126/science.ade3332

Brinker AE, Vivian CJ, Koestler DC, Tsue TT, Jensen RA, Welch DR. 2017. Mitochondrial haplotype alters mammary cancer tumorigenicity and metastasis in an oncogenic driver-dependent manner. *Cancer Res* **77**: 6941–6949. doi:10.1158/0008-5472.CAN-17-2194

Brown KK, Spinelli JB, Asara JM, Toker A. 2017. Adaptive reprogramming of de novo pyrimidine synthesis is a metabolic vulnerability in triple-negative breast cancer. *Cancer Discov* **7**: 391–399. doi:10.1158/2159-8290.CD-16-0611

Buzzai M, Jones RG, Amaravadi RK, Lum JJ, DeBerardinis RJ, Zhao F, Viollet B, Thompson CB. 2007. Systemic treatment with the antidiabetic drug metformin selectively impairs p53-deficient tumor cell growth. *Cancer Res* **67**: 6745–6752. doi:10.1158/0008-5472.CAN-06-4447

Cai H, Everett RS, Thakker DR. 2019. Efficacious dose of metformin for breast cancer therapy is determined by cation transporter expression in tumours. *Br J Pharmacol* **176**: 2724–2735. doi:10.1111/bph.14694

Campbell S, Mesaros C, Izzo L, Affronti H, Noji M, Schaffer BE, Tsang T, Sun K, Trefely S, Kruijning S, et al. 2021. Glutamine deprivation triggers NAGK-dependent hexosamine salvage. *eLife* **10**: e62644. doi:10.7554/eLife.62644

Cardaci S, Zheng L, Mackay G, Van Den Broek NJF, Mackenzie ED, Nixon C, Stevenson D, Tumanov S, Bulusu V, Kamphorst JJ, et al. 2015. Pyruvate carboxylation enables growth of SDH-deficient cells by supporting aspartate biosynthesis. *Nat Cell Biol* **17**: 1317–1326. doi:10.1038/ncb3233

Carrer A, Trefely S, Zhao S, Campbell SL, Norgard RJ, Schultz KC, Sidoli S, Parris JLD, Affronti HC, Sivanand S, et al. 2019. Acetyl-CoA metabolism supports multistep pancreatic tumorigenesis. *Cancer Discov* **9**: 416–435. doi:10.1158/2159-8290.CD-18-0567

Chakrabarty RP, Chandel NS. 2021. Mitochondria as signaling organelles control mammalian stem cell fate. *Cell Stem Cell* **28**: 394–408. doi:10.1016/j.stem.2021.02.011

Chandel NS, Avizonis D, Reczek CR, Weinberg SE, Menz S, Neuhaus R, Christian S, Haegebarth A, Algire C, Pollak M. 2016. Are metformin doses used in murine cancer models clinically relevant? *Cell Metab* **23**: 569–570. doi:10.1016/j.cmet.2016.03.010

Chapman NM, Zeng H, Nguyen TLM, Wang Y, Vogel P, Dhungana Y, Liu X, Neale G, Locasale JW, Chi H. 2018. mTOR coordinates transcriptional programs and mitochondrial metabolism of activated Treg subsets to protect tissue homeostasis. *Nat Commun* **9**: 1–15. doi:10.1038/s41467-018-04392-5

Chattopadhyay M, Jenkins EC, Lechuga-Vieco AV, Nie K, Fiel MI, Rialdi A, Guccione E, Enriquez JA, Sia D, Lujambio A, et al. 2022. The portrait of liver cancer is shaped by mitochondrial genetics. *Cell Rep* **38**: 110254. doi:10.1016/j.celrep.2021.110254

Chen YJ, Mahieu NG, Huang X, Singh M, Crawford PA, Johnson SL, Gross RW, Schaefer J, Patti GJ. 2016. Lactate metabolism is associated with mammalian mitochondria. *Nat Chem Biol* **12**: 937–943. doi:10.1038/nchembio.2172

Comerford SA, Huang Z, Du X, Wang Y, Cai L, Witkiewicz AK, Walters H, Tantawy MN, Fu A, Manning HC, et al. 2014. Acetate dependence of tumors. *Cell* **159**: 1591–1602. doi:10.1016/j.cell.2014.11.020

Correia-Melo C, Ichim G, Tait SWG, Passos JF. 2017. Depletion of mitochondria in mammalian cells through enforced mitophagy. *Nat Protoc* **12**: 183–194. doi:10.1038/nprot.2016.159

de Beauchamp L, Himonas E, Helgason GV. 2022. Mitochondrial metabolism as a potential therapeutic target in myeloid leukaemia. *Leukemia* **36**: 1–12. doi:10.1038/s41375-021-01416-w

DeBerardinis RJ, Chandel NS. 2020. We need to talk about the Warburg effect. *Nat Metab* **2**: 127–129. doi:10.1038/s42255-020-0172-2

Deuse T, Hu X, Agbor-Enoh S, Koch M, Spitzer MH, Gravina A, Alawi M, Marishta A, Peters B, Kosaloglu-Yalcin Z, et al. 2019. De novo mutations in mitochondrial DNA of iPSCs produce immunogenic neoepitopes in mice and humans. *Nat Biotechnol* **37**: 1137–1144. doi:10.1038/s41587-019-0227-7

Dong LF, Kovarova J, Bajzikova M, Bezawork-Geleta A, Svec D, Endaya B, Sachaphibulkij K, Coelho AR, Sebkova N, Ruzickova A, et al. 2017. Horizontal transfer of whole mitochondria restores tumorigenic potential in mitochondrial DNA-deficient cancer cells. *eLife* **6**: e22187. doi:10.7554/eLife.22187

Dong LF, Rohlena J, Zobalova R, Nahacka Z, Rodriguez AM, Berridge MV, Neuzil J. 2023. Mitochondria on the move: horizontal mitochondrial transfer in disease and health. *J Cell Biol* **222**: e202211044. doi:10.1083/jcb.202211044

Dzierzak E, Philipsen S. 2013. Erythropoiesis: development and differentiation. *Cold Spring Harb Perspect Med* **3**: a011601. doi:10.1101/cshperspect.a011601

Elia I, Rossi M, Stegen S, Broekaert D, Doglioni G, van Gorsel M, Boon R, Escalona-Noguero C, Torrekens S, Verfaillie C, et al. 2019. Breast cancer cells rely on environmental pyruvate to shape the metastatic niche. *Nature* **568**: 117–121. doi:10.1038/s41586-019-0977-x

Evans JMM, Donnelly LA, Emslie-Smith AM, Alessi DR, Morris AD. 2005. Metformin and reduced risk of cancer in diabetic patients. *Br Med J* **330**: 1304–1305. doi:10.1136/bmj.38415.708634.F7

Faubert B, Li KY, Cai L, Hensley CT, Kim J, Zacharias LG, Yang C, Do QN, Doucette S, Burguete D, et al. 2017. Lactate metabolism in human lung tumors. *Cell* **171**: 358–371.e9. doi:10.1016/j.cell.2017.09.019

Field CS, Baixauli F, Kyle RL, Puleston DJ, Cameron AM, Sanin DE, Hippen KL, Loschi M, Thangavelu G, Corrado M, et al. 2020. Mitochondrial integrity regulated by lipid metabolism is a cell-intrinsic checkpoint for Treg suppressive function. *Cell Metab* **31**: 422–437.e5. doi:10.1016/j.cmet.2019.11.021

Fletcher JW, Djulbegovic B, Soares HP, Siegel BA, Lowe VJ, Lyman GH, Coleman RE, Wahl R, Paschold JC, Avril N, et al. 2008. Recommendations on the use of 18F-FDG PET in oncology. *J Nucl Med* **49**: 480–508. doi:10.2967/jnumed.107.047787

Frauwirth KA, Riley JL, Harris MH, Parry RV, Rathmell JC, Plas DR, Elstrom RL, June CH, Thompson CB. 2002. The CD28 signaling pathway regulates glucose metabolism. *Immunity* **16**: 769–777. doi:10.1016/S1074-7613(02)00323-0

Frezza C, Zheng L, Folger O, Rajagopalan KN, MacKenzie ED, Jerby L, Micaroni M, Chaneton B, Adam J, Hedley A, et al. 2011. Haem oxygenase is synthetically lethal with the tumour suppressor fumarate hydratase. *Nature* **477**: 225–228. doi:10.1038/nature10363

Fu Z, Ye J, Dean JW, Bostick JW, Weinberg SE, Xiong L, Oliff KN, Chen ZE, Avram D, Chandel NS, et al. 2019. Requirement of mitochondrial transcription factor A in tissue-resident regulatory T cell maintenance and function. *Cell Rep* **28**: 159–171.e4. doi:10.1016/j.celrep.2019.06.024

Garcia-Bermudez J, Baudrier L, La K, Zhu XG, Fidelin J, Sviderskiy VO, Papagiannakopoulos T, Molina H, Snuderl M, Lewis CA, et al. 2018. Aspartate is a limiting metabolite for cancer cell proliferation under hypoxia and in tumours. *Nat Cell Biol* **20**: 775–781. doi:10.1038/s41556-018-0118-z

Garcia-Bermudez J, Badgley MA, Prasad S, Baudrier L, Liu Y, La K, Soula M, Williams RT, Yamaguchi N, Hwang RF, et al. 2022. Adaptive stimulation of macropinocytosis overcomes aspartate limitation in cancer cells under hypoxia. *Nat Metab* **4**: 724–738. doi:10.1038/s42255-022-00583-z

Gharpure KM, Pradeep S, Sans M, Rupaimoole R, Ivan C, Wu SY, Bayraktar E, Nagaraja AS, Mangala LS, Zhang X, et al. 2018. FABP4 as a key determinant of metastatic potential of ovarian cancer. *Nat Commun* **9**: 2923. doi:10.1038/s41467-018-04987-y

Ghergurovich JM, Lang JD, Levin MK, Briones N, Facista SJ, Mueller C, Cowan AJ, McBride MJ, Rodriguez ESR, Killian A, et al. 2021. Local production of lactate, ribose phosphate, and amino acids within human triple-negative breast cancer. *Med (NY)* **2**: 736–754. doi:10.1016/j.medj.2021.03.009

Gopal RK, Calvo SE, Shih AR, Chaves FL, McGuone D, Mick E, Pierce KA, Li Y, Garofalo A, Van Allen EM, et al. 2018. Early loss of mitochondrial complex I and rewiring of glutathione metabolism in renal oncocytoma. *Proc Natl Acad Sci* **115**: E6283–E6290. doi:10.1073/pnas.1711888115

Gorelick AN, Kim M, Chatila WK, La K, Hakimi AA, Berger MF, Taylor BS, Gammage PA, Reznik E. 2021. Respiratory complex and tissue lineage drive recurrent mutations in tumour mtDNA. *Nat Metab* **3**: 558–570. doi:10.1038/s42255-021-00378-8

Guo JY, Chen HY, Mathew R, Fan J, Strohecker AM, Karsli-Uzunbas G, Kamphorst JJ, Chen G, Lemons JMS, Karantza V, et al. 2011. Activated Ras requires autophagy to maintain oxidative metabolism and tumorigenesis. *Genes Dev* **25**: 460–470. doi:10.1101/gad.2016311

Han M, Bushong EA, Segawa M, Tiard A, Wong A, Brady MR, Momcilovic M, Wolf DM, Zhang R, Petcherski A, et al. 2023. Spatial mapping of mitochondrial networks and bioenergetics in lung cancer. *Nature* **615**: 712–719. doi:10.1038/s41586-023-05793-3

Hensley CT, Faubert B, Yuan Q, Lev-Cohain N, Jin E, Kim J, Jiang L, Ko B, Skelton R, Loudat L, et al. 2016. Metabolic heterogeneity in human lung tumors. *Cell* **164**: 681–694. doi:10.1016/j.cell.2015.12.034

Hirsch HA, Iliopoulos D, Tsichlis PN, Struhl K. 2009. Metformin selectively targets cancer stem cells, and acts together with chemotherapy to block tumor growth and prolong remission. *Cancer Res* **69**: 7507–7511. doi:10.1158/0008-5472.CAN-09-2994

Hui S, Ghergurovich JM, Morscher RJ, Jang C, Teng X, Lu W, Esparza LA, Reya T, Zhan L, Yanxiang Guo J, et al. 2017. Glucose feeds the TCA cycle via circulating lactate. *Nature* **551**: 115–118. doi:10.1038/nature24057

Inigo JR, Chandra D. 2022. The mitochondrial unfolded protein response (UPRmt): shielding against toxicity to mitochondria in cancer. *J Hematol Oncol* **15**: 98. doi:10.1186/s13045-022-01317-0

Iommarini L, Kurelac I, Capristo M, Calvaruso MA, Giorgio V, Bergamini C, Ghelli A, Nanni P, De Giovanni C, Carelli V, et al. 2014. Different mtDNA mutations modify tumor progression in dependence of the degree of respiratory complex I impairment. *Hum Mol Genet* **23**: 1453–1466. doi:10.1093/hmg/ddt533

Ishikawa K, Takenaga K, Akimoto M, Koshikawa N, Yamaguchi A, Imanishi H, Nakada K, Honma Y, Hayashi JI. 2008. ROS-generating mitochondrial DNA mutations can regulate tumor cell metastasis. *Science* **320**: 661–664. doi:10.1126/science.1156906

Jain IH, Calvo SE, Markhard AL, Skinner OS, To TL, Ast T, Mootha VK. 2020. Genetic screen for cell fitness in high or low oxygen highlights mitochondrial and lipid metabolism. *Cell* 181: 716–727.e11. doi:10.1016/j.cell.2020.03.029

Jiang L, Shestov AA, Swain P, Yang C, Parker SJ, Wang QA, Terada LS, Adams ND, McCabe MT, Pietrak B, et al. 2016. Reductive carboxylation supports redox homeostasis during anchorage-independent growth. *Nature* 532: 255–258. doi:10.1038/nature17393

Johnston K, Pachnis P, Tasdogan A, Faubert B, Zacharias LG, Vu HS, Rodgers-Augustyniak L, Johnson A, Huang F, Ricciardo S, et al. 2021. Isotope tracing reveals glycolysis and oxidative metabolism in childhood tumors of multiple histologies. *Med (NY)* 2: 395–410. doi:10.1016/j.medj.2021.01.002

Ju YS, Alexandrov LB, Gerstung M, Martincorena I, Nik-Zainal S, Ramakrishna M, Davies HR, Papaemmanuil E, Gundem G, Shlien A, et al. 2014. Origins and functional consequences of somatic mitochondrial DNA mutations in human cancer. *eLife* 3: e02935. doi:10.7554/eLife.02935

Kamphorst JJ, Cross JR, Fan J, de Stanchina E, Mathew R, White EP, Thompson CB, Rabinowitz JD. 2013. Hypoxic and Ras-transformed cells support growth by scavenging unsaturated fatty acids from lysophospholipids. *Proc Natl Acad Sci* 110: 8882–8887. doi:10.1073/pnas.1307237110

Kang BH, Siegelin MD, Plescia J, Raskett CM, Garlick DS, Dohi T, Lian JB, Stein GS, Languino LR, Altieri DC. 2010. Preclinical characterization of mitochondria-targeted small molecule Hsp90 inhibitors, gamitrinibs, in advanced prostate cancer. *Clin Cancer Res* 16: 4779–4788. doi:10.1158/1078-0432.CCR-10-1818

Karnkowska A, Vacek V, Zubáčová Z, Treitli SC, Petrželková R, Eme L, Novák L, Žárský V, Barlow LD, Herman EK, et al. 2016. A eukaryote without a mitochondrial organelle. *Curr Biol* 26: 1274–1284. doi:10.1016/j.cub.2016.03.053

Kenny TC, Gomez ML, Germain D. 2019. Mitohormesis, UPRMT, and the complexity of mitochondrial DNA landscapes in cancer. *Cancer Res* 79: 6057–6066. doi:10.1158/0008-5472.CAN-19-1395

Kim J, Hu Z, Cai L, Li K, Choi E, Faubert B, Bezwada D, Rodriguez-Canales J, Villalobos P, Lin YF, et al. 2017. CPS1 maintains pyrimidine pools and DNA synthesis in KRAS/LKB1-mutant lung cancer cells. *Nature* 546: 168–172. doi:10.1038/nature22359

Kim PK, Halbrook CJ, Kerk SA, Radyk M, Wisner S, Kremer DM, Sajjakulnukit P, Andren A, Hou SW, Trivedi A, et al. 2021. Hyaluronic acid fuels pancreatic cancer cell growth. *eLife* 10: e62645. doi:10.7554/eLife.62645

Kim M, Mahmood M, Reznik E, Gammage PA. 2022. Mitochondrial DNA is a major source of driver mutations in cancer. *Trends Cancer* 8: 1046–1059. doi:10.1016/j.trecan.2022.08.001

King MP, Attardi G. 1989. Human cells lacking mtDNA: repopulation with exogenous mitochondria by complementation. *Science* 246: 500–503. doi:10.1126/science.2814477

Kopinski PK, Singh LN, Zhang S, Lott MT, Wallace DC. 2021. Mitochondrial DNA variation and cancer. *Nat Rev Cancer* 21: 431–445. doi:10.1038/s41568-021-00358-w

Koundinya M, Sudhalter J, Courjaud A, Lionne B, Touyer G, Bonnet L, Menguy I, Schreiber I, Perrault C, Vougier S, et al. 2018. Dependence on the pyrimidine biosynthetic enzyme DHODH is a synthetic lethal vulnerability in mutant

KRAS-driven cancers. *Cell Chem Biol* 25: 705–717.e11. doi:10.1016/j.chembiol.2018.03.005

Krall AS, Mullen PJ, Surjono F, Momcilovic M, Schmid EW, Halbrook CJ, Thambundit A, Mittelman SD, Lyssiotis CA, Shackelford DB, et al. 2021. Asparagine couples mitochondrial respiration to ATF4 activity and tumor growth. *Cell Metab* 33: 1013–1026.e6. doi:10.1016/j.cmet.2021.02.001

Kuntz EM, Baquero P, Michie AM, Dunn K, Tardito S, Holyoake TL, Helgason GV, Gottlieb E. 2017. Targeting mitochondrial oxidative phosphorylation eradicates therapy-resistant chronic myeloid leukemia stem cells. *Nat Med* 23: 1234–1240. doi:10.1038/nm.4399

Ladds MJGW, Van Leeuwen IMM, Drummond CJ, Chu S, Healy AR, Popova G, Pastor Fernández A, Mollick T, Darekar S, Sedimbi SK, et al. 2018. A DHODH inhibitor increases p53 synthesis and enhances tumor cell killing by p53 degradation blockage. *Nat Commun* 9: 1–14. doi:10.1038/s41467-017-02088-w

Latorre-Pellicer A, Moreno-Loshuertos R, Lechuga-Vieco AV, Sánchez-Cabo F, Torroja C, Acín-Pérez R, Calvo E, Aix E, González-Guerra A, Logan A, et al. 2016. Mitochondrial and nuclear DNA matching shapes metabolism and healthy ageing. *Nature* 535: 561–565. doi:10.1038/nature18618

Le A, Lane AN, Hamaker M, Bose S, Gouw A, Barbi J, Tsukamoto T, Rojas CJ, Slusher BS, Zhang H, et al. 2012. Glucose-independent glutamine metabolism via TCA cycling for proliferation and survival in B cells. *Cell Metab* 15: 110–121. doi:10.1016/j.cmet.2011.12.009

Lee S, Lee H, Baek G, Kim JS. 2023. Precision mitochondrial DNA editing with high-fidelity DddA-derived base editors. *Nat Biotechnol* 41: 378–386. doi:10.1038/s41587-022-01486-w

Li L, Ng SR, Colón CI, Drapkin BJ, Hsu PP, Li Z, Nabel CS, Lewis CA, Romero R, Mercer KL, et al. 2019. Identification of DHODH as a therapeutic target in small cell lung cancer. *Sci Transl Med* 11: 7852. doi:10.1126/scitranslmed.aaw7852

Luengo A, Li Z, Gui DY, Sullivan LB, Zagorulya M, Do BT, Ferreira R, Naamati A, Ali A, Lewis CA, et al. 2021. Increased demand for NAD$^+$ relative to ATP drives aerobic glycolysis. *Mol Cell* 81: 691–707.e6. doi:10.1016/j.molcel.2020.12.012

Lussey-Lepoutre C, Hollinshead KER, Ludwig C, Menara M, Morin A, Castro-Vega LJ, Parker SJ, Janin M, Martinelli C, Ottolenghi C, et al. 2015. Loss of succinate dehydrogenase activity results in dependency on pyruvate carboxylation for cellular anabolism. *Nat Commun* 6: 1–9. doi:10.1038/ncomms9784

Ma EH, Verway MJ, Johnson RM, Roy DG, Steadman M, Hayes S, Williams KS, Sheldon RD, Samborska B, Kosinski PA, et al. 2019. Metabolic profiling using stable isotope tracing reveals distinct patterns of glucose utilization by physiologically activated CD8$^+$ T cells. *Immunity* 51: 856–870.e5. doi:10.1016/j.immuni.2019.09.003

Madera D, Vitale-Cross L, Martin D, Schneider A, Molinolo AA, Gangane N, Carey TE, McHugh JB, Komarck CM, Walline HM, et al. 2015. Prevention of tumor growth driven by *PIK3CA* and HPV oncogenes by targeting mTOR signaling with metformin in oral squamous carcinomas expressing OCT3. *Cancer Prev Res (Phila)* **8**: 197–207. doi:10.1158/1940-6207.CAPR-14-0348

Mahmood M, Liu EM, Shergold AL, Tolla E, Tait-Mulder J, Huerta-Uribe A, Shokry E, Young AL, Lilla S, Kim M, et al. 2024. Mitochondrial DNA mutations drive aerobic glycolysis to enhance checkpoint blockade response in melanoma. *Nat Cancer* doi:10.1038/s43018-023-00721-w

Martínez-Reyes I, Robles Cardona L, Kong H, Vasan K, Mcelroy GS, Werner M, Kihshen H, Reczek CR, Weinberg SE, Gao P, et al. 2020. Mitochondrial ubiquinol oxidation is necessary for tumour growth. *Nature* **585**: 288–292. doi:10.1038/s41586-020-2475-6

Mashimo T, Pichumani K, Vemireddy V, Hatanpaa KJ, Singh DK, Sirasanagandla S, Nannepaga S, Piccirillo SG, Kovacs Z, Foong C, et al. 2014. Acetate is a bioenergetic substrate for human glioblastoma and brain metastases. *Cell* **159**: 1603–1614. doi:10.1016/j.cell.2014.11.025

Mathur D, Stratikopoulos E, Ozturk S, Steinbach N, Pegno S, Schoenfeld S, Yong R, Murty VV, Asara JM, Cantley LC, et al. 2017. PTEN regulates glutamine flux to pyrimidine synthesis and sensitivity to dihydroorotate dehydrogenase inhibition. *Cancer Discov* **7**: 380–390. doi:10.1158/2159-8290.CD-16-0612

Mayers JR, Torrence ME, Danai LV, Papagiannakopoulos T, Davidson SM, Bauer MR, Lau AN, Ji BW, Dixit PD, Hosios AM, et al. 2016. Tissue of origin dictates branched-chain amino acid metabolism in mutant *Kras*-driven cancers. *Science* **353**: 1161–1165. doi:10.1126/science.aaf5171

Memmott RM, Mercado JR, Maier CR, Kawabata S, Fox SD, Dennis PA. 2010. Metformin prevents tobacco carcinogen-induced lung tumorigenesis. *Cancer Prev Res (Phila)* **3**: 1066–1076. doi:10.1158/1940-6207.CAPR-10-0055

Menk AV, Scharping NE, Moreci RS, Zeng X, Guy C, Salvatore S, Bae H, Xie J, Young HA, Wendell SG, et al. 2018. Early TCR signaling induces rapid aerobic glycolysis enabling distinct acute T cell effector functions. *Cell Rep* **22**: 1509–1521. doi:10.1016/j.celrep.2018.01.040

Metallo CM, Gameiro PA, Bell EL, Mattaini KR, Yang J, Hiller K, Jewell CM, Johnson ZR, Irvine DJ, Guarente L, et al. 2012. Reductive glutamine metabolism by IDH1 mediates lipogenesis under hypoxia. *Nature* **481**: 380–384. doi:10.1038/nature10602

Michl J, Wang Y, Monterisi S, Blaszczak W, Beveridge R, Bridges EM, Koth J, Bodmer WF, Swietach P. 2022. CRISPR-Cas9 screen identifies oxidative phosphorylation as essential for cancer cell survival at low extracellular pH. *Cell Rep* **38**: 110493. doi:10.1016/j.celrep.2022.110493

Mick E, Titov DV, Skinner OS, Sharma R, Jourdain AA, Mootha VK. 2020. Distinct mitochondrial defects trigger the integrated stress response depending on the metabolic state of the cell. *eLife* **9**: e49178. doi:10.7554/eLife.49178

Missiroli S, Perrone M, Genovese I, Pinton P, Giorgi C. 2020. Cancer metabolism and mitochondria: finding novel mechanisms to fight tumours. *EBioMed* **59**: 102943. doi:10.1016/j.ebiom.2020.102943

Mitchell P. 1961. Coupling of phosphorylation to electron and hydrogen transfer by a chemi-osmotic type of mechanism. *Nature* **191**: 144–148.

Mok BY, Kotrys AV, Raguram A, Huang TP, Mootha VK, Liu DR. 2022. CRISPR-free base editors with enhanced activity and expanded targeting scope in mitochondrial and

nuclear DNA. *Nat Biotechnol* **40**: 1378–1387. doi:10.1038/s41587-022-01256-8

Molina JR, Sun Y, Protopopova M, Gera S, Bandi M, Bristow C, McAfoos T, Morlacchi P, Ackroyd J, Agip ANA, et al. 2018. An inhibitor of oxidative phosphorylation exploits cancer vulnerability. *Nat Med* **24**: 1036–1046. doi:10.1038/s41591-018-0052-4

Momcilovic M, Jones A, Bailey ST, Waldmann CM, Li R, Lee JT, Abdelhady G, Gomez A, Holloway T, Schmid E, et al. 2019. In vivo imaging of mitochondrial membrane potential in non-small-cell lung cancer. *Nature* **575**: 380–384. doi:10.1038/s41586-019-1715-0

Mottis A, Herzig S, Auwerx J. 2019. Mitocellular communication: shaping health and disease. *Science* **366**: 827–832. doi:10.1126/science.aax3768

Mullen AR, Wheaton WW, Jin ES, Chen PH, Sullivan LB, Cheng T, Yang Y, Linehan WM, Chandel NS, Deberardinis RJ. 2012. Reductive carboxylation supports growth in tumour cells with defective mitochondria. *Nature* **481**: 385–388. doi:10.1038/nature10642

Naguib A, Mathew G, Reczek CR, Watrud K, Ambrico A, Herzka T, Salas IC, Lee MF, El-Amine N, Zheng W, et al. 2018. Mitochondrial complex I inhibitors expose a vulnerability for selective killing of Pten-null cells. *Cell Rep* **23**: 58–67. doi:10.1016/j.celrep.2018.03.032

Neinast MD, Jang C, Hui S, Murashige DS, Chu Q, Morscher RJ, Li X, Zhan L, White E, Anthony TG, et al. 2019. Quantitative analysis of the whole-body metabolic fate of branched-chain amino acids. *Cell Metab* **29**: 417–429.e4. doi:10.1016/j.cmet.2018.10.013

Nissanka N, Moraes CT. 2020. Mitochondrial DNA heteroplasmy in disease and targeted nuclease-based therapeutic approaches. *EMBO Rep* **21**: e49612. doi:10.15252/embr.201949612

Nwosu ZC, Ward MH, Sajjakulnukit P, Poudel P, Ragulan C, Kasperek S, Radyk M, Sutton D, Menjivar RE, Andren A, et al. 2023. Uridine-derived ribose fuels glucose-restricted pancreatic cancer. *Nature* **618**: 151–158. doi:10.1038/s41586-023-06073-w

Pachnis P, Wu Z, Faubert B, Tasdogan A, Gu W, Shelton S, Solmonson A, Rao AD, Kaushik AK, Rogers TJ, et al. 2022. In vivo isotope tracing reveals a requirement for the electron transport chain in glucose and glutamine metabolism by tumors. *Sci Adv* **8**: eabn9550. doi:10.1126/sciadv.abn9550

Pardee TS, Lee K, Luddy J, Maturo C, Rodriguez R, Isom S, Miller LD, Stadelman KM, Levitan D, Hurd D, et al. 2014. A phase I study of the first-in-class antimitochondrial metabolism agent, CPI-613, in patients with advanced hematologic malignancies. *Clin Cancer Res* **20**: 5255–5264. doi:10.1158/1078-0432.CCR-14-1019

Romero R, Sayin VI, Davidson SM, Bauer MR, Singh SX, Leboeuf SE, Karakousi TR, Ellis DC, Bhutkar A, Sánchez-Rivera FJ, et al. 2017. Keap1 loss promotes Kras-driven lung cancer and results in dependence on glutaminolysis. *Nat Med* **23**: 1362–1368. doi:10.1038/nm.4407

Rossiter NJ, Huggler KS, Adelmann CH, Keys HR, Soens RW, Sabatini DM, Cantor JR. 2021. CRISPR screens in physiologic medium reveal conditionally essential genes in human cells. *Cell Metab* **33**: 1248–1263.e9. doi:10.1016/j.cmet.2021.02.005

Rouault TA. 2015. Mammalian iron–sulphur proteins: novel insights into biogenesis and function. *Nat Rev Mol Cell Biol* **16:** 45–55. doi:10.1038/nrm3909

Sciacovelli M, Gonçalves E, Johnson TI, Zecchini VR, da Costa ASH, Gaude E, Drubbel AV, Theobald SJ, Abbo SR, Tran MGB, et al. 2016. Fumarate is an epigenetic modifier that elicits epithelial-to-mesenchymal transition. *Nature* **537:** 544–547. doi:10.1038/nature19353

Sena LA, Li S, Jairaman A, Prakriya M, Ezponda T, Hildeman DA, Wang CR, Schumacker PT, Licht JD, Perlman H, et al. 2013. Mitochondria are required for antigen-specific T cell activation through reactive oxygen species signaling. *Immunity* **38:** 225–236. doi:10.1016/j.immuni.2012.10.020

Shackelford DB, Abt E, Gerken L, Vasquez DS, Seki A, Leblanc M, Wei L, Fishbein MC, Czernin J, Mischel PS, et al. 2013. LKB1 inactivation dictates therapeutic response of non-small cell lung cancer to the metabolism drug phenformin. *Cancer Cell* **23:** 143–158. doi:10.1016/j.ccr.2012.12.008

Shi Y, Lim SK, Liang Q, Iyer SV, Wang HY, Wang Z, Xie X, Sun D, Chen YJ, Tabar V, et al. 2019. Gboxin is an oxidative phosphorylation inhibitor that targets glioblastoma. *Nature* **567:** 341–346. doi:10.1038/s41586-019-0993-x

Shim E-H, Livi CB, Rakheja D, Tan J, Benson D, Parekh V, Kho EY, Ghosh AP, Kirkman R, Velu S, et al. 2014. l-2-Hydroxyglutarate: an epigenetic modifier and putative oncometabolite in renal cancer. *Cancer Discov* **4:** 1290–1298. doi:10.1158/2159-8290.CD-13-0696

Shroff EH, Eberlin LS, Dang VM, Gouw AM, Gabay M, Adam SJ, Bellovin DI, Trand PT, Philbrick WM, Garcia-Ocana A, et al. 2015. MYC oncogene overexpression drives renal cell carcinoma in a mouse model through glutamine metabolism. *Proc Natl Acad Sci* **112:** 6539–6544. doi:10.1073/pnas.1507228112

Siegelin MD, Dohi T, Raskett CM, Orlowski GM, Powers CM, Gilbert CA, Ross AH, Plescia J, Altieri DC. 2011. Exploiting the mitochondrial unfolded protein response for cancer therapy in mice and human cells. *J Clin Invest* **121:** 1349–1360. doi:10.1172/JCI44855

Sivanand S, Vander Heiden MG. 2020. Emerging roles for branched-chain amino acid metabolism in cancer. *Cancer Cell* **37:** 147–156. doi:10.1016/j.cell.2019.12.011

Skinner OS, Blanco-Fernández J, Goodman RP, Kawakami A, Shen H, Kemény LV, Joesch-Cohen L, Rees MG, Roth JA, Fisher DE, et al. 2023. Salvage of ribose from uridine or RNA supports glycolysis in nutrient-limited conditions. *Nat Metab* **5:** 765–776. doi:10.1038/s42255-023-00774-2

Škrtić M, Sriskanthadevan S, Jhas B, Gebbia M, Wang X, Wang Z, Hurren R, Jitkova Y, Gronda M, Maclean N, et al. 2011. Inhibition of mitochondrial translation as a therapeutic strategy for human acute myeloid leukemia. *Cancer Cell* **20:** 674–688. doi:10.1016/j.ccr.2011.10.015

Spinelli JB, Yoon H, Ringel AE, Jeanfavre S, Clish CB, Haigis MC. 2017. Metabolic recycling of ammonia via glutamate dehydrogenase supports breast cancer biomass. *Science* **358:** 941–946. doi:10.1126/science.aam9305

Stuart SD, Schauble A, Gupta S, Kennedy AD, Keppler BR, Bingham PM, Zachar Z. 2014. A strategically designed small molecule attacks α-ketoglutarate dehydrogenase in tumor cells through a redox process. *Cancer Metab* **2:** 1–15. doi:10.1186/2049-3002-2-4

Sullivan LB, Gui DY, Hosios AM, Bush LN, Freinkman E, Vander Heiden MG. 2015. Supporting aspartate biosynthesis is an essential function of respiration in proliferating cells. *Cell* **162:** 552–563. doi:10.1016/j.cell.2015.07.017

Sullivan LB, Luengo A, Danai LV, Bush LN, Diehl FF, Hosios AM, Lau AN, Elmiligy S, Malstrom S, Lewis CA, et al. 2018. Aspartate is an endogenous metabolic limitation for tumour growth. *Nat Cell Biol* **20:** 782–788. doi:10.1038/s41556-018-0125-0

Sykes DB, Kfoury YS, Mercier FE, Wawer MJ, Law JM, Haynes MK, Lewis TA, Schajnovitz A, Jain E, Lee D, et al. 2016. Inhibition of dihydroorotate dehydrogenase overcomes differentiation blockade in acute myeloid leukemia. *Cell* **167:** 171–186.e15. doi:10.1016/j.cell.2016.08.057

Tajan M, Hock AK, Blagih J, Robertson NA, Labuschagne CF, Kruiswijk F, Humpton TJ, Adams PD, Vousden KH. 2018. A role for p53 in the adaptation to glutamine starvation through the expression of SLC1A3. *Cell Metab* **28:** 721–736.e6. doi:10.1016/j.cmet.2018.07.005

Tan JX, Finkel T. 2020. Mitochondria as intracellular signaling platforms in health and disease. *J Cell Biol* **219:** e202002179. doi:10.1083/jcb.202002179

Tan AS, Baty JW, Dong LF, Bezawork-Geleta A, Endaya B, Goodwin J, Bajzikova M, Kovarova J, Peterka M, Yan B, et al. 2015. Mitochondrial genome acquisition restores respiratory function and tumorigenic potential of cancer cells without mitochondrial DNA. *Cell Metab* **21:** 81–94. doi:10.1016/j.cmet.2014.12.003

Tan YQ, Zhang X, Zhang S, Zhu T, Garg M, Lobie PE, Pandey V. 2021. Mitochondria: the metabolic switch of cellular oncogenic transformation. *Biochim Biophys Acta* **1876:** 188534. doi:10.1016/j.bbcan.2021.188534

Tarasenko TN, Pacheco SE, Koenig MK, Gomez-Rodriguez J, Kapnick SM, Diaz F, Zerfas PM, Barca E, Sudderth J, DeBerardinis RJ, et al. 2017. Cytochrome c oxidase activity is a metabolic checkpoint that regulates cell fate decisions during T cell activation and differentiation. *Cell Metab* **25:** 1254–1268.e7. doi:10.1016/j.cmet.2017.05.007

Tasdogan A, Faubert B, Ramesh V, Ubellacker JM, Shen B, Solmonson A, Murphy MM, Gu Z, Gu W, Martin M, et al. 2020. Metabolic heterogeneity confers differences in melanoma metastatic potential. *Nature* **577:** 115–120. doi:10.1038/s41586-019-1847-2

Thomas LW, Esposito C, Morgan RE, Price S, Young J, Williams SP, Maddalena LA, McDermott U, Ashcroft M. 2021. Genome-wide CRISPR/Cas9 deletion screen defines mitochondrial gene essentiality and identifies routes for tumour cell viability in hypoxia. *Commun Biol* **4:** 1–12. doi:10.1038/s42003-021-02098-x

Tönjes M, Barbus S, Park YJ, Wang W, Schlotter M, Lindroth AM, Pleier SV, Bai AHC, Karra D, Piro RM, et al. 2013. BCAT1 promotes cell proliferation through amino acid catabolism in gliomas carrying wild-type IDH1. *Nat Med* **19:** 901–908. doi:10.1038/nm.3217

Van Vranken JG, Rutter J. 2015. You down with ETC? yeah, you know D!. *Cell* **162:** 471–473. doi:10.1016/j.cell.2015.07.027

Vasan K, Werner M, Chandel NS. 2020. Mitochondrial metabolism as a target for cancer therapy. *Cell Metab* **32:** 341–352. doi:10.1016/j.cmet.2020.06.019

Wang Y, Stancliffe E, Fowle-Grider R, Wang R, Wang C, Schwaiger-Haber M, Shriver LP, Patti GJ. 2022. Saturation of the mitochondrial NADH shuttles drives aerobic glycolysis in proliferating cells. *Mol Cell* **82:** 3270–3283.e9. doi:10.1016/j.molcel.2022.07.007

Warburg O. 1956. On the origin of cancer cells. *Science* **123:** 309–314. doi:10.1126/science.123.3191.309

Weinberg F, Hamanaka R, Wheaton WW, Weinberg S, Joseph J, Lopez M, Kalyanaraman B, Mutlu GM, Budinger GRS, Chandel NS. 2010. Mitochondrial metabolism and ROS generation are essential for Kras-mediated tumorigenicity. *Proc Natl Acad Sci* **107:** 8788–8793. doi:10.1073/pnas.1003428107

Weinberg SE, Singer BD, Steinert EM, Martinez CA, Mehta MM, Martínez-Reyes I, Gao P, Helmin KA, Abdala-Valencia H, Sena LA, et al. 2019. Mitochondrial complex III is essential for suppressive function of regulatory T cells. *Nature* **565:** 495–499. doi:10.1038/s41586-018-0846-z

Welch DR, Foster C, Rigoutsos I. 2022. Roles of mitochondrial genetics in cancer metastasis. *Trends Cancer* **8:** 1002–1018. doi:10.1016/j.trecan.2022.07.004

Wheaton WW, Weinberg SE, Hamanaka RB, Soberanes S, Sullivan LB, Anso E, Glasauer A, Dufour E, Mutlu GM, Scott Budinger GR, et al. 2014. Metformin inhibits mitochondrial complex I of cancer cells to reduce tumorigenesis. *eLife* **3:** e02242. doi:10.7554/eLife.02242

Wise DR, Ward PS, Shay JES, Cross JR, Gruber JJ, Sachdeva UM, Platt JM, DeMatteo RG, Simon MC, Thompson CB. 2011. Hypoxia promotes isocitrate dehydrogenase-dependent carboxylation of α-ketoglutarate to citrate to support cell growth and viability. *Proc Natl Acad Sci* **108:** 19611–19616. doi:10.1073/pnas.1117773108

Xiang Y, Stine ZE, Xia J, Lu Y, O'Connor RS, Altman BJ, Hsieh AL, Gouw AM, Thomas AG, Gao P, et al. 2015. Targeted inhibition of tumor-specific glutaminase diminishes cell-autonomous tumorigenesis. *J Clin Invest* **125:** 2293–2306. doi:10.1172/JCI75836

Yap TA, Daver N, Mahendra M, Zhang J, Kamiya-Matsuoka C, Meric-Bernstam F, Kantarjian HM, Ravandi F, Collins ME, Francesco MED, et al. 2023. Complex I inhibitor of oxidative phosphorylation in advanced solid tumors and acute myeloid leukemia: phase I trials. *Nat Med* **29:** 115–126. doi:10.1038/s41591-022-02103-8

Yuan Y, Ju YS, Kim Y, Li J, Wang Y, Yoon CJ, Yang Y, Martincorena I, Creighton CJ, Weinstein JN, et al. 2020. Comprehensive molecular characterization of mitochondrial genomes in human cancers. *Nat Genet* **52:** 342–352. doi:10.1038/s41588-019-0557-x

Zhang X, Dang CV. 2023. Time to hit pause on mitochondria-targeting cancer therapies. *Nat Med* **29:** 29–30. doi:10.1038/s41591-022-02129-y

Zhang G, Frederick DT, Wu L, Wei Z, Krepler C, Srinivasan S, Chae YC, Xu X, Choi H, Dimwamwa E, et al. 2016. Targeting mitochondrial biogenesis to overcome drug resistance to MAPK inhibitors. *J Clin Invest* **126:** 1834–1856. doi:10.1172/JCI82661

Zhang L, Yao Y, Zhang S, Liu Y, Guo H, Ahmed M, Bell T, Zhang H, Han G, Lorence E, et al. 2019. Metabolic reprogramming toward oxidative phosphorylation identifies a therapeutic target for mantle cell lymphoma. *Sci Transl Med* **11:** 1167. doi:10.1126/scitranslmed.aau1167

Zhang MS, Cui JD, Lee D, Yuen VWH, Chiu DKC, Goh CC, Cheu JWS, Tse APW, Bao MHR, Wong BPY, et al. 2022. Hypoxia-induced macropinocytosis represents a metabolic route for liver cancer. *Nat Commun* **13:** 954. doi:10.1038/s41467-022-28618-9

Zheng L, Zhu Z-R, Sneh T, Zhang WT, Wang Z-Y, Wu G-Y, He W, Qi H-G, Wang H, Wu X-Y, et al. 2023. Circulating succinate-modifying metabolites accurately classify and reflect the status of fumarate hydratase–deficient renal cell carcinoma. *J Clin Invest* **133:** e165028. doi:10.1172/JCI165028

Zhu XG, Chudnovskiy A, Baudrier L, Prizer B, Liu Y, Ostendorf BN, Yamaguchi N, Arab A, Tavora B, Timson R, et al. 2021. Functional genomics in vivo reveal metabolic dependencies of pancreatic cancer cells. *Cell Metab* **33:** 211–221.e6. doi:10.1016/j.cmet.2020.10.017

Isocitrate Dehydrogenase Mutations in Cancer: Mechanisms of Transformation and Metabolic Liability

Kathryn Gunn[1] and Julie-Aurore Losman[1,2]

[1]Division of Molecular and Cellular Oncology, Department of Medical Oncology, Dana-Farber Cancer Institute, Boston, Massachusetts 02215, USA

[2]Division of Hematology, Department of Medicine, Brigham and Women's Hospital, Boston, Massachusetts 02115, USA

Correspondence: julieaurore_losman@dfci.harvard.edu

Isocitrate dehydrogenase 1 and 2 (IDH1 and IDH2) are metabolic enzymes that interconvert isocitrate and 2-oxoglutarate (2OG). Gain-of-function mutations in *IDH1* and *IDH2* occur in a number of cancers, including acute myeloid leukemia, glioma, cholangiocarcinoma, and chondrosarcoma. These mutations cripple the wild-type activity of IDH and cause the enzymes to catalyze a partial reverse reaction in which 2OG is reduced but not carboxylated, resulting in production of the (R)-enantiomer of 2-hydroxyglutarate ((R)-2HG). (R)-2HG accumulation in *IDH-mutant* tumors results in profound dysregulation of cellular metabolism. The most well-characterized oncogenic effects of (R)-2HG involve the dysregulation of 2OG-dependent epigenetic tumor-suppressor enzymes. However, (R)-2HG has many other effects in *IDH-mutant* cells, some that promote transformation and others that induce metabolic dependencies. Herein, we review how cancer-associated *IDH* mutations impact epigenetic regulation and cellular metabolism and discuss how these effects can potentially be leveraged to therapeutically target *IDH-mutant* tumors.

Dysregulated cellular metabolism is a hallmark of cancer but, until recently, it was not clear whether dysregulated metabolism can, itself, drive tumorigenesis. The discovery of mutations in genes encoding the tricarboxylic acid (TCA) cycle enzymes *isocitrate dehydrogenase (IDH)*, *succinate dehydrogenase (SDH)*, and *fumarate hydratase (FH)* in cancer has provided critical insights into how dysregulated metabolism can directly promote cellular transformation (Laurenti and Tennant 2016). Cancer-associated *SDH* and *FH* mutations are loss-of-function mutations that result in accumulation of high levels of succinate and fumarate, respectively, oncometabolites that are hypothesized to transform cells by inhibiting 2-oxoglutarate (2OG)-dependent tumor-suppressor programs. *IDH* mutations were initially thought to likewise be loss-of-function (Yan et al. 2009). However, in a seminal study, Dang et al. (2009) reported that *IDH* mutations are, in fact, gain-of-function. The mutations alter the activity of IDH and cause the mutant enzymes to produce (R)-2-hydroxyglutarate ((R)-2-HG), a metabolite that is found at very low levels in normal cells but accumulates to high levels in *IDH-mutant* cells. Like succinate and fumarate, (R)-2HG is a 2OG analog that can dysregulate 2OG-dependent cellular processes. In this review, we will discuss the preclinical and clinical studies that have established (R)-2HG as an oncometabolite that directly mediates transformation by mutant IDH and will highlight the current gaps in our understanding of how mutant IDH and (R)-2HG promote tumorigenesis. We will also examine the current state of evidence regarding how (R)-2HG induces specific metabolic vulnerabilities that could represent novel therapeutic targets to treat patients with *IDH-mutant* tumors.

WILD-TYPE IDH ENZYMES PRODUCE 2-OXOGLUTARATE

IDH enzymes catalyze the oxidative decarboxylation of isocitrate to produce 2OG (Fig. 1; Alzial et al. 2022). Eukaryotic cells express three iso-forms of IDH: IDH1, IDH2, and IDH3. IDH3, the principal IDH isoform that contributes to the TCA cycle, is a heterotetrameric mitochondrial enzyme that uses nicotinamide adenine dinucleotide (NAD^+) as a cofactor. IDH3-derived 2OG is further metabolized to succinate and the NADH that is produced is used by the electron transport chain to generate ATP. IDH1 and IDH2 are structurally unrelated to IDH3 and function as homodimeric enzymes that use nicotinamide adenine dinucleotide phosphate ($NADP^+$) as a cofactor. IDH1 localizes to the cytoplasm and peroxisomes and IDH2 localizes to the mitochondria. IDH1 and IDH2 reactions are reversible and, under normal physiologic conditions, the "forward" reaction predominates. The 2OG produced by IDH1 and IDH2 contributes to mitochondrial and non-mitochondrial 2OG pools that, in addition to supporting the TCA cycle, also act as the principal carbon source for nitrogen assimilation reactions and support the activities of 2OG-dependent enzymes. The NADPH produced by IDH1 and IDH2 is used for lipid biosynthesis and provides critical reducing equivalents to counteract the accumulation of reac-

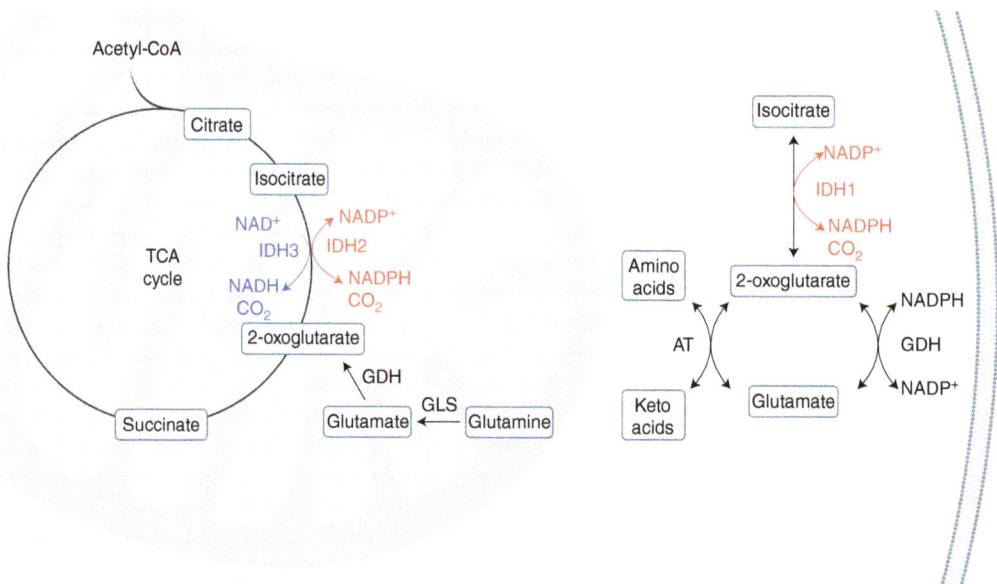

Figure 1. Overview of isocitrate dehydrogenase (IDH)-mediated 2OG metabolism. (TCA) Tricarboxylic acid, (GDH) glutamate dehydrogenase, (GLS) glutaminase, (AT) aminotransferase, (NAD(H)) nicotinamide adenine dinucleotide, (NADP(H)) nicotinamide adenine dinucleotide phosphate. (Figure generated with BioRender, biorender.com.)

tive oxygen species, thereby protecting cells from oxidative damage. Under conditions of cellular stress and hypoxia, the IDH1/2 "reverse" reaction predominates and glutamate-derived 2OG is converted to isocitrate, which can then be further metabolized to acetyl-CoA to rescue lipid and cholesterol biosynthesis when TCA cycle activity is compromised.

CANCER-ASSOCIATED MUTANT IDH ENZYMES PRODUCE (*R*)-2-HYDROXYGLUTARATE

Gain-of-function mutations in *IDH1* and *IDH2* are highly recurrent in a number of cancers (Fig. 2; Pirozzi and Yan 2021). *IDH1/2* mutations are disease-defining mutations in grade II/III adult astrocytoma and oligodendroglioma and in grade IV astrocytoma (previously known as "secondary glioblastoma") (Komori 2023). *IDH1/2* mutations are also highly prevalent in normal-karyotype acute myeloid leukemia (AML) and in secondary AML that arises from lower-grade myeloproliferative (MPN) and myelodysplastic (MDS) disorders. Several other cancers, including intrahepatic cholangiocarcinoma, central chondrosarcoma, sinonasal undifferentiated carcinoma (SNUC), and angioimmunoblastic T-cell lymphoma (AITL) have also been found to frequently harbor *IDH1/2* mutations.

Cancer-associated *IDH1/2* mutations occur at one of three conserved arginine residues in the active sites of the enzymes: R132 in IDH1 and R140 and R172 in IDH2 (Ward et al. 2010). The mutations result in substitution of any one of several shorter (histidine, lysine) and/or less basic

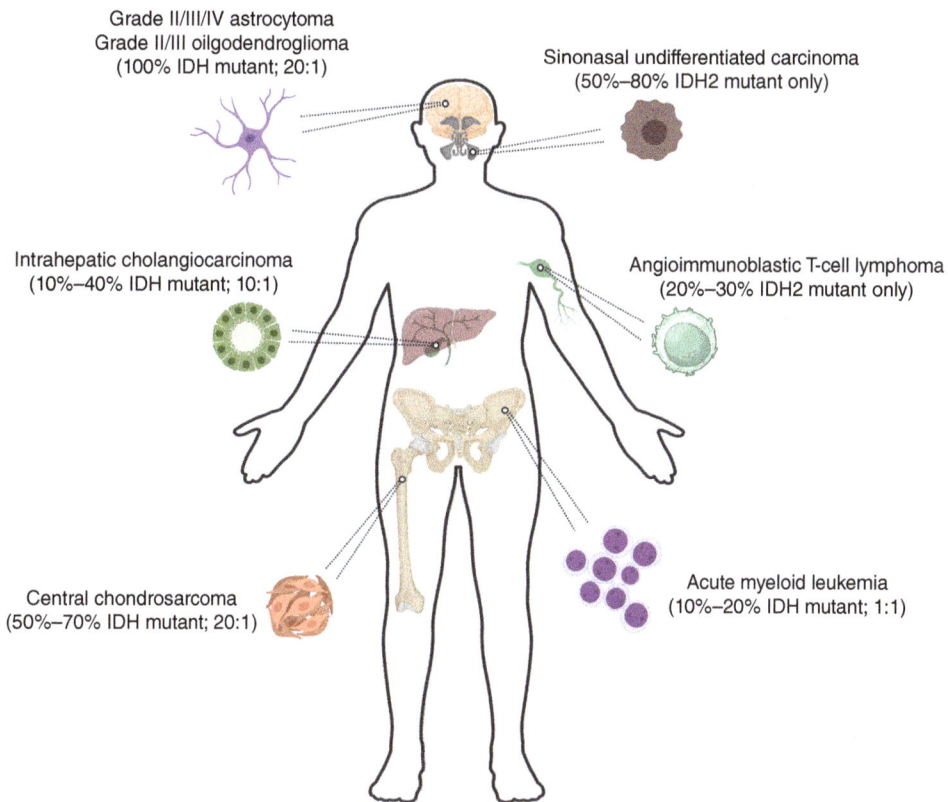

Figure 2. Isocitrate dehydrogenase (IDH) mutations are highly recurrent in a subset of human cancers. For each cancer type, the % that harbor *IDH* mutation, and the relative frequencies of *IDH1* and *IDH2* mutations (IDH1: IDH2) are indicated. (Figure generated with BioRender, biorender.com.)

(glutamine, cysteine, serine, leucine, glycine, methionine, tryptophan, proline, threonine) residues in the place of arginine. IDH1 R132, IDH2 R140, and IDH2 R172 residues form hydrogen bonds with the α and β carboxyl groups of isocitrate and promote isocitrate binding. The amino acid substitutions in the mutant enzymes decrease the affinity of IDH1/2 for isocitrate and increase its affinity for NADPH while still permitting 2OG binding. As a result, the "forward" oxidative decarboxylation activity of wild-type IDH1/2 is lost and the mutant enzymes can only catalyze a partial "reverse" reaction in which 2OG is reduced but not carboxylated, resulting in production of (R)-2HG. In *IDH-mutant* tumor cells, (R)-2HG can accumulate to levels as high as 30 mM (Dang et al. 2009; Gross et al. 2010).

2HG IN NORMAL CELLULAR METABOLISM

2HG is a five-carbon dicarboxylic acid with a chiral center at the second carbon atom that exists as one of two enantiomers, (R)-2HG (also known as (D)-2HG) and (S)-2HG (Fig. 3; also known as (L)-2HG). (R)- and (S)-2HG are both by-products of normal cellular metabolism. 2OG is reduced to (R)-2HG during conversion of γ-hydroxybutyrate to succinic semialdehyde by hydroxyacid-oxoacid transhydrogenase (HOT) (Struys et al. 2005b). (R)-2HG is also generated as a by-product of the oxidative degradation of 5-aminolevulinate by glyoxalase enzymes and by incomplete IDH1/2 "reverse" reactions in which 2OG is reduced but not carboxylated (Ježek 2020). Phosphoglycerate dehydrogenase (PHGDH) can also reduce 2OG to (R)-2HG when its preferred substrate, 3-phosphono-oxypyruvate, is limiting. Similarly, promiscuous reactions catalyzed by malate dehydrogenase (MDH) and lactate dehydrogenase (LDH) can produce (S)-2HG (Intlekofer et al. 2017).

(R)- and (S)-2HG are structurally identical to 2OG except that, at the second carbon atom, the ketone group is replaced with a hydroxyl group (Fig. 3). This structural similarity permits 2HG to bind in the place of 2OG and dysregulate 2OG-dependent cellular processes (Chowdhury et al. 2011; Xu et al. 2011; Koivunen et al. 2012; Lu et al. 2012). In eukaryotic cells, there are 70

2OG-dependent dioxygenases (2OGDDs) and an additional 30+ other enzymes that use 2OG as a cosubstrate (Table 1). These enzymes are involved in a wide range of cellular processes, including energy metabolism, metabolite biosynthesis, hypoxia signaling, and the epigenetic regulation of gene transcription. Although 2OGDDs have a higher affinity for 2OG than for (R)- or (S)-2HG, significant 2HG accumulation can disrupt 2OGDD activity. Two enzymes, (D)- and (L)-2-hydroxyglutarate dehydrogenase (D2HGDH and L2HGDH), prevent the accumulation of 2HG by converting (R)- and (S)-2HG, respectively, back to 2OG (Fig. 3; Struys et al. 2005a; Steenweg et al. 2010). The activities of D- and L2HGDH are sufficient to suppress 2HG levels to the low micromolar range under normal physiologic conditions. However, under acidic and hypoxic conditions, MDH, LDH, and PHGDH reactions become more promiscuous (Intlekofer et al. 2017). This results in increased production of (S)-2HG and, to a lesser extent, (R)-2HG. The increased production of (S)-2HG overwhelms the detoxification capacity of L2HGDH, resulting in accumulation of low-millimolar levels of (S)-2HG.

It is not known whether (R)-2HG plays a role in "stress" metabolism. However, (S)-2HG does appear to contribute to the physiologic response of cells to hypoxia (Intlekofer et al. 2015). (S)-2HG inhibits EGLN prolyl hydroxylases, 2OG- and oxygen-dependent enzymes that regulate the stability of hypoxia-inducible transcription factors HIF1α and HIF2α (Xu et al. 2011; Koivunen et al. 2012). Hypoxia-induced (S)-2HG results in more profound suppression of EGLN activity, and more profound induction of HIF activity, than would result from low oxygen levels alone. (S)-2HG also has EGLN- and HIF-independent effects on the hypoxia response by inhibiting 2OG-dependent epigenetic enzymes. In CD8[+] T cells, these pleiotropic effects of (S)-2HG result in enhanced cell proliferation and survival and increased effector T-cell activity (Tyrakis et al. 2016). As such, (S)-2HG functions as an immunometabolite to promote T-cell function. As discussed further below, tumor-derived (R)-2HG appears to have the opposite effect on T-cell function and may play a role in immune evasion of *IDH-mutant* tumors.

Cite this article as *Cold Spring Harb Perspect Med* doi: 10.1101/cshperspect.a041537

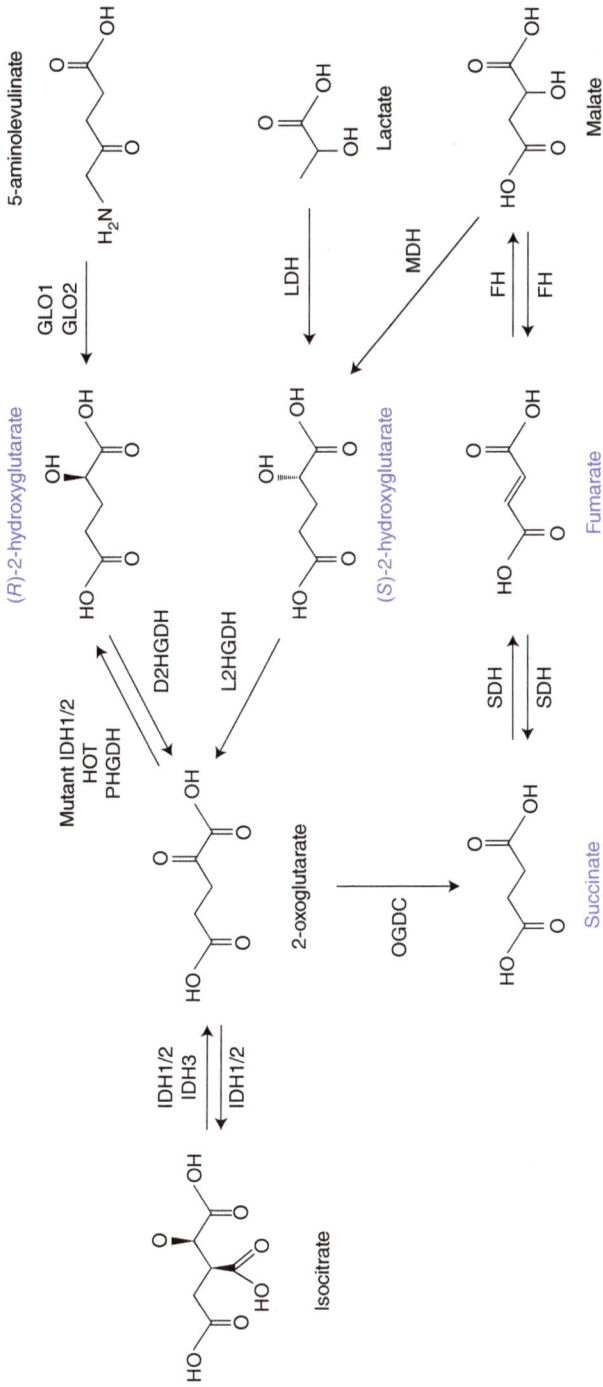

Figure 3. Metabolic pathways that produce oncometabolites. Oncometabolites (highlighted in blue) are by-products of normal cellular metabolism. (IDH) Isocitrate dehydrogenase, (HOT) hydroxyacid-oxoacid transhydrogenase, (PHGDH) phosphoglycerate dehydrogenase, ((D/L)2HGDH) (D/L)-2-hydroxyglutarate dehydrogenase, (OGDC) oxoglutarate dehydrogenase complex, (SDH) succinate dehydrogenase, (FH) fumarate hydratase, (MDH) malate dehydrogenase, (LDH) lactate dehydrogenase, (GLO) glyoxalase. (Figure generated with BioRender, biorender.com.)

Table 1. 2OG-dependent cellular enzymes

2OG-dependent dioxygenases		Other 2OG-dependent enzymes
ALKBH1/ABH1	**KDM4E**/KDM4DL/JMJD2E	**AASS**/LORSDH
ALKBH2/ABH2	**KDM4F**/JMJD2F	**ABAT**/GABAT
ALKBH3/ABH3/DEPC1	**KDM5A**/JARID1A/RBP2	**BCAT1**/BCT1
ALKBH4/ABH4	**KDM5B**/JARID1B/PLU1	**BCAT2**/BCT2/BCAM
ALKBH5/ABH5/OFOXD1	**KDM5C**/JARID1C/SMCX	**D2HGDH**
ALKBH6/ABH6	**KDM5D**/JARID1D/SMCY	**DHTKD1**/CMT2Q
ALKBH7/ABH7/SPATA11	**KDM6A**/UTX	**DLD**/LAD/GCSL
ALKBH8/ABH8/TRM9	**KDM6B**/JMJD3	**DLST**/DLTS/KGD2
ALKBH9/**FTO**	**KDM6C**/UTY	**GLUD1**/GLUD/GDH
ASPH/BAH	**KDM7A**/JHDM1D	**GLUD2**/GLUDP1
ASPHD1	KDM7B/**PHF8**/JHDM1F	**GOT1**/AST/SGOT
ASPHD2	KDM7C/**PHF2**/JHDM1E	**GOT2**/KYAT4/KAT4
BBOX1/BBH	**KDM8**/JMJD5	**GPT**/ALT/SGPT
BBOX2/**TMLHE**	**OGFOD1**/TPA1	**GPT2**/ALT2
EGLN1/PHD2	**OGFOD2**	HOT/**ADHFE1**/ADH8
EGLN2/PHD1	**OGFOD3**	**IDH1**
EGLN3/PHD3	**P3H1**/LEPRE1/GROS1	**IDH2**/D2HGA2
FBXL19/JHDM1C	**P3H2**/LEPREL1/MLAT4	**IDH3A**
HIF1AN/FIH1	**P3H3**/LEPREL2/GRCB	**IDH3B**/RP46
HR/ALUNC	**P4HA1**/P4HA	**KYAT1**/CCBL1/KAT1
HSPBAP1/PASS1	**P4HA2**	KYAT2/**AADAT**/KAT2
JARID2/JMJ/DIDDF	**P4HA3**	**KYAT3**/CCBL2/KAT3
JMJD4	**P4HB**/PO4DB/ERBA2L	**L2HGDH**
JMJD6/PTDSR	**P4HTM**/PHD4/EGLN4	**NIT1**
JMJD7	**PHYH**/PAHX	**NIT2**
JMJD8	**PHYHD1**	OAT/HOGA/GACR
KDM2A/JHDM1A/FBXL11	**PHYHIP**/DYRK1AP3	**OGDH**/OGDH2/KGD1
KDM2B/JHDM1B/FBXL10	**PLOD1**/LH1/LLH	**OGDHL1**
KDM3A/JHMD2A/JMJD1	**PLOD2**/LH2/TLH	**PHGDH**/PDG
KDM3B/JHDM2B/JMJD1B	**PLOD3**/LH3	**PSAT1**
KDM3C/**JMJD1C**/TRIP8	**RIOX1**/JMJD9/NO66	**TAT**
KDM4A/JHDM3A/JMJD2A	**RIOX2**/JMJD10/MINA	**TYW5**
KDM4B/JHDM3B/JMJD2B	**TET1**	
KDM4C/JMJD2C/GASC1	**TET2**	
KDM4D/JHDM3D/JMJD2D	**TET3**	

The Human Genome Organization (HUGO) gene symbols are indicated in bold.

(R)-2HG IS AN ONCOMETABOLITE

The "oncometabolite" model of tumorigenesis posits that, in certain cancers, specific metabolites accumulate to high levels and directly transform cells by acting as oncogenic signaling molecules (Yang et al. 2013; Shim et al. 2014). To date, four metabolites have been proposed to function as oncometabolites: (R)-2HG in IDH-mutant tumors, (S)-2HG in hypoxic renal tumors, succinate in SDH-mutant tumors, and fumarate in FH-mutant tumors. All four of these metabolites are 2OG analogs (Fig. 3), and they are all hypothesized to promote cellular transformation by dysregulating 2OG-dependent tumor-suppressor programs.

Evidence in support of the "oncometabolite" model of tumorigenesis is most compelling for (R)-2HG in IDH-mutant AML. (R)-2HG is both necessary and sufficient to phenocopy the effects of mutant IDH expression in a cell-based myeloid transformation assay (Losman et al. 2013). Moreover, mutant IDH inhibitors induce the differentiation and apoptosis of *IDH-mutant* AML cells in vitro and in patient-derived xenograft (PDX) models and have significant single-agent activity in patients with *IDH-mutant* AML (Losman et al. 2013; Wang et al. 2013; Stein et al. 2017; Yen et al. 2017). Finally, and perhaps most persuasively, a subset of patients with *IDH-mutant* AML who respond to mutant IDH inhibitor therapy relapse with mutations that restore (R)-2HG production, either by conferring drug resistance to mutant IDH or by mutating the other (wild-type) *IDH1/2* isoform (Harding et al. 2018; Intlekofer et al. 2018). Taken together, these findings strongly implicate (R)-2HG as the direct effector of mutant IDH-mediated transformation in AML.

In *IDH-mutant* solid tumors, the evidence that (R)-2HG is necessary and sufficient to mediate the oncogenic effects of mutant IDH is somewhat less conclusive. Although mutant IDH expression and treatment with cell-permeable (R)-2HG inhibit the differentiation of immortalized murine 3T3-L1 fibroblasts and murine 10T1/2 mesenchymal progenitor cells, it is not clear to what extent these cell lines reflect the biology of *IDH-mutant* tumors (Lu et al. 2012; Schvartzman et al. 2019). Many cancer cell lines generated from *IDH-mutant* solid tumors are not dependent on mutant IDH for growth in two-dimensional culture (Davis et al. 2014; Li et al. 2015; Johannessen et al. 2016; Saha et al. 2016). Moreover, many PDX models of *IDH-mutant* solid tumors are not sensitive to mutant IDH inhibitors (Tateishi et al. 2015; Kogiso et al. 2022). Consistent with these preclinical findings, the results of early-phase clinical trials of the mutant IDH1 inhibitor ivosidenib in *IDH1-mutant* solid tumors have been underwhelming. Even though ivosidenib significantly reduces plasma 2HG levels in patients with *IDH1-mutant* solid tumors, most patients with *IDH1-mutant* solid tumors treated with ivosidenib achieve, at best, a decrease in tumor growth rate, with very few patients experiencing tumor regression (Lowery et al. 2019; Fan et al. 2020; Mellinghoff et al. 2020; Tap et al. 2020). A follow-up phase I clinical trial of vorasidenib, a highly brain-penetrant dual mutant IDH1/2 inhibitor, in *IDH1-mutant* glioma found that, although

mutant IDH inhibition was able to induce sustained tumor shrinkage in a small subset of patients, most of the responders had low-grade, not high-grade, disease (Mellinghoff et al. 2021, 2023). It is possible that the same level of dependency on (R)-2HG is not present in *IDH-mutant* solid tumors as in *IDH-mutant* AML due to the presence of other oncogenic pathways that can compensate for loss of (R)-2HG. Alternatively, (R)-2HG may function as a "hit-and-run" oncometabolite in *IDH-mutant* solid tumors by inducing irreversible epigenetic changes that do not necessitate ongoing (R)-2HG production to maintain tumor-promoting cellular programs (Turcan et al. 2018). Arguing against these models and in support of an ongoing requirement for (R)-2HG in *IDH-mutant* solid tumors is the observation that some patients with *IDH1-mutant* cholangiocarcinoma develop drug-resistance mutations in mutant IDH1 after experiencing prolonged stable disease on ivosidenib (Harding et al. 2018; Lowery et al. 2019; Cleary et al. 2022). Perhaps the relative lack of efficacy of first-generation mutant IDH inhibitors in *IDH-mutant* solid tumors is because these drugs have suboptimal pharmacokinetic and/or pharmacodynamic properties. Further studies will be needed to determine whether more potent and more tissue-penetrant mutant IDH inhibitors can have greater clinical efficacy in *IDH-mutant* solid tumors.

PATTERNS OF *IDH* MUTATIONS IN DIFFERENT CANCERS

Although all cancer-associated IDH mutants produce (R)-2HG, the frequencies of *IDH1* and *IDH2* mutations, and the frequencies of specific amino acid substitutions, varies dramatically across different tumor types (Table 2; Pirozzi and Yan 2021). In low-grade gliomas, the ratio of *IDH1* to *IDH2* mutations is ~20:1, and IDH1 R132H is the single most common amino acid substitution. *IDH1* mutations also predominate in chondrosarcoma and intrahepatic cholangiocarcinoma, although in these tumors, the dominant substitution is IDH1 R132C. In AML, *IDH1* and *IDH2* are mutated at similar frequencies and IDH2 R140Q is the single most common IDH mutation, whereas in AITL and SNUC, mutations are exclusively

Table 2. Frequencies of IDH1 and IDH2 arginine substitutions in *IDH-mutant* tumors

Cancer type	IDH1/2 mutation frequency	IDH1:IDH2 ratio	Arginine substitutions	Allele frequencies
Grade II/III/IV astrocytoma Grade II/III oligodendroglioma	100%*	10:1–20:1	IDH1 R132H IDH1 R132C/S/L/G IDH2 R172K/M/W/S/G	85%–90% 5%–8% 3%–5%
Normal karyotype acute myeloid leukemia (NK-AML) AML secondary to myelodysplastic syndrome (MDS) and myeloproliferative neoplasms (MPN)	10%–20%	1:1–1:2	IDH1 R132H IDH1 R132C IDH1 R132S IDH1 R132L/G/P IDH2 R140Q IDH2 R140W/L IDH2 R172K IDH2 R172G/M	15%–20% 10%–15% 5% <5% 30%–50% <5% 10% <5%
Central chondrosarcoma	50%–70%	20:1	IDH1 R132C IDH1 R132G IDH1 R132H IDH1 R132L/S IDH2 R172S/T	40%–50% 20% 15%–20% 10%–15% 5%–10%
Intrahepatic cholangiocarcinoma (ICC)	10%–40%	10:1	IDH1 R132C IDH1 R132G/L IDH1 R132H/S IDH2 R172W	50%–65% 25%–40% 10% 10%
Angioimmunoblastic T-cell lymphoma (AITL)	20%–30%	IDH2 only	IDH2 R172K IDH2 R172M IDH2 R172G/T/S	60%–65% 15% 20%
Sinonasal undifferentiated carcinoma (SNUC)	50%–80%	IDH2 only	IDH2 R172S IDH2 R172T IDH2 R172M IDH2 R172G	60% 25% 10% 5%

The most common amino acid substitutions are indicated in red.

found in *IDH2* and are most frequently R172K and R172S substitutions, respectively.

It is not understood why the patterns of *IDH* mutations are so different in different tumor types, although several hypotheses have been proposed to explain this finding. Based on the observation that the catalytic activities of different IDH mutants vary significantly, it has been proposed that the threshold levels of (R)-2HG that are required for cellular transformation are different in different tumor types such that specific substitutions are selected for in a tissue-specific manner (Ward et al. 2013; Pusch et al. 2014). However, (R)-2HG levels in tumors that harbor the same *IDH* mutation can vary dramatically, and tumors of the same tissue type that harbor different *IDH* mutations do not appear to have specific characteristic (R)-2HG levels. It therefore seems unlikely that the distinct catalytic activities of the different IDH mutants fully explain the patterns of *IDH* mutations in different tumor types. Another possible explanation for why *IDH1* and *IDH2* mutations occur at starkly different frequencies in some cancer types is that, because IDH2 is a mitochondrial enzyme, IDH2 mutations result in very high levels of mitochondrial (R)-2HG. It is possible that (R)-2HG has "off-target" toxic effects on mitochondrial function that are poorly tolerated in some tumor types. This could explain why *IDH2* mutations are relatively rare in glioma, chondrosarcoma, and cholangiocarcinoma. In AITL and SNUC, on the other hand, it is possible that very high levels of mitochondrial (R)-2HG play a critical role in promoting cellular transformation, which could explain the lack of *IDH1* mutations in these diseases. It has also been speculated that IDH mutants have noncatalytic functions that contribute to cellular transformation. If so, these functions could be isoform- and/or substitution-specific and could result in different tissue-specific transformation capabilities of different IDH

Cite this article as *Cold Spring Harb Perspect Med* doi: 10.1101/cshperspect.a041537

mutants. However, there is little experimental evidence to suggest that mutant IDH has *(R)*-2HG-independent oncogenic functions. Finally, it is possible that the different frequencies of specific amino acid substitutions in IDH1/2 in different cancers are not due to tissue-specific selective pressure for specific mutant IDH variants but, rather, due to differences in the DNA damage and repair mechanisms that are engaged in different tumors that predispose to different nucleotide changes. Indeed, tissue-specific mutational processes have been found to contribute to the unique mutational signatures of many tumor types (Alexandrov et al. 2020; Yaacov et al. 2023). Although a similar phenomenon has not been reported in hematopoietic stem cells, it is perhaps notable that three of the four most common IDH substitutions in AML are all guanine (G) to adenine (A) mutations (R132H = CGT to CAT; R140Q = CGG to CAG; and R172K = AGG to AAG). This observation notwithstanding, it is unlikely, given the extraordinary diversity of *IDH* mutations in cancer, that tissue-specific mutational process-es are the sole explanation for why different mutant IDH variants predominate in different cancers. Further studies are needed to determine whether mutant IDH variants have tissue-specific cancer-promoting properties.

TUMOR-PROMOTING TARGETS OF *(R)*-2HG IN *IDH-MUTANT* CANCERS

Numerous studies have found that a wide range of 2OGDDs are inhibited by tumor-relevant concentrations of *(R)*-2HG in vitro (Table 3; Losman et al. 2020). This, combined with the observation that many 2OGDDs are recurrently silenced, deleted, or mutated in cancer, has led to the hypothesis that *(R)*-2HG functions as an oncometabolite by competitively inhibiting 2OGDD tumor suppressors.

TET Enzymes

Ten-eleven translocation (TET) enzymes TET1, TET2, and TET3 are 2OGDDs that hydroxylate the methyl group of 5-methylcytosine (5mC) to

Table 3. 2OG K_m values and *(R)*-2HG and *(S)*-2HG IC$_{50}$ values of 2OGDD enzymes

2OG-dependent dioxygenases	In vitro substrate(s)	2OG K_m (mM)	*(R)*-2HG IC$_{50}$ (mM)	*(S)*-2HG IC$_{50}$ (mM)
ALKBH2	1-methyladenine, 3-methylcytosine	0.004	0.40–0.50	0.15
ALKBH3	1-methyladenine, 3-methylcytosine	ND	0.50	ND
BBOX1	γ-butyrobetaine	0.01	0.01–0.2	0.14
EGLN2	HIF1α, HIF2α (proline)	0.002	NA—cofactor	0.63
EGLN1	HIF1α, HIF2α (proline)	0.001–0.27	NA—cofactor	0.42–1.15
EGLN3	HIF1α, HIF2α (proline)	0.12	NA	0.09
HIF1AN	HIF1α (asparagine)	0.15–0.25	1.1–1.5	0.19–0.30
KDM2A	H3K36me2	ND	0.11	0.48
KDM4A	H3K9me3, H3K36me3	0.006–0.025	0.02–0.16	0.26–0.29
KDM4B	H3K9me3	0.006	0.15	0.45
KDM4C	H3K9me3, H3K36me3	0.004–0.012	0.08	0.97
KDM5A	H3K4me3, H3K4me2	0.005	0.93	0.15
KDM5B	H3K4me3, H3K4me2, H3K4me1	0.01	3.6–10.9	0.63–1.60
KDM5C	H3K4me3, H3K4me2	0.003–0.005	0.67	0.20
KDM5D	H3K4me3, H3K4me2	0.004	0.80	0.31
KDM6A	H3K27me3, H3K27me2	0.008–0.01	0.18	0.18
KDM6B	H3K27me3, H3K27me2	0.008–0.05	0.35	0.75
P4HA1	Collagen (proline)	0.20	1.8	0.31
TET1	5-methylcytosine, 5-formylcytosine, 5-carboxycytosine	0.06	4.0	1.0
TET2	5-methylcytosine, 5-formylcytosine, 5-carboxycytosine	0.06	5.0	1.6

produce 5-hydroxymethycytosine (5hmC) (Tahiliani et al. 2009). 5hmC can then be further oxidized by TET enzymes to produce 5-formylcytosine (5fC) and 5-carboxylcytosine (5caC) (Ito et al. 2011). In addition to being substrates of the base-excision repair pathway that mediates active DNA demethylation, 5hmC, 5fC, and 5caC are stable epigenetic marks that regulate numerous cellular processes, including stem cell pluripotency, enhancer poising, and DNA and RNA polymerase fidelity (He et al. 2011; Koh et al. 2011; Song et al. 2013; Ji et al. 2014; You et al. 2014; Caldwell et al. 2021).

Dysregulation of TET function is a common finding in many cancers. However, of the three TET family members, only *TET2* is an established, bona fide tumor-suppressor gene. Somatic loss-of-function mutations in *TET2*, including chromosomal microdeletions and missense, nonsense, and frameshift mutations, are highly recurrent across the entire spectrum of clonal myeloid disorders, from clonal hematopoiesis of indeterminate potential (CHIP), to MPN, MDS, and AML (Bowman and Levine 2017). *TET2* is also recurrently mutated in T-cell lymphoma and acute lymphoblastic leukemia. In individuals with CHIP, heterozygous *TET2* mutations are frequently the only detectable mutation, and many *TET2* mutations in clonal myeloid disorders are point mutations in the catalytic domain that abolish catalytic activity (Busque et al. 2012; Jaiswal et al. 2014). Taken together, these findings suggest that haploinsufficient loss of TET2 catalytic activity is sufficient to drive clonal hematopoiesis.

Several lines of evidence that suggest that TET2 is a functionally important target of (*R*)-2HG in *IDH-mutant* AML. Tumor-relevant concentrations of (*R*)-2HG inhibit TET2 activity in vitro (Table 3), and *IDH-mutant* AML cells have significantly decreased 5hmC levels when compared to *IDH-* and *TET2-wild-type* AML cells (Figueroa et al. 2010; Xu et al. 2011; Koivunen et al. 2012; Kroeze et al. 2014). Moreover, shRNA-mediated knockdown of *TET2* expression phenocopies mutant IDH expression in a cell-based myeloid transformation assay (Losman et al. 2013). Finally, and most compellingly, loss-of-function mutations in *TET2* and gain-of-function mutations in

IDH1/2 are largely mutually exclusive in normal karyotype AML (Figueroa et al. 2010). Taken together, these observations provide strong evidence that mutant IDH and (*R*)-2HG promote leukemogenesis at least in part by inhibiting TET2 activity.

The role of TET2 as a functional target of (*R*)-2HG is less well-established in other *IDH-mutant* tumor types. Although shRNA-mediated knockdown of *TET2* expression phenocopies mutant IDH expression in a cell-based glial transformation assay, *TET2* mutations have not been described in brain tumors (Koivunen et al. 2012; Kraus et al. 2015). Moreover, *IDH-mutant* gliomas do not have lower 5hmC levels than *IDH-wild-type* gliomas (Kraus et al. 2012, 2015; Orr et al. 2012; Gunn et al. 2023). Although this would seem to suggest that TET2 is not inhibited in *IDH-mutant* gliomas, it is important to note that 5hmC levels are profoundly decreased in glioma tissue compared to normal brain tissue irrespective of *IDH* mutation status. TET activity appears to be suppressed by other mechanisms in *IDH-wild-type* gliomas, including genomic deletion and nuclear exclusion of TET1 and transcriptional silencing of *TET2* (Kim et al. 2011; Müller et al. 2012; Forloni et al. 2016; Stasik et al. 2020). This suggests that *TET1* and *TET2* are indeed glial tumor-suppressor genes, and that loss of TET function, either by (*R*)-2HG-mediated inhibition of TET activity or by other genetic and epigenetic mechanisms, plays an important role in gliomagenesis. In other types of solid tumors that harbor *IDH* mutations, including chondrosarcoma and cholangiocarcinoma, *TET* genes are likewise not recurrently mutated, and it is not clear what role (*R*)-2HG-mediated inhibition of TET activity plays in the pathophysiology of these cancers.

AITL is the only other tumor type besides myeloid malignancies in which both *IDH2* and *TET2* are known to be frequently mutated. *TET2* mutations are found in ~80% of cases and *IDH2* mutations are found in 20%–30% of cases (Cairns et al. 2012; Odejide et al. 2014; Yu and Zhang 2021). Unlike in AML, *TET2*, and *IDH2* mutations frequently co-occur in AITL, with 70%–90% of *IDH2-mutant* cases also harboring a *TET2* mutation. Although it is possible that the

Cite this article as *Cold Spring Harb Perspect Med* doi: 10.1101/cshperspect.a041537

IDH2 and *TET2* mutations in AITL are present in different subclones, the very high frequency of co-occurrence of the mutations suggests that they act synergistically in this disease. One possible explanation for why genetic loss and chemical inhibition of TET2 are both selected for in AITL is that TET2 has both catalytic and non-catalytic tumor-suppressor functions in AITL such that acquisition of an *IDH2* mutation does not functionally recapitulate acquisition of a *TET2* mutation (Chen et al. 2013; Zhang et al. 2015). But if that is the case, what would be the basis for the selective pressure to acquire an *IDH2* mutation in *TET2* mutant cells? Perhaps mutant IDH2 has other tumor-suppressor targets that contribute to transformation in AITL, or perhaps (R)-2HG has non-cell-autonomous effects on the tumor microenvironment that promote lymphomagenesis. Consistent with these hypotheses, introduction of an *Idh2 R172K* knock-in allele into a *Tet2* knockout mouse model of AITL results in dysregulation of B-cell function and a more aggressive disease phenotype (Leca et al. 2023).

JmjC-KDM Enzymes

JmjC-domain-containing histone lysine demethylases (JmjC-KDM) are 2OGDDs that play a critical role in the epigenetic regulation of gene transcription by regulating the methylation states of activating (H3K4, H3K36, H3K79) and repressive (H3K9, H3K27) histone methylation marks (Dimitrova et al. 2015). A number of JmjC-KDM enzymes are dysregulated in cancer by epigenetic silencing, deletion, or mutation, and (R)-2HG can inhibit many of these same KDM enzymes in vitro (Table 3; Losman et al. 2020). It therefore seems reasonable to assume that (R)-2HG-mediated inhibition of JmjC-KDM tumor-suppressor enzymes contributes to mutant IDH-mediated transformation. But which JmjC-KDM enzymes are functionally relevant targets of (R)-2HG, and are different JmjC-KDM enzymes functionally relevant in different *IDH-mutant* tumors?

KDM5 enzymes are JmjC-domain-containing H3K4 histone lysine demethylases that are inhibited by tumor-relevant concentrations of (R)-2HG in vitro, and there are several lines of evidence that suggest that three members of the KDM5 family, KDM5A, KDM5C, and KDM5D, are functionally important targets of (R)-2HG in *IDH-mutant* AML and *IDH-mutant* glioma. In the context of AML, myeloid cells from *Idh1 R132H* knock-in mice and primary normal karyotype *IDH-mutant* AML cells from patients display increased trimethyl-H3K4 levels when compared to their *IDH-wild-type* counterparts (Sasaki et al. 2012b; Gunn et al. 2023). Moreover, CRISPR-Cas9-mediated codeletion of *KDM5A*, *KDM5C*, and *KDM5D* and treatment with a pan-KDM5 inhibitor both phenocopy mutant IDH expression in a myeloid transformation assay (Gunn et al. 2023). In the context of glioma, patient-derived *IDH-mutant* glioma multicellular tumor spheroid (MCTS) lines have significantly increased trimethyl-H3K4 levels when compared to *IDH-wild-type* glioma MCTS lines and small-molecule inhibition of KDM5 activity phenocopies mutant IDH expression in a glial transformation assay. These findings suggest that, in AML and glioma, (R)-2HG-mediated inhibition of KDM5 activity contributes to mutant IDH-mediated transformation. Interestingly, in many cancer types in which *IDH1* and *IDH2* are not mutated, *KDM5A* and *KDM5B* are amplified and overexpressed and promote malignant phenotypes (Lin et al. 2011; Teng et al. 2013; Yamamoto et al. 2014; McBrayer et al. 2018b). If KDM5 activity is indeed a dependency in these cancers, it is possible that *IDH* mutations are selected against. Such context-specific antitumor effects of (R)-2HG could explain, at least in part, why *IDH* mutations are found in only a limited number of cancer types (Fig. 2).

The KDM4 family of H3K9 histone lysine demethylases has also been implicated in transformation by mutant IDH. In immortalized murine 3T3-L1 fibroblasts, shRNA-mediated inhibition of *KDM4C* expression is sufficient to phenocopy mutant IDH expression and block adipocyte differentiation (Lu et al. 2012); and in murine 10T1/2 mesenchymal progenitor cells, (R)-2HG-mediated dysregulation of H3K9 methylation blocks MyoD-induced myocyte differentiation (Schvartzman et al. 2019). The ob-

K. Gunn and J.-A. Losman

servation that KDM4 inhibition can block the differentiation of mesenchymal cells suggests that KDM4 enzymes are soft tissue tumor suppressors that contribute to (R)-2HG-mediated transformation in *IDH-mutant* chondrosarcoma. It is not known what role, if any, KDM4 enzymes play in other *IDH-mutant* tumors. However, it is interesting to note that KDM4C is actually a dependency in *MLL-translocated* and *MOZ-TIF2-translocated* AML (Cheung et al. 2016; Agger et al. 2019). Although this would seem to suggest that KDM4C is not a myeloid tumor suppressor, it is possible that *KDM4C* has distinct functions in different subtypes of AML, functioning as a tumor-suppressor gene in *IDH-mutant* AML and an oncogene in translocation-positive AML. Indeed, this could explain, at least in part, why *IDH* mutations are predominantly found in normal karyotype AML and are rarely, if ever, present in *MLL-translocated* AML.

Given that many JmjC-KDM enzymes have tumor-promoting functions and given that different histone methylation marks reciprocally regulate the transcription of the same genes, it seems unlikely that (R)-2HG acts as a pan-KDM inhibitor in *IDH-mutant* tumors. This begs the question, is there any selectivity to the effects of (R)-2HG on JmjC-KDM enzymes in mutant IDH-transformed cells? If disruption of certain histone methylation marks is antithetical to mutant IDH-mediated transformation, how do *IDH-mutant* cells "protect" those histone methylation marks from (R)-2HG-mediated dysregulation? *IDH-mutant* cells could engage compensatory pathways that "repair" any damaging effects of (R)-2HG on histone lysine methylation by, for example, down-regulating the expression and/or activities of specific histone lysine methyltransferases. Alternatively, *IDH-mutant* cells could regulate how (R)-2HG affects JmjC-KDM activity such that tumor-suppressor JmjC-KDM enzymes are inhibited and tumor-promoting JmjC-KDM enzymes are protected from inhibition. Several mechanisms that regulate JmjC-KDM enzyme activity have been identified, including modulation of demethylase expression, modulation of demethylase recruitment to different macromolecular complexes, and modulation of chromatin accessibility (Lan

et al. 2008). It has also been hypothesized that posttranslational modifications of JmjC-KDM enzymes can regulate demethylase activity (Separovich and Wilkins 2021). Although it is not known whether any of these mechanisms play a role in regulating histone lysine methylation in *IDH-mutant* cells, the observation that histone methylation marks are not universally increased in *IDH-mutant* cells suggests that there is some degree of regulation of the effects of (R)-2HG on histone lysine methylation (Sasaki et al. 2012a,b; Pekmezci et al. 2020).

EGLN Enzymes

EGLN prolyl-4 hydroxylases are 2OGDDs that act as cellular oxygen sensors by regulating the stability of HIF1α and HIF2α (Kaelin and Ratcliffe 2008). Unlike other 2OGDDs, EGLN enzymes are not inhibited by (R)-2HG. Rather, (R)-2HG acts as an alternative cosubstrate and potentiates EGLN activity (Koivunen et al. 2012). Consistent with this observation, HIFα levels are lower in *IDH-mutant* gliomas than *IDH-wild-type* gliomas, and HIFα levels are suppressed in T cells exposed to cell-permeable (R)-2HG (Williams et al. 2011; Koivunen et al. 2012; Böttcher et al. 2018). Interestingly, both overexpression of EGLN1 and shRNA-mediated knockdown of *HIF1A* are each sufficient to promote soft-agar colony formation in a glial transformation assay, and *Hif1a* deletion potentiates tumor growth in a mouse model of *IDH-wild-type* glioma (Blouw et al. 2003; Koivunen et al. 2012). These observations suggest that *HIF1A* functions as a tumor-suppressor gene in glioma and that (R)-2HG-mediated stimulation of EGLN activity, by down-regulating HIF1α activity, contributes to mutant IDH-mediated gliomagenesis. Whether (R)-2HG-mediated stimulation of EGLN activity plays a role in other *IDH-mutant* tumors is not known.

METABOLIC VULNERABILITIES INDUCED BY MUTANT IDH

The metabolic consequences of *IDH1/2* mutations are not confined to the protumorigenic effects of (R)-2HG on 2OGDDs. (R)-2HG also has direct effects on other 2OG-dependent cellular processes that promote cell proliferation and survival (Fack et al. 2017). In addition, the catalytic activity of mutant IDH, by consuming NADPH, can disrupt the redox balance of cells (Gelman et al. 2018). Given the pleiotropic effects of mutant IDH on cellular metabolism, there has been a great deal of interest in identifying detrimental effects of mutant IDH and (R)-2HG that could represent therapeutic opportunities to target IDH-mutant tumors.

DNA Damage Repair and Redox Homeostasis

There is extensive preclinical and clinical data to suggest that DNA damage repair pathways and redox homeostasis are defective in IDH-mutant cancer cells, and several different mechanisms have been invoked to explain these defects (Shi et al. 2023). One proposed mechanism is that millimolar quantities of 2OG and NADPH are consumed by mutant IDH to produce equimolar quantities of (R)-2HG, resulting in a decrease in the NADPH:NADP$^+$ ratio in IDH-mutant cells (Bleeker et al. 2010; Badur et al. 2018). Because NADPH is required to recycle oxidized glutathione to reduced glutathione, depletion of NADPH compromises the ability of IDH-mutant cells to respond to DNA damage.

The defective DNA damage repair in IDH-mutant cells has also been linked to (R)-2HG-mediated dysregulation of H3K9 methylation. One study found that (R)-2HG-mediated inhibition of KDM4B results in aberrant H3K9 hypermethylation at sites of double-strand DNA breaks, which disrupts homologous recombination-mediated DNA repair and induces sensitivity of IDH-mutant cells to poly(ADP)-ribose polymerase (PARP) inhibitors (Sulkowski et al. 2017). A different study found that the enhanced dependence of IDH-mutant cells on PARP is due to (R)-2HG-induced accumulation of H3K9-methylated heterochromatin, which requires PARP activity to overcome heterochromatin-related replication stress (Schvartzman et al. 2023). Yet another study found that (R)-2HG-mediated inhibition of H3K9 demethylation results in silencing of ataxia telangiectasia mutated (ATM), which results in defective cell cycle checkpoint signaling (Sulkowski et al. 2020).

The BCAT family of branched-chain amino acid transaminases have also been found to be direct targets of (R)-2HG that contribute to the redox imbalance and defective DNA repair of IDH-mutant cells (McBrayer et al. 2018a). BCAT enzymes catalyze the transamination of branched-chain α-keto acids to produce branched-chain L-amino acids in a reversible redox reaction that interconverts glutamate and 2OG (Fig. 1). Tumor-relevant concentrations of (R)-2HG inhibit BCAT reductive activity, resulting in decreased conversion of 2OG to glutamate. Glutamate is a critical cellular metabolite that is required for the synthesis of glutathione, an endogenous antioxidant. Suppression of BCAT-mediated glutamate production by (R)-2HG decreases glutathione levels in IDH-mutant cells. To maintain glutamate levels and rescue glutathione synthesis, IDH-mutant cells up-regulate the activity of glutaminase (GLS), an enzyme that converts glutamine to glutamate. This enhanced requirement for GLS in IDH-mutant cells causes the cells to be hypersensitive to GLS inhibition under conditions of oxidative stress.

Non-tumor-promoting metabolic effects of mutant IDH have the potential to represent cancer-specific vulnerabilities that can be exploited therapeutically. Indeed, based on the preclinical findings described above, clinical trials are currently underway to test the safety and efficacy of the PARP inhibitor olaparib in patients with IDH-mutant AML and IDH-mutant glioma, and the GLS inhibitor telaglenastat in patients with IDH-mutant glioma.

Fatty Acid Biosynthesis

In addition to its role in redox regulation, NADPH also plays a critical role in reductive biosynthesis reactions, including de novo fatty acid biosynthesis (Gelman et al. 2018). Fatty acid biosynthesis occurs exclusively in the cytoplasm and is dependent on cytoplasmic NADPH pools, which are regenerated from cytoplasmic NADP$^+$ by four mechanisms: IDH1-mediated oxidative decarboxylation of isocitrate, malic enzyme 1 (ME1)-mediated oxidative decarboxylation of pyruvate, one-carbon serine and glycine metabolism, and the pentose-phosphate pathway (Martínez-Reyes and Chandel 2014; Liu et al. 2016). In *IDH1-mutant* cells, the shunting of cytoplasmic NADPH away from fatty acid production and into (*R*)-2HG production, along with wild-type IDH1 haploinsufficiency, results in defective de novo lipid biosynthesis and compensatory up-regulation of acetyl CoA carboxylase 1 (ACC1)-dependent fatty acid β-oxidation (Thomas et al. 2023). This enhanced requirement for ACC1 in *IDH1-mutant* cells causes the cells to be hypersensitive to ACC1 inhibition under conditions of lipid deprivation. In preclinical models, pharmacologic targeting of ACC1 has been found to sensitize *IDH1-mutant* AML cells to the BCL2 inhibitor, venetoclax.

Apoptosis

(*R*)-2HG, in addition to its effects on 2OG-dependent cellular processes, has also been reported to directly inhibit the activities of the electron transport chain components cytochrome *c* oxidase (COX, also known as complex IV) and ATP synthase (also known as complex V) (Chan et al. 2015; Fu et al. 2015). COX transfers electrons from reduced cytochrome *c* to molecular oxygen and pumps protons across the inner mitochondrial membrane to generate the mitochondrial proton gradient. ATP synthase allows protons to flow back into the mitochondrial matrix and uses the released free energy to synthesize ATP from ADP. In *IDH-mutant* AML cells, (*R*)-2HG-mediated inhibition of COX activity has been shown to activate the proapoptotic proteins BAX and BAK and enhance the dependence of the cells on BCL-2 (Chan et al. 2015). In *IDH-mutant* glial cells, (*R*)-2HG-mediated inhibition of ATP synthase activity has been shown to suppress ATP production, which activates 5′ AMP-activated protein kinase (AMPK) and down-regulates protein synthesis (Fu et al. 2015). This results in decreased MCL-1 expression and enhanced dependence of *IDH-mutant* cells on BCL-XL. These complementary findings suggest that inhibitors of BCL-2 and/or BCL-XL could have clinical efficacy against *IDH-mutant* tumors.

NON-CELL-AUTONOMOUS EFFECTS OF (*R*)-2HG

An interesting observation was made during the initial phase I/II clinical trial of the mutant IDH2 inhibitor enasidenib in patients with *IDH2-mutant* AML. There appeared to be no association between the patients' baseline, pretreatment *mutant IDH2* variant allele frequency (VAF) and their probability of achieving a complete response to therapy (Amatangelo et al. 2017). Indeed, patients who achieved complete responses had baseline *mutant IDH2* VAFs that ranged from <5% to >40%, suggesting that, in these patients, enasidenib was able to target both the *IDH2-mutant* and the *IDH2-wild-type* AML blast cells. Subsequent clinical studies of enasidenib and ivosidenib in *IDH2-* and *IDH1-mutant* AML, respectively, further confirmed that patients with subclonal *IDH* mutations can achieve complete responses to mutant IDH inhibitors (Stein et al. 2019; Roboz et al. 2020; DiNardo et al. 2021).

Given that mutant IDH inhibitors do not have activity against *IDH-wild-type* AML, how can they have activity against *IDH-wild-type* AML subclones in patients with *IDH-mutant* AML? One possibility is that the (*R*)-2HG produced by *IDH-mutant* AML subclones is taken up by surrounding preleukemic *IDH-wild-type* subclones, which are then fully transformed by (*R*)-2HG and become dependent on mutant IDH activity. Consistent with this hypothesis, daily intraperitoneal injections of (*R*)-2HG can accelerate the development of full-blown AML in a mouse model of *HoxA9*-transformed monocytic leukemia (Chaturvedi et al. 2016). Although it is not clear how the bone marrow (*R*)-2HG levels achieved in this mouse study compare to bone marrow (*R*)-2HG levels in patients with subclonal *IDH-mutant* AML, these results do suggest that (*R*)-2HG can have paracrine transforming effects on myeloid cells. Another model that could explain the mutant IDH-dependence of *IDH-wild-type* subclones in *IDH-mutant* AML patients is that (*R*)-2HG has effects on the bone marrow microenvironment that make it more hospitable to AML cells irrespective of their *IDH* mutation status. Indeed,

Cite this article as *Cold Spring Harb Perspect Med* doi: 10.1101/cshperspect.a041537

(R)-2HG has been found to induce extracellular signal-regulated kinase (ERK) signaling in bone marrow stromal cells, which results in activation of NF-κB and up-regulation of expression of cytokines, including IL-6 and IL-8, that stimulate the proliferation of both *IDH-wild-type* and *IDH-mutant* AML cells (Chen et al. 2016). Finally, there is a growing body of evidence that suggests that, unlike (S)-2HG, (R)-2HG impairs T-cell function and reshapes the immune microenvironment to down-regulate antitumor immunity. In glioma and cholangiocarcinoma, *IDH* mutation positivity is associated with significantly lower numbers of tumor-infiltrating lymphocytes (TILs) and decreased T-cell effector function (Amankulor et al. 2017; Bunse et al. 2018; Han et al. 2019; Notarangelo et al. 2022; Wu et al. 2022). This blunted T-cell activity is due, at least in part, to the uptake by $CD4^+$ and $CD8^+$ T cells of (R)-2HG, which accumulates to low millimolar levels in the cells and alters their metabolism. This altered metabolism results in impaired T-cell receptor signaling, decreased T-cell cytotoxicity, and decreased PD-1 expression. Treatment with mutant IDH inhibitors reverses these phenotypes and enhances antitumor immunity (Bunse et al. 2018). These findings have led to the initiation of several clinical trials combining mutant IDH inhibitors and immune checkpoint inhibitors for the treatment of *IDH-mutant* solid tumors.

CONCLUDING REMARKS

The discovery of *IDH* mutations in cancer represents a major advance in the field of oncology, and significant progress has been made over the last several years in defining the mechanisms by which *IDH* mutations promote tumorigenesis. However, our understanding of the pleiotropic effects of mutant IDH in tumor cells is still incomplete. Moreover, although mutant IDH inhibitors have been developed that have considerable activity against *IDH-mutant* AML, there has been less progress in developing effective treatments for patients with *IDH-mutant* solid tumors. Several novel therapeutic strategies, including exploiting the many detrimental metabolic consequences of mutant IDH activity in tumor cells and exploiting the non-cell-autonomous effects of (R)-2HG on the tumor microenvironment, have the potential to effectively target *IDH-mutant* cancers. Further studies are needed to dissect the complex effects of (R)-2HG on tumor cells and the tumor microenvironment to fully realize the potential for therapeutic targeting of mutant IDH biology.

REFERENCES

Agger K, Nishimura K, Miyagi S, Messling JE, Rasmussen KD, Helin K. 2019. The KDM4/JMJD2 histone demethylases are required for hematopoietic stem cell maintenance. *Blood* **134:** 1154–1158. doi:10.1182/blood.2019000855

Alexandrov LB, Kim J, Haradhvala NJ, Huang MN, Tian Ng AW, Wu Y, Boot A, Covington KR, Gordenin DA, Bergstrom EN, et al. 2020. The repertoire of mutational signatures in human cancer. *Nature* **578:** 94–101. doi:10.1038/s41586-020-1943-3

Alzial G, Renoult O, Paris F, Gratas C, Clavreul A, Pecqueur C. 2022. Wild-type isocitrate dehydrogenase under the spotlight in glioblastoma. *Oncogene* **41:** 613–621. doi:10.1038/s41388-021-02056-1

Amankulor NM, Kim Y, Arora S, Kargl J, Szulzewsky F, Hanke M, Margineantu DH, Rao A, Bolouri H, Delrow J, et al. 2017. Mutant IDH1 regulates the tumor-associated immune system in gliomas. *Genes Dev* **31:** 774–786. doi:10.1101/gad.294991.116

Amatangelo MD, Quek L, Shih A, Stein EM, Roshal M, David MD, Marteyn B, Farnoud NR, de Botton S, Bernard OA, et al. 2017. Enasidenib induces acute myeloid leukemia cell differentiation to promote clinical response. *Blood* **130:** 732–741. doi:10.1182/blood-2017-04-779447

Badur MG, Muthusamy T, Parker SJ, Ma S, McBrayer SK, Cordes T, Magana JH, Guan KL, Metallo CM. 2018. Oncogenic R132 IDH1 mutations limit NADPH for de novo lipogenesis through (D)2-hydroxyglutarate production in fibrosarcoma cells. *Cell Rep* **25:** 1680. doi:10.1016/j.celrep.2018.10.099

Bleeker FE, Atai NA, Lamba S, Jonker A, Rijkeboer D, Bosch KS, Tigchelaar W, Troost D, Vandertop WP, Bardelli A, et al. 2010. The prognostic *IDH1^{R132}* mutation is associated with reduced $NADP^+$-dependent IDH activity in glioblastoma. *Acta Neuropathol* **119:** 487–494. doi:10.1007/s00401-010-0645-6

Blouw B, Song H, Tihan T, Bosze J, Ferrara N, Gerber HP, Johnson RS, Bergers G. 2003. The hypoxic response of tumors is dependent on their microenvironment. *Cancer Cell* **4:** 133–146. doi:10.1016/S1535-6108(03)00194-6

Böttcher M, Renner K, Berger R, Mentz K, Thomas S, Cardenas-Conejo ZE, Dettmer K, Oefner PJ, Mackensen A, Kreutz M, et al. 2018. D-2-hydroxyglutarate interferes with HIF-1α stability skewing T-cell metabolism towards oxidative phosphorylation and impairing Th17 polarization. *Oncoimmunology* **7:** e1445454. doi:10.1080/2162402X.2018.1445454

Bowman RL, Levine RL. 2017. TET2 in normal and malignant hematopoiesis. *Cold Spring Harb Perspect Med* 7: a026518. doi:10.1101/cshperspect.a026518

Bunse L, Pusch S, Bunse T, Sahm F, Sanghvi K, Friedrich M, Alansary D, Sonner JK, Green E, Deumelandt K, et al. 2018. Suppression of antitumor T cell immunity by the oncometabolite (R)-2-hydroxyglutarate. *Nat Med* 24: 1192–1203. doi:10.1038/s41591-018-0095-6

Busque L, Patel JP, Figueroa ME, Vasanthakumar A, Provost S, Hamilou Z, Mollica L, Li J, Viale A, Heguy A, et al. 2012. Recurrent somatic TET2 mutations in normal elderly individuals with clonal hematopoiesis. *Nat Genet* 44: 1179–1181. doi:10.1038/ng.2413

Cairns RA, Iqbal J, Lemonnier F, Kucuk C, de Leval L, Jais JP, Parrens M, Martin A, Xerri L, Brousset P, et al. 2012. IDH2 mutations are frequent in angioimmunoblastic T-cell lymphoma. *Blood* 119: 1901–1903. doi:10.1182/blood-2011-11-391748

Caldwell BA, Liu MY, Prasasya RD, Wang T, DeNizio JE, Leu NA, Amoh NYA, Krapp C, Lan Y, Shields EJ, et al. 2021. Functionally distinct roles for TET-oxidized 5-methylcytosine bases in somatic reprogramming to pluripotency. *Mol Cell* 81: 859–869.e8. doi:10.1016/j.molcel.2020.11.045

Chan SM, Thomas D, Corces-Zimmerman MR, Xavy S, Rastogi S, Hong WJ, Zhao F, Medeiros BC, Tyvoll DA, Majeti R. 2015. Isocitrate dehydrogenase 1 and 2 mutations induce BCL-2 dependence in acute myeloid leukemia. *Nat Med* 21: 178–184. doi:10.1038/nm.3788

Chaturvedi A, Araujo Cruz MM, Jyotsana N, Sharma A, Goparaju R, Schwarzer A, Gorlich K, Schottmann R, Struys EA, Jansen EE, et al. 2016. Enantiomer-specific and paracrine leukemogenicity of mutant IDH metabolite 2-hydroxyglutarate. *Leukemia* 30: 1708–1715. doi:10.1038/leu.2016.71

Chen Q, Chen Y, Bian C, Fujiki R, Yu X. 2013. TET2 promotes histone O-GlcNAcylation during gene transcription. *Nature* 493: 561–564. doi:10.1038/nature11742

Chen JY, Lai YS, Tsai HJ, Kuo CC, Yen BL, Yeh SP, Sun HS, Hung WC. 2016. The oncometabolite R-2-hydroxyglutarate activates NF-κB-dependent tumor-promoting stromal niche for acute myeloid leukemia cells. *Sci Rep* 6: 32428. doi:10.1038/srep32428

Cheung N, Fung TK, Zeisig BB, Holmes K, Rane JK, Mowen KA, Finn MG, Lenhard B, Chan LC, So CW. 2016. Targeting aberrant epigenetic networks mediated by PRMT1 and KDM4C in acute myeloid leukemia. *Cancer Cell* 29: 32–48. doi:10.1016/j.ccell.2015.12.007

Chowdhury R, Yeoh KK, Tian YM, Hillringhaus L, Bagg EA, Rose NR, Leung IK, Li XS, Woon EC, Yang M, et al. 2011. The oncometabolite 2-hydroxyglutarate inhibits histone lysine demethylases. *EMBO Rep* 12: 463–469. doi:10.1038/embor.2011.43

Cleary JM, Rouaisnel B, Daina A, Raghavan S, Roller LA, Huffman BM, Singh H, Wen PY, Bardeesy N, Zoete V, et al. 2022. Secondary IDH1 resistance mutations and oncogenic IDH2 mutations cause acquired resistance to ivosidenib in cholangiocarcinoma. *NPJ Precis Oncol* 6: 61. doi:10.1038/s41698-022-00304-5

Dang L, White DW, Gross S, Bennett BD, Bittinger MA, Driggers EM, Fantin VR, Jang HG, Jin S, Keenan MC, et al. 2009. Cancer-associated IDH1 mutations produce 2-hydroxyglutarate. *Nature* 462: 739–744. doi:10.1038/nature08617

Davis MI, Gross S, Shen M, Straley KS, Pragani R, Lea WA, Popovici-Muller J, DeLaBarre B, Artin E, Thorne N, et al. 2014. Biochemical, cellular, and biophysical characterization of a potent inhibitor of mutant isocitrate dehydrogenase IDH1. *J Biol Chem* 289: 13717–13725. doi:10.1074/jbc.M113.511030

Dimitrova E, Turberfield AH, Klose RJ. 2015. Histone demethylases in chromatin biology and beyond. *EMBO Rep* 16: 1620–1639. doi:10.15252/embr.201541113

DiNardo CD, Stein AS, Stein EM, Fathi AT, Frankfurt O, Schuh AC, Döhner H, Martinelli G, Patel PA, Raffoux E, et al. 2021. Mutant isocitrate dehydrogenase 1 inhibitor ivosidenib in combination with azacitidine for newly diagnosed acute myeloid leukemia. *J Clin Oncol* 39: 57–65. doi:10.1200/JCO.20.01632

Fack F, Tardito S, Hochart G, Oudin A, Zheng L, Fritah S, Golebiewska A, Nazarov PV, Bernard A, Hau AC, et al. 2017. Altered metabolic landscape in IDH-mutant gliomas affects phospholipid, energy, and oxidative stress pathways. *EMBO Mol Med* 9: 1681–1695. doi:10.15252/emmm.201707729

Fan B, Mellinghoff IK, Wen PY, Lowery MA, Goyal L, Tap WD, Pandya SS, Manyak E, Jiang L, Liu G, et al. 2020. Clinical pharmacokinetics and pharmacodynamics of ivosidenib, an oral, targeted inhibitor of mutant IDH1, in patients with advanced solid tumors. *Invest New Drugs* 38: 433–444. doi:10.1007/s10637-019-00771-x

Figueroa ME, Abdel-Wahab O, Lu C, Ward PS, Patel J, Shih A, Li Y, Bhagwat N, Vasanthakumar A, Fernandez HF, et al. 2010. Leukemic IDH1 and IDH2 mutations result in a hypermethylation phenotype, disrupt TET2 function, and impair hematopoietic differentiation. *Cancer Cell* 18: 553–567. doi:10.1016/j.ccr.2010.11.015

Forloni M, Gupta R, Nagarajan A, Sun LS, Dong Y, Pirazzoli V, Toki M, Wurtz A, Melnick MA, Kobayashi S, et al. 2016. Oncogenic EGFR represses the TET1 DNA demethylase to induce silencing of tumor suppressors in cancer cells. *Cell Rep* 16: 457–471. doi:10.1016/j.celrep.2016.05.087

Fu X, Chin RM, Vergnes L, Hwang H, Deng G, Xing Y, Pai MY, Li S, Ta L, Fazlollahi F, et al. 2015. 2-Hydroxyglutarate inhibits ATP synthase and mTOR signaling. *Cell Metab* 22: 508–515. doi:10.1016/j.cmet.2015.06.009

Gelman SJ, Naser F, Mahieu NG, McKenzie LD, Dunn GP, Chheda MG, Patti GJ. 2018. Consumption of NADPH for 2-HG synthesis increases pentose phosphate pathway flux and sensitizes cells to oxidative stress. *Cell Rep* 22: 512–522. doi:10.1016/j.celrep.2017.12.050

Gross S, Cairns RA, Minden MD, Driggers EM, Bittinger MA, Jang HG, Sasaki M, Jin S, Schenkein DP, Su SM, et al. 2010. Cancer-associated metabolite 2-hydroxyglutarate accumulates in acute myelogenous leukemia with isocitrate dehydrogenase 1 and 2 mutations. *J Exp Med* 207: 339–344. doi:10.1084/jem.20092506

Gunn K, Myllykoski M, Cao JZ, Ahmed M, Huang B, Rouaisnel B, Diplas BH, Levitt MM, Looper R, Doench JG, et al. 2023. (R)-2-hydroxyglutarate inhibits KDM5 histone lysine demethylases to drive transformation in *IDH*-mutant cancers. *Cancer Discov* 13: 1478–1497. doi:10.1158/2159-8290.CD-22-0825

Han CJ, Zheng JY, Sun L, Yang HC, Cao ZQ, Zhang XH, Zheng LT, Zhen XC. 2019. The oncometabolite 2-hydroxyglutarate inhibits microglial activation via the AMPK/mTOR/NF-κB pathway. *Acta Pharmacol Sin* **40:** 1292–1302. doi:10.1038/s41401-019-0225-9

Harding JJ, Lowery MA, Shih AH, Schvartzman JM, Hou S, Famulare C, Patel M, Roshal M, Do RK, Zehir A, et al. 2018. Isoform switching as a mechanism of acquired resistance to mutant isocitrate dehydrogenase inhibition. *Cancer Discov* **8:** 1540–1547. doi:10.1158/2159-8290.CD-18-0877

He YF, Li BZ, Li Z, Liu P, Wang Y, Tang Q, Ding J, Jia Y, Chen Z, Li L, et al. 2011. Tet-mediated formation of 5-carboxylcytosine and its excision by TDG in mammalian DNA. *Science* **333:** 1303–1307. doi:10.1126/science.1210944

Intlekofer AM, Dematteo RG, Venneti S, Finley LW, Lu C, Judkins AR, Rustenburg AS, Grinaway PB, Chodera JD, Cross JR, et al. 2015. Hypoxia induces production of l-2-hydroxyglutarate. *Cell Metab* **22:** 304–311. doi:10.1016/j.cmet.2015.06.023

Intlekofer AM, Wang B, Liu H, Shah H, Carmona-Fontaine C, Rustenburg AS, Salah S, Gunner MR, Chodera JD, Cross JR, et al. 2017. L-2-Hydroxyglutarate production arises from noncanonical enzyme function at acidic pH. *Nat Chem Biol* **13:** 494–500. doi:10.1038/nchembio.2307

Intlekofer AM, Shih AH, Wang B, Nazir A, Rustenburg AS, Albanese SK, Patel M, Famulare C, Correa FM, Takemoto N, et al. 2018. Acquired resistance to IDH inhibition through *trans* or *cis* dimer-interface mutations. *Nature* **559:** 125–129. doi:10.1038/s41586-018-0251-7

Ito S, Shen L, Dai Q, Wu SC, Collins LB, Swenberg JA, He C, Zhang Y. 2011. Tet proteins can convert 5-methylcytosine to 5-formylcytosine and 5-carboxylcytosine. *Science* **333:** 1300–1303. doi:10.1126/science.1210597

Jaiswal S, Fontanillas P, Flannick J, Manning A, Grauman PV, Mar BG, Lindsley RC, Mermel CH, Burtt N, Chavez A, et al. 2014. Age-related clonal hematopoiesis associated with adverse outcomes. *N Engl J Med* **371:** 2488–2498. doi:10.1056/NEJMoa1408617

Ježek P. 2020. 2-Hydroxyglutarate in cancer cells. *Antioxid Redox Signal* **33:** 903–926. doi:10.1089/ars.2019.7902

Ji D, You C, Wang P, Wang Y. 2014. Effects of tet-induced oxidation products of 5-methylcytosine on DNA replication in mammalian cells. *Chem Res Toxicol* **27:** 1304–1309. doi:10.1021/tx500169u

Johannessen TA, Mukherjee J, Viswanath P, Ohba S, Ronen SM, Bjerkvig R, Pieper RO. 2016. Rapid conversion of mutant IDH1 from driver to passenger in a model of human gliomagenesis. *Mol Cancer Res* **14:** 976–983. doi:10.1158/1541-7786.MCR-16-0141

Kaelin WG Jr, Ratcliffe PJ. 2008. Oxygen sensing by metazoans: the central role of the HIF hydroxylase pathway. *Mol Cell* **30:** 393–402. doi:10.1016/j.molcel.2008.04.009

Kim YH, Pierscianek D, Mittelbronn M, Vital A, Mariani L, Hasselblatt M, Ohgaki H. 2011. *TET2* promoter methylation in low-grade diffuse gliomas lacking *IDH1/2* mutations. *J Clin Pathol* **64:** 850–852. doi:10.1136/jclinpath-2011-200133

Kogiso M, Qi L, Du Y, Braun FK, Zhang H, Huang LF, Guo L, Huang Y, Teo WY, Lindsay H, et al. 2022. Synergistic antitumor efficacy of mutant isocitrate dehydrogenase 1 inhibitor SYC-435 with standard therapy in patient-derived xenograft mouse models of glioma. *Transl Oncol* **18:** 101368. doi:10.1016/j.tranon.2022.101368

Koh KP, Yabuuchi A, Rao S, Huang Y, Cunniff K, Nardone J, Laiho A, Tahiliani M, Sommer CA, Mostoslavsky G, et al. 2011. Tet1 and Tet2 regulate 5-hydroxymethylcytosine production and cell lineage specification in mouse embryonic stem cells. *Cell Stem Cell* **8:** 200–213. doi:10.1016/j.stem.2011.01.008

Koivunen P, Lee S, Duncan CG, Lopez G, Lu G, Ramkissoon S, Losman JA, Joensuu P, Bergmann U, Gross S, et al. 2012. Transformation by the (R)-enantiomer of 2-hydroxyglutarate linked to EGLN activation. *Nature* **483:** 484–488. doi:10.1038/nature10898

Komori T. 2023. Update of the 2021 WHO classification of tumors of the central nervous system: adult diffuse gliomas. *Brain Tumor Pathol* **40:** 1–3. doi:10.1007/s10014-022-00446-1

Kraus TF, Globisch D, Wagner M, Eigenbrod S, Widmann D, Münzel M, Müller M, Pfaffeneder T, Hackner B, Feiden W, et al. 2012. Low values of 5-hydroxymethylcytosine (5hmC), the "sixth base," are associated with anaplasia in human brain tumors. *Int J Cancer* **131:** 1577–1590. doi:10.1002/ijc.27429

Kraus TF, Greiner A, Steinmaurer M, Dietinger V, Guibourt V, Kretzschmar HA. 2015. Genetic characterization of ten-eleven-translocation methylcytosine dioxygenase alterations in human glioma. *J Cancer* **6:** 832–842. doi:10.7150/jca.12010

Kroeze LI, Aslanyan MG, van Rooij A, Koorenhof-Scheele TN, Massop M, Carell T, Boezeman JB, Marie JP, Halkes CJ, de Witte T, et al. 2014. Characterization of acute myeloid leukemia based on levels of global hydroxymethylation. *Blood* **124:** 1110–1118. doi:10.1182/blood-2013-08-518514

Lan F, Nottke AC, Shi Y. 2008. Mechanisms involved in the regulation of histone lysine demethylases. *Curr Opin Cell Biol* **20:** 316–325. doi:10.1016/j.ceb.2008.03.004

Laurenti G, Tennant DA. 2016. Isocitrate dehydrogenase (IDH), succinate dehydrogenase (SDH), fumarate hydratase (FH): three players for one phenotype in cancer? *Biochem Soc Trans* **44:** 1111–1116. doi:10.1042/BST20160099

Leca J, Lemonnier F, Meydan C, Foox J, El Ghamrasni S, Mboumba DL, Duncan GS, Fortin J, Sakamoto T, Tobin C, et al. 2023. IDH2 and TET2 mutations synergize to modulate T follicular helper cell functional interaction with the AITL microenvironment. *Cancer Cell* **41:** 323–339.e10. doi:10.1016/j.ccell.2023.01.003

Li L, Paz AC, Wilky BA, Johnson B, Galoian K, Rosenberg A, Hu G, Tinoco G, Bodamer O, Trent JC. 2015. Treatment with a small molecule mutant IDH1 inhibitor suppresses tumorigenic activity and decreases production of the oncometabolite 2-hydroxyglutarate in human chondrosarcoma cells. *PLoS ONE* **10:** e0133813. doi:10.1371/journal.pone.0133813

Lin W, Cao J, Liu J, Beshiri ML, Fujiwara Y, Francis J, Cherniack AD, Geisen C, Blair LP, Zou MR, et al. 2011. Loss of the retinoblastoma binding protein 2 (RBP2) histone demethylase suppresses tumorigenesis in mice lacking *Rb1* or *Men1*. *Proc Natl Acad Sci* **108:** 13379–13386. doi:10.1073/pnas.1110104108

Liu L, Shah S, Fan J, Park JO, Wellen KE, Rabinowitz JD. 2016. Malic enzyme tracers reveal hypoxia-induced switch in adipocyte NADPH pathway usage. *Nat Chem Biol* **12:** 345–352. doi:10.1038/nchembio.2047

Losman JA, Looper R, Koivunen P, Lee S, Schneider RK, McMahon C, Cowley G, Root D, Ebert BL, Kaelin WG Jr. 2013. (R)-2-hydroxyglutarate is sufficient to promote leukemogenesis and its effects are reversible. *Science* **339:** 1621–1625. doi:10.1126/science.1231677

Losman JA, Koivunen P, Kaelin WG Jr. 2020. 2-Oxoglutarate-dependent dioxygenases in cancer. *Nat Rev Cancer* **20:** 710–726. doi:10.1038/s41568-020-00303-3

Lowery MA, Burris HA, Janku F, Shroff RT, Cleary JM, Azad NS, Goyal L, Maher EA, Gore L, Hollebecque A, et al. 2019. Safety and activity of ivosidenib in patients with IDH1-mutant advanced cholangiocarcinoma: a phase 1 study. *Lancet Gastroenterol Hepatol* **4:** 711–720. doi:10.1016/S2468-1253(19)30189-X

Lu C, Ward PS, Kapoor GS, Rohle D, Turcan S, Abdel-Wahab O, Edwards CR, Khanin R, Figueroa ME, Melnick A, et al. 2012. IDH mutation impairs histone demethylation and results in a block to cell differentiation. *Nature* **483:** 474–478. doi:10.1038/nature10860

Martínez-Reyes I, Chandel NS. 2014. Mitochondrial one-carbon metabolism maintains redox balance during hypoxia. *Cancer Discov* **4:** 1371–1373. doi:10.1158/2159-8290.CD-14-1228

McBrayer SK, Mayers JR, DiNatale GJ, Shi DD, Khanal J, Chakraborty AA, Sarosiek KA, Briggs KJ, Robbins AK, Sewastianik T, et al. 2018a. Transaminase inhibition by 2-hydroxyglutarate impairs glutamate biosynthesis and redox homeostasis in glioma. *Cell* **175:** 101–116.e25. doi:10.1016/j.cell.2018.08.038

McBrayer SK, Olenchock BA, DiNatale GJ, Shi DD, Khanal J, Jennings RB, Novak JS, Oser MG, Robbins AK, Modiste R, et al. 2018b. Autochthonous tumors driven by *Rb1* loss have an ongoing requirement for the RBP2 histone demethylase. *Proc Natl Acad Sci* **115:** E3741–E3748. doi:10.1073/pnas.1716029115

Mellinghoff IK, Ellingson BM, Touat M, Maher E, De La Fuente MI, Holdhoff M, Cote GM, Burris H, Janku F, Young RJ, et al. 2020. Ivosidenib in isocitrate dehydrogenase 1-mutated advanced glioma. *J Clin Oncol* **38:** 3398–3406. doi:10.1200/JCO.19.03327

Mellinghoff IK, Penas-Prado M, Peters KB, Burris HA, Maher EA, Janku F, Cote GM, de la Fuente MI, Clarke JL, Ellingson BM, et al. 2021. Vorasidenib, a dual inhibitor of mutant IDH1/2, in recurrent or progressive glioma; results of a first-in-human phase I trial. *Clin Cancer Res* **27:** 4491–4499. doi:10.1158/1078-0432.CCR-21-0611

Mellinghoff IK, Lu M, Wen PY, Taylor JW, Maher EA, Arrillaga-Romany I, Peters KB, Ellingson BM, Rosenblum MK, Chun S, et al. 2023. Vorasidenib and ivosidenib in IDH1-mutant low-grade glioma: a randomized, perioperative phase 1 trial. *Nat Med* **29:** 615–622. doi:10.1038/s41591-022-02141-2

Müller T, Gessi M, Waha A, Isselstein LJ, Luxen D, Freihoff D, Freihoff J, Becker A, Simon M, Hammes J, et al. 2012. Nuclear exclusion of TET1 is associated with loss of 5-hydroxymethylcytosine in IDH1 wild-type gliomas. *Am J Pathol* **181:** 675–683. doi:10.1016/j.ajpath.2012.04.017

Notarangelo G, Spinelli JB, Perez EM, Baker GJ, Kurmi K, Elia I, Stopka SA, Baquer G, Lin JR, Golby AJ, et al. 2022. Oncometabolite d-2HG alters T cell metabolism to impair CD8[+] T cell function. *Science* **377:** 1519–1529. doi:10.1126/science.abj5104

Odejide O, Weigert O, Lane AA, Toscano D, Lunning MA, Kopp N, Kim S, van Bodegom D, Bolla S, Schatz JH, et al. 2014. A targeted mutational landscape of angioimmunoblastic T-cell lymphoma. *Blood* **123:** 1293–1296. doi:10.1182/blood-2013-10-531509

Orr BA, Haffner MC, Nelson WG, Yegnasubramanian S, Eberhart CG. 2012. Decreased 5-hydroxymethylcytosine is associated with neural progenitor phenotype in normal brain and shorter survival in malignant glioma. *PLoS ONE* **7:** e41036. doi:10.1371/journal.pone.0041036

Pekmezci M, Phillips JJ, Dirilenoglu F, Atasever-Rezanko T, Tihan T, Solomon D, Bollen A, Perry A. 2020. Loss of H3K27 trimethylation by immunohistochemistry is frequent in oligodendroglioma, IDH-mutant and 1p/19q-codeleted, but is neither a sensitive nor a specific marker. *Acta Neuropathol* **139:** 597–600. doi:10.1007/s00401-019-02123-8

Pirozzi CJ, Yan H. 2021. The implications of IDH mutations for cancer development and therapy. *Nat Rev Clin Oncol* **18:** 645–661. doi:10.1038/s41571-021-00521-0

Pusch S, Schweizer L, Beck AC, Lehmler JM, Weissert S, Balss J, Miller AK, von Deimling A. 2014. D-2-hydroxyglutarate producing neo-enzymatic activity inversely correlates with frequency of the type of isocitrate dehydrogenase 1 mutations found in glioma. *Acta Neuropathol Commun* **2:** 19. doi:10.1186/2051-5960-2-19

Roboz GJ, DiNardo CD, Stein EM, de Botton S, Mims AS, Prince GT, Altman JK, Arellano ML, Donnellan W, Erba HP, et al. 2020. Ivosidenib induces deep durable remissions in patients with newly diagnosed IDH1-mutant acute myeloid leukemia. *Blood* **135:** 463–471. doi:10.1182/blood.2019002140

Saha SK, Gordan JD, Kleinstiver BP, Vu P, Najem MS, Yeo JC, Shi L, Kato Y, Levin RS, Webber JT, et al. 2016. Isocitrate dehydrogenase mutations confer dasatinib hypersensitivity and SRC dependence in intrahepatic cholangiocarcinoma. *Cancer Discov* **6:** 727–739. doi:10.1158/2159-8290.CD-15-1442

Sasaki M, Knobbe CB, Itsumi M, Elia AJ, Harris IS, Chio II, Cairns RA, McCracken S, Wakeham A, Haight J, et al. 2012a. D-2-hydroxyglutarate produced by mutant IDH1 perturbs collagen maturation and basement membrane function. *Genes Dev* **26:** 2038–2049. doi:10.1101/gad.198200.112

Sasaki M, Knobbe CB, Munger JC, Lind EF, Brenner D, Brüstle A, Harris IS, Holmes R, Wakeham A, Haight J, et al. 2012b. IDH1(R132H) mutation increases murine haematopoietic progenitors and alters epigenetics. *Nature* **488:** 656–659. doi:10.1038/nature11323

Schvartzman JM, Reuter VP, Koche RP, Thompson CB. 2019. 2-hydroxyglutarate inhibits MyoD-mediated differentiation by preventing H3K9 demethylation. *Proc Natl Acad Sci* **116:** 12851–12856. doi:10.1073/pnas.1817662116

Schvartzman JM, Forsyth G, Walch H, Chatila W, Taglialatela A, Lee BJ, Zhu X, Gershik S, Cimino FV, Santella A, et al. 2023. Oncogenic IDH mutations increase heterochromatin-related replication stress without impacting homologous recombination. *Mol Cell* **83**: 2347–2356.e8. doi:10.1016/j.molcel.2023.05.026

Separovich RJ, Wilkins MR. 2021. Ready, SET, go: post-translational regulation of the histone lysine methylation network in budding yeast. *J Biol Chem* **297**: 100939. doi:10.1016/j.jbc.2021.100939

Shi DD, Anand S, Abdullah KG, McBrayer SK. 2023. DNA damage in IDH-mutant gliomas: mechanisms and clinical implications. *J Neurooncol* **162**: 515–523. doi:10.1007/s11060-022-04172-8

Shim EH, Livi CB, Rakheja D, Tan J, Benson D, Parekh V, Kho EY, Ghosh AP, Kirkman R, Velu S, et al. 2014. L-2-hydroxyglutarate: an epigenetic modifier and putative oncometabolite in renal cancer. *Cancer Discov* **4**: 1290–1298. doi:10.1158/2159-8290.CD-13-0696

Song CX, Szulwach KE, Dai Q, Fu Y, Mao SQ, Lin L, Street C, Li Y, Poidevin M, Wu H, et al. 2013. Genome-wide profiling of 5-formylcytosine reveals its roles in epigenetic priming. *Cell* **153**: 678–691. doi:10.1016/j.cell.2013.04.001

Stasik S, Juratli TA, Petzold A, Richter S, Zolal A, Schackert G, Dahl A, Krex D, Thiede C. 2020. Exome sequencing identifies frequent genomic loss of TET1 in IDH-wild-type glioblastoma. *Neoplasia* **22**: 800–808. doi:10.1016/j.neo.2020.10.010

Steenweg ME, Jakobs C, Errami A, van Dooren SJ, Adeva Bartolomé MT, Aerssens P, Augoustides-Savvapoulou P, Baric I, Baumann M, Bonafé L, et al. 2010. An overview of L-2-hydroxyglutarate dehydrogenase gene (L2HGDH) variants: a genotype-phenotype study. *Hum Mutat* **31**: 380–390. doi:10.1002/humu.21197

Stein EM, DiNardo CD, Pollyea DA, Fathi AT, Roboz GJ, Altman JK, Stone RM, DeAngelo DJ, Levine RL, Flinn IW, et al. 2017. Enasidenib in mutant IDH2 relapsed or refractory acute myeloid leukemia. *Blood* **130**: 722–731. doi:10.1182/blood-2017-04-779405

Stein EM, DiNardo CD, Fathi AT, Pollyea DA, Stone RM, Altman JK, Roboz GJ, Patel MR, Collins R, Flinn IW, et al. 2019. Molecular remission and response patterns in patients with mutant-IDH2 acute myeloid leukemia treated with enasidenib. *Blood* **133**: 676–687. doi:10.1182/blood-2018-08-869008

Struys EA, Salomons GS, Achouri Y, Van Schaftingen E, Grosso S, Craigen WJ, Verhoeven NM, Jakobs C. 2005a. Mutations in the D-2-hydroxyglutarate dehydrogenase gene cause D-2-hydroxyglutaric aciduria. *Am J Hum Genet* **76**: 358–360. doi:10.1086/427890

Struys EA, Verhoeven NM, Ten Brink HJ, Wickenhagen WV, Gibson KM, Jakobs C. 2005b. Kinetic characterization of human hydroxyacid–oxoacid transhydrogenase: relevance to D-2-hydroxyglutaric and γ-hydroxybutyric acidurias. *J Inherit Metab Dis* **28**: 921–930. doi:10.1007/s10545-005-0114-x

Sulkowski PL, Corso CD, Robinson ND, Scanlon SE, Purshouse KR, Bai H, Liu Y, Sundaram RK, Hegan DC, Fons NR, et al. 2017. 2-hydroxyglutarate produced by neomorphic IDH mutations suppresses homologous recombination and induces PARP inhibitor sensitivity. *Sci Transl Med* **9**: eaal246. doi:10.1126/scitranslmed.aal2463

Sulkowski PL, Oeck S, Dow J, Economos NG, Mirfakhraie L, Liu Y, Noronha K, Bao X, Li J, Shuch BM, et al. 2020. Oncometabolites suppress DNA repair by disrupting lo-cal chromatin signalling. *Nature* **582**: 586–591. doi:10.1038/s41586-020-2363-0

Tahiliani M, Koh KP, Shen Y, Pastor WA, Bandukwala H, Brudno Y, Agarwal S, Iyer LM, Liu DR, Aravind L, et al. 2009. Conversion of 5-methylcytosine to 5-hydroxyme-thylcytosine in mammalian DNA by MLL partner TET1. *Science* **324**: 930–935. doi:10.1126/science.1170116

Tap WD, Villalobos VM, Cote GM, Burris H, Janku F, Mir O, Beeram M, Wagner AJ, Jiang L, Wu B, et al. 2020. Phase I study of the mutant IDH1 inhibitor ivosidenib: safety and clinical activity in patients with advanced chondrosarcoma. *J Clin Oncol* **38**: 1693–1701. doi:10.1200/JCO.19.02492

Tateishi K, Wakimoto H, Iafrate AJ, Tanaka S, Loebel F, Lelic N, Wiederschain D, Bedel O, Deng G, Zhang B, et al. 2015. Extreme vulnerability of IDH1 mutant cancers to NAD$^+$ depletion. *Cancer Cell* **28**: 773–784. doi:10.1016/j.ccell.2015.11.006

Teng YC, Lee CF, Li YS, Chen YR, Hsiao PW, Chan MY, Lin FM, Huang HD, Chen YT, Jeng YM, et al. 2013. Histone demethylase RBP2 promotes lung tumorigenesis and cancer metastasis. *Cancer Res* **73**: 4711–4721. doi:10.1158/0008-5472.CAN-12-3165

Thomas D, Wu M, Nakauchi Y, Zheng M, Thompson-Peach CAL, Lim K, Landberg N, Köhnke T, Robinson N, Kaur S, et al. 2023. Dysregulated lipid synthesis by oncogenic IDH1 mutation is a targetable synthetic lethal vulnerability. *Cancer Discov* **13**: 496–515. doi:10.1158/2159-8290.CD-21-0218

Turcan S, Makarov V, Taranda J, Wang Y, Fabius AWM, Wu W, Zheng Y, El-Amine N, Haddock S, Nanjangud G, et al. 2018. Mutant-IDH1-dependent chromatin state reprogramming, reversibility, and persistence. *Nat Gen* **50**: 62–72. doi:10.1038/s41588-017-0001-z

Tyrakis PA, Palazon A, Macias D, Lee KL, Phan AT, Veliça P, You J, Chia GS, Sim J, Doedens A, et al. 2016. S-2-hydroxyglutarate regulates CD8$^+$ T-lymphocyte fate. *Nature* **540**: 236–241. doi:10.1038/nature20165

Wang F, Travins J, de la Barre B, Lacronique-Penard V, Schalm S, Hansen E, Straley KS, Kernytsky A, Liu W, Gliser C, et al. 2013. Targeted inhibition of mutant IDH2 in leukemia cells induces cellular differentiation. *Science* **340**: 622–626. doi:10.1126/science.1234769

Ward PS, Patel J, Wise DR, Abdel-Wahab O, Bennett BD, Coller HA, Cross JR, Fantin VR, Hedvat CV, Perl AE, et al. 2010. The common feature of leukemia-associated IDH1 and IDH2 mutations is a neomorphic enzyme activity converting α-ketoglutarate to 2-hydroxygluta-rate. *Cancer Cell* **17**: 225–234. doi:10.1016/j.ccr.2010.01.020

Ward PS, Lu C, Cross JR, Abdel-Wahab O, Levine RL, Schwartz GK, Thompson CB. 2013. The potential for isocitrate dehydrogenase mutations to produce 2-hydrox-yglutarate depends on allele specificity and subcellular compartmentalization. *J Biol Chem* **288**: 3804–3815. doi:10.1074/jbc.M112.435495

Williams SC, Karajannis MA, Chiriboga L, Golfinos JG, von Deimling A, Zagzag D. 2011. R132H-mutation of isocitrate dehydrogenase-1 is not sufficient for HIF-1α up-regulation in adult glioma. *Acta Neuropathol* **121**: 279–281. doi:10.1007/s00401-010-0790-y

Wu MJ, Shi L, Dubrot J, Merritt J, Vijay V, Wei TY, Kessler E, Olander KE, Adil R, Pankaj A, et al. 2022. Mutant IDH inhibits IFNγ–TET2 signaling to promote immunoevasion and tumor maintenance in cholangiocarcinoma. *Cancer Discov* **12:** 812–835. doi:10.1158/2159-8290.CD-21-1077

Xu W, Yang H, Liu Y, Yang Y, Wang P, Kim SH, Ito S, Yang C, Wang P, Xiao MT, et al. 2011. Oncometabolite 2-hydroxyglutarate is a competitive inhibitor of α-ketoglutarate-dependent dioxygenases. *Cancer Cell* **19:** 17–30. doi:10.1016/j.ccr.2010.12.014

Yaacov A, Rosenberg S, Simon I. 2023. Mutational signatures association with replication timing in normal cells reveals similarities and differences with matched cancer tissues. *Sci Rep* **13:** 7833. doi:10.1038/s41598-023-34631-9

Yamamoto S, Wu Z, Russnes HG, Takagi S, Peluffo G, Vaske C, Zhao X, Moen Vollan HK, Maruyama R, Ekram MB, et al. 2014. JARID1B is a luminal lineage-driving oncogene in breast cancer. *Cancer Cell* **25:** 762–777. doi:10.1016/j.ccr.2014.04.024

Yan H, Parsons DW, Jin G, McLendon R, Rasheed BA, Yuan W, Kos I, Batinic-Haberle I, Jones S, Riggins GJ, et al. 2009. IDH1 and IDH2 mutations in gliomas. *N Engl J Med* **360:** 765–773. doi:10.1056/NEJMoa0808710

Yang M, Soga T, Pollard PJ. 2013. Oncometabolites: linking altered metabolism with cancer. *J Clin Invest* **123:** 3652–3658. doi:10.1172/JCI67228

Yen K, Travins J, Wang F, David MD, Artin E, Straley K, Padyana A, Gross S, DeLaBarre B, Tobin E, et al. 2017. AG-221, a first-in-class therapy targeting acute myeloid leukemia harboring oncogenic *IDH2* mutations. *Cancer Discov* **7:** 478–493. doi:10.1158/2159-8290.CD-16-1034

You C, Ji D, Dai X, Wang Y. 2014. Effects of Tet-mediated oxidation products of 5-methylcytosine on DNA transcription in vitro and in mammalian cells. *Sci Rep* **4:** 7052. doi:10.1038/srep07052

Yu DD, Zhang J. 2021. Update on recurrent mutations in angioimmunoblastic T-cell lymphoma. *Int J Clin Exp Pathol* **14:** 1108–1118.

Zhang Q, Zhao K, Shen Q, Han Y, Gu Y, Li X, Zhao D, Liu Y, Wang C, Zhang X, et al. 2015. Tet2 is required to resolve inflammation by recruiting Hdac2 to specifically repress IL-6. *Nature* **525:** 389–393. doi:10.1038/nature15252

Knowledge-Based Therapeutics for Tricarboxylic Acid (TCA) Cycle-Deficient Cancers

Daniel Peled,[1] Ruth Casey,[2] and Eyal Gottlieb[3]

[1]Department of Cell Biology and Cancer Science, Rappaport Faculty of Medicine, Technion - Israel Institute of Technology, Haifa 3525433, Israel

[2]Department of Medical Genetics, NIHR Cambridge Biomedical Research Centre, Cancer Research UK Cambridge Centre, Cambridge Biomedical Campus, University of Cambridge, Cambridge CB2 0QQ, United Kingdom

[3]Department of Cancer Biology, University of Texas MD Anderson Cancer Center, Houston, Texas 77030, USA

Correspondence: EGottlieb@mdanderson.org

With the foundation pre-laid, research in the new millennium has readily excavated and expanded upon the architectural framework laid out by Otto Warburg's seminal work in a new wave of "westward expansion," ever widening our understanding of cancer metabolism beyond the telescopic vision seen over a century ago. On this path, the unique circuitry of the cancer metabolic program has been elucidated, illuminating mutations of conserved cellular pathways implicated in tumorigenesis. Paramount among these are mutations in tricarboxylic acid cycle enzymes, succinate dehydrogenase, and fumarate hydratase, leading to deleterious accumulations in metabolic intermediates, "oncometabolites," the pilots of the disease process. In this work, we seek to reflect on the advancements in the field in recent years, updating knowledge on the exact biochemical mechanisms at the helm of the tumor, providing rationale for clinical trials currently underway, and anticipating directions for the future on this expansive frontier.

Nearly a century since its inception, the idea that cancer cells can alter their functional phenotype has been ratified and lately has become a revived topic of interest in the field of metabolism. Through a lull since Otto Warburg's discovery at the beginning of the twentieth century, numerous mutations in metabolic enzymes have been cataloged in recent years to show that either loss- or gain-of-function of specific metabolic enzymes play a critical role in tumorigenesis (Warburg et al. 1927). It was recognized that up- or down-regulation of metabolic enzymes across the cell's functional network are implicated in tumors' metabolic rewiring, yet none are so interwoven into the cellular regulatory system as those of the tricarboxylic acid (TCA) cycle. This amphibolic enzymatic process is the crossroads of the cell's energetic and biosynthetic capacity. The TCA cycle is involved in anabolism, heme and iron–sulfur complex biosynthesis, urea cycle, as well as in the metabolism of fatty, amino, and nucleic acids (Arnold and Finley 2023). Among the many enzymes in this pathway, three are paradigms to discussion: succinate dehydrogenase (SDH), fumarate hydratase (FH), and isocitrate dehydrogenase (IDH) (the latter is discussed in Gunn and Losman 2023). The genes coding these enzymes are critical to cell survival. Therefore, gain- or loss-of-function mutations distinctly impede their activity and are detrimental to cellular and organismal fate. If humans inherit maternal and paternal loss-of-function mutated alleles of these critical genes, they are prone to severely deleterious pathologies. Leigh syndrome, neonatal dilated cardiomyopathy, and neurodegeneration with ataxia and late-onset optic atrophy (NDAXOA) are examples of inborn errors of metabolism caused by biallelic germline mutations in human SDHA, one of the four subunits of the SDH enzyme. As opposed to biallelic genetic disorders, in cancer predisposition syndromes, patients are born with one mutant and one normal allele of a tumor suppressor gene and then suffer a second somatic "hit" (Knudsonian two-hit hypothesis), by which cells lose their heterozygosity and become susceptible to a multitude of cancers (Knudson 1971). Forming the basis of this work, SDH and FH will serve as the paradigm for our understanding of the consequences of mutations in metabolic tumor suppressor genes. The tumorigenic processes associated with SDH- and FH-related syndromes act in a multifactorial mode, culminating in a cancer phenotype, via (1) pseudohypoxia, the process by which hypoxia-response genes are transcribed irrespective of the presence of true hypoxia, (2) DNA and histone hypermethylation, and (3) reactive oxygen species (ROS). Mutations in SDH and FH result in deleterious amassments of succinate and fumarate, respectively. These accretions of TCA cycle intermediates are highly correlated with incidence of specific cancers, thus earning the moniker "oncometabolites" (Chowdhury et al. 2011). Of note, IDH-related cancers are not associated with hereditary syndromes and only one allele is somatically mutated, thus presenting with a gain-of-function phenotype (Parker and Metallo 2015).

Oncometabolites generally act as competitive inhibitors of dioxygenases, a family of enzymes that split molecular oxygen (O_2) into a hydroxyl group (-OH) on their substrates (Fig. 1) while the second oxygen atom oxidizes α-ketoglutarate (αKG) to

succinate (McNeill et al. 2002; Nguyen and Durán 2016). Some dioxygenases are functionally attuned to molecular oxygen sensing and their inhibition acclimates the cell to pseudohypoxia, while other dioxygenases act as histone or DNA demethylases (Losman et al. 2020). Pseudohypoxia is mediated by the hypoxia-independent stabilization of the labile α subunits of hypoxia-inducible factors (HIFs) HIF1A and HIF2A. The levels of these proteins are tightly controlled posttranslationally through the hydroxylation of specific proline residues within their oxygen-dependent degradation domain via the oxygen sensor dioxygenases known as HIF-prolyl hydroxylases (PHDs) (Marxsen et al. 2004). HIF hydroxylation enables the binding of the E3 ubiquitin ligase von Hippel–Landau (VHL), which consequently targets HIF for degradation in an oxygen-dependent manner (Hayashi et al. 2019). Dysfunctions of this pathway can occur at many levels. One example is the classic VHL disease, caused by the germline loss of function of the VHL gene, leading to unadulterated HIF expression. In the case of SDH or FH loss of function, the inhibition of PHDs by succinate and fumarate, respectively, prevents VHL binding to HIF, and results in pseudohypoxia.

At large, chromatin (structured DNA and histones) remodeling is achieved by chemical alterations, regulating the accessibility of the chromatin to the transcriptional machinery of the cell. These include DNA cytosine-methylation, and many histone modifications such as lysine and arginine-methylation, acetylation, ubiquitylation, ADP-ribosylation, and SUMOylation (Sulkowski et al. 2020). In a similar fashion to PHD inhibition, the burgeoning tides of oncometabolites also block demethylation pathways, resulting in hypercytosine methylation on DNA and hyperlysine methylation on histones (Nowicki and Gottlieb 2015). The equilibrium of DNA methylation is balanced by the ebb and flow of DNA methyltransferases (DNMTs) and DNA demethylases, 10-11-translocation methylcytosine dioxygenases (TETs). TETs catalyze the αKG-dependent hydroxylation reaction of 5-methylcytosine to 5-hydroxymethylcytosine (5-hmc), and further into unmethylated cytosine and methanol (Inoue et al. 2016). As αKG-dependent dioxygenases, TETs can be inhibited by

Cite this article as *Cold Spring Harb Perspect Med* doi: 10.1101/cshperspect.a041536

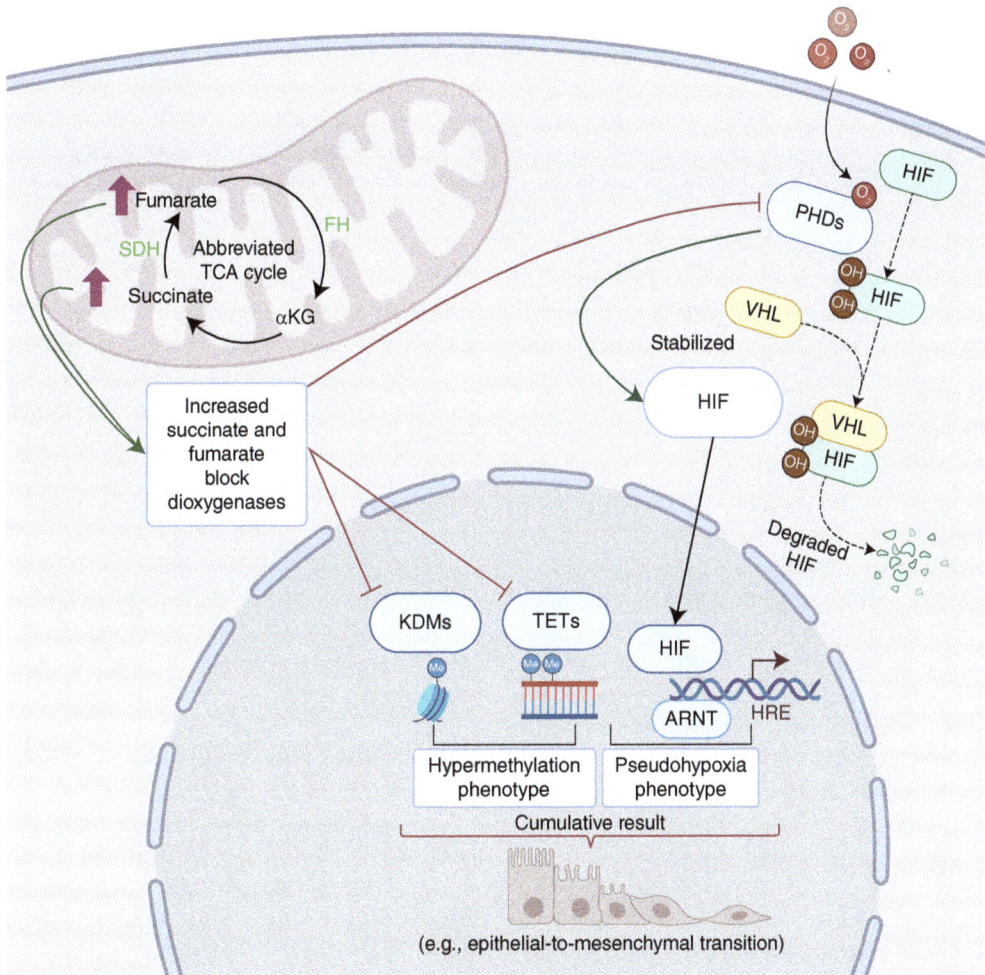

Figure 1. Schematic representation of oncometabolite-driven gene-expression changes. Accumulations of succinate and fumarate, due to succinate dehydrogenase (SDH) or fumarate hydratase (FH) deficiencies, respectively, result in aberrant dioxygenases functioning, which causes two major changes in the cancer cell, which further feed into one another, propelling the cell to epithelial–mesenchymal transition. (1) Hypermethylation—both histone hypermethylation via inhibited KDMs and DNA hypermethylation via inhibited TETs. (2) Pseudohypoxia—via inhibited prolyl hydroxylases (PHDs), leading to constitutively stabilized hypoxia-inducible factor (HIF) and subsequently induced hypoxia-response element (HRE)-regulated genes. (Figure generated with BioRender, https://biorender.com.)

oncometabolites, thus disturbing the balance of DNA methylation. Importantly, TET 1 and TET2 are known tumor suppressors, whose direct genetic loss of function leads to tumorigenic processes, particularly of mixed lineage leukemia (MLL) and acute myelogenous leukemia (AML), respectively (Huang et al. 2013; Tulstrup et al. 2021). Similar to DNA, histone methylation programs are orchestrated by the contrasting activities of histone methyltransferases and histone lysine and arginine demethylases. Of note, many lysine demethylases, especially those containing the Jumonji-like domain—JMJ, are αKG-dependent dioxygenases (Pollard et al. 2008; Johansson et al. 2014).

Multiple theories have also been put forward to answer how ROS may contribute to HIF-A stabilization under normoxic conditions, specifically in the context of SDH and FH mutations. It was suggested that ROS induces oxidation of iron cofactors of PHDs, while others suggest that ROS results in the up-regulation of HIF-A protein translation (Movafagh et al. 2015). Micro-RNAs (miRs) also take part in the hypoxia regulatory circuits. MiR-210, a HIF target, was shown to alter levels of iron-sulfur scaffold protein, ISCU, and subsequently induce ROS (Favaro et al. 2010). Furthermore, under acute hypoxia, HIF1 and HIF2 employ miR-210 to reduce the accumulation of HIF3, a dominant-negative regulator of HIF1 (Serocki et al. 2018). Similarly, miR-147 was shown in vitro to stabilize HIF1 via targeting of HIF3 (Wang et al. 2016). Taken together, the tumorigenic mechanism behind these cancers is the intersection between altered metabolism and aberrant gene expression.

While downstream mechanistic contribution of SDH or FH loss (and of IDH oncogenic mutations) to cancer converge on rather similar outcomes such as pseudohypoxia and hypermethylation phenotypes, there are apparent differences in the tissue of origin from which tumors with these different mutations arise. These differences can be the result of multiple factors. First, varied oncometabolites may have different effects on specific dioxygenases, and with that, on the transcriptomic and phenotypic outcome. Second, beyond their inhibitory effect on dioxygenases, the consequences of specific genetic alterations may have different metabolic adaptations and/or biochemical outcomes. Third, considering the housekeeping functions of the metabolic tumor suppressor genes, the ability of specific tissues to survive their genetic losses would dictate the ability of those tissues to feel and respond to the oncogenic effects of the accumulated oncometabolites.

THE BIOCHEMISTRY AND PATHOPHYSIOLOGY OF SUCCINATE DEHYDROGENASE

SDH, otherwise known as complex II of the electron transport chain (ETC), is an enzyme that serves as part of the oxidative phosphorylation machinery. It is a heterotetrameric protein complex that consists of two main components: (1) a catalytic core in the mitochondrial matrix, which is formed by two subunits, SDHA (c5p15.33) and SDHB (c1p36.13), as well as (2) a membrane component, formed by two additional subunits, SDHC (c1q23.3) and SDHD (c11q23.1), which anchor the enzyme complex to the inner mitochondrial membrane (Rutter et al. 2010; Bardella et al. 2011). The catalytic core of the enzyme aids in the organized transfer of electrons to ubiquinone. The membrane component works to stabilize the binding of ubiquinone to the enzyme via histidine ligands and a heme *b* moiety. Together with SDH assembly factors 1 and 2 (SDHAF1 [c19q13.12] and SDHAF2 [c11q12.2]), all of the above genes fall under the term SDHx (Dubard Gault et al. 2018).

Aberrations of each of the aforementioned enzyme subunits and their assembly factors are associated with specific cancer pathologies, namely, paraganglioma (PGL), pheochromocytoma (PHEO), gastrointestinal stromal tumors (GIST), renal cell carcinoma (RCC), and pituitary tumors (Pawlu et al. 2005; Fang et al. 2021; Loughrey et al. 2022). Of note, SDHB-associated tumors present with the most aggressive disease course and mortality (Amar et al. 2007). SDHC-related pathologies have been less extensively studied; however, a recent case series from across the United Kingdom details the mutation's relation to head and neck PGL, extra-adrenal PGL, and PHEO (Williams et al. 2022). SDHD is unique in that it is maternally imprinted, meaning that the maternal allele is silenced while the paternal allele is activated, which presents an interesting caveat to loss of heterozygosity in SDH-deficient cancers (Hensen et al. 2004; Bayley et al. 2014; Burnichon et al. 2017). Additionally, SDHD mutation is associated with more head and neck PGL than SDHB (Pawlu et al. 2005). Mutations of SDHA, unlike other SDHx genes, are rarely associated with hereditary PGL or PHEO (Burnichon et al. 2010). Rather, they are more often linked to GIST (Casey et al. 2017).

THE BIOCHEMISTRY AND PATHOPHYSIOLOGY OF FUMARATE HYDRATASE

The 10-exon-long FH gene is located at 1q42.1 in the human genome (Schmidt et al. 2020). It is formed by 510 amino acids folded into a structure with three functional domains: Central, amino-terminal lyase 1, and carboxyl-terminal fumarase C (Allegri et al. 2010). FH can be divided into two classes. Class I is dimeric and iron-dependent with an accompanying iron sulfur cluster, whereas class II is homotetrameric and iron-independent, mainly found in humans (Feliciano et al. 2016). Expression of this gene is differentially processed to form either a mitochondrial or cytosolic protein, distinguishable by pyroglutamic acid on the mitochondrial form and *N*-acetylalanine on the cytosolic form (Picaud et al. 2011). The mitochondrial isoform is of interest due to its utility in the TCA cycle and the cytosolic isoform is important due to its ability to metabolize fumarate from various metabolic processes like the urea cycle, and purine metabolism. Fumarate itself, a chemically reactive molecule, modifies cysteine residues on proteins and peptides like glutathione (Zheng et al. 2015). Germline mutations in the FH gene have been associated with hereditary leiomyomatosis and renal cell cancer (HLRCC), mainly type 2 renal papillary cancer (PRCC2), as well as cutaneous leiomyomas and uterine fibroids, which can be the presenting feature in women (Casey et al. 2020).

EMPLOYING KNOWLEDGE-BASED THERAPEUTICS

Many of the biochemical consequences of FH and SDH deficiency are alike. Therefore, similar therapeutic approaches related to general bioenergetic status or to the consequences of oncometabolite accumulation within these tumors should be considered. Nonetheless, there are major differences between the metabolic activities outside the mitochondria with FH and SDH. While SDH is relegated to the TCA cycle and ETC functions, FH has additional cytosolic and nuclear activities and, unlike succinate, fumarate itself is both substrate and product in many catalytic and noncatalytic, non-TCA cycle reactions (Yang et al. 2012a; Jiang et al. 2015; Eniafe and Jiang 2021; Solaimuthu et al. 2022). These unique traits may generate further diagnostic and therapeutic opportunities in the management of FH-deficient cancers.

Unfortunately, to date, no clinically specific targeted therapies have been approved for use in FH- and SDH-deficient cancers; however, the next section will recount where the current clinical entry points stand. To elaborate on these opportunities, the following will focus on targeted strategies toward (1) metabolic remodeling unique to these cancers, (2) oncometabolite-induced rewiring of the transcriptome, and (3) the biochemical consequences of nonenzymatic reactions due to increased fumarate in the cell.

METABOLIC REMODELING

Cancers are able to adapt their metabolism to feed the ever-growing tumor. In this light, TCA cycle-deficient cells specifically modulate the activities of energetic processes, particularly glycolytic flux, for the purpose of supporting energetic demands, enhanced cellular growth, and proliferation (Yang et al. 2012b). An effective way to target fermentative glycolysis and cytosolic NAD^+ recycling (required for effective glycolysis within the tumor) is to inhibit pyruvate reduction to lactate via lactate dehydrogenase (LDH) (Vazquez et al. 2016). Indeed, when LDH activity was genetically silenced with shRNA in xenografted FH-deficient tumors made from human cancer cells, a significant decrease in proliferation rate and tumor size was recorded (Xie et al. 2009). Nevertheless, despite many approaches and successful preclinical reports, LDH inhibitors did not yet progress to clinical use (Sharma et al. 2022). In addition to the increased glycolysis, TCA cycle-deficient cancers display other metabolic alterations. For example, decreased activity of the energy-sensing enzyme AMP-dependent protein kinase (AMPK) and subsequent decreased phosphorylation of acetyl CoA carboxylase, leads to increased fatty acid synthesis (Linehan and Rouault 2013). Whether such metabolic alterations create therapeutic opportunities is yet to be evaluated preclinically. Fatty acid synthesis inhibitors have been tested clinically (NCT03179904), but not in the context of SDH or FH deficiency.

Glutamine metabolism is a hallmark of cancer metabolism, by way of its sheer abundance and centrality in the donation of carbon and nitrogen to biosynthetic pathways critical to proliferation of the tumor (for example, amino, fatty, and nucleic acid synthesis), leading some cancer cells to become "glutamine addicted" (Masisi et al. 2020). Additionally, glutamine is implicated in ROS management via glutathione synthesis. Glutaminase plays an integral role in the production of glutamate from glutamine, which can further be modified to αKG to fuel the TCA cycle (Chen and Cui 2015). With all of these implicated pathways, therapeutic approaches under development target glutaminase in multiple cancers, including SDHB-associated PGLs and PHEOs (Table 1). In an in vitro PHEO model, a significantly increased GLS-1 expression in cells depleted of SDH function was reported (Sarkadi et al. 2020). Furthermore the selective GLS-1 inhibitor, bis-2-(5-phenylacetamido-1,3,4-thiadiazol-2-yl)ethyl sulfide (BPTES) decreased the number of proliferating, SDH-abrogated cells. In support of this in vitro study, SDHB-related cancers display up-regulated glutamine metabolism (Lussey-Lepoutre et al. 2015). In SDH-deficient tumors, glutaminolysis can further support succinate production, and its oncometabolic functions (Moreno et al. 2020). To this end, a small molecule, allosteric and selective glutaminase inhibitor, telaglenastat (formerly known as CB-839), was investigated in SDH-deficient tumors, among other solid tumors, in a clinical trial (NCT02071862). Telaglenastat was well tolerated and showed signs of anticancer activity in a limited cohort of SDH-deficient tumors; however, the current cohort was too small to draw significant conclusions (Harding et al. 2021). Recent literature also points to the added tumor-reducing benefit of combining GLS-1 inhibition with disruption of either (1) mTOR with everolimus, or (2) VEGF/MET/AXL with cabozantinib (Yang et al. 2019). It was suggested that such combination therapy reduced overall consumption of glucose and glutamine, resulting in antiproliferative effects, culminating in decreased production of ATP and cellular building blocks (Emberley et al. 2021). CANTATA (NCT03428217), a randomized, clinical, placebo-controlled, double-blind trial studied the synergy between telaglenastat and cabozantinib in RCC (Tannir et al. 2022). While preclinical studies showed promising results, the aforementioned combination failed to promote the efficacy of both agents in the context of RCC regression in general, showing equal progression-free survival in telaglenastat + carbozantinib versus placebo + carbozantinib. However, no separate analysis for SDH-deficient RCC was performed and numbers of SDH-deficient RCC were low (Tannir et al. 2022). ENTRATA (NCT03163667) studied the concomitant effect of everolimus and telaglenastat in RCC (Lee et al. 2022). The combination was well tolerated and improved progression-free survival. Nevertheless, no GLS-1 therapies (monotherapy or combined therapy) are known to benefit TCA cycle-deficient RCC to date.

Urea cycle is also dysregulated in FH-deficient cancers. Normally, arginosuccinate lyase (ASL) functions to create fumarate and arginine from arginosuccinate. However, in the context of high fumarate levels, the reaction is reversed by Le-Chatelierian equilibrium principles, resulting in a flux toward the precursor arginosuccinate (Vazquez et al. 2016). The arginine shunted into arginosuccinate production is taken from exogenous sources, while the fumarate is abundant due to the nature of the FH deficiency. This mechanism aids to sequester fumarate in the tumor cell in arginosuccinate and prevent it from reaching toxic levels, allowing permissive tumor growth. This delineates exogenous arginine as a limiting factor in the reaction. Therefore, it is targetable by way of either circulating arginine depletion or its import blockade for the obligate-arginine-auxotrophic tumor. To this end, pegylated arginine deiminase (ADI-PEG 20) was used in vitro to deplete extracellular arginine and the subsequent formation of arginosuccinate, resulting in decreased cellular proliferation of FH-deficient cancer cells (Zheng et al. 2013). Recently, ADI-PEG 20, when combined with spermidine analog GC7, N1-guanyl-1,7-diaminoheptane, was shown to prevent resistance to ADI-PEG 20 treatment through GC7-based TCA cycle inhibition (Carpentier et al. 2023). Furthering this to patients, there was a phase II/III clinical trial (NCT02709512) that adds ADI-PEG 20 to SOC (therapy including combination of permetrexed and cisplatin) treatment to patients with nonepithelioid malignant pleural mesothelioma portends to starve tumor cells of arginine, leading to cell death (Szlosarek et al. 2023). Hence, it is of interest to explore this therapy in the context of TCA cycle-deficient tumors, as these tumors may have defunct arginine production and, therefore, clinical use, providing a tolerable side effect profile in this specific patient population.

A potentially effective cancer therapeutic strategy identifies genes that become essential following a loss of a specific tumor suppressor, an approach known as "synthetic lethality." Considering the major metabolic consequences of FH loss and fumarate level induction, several synthetic lethal approaches were theorized for targeted therapy. One of the major metabolic consequences of FH loss is increased redox stress, exacerbated by glutathione succination (generated by a chemical reaction between fumarate and reduced thiol [-SH]) and managed by Nrf2 induction (Fig. 2B; Sullivan et al. 2013; Zheng et al. 2015). Additionally, SDHB-silenced tumors showed similar reliance on Nrf2-led expression profile to combat increased redox stress (Liu et al. 2020). This state allows for the therapeutic exploitation via synthetic lethality of several redox mediators. It was demonstrated that heme oxygenase (HO-1, enzyme and HMOX1, gene) is synthetically lethal with FH (www.ncbi.nlm.nih.gov/gene/3162#bibliography). HMOX1 is itself an Nrf2 target gene and, as such, an important antioxidant. Hence, selective killing of FH-deficient cancer cells can be achieved by specific inhibition of HO-1 (Frezza et al. 2011; Podkalicka et al. 2020). Another important Nrf2 target is the cystine transporter and ferroptosis mitigator, SLC7A11 (Koppula et al. 2021). Ferroptosis is a unique type of nonapoptotic, programmed cell death that is iron-dependent. Cystine, comprised of two oxidized cysteine molecules, is a plasma-circulating molecule that is uptaken by Nrf2-activated cells and subsequently reduced intracellularly to its constituent molecules, supporting glutathione biosynthesis (Vazquez et al. 2016). Indeed, it was demonstrated that FH-deficient cells in which glutathione is succinated and Nrf2 is induced, are dependent on SLC7A11 (Kerins et al. 2018). Despite the potential sensitization of FH-deficient cells to redox induction and ferroptosis-

inducing agents, to our knowledge, there are no ongoing clinical studies with HO-1 or SLC7A11 inhibitors.

Importantly, cells with a TCA cycle-deficient phenotype partially compensate for their telescoped TCA cycle through an altered production of the nonessential amino acid, aspartate, via pyruvate carboxylase that produces oxaloacetate, the precursor for aspartate, directly from pyruvate (Mullen et al. 2014; Cardaci et al. 2015). A small molecule tool compound, ZY-444, is a pyruvate carboxylate inhibitor, which demonstrated effective tumor growth inhibition in a preclinical model for breast cancer (Lin et al. 2020). By extension, this or similar pyruvate carboxylate inhibitors may have use in the targeting of TCA cycle-deficient tumors.

Cells under perpetual redox stress depend on NADPH production for the maintenance of reduced glutathione and for surviving redox stress. The oxidative pentose phosphate pathway (oxPPP) is a major player in the reduction of $NADP^+$ to NADPH. In line with that, FH-deficient cells demonstrate dependency on oxPPP (Adam et al. 2011; Yang et al. 2013). Targeting glucose-6-phosphatase dehydrogenase (G6PD), the first and rate-limiting enzyme of the oxPPP, has been explored as a potential therapeutic opportunity. Until recently, DHEA, an endogenous steroid, was thought to act as an inhibitor of G6PD; however, this is not the case (Ghergurovich et al. 2020). To the best of our knowledge, no further inhibitors of G6PD have been tested in the clinic, especially not within the context of TCA cycle-deficient cancers.

THERAPEUTIC OPPORTUNITIES DUE TO ONCOMETABOLITES

Accretions of oncometabolites elaborate unique phenotypes in SDH- and FH-deficient cancers, hinging on chromatin modification and genetic reprogramming. Targeted therapies and clinical trials, informed by twenty-first century scientific advances, have been elaborated to improve outcomes in these TCA cycle-deficient cancers. At first, tyrosine-kinase inhibitors (TKIs) had been highlighted as a therapeutic option for SDH-deficient GIST (Nannini et al. 2021). This is thought to

Table 1. Clinical trials for tricarboxylic acid (TCA) cycle-deficient cancers mentioned in the text

Disease	Trial ID	Title	Summary	Dates	Progress
FH-def (general) SDH-def (general) SDH-def GIST	NCT02071862	Study of the glutaminase inhibitor CB-839 in solid tumors	Exploiting tumors' dependence on glutamine, CB-839 used to inhibit tumors' glutaminase. Among other cancers, FH-deficient tumors, SDH-deficient GIST, and SDH-deficient non-GIST cancers were treated.	Feb 26, 2014– Jul 20, 2022	Completed
FH-def RCC SDH-def RCC	NCT04068831	Talazoparib and avelumab in participants with metastatic renal cell carcinoma	Patients received talazoparib (PARPi) and avelumab in context of either VHL-, SDH-, or FH-deficient RCC.	Aug 28, 2019– ongoing	Active, not recruiting
FH-def RCC	NCT04387500	Sintilimab injection combined with inlyta in fumarate hydratase- deficient renal cell carcinoma	Examining ORR and PFS (over 3 yr each) in response to sintilimab (PD-1i) injection and treatment with inlyta (tyrosine kinase inhibitor) in FH-deficient RCC.	May 14, 2020– ongoing	Active, recruiting
Nonspecific	NCT03428217	CANTATA: CB-839 with cabozantinib vs. cabozantinib with placebo in patients with metastatic renal cell carcinoma (CANTATA)	Nongenotyped RCC treatment with cabozantinib and either CB-839 or placebo to see differences between PFS in 18 mo, and OS in 36 mo.	Feb 9, 2018– Aug 23, 2021	Completed
Nonspecific	NCT03163667	CB-839 with everolimus vs. placebo with everolimus in participants with renal cell carcinoma (RCC) (ENTRATA)	Nongenotyped ccRCC treatment with everolimus and either CB-839 or placebo to see differences between PFS in 11.2 mo, and OS in 30.4 mo.	May 23, 2017– Sep 15, 2022	Completed
SDH-def GIST	NCT03556384	Temozolomide (TMZ) in advanced succinate dehydrogenase (SDH)-mutant/deficient gastrointestinal stromal tumor (GIST)	Examine the efficacy of TMZ in advanced SDH-deficient GIST via measures of ORR in 6 mo and PFS in 4 yr, OS in 4 yr, and detailed summary of adverse events over 6 mo.	June 14, 2018– ongoing	Recruiting

Continued

Table 1. *Continued*

Disease	Trial ID	Title	Summary	Dates	Progress
Nonspecific	NCT04394858	Testing the addition of an anticancer drug, olaparib, to the usual chemotherapy (temozolomide) for advanced neuroendocrine cancer	Nongenotyped neuroendocrine tumors (with future intention to segregate SDH deficiency) treated with temozolomide (tyrosine kinase inhibitor) plus olaparib (PARP-i) to observe PFS, OS, OR, and incidence of adverse events over 5 yr.	May 20, 2020–ongoing	Recruiting

be due to the lack of SDH, driving a hypoxic response via HIF-dependent transcription and consequent angiogenic cascade mediated by the vascular endothelial growth factor (VEGF) pathway. This hypothesis was initially confirmed in cells treated with sunitinib, a tyrosine kinase inhibitor with antiangiogenic properties via VEGFR inhibition (Cassol et al. 2014; Boikos et al. 2016). Within GIST, angiogenic genes were found to be up-regulated, suggesting that targeted therapies to VEGF and its receptors may have clinical utility (Favier et al. 2012). Of note, the first-line therapy for GIST overall, imatinib, serving as a c-kit inhibitor, is relatively ineffective in treating wild-type c-kit or PDGFR tumors (WT-GIST), half of which are SDH-deficient (Belinsky et al. 2017; Nannini et al. 2021). Therefore, specific therapies for TCA cycle-deficient cancers were tested based upon the up-regulation of angiogenic genes. Time to tumor progression was lengthened and multiple instances of disease stabilization were achieved upon treatment with sunitinib versus imatinib (Janeway et al. 2009). An observational study supported these findings by showing that four patients who experienced disease progression while under monotherapy with imatinib were stabilized with sunitinib and achieved disease control of their GIST (Liu et al. 2017). In agreement with the oncometabolic role of succinate, transcriptome analysis highlighted that the HIF2a transcriptional signature was up-regulated in SDH-

deficient PHEO and PGL (Favier et al. 2012). This is clinically significant, as targeted therapies to nullify the above transcription factor's response to the pseudohypoxic tumor microenvironment may prove useful. Belzutifan, an FDA-approved drug that impedes the interaction between HIF2a and its cotranscription factor ARNT/HIF1B, decreases tumor burden in VHL-deficient renal cancer (Courtney et al. 2018; Moog et al. 2020; Jonasch et al. 2021). Considering the pseudohypoxic phenotype, it is important to research the effects of this drug on TCA cycle-deficient tumors. Currently underway (NCT04924075) is a phase II study testing belzuitfan in advanced PGL, advanced GIST, and solid tumors, all with pseudohypoxia-related genetic alterations.

The importance of TET inhibition by oncometabolites has been typified in TCA cycle-deficient tumors in our understanding of the hypermethylation phenotype. Succinate- or fumarate-mediated HIF2a activation and TET2 inhibition generates a positive feedback loop between pseudohypoxia and hypermethylation (Fig. 1), in which HIF2a stimulates methylation processes while TET2 inhibition by the oncometabolites maintain an hypermethylation state that enables epithelial-to-mesenchymal transition (EMT)-mediated by HIF (Sciacovelli et al. 2016; Morin et al. 2020). O^6-methylguanine-DNA methyltransferase (MGMT) functions to repair DNA via the removal of alkyl groups from nucle-

A

Fumarate   +   Cysteine   2SC

B

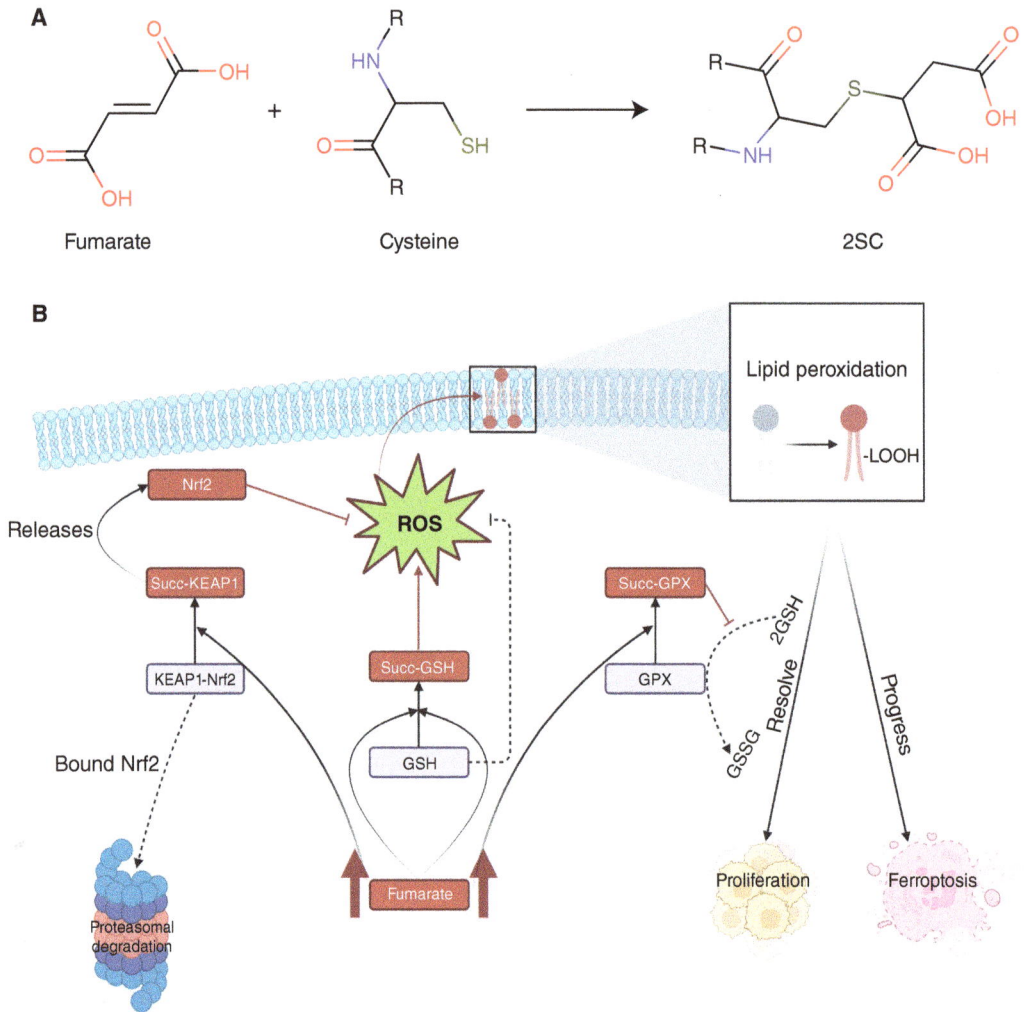

Figure 2. Schematic representation of molecular and cellular level changes caused by succination. (*A*) Chemical structure of succination: fumarate and cysteine combining to form *S*-(2-succinic)cysteine (2-SC). (*B*) Model of cellular pathways impacted by succination: Succination of glutathione and KEAP1 balances intracellular reactive oxygen species (ROS) levels through Nrf2 induction. GPX4 succination prevents efficient management of lipid peroxidation, sensitizing cells to ferroptosis. Dotted lines correspond to reactions that are inhibited by succination. (Figure generated with BioRender, https://biorender.com.)

otides, usually guanine. Without this important function, cells are vulnerable to alkylating agents. Extensive hypermethylation, particularly of the *MGMT* promoter region in glioblastoma, has been associated with increased sensitivity to temozolomide, an alkylating chemotherapeutic (Hegi et al. 2005; Ravegnini and Ricci 2019; Giger et al. 2022). There are ongoing studies to identify induced vulnerabilities associated with hypermethylation phenotype mediated by TET inhibi-

tion (Morin et al. 2020). However, temozolomide sensitivity in SDHx-deficient PHEO and PARA was assessed in a retrospective study detailing that temozolomide had limited efficacy (Perez et al. 2022). Interestingly, it has been reported that in SDH-deficient GIST, similarly to glioblastoma, MGMT hypermethylation of the promoter's CpG island is associated with lower expression of MGMT (Hadoux et al. 2014). Such a hypermethylation phenotype is likely associated with

TET and JmJ domain-containing histone demethylase inhibition by succinate (Letouzé et al. 2013). Therefore, NCT03556384, a phase 2 clinical study, assesses the efficacy of temozolomide on advanced SDH-deficient GIST with fulfillment of primary objectives expected in 2023.

Syrosingopine, an inhibitor of the monocarboxylate transporters 1 (MCT1) and MCT4, was used in conjunction with metformin, a mild oxidative phosphorylation inhibitor, to induce synthetic lethality via accumulation of lactate intracellularly (Benjamin et al. 2018). A similar approach has been taken to clinical trial via the MCT1 inhibitor AZD-3965 (NCT01791595) to induce intracellular lactate, thereby decreasing intracellular pH and disrupting the feedback networks of glycolysis (McNeillis et al. 2020). While these drugs have not yet been studied in the context of TCA cycle-deficient cancers, their mechanistic approach may be exploited.

An additional reported role for oncometabolites is their direct role in inducing DNA damage. Oncometabolites can inhibit homology-directed repair (HDR) pathways via the inhibition of KDM4B, a lysine demethylase, leading to increased hypermethylation of histone 3 lysine 9 (H3K9) (Sulkowski et al. 2018). Subsequently, the augmented hypermethylation of H3K9 adjacent to DNA damage sites disguises the signal needed for synchronous HDR function (Sulkowski et al. 2020). It has been suggested that Tip-60 is activated at double-strand break (DSB) sites where it complexes with ATM to repair DNA damage, and increased levels of oncometabolites make ATM less active (Sun et al. 2005). It was theorized that oncometabolites increase the methylation status of H3K9m3e3 so that the spike needed at DSBs is not detected above the new high threshold (Sulkowski et al. 2020). With disordered HDR mechanisms, cells become increasingly sensitive to PARP inhibitors such as olaparib and BMN-673 (Sulkowski et al. 2018). To this end, PARP inhibitors are currently being used in the clinic for PHEO and PGL in TCA cycle-deficient tumors (NCT04394858).

In recent years, our understanding of miRs has guided new and innovative therapies. For example, targeted reduction of the oncogenic miR-155 by the oligonucleotide anti-miR-155, cobomarsen, was shown to reduce tumor burden in cutaneous T-cell lymphoma and was therefore put to the test in subsequent clinical trials (Bartolucci et al. 2022). PHEO and PGLs associated with germline SDHx mutations were found to overexpress the HIF target, miR-210, both in vitro and in patient samples (Tsang et al. 2014). This is useful because it identifies miR-210 as a marker for pseudohypoxia within these TCA cycle-deficient cancers. MiR-210 functions by controlling certain vascular remodeling genes such as ephrin A3 (a ligand for ephrin receptor, associated with angiogenesis) (Hu et al. 2010). The sheer abundance of miR-210 may serve as reason enough to explore its essentiality in TCA cycle-deficient cells and to develop anti-miR-210 therapies for these tumors.

Many RNA epitranscriptome modulators (RNA demethylases) may also be affected by increased levels of oncometabolites (Mauer et al. 2019). These modulators act on RNA molecules and manage the dynamics of translation. For example, oncometabolites resulting from FH mutation inhibit FTO (fat mass and obesity-associated protein), the RNA demethylase acting on N^6-methyladenosine, whereas other RNA demethylases are spared, including those acting on N^1-methyladenosine and 5-formylcytosine (researchfestival.nih.gov/2023/posters/rewiring-rna-methylation-oncometabolite-fumarate-renal-cell-carcinoma). While FTO has been implicated in cancer, the mechanistic understanding underlying potential therapeutic opportunities is yet to be fully elucidated.

NONENZYMATIC ONCOMETABOLIC ROLE OF FUMARATE

FH-deficient cells accumulate fumarate and succinate and may present with dysfunction of complexes I and II of the ETC (Tyrakis et al. 2017). On the one hand, high levels of intracellular fumarate cause FH-deficient tumors to operate similarly to SDH-deficient tumors via pseudohypoxia and hypermethylation (Navarro et al. 2022). However, an important complexity to note is that fumarate is an inherently more reactive molecule than succinate.

Fumarate has been found to disrupt normal cellular function via the nonenzymatic covalent modification of cellular proteins (Fig. 2A) to form S-(2-succinyl)cysteine (aka 2-succinocysteine [2SC]) in a posttranslational process aptly named "succination" (Alderson et al. 2006). These processes induce perturbations of multiple reactions that generate potential biomarkers for FH-deficient tumors. Of note, a recent study discovered unique fumarate-altered metabolites in the circulation of patients harboring FH-deficient RCC (Zheng et al. 2023). These metabolites, succinyl-adenosine and succinic-cysteine (in a free amino acid format, not as a posttranslational protein decoration), enable disease detection at early respectable stages, and, therefore, effective monitoring of liquid biopsies may become a lifesaving clinical practice. Immunohistochemical staining of 2SC-decorated proteins is a useful diagnostic technique in the pathological confirmation of FH-deficient cancers (Trpkov et al. 2016). However, unlike periodic monitoring of plasma metabolites, the visualization diagnostic approach depends on attaining biopsies and cannot be used for early detection or to monitor disease progression. Nevertheless, nonenzymatic protein succination can play a mechanistic role in the tumorigenic process and may expose vulnerabilities of FH-deficient tumors. For instance, the inhibition via succination of the E3 ubiquitin ligase kelch-like ECH-associated protein 1 (KEAP1) prevents the degradation of Nrf2 and then acts via a "feedforward" mechanism to reinforce an antioxidant environment ideal for tumor growth (Adam et al. 2011; Sullivan et al. 2013; Sourbier et al. 2019; Rogerson et al. 2023). From an immune standpoint, Nrf2 has been shown to inhibit interferon β and quells the innate immune response, setting an anti-inflammatory scene for the tumor to grow (Ryan et al. 2022). Nrf2-inhibitors have been elaborated to induce a proapoptotic response (Pouremamali et al. 2022). With this knowledge, investigators have sought to systematically attack FH-deficient tumors with ROS-based therapies. Bortezamib, a potent ROS inducer via proteasomal dysfunction, has been shown to counteract the innate antioxidant mechanisms of FH-deficient cancers and lower tumor burden when combined with cisplatin in preclinical studies (Sourbier et al. 2010). Succinated, therefore defunct, glutathione peroxidase 4 (GPX4) is also seen in FH-deficient cells (Kerins et al. 2018). GPX4 normally protects cells from lipid peroxidation, as such, its succination by fumarate further sensitizes cells to ferroptosis (Kerins et al. 2018; Stockwell 2019). Counterintuitively though, FH-deficient cells express increased levels of GPX4 and are hypersensitive to direct GPX4 inhibitors RSL3 and ML162 (Kerins et al. 2018). Fumarate accumulation has also been linked to inhibition of PTEN via posttranslational succination at its cysteine 211, precluding the succinated PTEN moiety from anchoring to the plasma membrane, thereby leading to up-regulation of phosphoinositide 3-kinase (PI3K)/protein kinase B (AKT) signaling pathway (Ge et al. 2022). This allows for potential therapeutics targeting the deregulated PI3K/AKT signaling via PI3K and AKT inhibitors. To date, AKT inhibitors have not shown much promise due to toxic side effects (Duan et al. 2020). However, PI3K inhibitors have been tried preclinically and showed efficacy (Van Looy et al. 2014). Nevertheless, treatment with PI3K inhibitors induced adaptive mutations in *PTEN* that nullified the treatment efficacy (Papa and Pandolfi 2019). It would be of interest to learn whether PI3K activation via PTEN cysteine succination would be more sensitive to PI3K inhibitors and less likely to develop resistance.

METABOLITES AS DIAGNOSTIC BIOMARKERS

Through the above discussion, we have elaborated on the link between genetic deficiencies of the TCA cycle and the unique metabolic landscape of the tumor and circulation. Such dramatic metabolic changes can be harnessed to monitor tumor burden and, with that, treatment efficacy. Magnetic resonance spectroscopy has been used serially to monitor metabolites in vivo, specifically succinate and fumarate levels in patients with SDH and FH deficiency, respectively (Lussey-Lepoutre et al. 2020; Wu et al. 2022). This works by detecting peaks of compounds of interest that do not overlap with other compounds to identify a clear signal, correlated to the compound of interest. This method has been proven compatible within a diverse array of TCA cycle-deficient cancers (Branzoli et al. 2023). Beyond traditional measures of tumor size, longitudinal metabolic imaging analyses may offer a noninvasive approach to record response to treatment (Moog et al. 2022). Beyond metabolic imaging, circulating metabolites may also be used as diagnostic biomarkers to monitor tumor burden and pharmacodynamic biomarkers to monitor treatment efficacy. Indeed, succinyladenosine and succinocysteine, the two circulating metabolites mentioned above, normally serve as classifiers for FH-deficient RCC, and were also used to effectively monitor disease progression and treatment response (Zheng et al. 2023).

DISCUSSION

Succinate dehydrogenase and fumarate hydratase are two key enzymes involved in the TCA cycle. Mutations in these enzymes have been associated with the development of various types of cancer, including paragangliomas, pheochromocytomas, renal cell carcinoma, and leiomyomas. The mutations in these enzymes lead to the accumulation of succinate and fumarate, respectively, which can have profound effects on cellular metabolism and lead to a variety of oncometabolic changes, including but not limited to the reconstruction of the tumor cell's vital metabolic processes, the adaptation of its expression profile, and the deleterious accumulation of reactive intermediates in the cell. Clinical trials have been conducted to explore the potential of targeting these oncometabolic changes for therapeutic purposes. Notable approaches include the targeting of glycolytic flux, glutamine metabolism, ferroptosis, TET inhibition, among others. Current therapies for tumors with SDH and FH mutations are limited. Surgical resection is often the first-line treatment for localized tumors, and there are no specific targeted therapies approved for TCA cycle-deficient cancers. However, advances in our understanding of the oncometabolic changes associated with SDH and FH mutations may lead to the development of more effective targeted therapies in the future.

CONCLUSION

Through the lens of this review, we wish to bring to the forefront the most recent advances in both the biological underpinnings of TCA cycle-deficient cancers, the rationale for clinical trials targeting vulnerabilities in these cancers as they stand in the early 2020s, and future prospects for therapeutic developments in avenues yet to be explored in-clinic. To date, there are currently no targeted therapies approved for tumors with SDH and FH mutations and many of our treatment options currently swing with the surgical knife, rather than tried and proven biological remedies. With hope for the future, advances in our understanding of the underlying oncometabolic changes associated with mutations of TCA cycle-deficient cancers may lead to the development of more effective combined therapeutic approaches, improving outcomes for afflicted patients.

REFERENCES

*Reference is also in this subject collection.

Adam J, Hatipoglu E, O'Flaherty L, Ternette N, Sahgal N, Lockstone H, Baban D, Nye E, Stamp GW, Wolhuter K, et al. 2011. Renal cyst formation in Fh1-deficient mice is independent of the Hif/Phd pathway: roles for fumarate in KEAP1 succination and Nrf2 signaling. *Cancer Cell* **20**: 524–537 doi:10.1016/j.ccr.2011.09.006

Alderson NL, Wang Y, Blatnik M, Frizzell N, Walla MD, Lyons TJ, Alt N, Carson JA, Nagai R, Thorpe SR, et al. 2006. S-(2-succinyl)cysteine: a novel chemical modification of tissue proteins by a Krebs cycle intermediate. *Arch Biochem Biophys* **450**: 1–8. doi:10.1016/j.abb.2006.03.005

Allegri G, Fernandes MJ, Scalco FB, Correia P, Simoni RE, Llerena JC Jr, de Oliveira ML. 2010. Fumaric aciduria: an overview and the first Brazilian case report. *J Inherit Metab Dis* **33**: 411–419. doi:10.1007/s10545-010-9134-2

Amar L, Baudin E, Burnichon N, Peyrard S, Silvera S, Bertherat J, Bertagna X, Schlumberger M, Jeunemaitre X, Gimenez-Roqueplo AP, et al. 2007. Succinate dehydrogenase B gene mutations predict survival in patients with malignant pheochromocytomas or paragangliomas. *J Clin Endocrinol Metab* **92**: 3822–3828. doi:10.1210/jc.2007-0709

Arnold PK, Finley LWS. 2023. Regulation and function of the mammalian tricarboxylic acid cycle. *J Biol Chem* **299**: 102838. doi:10.1016/j.jbc.2022.102838

Bardella C, Pollard PJ, Tomlinson I. 2011. SDH mutations in cancer. *Biochim Biophys Acta* **1807**: 1432–1443. doi:10.1016/j.bbabio.2011.07.003

Bartolucci D, Pession A, Hrelia P, Tonelli R. 2022. Precision anti-cancer medicines by oligonucleotide therapeutics in clinical research targeting undruggable proteins and non-coding RNAs. *Pharmaceutics* **14**: 1453. doi:10.3390/phar maceutics14071453

Bayley JP, Oldenburg RA, Nuk J, Hoekstra AS, van der Meer CA, Korpershoek E, McGillivray B, Corssmit EPM, Dinjens WNM, de Krijger RR, et al. 2014. Paraganglioma and pheochromocytoma upon maternal transmission of SDHD mutations. *BMC Med Genet* **15**: 111. doi:10.1186/s12881-014-0111-8

Belinsky MG, Cai KQ, Zhou Y, Luo B, Pei J, Rink L, von Mehren M. 2017. Succinate dehydrogenase deficiency in a PDGFRA mutated GIST. *BMC Cancer* **17**: 512. doi:10.1186/s12885-017-3499-7

Benjamin D, Robay D, Hindupur SK, Pohlmann J, Colombi M, El-Shemerly MY, Maira SM, Moroni C, Lane HA, Hall MN. 2018. Dual inhibition of the lactate transporters MCT1 and MCT4 is synthetic lethal with metformin due to NAD⁺ depletion in cancer cells. *Cell Rep* **25**: 3047–3058. e4. doi:10.1016/j.celrep.2018.11.043

Boikos SA, Pappo AS, Killian JK, LaQuaglia MP, Weldon CB, George S, Trent JC, von Mehren M, Wright JA, Schiffman JD, et al. 2016. Molecular subtypes of *KIT/PDGFRA* wild-type gastrointestinal stromal tumors: a report from the National Institutes of Health Gastrointestinal Stromal Tumor Clinic. *JAMA Oncol* **2**: 922–928. doi:10.1001/jamaoncol.2016.0256

Branzoli F, Salgues B, Marjańska M, Laloi-Michelin M, Herman P, Le Collen L, Delemer B, Riancho J, Kuhn E, Jublanc C, et al. 2023. SDHx mutation and pituitary adenoma: can in vivo 1H-MR spectroscopy unravel the link? *Endocr Relat Cancer* **30**: e220198. doi:10.1530/ERC-22-0198

Burnichon N, Brière JJ, Libé R, Vescovo L, Rivière J, Tissier F, Jouanno E, Jeunemaitre X, Bénit P, Tzagoloff A, et al. 2010. SDHA is a tumor suppressor gene causing paraganglioma. *Hum Mol Genet* **19**: 3011–3020. doi:10.1093/hmg/ddq206

Burnichon N, Mazzella JM, Drui D, Amar L, Bertherat J, Coupier I, Delemer B, Guilhem I, Herman P, Kerlan V, et al. 2017. Risk assessment of maternally inherited *SDHD* paraganglioma and phaeochromocytoma. *J Med Genet* **54**: 125–133. doi:10.1136/jmedgenet-2016-104297

Cardaci S, Zheng L, MacKay G, van den Broek NJF, MacKenzie ED, Nixon C, Stevenson D, Tumanov S, Bulusu V, Kamphorst JJ, et al. 2015. Pyruvate carboxylation enables growth of SDH-deficient cells by supporting aspartate biosynthesis. *Nat Cell Biol* **17**: 1317–1326. doi:10.1038/ncb3233

Carpentier J, Szlosarek PW, Martin SA. 2023. Abstract 1760: ADI-PEG20 and GC7 as a novel anti-metabolite strategy for the treatment of malignant pleural mesothelioma. *Cancer Res* **83**: 1760–1760. doi:10.1158/1538-7445.AM2023-1760

Casey RT, Ascher DB, Rattenberry E, Izatt L, Andrews KA, Simpson HL, Challis B, Park SM, Bulusu VR, Lalloo F, et al. 2017. SDHA related tumorigenesis: a new case series and literature review for variant interpretation and pathogenicity. *Mol Genet Genomic Med* **5**: 237–250. doi:10.1002/mgg3.279

Casey RT, McLean MA, Challis BG, McVeigh TP, Warren AY, Mendil L, Houghton R, De Sanctis S, Kosmoliaptsis V, Sandford RN, et al. 2020. Fumarate metabolic signature for the detection of reed syndrome in humans. *Clin Cancer Res* **26**: 391–396. doi:10.1158/1078-0432.CCR-19-1729

Cassol CA, Winer D, Liu W, Guo M, Ezzat S, Asa SL. 2014. Tyrosine kinase receptors as molecular targets in pheochromocytomas and paragangliomas. *Mod Pathol* **27**: 1050–1062. doi:10.1038/modpathol.2013.233

Chen L, Cui H. 2015. Targeting glutamine induces apoptosis: a cancer therapy approach. *Int J Mol Sci* **16**: 22830–22855. doi:10.3390/ijms160922830

Chowdhury R, Yeoh KK, Tian YM, Hillringhaus L, Bagg EA, Rose NR, Leung IKH, Li XS, Woon ECY, Yang M, et al. 2011. The oncometabolite 2-hydroxyglutarate inhibits histone lysine demethylases. *EMBO Rep* **12**: 463–469. doi:10.1038/embor.2011.43

Courtney KD, Infante JR, Lam ET, Figlin RA, Rini BI, Brugarolas J, Zojwalla NJ, Lowe AM, Wang K, Wallace EM, et al. 2018. Phase I dose-escalation trial of PT2385, a first-in-class hypoxia-inducible factor-2α antagonist in patients with previously treated advanced clear cell renal cell carcinoma. *J Clin Oncol* **36**: 867–874. doi:10.1200/JCO.2017.74.2627

Duan Y, Haybaeck J, Yang Z. 2020. Therapeutic potential of PI3K/AKT/mTOR pathway in gastrointestinal stromal tumors: rationale and progress. *Cancers (Basel)* **12**: 2972. doi:10.3390/cancers12102972

Dubard Gault M, Mandelker D, DeLair D, Stewart CR, Kemel Y, Sheehan MR, Siegel B, Kennedy J, Marcell V, Arnold A, et al. 2018. Germline *SDHA* mutations in children and adults with cancer. *Cold Spring Harb Mol Case Stud* **4**: a002584. doi:10.1101/mcs.a002584

Emberley E, Pan A, Chen J, Dang R, Gross M, Huang T, Li W, MacKinnon A, Singh D, Sotirovska N, et al. 2021. The glutaminase inhibitor telaglenastat enhances the antitumor activity of signal transduction inhibitors everolimus and cabozantinib in models of renal cell carcinoma. *PLoS ONE* **16**: e0259241. doi:10.1371/journal.pone.0259241

Eniafe J, Jiang S. 2021. The functional roles of TCA cycle metabolites in cancer. *Oncogene* **40**: 3351–3363. doi:10.1038/s41388-020-01639-8

Fang Z, Sun Q, Yang H, Zheng J. 2021. SDHB suppresses the tumorigenesis and development of ccRCC by inhibiting glycolysis. *Front Oncol* **11**: 639408. doi:10.3389/fonc.2021.639408

Favaro E, Ramachandran A, McCormick R, Gee H, Blancher C, Crosby M, Devlin C, Blick C, Buffa F, Li JL, et al. 2010. MicroRNA-210 regulates mitochondrial free radical response to hypoxia and Krebs cycle in cancer cells by targeting iron sulfur cluster protein ISCU. *PLoS ONE* **5**: e10345. doi:10.1371/journal.pone.0010345

Favier J, Igaz P, Burnichon N, Amar L, Libé R, Badoual C, Tissier F, Bertherat J, Plouin PF, Jeunemaitre X, et al. 2012. Rationale for anti-angiogenic therapy in pheochromocytoma and paraganglioma. *Endocr Pathol* **23**: 34–42. doi:10.1007/s12022-011-9189-0

Feliciano PR, Drennan CL, Nonato MC. 2016. Crystal structure of an Fe-S cluster-containing fumarate hydratase enzyme from *Leishmania major* reveals a unique protein fold. *Proc Natl Acad Sci* **113**: 9804–9809. doi:10.1073/pnas.1605031113

Frezza C, Zheng L, Folger O, Rajagopalan KN, MacKenzie ED, Jerby L, Micaroni M, Chaneton B, Adam J, Hedley A, et al. 2011. Haem oxygenase is synthetically lethal with the tumour suppressor fumarate hydratase. *Nature* **477**: 225–228. doi:10.1038/nature10363

Cite this article as *Cold Spring Harb Perspect Med* doi: 10.1101/cshperspect.a041536

Ge X, Li M, Yin J, Shi Z, Fu Y, Zhao N, Chen H, Meng L, Li X, Hu Z, et al. 2022. Fumarate inhibits PTEN to promote tumorigenesis and therapeutic resistance of type2 papillary renal cell carcinoma. *Mol Cell* **82:** 1249–1260.e7. doi:10.1016/j.molcel.2022.01.029

Ghergurovich JM, García-Cañaveras JC, Wang J, Schmidt E, Zhang Z, TeSlaa T, Patel H, Chen L, Britt EC, Piqueras-Nebot M, et al. 2020. A small molecule G6PD inhibitor reveals immune dependence on pentose phosphate pathway. *Nat Chem Biol* **16:** 731–739. doi:10.1038/s41589-020-0533-x

Giger OT, Ten Hoopen R, Shorthouse D, Abdullahi S, Bulusu VR, Jadhav S, Maher ER, Casey RT. 2022. Preferential *MGMT* hypermethylation in SDH-deficient wild-type GIST. *J Clin Pathol* jcp-2022-208462. doi:10.1136/jcp-2022-208462

* Gunn K, Losman JA. 2023. Isocitrate dehydrogenase mutations in cancer: mechanisms of transformation and metabolic liability. *Cold Spring Harb Perspect Med* doi:10.1101/cshperspect.a041537

Hadoux J, Favier J, Scoazec JY, Leboulleux S, Al Ghuzlan A, Caramella C, Déandreis D, Borget I, Loriot C, Chougnet C, et al. 2014. *SDHB* mutations are associated with response to temozolomide in patients with metastatic pheochromocytoma or paraganglioma. *Int J Cancer* **135:** 2711–2720. doi:10.1002/ijc.28913

Harding M, Telli M, Munster P, Voss MH, Infante JR, De-Michele A, Dunphy M, Le MH, Molineaux C, Orford K, et al. 2021. A phase I dose-escalation and expansion study of telaglenastat in patients with advanced or metastatic solid tumors. *Clin Cancer Res* **27:** 4994–5003.

Hayashi Y, Yokota A, Harada H, Huang G. 2019. Hypoxia/pseudohypoxia-mediated activation of hypoxia-inducible factor-1α in cancer. *Cancer Sci* **110:** 1510–1517. doi:10.1111/cas.13990

Hegi ME, Diserens AC, Gorlia T, Hamou MF, de Tribolet N, Weller M, Kros JM, Hainfellner JA, Mason W, Mariani L, et al. 2005. *MGMT* gene silencing and benefit from temozolomide in glioblastoma. *N Engl J Med* **352:** 997–1003. doi:10.1056/NEJMoa043331

Hensen EF, Jordanova ES, van Minderhout IJ, Hogendoorn PC, Taschner PE, van der Mey AG, Devilee P, Cornelisse CJ. 2004. Somatic loss of maternal chromosome 11 causes parent-of-origin-dependent inheritance in SDHD-linked paraganglioma and phaeochromocytoma families. *Oncogene* **23:** 4076–4083. doi:10.1038/sj.onc.1207591

Hu S, Huang M, Li Z, Jia F, Ghosh Z, Lijkwan MA, Fasanaro P, Sun N, Wang X, Martelli F, et al. 2010. MicroRNA-210 as a novel therapy for treatment of ischemic heart disease. *Circulation* **122:** S124–S131.

Huang H, Jiang X, Li Z, Li Y, Song CX, He C, Sun M, Chen P, Gurbuxani S, Wang J, et al. 2013. TET1 plays an essential oncogenic role in MLL-rearranged leukemia. *Proc Natl Acad Sci* **110:** 11994–11999. doi:10.1073/pnas.1310656110

Inoue S, Lemonnier F, Mak TW. 2016. Roles of IDH1/2 and TET2 mutations in myeloid disorders. *Int J Hematol* **103:** 627–633. doi:10.1007/s12185-016-1973-7

Janeway KA, Albritton KH, Van Den Abbeele AD, D'Amato GZ, Pedrazzoli P, Siena S, Picus J, Butrynski JE, Schlemmer M, Heinrich MC, et al. 2009. Sunitinib treatment in pediatric patients with advanced GIST following failure of imatinib. *Pediatr Blood Cancer* **52:** 767–771. doi:10.1002/pbc.21909

Jiang Y, Qian X, Shen J, Wang Y, Li X, Liu R, Xia Y, Chen Q, Peng G, Lin SY, et al. 2015. Local generation of fumarate promotes DNA repair through inhibition of histone H3 demethylation. *Nat Cell Biol* **17:** 1158–1168. doi:10.1038/ncb3209

Johansson C, Tumber A, Che K, Cain P, Nowak R, Gileadi C, Oppermann U. 2014. The roles of Jumonji-type oxygenases in human disease. *Epigenomics* **6:** 89–120. doi:10.2217/epi.13.79

Jonasch E, Donskov F, Iliopoulos O, Rathmell WK, Narayan VK, Maughan BL, Oudard S, Else T, Maranchie JK, Welsh SJ, et al. 2021. Belzutifan for renal cell carcinoma in von Hippel–Lindau disease. *N Engl J Med* **385:** 2036–2046. doi:10.1056/NEJMoa2103425

Kerins MJ, Milligan J, Wohlschlegel JA, Ooi A. 2018. Fumarate hydratase inactivation in hereditary leiomyomatosis and renal cell cancer is synthetic lethal with ferroptosis induction. *Cancer Sci* **109:** 2757–2766. doi:10.1111/cas.13701

Knudson AG. 1971. Mutation and cancer: statistical study of retinoblastoma. *Proc Natl Acad Sci* **68:** 820–823. doi:10.1073/pnas.68.4.820

Koppula P, Zhuang L, Gan B. 2021. Cystine transporter SLC7A11/xCT in cancer: ferroptosis, nutrient dependency, and cancer therapy. *Protein Cell* **12:** 599–620. doi:10.1007/s13238-020-00789-5

Lee CH, Motzer R, Emamekhoo H, Matrana M, Percent I, Hsieh JJ, Hussain A, Vaishampayan U, Liu S, McCune S, et al. 2022. Telaglenastat plus everolimus in advanced renal cell carcinoma: a randomized, double-blinded, placebo-controlled, phase II ENTRATA trial. *Clin Cancer Res* **28:** 3248–3255. doi:10.1158/1078-0432.CCR-22-0061

Letouzé E, Martinelli C, Loriot C, Burnichon N, Abermil N, Ottolenghi C, Janin M, Menara M, Nguyen AT, Benit P, et al. 2013. SDH mutations establish a hypermethylator phenotype in paraganglioma. *Cancer Cell* **23:** 739–752. doi:10.1016/j.ccr.2013.04.018

Lin Q, He Y, Wang X, Zhang Y, Hu M, Guo W, He Y, Zhang T, Lai L, Sun Z, et al. 2020. Targeting pyruvate carboxylase by a small molecule suppresses breast cancer progression. *Adv Sci* **7:** 1903483. doi:10.1002/advs.201903483

Linehan WM, Rouault TA. 2013. Molecular pathways: fumarate hydratase-deficient kidney cancer—targeting the Warburg effect in cancer. *Clin Cancer Res* **19:** 3345–3352. doi:10.1158/1078-0432.CCR-13-0304

Liu W, Zeng X, Wu X, He J, Gao J, Shuai X, Wang G, Zhang P, Tao K. 2017. Clinicopathologic study of succinate-dehydrogenase-deficient gastrointestinal stromal tumors: a single-institutional experience in China. *Medicine (Baltimore)* **96:** e7668. doi:10.1097/MD.0000000000007668

Liu Y, Pang Y, Caisova V, Ding J, Yu D, Zhou Y, Huynh TT, Ghayee H, Pacak K, Yang C. 2020. Targeting NRF2-governed glutathione synthesis for SDHB-mutated pheochromocytoma and paraganglioma. *Cancers (Basel)* **12:** 280. doi:10.3390/cancers12020280

Losman JA, Koivunen P, Kaelin WG. 2020. 2-Oxoglutarate-dependent dioxygenases in cancer. *Nat Rev Cancer* **20:** 710–726. doi:10.1038/s41568-020-00303-3

Loughrey PB, Roncaroli F, Healy E, Weir P, Basetti M, Casey RT, Hunter SJ, Korbonits M. 2022. Succinate dehydrogenase and MYC-associated factor X mutations in pituitary neuroendocrine tumours. *Endocr Relat Cancer* **29**: R157–R172. doi:10.1530/ERC-22-0157

Lussey-Lepoutre C, Hollinshead KER, Ludwig C, Menara M, Morin A, Castro-Vega LJ, Parker SJ, Janin M, Martinelli C, Ottolenghi C, et al. 2015. Loss of succinate dehydrogenase activity results in dependency on pyruvate carboxylation for cellular anabolism. *Nat Commun* **6**: 8784. doi:10.1038/ncomms9784

Lussey-Lepoutre C, Bellucci A, Burnichon N, Amar L, Buffet A, Drossart T, Fontaine S, Clement O, Benit P, Rustin P, et al. 2020. Succinate detection using in vivo 1H-MR spectroscopy identifies germline and somatic SDHx mutations in paragangliomas. *Eur J Nucl Med Mol Imaging* **47**: 1510–1517 doi:10.1007/s00259-019-04633-9

Marxsen JH, Stengel P, Doege K, Heikkinen P, Jokilehto T, Wagner T, Jelkmann W, Jaakkola P, Metzen E. 2004. Hypoxia-inducible factor-1 (HIF-1) promotes its degradation by induction of HIF-α-prolyl-4-hydroxylases. *Biochem J* **381**: 761–767. doi:10.1042/BJ20040620

Masisi BK, El Ansari R, Alfarsi L, Rakha EA, Green AR, Craze ML. 2020. The role of glutaminase in cancer. *Histopathology* **76**: 498–508. doi:10.1111/his.14014

Mauer J, Sindelar M, Despic V, Guez T, Hawley BR, Vasseur JJ, Rentmeister A, Gross SS, Pellizzoni L, Debart F, et al. 2019. FTO controls reversible m6Am RNA methylation during snRNA biogenesis. *Nat Chem Biol* **15**: 340–347. doi:10.1038/s41589-019-0231-8

McNeill LA, Hewitson KS, Gleadle JM, Horsfall LE, Oldham NJ, Maxwell PH, Pugh CW, Ratcliffe PJ, Schofield CJ. 2002. The use of dioxygen by HIF prolyl hydroxylase (PHD1). *Bioorg Med Chem Lett* **12**: 1547–1550. doi:10.1016/s0960-894x(02)00219-6

McNeillis R, Greystoke A, Walton J, Bacon C, Keun H, Siskos A, Petrides G, Leech N, Jenkinson F, Bowron A, et al. 2020. A case of malignant hyperlactaemic acidosis appearing upon treatment with the mono-carboxylase transporter 1 inhibitor AZD3965. *Br J Cancer* **122**: 1141–1145. doi:10.1038/s41416-020-0727-8

Moog S, Lussey-Lepoutre C, Favier J. 2020. Epigenetic and metabolic reprogramming of SDH-deficient paragangliomas. *Endocr Relat Cancer* **27**: R451–R463. doi:10.1530/ERC-20-0346

Moog S, Salgues B, Braik-Djellas Y, Viel T, Balvay D, Autret G, Robidel E, Gimenez-Roquepló AP, Tavitian B, Lussey-Lepoutre C, et al. 2022. Preclinical evaluation of targeted therapies in Sdhb-mutated tumors. *Endocr Relat Cancer* **29**: 375–388. doi:10.1530/ERC-22-0030

Moreno C, Santos RM, Burns R, Zhang WC. 2020. Succinate dehydrogenase and ribonucleic acid networks in cancer and other diseases. *Cancers (Basel)* **12**: 3237. doi:10.3390/cancers12113237

Morin A, Goncalves J, Moog S, Castro-Vega LJ, Job S, Buffet A, Fontenille MJ, Woszczyk J, Gimenez-Roquepló AP, Letouzé E, et al. 2020. TET-mediated hypermethylation primes SDH-deficient cells for HIF2α-driven mesenchymal transition. *Cell Rep* **30**: 4551–4566.e7. doi:10.1016/j.celrep.2020.03.022

Movafagh S, Crook S, Vo K. 2015. Regulation of hypoxia-inducible factor-1a by reactive oxygen species: new developments in an old debate. *J Cell Biochem* **116**: 696–703. doi:10.1002/jcb.25074

Mullen AR, Hu Z, Shi X, Jiang L, Boroughs LK, Kovacs Z, Boriack R, Rakheja D, Sullivan LB, Linehan WM, et al. 2014. Oxidation of α-ketoglutarate is required for reductive carboxylation in cancer cells with mitochondrial defects. *Cell Rep* **7**: 1679–1690. doi:10.1016/j.celrep.2014.04.037

Nannini M, Rizzo A, Indio V, Schipani A, Astolfi A, Pantaleo MA. 2021. Targeted therapy in *SDH*-deficient GIST. *Ther Adv Med Oncol* **13**: 1758835921102232. doi:10.1177/17588359211023278

Navarro C, Ortega Á, Santeliz R, Garrido B, Chacín M, Galban N, Vera I, De Sanctis JB, Bermúdez V. 2022. Metabolic reprogramming in cancer cells: emerging molecular mechanisms and novel therapeutic approaches. *Pharmaceutics* **14**: 1303. doi:10.3390/pharmaceutics14061303

Nguyen TL, Durán RV. 2016. Prolyl hydroxylase domain enzymes and their role in cell signaling and cancer metabolism. *Int J Biochem Cell Biol* **80**: 71–80. doi:10.1016/j.biocel.2016.09.026

Nowicki S, Gottlieb E. 2015. Oncometabolites: tailoring our genes. *FEBS J* **282**: 2796–2805. doi:10.1111/febs.13295

Papa A, Pandolfi PP. 2019. The PTEN–PI3K axis in cancer. *Biomolecules* **9**: 153. doi:10.3390/biom9040153

Parker SJ, Metallo CM. 2015. Metabolic consequences of oncogenic IDH mutations. *Pharmacol Ther* **152**: 54–62. doi:10.1016/j.pharmthera.2015.05.003

Pawlu C, Bausch B, Neumann HP. 2005. Mutations of the SDHB and SDHD genes. *Fam Cancer* **4**: 49–54. doi:10.1007/s10689-004-4227-4

Perez K, Jacene H, Hornick JL, Ma C, Vaz N, Brais LK, Alexander H, Baddoo W, Astone K, Esplin ED, et al. 2022. SDHx mutations and temozolomide in malignant pheochromocytoma and paraganglioma. *Endocr Relat Cancer* **29**: 533–544. doi:10.1530/ERC-21-0392

Picaud S, Kavanagh KL, Yue WW, Lee WH, Muller-Knapp S, Gileadi O, Sacchettini J, Oppermann U. 2011. Structural basis of fumarate hydratase deficiency. *J Inherit Metab Dis* **34**: 671–676. doi:10.1007/s10545-011-9294-8

Podkalicka P, Mucha O, Kruczek S, Biela A, Andrysiak K, Stępniewski J, Mikulski M, Gałęzowski M, Sitarz K, Brzózka K, et al. 2020. Synthetically lethal interactions of heme oxygenase-1 and fumarate hydratase genes. *Biomolecules* **10**: 143. doi:10.3390/biom10010143

Pollard PJ, Loenarz C, Mole DR, McDonough MA, Gleadle JM, Schofield CJ, Ratcliffe PJ. 2008. Regulation of Jumonji-domain-containing histone demethylases by hypoxia-inducible factor (HIF)-1α. *Biochem J* **416**: 387–394. doi:10.1042/BJ20081238

Pouremamali F, Pouremamali A, Dadashpour M, Soozangar N, Jeddi F. 2022. An update of Nrf2 activators and inhibitors in cancer prevention/promotion. *Cell Commun Signal* **20**: 100. doi:10.1186/s12964-022-00906-3

Ravegnini G, Ricci R. 2019. Succinate dehydrogenase-deficient gastrointestinal stromal tumors: small steps toward personalized medicine? *Epigenet Insights* **12**: 2516865719842534. doi:10.1177/2516865719842534

Rogerson C, Sciacovelli M, Maddalena LA, Pouikli A, Segarra-Mondejar M, Valcarcel-Jimenez L, Schmidt C, Yang M, Ivanova E, Kent J, et al. 2023. FOXA2 controls the antioxidant response in FH-deficient cells. *Cell Rep* **42**: 112751. doi:10.1016/j.celrep.2023.112751

Cite this article as *Cold Spring Harb Perspect Med* doi: 10.1101/cshperspect.a041536

Rutter J, Winge DR, Schiffman JD. 2010. Succinate dehydro-genase—assembly, regulation and role in human disease. *Mitochondrion* **10:** 393–401. doi:10.1016/j.mito.2010.03.001

Ryan DG, Knatko EV, Casey AM, Hukelmann JL, Dayalan Naidu S, Brenes AJ, Ekkunagul T, Baker C, Higgins M, Tronci L, et al. 2022. Nrf2 activation reprograms macrophage intermediary metabolism and suppresses the type I interferon response. *iScience* **25:** 103827. doi:10.1016/j.isci.2022.103827

Sarkadi B, Meszaros K, Krencz I, Canu L, Krokker L, Zakarias S, Barna G, Sebestyen A, Papay J, Hujber Z, et al. 2020. Glutaminases as a novel target for SDHB-associated pheochromocytomas/paragangliomas. *Cancers (Basel)* **12:** 599. doi:10.3390/cancers12030599

Schmidt C, Sciacovelli M, Frezza C. 2020. Fumarate hydratase in cancer: a multifaceted tumour suppressor. *Semin Cell Dev Biol* **98:** 15–25. doi:10.1016/j.semcdb.2019.05.002

Sciacovelli M, Gonçalves E, Johnson TI, Zecchini VR, da Costa ASH, Gaude E, Drubbel AV, Theobald SJ, Abbo SR, Tran MGB, et al. 2016. Fumarate is an epigenetic modifier that elicits epithelial-to-mesenchymal transition. *Nature* **537:** 544–547. doi:10.1038/nature19353

Serocki M, Bartoszewska S, Janaszak-Jasiecka A, Ochocka RJ, Collawn JF, Bartoszewski R. 2018. miRNAs regulate the HIF switch during hypoxia: a novel therapeutic target. *Angiogenesis* **21:** 183–202. doi:10.1007/s10456-018-9600-2

Sharma D, Singh M, Rani R. 2022. Role of LDH in tumor glycolysis: regulation of LDHA by small molecules for cancer therapeutics. *Semin Cancer Biol* **87:** 184–195. doi:10.1016/j.semcancer.2022.11.007

Solaimuthu B, Lichtenstein M, Hayashi A, Khatib A, Plaschkes I, Nevo Y, Tanna M, Pines O, Shaul YD. 2022. Depletion of fumarate hydratase, an essential TCA cycle enzyme, drives proliferation in a two-step model. *Cancers (Basel)* **14:** 5508. doi:10.3390/cancers14225508

Sourbier C, Valera-Romero V, Giubellino A, Yang Y, Sudarshan S, Neckers L, Linehan WM. 2010. Increasing reactive oxygen species as a therapeutic approach to treat hereditary leiomyomatosis and renal cell cancer. *Cell Cycle* **9:** 4183–4189. doi:10.4161/cc.9.20.13458

Sourbier C, Ricketts CJ, Liao PJ, Matsumoto S, Wei D, Lang M, Railkar R, Yang Y, Wei MH, Agarwal P, et al. 2019. Proteasome inhibition disrupts the metabolism of fumarate hydratase- deficient tumors by downregulating p62 and c-Myc. *Sci Rep* **9:** 18409. doi:10.1038/s41598-019-55003-2

Stockwell BR. 2019. A powerful cell-protection system prevents cell death by ferroptosis. *Nature* **575:** 597–598. doi:10.1038/d41586-019-03145-8

Sulkowski PL, Sundaram RK, Oeck S, Corso CD, Liu Y, Noorbakhsh S, Niger M, Boeke M, Ueno D, Kalathil AN, et al. 2018. Krebs-cycle-deficient hereditary cancer syndromes are defined by defects in homologous-recombination DNA repair. *Nat Genet* **50:** 1086–1092. doi:10.1038/s41588-018-0170-4

Sulkowski PL, Oeck S, Dow J, Economos NG, Mirfakhraie L, Liu Y, Noronha K, Bao X, Li J, Shuch BM, et al. 2020. Oncometabolites suppress DNA repair by disrupting local chromatin signalling. *Nature* **582:** 586–591. doi:10.1038/s41586-020-2363-0

Sullivan LB, Martinez-Garcia E, Nguyen H, Mullen AR, Dufour E, Sudarshan S, Licht JD, Deberardinis RJ, Chandel NS. 2013. The proto-oncometabolite fumarate binds glutathione to amplify ROS-dependent signaling. *Mol Cell* **51:** 236–248. doi:10.1016/j.molcel.2013.05.003

Sun Y, Jiang X, Chen S, Fernandes N, Price BD. 2005. A role for the Tip60 histone acetyltransferase in the acetylation and activation of ATM. *Proc Natl Acad Sci* **102:** 13182–13187. doi:10.1073/pnas.0504211102

Szlosarek PW, Creelan B, Sarkodie T, Nolan L, Taylor P, Olevsky O, Grosso F, Cortinovis D, Chitnis M, Roy A, et al. 2023. Abstract CT007: phase 2-3 trial of pegargiminase plus chemotherapy versus placebo plus chemotherapy in patients with non-epithelioid pleural mesothelioma. *Cancer Res* **83:** CT007. doi:10.1158/1538-7445.AM2023-CT007

Tannir NM, Agarwal N, Porta C, Lawrence NJ, Motzer R, McGregor B, Lee RJ, Jain RK, Davis N, Appleman LJ, et al. 2022. Efficacy and safety of telaglenastat plus cabozantinib vs placebo plus cabozantinib in patients with advanced renal cell carcinoma: the CANTATA randomized clinical trial. *JAMA Oncol* **8:** 1411–1418. doi:10.1001/jamaoncol.2022.3511

Trpkov K, Hes O, Agaimy A, Bonert M, Martinek P, Magi-Galluzzi C, Kristiansen G, Lüders C, Nesi G, Compérat E, et al. 2016. Fumarate hydratase-deficient renal cell carcinoma is strongly correlated with fumarate hydratase mutation and hereditary leiomyomatosis and renal cell carcinoma syndrome. *Am J Surg Pathol* **40:** 865–875. doi:10.1097/PAS.0000000000000617

Tsang VHM, Dwight T, Benn DE, Meyer-Rochow GY, Gill AJ, Sywak M, Sidhu S, Veivers D, Sue CM, Robinson BG, et al. 2014. Overexpression of miR-210 is associated with SDH-related pheochromocytomas, paragangliomas, and gastrointestinal stromal tumours. *Endocr Relat Cancer* **21:** 415–426. doi:10.1530/ERC-13-0519

Tulstrup M, Soerensen M, Hansen JW, Gillberg L, Needhamsen M, Kaastrup K, Helin K, Christensen K, Weischenfeldt J, Grønbæk K. 2021. TET2 mutations are associated with hypermethylation at key regulatory enhancers in normal and malignant hematopoiesis. *Nat Commun* **12:** 6061. doi:10.1038/s41467-021-26093-2

Tyrakis PA, Yurkovich ME, Sciacovelli M, Papachristou EK, Bridges HR, Gaude E, Schreiner A, D'Santos C, Hirst J, Hernandez-Fernaud J, et al. 2017. Fumarate hydratase loss causes combined respiratory chain defects. *Cell Rep* **21:** 1036–1047. doi:10.1016/j.celrep.2017.09.092

Van Looy T, Wozniak A, Floris G, Sciot R, Li H, Wellens J, Vanleeuw U, Fletcher JA, Manley PW, Debiec-Rychter M, et al. Phosphoinositide 3-kinase inhibitors combined with imatinib in patient-derived xenograft models of gastrointestinal stromal tumors: rationale and efficacy. *Clin Cancer Res* **20:** 6071–6082. doi:10.1158/1078-0432.CCR-14-1823

Vazquez A, Kamphorst JJ, Markert EK, Schug ZT, Tardito S, Gottlieb E. 2016. Cancer metabolism at a glance. *J Cell Sci* **129:** 3367–3373. doi:10.1242/jcs.181016

Wang F, Zhang H, Xu N, Huang N, Tian C, Ye A, Hu G, He J, Zhang Y. 2016. A novel hypoxia-induced miR-147a regulates cell proliferation through a positive feedback loop of stabilizing HIF-1α. *Cancer Biol Ther* **17:** 790–798. doi:10.1080/15384047.2016.1195040

Warburg O, Wind F, Negelein E. 1927. The metabolism of tumors in the body. *J Gen Physiol* **8:** 519–530. doi:10.1085/jgp.8.6.519

Williams ST, Chatzikyriakou P, Carroll PV, McGowan BM, Velusamy A, White G, Obholzer R, Akker S, Tufton N, Casey RT, et al. 2022. SDHC phaeochromocytoma and paraganglioma: a UK-wide case series. *Clin Endocrinol* **96:** 499–512. doi:10.1111/cen.14594

Wu G, Liu G, Wang J, Pan S, Luo Y, Xu Y, Kong W, Sun P, Xu J, Xue W, et al. 2022. MR spectroscopy for detecting fumarate hydratase deficiency in hereditary leiomyomatosis and renal cell carcinoma syndrome. *Radiology* **305:** 631–639. doi:10.1148/radiol.212984

Xie H, Valera VA, Merino MJ, Amato AM, Signoretti S, Linehan WM, Sukhatme VP, Seth P. 2009. LDH-A inhibition, a therapeutic strategy for treatment of hereditary leiomyomatosis and renal cell cancer. *Mol Cancer Ther* **8:** 626–635. doi:10.1158/1535-7163.MCT-08-1049

Yang M, Soga T, Pollard PJ, Adam J. 2012a. The emerging role of fumarate as an oncometabolite. *Front Oncol* **2:** 85. doi:10.3389/fonc.2012.00085

Yang Y, Valera V, Sourbier C, Vocke CD, Wei M, Pike L, Huang Y, Merino MA, Bratslavsky G, Wu M, et al. 2012b. A novel fumarate hydratase-deficient HLRCC kidney cancer cell line, UOK268: a model of the Warburg effect in cancer. *Cancer Genet* **205:** 377–390. doi:10.1016/j.cancergen.2012.05.001

Yang Y, Lane AN, Ricketts CJ, Sourbier C, Wei MH, Shuch B, Pike L, Wu M, Rouault TA, Boros LG, et al. 2013. Metabolic reprogramming for producing energy and reducing power in fumarate hydratase null cells from hereditary leiomyomatosis renal cell carcinoma. *PLoS ONE* **8:** e72179. doi:10.1371/journal.pone.0072179

Yang J, Guo Y, Seo W, Zhang R, Lu C, Wang Y, Luo L, Paul B, Yan W, Saxena D, et al. 2019. Targeting cellular metabolism to reduce head and neck cancer growth. *Sci Rep* **9:** 4995. doi:10.1038/s41598-019-41523-4

Zheng L, MacKenzie ED, Karim SA, Hedley A, Blyth K, Kalna G, Watson DG, Szlosarek P, Frezza C, Gottlieb E. 2013. Reversed argininosuccinate lyase activity in fumarate hydratase-deficient cancer cells. *Cancer Metab* **1:** 12. doi:10.1186/2049-3002-1-12

Zheng L, Cardaci S, Jerby L, MacKenzie ED, Sciacovelli M, Johnson TI, Gaude E, King A, Leach JD, Edrada-Ebel R, et al. 2015. Fumarate induces redox-dependent senescence by modifying glutathione metabolism. *Nat Commun* **6:** 6001. doi:10.1038/ncomms7001

Zheng L, Zhu ZR, Sneh T, Zhang WT, Wang ZY, Wu GY, He W, Qi HG, Wang H, Wu XY, et al. 2023. Circulating succinate-modifying metabolites accurately classify and reflect the status of fumarate hydratase-deficient renal cell carcinoma. *J Clin Invest* **133:** e165028. doi:10.1172/JCI165028

Cite this article as *Cold Spring Harb Perspect Med* doi: 10.1101/cshperspect.a041536

Interactions of Fatty Acid and Cholesterol Metabolism with Cellular Stress Response Pathways in Cancer

Alina M. Winkelkotte,[1] Kamal Al-Shami,[1] Adriano B. Chaves-Filho,[1,2] Felix C.E. Vogel,[1] and Almut Schulze[1]

[1]Division of Tumor Metabolism and Microenvironment, German Cancer Research Center (DKFZ), 69120 Heidelberg, Germany

[2]Institute of Chemistry, University of São Paulo, 05508000 São Paulo, Brazil

Correspondence: almut.schulze@dkfz-heidelberg.de

Lipids have essential functions as structural components of cellular membranes, as efficient energy storage molecules, and as precursors of signaling mediators. While deregulated glucose and amino acid metabolism in cancer have received substantial attention, the roles of lipids in the metabolic reprogramming of cancer cells are less well understood. However, since the first description of de novo fatty acid biosynthesis in cancer tissues almost 70 years ago, numerous studies have investigated the complex functions of altered lipid metabolism in cancer. Here, we will summarize the mechanisms by which oncogenic signaling pathways regulate fatty acid and cholesterol metabolism to drive rapid proliferation and protect cancer cells from environmental stress. The review also discusses the role of fatty acid metabolism in metabolic plasticity required for the adaptation to changing microenvironments during cancer progression and the connections between fatty acid and cholesterol metabolism and ferroptosis.

Lipids play multiple biological roles as they constitute the major structural components of cellular membranes and serve as precursors for the synthesis of several cofactors, vitamins, hormones, and signaling molecules. Additionally, lipids can also be used as a fuel source to generate ATP and/or, conversely, as a substrate for energy storage. According to the LIPID MAPS classification system (www.lipidmaps.org), lipids can be categorized into seven main classes: fatty acids, glycerolipids, glycerophospholipids, sphingolipids, sterols lipids, prenol lipids, and polyketides (Fahy et al. 2005; Liebisch et al. 2020). The modular structure of lipid molecules results in tremendous complexity, posing a challenge to analytical technologies (Shevchenko and Simons 2010). Glycerophospholipids and sphingolipids are structural components of cellular membranes (Harayama and Riezman 2018). Glycerolipids, most notably triacylglycerides, function as energy storage molecules and are localized to lipid droplets, unique cellular organelles. Glycerolipids, glycerophospholipids, and sphingolipids are synthesized from fatty acids that are linked to either a glycerol or a sphingosine backbone through either ester or ether bonds (Nohturfft and Zhang 2009). The length and number of double bonds of the fatty acid chains determine the biophysical properties of the lipid molecule.

In addition to their function as building blocks of complex lipids, fatty acids can also function as substrates for the posttranslational modification of proteins (Resh 2013) and as precursors for the synthesis of important signaling molecules involved in autocrine and paracrine signaling (Wang and Dubois 2010). Sterol lipids are structurally distinct from other lipids, as they consist of four linked hydrocarbon rings. Cholesterol, the most prominent member of this class, is a component of cellular membranes, where it plays a crucial role in determining fluidity. Furthermore, cholesterol is also a precursor for the synthesis of steroid hormones and bile acids. Due to its vital role in the maintenance of cell integrity, the synthesis of cholesterol has to be tightly regulated. Moreover, the cholesterol biosynthesis pathway produces several metabolic intermediates with essential functions. Recent work has revealed that cancer cells show distinct alteration in the synthesis and modification of fatty acids as well as cholesterol biosynthesis (Mullen et al. 2016; Röhrig and Schulze 2016; Koundouros and Poulogiannis 2020; Snaebjornsson et al. 2020). These alterations promote rapid cell proliferation and increase stress resistance (Peck and Schulze 2019; Broadfield et al. 2021). It is, therefore, vital to uncover the specific mechanisms by which oncogenic signaling impacts fatty acid metabolism to support the transformed phenotype.

TRANSCRIPTIONAL REGULATION OF FATTY ACID AND CHOLESTEROL SYNTHESIS

Many of the enzymes required for de novo fatty acid synthesis are under the control of the sterol regulatory element-binding protein 1 (*SREBF1*/SREBP1), a helix–loop–helix transcription factor that is regulated via proteolytic processing downstream from a lipid-sensing mechanism (Fig. 1; Shimano and Sato 2017). SREBPs are initially

translated as inactive precursors that reside as transmembrane proteins in the endoplasmic reticulum (ER), where they form complexes with the SREBP cleavage activating protein (SCAP). When intracellular sterol levels drop below a certain threshold, the SREBP/SCAP complex translocates to the Golgi via COPII-mediated transport. In the Golgi, a two-step proteolytic cleavage process releases the amino-terminal half of the SREBP protein, which can then enter the nucleus and bind to the sterol regulatory elements (SREs) in the promoters of its target genes (DeBose-Boyd and Ye 2018). The mature forms of SREBP contain both the DNA binding and transactivation domains. It is worth noting that SREBP1 exists in two splice variants (SREBP1a and SREBP1c), which differ in the sequence of their transactivation domain and exhibit tissue-specific expression patterns (Shimano and Sato 2017). For simplicity, this review does not discriminate between SREBP1a and SREBP1c.

In the nucleus, mature SREBPs are subjected to further regulation through posttranslational mechanisms. It has been shown that the glycogen synthase kinase 3 (GSK3) can phosphorylate mature SREBP at several highly conserved serine and threonine residues (Sundqvist et al. 2005). This phosphorylation facilitates binding by the F-Box and WD repeat domain-containing protein 7 (FBXW7) ubiquitin ligase, leading to ubiquitylation and subsequent degradation of mature SREBP. Interestingly, this form of regulation was shown to be dependent on DNA binding (Sundqvist and Ericsson 2003), suggesting a role in the turnover of transcription factor complexes. In addition, SREBPs are activated in response to mitotic stimuli via the PI3-kinase/Akt/mTORC1 axis and contribute to cell growth and cell proliferation in cancer (Porstmann et al. 2008; Düvel et al. 2010; Peterson et al. 2011). Multiple mechanisms have been shown to contribute to the activation of SREBP by mechanistic target of rapamycin complex 1 (mTORC1). One of these mechanisms involves the regulation of nuclear localization of mature SREBP1 by the phosphatidate phosphatase LPIN1. LPIN1 sequesters mature SREBP1 to the nuclear periphery, thereby preventing its ability to function as a transcriptional regulator. Phosphorylation of

Cite this article as *Cold Spring Harb Perspect Med* doi: 10.1101/cshperspect.a041548

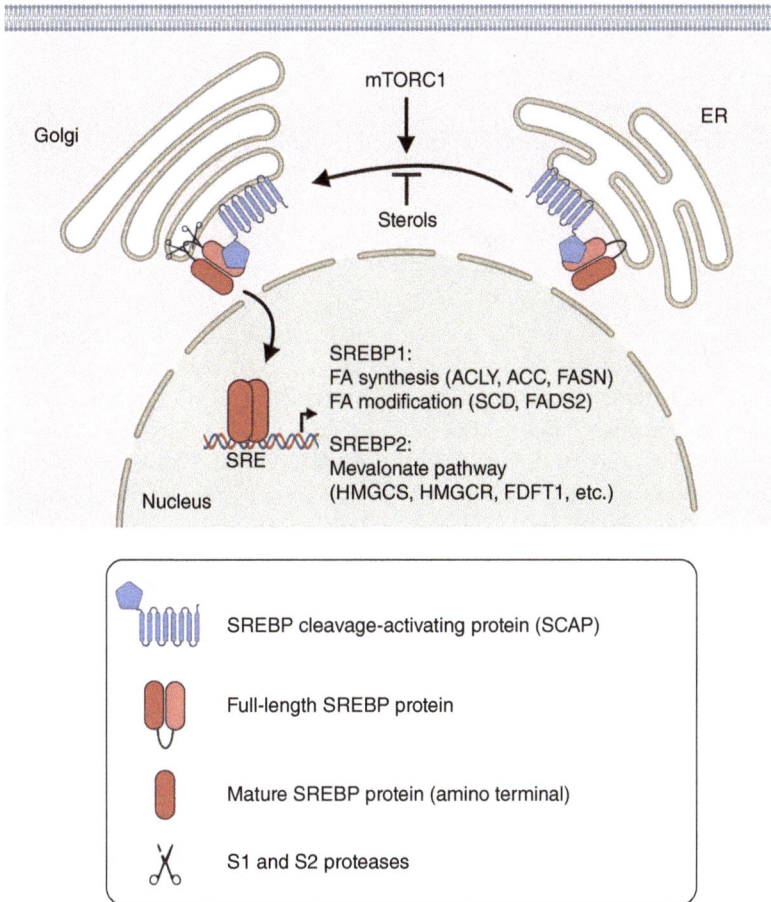

Figure 1. Mechanism of regulation of sterol regulatory element-binding protein (SREBP) by sterols and oncogenic signaling. SREBPs are translated as inactive precursors and localize to the endoplasmic reticulum (ER)-membrane where they interact with the SREBP cleavage-activating protein (SCAP). In the presence of low intracellular sterol levels or oncogenic signaling by the mechanistic target of rapamycin complex 1 (mTORC1), the SREBP/SCAP complex is transported via COPII vesicles to the Golgi, where a two-step proteolytic cleavage process releases the amino-terminal half of the SREBP. This mature form of SREBP contains the transactivation and DNA-binding domains and translocates to the nucleus, where it binds to sterol regulatory elements (SREs) in the promoter regions of its target genes. SREBP1 preferentially binds to genes involved in fatty acid synthesis and modification while SREBP2 preferentially regulates genes coding for enzymes of the mevalonate pathway. (ACLY) ATP-citrate lyase, (ACC) acetyl-CoA carboxylase, (FASN) fatty acid synthase, (SCD) stearoyl-CoA desaturase, (FADS2) fatty acid desaturase 2, (HMGCS) HMG-CoA synthase, (HMGCR) HMG-CoA reductase, (FDFT1) farnesyl-diphosphate farnesyltransferase 1. (Figure created in BioRender.)

LPIN1 by mTORC1 results in its cytoplasmic retention, thereby allowing mature SREBP1 to bind to its target genes (Peterson et al. 2011). In addition, mTORC1 phosphorylates the CREB-regulated transcription coactivator 2 (CRTC2) to promote the ER-to-Golgi translocation of SREBP1 (Han et al. 2015). Finally, Akt-dependent down-regulation of the insulin-induced gene 2a also promotes SREBP1 activation (Yecies et al. 2011). These findings show the close interactions between cellular signaling networks and the transcriptional regulation of fatty acid and cholesterol biosynthesis that can lead to their deregulation in cancer.

FATTY ACID SYNTHESIS IN CELL GROWTH AND STRESS RESISTANCE

Mammals can generate saturated fatty acids (SFAs) and monounsaturated fatty acids (MUFAs) from de novo synthesis using acetyl-CoA as a substrate. The sequential condensation of two-carbon units by the enzyme fatty acid synthase (FASN) generates the 16-carbon SFA palmitic acid, which is further elongated and desaturated to produce MUFA, including palmitoleic acid and oleic acid. SFA and MUFA can also be obtained through the uptake of free fatty acids or fatty acid–containing lipids. Polyunsaturated fatty acids (PUFAs), on the other hand, cannot be synthesized de novo but must be derived from dietary ω-3 and ω-6 essential fatty acids. The most abundant essential dietary fatty acids are linoleic acid and α-linolenic acid, which are further modified by elongation and desaturation. The composition of the intracellular fatty acid pool of a cancer cell, therefore, depends on cell intrinsic enzymatic activities and the availability of specific lipids within the tumor microenvironment.

Activation of SREBP1 by Akt and mTORC1 also induces the expression of stearoyl-CoA desaturase (SCD) and fatty acid desaturase 2 (FADS2), two desaturases that introduce double bonds into the hydrocarbon chains of fatty acids (at the Δ9 or Δ6 positions, respectively), through an SREBP1-dependent mechanism (Griffiths et al. 2013; Triki et al. 2020). Inhibition of SREBP1 in primary pigment epithelial cells and cancer cells causes aberrant accumulation of SFAs, leading to lipotoxicity, endoplasmic reticulum stress (ER-stress), and cell death (Griffiths et al. 2013; Williams et al. 2013). A similar phenotype was observed in mouse embryonic fibroblasts when mTORC1 signaling was activated under tumor-like metabolic stress, involving serum and oxygen depletion (Young et al. 2013). Furthermore, cancer cells rely on sufficient de novo MUFA biosynthesis to prevent ER stress (Peck and Schulze 2016; Ackerman and Simon 2024). Additionally, FADS2 was shown to catalyze the Δ6 desaturation of palmitic acid to generate sapienic acid, a MUFA usually only found in sebocytes. The formation of sapienic acid by FADS2 was sufficient to support survival in cancer cells when SCD is inhibited (Vriens et al. 2019).

Fatty acid synthesis is also regulated by the liver X receptors (LXRs) and the significance of LXR for cancer biology has already been recognized (Lin and Gustafsson 2015). For instance, targeting LXR1 through an inverse-agonist inhibitor exhibits a broad antitumor activity by blocking fatty acid synthesis and lowering glycolysis (Flaveny et al. 2015). However, aberrant activation of LXR can also be detrimental to cancer cells as it was shown to block SREBP1 and accelerate cholesterol efflux in glioblastoma (Guo et al. 2011; Villa et al. 2016). Furthermore, Rudalska et al. (2021) showed that combined activation of LXR and inhibition of Raf induce lethal lipotoxicity in liver cancer. More recently, it has been reported that cancer cells that metastasize to the lipid-poor microenvironment of the brain show a high dependency on SREBP1 expression to support de novo fatty acid biosynthesis and desaturation (Jin et al. 2020; Ferraro et al. 2021). Inhibition of fatty acid synthesis by blocking FASN in breast cancer cells had only a minimal effect on primary tumors, presumably because the breast tissue provides sufficient amounts of exogenous fatty acids. In contrast, genetic deletion or chemical inhibition of FASN efficiently reduced the growth of breast cancer cells in the microenvironment of the brain after intracranial injection (Ferraro et al. 2021), highlighting the importance of the tumor microenvironment in defining the metabolic vulnerabilities of cancer cells.

THE MEVALONATE PATHWAY AS METABOLIC HUB IN CANCER CELLS

The synthesis of cholesterol and other sterol lipids involves a series of reactions that catalyze the sequential linkage of carbon units to form isoprenoid molecules. These are then circularized to form a backbone of hydrocarbon rings, which are subsequently extensively modified through either the Bloch or the Kandutsch–Russel pathway (Bloch 1952). The first part of cholesterol biosynthesis is also known as the mevalonate pathway, named after its key intermediate (Mullen et al. 2016). Its central enzyme is HMG-CoA reductase (Gold-stein and Brown 1973), which is also the target of statins, a class of cholesterol-lowering drugs.

The mevalonate pathway produces a number of metabolic intermediates that are crucial for important cellular processes (Mullen et al. 2016). One of them is farnesyl-pyrophosphate, which serves as a substrate for protein prenylation (Wang and Casey 2016). Several small GTPases, including K-Ras and Rho, require prenylation for their correct subcellular localization and activity. Deregulation of the mevalonate pathway has been linked to aberrant activation of N-Ras in response to inactivation of Rb (Shamma et al. 2009). Far-nesyl-pyrophosphate also functions as a substrate for the production of ubiquinone, an essential electron transport molecule that forms part of the mitochondrial electron transport chain (ETC). Inhibition of the mevalonate pathway in p53-deficient cancer cells not only blocked mito-chondrial electron transport but also lowered the activity of dihydroorotate dehydrogenase (DHODH), an enzyme of the pyrimidine biosyn-thesis pathway (Kaymak et al. 2020). Moreover, it has been demonstrated that statins reduce ubi-quinone levels, leading to oxidative stress and cancer cell death in vitro and in vivo (McGregor et al. 2020). Another metabolic intermediate of the mevalonate pathway is squalene, which is formed by the condensation of two molecules of farnesyl-pyrophosphate by farnesyl-diphos-phate farnesyltransferase 1 (FDFT1). Interesting-ly, accumulation of squalene due to genetic loss of FDFT1 in ALK$^+$ anaplastic large cell lymphomas resulted in oxidative stress resistance but ren-dered these cancers highly sensitive to the inhibi-tion of cholesterol uptake (Garcia-Bermudez et al. 2019). However, it should be noted that accumulation of squalene has also been associat-ed with enhanced toxicity, as squalene epoxidase (SQLE), which converts squalene to 2,3-oxidos-qualene, was identified in a chemical screen of neuroendocrine tumor cells (Mahoney et al. 2019). It is likely that the potential cytoprotective and cytotoxic functions of squalene depend on the cellular context or the level of accumulation. Interestingly, deregulation of the mevalonate pathway can also have non-cell-autonomous ef-fects. Phosphorylated derivates of mevalonate,

such as isopentenyl-pyrophosphate, act as danger signals and are recognized by innate-like γ/δ T cells (Thurnher and Gruenbacher 2015).

Expression of most enzymes in the mevalo-nate pathway is controlled by sterol regulatory element-binding protein 2 (*SREBF2*/SREBP2), which is closely related to SREBP1 and con-trolled via similar posttranslational mechanisms (Shimano and Sato 2017). Activation of SREBP2 in cancer cells increases cholesterol biosynthesis to modulate cell membrane fluidity and lipid raft formation, favoring an invading and metastasiz-ing phenotype. For instance, the activation of SREBP2 by mutant p53 disrupts normal tissue architecture in breast cancer (Fig. 2A; Freed-Pas-tor et al. 2012). Interestingly, the readdition of the mevalonate pathway product geranylgeranyl-pyrophosphate rescued breast cancer cell inva-siveness in the presence of statins, suggesting a direct link between the mevalonate pathway and protein prenylation in cancer (Freed-Pastor et al. 2012). In contrast, wild-type p53 can repress SREBP2 through transcriptional induction of the ABCA1 cholesterol transporter (Moon et al. 2019). Enhanced ABCA1 expression blocked SREBP2 maturation and reduced the activity of the mevalonate pathway, thereby preventing tu-morigenesis in liver cancer (Fig. 2B; Moon et al. 2019). A second mechanism for the inhibition of the mevalonate pathway downstream from p53 involves the activation of GSK3, which promotes phosphorylation and degradation of mature SREBP2. Loss of p53 stabilized SREBP2, leading to the induction of mevalonate pathway enzymes and promoting pyrimidine synthesis in p53-de-ficient colon cancer cells (Fig. 2C; Kaymak et al. 2020). Furthermore, the deubiquitinating en-zyme ubiquitin-specific peptidase 28 (USP28) was found to stabilize mature SREBP2 by remov-ing ubiquitin moieties (Maier et al. 2023). Dele-tion of USP28 or SREBP2 reduced tumor load in a mouse model of squamous lung carcinoma (Prieto-Garcia et al. 2020; Maier et al. 2023).

FATTY ACID UPTAKE AND OXIDATION AS DRIVERS OF METASTASIS FORMATION

Fatty acid uptake can occur through passive dif-fusion (flip-in) or the action of various trans-

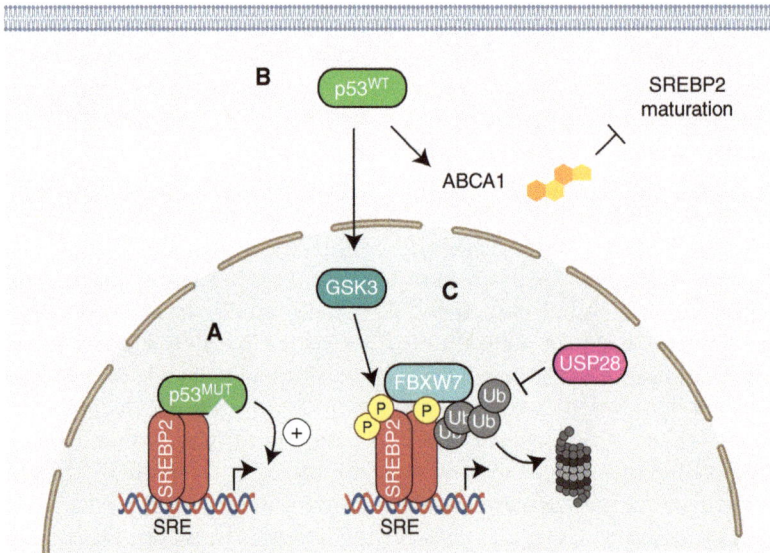

Figure 2. Regulation of sterol regulatory element-binding protein 2 (SREBP2) by p53. (*A*) Mutant p53 can bind to SREBP2 at the promoters of its target genes. This mediates the activation of transcription and enhances the expression of mevalonate pathway enzymes to promote cancer cell migration and invasion. (*B*) Wild-type p53 blocks SREBP2 activation by inducing the expression of the cholesterol transporter ATP-binding cassette subfamily A member 1 (ABCA1). This increases intracellular sterol levels and blocks SREBP2 maturation. Loss of p53 of ablation of ABCA1 increases SREBP2 maturation in liver cancer. (*C*) Wild-type p53 also enhances the stability of mature SREBP2 through a mechanism dependent on the glycogen synthase kinase 3 (GSK3). GSK3 phosphorylates SREBP2 on several conserved residues. This phosphorylation induces binding of the F-Box and WD repeat domain-containing protein 7 (FBXW7), resulting in ubiquitylation and proteasome-dependent degradation of mature SREBP2. Loss of p53 inhibits GSK3 activity, leading to enhanced protein stability of SREBP2 and elevated expression of mevalonate pathway enzymes. SREBP2 ubiquitylation is also counteracted by the ubiquitin-specific peptidase 28 (USP28). (Ub) Ubiquitin, (P) phosphate, (SRE) sterol regulatory element. (Figure created in BioRender.)

membrane proteins acting as fatty acid transporters. The most prominent fatty acid transporter is the scavenging receptor CD36 (also known as thrombospondin receptor or fatty acid translocase). Its crystal structure reveals a central tunnel that could mediate the movement of fatty acids (Hsieh et al. 2016). However, it is not yet clear whether CD36 is directly involved in transporter activity or if it mediates fatty acid uptake by stimulating endocytosis (Hao et al. 2020). Interestingly, CD36 has been found to be highly expressed in metastasis-initiating stem-like cells in oral squamous carcinoma, linking fatty acid uptake to metastasis formation (Pascual et al. 2017). The family of fatty acid transport proteins (FATPs) consists of six members (SLC27A1–6) with tissue-specific expression and different substrate specificity and there is evidence for the overexpression of several FATPs in cancer (Acharya et al. 2023). Fatty acid uptake is also facilitated by the expression of fatty acid-binding proteins (FABPs). For example, FABP3 and FABP7 have been shown to be induced in hypoxic cells to promote fatty acid uptake and triglyceride storage, providing bioenergetic substrates during reoxygenation (Bensaad et al. 2014). Furthermore, it was shown that hypoxic or Ras-transformed cancer cells selectively take up lysophospholipids to scavenge unsaturated fatty acids (Kamphorst et al. 2013). Finally, the accumulation of cholesterylesters via sterol *O*-acyltransferase 1 (SOAT1, also known as ACAT-1) was shown to drive aggressiveness in prostate cancer by maintaining low

Cite this article as *Cold Spring Harb Perspect Med* doi: 10.1101/cshperspect.a041548

intracellular concentrations of free cholesterol. This allows for SREBP2-dependent expression of the low-density lipoprotein receptor (LDLR), supporting the uptake of essential fatty acids (Yue et al. 2014).

Numerous studies have reported that enhanced fatty acid metabolism via β-oxidation is generally associated with cancer cell dissemination and metastasis formation (Martin-Perez et al. 2021, 2022). While fatty acid synthesis takes place in the cytoplasm, fatty acid degradation via β-oxidation is localized to the mitochondria. Synthesis and degradation of fatty acids are usually mutually exclusive, due to the inhibition of carnitine-palmitoyl transferase (CPT1), the enzyme required for the transfer of fatty acid into the mitochondrial matrix, by malonyl-CoA, the first metabolite generated as part of the fatty acid synthesis process (Carracedo et al. 2013). CPT1C is highly expressed in cancers that have undergone epithelial to mesenchymal transition (EMT) (Nath and Chan 2016), while inhibition of CPT1A prevents breast cancer metastasis (Loo et al. 2021), suggesting that enhanced fatty acid oxidation is a common feature of metastatic cancer cells. Indeed, single-cell RNA sequencing and metabolomics analysis comparing primary tumors to micrometastases from different sites revealed a global shift from glycolysis to fatty acid metabolism in breast cancer (Davis et al. 2020). However, fatty acid metabolism not only provides cancer cells with a readily available nutrient source but can also impact regulatory processes. It was recently shown that CPT1a dependent oxidation of palmitate induces prometastatic NF-κB signaling in breast cancer by providing acetyl-CoA as substrate for the lysine acetyltransferase 2a (KAT2a), which acetylates the p65 subunit of NF-κB. Silencing of either CPT1a or KAT2a prevented palmitate-induced spheroid growth and impaired lung metastasis formation (Altea-Manzano et al. 2023). This demonstrates that a metabolic shift toward fatty acid metabolism impacts regulatory mechanisms that promote cancer progression.

The uptake of fatty acids naturally depends on the local availability of either free or esterified fatty acids within the tumor microenvironment. Lipid-rich microenvironments, such as breast,

liver, and adipose tissue, are likely to supply sufficient amounts of fatty acids as an energy source for cancer cells. In fact, cancer cells can also actively remodel their environment, for example, by inducing adipocytes to secrete fatty acids. Such mechanisms of metabolic cross talk have been described for metastatic ovarian and breast cancer (Dirat et al. 2011; Nieman et al. 2011) and in melanoma (Zhang et al. 2018). As mentioned above, some tissues may not provide sufficient amounts of exogenous lipids, making metastatic cancer cells highly dependent on de novo fatty acid synthesis and modification (Jin et al. 2020; Ferraro et al. 2021). The high plasticity and flexibility of cancer metabolism must be considered when devising therapeutic strategies targeting fatty acid metabolism (Bergers and Fendt 2021).

FATTY ACID AND CHOLESTEROL METABOLISM AS DRIVERS OF FERROPTOSIS RESISTANCE IN CANCER

Altered lipid metabolism in cancer cells is intricately linked to their sensitivity toward an iron-mediated form of cell death, termed ferroptosis (Dixon et al. 2012). Ferroptosis is induced by the toxic accumulation of lipid peroxides, which leads to irreversible damage and rupture of the plasma membrane (Yang and Stockwell 2016; Friedmann Angeli et al. 2019). Ferroptosis is strongly modulated by cellular intermediate metabolism and nutritional cues (Mishima and Conrad 2022).

Numerous intracellular processes counteract lipid peroxidation and prevent ferroptosis. One of these involves the action of glutathione peroxidase 4 (GPX4), which uses glutathione as a cofactor to convert lipid peroxides into nontoxic lipid alcohols (Conrad et al. 2018; Dixon and Stockwell 2019). Initial work by the Conrad group revealed that genetic deletion of GPX4 caused a nonapoptotic form of cell death that could be rescued by lipid-targeted antioxidants (e.g., liproxstatin) or by overexpression of components of the cystine transporter system Xc^- (Banjac et al. 2008; Seiler et al. 2008). Later work by Stockwell and colleagues identified a similar mechanism of cell death triggered by a class of compounds that block the activity of Xc^-

in Ras-transformed cancer cells, and coined the term ferroptosis (Dixon et al. 2012). Since then, numerous studies have demonstrated the importance of cystine uptake, glutathione biosynthesis, and GPX4 activity for ferroptosis prevention (for review, see Stockwell 2022). More recently, a second major antiferroptotic mechanism involving the ferroptosis suppressor protein 1 (FSP1) has been identified (Bersuker et al. 2019; Doll et al. 2019). FSP1 localizes to the plasma membrane via a myristate moiety where it facilitates the reduction of ubiquinone to maintain its action as lipophilic antioxidant that prevents lipid peroxidation. Since this discovery, numerous efforts have been undertaken to identify compounds that block the activity of FSP1 to target ferroptosis resistance in cancer (Yoshioka et al. 2022; Hendricks et al. 2023). FSP1 is also up-regulated in cells expressing oncogenic K-Ras and prevents ferroptosis during tumor initiation (Müller et al. 2023). Moreover, it was recently shown that FSP1 also facilitates the reduction of vitamin K to maintain its potent antioxidant function (Mishima et al. 2022).

Importantly, lipids differ in their relative susceptibility to peroxidation, as this reaction requires the introduction of a peroxyl group instead of a hydrogen atom in the fatty acid chain. PUFAs are highly susceptible to peroxidation and mechanisms that mediate the formation of PUFA-containing membrane lipids increase ferroptosis sensitivity. For instance, the expression of the acyl-CoA synthetase long-chain family member 4 (ACSL4), which primarily activates long-chain PUFA for their incorporation into membrane lipids, was required for ferroptosis sensitivity in basal breast cancer cells (Doll et al. 2017). ACSL4 was also involved in the formation of phosphatidylethanolamine (PE) species containing the PUFA arachidonic or adrenic acid (Kagan et al. 2017). Moreover, the remodeling of membrane lipids by the inducible phospholipase A2 β (PLA2G6), which removes highly peroxidizable PUFA from membrane lipids, functions to suppress ferroptosis (Chen et al. 2021). Conversely, enhanced lipid remodeling in response to exogenous PUFA can also enhance ferroptosis sensitivity (Fig. 3A). Treatment with α-eleostearic acid (αESA), a PUFA

naturally found in tung oil, was found to promote lipid peroxidation and ferroptosis sensitivity in cancer cells, and dietary administration of tung oil reduced tumor growth and metastasis formation in triple-negative breast cancer xenografts (Beatty et al. 2021).

While PUFA generally enhances ferroptosis sensitivity, increasing the amounts of MUFA in membrane lipids reduces the susceptibility of cells toward lipid peroxidation and ferroptosis (Fig. 3B). Addition of exogenous MUFA, particularly oleic acid, was shown to reduce the amounts of oxidizable PUFA in the plasma membrane and drive cells into a ferroptosis-resistant state (Magtanong et al. 2019). Moreover, the oleic acid present in the lymphatic fluid protects metastatic melanoma cells from ferroptosis and promotes cancer dissemination via the lymphatic route (Ubellacker et al. 2020). The activation of de novo fatty acid synthesis in cancer cells generally leads to an increased proportion of MUFA compared to PUFA in membrane lipids and protects them from damage by free radicals (Rysman et al. 2010). Moreover, a global analysis of the metabolic landscape of 928 cancer cell lines (Cancer Cell Line Encyclopedia [CCLE]) showed that cells with a high proportion of PUFA in their lipidome (PUFA^{high}) are strongly dependent on the expression of GPX4, presumably to prevent lipid peroxidation and ferroptosis. In contrast, PUFA^{low} cancer cells were highly sensitive toward depletion of SCD, most likely to prevent ER-stress and lipotoxicity (Li et al. 2019). Moreover, the activation of SREBP1 downstream from the PI3-kinase/Akt/mTORC1 signaling axis prevents ferroptosis in cancer cells by promoting fatty acid synthesis and SCD-dependent MUFA formation (Yi et al. 2020). On the other hand, the transcription factor BACH1 was shown to repress SCD-mediated MUFA synthesis in esophageal carcinoma, thereby only allowing cancer cell dissemination primarily via the lymphatic system (Xie et al. 2023). Increased expression of SCD in cancer cells and FABP4 in cells of the tumor microenvironment also induces ferroptosis resistance to promote tumor recurrence (Luis et al. 2021). Similarly, ovarian cancer cells with a mesenchymal phenotype show enhanced expression of SCD and decreased

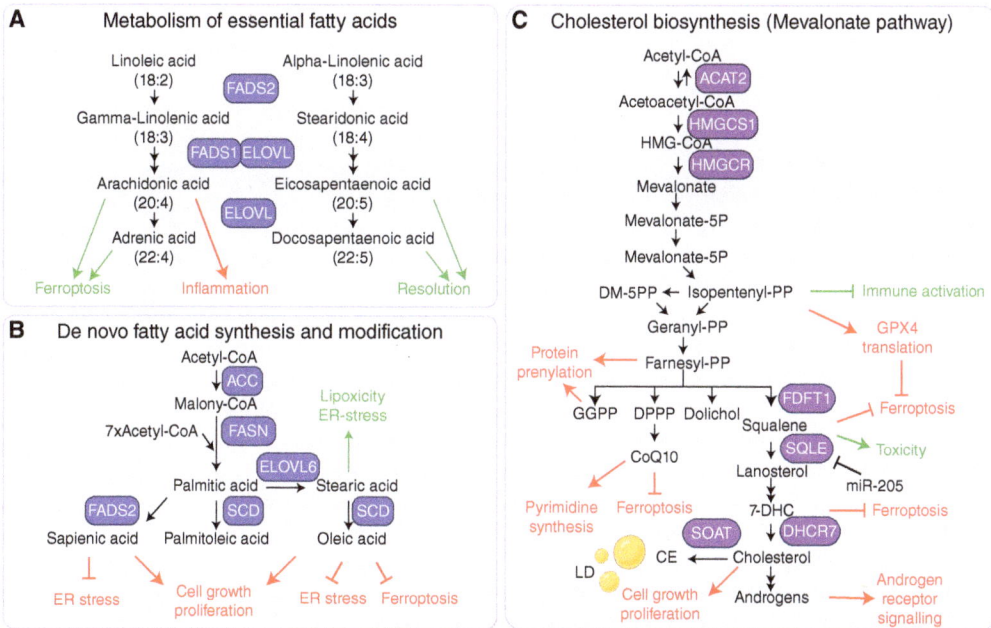

Figure 3. Interactions of fatty acid and cholesterol biosynthesis with cellular stress response and ferroptosis pathways. (*A*) Metabolism of the ω-6 essential fatty acid, linoleic acid, produces arachidonic acid and adrenic acid, two polyunsaturated fatty acids (PUFAs) that promote ferroptosis when incorporated into membrane lipids. Arachidonic acid is also the precursor for the synthesis of proinflammatory eicosanoids, including prostaglandin E2 (PGE2). Anti-inflammatory eicosanoids are produced from the ω-3 essential fatty acid α-linoleic acid. (*B*) De novo fatty acid synthesis and desaturation produce monounsaturated fatty acids (sapienic, palmitoleic, and oleic acid) that are essential for cell proliferation and prevent endoplasmic reticulum stress (ER-stress) and ferroptosis. Aberrant accumulation of saturated fatty acids (stearic acid), for example, due to inhibition of stearoyl-CoA desaturase (SCD), leads to ER-stress and lipotoxicity. (*C*) Cholesterol biosynthesis via the mevalonate pathway (the Kandutsch–Russell and Bloch pathways are simplified). Isopentenyl-pyrophosphate (Isopentenyl-PP) produced by the mevalonate pathway is required for the translation of glutathione peroxidase 4 (GPX4) to protect cells from ferroptosis. Farnesyl-pyrophosphate (Farnesyl-PP) and geranylgeranyl-pyrophosphate (GGPP) promote the prenylation of small G-proteins. Farnesyl-PP also serves as a substrate for the synthesis of ubiquinone (CoQ10), an electron transfer protein required for pyrimidine synthesis at the inner mitochondrial membrane. Within the plasma membrane, CoQ10 functions as a lipophilic antioxidant to counteract lipid peroxidation downstream from the ferroptosis suppressor protein 1 (FSP1). Squalene prevents lipid peroxidation but can also accumulate to toxic levels. Further downstream, 7-dehydroxycholesterol has also antioxidant function, demonstrating that multiple intermediates of cholesterol synthesis prevent ferroptosis. Cholesterol is an important component of cellular membranes and is esterified to be stored together with triglycerides in lipid droplets. (ACC) Acetyl-CoA carboxylase, (CE) cholesteryl ester, (FASN) fatty acid synthase, (ELOVL6) fatty acid elongase 6, (FADS2) fatty acid desaturase 2, (FADS1) fatty acid desaturase 1, (ACAT2) acetyl-CoA acetyltransferase 2, (HMGCS1) HMG-CoA synthase 1, (HMGCR) HMG-CoA reductase, (FDFT1) farnesyl-diphosphate farnesyltransferase 1, (SQLE) squalene epoxidase, (DHCR7) 7-dehydrocholesterol reductase, (SOAT) sterol O-acyltransferase, (7-DHC) 7-dehydrocholesterol, (LD) lipid droplets. (Figure created in BioRender.)

sensitivity to ferroptosis (Tesfay et al. 2019). Another study reported that colorectal cancer lung metastases in mice could be diminished by blocking Scd1 expression as a result of targeting transcriptional regulation via Srebf1 with a novel compound trichothecin (Liao et al. 2020). This indicates that direct or indirect inhibition of SCD and consequently altering cellular MUFA–PUFA balance represents a potential therapeutic target to enhance lipid peroxidation and induce ferroptosis during metastatic spread. Reduced fatty acid metabolism can also promote ferroptosis sensitivity in cancer cells. For example, it was shown that VHL-mutant clear cell renal cell carcinoma (ccRCC) cells are highly dependent on cystine uptake and glutathione biosynthesis to prevent ferroptosis caused by lipid accumulation, a hallmark of the clear cell phenotype (Miess et al. 2018). Moreover, it was shown that constitute activation of HIF-1α prevents lipolysis in ccRCC cells, thereby leading to lipid accumulation and enhanced ferroptosis sensitivity (Zou et al. 2019). Taken together, these findings highlight the importance of cell intrinsic and extrinsic factors that shape lipid metabolism and fatty acid composition and consequently define ferroptosis sensitivity in cancer cells.

While fatty acid metabolism regulates the susceptibility of membrane lipids toward oxidative damage, components of the mevalonate pathway mostly participate in the regulation of antiferroptotic mechanisms (Fig. 3C). One crucial connection between the mevalonate pathway and ferroptosis comes from the fact that translation of GPX4, a selenocysteine (Sec) protein, requires isoprenylation of the Sec-charged tRNA using isopentenylpyrophosphate as a substrate (Warner et al. 2000). As a consequence, inhibiting the mevalonate pathway by using statins can reduce GPX4 expression and induce ferroptosis, as shown for therapy-resistant mesenchymal cancer cells (Viswanathan et al. 2017). In contrast, a ferroptosis-opposing function of the mevalonate pathway was found during the characterization of the ferroptosis-inducing compound FIN56 (Shimada et al. 2016). This compound was found to activate FDFT1 (also known as squalene synthase). Importantly, induction of ferroptosis by FIN56 could be blocked by inhibition of FDFT1 or SQLE, or by the addition of idebenone, a hydrophilic CoQ10 analog (Shimada et al. 2016). This suggests that FIN56 induces ferroptosis by depleting the available pool of farnesylpyrophosphate, thereby preventing the synthesis of the lipophilic antioxidant ubiquinone. In addition, FIN56 also reduces GPX4 protein levels (Shimada et al. 2016), potentially by inducing GPX4 degradation through an autophagic mechanism (Sun et al. 2021), implying a dual function as ferroptosis inducer. As mentioned above, the accumulation of squalene, the product of FDFT1, was

shown to prevent ferroptosis in lymphoma (Garcia-Bermudez et al. 2019). Finally, 7-dehydrocholesterol reductase (DHCR7) was shown to promote ferroptosis in cancer cells, suggesting that its substrate, 7-dehydrocholesterol (7-DHC), has an antiferroptotic function (see Freitas et al. 2024; Yamada et al. 2024). These studies emphasize that modulation of different reactions of the mevalonate pathway can have either pro or antiferroptotic effects. Global up-regulation of mevalonate pathway enzymes by SREBP2 most likely promotes ferroptosis resistance, as it should increase the availability of all metabolic intermediates. Furthermore, SREBP2 also directly mediates the transcription of the iron carrier transferrin (TF) to reduce the intracellular iron pool, leading to reduced lipid peroxidation and ferroptosis (Hong et al. 2021).

TARGETING FATTY ACID AND CHOLESTEROL METABOLISM FOR CANCER TREATMENT

While deregulated fatty acid and cholesterol metabolism is well established, successful strategies to target these processes for cancer therapy are mostly lacking. Extensive work over the past decades demonstrating the efficacy of lipid metabolism inhibitors in preclinical studies has been reviewed recently (Broadfield et al. 2021).

Early inhibitors of FASN showed dose-limiting toxicity due to anorexia (Loftus et al. 2000). The more recently developed orally available compound TVB-2640 has shown potent target inhibition and safety profile in a phase I dose-escalating study (Falchook et al. 2021) and is currently undergoing clinical trial for several tumor types (ClinicalTrials.gov), including relapsed high-grade astrocytoma (Kelly et al. 2023). In contrast, compounds of the statin family of HMGCR inhibitors targeting the mevalonate pathway have a long clinical history in the treatment of hypercholesterolemia, and their use as anticancer agents is frequently discussed (Longo et al. 2020). Indeed, there are currently over 30 clinical trials investigating the effect of statins in the prevention or treatment of malignancies (ClinicalTrials.gov). Several other compounds that target enzymes of the mevalonate pathway, such as inhibitors of FDFT1 or SQLE, are already in clinical use for other diseases and could be repurposed for their use as anticancer agents.

A major challenge when targeting lipid metabolism is posed by the high plasticity and flexibility, as cancer cells can rapidly switch from de novo synthesis to lipid uptake in response to targeting strategies. It is, therefore, important to exploit selective metabolic vulnerabilities, for example, by targeting therapeutic strategies to conditions that limit this metabolic flexibility. One example of such selective targeting is the metabolic vulnerability of metastatic cancer cells induced by the lipid-poor environment of the brain (Jin et al. 2020; Ferraro et al. 2021). Under these conditions, cancer cells become highly sensitive toward inhibition of fatty acid synthesis and desaturation, making the development of effective inhibitions of SCD activity a therapeutic priority. A similar dependency on SCD was also observed in acute lymphoblastic leukemia (ALL) cells infiltrating the central nervous system (CNS), demonstrating the potential general application of this concept (Savino et al. 2020). Additionally, inhibition of SCD or FADS2 also synergized with temozolomide in recurrent glioblastoma (Parik et al. 2022). In this context, the development of inhibitors for FASN, SCD, or FADS2 that permeate the blood–brain barrier, such as the FASN inhibitor BI-99179 (Kley et al. 2011), is of central importance. In contrast, cancer cells growing in lipid-rich microenvironments, such as the mammary gland or liver, may be more susceptible to inhibition of fatty acid uptake. The fatty acid transporter CD36 is localized to the cell surface, making inhibition by blocking antibodies a therapeutic option (Pascual et al. 2017). CD36 is generally associated with metastasis-initiating stem cells (Pascual et al. 2017) or treatment-resistant minimal residual disease (Rambow et al. 2018) and may thus represent a target to treat advanced cancers.

Therapeutic strategies can also exploit the induction of cellular stress pathways resulting from the modulation of lipid metabolism. One such strategy involves inducing of lethal lipotoxicity by combining the activation of de novo fatty acid synthesis with the inhibition of fatty acid desaturation. This approach was demonstrated through LXR activation by the multikinase inhibitor sorafenib in liver cancer. Combined LXR activation and inhibition of Raf-1 led to the destabilization of SCD protein, causing the toxic accumulation of SFAs and ultimately cell death due to ER-stress (Rudalska et al. 2021). In addition, the transcriptional programs induced downstream from the ER-stress pathway can also induce the expression of genes involved in fatty acid and lipid biosynthesis (Moncan et al. 2021). This suggests that combined targeting of lipid metabolism with modulators of the ER-stress pathway (Maas and Diehl 2015) could also be a potentially effective therapeutic approach. It this context, the effect of the tumor microenvironment must also be considered. For instance, tumor-derived lipids have recently been shown to induce ER-stress and M2 polarization in macrophages (Di Conza et al. 2021).

Another strategy to target cancer cells involves selectively altering membrane lipid remodeling to enhance lipid peroxidation and ferroptosis. One of these strategies is to block phospholipases to prevent the selective removal of PUFA from membrane lipids. For example, it was recently demonstrated that darapladib, an inhibitor of the lipoprotein-associated phospholipase A2 (PLA2G7), sensitizes cancer cells to ferroptosis (Oh et al. 2023). Drugs that target lipid metabolism that have been developed to treat metabolic syndrome and obesity are also investigated for their efficacy as anticancer agents. For example, LCQ-908 (pradigastat), an inhibitor of diacylglycerol acyltransferase 1 (DGAT1), an enzyme required for the synthesis of triacylglycerol, is currently evaluated for the treatment of hypertriglyceridemia. Such compounds could also be considered for the treatment of cancer, as a recent study has shown that genetic deletion of DGAT1 induced apoptosis in glioblastoma cancer cells in vitro and in xenograft models by increasing fat catabolism and inducing oxidative stress (Cheng et al. 2020).

Drugs that target cholesterol metabolism are also being investigated for their potential as anticancer agents. In particular, blocking the mevalonate pathway by statins or other compounds depletes essential metabolic intermediates that cannot be provided through uptake. Strategies to target the mevalonate pathway for cancer therapy have to consider the negative feedback mechanism by which inhibition of cholesterol synthesis will lead to a compensatory activation of SREBP2 processing (Sakai et al. 1996). It is, therefore, likely that statins have to be used in combination with other drugs that prevent SREBP activation (Pandyra et al. 2014) and thereby sensitize cancer cells to statin treatment. Several compounds that potentiate the effects of statins have been recently identified using a pharmacogenomic approach (van Leeuwen et al. 2022). Nevertheless, some cancer types may still be particularly susceptible to the inhibition of cholesterol synthesis due to their increased demand for sterols. For example, we have shown that inhibition of SQLE is highly effective in eliminating prostate cancer cells in vitro and in vivo (Kalogirou et al. 2021). SQLE is up-regulated in advanced prostate cancer due to the loss of miR-205, resulting in elevated cholesterol synthesis and activation of the androgen receptor. Inhibition of SQLE by the FDA-approved antifungal drug terbinafine blocked biochemical progression in end-stage prostate cancer patients (Kalogirou et al. 2021), suggesting that targeting of this enzyme could have a clinical benefit. Targeting SQLE may also produce fewer side effects compared to inhibition of HMGCR, as only the lower part of the cholesterol biosynthesis pathway is blocked. The close link between cholesterol biosynthesis and ferroptosis may also offer additional therapeutic avenues for the elimination of cancer cells.

CONCLUSIONS AND OUTLOOK

Altered lipid metabolism is now well established as an important feature of cancer cells. While important mechanisms by which oncogenic signaling pathways regulate fatty acid and cholesterol biosynthesis have been identified, many of the functions by which lipids promote tumor development and progression remain to be elucidated. The emerging links between altered lipid metabolism, oxidative stress, and ferroptosis in cancer may offer new avenues for therapeutic intervention. Indeed, cancer drugs that exert their function by inducing oxidative stress may be more effective in combination with inhibitors of fatty acid desaturation or ubiqui-

none production. Another aspect to consider is the role of lipids in the complex interactions between cancer cells and the microenvironment. Lipid mediators, including lysophosphatidic acid (LPA), participate in cell–cell communication and can drive cancer cell migration and invasion. The secreted extracellular lysophospholipase D (ENPP2, also known as autotaxin, ATX) promotes the formation of LPA in the tumor microenvironment. It was shown that ATX secreted by pancreatic cancer cells produces LPA from lipids secreted by pancreatic stellate cells to drive cancer progression. In addition, ATX secreted by cancer cells repels tumor-infiltrating T cells to prevent anticancer immunity (Matas-Rico et al. 2021). Given the significance of stromal cells in shaping the lipidome of the tumor microenvironment, studies to investigate the effect of targeting lipid metabolism have to be conducted in fully immune-competent in vivo models. This complexity is even further increased by lipids derived from microbiota, which are increasingly found to have a major impact on tumor development (Loo et al. 2017). When targeting lipid metabolism, it is also imperative to consider the effect of diet. Indeed, exposure to a ketogenic diet rich in palm oil was shown to inhibit tumor growth by inducing the accumulation of SFA. In contrast, the addition of lard, which also provides MUFA, prevented the inhibitory effect of caloric restriction on tumor growth (Lien et al. 2021). It can, therefore, be envisioned that successful treatment strategies targeting lipid metabolism will also involve strict dietary regimens. Adverse effects of targeting lipid metabolism on immune cell function must also be avoided. Finally, drugs that modulate lipid metabolism may also not be tolerated in patients with advanced disease, as they can exacerbate systemic morbidity and cancer cachexia. A detailed understanding of lipid metabolism at the cellular and systemic level is, therefore, essential to develop successful treatment strategies.

ACKNOWLEDGMENTS

The authors thank the members of the Division of Tumor Metabolism and Microenvironment for helpful discussions. The authors also acknowledge support from the German Research Foundation (SCHU2670 and SPP2306). A.B.C.F.

is funded by a fellowship from the São Paulo Research Foundation (FAPESP). All authors contributed to the manuscript and figures. The authors declare no competing interests.

REFERENCES

Acharya R, Shetty SS, Kumari NS. 2023. Fatty acid transport proteins (FATPs) in cancer. *Chem Phys Lipids* **250:** 105269. doi:10.1016/j.chemphyslip.2022.105269

Ackerman D, Simon MC. 2014. Hypoxia, lipids, and cancer: surviving the harsh tumor microenvironment. *Trends Cell Biol* **24:** 472–478. doi:10.1016/j.tcb.2014.06.001

Altea-Manzano P, Doglioni G, Liu Y, Cuadros AM, Nolan E, Fernández-García J, Wu Q, Planque M, Laue KJ, Cidre-Aranaz F, et al. 2023. A palmitate-rich metastatic niche enables metastasis growth via p65 acetylation resulting in pro-metastatic NF-κB signaling. *Nat Cancer* **4:** 344–364. doi:10.1038/s43018-023-00513-2

Banjac A, Perisic T, Sato H, Seiler A, Bannai S, Weiss N, Kölle P, Tschoep K, Issels RD, Daniel PT, et al. 2008. The cystine/cysteine cycle: a redox cycle regulating susceptibility versus resistance to cell death. *Oncogene* **27:** 1618–1628. doi:10.1038/sj.onc.1210796

Beatty A, Singh T, Tyurina YY, Tyurin VA, Samovich S, Nicolas E, Maslar K, Zhou Y, Cai KQ, Tan Y, et al. 2021. Ferroptotic cell death triggered by conjugated linolenic acids is mediated by ACSL1. *Nat Commun* **12:** 2244. doi:10.1038/s41467-021-22471-y

Bensaad K, Favaro E, Lewis CA, Peck B, Lord S, Collins JM, Pinnick KE, Wigfield S, Buffa FM, Li JL, et al. 2014. Fatty acid uptake and lipid storage induced by HIF-1α contribute to cell growth and survival after hypoxia-reoxygenation. *Cell Rep* **9:** 349–365. doi:10.1016/j.celrep.2014.08.056

Bergers G, Fendt SM. 2021. The metabolism of cancer cells during metastasis. *Nat Rev Cancer* **21:** 162–180. doi:10.1038/s41568-020-00320-2

Bersuker K, Hendricks JM, Li Z, Magtanong L, Ford B, Tang PH, Roberts MA, Tong B, Maimone TJ, Zoncu R, et al. 2019. The CoQ oxidoreductase FSP1 acts parallel to GPX4 to inhibit ferroptosis. *Nature* **575:** 688–692. doi:10.1038/s41586-019-1705-2

Bloch K. 1952. Biological synthesis of cholesterol. *Harvey Lect* **48:** 68–88.

Broadfield LA, Pane AA, Talebi A, Swinnen JV, Fendt SM. 2021. Lipid metabolism in cancer: new perspectives and emerging mechanisms. *Dev Cell* **56:** 1363–1393. doi:10.1016/j.devcel.2021.04.013

Carracedo A, Cantley LC, Pandolfi PP. 2013. Cancer metabolism: fatty acid oxidation in the limelight. *Nat Rev Cancer* **13:** 227–232. doi:10.1038/nrc3483

Chen D, Chu B, Yang X, Liu Z, Jin Y, Kon N, Rabadan R, Jiang X, Stockwell BR, Gu W. 2021. iPLA2β-mediated lipid detoxification controls p53-driven ferroptosis independent of GPX4. *Nat Commun* **12:** 3644. doi:10.1038/s41467-021-23902-6

Cheng X, Geng F, Pan M, Wu X, Zhong Y, Wang C, Tian Z, Cheng C, Zhang R, Puduvalli V, et al. 2020. Targeting DGAT1 ameliorates glioblastoma by increasing fat catabolism and oxidative stress. *Cell Metab* **32:** 229–242.e8. doi:10.1016/j.cmet.2020.06.002

Conrad M, Kagan VE, Bayir H, Pagnussat GC, Head B, Traber MG, Stockwell BR. 2018. Regulation of lipid peroxidation and ferroptosis in diverse species. *Genes Dev* **32:** 602–619. doi:10.1101/gad.314674.118

Davis RT, Blake K, Ma D, Gabra MBI, Hernandez GA, Phung AT, Yang Y, Maurer D, Lefebvre A, Alshetaiwi H, et al. 2020. Transcriptional diversity and bioenergetic shift in human breast cancer metastasis revealed by single-cell RNA sequencing. *Nat Cell Biol* **22:** 310–320. doi:10.1038/s41556-020-0477-0

DeBose-Boyd RA, Ye J. 2018. SREBPs in lipid metabolism, insulin signaling, and beyond. *Trends Biochem Sci* **43:** 358–368. doi:10.1016/j.tibs.2018.01.005

Di Conza G, Tsai CH, Gallart-Ayala H, Yu YR, Franco F, Zaffalon L, Xie X, Li X, Xiao Z, Raines LN, et al. 2021. Tumor-induced reshuffling of lipid composition on the endoplasmic reticulum membrane sustains macrophage survival and pro-tumorigenic activity. *Nat Immunol* **22:** 1403–1415. doi:10.1038/s41590-021-01047-4

Dirat B, Bochet L, Dabek M, Daviaud D, Dauvillier S, Majed B, Wang YY, Meulle A, Salles B, Le Gonidec S, et al. 2011. Cancer-associated adipocytes exhibit an activated phenotype and contribute to breast cancer invasion. *Cancer Res* **71:** 2455–2465. doi:10.1158/0008-5472.CAN-10-3323

Dixon SJ, Stockwell BR. 2019. The hallmarks of ferroptosis. *Annu Rev Cancer Biol* **3:** 35–54. doi:10.1146/annurev-cancerbio-030518-055844

Dixon SJ, Lemberg KM, Lamprecht MR, Skouta R, Zaitsev EM, Gleason CE, Patel DN, Bauer AJ, Cantley AM, Yang WS, et al. 2012. Ferroptosis: an iron-dependent form of nonapoptotic cell death. *Cell* **149:** 1060–1072. doi:10.1016/j.cell.2012.03.042

Doll S, Proneth B, Tyurina YY, Panzilius E, Kobayashi S, Ingold I, Irmler M, Beckers J, Aichler M, Walch A, et al. 2017. ACSL4 dictates ferroptosis sensitivity by shaping cellular lipid composition. *Nat Chem Biol* **13:** 91–98. doi:10.1038/nchembio.2239

Doll S, Freitas FP, Shah R, Aldrovandi M, da Silva MC, Ingold I, Goya Grocin A, Xavier da Silva TN, Panzilius E, Scheel CH, et al. 2019. FSP1 is a glutathione-independent ferroptosis suppressor. *Nature* **575:** 693–698. doi:10.1038/s41586-019-1707-0

Düvel K, Yecies JL, Menon S, Raman P, Lipovsky AI, Souza AL, Triantafellow E, Ma Q, Gorski R, Cleaver S, et al. 2010. Activation of a metabolic gene regulatory network downstream of mTOR complex 1. *Mol Cell* **39:** 171–183. doi:10.1016/j.molcel.2010.06.022

Fahy E, Subramaniam S, Brown HA, Glass CK, Merrill AH, Murphy RC, Raetz CR, Russell DW, Seyama Y, Shaw W, et al. 2005. A comprehensive classification system for lipids. *J Lipid Res* **46:** 839–861. doi:10.1194/jlr.E400004-JLR200

Falchook G, Infante J, Arkenau HT, Patel MR, Dean E, Borazanci E, Brenner A, Cook N, Lopez J, Pant S, et al. 2021. First-in-human study of the safety, pharmacokinetics, and pharmacodynamics of first-in-class fatty acid synthase inhibitor TVB-2640 alone and with a taxane in advanced tumors. *EClinicalMedicine* **34:** 100797. doi:10.1016/j.eclinm.2021.100797

Ferraro GB, Ali A, Luengo A, Kodack DP, Deik A, Abbott KL, Bezwada D, Blanc L, Prideaux B, Jin X, et al. 2021. Fatty acid synthesis is required for breast cancer brain metastasis. *Nat Cancer* **2:** 414–428. doi:10.1038/s43018-021-00183-y

Flaveny CA, Griffett K, El-Gendy Bel D, Kazantzis M, Sengupta M, Amelio AL, Chatterjee A, Walker J, Solt LA, Kamenecka TM, et al. 2015. Broad anti-tumor activity of a small molecule that selectively targets the Warburg effect and lipogenesis. *Cancer Cell* **28:** 42–56. doi:10.1016/j.ccell.2015.05.007

Freed-Pastor WA, Mizuno H, Zhao X, Langerød A, Moon SH, Rodriguez-Barrueco R, Barsotti A, Chicas A, Li W, Polotskaia A, et al. 2012. Mutant p53 disrupts mammary tissue architecture via the mevalonate pathway. *Cell* **148:** 244–258. doi:10.1016/j.cell.2011.12.017

Friedmann Angeli JP, Miyamoto S, Schulze A. 2019. Ferroptosis: the greasy side of cell death. *Chem Res Toxicol* **32:** 362–369. doi:10.1021/acs.chemrestox.8b00349

Freitas FP, et al. 2024. 7-Dehydrocholesterol is an endogenous suppressor of ferroptosis. *Nature* **626:** 401–410. doi:10.21203/rs.3.rs-943221/v1

Garcia-Bermudez J, Baudrier L, Bayraktar EC, Shen Y, La K, Guarecuco R, Yucel B, Fiore D, Tavora B, Freinkman E, et al. 2019. Squalene accumulation in cholesterol auxotrophic lymphomas prevents oxidative cell death. *Nature* **567:** 118–122. doi:10.1038/s41586-019-0945-5

Goldstein JL, Brown MS. 1973. Familial hypercholesterolemia: identification of a defect in the regulation of 3-hydroxy-3-methylglutaryl coenzyme A reductase activity associated with overproduction of cholesterol. *Proc Natl Acad Sci* **70:** 2804–2808. doi:10.1073/pnas.70.10.2804

Griffiths B, Lewis CA, Bensaad K, Ros S, Zhang Q, Ferber EC, Konisti S, Peck B, Miess H, East P, et al. 2013. Sterol regulatory element binding protein-dependent regulation of lipid synthesis supports cell survival and tumor growth. *Cancer Metab* **1:** 3. doi:10.1186/2049-3002-1-3

Guo D, Reinitz F, Youssef M, Hong C, Nathanson D, Akhavan D, Kuga D, Amzajerdi AN, Soto H, Zhu S, et al. 2011. An LXR agonist promotes glioblastoma cell death through inhibition of an EGFR/AKT/SREBP-1/LDLR-dependent pathway. *Cancer Discov* **1:** 442–456. doi:10.1158/2159-8290.CD-11-0102

Han J, Li E, Chen L, Zhang Y, Wei F, Liu J, Deng H, Wang Y. 2015. The CREB coactivator CRTC2 controls hepatic lipid metabolism by regulating SREBP1. *Nature* **524:** 243–246. doi:10.1038/nature14557

Hao JW, Wang J, Guo H, Zhao YY, Sun HH, Li YF, Lai XY, Zhao N, Wang X, Xie C, et al. 2020. CD36 facilitates fatty acid uptake by dynamic palmitoylation-regulated endocytosis. *Nat Commun* **11:** 4765. doi:10.1038/s41467-020-18565-8

Harayama T, Riezman H. 2018. Understanding the diversity of membrane lipid composition. *Nat Rev Mol Cell Biol* **19:** 281–296. doi:10.1038/nrm.2017.138

Hendricks JM, Doubravsky CE, Wehri E, Li Z, Roberts MA, Deol KK, Lange M, Lasheras-Otero I, Momper JD, Dixon SJ, et al. 2023. Identification of structurally diverse FSP1 inhibitors that sensitize cancer cells to ferroptosis. *Cell Chem Biol* **30:** 1090–1103.e7. doi:10.1016/j.chembiol.2023.04.007

Hong X, Roh W, Sullivan RJ, Wong KHK, Wittner BS, Guo H, Dubash TD, Sade-Feldman M, Wesley B, Horwitz E, et al. 2021. The lipogenic regulator SREBP2 induces transferrin

in circulating melanoma cells and suppresses ferroptosis. *Cancer Discov* **11:** 678–695. doi:10.1158/2159-8290.CD-19-1500

Hsieh FL, Turner L, Bolla JR, Robinson CV, Lavstsen T, Higgins MK. 2016. The structural basis for CD36 binding by the malaria parasite. *Nat Commun* **7:** 12837. doi:10.1038/ncomms12837

Jin X, Demere Z, Nair K, Ali A, Ferraro GB, Natoli T, Deik A, Petronio L, Tang AA, Zhu C, et al. 2020. A metastasis map of human cancer cell lines. *Nature* **588:** 331–336. doi:10.1038/s41586-020-2969-2

Kagan VE, Mao G, Qu F, Angeli JP, Doll S, Croix CS, Dar HH, Liu B, Tyurin VA, Ritov VB, et al. 2017. Oxidized arachidonic and adrenic PEs navigate cells to ferroptosis. *Nat Chem Biol* **13:** 81–90. doi:10.1038/nchembio.2238

Kalogirou C, Linxweiler J, Schmucker P, Snaebjornsson MT, Schmitz W, Wach S, Krebs M, Hartmann E, Puhr M, Müller A, et al. 2021. MiR-205-driven downregulation of cholesterol biosynthesis through SQLE-inhibition identifies therapeutic vulnerability in aggressive prostate cancer. *Nat Commun* **12:** 5066. doi:10.1038/s41467-021-25325-9

Kamphorst JJ, Cross JR, Fan J, de Stanchina E, Mathew R, White EP, Thompson CB, Rabinowitz JD. 2013. Hypoxic and Ras-transformed cells support growth by scavenging unsaturated fatty acids from lysophospholipids. *Proc Natl Acad Sci* **110:** 8882–8887. doi:10.1073/pnas.1307237110

Kaymak I, Maier CR, Schmitz W, Campbell AD, Dankworth B, Ade CP, Walz S, Paauwe M, Kalogirou C, Marouf H, et al. 2020. Mevalonate pathway provides ubiquinone to maintain pyrimidine synthesis and survival in p53-deficient cancer cells exposed to metabolic stress. *Cancer Res* **80:** 189–203. doi:10.1158/0008-5472.CAN-19-0650

Kelly W, Diaz Duque AE, Michalek J, Konkel B, Caflisch L, Chen Y, Pathuri SC, Madhusudanannair-Kunnuparampil V, Floyd J, Brenner A. 2023. Phase II investigation of TVB-2640 (Denifanstat) with bevacizumab in patients with first relapse high-grade astrocytoma. *Clin Cancer Res* **29:** 2419–2425. doi:10.1158/1078-0432.CCR-22-2807

Kley JT, Mack J, Hamilton B, Scheuerer S, Redemann N. 2011. Discovery of BI 99179, a potent and selective inhibitor of type I fatty acid synthase with central exposure. *Bioorg Med Chem Lett* **21:** 5924–5927. doi:10.1016/j.bmcl.2011.07.083

Koundouros N, Poulogiannis G. 2020. Reprogramming of fatty acid metabolism in cancer. *Br J Cancer* **122:** 4–22. doi:10.1038/s41416-019-0650-z

Li H, Ning S, Ghandi M, Kryukov GV, Gopal S, Deik A, Souza A, Pierce K, Keskula P, Hernandez D, et al. 2019. The landscape of cancer cell line metabolism. *Nat Med* **25:** 850–860. doi:10.1038/s41591-019-0404-8

Liao C, Li M, Li X, Li N, Zhao X, Wang X, Song Y, Quan J, Cheng C, Liu J, et al. 2020. Trichothecin inhibits invasion and metastasis of colon carcinoma associating with SCD-1-mediated metabolite alteration. *Biochim Biophys Acta Mol Cell Biol Lipids* **1865:** 158540. doi:10.1016/j.bbalip.2019.158540

Liebisch G, Fahy E, Aoki J, Dennis EA, Durand T, Ejsing CS, Fedorova M, Feussner I, Griffiths WJ, Köeler H, et al. 2020. Update on LIPID MAPS classification, nomenclature, and shorthand notation for MS-derived lipid structures. *J Lipid Res* **61:** 1539–1555. doi:10.1194/jlr.S120001025

 Cite this article as *Cold Spring Harb Perspect Med* doi: 10.1101/cshperspect.a041548

Lien EC, Westermark AM, Zhang Y, Yuan C, Li Z, Lau AN, Sapp KM, Wolpin BM, Vander Heiden MG. 2021. Low glycaemic diets alter lipid metabolism to influence tumour growth. *Nature* 599: 302–307. doi:10.1038/s41586-021-04049-2

Lin CY, Gustafsson JA. 2015. Targeting liver X receptors in cancer therapeutics. *Nat Rev Cancer* 15: 216–224. doi:10.1038/nrc3912

Loftus TM, Jaworsky DE, Frehywot GL, Townsend CA, Ronnett GV, Lane MD, Kuhajda FP. 2000. Reduced food intake and body weight in mice treated with fatty acid synthase inhibitors. *Science* 288: 2379–2381. doi:10.1126/science.288.5475.2379

Longo J, van Leeuwen JE, Elbaz M, Branchard E, Penn LZ. 2020. Statins as anticancer agents in the era of precision medicine. *Clin Cancer Res* 26: 5791–5800. doi:10.1158/1078-0432.CCR-20-1967

Loo TM, Kamachi F, Watanabe Y, Yoshimoto S, Kanda H, Arai Y, Nakajima-Takagi Y, Iwama A, Koga T, Sugimoto Y, et al. 2017. Gut microbiota promotes obesity-associated liver cancer through PGE2-mediated suppression of antitumor immunity. *Cancer Discov* 7: 522–538. doi:10.1158/2159-8290.CD-16-0932

Loo SY, Toh LP, Xie WH, Pathak E, Tan W, Ma S, Lee MY, Shatishwaran S, Yeo JZZ, Yuan J, et al. 2021. Fatty acid oxidation is a druggable gateway regulating cellular plasticity for driving metastasis in breast cancer. *Sci Adv* 7: eabh2443. doi:10.1126/sciadv.abh2443

Luis G, Godfroid A, Nishiumi S, Cimino J, Blacher S, Maquoi E, Wery C, Collignon A, Longuespée R, Montero-Ruiz L, et al. 2021. Tumor resistance to ferroptosis driven by Stearoyl-CoA Desaturase-1 (SCD1) in cancer cells and fatty acid biding protein-4 (FABP4) in tumor microenvironment promote tumor recurrence. *Redox Biol* 43: 102006. doi:10.1016/j.redox.2021.102006

Maas NL, Diehl JA. 2015. Molecular pathways: the PERKs and pitfalls of targeting the unfolded protein response in cancer. *Clin Cancer Res* 21: 675–679. doi:10.1158/1078-0432.CCR-13-3239

Magtanong L, Ko PJ, To M, Cao JY, Forcina GC, Tarangelo A, Ward CC, Cho K, Patti GJ, Nomura DK, et al. 2019. Exogenous monounsaturated fatty acids promote a ferroptosis-resistant cell state. *Cell Chem Biol* 26: 420–432.e9. doi:10.1016/j.chembiol.2018.11.016

Mahoney CE, Pirman D, Chubukov V, Sleger T, Hayes S, Fan ZP, Allen EL, Chen Y, Huang L, Liu M, et al. 2019. A chemical biology screen identifies a vulnerability of neuroendocrine cancer cells to SQLE inhibition. *Nat Commun* 10: 96. doi:10.1038/s41467-018-07959-4

Maier CR, Hartmann O, Prieto-Garcia C, Al-Shami KM, Schlicker L, Vogel FCE, Haid S, Klann K, Buck V, Münch C, et al. 2023. USP28 controls SREBP2 and the mevalonate pathway to drive tumour growth in squamous cancer. *Cell Death Differ* 30: 1710–1725. doi:10.1038/s41418-023-01173-6

Martin-Perez M, Urdiroz-Urricelqui U, Bigas C, Benitah SA. 2021. Lipid metabolism in metastasis and therapy. *Curr Opin Styst Biol* 28: 100401.

Martin-Perez M, Urdiroz-Urricelqui U, Bigas C, Benitah SA. 2022. The role of lipids in cancer progression and metastasis. *Cell Metab* 34: 1675–1699. doi:10.1016/j.cmet.2022.09.023

Matas-Rico E, Frijlink E, van der Haar Àvila I, Menegakis A, van Zon M, Morris AJ, Koster J, Salgado-Polo F, de Kivit S, Lança T, et al. 2021. Autotaxin impedes anti-tumor immunity by suppressing chemotaxis and tumor infiltration of CD8[+] T cells. *Cell Rep* 37: 110013. doi:10.1016/j.celrep.2021.110013

McGregor GH, Campbell AD, Fey SK, Tumanov S, Sumpton D, Blanco GR, Mackay G, Nixon C, Vazquez A, Sansom OJ, et al. 2020. Targeting the metabolic response to statin-mediated oxidative stress produces a synergistic antitumor response. *Cancer Res* 80: 175–188. doi:10.1158/0008-5472.CAN-19-0644

Miess H, Dankworth B, Gouw AM, Rosenfeldt M, Schmitz W, Jiang M, Saunders B, Howell M, Downward J, Felsher DW, et al. 2018. The glutathione redox system is essential to prevent ferroptosis caused by impaired lipid metabolism in clear cell renal cell carcinoma. *Oncogene* 37: 5435–5450. doi:10.1038/s41388-018-0315-z

Mishima E, Conrad M. 2022. Nutritional and metabolic control of ferroptosis. *Annu Rev Nutr* 42: 275–309. doi:10.1146/annurev-nutr-062320-114541

Mishima E, Ito J, Wu Z, Nakamura T, Wahida A, Doll S, Tonnus W, Nepachalovich P, Eggenhofer E, Aldrovandi M, et al. 2022. A non-canonical vitamin K cycle is a potent ferroptosis suppressor. *Nature* 608: 778–783. doi:10.1038/s41586-022-05022-3

Moncan M, Mnich K, Blomme A, Almanza A, Samali A, Gorman AM. 2021. Regulation of lipid metabolism by the unfolded protein response. *J Cell Mol Med* 25: 1359–1370. doi:10.1111/jcmm.16255

Moon SH, Huang CH, Houlihan SL, Regunath K, Freed-Pastor WA, Morris JP, Tschaharganeh DF, Kastenhuber ER, Barsotti AM, Culp-Hill R, et al. 2019. P53 represses the mevalonate pathway to mediate tumor suppression. *Cell* 176: 564–580.e19. doi:10.1016/j.cell.2018.11.011

Mullen PJ, Yu R, Longo J, Archer MC, Penn LZ. 2016. The interplay between cell signalling and the mevalonate pathway in cancer. *Nat Rev Cancer* 16: 718–731. doi:10.1038/nrc.2016.76

Müller F, Lim JKM, Bebber CM, Seidel E, Tishina S, Dahlhaus A, Stroh J, Beck J, Yapici FI, Nakayama K, et al. 2023. Elevated FSP1 protects KRAS-mutated cells from ferroptosis during tumor initiation. *Cell Death Differ* 30: 442–456. doi:10.1038/s41418-022-01096-8

Nath A, Chan C. 2016. Genetic alterations in fatty acid transport and metabolism genes are associated with metastatic progression and poor prognosis of human cancers. *Sci Rep* 6: 18669. doi:10.1038/srep18669

Nieman KM, Kenny HA, Penicka CV, Ladanyi A, Buell-Gutbrod R, Zillhardt MR, Romero IL, Carey MS, Mills GB, Hotamisligil GS, et al. 2011. Adipocytes promote ovarian cancer metastasis and provide energy for rapid tumor growth. *Nat Med* 17: 1498–1503. doi:10.1038/nm.2492

Nohturfft A, Zhang SC. 2009. Coordination of lipid metabolism in membrane biogenesis. *Annu Rev Cell Dev Biol* 25: 539–566. doi:10.1146/annurev.cellbio.24.110707.175344

Oh M, Jang SY, Lee JY, Kim JW, Jung Y, Seo J, Han TS, Jang E, Son HY, Kim D, et al. 2023. The lipoprotein-associated phospholipase A2 inhibitor Darapladib sensitises cancer cells to ferroptosis by remodeling lipid metabolism. *Nat Commun* 14: 5728. doi:10.1038/s41467-023-41462-9

Pandyra A, Mullen PJ, Kalkat M, Yu R, Pong JT, Li Z, Trudel S, Lang KS, Minden MD, Schimmer AD, et al. 2014. Immediate utility of two approved agents to target both the metabolic mevalonate pathway and its restorative feedback loop. *Cancer Res* **74:** 4772–4782. doi:10.1158/0008-5472.CAN-14-0130

Parik S, Fernández-García J, Lodi F, De Vlaminck K, Derweduwe M, De Vleeschouwer S, Sciot R, Geens W, Weng L, Bosisio FM, et al. 2022. GBM tumors are heterogeneous in their fatty acid metabolism and modulating fatty acid metabolism sensitizes cancer cells derived from recurring GBM tumors to temozolomide. *Front Oncol* **12:** 988872. doi:10.3389/fonc.2022.988872

Pascual G, Avgustinova A, Mejetta S, Martín M, Castellanos A, Attolini CS, Berenguer A, Prats N, Toll A, Hueto JA, et al. 2017. Targeting metastasis-initiating cells through the fatty acid receptor CD36. *Nature* **541:** 41–45. doi:10.1038/nature20791

Peck B, Schulze A. 2016. Lipid desaturation—the next step in targeting lipogenesis in cancer? *FEBS J* **283:** 2767–2778. doi:10.1111/febs.13681

Peck B, Schulze A. 2019. Lipid metabolism at the nexus of diet and tumor microenvironment. *Trends Cancer* **5:** 693–703. doi:10.1016/j.trecan.2019.09.007

Peterson TR, Sengupta SS, Harris TE, Carmack AE, Kang SA, Balderas E, Guertin DA, Madden KL, Carpenter AE, Finck BN, et al. 2011. mTOR complex 1 regulates lipin 1 localization to control the SREBP pathway. *Cell* **146:** 408–420. doi:10.1016/j.cell.2011.06.034

Portstmann T, Santos CR, Griffiths B, Cully M, Wu M, Leevers S, Griffiths JR, Chung YL, Schulze A. 2008. SREBP activity is regulated by mTORC1 and contributes to Akt-dependent cell growth. *Cell Metab* **8:** 224–236. doi:10.1016/j.cmet.2008.07.007

Prieto-Garcia C, Hartmann O, Reissland M, Braun F, Fischer T, Walz S, Schülein-Völk C, Eilers U, Ade CP, Calzado MA, et al. 2020. Maintaining protein stability of ΔNp63 via USP28 is required for squamous cancer cells. *EMBO Mol Med* **12:** e11101. doi:10.15252/emmm.201911101

Rambow F, Rogiers A, Marin-Bejar O, Aibar S, Femel J, Dewaele M, Karras P, Brown D, Chang YH, Debiec-Rychter M, et al. 2018. Toward minimal residual disease-directed therapy in melanoma. *Cell* **174:** 843–855.e19. doi:10.1016/j.cell.2018.06.025

Resh MD. 2013. Covalent lipid modifications of proteins. *Curr Biol* **23:** R431–R435. doi:10.1016/j.cub.2013.04.024

Röhrig F, Schulze A. 2016. The multifaceted roles of fatty acid synthesis in cancer. *Nat Rev Cancer* **16:** 732–749. doi:10.1038/nrc.2016.89

Rudalska R, Harbig J, Snaebjornsson MT, Klotz S, Zwirner S, Taranets L, Heinzmann F, Kronenberger T, Forster M, Cui W, et al. 2021. LXRα activation and Raf inhibition trigger lethal lipotoxicity in liver cancer. *Nat Cancer* **2:** 201–217. doi:10.1038/s43018-020-00168-3

Rysman E, Brusselmans K, Scheys K, Timmermans L, Derua R, Munck S, Van Veldhoven PP, Waltregny D, Daniëls VW, Machiels J, et al. 2010. De novo lipogenesis protects cancer cells from free radicals and chemotherapeutics by promoting membrane lipid saturation. *Cancer Res* **70:** 8117–8126. doi:10.1158/0008-5472.CAN-09-3871

Sakai J, Duncan EA, Rawson RB, Hua X, Brown MS, Goldstein JL. 1996. Sterol-regulated release of SREBP-2 from cell membranes requires two sequential cleavages, one within a transmembrane segment. *Cell* **85:** 1037–1046. doi:10.1016/S0092-8674(00)81304-5

Savino AM, Fernandes SI, Olivares O, Zemlyansky A, Cousins A, Markert EK, Barel S, Geron I, Frishman L, Birger Y, et al. 2020. Metabolic adaptation of acute lymphoblastic leukemia to the central nervous system microenvironment is dependent on Stearoyl CoA desaturase. *Nat Cancer* **1:** 998–1009. doi:10.1038/s43018-020-00115-2

Seiler A, Schneider M, Förster H, Roth S, Wirth EK, Culmsee C, Plesnila N, Kremmer E, Rådmark O, Wurst W, et al. 2008. Glutathione peroxidase 4 senses and translates oxidative stress into 12/15-lipoxygenase dependent- and AIF-mediated cell death. *Cell Metab* **8:** 237–248. doi:10.1016/j.cmet.2008.07.005

Shamma A, Takegami Y, Miki T, Kitajima S, Noda M, Obara T, Okamoto T, Takahashi C. 2009. Rb regulates DNA damage response and cellular senescence through E2F-dependent suppression of N-ras isoprenylation. *Cancer Cell* **15:** 255–269. doi:10.1016/j.ccr.2009.03.001

Shevchenko A, Simons K. 2010. Lipidomics: coming to grips with lipid diversity. *Nat Rev Mol Cell Biol* **11:** 593–598. doi:10.1038/nrm2934

Shimada K, Skouta R, Kaplan A, Yang WS, Hayano M, Dixon SJ, Brown LM, Valenzuela CA, Wolpaw AJ, Stockwell BR. 2016. Global survey of cell death mechanisms reveals metabolic regulation of ferroptosis. *Nat Chem Biol* **12:** 497–503. doi:10.1038/nchembio.2079

Shimano H, Sato R. 2017. SREBP-regulated lipid metabolism: convergent physiology—divergent pathophysiology. *Nat Rev Endocrinol* **13:** 710–730. doi:10.1038/nrendo.2017.91

Snaebjornsson MT, Janaki-Raman S, Schulze A. 2020. Greasing the wheels of the cancer machine: the role of lipid metabolism in cancer. *Cell Metab* **31:** 62–76. doi:10.1016/j.cmet.2019.11.010

Stockwell BR. 2022. Ferroptosis turns 10: emerging mechanisms, physiological functions, and therapeutic applications. *Cell* **185:** 2401–2421. doi:10.1016/j.cell.2022.06.003

Sun Y, Berleth N, Wu W, Schlütermann D, Deitersen J, Stuhldreier F, Berning L, Friedrich A, Akgün S, Mendiburo MJ, et al. 2021. Fin56-induced ferroptosis is supported by autophagy-mediated GPX4 degradation and functions synergistically with mTOR inhibition to kill bladder cancer cells. *Cell Death Dis* **12:** 1028. doi:10.1038/s41419-021-04306-2

Sundqvist A, Ericsson J. 2003. Transcription-dependent degradation controls the stability of the SREBP family of transcription factors. *Proc Natl Acad Sci* **100:** 13833–13838. doi:10.1073/pnas.2335135100

Sundqvist A, Bengoechea-Alonso MT, Ye X, Lukiyanchuk V, Jin J, Harper JW, Ericsson J. 2005. Control of lipid metabolism by phosphorylation-dependent degradation of the SREBP family of transcription factors by SCF(Fbw7). *Cell Metab* **1:** 379–391. doi:10.1016/j.cmet.2005.04.010

Tesfay L, Paul BT, Konstorum A, Deng Z, Cox AO, Lee J, Furdui CM, Hegde P, Torti FM, Torti SV. 2019. Stearoyl-CoA desaturase 1 protects ovarian cancer cells from ferroptotic cell death. *Cancer Res* **79:** 5355–5366. doi:10.1158/0008-5472.CAN-19-0369

Thurnher M, Gruenbacher G. 2015. T lymphocyte regulation by mevalonate metabolism. *Sci Signal* **8:** re4. doi:10.1126/scisignal.2005970

Triki M, Rinaldi G, Planque M, Broekaert D, Winkelkotte AM, Maier CR, Janaki Raman S, Vandekeere A, Van Elsen J, Orth MF, et al. 2020. mTOR signaling and SREBP activity increase FADS2 expression and can activate sapienate biosynthesis. *Cell Rep* **31**: 107806. doi:10.1016/j.celrep .2020.107806

Ubellacker JM, Tasdogan A, Ramesh V, Shen B, Mitchell EC, Martin-Sandoval MS, Gu Z, McCormick ML, Durham AB, Spitz DR, et al. 2020. Lymph protects metastasizing melanoma cells from ferroptosis. *Nature* **585**: 113–118. doi:10.1038/s41586-020-2623-z

van Leeuwen JE, Ba-Alawi W, Branchard E, Cruickshank J, Schormann W, Longo J, Silvester J, Gross PL, Andrews DW, Cescon DW, et al. 2022. Computational pharmacogenomic screen identifies drugs that potentiate the anti-breast cancer activity of statins. *Nat Commun* **13**: 6323. doi:10.1038/s41467-022-33144-9

Villa GR, Hulce JJ, Zanca C, Bi J, Ikegami S, Cahill GL, Gu Y, Lum KM, Masui K, Yang H, et al. 2016. An LXR-cholesterol axis creates a metabolic co-dependency for brain cancers. *Cancer Cell* **30**: 683–693. doi:10.1016/j.ccell .2016.09.008

Viswanathan VS, Ryan MJ, Dhruv HD, Gill S, Eichhoff OM, Seashore-Ludlow B, Kaffenberger SD, Eaton JK, Shimada K, Aguirre AJ, et al. 2017. Dependency of a therapy-resistant state of cancer cells on a lipid peroxidase pathway. *Nature* **547**: 453–457. doi:10.1038/nature23007

Vriens K, Christen S, Parik S, Broekaert D, Yoshinaga K, Talebi A, Dehairs J, Escalona-Noguero C, Schmieder R, Cornfield T, et al. 2019. Evidence for an alternative fatty acid desaturation pathway increasing cancer plasticity. *Nature* **566**: 403–406. doi:10.1038/s41586-019-0904-1

Wang M, Casey PJ. 2016. Protein prenylation: unique fats make their mark on biology. *Nat Rev Mol Cell Biol* **17**: 110–122. doi:10.1038/nrm.2015.11

Wang D, Dubois RN. 2010. Eicosanoids and cancer. *Nat Rev Cancer* **10**: 181–193. doi:10.1038/nrc2809

Warner GJ, Berry MJ, Moustafa ME, Carlson BA, Hatfield DL, Faust JR. 2000. Inhibition of selenoprotein synthesis by selenocysteine tRNA[Ser]Sec lacking isopentenyladenosine. *J Biol Chem* **275**: 28110–28119. doi:10.1074/jbc .M001280200

Williams KJ, Argus JP, Zhu Y, Wilks MQ, Marbois BN, York AG, Kidani Y, Pourzia AL, Akhavan D, Lisiero DN, et al. 2013. An essential requirement for the SCAP/SREBP signaling axis to protect cancer cells from lipotoxicity. *Cancer Res* **73**: 2850–2862. doi:10.1158/0008-5472.CAN-13-0382-T

Xie X, Tian L, Zhao Y, Liu F, Dai S, Gu X, Ye Y, Zhou L, Liu X, Sun Y, et al. 2023. BACH1-induced ferroptosis drives lymphatic metastasis by repressing the biosynthesis of mono-unsaturated fatty acids. *Cell Death Dis* **14**: 48. doi:10.1038/ s41419-023-05571-z

Yamada N, Karasawa T, Komada T, Matsumura T, Baatarjav C, Ito J, Nakagawa K, Yamamuro D, Ishibashi S, Miura K, et al. 2024. Inhibition of 7-dehydrocholesterol reductase prevents hepatic ferroptosis under an active state of sterol synthesis. *Nat Commun* **15**: 2195. doi:10.1038/s41467-024-46386-6

Yang WS, Stockwell BR. 2016. Ferroptosis: death by lipid peroxidation. *Trends Cell Biol* **26**: 165–176. doi:10.1016/j .tcb.2015.10.014

Yecies JL, Zhang HH, Menon S, Liu S, Yecies D, Lipovsky AI, Gorgun C, Kwiatkowski DJ, Hotamisligil GS, Lee CH, et al. 2011. Akt stimulates hepatic SREBP1c and lipogenesis through parallel mTORC1-dependent and independent pathways. *Cell Metab* **14**: 21–32. doi:10.1016/j.cmet.2011 .06.002

Yi J, Zhu J, Wu J, Thompson CB, Jiang X. 2020. Oncogenic activation of PI3K-AKT-mTOR signaling suppresses ferroptosis via SREBP-mediated lipogenesis. *Proc Natl Acad Sci* **117**: 31189–31197. doi:10.1073/pnas.2017152117

Yoshioka H, Kawamura T, Muroi M, Kondoh Y, Honda K, Kawatani M, Aono H, Waldmann H, Watanabe N, Osada H. 2022. Identification of a small molecule that enhances ferroptosis via inhibition of ferroptosis suppressor protein 1 (FSP1). *ACS Chem Biol* **17**: 483–491. doi:10.1021/ac schembio.2c00028

Young RM, Ackerman D, Quinn ZL, Mancuso A, Gruber M, Liu L, Giannoukos DN, Bobrovnikova-Marjon E, Diehl JA, Keith B, et al. 2013. Dysregulated mTORC1 renders cells critically dependent on desaturated lipids for survival under tumor-like stress. *Genes Dev* **27**: 1115–1131. doi:10 .1101/gad.198630.112

Yue S, Li J, Lee SY, Lee HJ, Shao T, Song B, Cheng L, Masterson TA, Liu X, Ratliff TL, et al. 2014. Cholesteryl ester accumulation induced by PTEN loss and PI3K/AKT activation underlies human prostate cancer aggressiveness. *Cell Metab* **19**: 393–406. doi:10.1016/j.cmet.2014.01.019

Zhang M, Di Martino JS, Bowman RL, Campbell NR, Baksh SC, Simon-Vermot T, Kim IS, Haldeman P, Mondal C, Yong-Gonzales V, et al. 2018. Adipocyte-derived lipids mediate melanoma progression via FATP proteins. *Cancer Discov* **8**: 1006–1025. doi:10.1158/2159-8290.CD-17-1371

Zou Y, Palte MJ, Deik AA, Li H, Eaton JK, Wang W, Tseng YY, Deasy R, Kost-Alimova M, Dančík V, et al. 2019. A GPX4-dependent cancer cell state underlies the clear-cell morphology and confers sensitivity to ferroptosis. *Nat Commun* **10**: 1617. doi:10.1038/s41467-019-09277-9

From the Inside Out: Exposing the Roles of Urea Cycle Enzymes in Tumors and Their Micro and Macro Environments

Emma Hajaj,[1] Sabina Pozzi,[1] and Ayelet Erez

Department of Molecular Cell Biology, Weizmann Institute of Science, Rehovot 7610001, Israel

Correspondence: ayelet.erez@weizmann.ac.il

Catabolic pathways change in anabolic diseases such as cancer to maintain metabolic homeostasis. The liver urea cycle (UC) is the main catabolic pathway for disposing excess nitrogen. Outside the liver, the UC enzymes are differentially expressed based on each tissue's needs for UC intermediates. In tumors, there are changes in the expression of UC enzymes selected for promoting tumorigenesis by increasing the availability of essential UC substrates and products. Consequently, there are compensatory changes in the expression of UC enzymes in the cells that compose the tumor microenvironment. Moreover, extrahepatic tumors induce changes in the expression of the liver UC, which contribute to the systemic manifestations of cancer, such as weight loss. Here, we review the multilayer changes in the expression of UC enzymes throughout carcinogenesis. Understanding the changes in UC expression in the tumor and its micro and macro environment can help identify biomarkers for early cancer diagnosis and vulnerabilities that can be targeted for therapy.

THE UREA CYCLE ENZYMES AND METABOLITES IN PHYSIOLOGICAL STATES

The urea cycle (UC) operates in hepatocytes to convert two nitrogen molecules from ammonia and aspartate into one urea molecule (Fig. 1; Watford 2003). The process involves two transporters, five enzymes, and one cofactor-producing enzyme, N-acetylglutamate synthetase (NAGS), to dispose of 85%–95% of the body's waste nitrogen as urea in the urine (Hoffer 2016).

In the first step, carbamoyl phosphate synthetase 1 (CPS1) catalyzes the synthesis of car-bamoyl phosphate (CP) from ATP and bicarbonate, using ammonia as a nitrogen source and NAG as a co-factor. Next, ornithine trans-carbamylase (OTC) creates citrulline from ornithine and CP. These two steps occur in the mitochondria, followed by citrulline transport to the cytosol by the ornithine transporter 1 (ORNT1). In the cytosolic reactions, citrulline is condensed with aspartate by argininosuccinate synthase (ASS1) to form argininosuccinate. The second mitochondrial transporter citrin (SLC25A13) provides mitochondrial aspartate to the cytosol for this reaction. Argininosuccinate is then broken down by argininosuccinate

---

Cite this article as *Cold Spring Harb Perspect Med* doi: 10.1101/cshperspect.a041538

lyase (ASL) into arginine and fumarate. Finally, arginine is hydrolyzed into urea and ornithine by arginase 1 (ARG1), regenerating the ornithine for another round of the cycle (Fig. 1; Watford 2003). Hence, there is no net synthesis of UC intermediates for usage in the liver other than ammonia disposal. Nevertheless, some metabolites, such as argininosuccinate and urea, are secreted from the UC, and other metabolites, such as aspartate and fumarate, are exchanged with the tricarboxylic acid (TCA) cycle (Fig. 1).

Outside the liver, different UC enzymes are expressed in accordance with the cellular needs for UC metabolites. In kidney cells, the expression of ASL and ASS1 makes the kidney the leading site for systemic de novo arginine generation from citrulline that is produced in the small intestine (Blachier et al. 1993; De Jonge et al. 1998). Since

arginine is a semi-essential amino acid, most cells can independently synthesize arginine via the arginine–citrulline cycle under arginine deprivation states (Husson et al. 2003; van de Poll et al. 2007). In this cycle, arginine is converted to citrulline by nitric oxide (NO) synthase (NOS), and NO is released. Citrulline can then be recycled to arginine by ASS1 and ASL, forming the citrulline–NO cycle (Fig. 1). Arginine is fundamental for the survival of multiple cell types because it can be used as a substrate for generating essential metabolites, such as the synthesis of ornithine by ARG2 (Nagamani et al. 2012). ARG2, a mitochondrial enzyme ubiquitously expressed in extrahepatic tissues, synthesizes ornithine when there is a cellular need for ornithine downstream metabolites polyamine, proline, and glutamate (Fig. 1; Cederbaum et al. 2004).

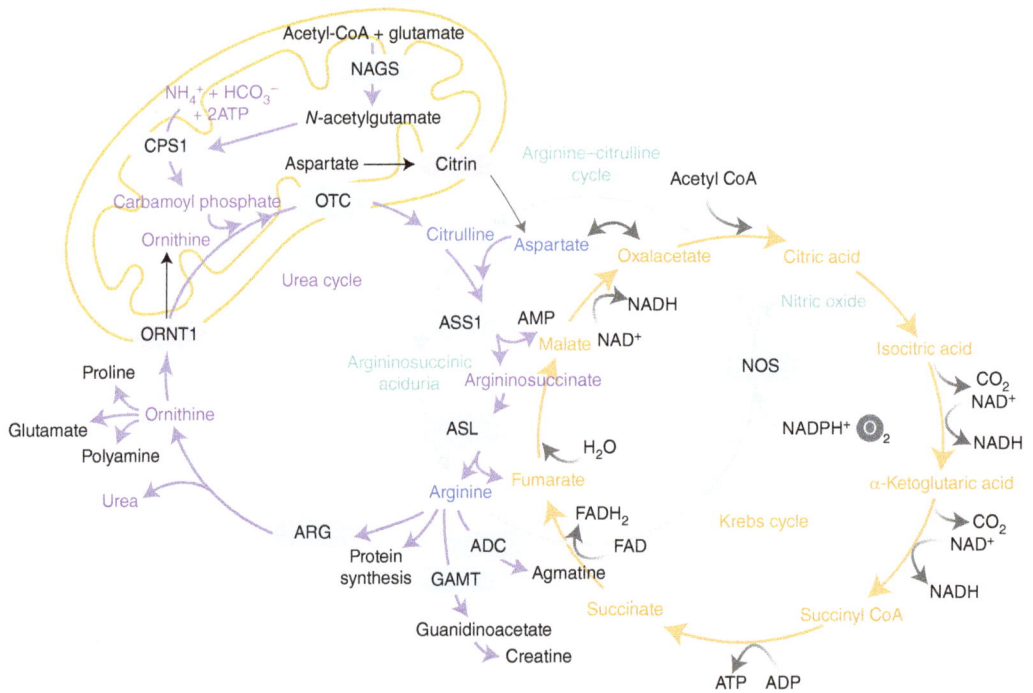

Figure 1. The urea cycle (UC) enzymes and metabolites in the liver and extrahepatic tissues. A schematic representation of UC enzymes/transporters, a cofactor-producing enzyme, N-acetylglutamate synthetase (NAGS), and metabolites that are produced by hepatocytes. (CPS1) Carbamoyl phosphate synthetase 1, (ASS1) argininosuccinate synthase, (ASL) argininosuccinate lyase, (ARG) arginase, (OTC) ornithine transcarbamylase, (ORNT1) ornithine transporter 1, (SLC25A13) citrin. ASS1, ASL, and NOS participate in the arginine–citrulline cycle in extrahepatic tissues to generate nitric oxide (NO) and arginine. The potential metabolic fates of UC metabolites are also depicted. Aspartate and fumarate are exchanged between the UC and the Krebs cycle. (Created with BioRender.com.)

The importance of UC to normal physiology is further highlighted by the severe clinical presentation of children born with malfunctioning UC due to germline mutations in one of the UC enzymes (Erez and DeBerardinis 2015). In extremely severe cases of UC disorders, ammonia accumulates in the brain right after birth and may lead to brain edema and sometimes death (Erez et al. 2011). Interestingly, children with mild and moderate UC disorders demonstrate chronic long-term complications such as hypertension and cognitive delays, even after liver transplant, emphasizing the crucial roles of UC enzymes outside the liver (Erez et al. 2011; Lerner et al. 2019).

The essentiality of UC metabolites for cell proliferation and survival makes them beneficial for cancer growth. Indeed, UC intermediates were described to affect cancer hallmarks as uncontrolled proliferation, mutagenesis, and immune evasion (Lee et al. 2018; Keshet et al. 2020).

UC-RELATED METABOLIC CHANGES WITHIN THE TUMOR

Tumor cells, emerging from various cell origins, have been shown to dysregulate the expression of UC enzymes in a nonrandon direction that is independent from UC expression in the tissue of origin, selected for benefiting carcinogenesis and resulting in worsening cancer patients' outcomes (Fig. 2).

There are three main mechanisms by which UC rewiring in the tumors supports cancer proliferation, growth, and survival.

Elevated Tumor Levels of Arginine and Its Downstream Metabolites

Arginine is required for cancer growth and survival. In hepatocellular carcinoma (HCC), experimental inhibition of the arginine transporter SLC7A1 slows cell growth in vitro and in vivo by inducing a stress response that promotes HCC

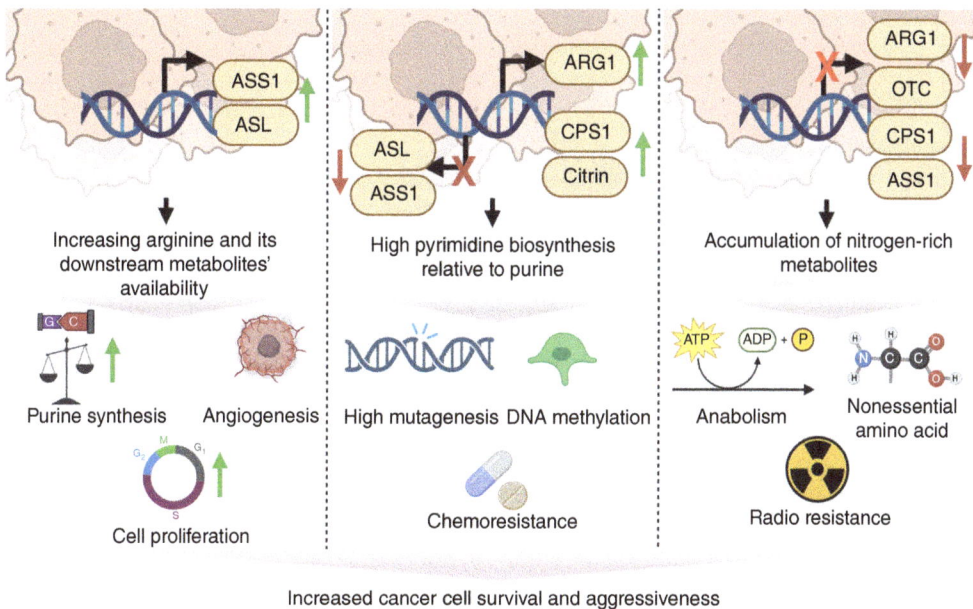

Figure 2. Alterations in the expression of the urea cycle (UC) enzymes increase tumorigenesis. Tumor cells are selected to enhance or repress the expression of UC enzymes to benefit tumorigenic properties by three main mechanisms. (*Left* panel) Overexpressing ASS1 and argininosuccinate lyase (ASL) increases arginine levels, which can be used for nitric oxide (NO) or polyamine synthesis. (*Middle* panel) Overexpression of ARG1, CPS1, and citrin and the down-regulation of ASS1 and ASL lead to increased biosynthesis of pyrimidines relative to purines, enhancing several tumorigenic phenotypes. (*Right* panel) The down-regulation of ARG1, OTC, CPS1, and ASS1 increases the accumulation of nitrogen-rich metabolites such as ammonia and glutamine. Together and each by itself, these mechanisms lead to enhanced cancer aggressiveness. (Created with BioRender.com.)

cell-cycle arrest and quiescence (Missiaen et al. 2022). High expression of ASS1 and ASL increase arginine levels, promoting either or both NO and polyamine synthesis. Indeed, high ASS1 expression levels were observed in a significant cohort of cancers, including ovarian, thyroid, pancreatic, colorectal, gastric, esophageal, cervical, and squamous cell carcinoma of the lung, and associated with poor survival (Fig. 2; Szlosarek et al. 2007; Delage et al. 2010; Huang et al. 2013b, 2015, 2017; Shan et al. 2015; Bateman et al. 2017; Tsai et al. 2018; Gong et al. 2019; Keshet et al. 2020). In many of these cancers, ASS1 up-regulation was induced by p53 (Miyamoto et al. 2017).

The up-regulation of ASL and ASS1 in cancer can increase the cellular availability of NO, which can be a friend or foe; on the one hand, it is protumorigenic through the activation of angiogenic, mitogenic (ERK, EGFR), and oncogenic signaling cascades (mTOR, WNT, p53). On the other hand, NO has antitumorigenic effects through apoptosis activation, tumor growth restriction, and up-regulation of the immune response against cancer cells (Jenkins et al. 1995; Albaugh et al. 2017; Keshet and Erez 2018). Specifically, under conditions of glucose deprivation, high NO resulting from elevated ASS1 levels was demonstrated to contribute to cancer survival in vitro and in vivo via increasing the S-nitrosylation of both pyruvate carboxylase and phosphoenolpyruvate carboxykinase 2, promoting truncated gluconeogenesis, and consequently the levels of serine-glycine and purine synthesis (Keshet et al. 2020). The intensified generation of purine contributed to a purine-rich mutational bias, the generation of less immunogenic peptides, and a poor response to immunotherapy. Indeed, when high-ASS1 expressing cancer cells were treated with a purine synthesis inhibitor—mizoribine—which reversed the purine-to-pyrimidine ratio to favor pyrimidines, the sensitivity to anti-programmed cell death 1 (PD-1) therapy was enhanced. Even in human cancers previously reported to be unresponsive to immune checkpoint therapy, treatment with mizoribine induced a response from the patient's autologous T cells (Keshet et al. 2020).

ARG1 and ARG2 compete with NOS over arginine to be used for ornithine synthesis, affecting cancer development and progression. ARG1 up-regulation decreases arginine levels and has been associated with poor prognosis in colorectal cancer (CRC) (Ma et al. 2019; Krzystek-Korpacka et al. 2020; Wang et al. 2023). In vitro and in vivo studies showed that ARG1 is essential for HCC and CRC cells for the epithelial-to-mesenchymal transition and that its expression increased cell migration and invasion (You et al. 2018; Wang et al. 2023). ARG2 up-regulation is described in breast basal-like cells and occasionally in Her2$^+$ cancer cells, malignant follicular thyroid lesions, gastric adenocarcinomas, and acute myeloid leukemia (AML) (Takenawa et al. 2004; Cerutti et al. 2006; Mussai et al. 2013; Roci et al. 2019). In prostate cancer cells, both ARG1 and ARG2 expression were found to be affected by androgen secretion (Mumenthaler et al. 2008; Gannon et al. 2010; Jang et al. 2018; Weis-Banke et al. 2020). The silencing of ARG1 and ARG2 in LNCaP prostate cancer cells impaired cell proliferation without affecting NO levels (Gannon et al. 2010). Indeed, in several cancer types, arginine is used to increase ornithine levels for polyamine synthesis. Arginine uptake and ornithine synthesis are among the main metabolic reactions differentially active during the G_2/M phase in cancer cells compared to nontransformed cells. In support, the knockdown of ARG2 in cancer cells impairs polyamine synthesis and arrests proliferation in G_2/M (Roci et al. 2019). Uniquely, in clear cell renal carcinoma (ccRCC), reduced ARG2 expression promotes tumor growth by maintaining the pool of intracellular pyridoxal phosphate cofactor for multiple biosynthetic reactions that contribute to increased biomass and cell division and preventing toxic polyamine accumulation (Ochocki et al. 2018).

High Pyrimidine Biosynthesis

CPS1 expression is up-regulated in several cancer types, including rectal, stomach, melanoma, sarcoma, lung carcinoma, glioma, glioblastoma, and B-cell lymphoma (Lee et al. 2014, 2018). Up-regulation of CPS1 was linked to p53 loss in colon cancer and hepatoblastoma cells (Li et al. 2019). In non-small-cell lung cancers (NSCLCs), the mechanism by which high CPS1 promotes tumorigenesis was described to be caused by the consequently increased synthesis of CP, which is also a substrate for pyrimidine biosynthesis via CPS2, aspartate transcarbamylase, and dihydroorotase (CAD) enzyme (Kim et al. 2017). High CP leaks from the mitochondria to the cytosol and increases the substrate availability required for a high rate of pyrimidine biosynthesis (Fig. 3). Indeed, overexpression of CPS1 was an adverse prognostic factor in rectal cancer treated with chemoradiation (Lee et al. 2014). Furthermore, silencing of

CPS1 in cancer cells with high CPS1 expression resulted in cell death in vitro and inhibited tumor growth in vivo due to the depletion of pyrimidine synthesis (Kim et al. 2017).

In deference to the elevation in CPS1 expression, multiple tumor types display reduced expression of ASS1 and, to a lesser extent, of ASL, including mesothelioma, myxofibrosarcoma, HCC, bladder, lung, ovarian, pancreas, and renal cell carcinoma (Delage et al. 2010; Kelly et al. 2012; Huang et al. 2013a; Syed et al. 2013; Allen et al. 2014; Cao et al. 2019; Kim et al. 2020; Khare et al. 2021). In these cancers, the down-regulation of ASS1 and ASL is attributed to promoter hypermethylation (Huang et al. 2013a; Syed et al.

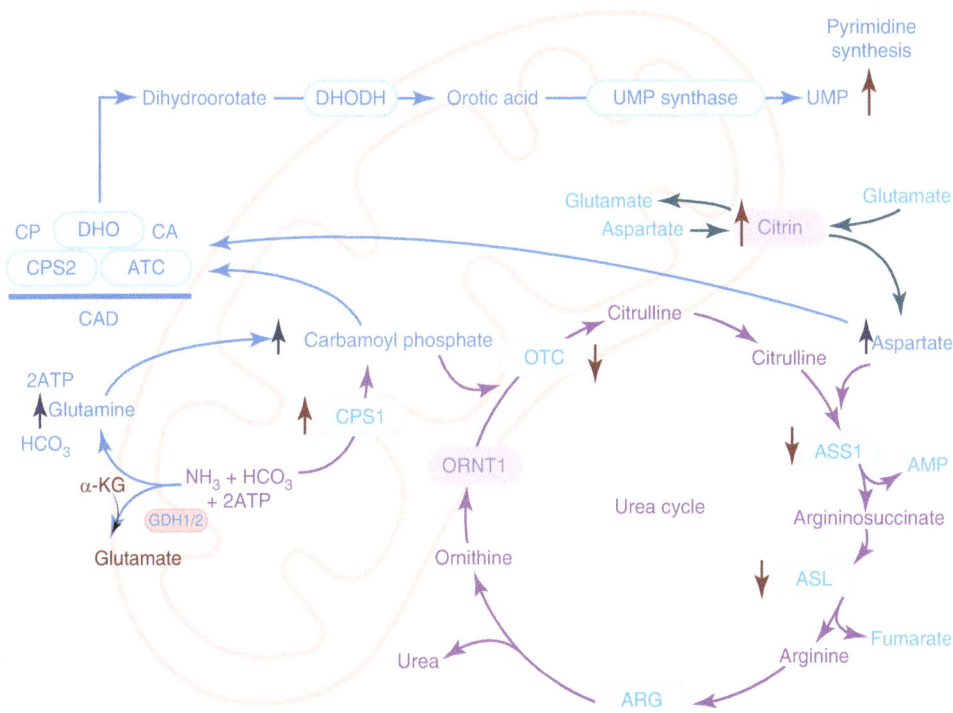

Figure 3. Specific alterations in the expression of urea cycle (UC) proteins increase substrate availability for CAD de novo synthesis of pyrimidines. The trifunctional enzyme CAD (carbamoyl phosphate synthetase 2 [CPS2], aspartate transcarbamylase [ATC], and dihydroorotase [DHO]) is the bottleneck enzyme for pyrimidine synthesis. The synthesis involves the generation of the intermediates carbamoyl phosphate (CP) and carbamoyl aspartate (CA) following the addition of aspartate for dihydroorotate production. The mitochondrial inner membrane protein DHODH oxidizes dihydroorotase to orotic acid and then phosphorylated to produce UMP by UMP synthase. Reduced activity of ornithine transcarbamylase (OTC), argininosuccinate lyase (ASL), and argininosuccinate synthase (ASS1) or up-regulation of citrin, CSP1, and CP increase substrate availability for CAD and, therefore, de novo pyrimidine production. Ammonia can also contribute to the production of glutamate via glutamate dehydrogenase 2 (GDH2). (Created with BioRender.com.)

2013; Allen et al. 2014). Like CPS1, decreased activity of ASS1 in cancers supports proliferation by facilitating pyrimidine synthesis by CAD through the increased availability of another one of its substrates, aspartate (Rabinovich et al. 2015). Indeed, in several cancer types, the down-regulation of ASS1 and ASL correlates with high proliferation, high rate of migration, and a worse prognosis (Kobayashi et al. 2010; Allen et al. 2014; Tan et al. 2014; Tao et al. 2019; Khare et al. 2021). For instance, in endometrioid carcinoma specimens, peripheral tumor cells decrease ASS1 expression to facilitate tumor invasion by activating mTOR via inhibition of DEP domain-containing mTOR-interacting protein (DEPTOR) (Ohshima et al. 2017).

In addition to supporting cancer proliferation in HCC and ovarian cancers, the down-regulation of ASS1 leads to resistance to platinum-based chemotherapies (Nicholson et al. 2009; McAlpine et al. 2014). Cisplatin is the first-choice chemotherapeutic agent in ovarian cancer; hence, resistance to its effect may be crucial for these cancer patients. Cisplatin affects purine/pyrimidine metabolism (von Stechow et al. 2013), and its binding to the DNA is biased toward purines (Zeng et al. 2019). Therefore, the increased pyrimidine synthesis following ASS1 down-regulation increases the number of transversion mutations in which purine is replaced by pyrimidine. Consequently, there is less purine available for binding, which may contribute to cancer resistance to cisplatin.

Among multiple cancer types, the transporter citrin is up-regulated, increasing cytosolic aspartate availability (Lee et al. 2018; Rabinovich et al. 2020). In ASS1-deficient osteosarcoma cells, induced silencing of citrin restricts aspartate availability for pyrimidine biosynthesis and reduces mTOR-dependent activating phosphorylation of CAD, thus restricting pyrimidine synthesis and proliferation (Rabinovich et al. 2015). As part of the malate–aspartate shuttle, citrin regulates other metabolic pathways, including glycolysis, oxidative phosphorylation (OXPHOS), mitophagy, and invasiveness through intraorganelle regulation of the NAD:NADH ratio (Rabinovich et al. 2020).

Notably, the alterations in the expression of the UC proteins described herein are selected for a specific rewiring that increases substrate availability for CAD (Fig. 3). Thus, when dysregulation exists in the expression of multiple UC enzymes (urea cycle disorder [UCD]) to promote CAD activation, the consequent proliferation and mutation phenotypes are more robust than those induced by a single enzymatic change (Lee et al. 2018).

Accumulation of Nitrogen-Rich Metabolites

In contrast to normal cells, cancer cells recycle excess ammonia to synthesize amino acids and nucleic acids as building blocks for cancer proliferation (Tardito et al. 2015; Spinelli et al. 2017). In addition, under glutamine depletion, ammonia can be scavenged together with α-KG for the synthesis of glutamate by glutamate dehydrogenase 1/2 (GDH1/2), stimulating the mTORC1 pathway and promoting cell proliferation (Takeuchi et al. 2018; Dai et al. 2022).

In human HepG2-derived cell lines, the malfunctioning of ARG1 and OTC results in excess ammonia (Mavri-Damelin et al. 2007). Similarly, acute lymphocytic leukemia cells have excess ammonia because of the down-regulation of OTC expression (De Santo et al. 2018). In HCC cells, CPS1 deficiency, leading to excess ammonia, was also related to resistance to radiotherapy and a worse prognosis. Resistance to radiotherapy was influenced by reduced cell apoptosis and induction of a cell-cycle arrest achieved by stabilization of the oncoprotein c-Myc at the post-transcriptional level and by the up-regulation of cyclinA2 and cyclinD1 expression (Zhang et al. 2023b).

ASS1-depleted tumor cells have higher levels of ammonia and glutamine. Since both these metabolites are alkaline, their accumulation helps the cancer cells maintain an alkalic intracellular pH (Silberman et al. 2019). Thus, in addition to supporting proliferation, high ammonia and glutamine levels counteract the high lactate levels produced by the enhanced glycolysis of the highly proliferating cancer cells.

As described above, the UC enzymes' expression is dynamic and can either be up-regulated or down-regulated in correspondence with the cell state and its needs for UC intermediates (Fig. 2). As the tumor grows, the increased requirement for UC metabolites leads to changes in UC enzymes' expression within the tumor microenvironment (TME). The changes in the TME can compensate for deficiencies in UC intermediates that result from the metabolic rewiring of UC enzymes' expression in the tumor.

UC CHANGES WITHIN THE TUMOR MICROENVIRONMENT (TME)

The TME supports tumor growth by supplying a continuous exchange of metabolites and nutrients between the tumor and cells in the microenvironment during tumor progression. These metabolic interactions are essential to sustain tumor

development, angiogenesis, and metastasis. Eventually, the TME becomes more and more hostile, characterized by reduced oxygen supply, elevated levels of reactive oxygen species (ROS), low glucose induced by tumor-enhanced glycolysis, and limited sources of amino acids (such as arginine, cysteine, and tryptophan). Consequently, the UC enzymes and metabolites are altered in tumor cells and within the cells of the TME to supply the tumor demands for nutrients and restrict nutrient availability for the antitumor response (Figs. 4 and 5; Feng et al. 2022).

The Cross Talk of Immune and Tumor Cells via the UC

While cancer cells can up-regulate ASS1 expression and survive in an arginine-depleted

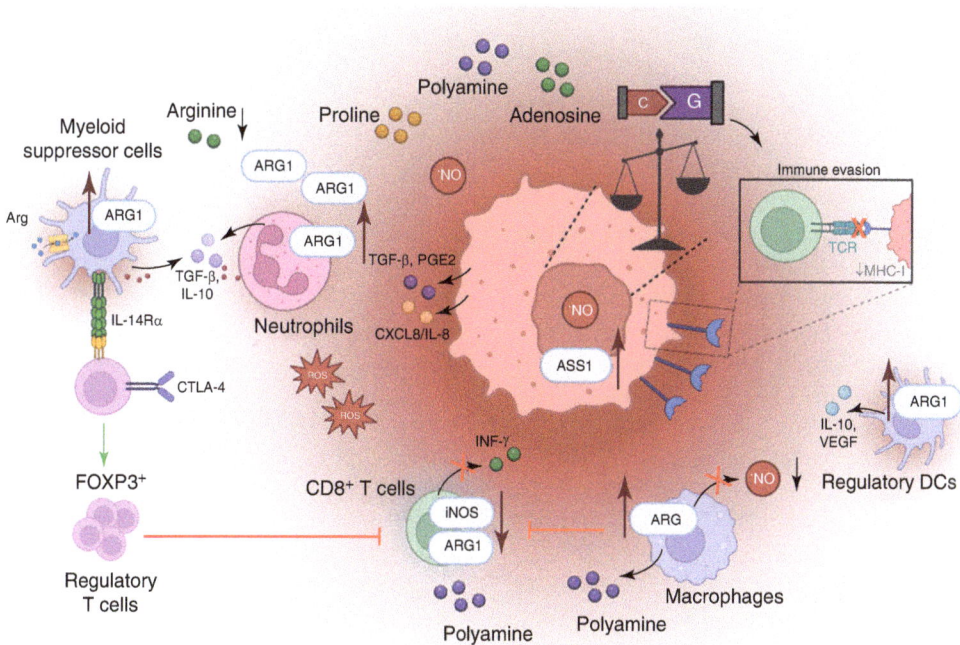

Figure 4. Dysregulation of the urea cycle (UC) enzymes in the tumor microenvironment (TME) sustains tumor growth by promoting immune suppression. A schematic depiction of the TME and tumors' cross talks when the tumor cells overexpress argininosuccinate synthase (ASS1) and the immune cells express arginase 1 (ARG1). In tumors expressing high ASS1, arginine synthesis promotes high nitric oxide (NO) levels and the production of polyamines, proline, and adenosine monophosphate (AMP), stimulating the onset of the immune-suppressive microenvironment. Unlike tumor cells, T cells cannot produce de novo arginine and have reduced activity in an arginine-depleted TME. ARG1-expressing and -secreting immune cells further deplete arginine from the TME, increasing proline and polyamine availability for tumor proliferation while decreasing NO availability for antitumor immune response. (Created with BioRender.com.)

tumor environment (TME), most immune system cells are auxotrophic for multiple amino acids, including arginine, requiring an external source to sustain their protein biosynthesis (Murray 2016; Apiz-Saab et al. 2022). Arginine deprivation in the TME results in poor activation and decreased cytotoxicity properties of T cells expressing low ASS1 levels (Bronte et al. 2005; Apiz-Saab et al. 2022). Moreover, arginine deficiency was shown to cause a reduction of central memory T cells (Tcm) and reduced antitumor activity in a mouse model of B16-OVA melanoma (Geiger et al. 2016). Indeed, multiple cancer types up-regulate ASS1 by stabilizing the binding of ATF4 and CEBPβ on ASS1 enhancers while reducing repressive histone methylation (Crump et al. 2021) in T cells; arginine starvation causes genome-wide chromatin compaction, which prevents the binding of ATF4 and CEBPβ to the consensus region and blocks ASS1 transcription (Thevenot et al. 2014).

In addition to the metabolic benefits ASS1 expression provides tumors by increasing arginine levels, tumors expressing ASS1 produce high levels of adenosine monophosphate (AMP) in the reaction that generates argininosuccinate from aspartate and citrulline (Fig. 1). AMP and adenosine can interchange based on cellular needs (Fenouillet et al. 2019). High adenosine levels shift the cytokine and cellular profile of the TME away from the cytotoxic CD8 T cells and natural killer (NK) milieu toward immune tolerance and suppression (Raskovalova et al. 2005; Borea et al. 2018). Stimulation by adenosine skews dendritic cell (DC) differentiation toward a distinct cell population characterized by the expression of both DC and monocyte/macrophage cell surface markers of immune suppression, tolerance, and angiogenesis (Novitskiy et al. 2008). In regulatory T cells (Tregs), high levels of adenosine induce immunosuppression and suppress the function of effector T cells (Fig. 4; Mandapathil et al. 2010). Several genes regulating extracellular adenosine metabolism and signaling have been identified as direct targets of hypoxia-inducible factors (HIFs) (Li et al. 2017). In melanoma, adenosine signaling is an established mechanism for immune evasion, leading the rationale to enhance the successful outcomes of anti-checkpoint therapy by combining it with adenosine signaling inhibitors (Passarelli et al. 2019; Augustin et al. 2022).

As the availability of nutrients in the TME becomes limiting, the TME gradually turns into an immune-suppressive and protumorigenic environment, with increasing infiltration of Tregs, myeloid-derived suppressor cells (MDSCs), macrophages, neutrophils, and DCs. Specifically, it was shown that the overexpression of ASS1 in ovarian cancer reprogrammed the immune TME to enhance the production of IFN-α and TNF-α signaling, leading to the recruitment of N2 neutrophils with an immunosuppressive phenotype (Feng et al. 2022). This generates a vicious cycle in which the decreased antitumor immune response enables tumor growth, depleting more nutrients from the TME, thus augmenting the immunosuppressive phenotype.

Notably, tumor-secreted molecules can induce the expression of ARG1 on different immune cells, contributing to multiple immune-suppressive mechanisms by decreasing NO and promoting tumor progression (Rotondo et al. 2009; Feng et al. 2022). In 3LL lung cancer, secreted TGF-β and PGE2 induced ARG1 expression in regulatory DCs, inhibiting CD4 T helper cell proliferation in vitro and in vivo and suppressing CD8 T-cell response. Similar results were shown in BALB/C breast cancer models (Liu et al. 2009; Norian et al. 2009). In ovarian cancer cells and an NSCLC model, secretion of CXCL8 and ROS by the tumor cells increased ARG1-expressing neutrophil levels (Feng et al. 2022). The stimulated neutrophils increased the secretion of ARG1, sequestering arginine from the TME and impairing the functionality of T cells (Rotondo et al. 2009). Similarly, MDSCs in human renal carcinoma were found to deplete arginine and induce immune suppression in the TME by expressing and secreting ARG1 (Rodriguez et al. 2004, 2009). In addition, ARG1 expressing MDSCs could induce T-cell anergy by cross-presenting tumor antigens (IL-14Rα expression) to Tregs, encouraging the expansion of the preexisting natural Tregs (FOXP3[+]) (Curti et al. 2007; Serafini et al. 2008).

Cite this article as *Cold Spring Harb Perspect Med* doi: 10.1101/cshperspect.a041538

The increased expression of ARG1 together with the expression of immune-suppressive markers (i.e., programmed cell death ligand 1 [PD-L1], IL-11Rα, AHR, CD209, DPP4, XCR1, GPR44), and the antiapoptotic signal (B-cell lymphoma 2 [BCL2]) were all demonstrated to be driven by enhanced expression of the β2-adrenergic receptor (β2-AR) following adrenergic stress created by nerve fibers releasing catecholamines in the TME (Mohammadpour et al. 2019). The adrenergic stress reduced T-cell activation by lowering the levels of IFN-γ in CD8 T cells and harmed DC maturation (Bucsek et al. 2017; Mohammadpour et al. 2018).

In addition to depleting arginine from the TME, ARG1 expression in immune cells can support tumorigenesis by increasing ornithine availability for polyamines and proline synthesis, which is essential for cancer proliferation and tissue remodeling (Matos et al. 2021). Indeed, ARG1 generation in macrophages supplied tumor cells with polyamines and decreased NO production by competing with inducible nitric oxide synthase (iNOS) for arginine substrate. Consequently, tumor growth was supported by the polyamines and by the decreased macrophage production of NO, which reduced their cytotoxicity against breast cancer tumor cells (Chang et al. 2001).

These studies highlight the survival benefits that the expression of UC enzymes provide the tumor by enabling endogenous arginine synthesis when the TME is arginine deficient. The ability to synthesize arginine tilts the metabolic equation to favor cancer over immune cell survival and determines, at least in part, cancer outcomes.

The Cooperation of Stromal Cells and Tumor Cells in UC Rewiring

Several studies pointed out the crucial metabolic roles of cancer-associated fibroblasts (CAFs) in supporting tumor cell growth, development, and metastasis by providing the tumor with nutrients (Yang et al. 2016; Lu et al. 2019; Ogando et al. 2019; Mestre-Farrera et al. 2021). CAFs expressing high levels of ARG2 provide ornithine, proline, and polyamines, which are vital for cancer cell growth and proliferation (Ino et al. 2013). In parallel, the overexpression of ARG2 in CAFs depletes arginine from the TME, decreasing T-cell infiltration and promoting immunologically cold tumor phenotype associated with poor prognosis (e.g., in patients with NSCLC) (Fig. 5; Giatromanolaki et al. 2021).

Cancer cells and fibroblasts increase the expression of SLC4A11, a sensitive H$^+$ channel-like membrane transporter for ammonia, enabling the consumption of higher amounts of glutamine (Ogando et al. 2019). Additionally, ammonia secreted by cancer cells was shown to activate the CAFs through MYC and reprogram metabolic pathways that increase glutamine secretion when the TME is glutamine-poor (Yan et al. 2018). In a model of HCC, enzymes involved in ammonia assimilation, such as GDH1 and glutamine synthetase (GS), were up-regulated in normal liver tissue compared to HCC. Furthermore, the elevated ammonia produced by the HCC cells was converted to urea by the UC in the healthy portion of the liver (Bai et al. 2021).

Another critical cooperation between tumor cells and the TME occurs in a glutamine-limiting environment. Glutamine is essential for cancer survival and proliferation. Among other contributions to tumorigenesis, glutamine is a necessary precursor for the synthesis of macromolecules and is a substrate for the de novo synthesis of pyrimidine and nonessential amino acids such as aspartate and arginine (Hensley et al. 2013). Different types of stromal cells in the TME can provide cancer cells with glutamine, such as astrocytes in glioblastoma (Lyssiotis and Kimmelman 2017), adipocytes in acute lymphoblastic leukemia (Ehsanipour et al. 2013), and CAFs in ovarian and prostate cancers (Yang et al. 2016; Mishra et al. 2018). In addition, in a glutamine-deprived environment, tumor cells can uptake by micropinocytosis aspartate and arginine to sustain their proliferation and survival (Tajan et al. 2018; Lowman et al. 2019).

The supply of nutrients is not limited to glutamine. Indeed, CAFs can supply cancer cells with asparagine, glutamate, or aspartate to sustain cancer cells' growth and functions (Pavlova et al. 2018; Bertero et al. 2019). Tumors can also induce cell autophagy and mitophagy in CAFs to increase the availability of nutrients (Lisanti et al. 2010). In pancreatic ductal adenocarcino-

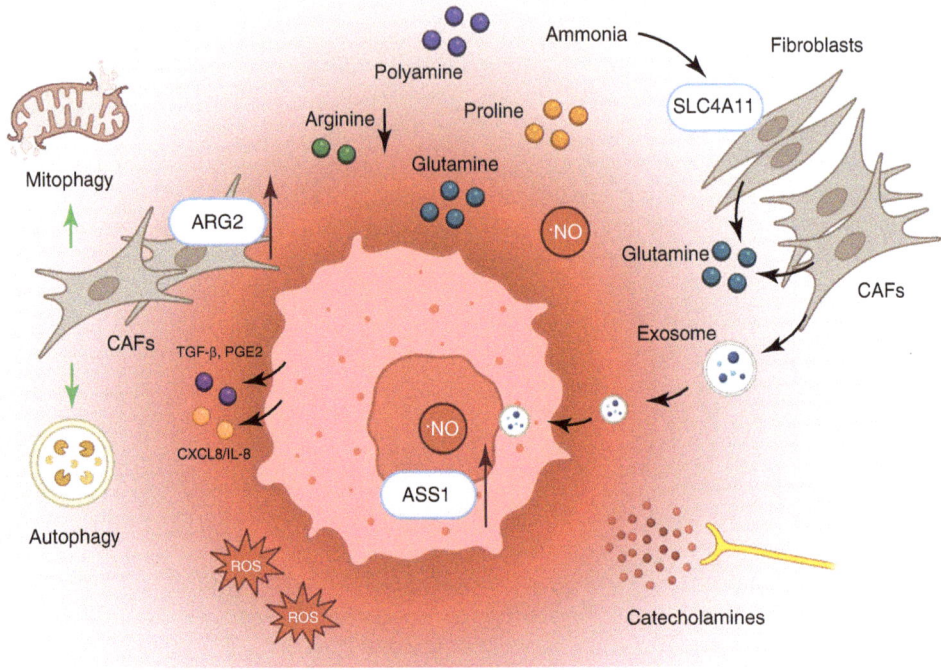

Figure 5. Dysregulation of the urea cycle (UC) in the tumor microenvironment (TME) stromal cells sustains tumor growth. A schematic depiction of the TME and tumors' cross talks when the tumor cells overexpress argininosuccinate synthase (ASS1) and the stromal cells express arginase 2 (ARG2). To sustain tumor needs, the stromal (cancer-associated fibroblasts [CAFs] and fibroblasts) microenvironment supplies the tumor with proline and polyamine, and is also undergoing autophagy and mitophagy, providing the tumor with nutrients that are either secreted or stored and released via exosomes. (Created with BioRender.com.)

ma (PDAC), it was demonstrated that pancreatic stellate stromal cells undergo autophagy to increase the secretion of nonessential amino acids, including alanine, which provides an alternative carbon fuel for the TCA cycle and decreases the tumor's dependence on glucose (Sousa et al. 2016).

Thus, rewired tumor metabolism directly affects CAFs metabolism to supplement the tumor with the consequent deficient nutrients involving UC enzymes and metabolites. The dysregulation in the expression of UC enzymes can co-occur in both cell types in a similar or complementary direction (Hinow et al. 2021).

TRANSLATION INTO THE CLINIC

As dysregulations in UC enzymes' expression are selected to benefit the tumor, it is logical to try and exploit the rewired pathways for anticancer therapy. One approach is to target the dysregulated enzyme or block its activity directly. Such an approach showed promising results using a CPS1 inhibitor that restricted pyrimidine biosynthesis in cancer cells that express high CPS1 levels (Yao et al. 2020; Zhang et al. 2023a). In the case of NSCLC refractory to standard EGFR inhibitors, the inactivation of CPS1 synergized with gemcitabine, pemetrexed, and AZD7762 treatments in restricting tumor growth (Çeliktaş et al. 2017).

Another treatment modality is to target the missing or excess metabolite due to UC dysregulation. An example is the strategy to increase the antitumor immune response by overcoming arginine depletion in the TME, using ARG inhibitors alone or in combination with other drugs to increase arginine levels (Martinenaite et al. 2019; Grzywa et al. 2020). Encouragingly, CAR T cells engineered to express ASS1 and

Cite this article as *Cold Spring Harb Perspect Med* doi: 10.1101/cshperspect.a041538

OTC increased arginine levels, enabled proliferation, and increased T cells' cytotoxicity. Consequently, the modified CAR T cells improved mice survival in a model of AML and restored the arginine level in the plasma (Fultang et al. 2020). Additionally, immunotherapy with vaccines against ARG1 was shown to mediate ARG1-expressing cell death and attain stable disease in cancer patients with solid tumors for several months (Weis-Banke et al. 2020).

The discovery that tumors with loss of ASS1 expression are arginine auxotrophic led to the emergence of therapies that can selectively induce arginine deprivation in cancer and not in nontumor normal cells that express ASS1. Mycoplasma-derived arginine deiminase (ADI-PEG20), a cloned arginine-degrading enzyme conjugated with polyethylene glycol (PEG), was found to be a very promising drug in extensive in vitro studies and phase 1 trials for multiple cancer types, both as a single drug and in combination with chemotherapy or immunotherapy (Thongkum et al. 2017; Harding et al. 2018; Chang et al. 2021). Interestingly, two recent phase 2 clinical trial studies for advanced HCC and refractory SCLC failed to show the benefit of the treatment (Hall et al. 2020; Harding et al. 2021), while a clinical trial treating cancer patients with mesothelioma has demonstrated clinical benefits (Szlosarek et al. 2020). Another agent used to generate arginine deprivation is pegylated human ARG1 (rhArg1peg5000, BCT-100). BCT-100 was preclinically tested and showed efficacy against ASS1-low solid and hematological cancers, as well as in several phase 1 clinical trials (De Santo et al. 2018; Yau et al. 2022). Thus, more research is needed to evaluate the clinical advantages of treating cancer patients with a combination of arginine-depleting agents and chemotherapy.

CONCLUDING REMARKS AND FUTURE PERSPECTIVES

In the emerging era of personalized medicine, one of the biggest challenges is to tailor a treatment regimen for each patient based on tumor and host-specific characteristics (i.e., biomarkers and signatures are much needed for clinical decision-making). In multiple cancer types, UCD, calculated as a score based on the enzymes with rewired expression, was associated with worse outcomes, immune infiltration, and a better response to immunotherapy (Lee et al. 2018; Guo et al. 2022; Zhao et al. 2022). Similarly, a combined score of high CAD and low CPS1 expression was found to be an independent prognostic marker for survival in HCC patients. These cancer patients might benefit from inhibiting pyrimidine synthesis, for example, by 5-Fluorouracil (Ridder et al. 2021). Thus, the knowledge gathered regarding the dysregulation of the UC in the tumor and the TME can be exploited to direct clinical decisions and treatment choices.

Zooming out from the tumor and the TME, the tumor connects with the host via secreted molecules, vessels, and nerves. Since it is well established that metabolic disorders such as diabetes and obesity affect tumor development, it is logical to assume that tumorigenesis will affect liver metabolism and the expression of the UC enzymes. Recently, we found systemic inflammation induced by extrahepatic cancers, such as breast and pancreas, leads to liver infiltration of innate immune cells. Consequently, there are transcriptional perturbations in hepatocytes, resulting in the depletion of HNF4α, a key regulator of liver metabolism. As a result, multiple liver metabolic pathways such as the UC, albumin, and fatty acid synthesis are dysfunctional, contributing to the development of systemic manifestations such as weight loss (Lee et al. 2018; Goldman et al. 2023). Interestingly, preserving liver metabolism by maintaining HNF4α levels restricts weight loss and preserves body composition in pancreatic tumor-bearing mice.

Thus, tumors can extend metabolic effects beyond the vicinity of the TME and may contribute to systemic complications accompanying carcinogenesis, such as metastasis, resistance to therapy, and cachexia, by regulating liver metabolism, including the UC. Understanding the cancer-induced changes in systemic metabolism in general and in the UC can potentially improve cancer diagnosis and advance cancer patient management. Furthermore, it may provide new treatment approaches to improve cancer patients' survival and quality of life.

ACKNOWLEDGMENTS

A.E. is supported by research grants from the European research program (ERC818943), the Israel Science Foundation (860/18), and The Israel Cancer Research Fund (837124). A.E. received additional support from The Moross Integrated Cancer Center, Blumberg Family Research Fellow Chair in Honor of Talia Lynn Steckman, from Manya and Adolph Zarovinsky, and the Koret Foundation. S.P. is funded by the Sergio Lombroso Postdoctoral Fellowship. We have a paid license to use BioRender through the Weizmann Institute.

REFERENCES

Albaugh VL, Pinzon-Guzman C, Barbul A. 2017. Arginine —dual roles as an onconutrient and immunonutrient. *J Surg Oncol* **115:** 273–280. doi:10.1002/jso.24490

Allen MD, Luong P, Hudson C, Leyton J, Delage B, Ghazaly E, Cutts R, Yuan M, Syed N, Lo Nigro C, et al. 2014. Prognostic and therapeutic impact of argininosuccinate synthetase 1 control in bladder cancer as monitored longitudinally by PET imaging. *Cancer Res* **74:** 896–907. doi:10.1158/0008-5472.CAN-13-1702

Apiz-Saab JJ, Dzierozynski LN, Jonker PB, Zhu Z, Chen RN, Oh M, Sheehan C, Macleod KF, Weber CR, Muir A. 2022. Pancreatic tumors activate arginine biosynthesis to adapt to myeloid-driven amino acid stress. bioRxiv doi:10.1101/2022.06.21.497008

Augustin RC, Leone RD, Naing A, Fong L, Bao R, Luke JJ. 2022. Next steps for clinical translation of adenosine pathway inhibition in cancer immunotherapy. *J Immunother Cancer* **10:** e004089. doi:10.1136/jitc-2021-004089

Bai C, Wang H, Dong D, Li T, Yu Z, Guo J, Zhou W, Li D, Yan R, Wang L, et al. 2021. Urea as a by-product of ammonia metabolism can be a potential serum biomarker of hepatocellular carcinoma. *Front Cell Dev Biol* **9:** 650748. doi:10.3389/fcell.2021.650748

Bateman LA, Ku WM, Heslin MJ, Contreras CM, Skibola CF, Nomura DK. 2017. Argininosuccinate synthase 1 is a metabolic regulator of colorectal cancer pathogenicity. *ACS Chem Biol* **12:** 905–911. doi:10.1021/acschembio .6b01158

Bertero T, Oldham WM, Grasset EM, Bourget I, Boulter E, Pisano S, Hofman P, Bellvert F, Meneguzzi G, Bulavin DV, et al. 2019. Tumor-stroma mechanics coordinate amino acid availability to sustain tumor growth and malignancy. *Cell Metab* **29:** 124–140.e10. doi:10.1016/j.cmet .2018.09.012

Blachier F, Mrabettouil H, Posho L, Darcyvrillon B, Duee PH. 1993. Intestinal arginine metabolism during development. Evidence for de novo synthesis of l-arginine in newborn pig enterocytes. *Eur J Biochem* **216:** 109–117. doi:10.1111/j.1432-1033.1993.tb18122.x

Borea PA, Gessi S, Merighi S, Vincenzi F, Varani K. 2018. Pharmacology of adenosine receptors: the state of the art. *Physiol Rev* **98:** 1591–1625. doi:10.1152/physrev.00049 .2017

Bronte V, Kasic T, Gri G, Gallana K, Borsellino G, Marigo I, Battistini L, Iafrate M, Prayer-Galetti T, Pagano F, et al. 2005. Boosting antitumor responses of T lymphocytes infiltrating human prostate cancers. *J Exp Med* **201:** 1257–1268. doi:10.1084/jem.20042028

Bucsek MJ, Qiao G, MacDonald CR, Giridharan T, Evans L, Niedzwecki B, Liu H, Kokolus KM, Eng JWL, Messmer MN, et al. 2017. β-Adrenergic signaling in mice housed at standard temperatures suppresses an effector phenotype in CD8+ T cells and undermines checkpoint inhibitor therapy β-blockers increase T-cell effectors and anti-PD-1 efficacy. *Cancer Res* **77:** 5639–5651. doi:10.1158/ 0008-5472.CAN-17-0546

Cao Y, Ding W, Zhang J, Gao Q, Yang H, Cao W, Wang Z, Fang L, Du R. 2019. Significant down-regulation of urea cycle generates clinically relevant proteomic signature in hepatocellular carcinoma patients with macrovascular invasion. *J Proteome Res* **18:** 2032–2044. doi:10.1021/acs .jproteome.8b00921

Cederbaum SD, Yu H, Grody WW, Kern RM, Yoo P, Iyer RK. 2004. Arginases I and II: do their functions overlap? *Mol Genet Metab* **81:** 38–44. doi:10.1016/j.ymgme.2003 .10.012

Çeliktaş M, Tanaka I, Chandra Tripathi S, Fahrmann JF, Aguilar-Bonavides C, Villalobos P, Delgado O, Dhillon D, Dennison JB, Ostrin EJ, et al. 2017. Role of CPS1 in cell growth, metabolism, and prognosis in LKB1-inactivated lung adenocarcinoma. *J Natl Cancer Inst* **109:** 1–9. doi:10 .1093/jnci/djw231

Cerutti JM, Latini FR, Nakabashi C, Delcelo R, Andrade VP, Amadei MJ, Maciel RM, Hojaij FC, Hollis D, Shoemaker J, et al. 2006. Diagnosis of suspicious thyroid nodules using four protein biomarkers. *Clinical Cancer Res* **12:** 3311–3318. doi:10.1158/1078-0432.CCR-05-2226

Chang CI, Liao JC, Kuo L. 2001. Macrophage arginase promotes tumor cell growth and suppresses nitric oxide-mediated tumor cytotoxicity. *Cancer Res* **61:** 1100–1106.

Chang KY, Chiang NJ, Wu SY, Yen CJ, Chen SH, Yeh YM, Li CF, Feng X, Wu K, Johnston A, et al. 2021. Phase 1b study of pegylated arginine deiminase (ADI-PEG 20) plus Pembrolizumab in advanced solid cancers. *Oncoimmunology* **10:** 1943253. doi:10.1080/2162402X.2021.1943253

Crump NT, Hadjinicolaou AV, Xia M, Walsby-Tickle J, Gileadi U, Chen JL, Setshedi M, Olsen LR, Lau IJ, Godfrey L, et al. 2021. Chromatin accessibility governs the differential response of cancer and T cells to arginine starvation. *Cell Rep* **35:** 109101. doi:10.1016/j.celrep.2021.109101

Curti A, Pandolfi S, Valzasina B, Aluigi M, Isidori A, Ferri E, Salvestrini V, Bonanno G, Rutella S, Durelli I, et al. 2007. Modulation of tryptophan catabolism by human leukemic cells results in the conversion of CD25− into CD25+ T regulatory cells. *Blood* **109:** 2871–2877. doi:10.1182/ blood-2006-07-036863

Dai W, Shen J, Yan J, Bott AJ, Maimouni S, Daguplo HQ, Wang Y, Khayati K, Guo JY, Zhang L, et al. 2022. Glutamine synthetase limits β-catenin–mutated liver cancer growth by maintaining nitrogen homeostasis and suppressing mTORC1. *J Clin Invest* 132: e161408. doi:10.1172/JCI161408

de Jonge WJ, Dingemanse MA, de Boer PA, Lamers WH, Moorman AF. 1998. Arginine-metabolizing enzymes in the developing rat small intestine. *Pediatr Res* 43: 442–451. doi:10.1203/00006450-199804000-00002

Delage B, Fennell DA, Nicholson L, McNeish I, Lemoine NR, Crook T, Szlosarek PW. 2010. Arginine deprivation and argininosuccinate synthetase expression in the treatment of cancer. *Int J Cancer* 126: 2762–2772.

De Santo C, Booth S, Vardon A, Cousins A, Tubb V, Perry T, Noyvert B, Beggs A, Ng M, Halsey C, et al. 2018. The arginine metabolome in acute lymphoblastic leukemia can be targeted by the pegylated-recombinant arginase I BCT-100. *Int J Cancer* 142: 1490–1502. doi:10.1002/ijc.31170

Ehsanipour EA, Sheng X, Behan JW, Wang X, Butturini A, Avramis VI, Mittelman SD. 2013. Adipocytes cause leukemia cell resistance to L-asparaginase via release of glutamine. *Cancer Res* 73: 2998–3006. doi:10.1158/0008-5472.CAN-12-4402

Erez A, DeBerardinis RJ. 2015. Metabolic dysregulation in monogenic disorders and cancer—finding method in madness. *Nat Rev Cancer* 15: 440–448. doi:10.1038/nrc3949

Erez A, Nagamani SC, Shchelochkov OA, Premkumar MH, Campeau PM, Chen Y, Garg HK, Li L, Mian A, Bertin TK, et al. 2011. Requirement of argininosuccinate lyase for systemic nitric oxide production. *Nat Med* 17: 1619–1626. doi:10.1038/nm.2544

Feng X, Ji Z, Yang G. 2022. ASS1 regulates immune microenvironment via CXCL8 signaling in ovarian cancer. *Biochem Biophys Res Commun* 631: 86–92. doi:10.1016/j.bbrc.2022.08.045

Fenouillet E, Mottola G, Kipson N, Paganelli F, Guieu R, Ruf J. 2019. Adenosine receptor profiling reveals an association between the presence of spare receptors and cardiovascular disorders. *Int J Mol Sci* 20: 5964. doi:10.3390/ijms20235964

Fultang L, Booth S, Yogev O, Martins da Costa B, Tubb V, Panetti S, Stavrou V, Scarpa U, Jankevics A, Lloyd G, et al. 2020. Metabolic engineering against the arginine microenvironment enhances CAR-T cell proliferation and therapeutic activity. *Blood* 136: 1155–1160. doi:10.1182/blood.2019004500

Gannon PO, Godin-Ethier J, Hassler M, Delvoye N, Aversa M, Poisson AO, Péant B, Alam Fahmy M, Saad F, Lapointe R, et al. 2010. Androgen-regulated expression of arginase 1, arginase 2 and interleukin-8 in human prostate cancer. *PLoS ONE* 5: e12107. doi:10.1371/journal.pone.0012107

Geiger R, Rieckmann JC, Wolf T, Basso C, Feng Y, Fuhrer T, Kogadeeva M, Picotti P, Meissner F, Mann M, et al. 2016. L-arginine modulates T cell metabolism and enhances survival and antitumor activity. *Cell* 167: 829–842.e13. doi:10.1016/j.cell.2016.09.031

Giatromanolaki A, Harris AL, Koukourakis MI. 2021. The prognostic and therapeutic implications of distinct patterns of argininosuccinate synthase 1 (ASS1) and arginase-2 (ARG2) expression by cancer cells and tumor stroma in non-small-cell lung cancer. *Cancer Metab* 9: 1–10. doi:10.1186/s40170-021-00264-7

Goldman O, Adler LN, Hajaj E, Croese T, Darzi N, Galai S, Tishler H, Ariav Y, Lavie D, Fellus-Alyagor L, et al. 2023. Early infiltration of innate immune cells to the liver depletes HNF4a and promotes extrahepatic carcinogenesis. *Cancer Discov* doi:10.1158/2159-8290.CD-22-1062

Gong R, He L, Zhou H, Cheng S, Ren F, Chen J, Ren J. 2019. Down-regulation of argininosuccinate lyase induces hepatoma cell apoptosis through activating Bax signaling pathway. *Genes Dis* 6: 296–303. doi:10.1016/j.gendis.2018.11.003

Grzywa TM, Sosnowska A, Matryba P, Rydzynska Z, Jasinski M, Nowis D, Golab J. 2020. Myeloid cell-derived arginase in cancer immune response. *Front Immunol* 11: 938. doi:10.3389/fimmu.2020.00938

Guo H, Wang Y, Gou L, Wang X, Tang Y, Wang X. 2022. A novel prognostic model based on urea cycle-related gene signature for colorectal cancer. *Front Surg* 9: 1027655. doi:10.3389/fsurg.2022.1027655

Hall PE, Ready N, Johnston A, Bomalaski JS, Venhaus RR, Sheaff M, Krug L, Szlosarek PW. 2020. Phase II study of arginine deprivation therapy with pegargiminase in patients with relapsed sensitive or refractory small-cell lung cancer. *Clin Lung Cancer* 21: 527–533. doi:10.1016/j.cllc.2020.07.012

Harding JJ, Do RK, Dika IE, Hollywood E, Uhlitskykh K, Valentino E, Wan P, Hamilton C, Feng X, Johnston A, et al. 2018. A phase 1 study of ADI-PEG 20 and modified FOLFOX6 in patients with advanced hepatocellular carcinoma and other gastrointestinal malignancies. *Cancer Chemother Pharmacol* 82: 429–440. doi:10.1007/s00280-018-3635-3

Harding JJ, Yang TS, Chen YY, Feng YH, Yen CJ, Ho CL, Huang WT, El Dika I, Akce M, Tan B, et al. 2021. Assessment of pegylated arginine deiminase and modified FOLFOX6 in patients with advanced hepatocellular carcinoma: results of an international, single-arm, phase 2 study. *Cancer* 127: 4585–4593. doi:10.1002/cncr.33870

Hensley CT, Wasti AT, DeBerardinis RJ. 2013. Glutamine and cancer: cell biology, physiology, and clinical opportunities. *J Clin Invest* 123: 3678–3684. doi:10.1172/JCI69600

Hinow P, Pinter G, Yan W, Wang SE. 2021. Modeling the bidirectional glutamine/ammonium conversion between cancer cells and cancer-associated fibroblasts. *PeerJ* 9: e10648. doi:10.7717/peerj.10648

Hoffer LJ. 2016. Human protein and amino acid requirements. *JPEN J Parenter Enteral Nutr* 40: 460–474. doi:10.1177/0148607115624084

Huang HY, Wu WR, Wang YH, Wang JW, Fang FM, Tsai JW, Li SH, Hung HC, Yu SC, Lan J, et al. 2013a. ASS1 as a novel tumor suppressor gene in myxofibrosarcomas: aberrant loss via epigenetic DNA methylation confers aggressive phenotypes, negative prognostic impact, and therapeutic relevance ASS1 deficiency in myxofibrosarcomas. *Clin Cancer Res* 19: 2861–2872. doi:10.1158/1078-0432.CCR-12-2641

Huang HL, Hsu HP, Shieh SC, Chang YS, Chen WC, Cho CY, Teng CF, Su IJ, Hung WC, Lai MD. 2013b. Attenuation of argininosuccinate lyase inhibits cancer growth via cyclin A2 and nitric oxide. *Mol Cancer Therapeut* **12**: 2505–2516. doi:10.1158/1535-7163.MCT-12-0863

Huang HL, Chen WC, Hsu HP, Cho CY, Hung YH, Wang CY, Lai MD. 2015. Argininosuccinate lyase is a potential therapeutic target in breast cancer. *Oncol Rep* **34**: 3131–3139. doi:10.3892/or.2015.4280

Huang HL, Chen WC, Hsu HP, Cho CY, Hung YH, Wang CY, Lai MD. 2017. Silencing of argininosuccinate lyase inhibits colorectal cancer formation. *Oncol Rep* **37**: 163–170. doi:10.3892/or.2016.5221

Husson A, Brasse-Lagnel C, Fairand A, Renouf S, Lavoinne A. 2003. Argininosuccinate synthetase from the urea cycle to the citrulline–NO cycle. *Eur J Biochem* **270**: 1887–1899. doi:10.1046/j.1432-1033.2003.03559.x

Ino Y, Yamazaki-Itoh R, Oguro S, Shimada K, Kosuge T, Zavada J, Kanai Y, Hiraoka N. 2013. Arginase II expressed in cancer-associated fibroblasts indicates tissue hypoxia and predicts poor outcome in patients with pancreatic cancer. *PLoS ONE* **8**: e55146. doi:10.1371/journal.pone.0055146

Jang TJ, Kim SA, Kim MK. 2018. Increased number of arginase 1-positive cells in the stroma of carcinomas compared to precursor lesions and nonneoplastic tissues. *Pathol Res Pract* **214**: 1179–1184. doi:10.1016/j.prp.2018.06.016

Jenkins DC, Charles IG, Thomsen LL, Moss DW, Holmes LS, Baylis SA, Rhodes P, Westmore K, Emson PC, Moncada S. 1995. Roles of nitric oxide in tumor growth. *Proc Natl Acad Sci* **92**: 4392–4396. doi:10.1073/pnas.92.10.4392

Kelly MP, Jungbluth AA, Wu BW, Bomalaski J, Old LJ, Ritter G. 2012. Arginine deiminase PEG20 inhibits growth of small cell lung cancers lacking expression of argininosuccinate synthetase. *Br J Cancer* **106**: 324–332. doi:10.1038/bjc.2011.524

Keshet R, Erez A. 2018. Arginine and the metabolic regulation of nitric oxide synthesis in cancer. *Disease Models Mech* **11**: dmm033332. doi:10.1242/dmm.033332

Keshet R, Lee JS, Adler L, Iraqi M, Ariav Y, Lim LQJ, Lerner S, Rabinovich S, Oren R, Katzir R, et al. 2020. Targeting purine synthesis in ASS1-expressing tumors enhances the response to immune checkpoint inhibitors. *Nat Cancer* **1**: 894–908. doi:10.1038/s43018-020-0106-7

Khare S, Kim LC, Lobel G, Doulias PT, Ischiropoulos H, Nissim I, Keith B, Simon MC. 2021. ASS1 and ASL suppress growth in clear cell renal cell carcinoma via altered nitrogen metabolism. *Cancer Metab* **9**: 1–16. doi:10.1186/s40170-021-00271-8

Kim J, Hu Z, Cai L, Li K, Choi E, Faubert B, Bezwada D, Rodriguez-Canales J, Villalobos P, Lin YF, et al. 2017. CPS1 maintains pyrimidine pools and DNA synthesis in KRAS/LKB1-mutant lung cancer cells. *Nature* **546**: 168–172. doi:10.1038/nature22359

Kim SS, Cui J, Xu S, Poddar S, Le TM, Li L, Wu N, Moore A, Zhou L, Yu A, et al. 2020. Histone deacetylase inhibition is synthetically lethal with arginine deprivation in pancreatic cancers with low argininosuccinate synthetase 1 expression. *Cancer Res* **80**(16_Suppl.): 554–554. doi:10.1158/1538-7445.AM2020-554

Kobayashi E, Masuda M, Nakayama R, Ichikawa H, Satow R, Shitashige M, Honda K, Yamaguchi U, Shoji A, Tochigi

N, et al. 2010. Reduced argininosuccinate synthetase is a predictive biomarker for the development of pulmonary metastasis in patients with osteosarcoma. *Mol Cancer Therapeut* **9**: 535–544. doi:10.1158/1535-7163.MCT-09-0774

Krzystek-Korpacka M, Szczęśniak-Sięga B, Szczuka I, Fortuna P, Zawadzki M, Kubiak A, Mierzchała-Pasierb M, Fleszar MG, Lewandowski Ł, Serek P, et al. 2020. L-arginine/nitric oxide pathway is altered in colorectal cancer and can be modulated by novel derivatives from oxicam class of non-steroidal anti-inflammatory drugs. *Cancers (Basel)* **12**: 2594. doi:10.3390/cancers12092594

Lee YY, Li CF, Lin CY, Lee SW, Sheu MJ, Lin LC, Chen TJ, Wu TF, Hsing CH. 2014. Overexpression of CPS1 is an independent negative prognosticator in rectal cancers receiving concurrent chemoradiotherapy. *Tumour Biol* **35**: 11097–11105. doi:10.1007/s13277-014-2425-8

Lee JS, Adler L, Karathia H, Carmel N, Rabinovich S, Auslander N, Keshet R, Stettner N, Silberman A, Agemy L, et al. 2018. Urea cycle dysregulation generates clinically relevant genomic and biochemical signatures. *Cell* **174**: 1559–1570.e22. doi:10.1016/j.cell.2018.07.019

Lerner S, Anderzhanova E, Verbitsky S, Eilam R, Kuperman Y, Tsoory M, Kuznetsov Y, Brandis A, Mehlman T, Mazkereth R, et al. 2019. ASL metabolically regulates tyrosine hydroxylase in the nucleus locus coeruleus. *Cell Rep* **29**: 2144–2153.e7. doi:10.1016/j.celrep.2019.10.043

Li J, Wang L, Chen X, Li L, Li Y, Ping Y, Huang L, Yue D, Zhang Z, Wang F, et al. 2017. CD39/CD73 upregulation on myeloid-derived suppressor cells via TGF-β-mTOR-HIF-1 signaling in patients with non-small cell lung cancer. *Oncoimmunology* **6**: e1320011. doi:10.1080/2162402X.2017.1320011

Li L, Mao Y, Zhao L, Li L, Wu J, Zhao M, Du W, Yu L, Jiang P. 2019. P53 regulation of ammonia metabolism through urea cycle controls polyamine biosynthesis. *Nature* **567**: 253–256. doi:10.1038/s41586-019-0996-7

Lisanti MP, Martinez-Outschoorn UE, Chiavarina B, Pavlides S, Whitaker-Menezes D, Tsirigos A, Witkiewicz AK, Lin Z, Balliet RM, Howell A, et al. 2010. Understanding the "lethal" drivers of tumor-stroma co-evolution: emerging role(s) for hypoxia, oxidative stress and autophagy/mitophagy in the tumor microenvironment. *Cancer Biol Ther* **10**: 537–542. doi:10.4161/cbt.10.6.13370

Liu Q, Zhang C, Sun A, Zheng Y, Wang L, Cao X. 2009. Tumor-educated CD11bhighIalow regulatory dendritic cells suppress T cell response through arginase I. *J Immunol* **182**: 6207–6216. doi:10.4049/jimmunol.0803926

Lowman XH, Hanse EA, Yang Y, Gabra MBI, Tran TQ, Li H, Kong M. 2019. P53 promotes cancer cell adaptation to glutamine deprivation by upregulating Slc7a3 to increase arginine uptake. *Cell Rep* **26**: 3051–3060.e4. doi:10.1016/j.celrep.2019.02.037

Lu Y, Wang L, Ding W, Wang D, Wang X, Luo Q, Zhu L. 2019. Ammonia mediates mitochondrial uncoupling and promotes glycolysis via HIF-1 activation in human breast cancer MDA-MB-231 cells. *Biochem Biophys Res Commun* **519**: 153–159. doi:10.1016/j.bbrc.2019.08.152

Lyssiotis CA, Kimmelman AC. 2017. Metabolic interactions in the tumor microenvironment. *Trends Cell Biol* **27**: 863–875. doi:10.1016/j.tcb.2017.06.003

Cite this article as *Cold Spring Harb Perspect Med* doi: 10.1101/cshperspect.a041538

Ma Z, Lian J, Yang M, Wuyang J, Zhao C, Chen W, Liu C, Zhao Q, Lou C, Han J, et al. 2019. Overexpression of Arginase-1 is an indicator of poor prognosis in patients with colorectal cancer. *Pathol Res Pract* **215**: 152383. doi:10.1016/j.prp.2019.03.012

Mandapathil M, Hilldorfer B, Szczepanski MJ, Czystowska M, Szajnik M, Ren J, Lang S, Jackson EK, Gorelik E, Whiteside TL. 2010. Generation and accumulation of immunosuppressive adenosine by human CD4[+] CD25[high]FOXP3[+] regulatory T cells. *J Biol Chem* **285**: 7176–7186. doi:10.1074/jbc.M109.047423

Martinenaite E, Ahmad SM, Bendtsen SK, Jørgensen MA, Weis-Banke SE, Svane IM, Andersen MH. 2019. Arginase-1-based vaccination against the tumor microenvironment: the identification of an optimal T-cell epitope. *Cancer Immunol Immunother* **68**: 1901–1907. doi:10.1007/s00262-019-02425-6

Matos A, Carvalho M, Bicho M, Ribeiro R. 2021. Arginine and arginases modulate metabolism, tumor microenvironment and prostate cancer progression. *Nutrients* **13**: 4503. doi:10.3390/nu13124503

Mavri-Damelin D, Eaton S, Damelin LH, Rees M, Hodgson HJ, Selden C. 2007. Ornithine transcarbamylase and arginase I deficiency are responsible for diminished urea cycle function in the human hepatoblastoma cell line HepG2. *Int J Biochem Cell Biol* **39**: 555–564. doi:10.1016/j.biocel.2006.10.007

McAlpine JA, Lu HT, Wu KC, Knowles SK, Thomson JA. 2014. Down-regulation of argininosuccinate synthetase is associated with cisplatin resistance in hepatocellular carcinoma cell lines: implications for PEGylated arginine deiminase combination therapy. *BMC Cancer* **14**: 1–12. doi:10.1186/1471-2407-14-621

Mestre-Farrera A, Bruch-Oms M, Peña R, Rodríguez-Morató J, Alba-Castellón L, Comerma L, Quintela-Fandino M, Duñach M, Baulida J, Pozo ÓJ, et al. 2021. Glutamine-directed migration of cancer-activated fibroblasts facilitates epithelial tumor invasion. *Cancer Res* **81**: 438–451. doi:10.1158/0008-5472.CAN-20-0622

Mishra R, Haldar S, Placencio V, Madhav A, Rohena-Rivera K, Agarwal P, Duong F, Angara B, Tripathi M, Liu Z, et al. 2018. Stromal epigenetic alterations drive metabolic and neuroendocrine prostate cancer reprogramming. *J Clin Invest* **128**: 4472–4484. doi:10.1172/JCI99397

Missiaen R, Anderson NM, Kim LC, Nance B, Burrows M, Skuli N, Carens M, Riscal R, Steensels A, Li F, et al. 2022. GCN2 inhibition sensitizes arginine-deprived hepatocellular carcinoma cells to senolytic treatment. *Cell Metab* **34**: 1151–1167.e7. doi:10.1016/j.cmet.2022.06.010

Miyamoto T, Lo PHY, Saichi N, Ueda K, Hirata M, Tanikawa C, Matsuda K. 2017. Argininosuccinate synthase 1 is an intrinsic Akt repressor transactivated by p53. *Sci Adv* **3**: e1603204. doi:10.1126/sciadv.1603204

Mohammadpour H, O'Neil R, Qiu J, McCarthy PL, Repasky EA, Cao X. 2018. Blockade of host β2-adrenergic receptor enhances graft-versus-tumor effect through modulating APCs. *J Immunol* **200**: 2479–2488. doi:10.4049/jimmunol.1701752

Mohammadpour H, MacDonald CR, Qiao G, Chen M, Dong B, Hylander BL, McCarthy PL, Abrams SI, Repasky EA. 2019. B2 adrenergic receptor–mediated signaling regulates the immunosuppressive potential of myeloid-de-rived suppressor cells. *J Clin Invest* **129**: 5537–5552. doi:10.1172/JCI129502

Mumenthaler SM, Yu H, Tze S, Cederbaum SD, Pegg AE, Seligson DB, Grody WW. 2008. Expression of arginase II in prostate cancer. *Int J Oncol* **32**: 357–365.

Murray PJ. 2016. Amino acid auxotrophy as a system of immunological control nodes. *Nat Immunol* **17**: 132–139. doi:10.1038/ni.3323

Mussai F, De Santo C, Abu-Dayyeh I, Booth S, Quek L, McEwen-Smith RM, Qureshi A, Dazzi F, Vyas P, Cerundolo V. 2013. Acute myeloid leukemia creates an arginase-dependent immunosuppressive microenvironment. *Blood* **122**: 749–758. doi:10.1182/blood-2013-01-480129

Nagamani SC, Erez A, Lee B. 2012. Argininosuccinate lyase deficiency. *Genet Med* **14**: 501–507. doi:10.1038/gim.2011.1

Nicholson LJ, Smith PR, Hiller L, Szlosarek PW, Kimberley C, Sehouli J, Koensgen D, Mustea A, Schmid P, Crook T. 2009. Epigenetic silencing of argininosuccinate synthetase confers resistance to platinum-induced cell death but collateral sensitivity to arginine auxotrophy in ovarian cancer. *Int J Cancer* **125**: 1454–1463. doi:10.1002/ijc.24546

Norian LA, Rodriguez PC, O'Mara LA, Zabaleta J, Ochoa AC, Cella M, Allen PM. 2009. Tumor-infiltrating regulatory dendritic cells inhibit CD8[+] T cell function via L-arginine metabolism. *Cancer Res* **69**: 3086–3094. doi:10.1158/0008-5472.CAN-08-2826

Novitskiy SV, Ryzhov S, Zaynagetdinov R, Goldstein AE, Huang Y, Tikhomirov OY, Blackburn MR, Biaggioni I, Carbone DP, Feoktistov I, et al. 2008. Adenosine receptors in regulation of dendritic cell differentiation and function. *Blood* **112**: 1822–1831. doi:10.1182/blood-2008-02-136325

Ochocki JD, Khare S, Hess M, Ackerman D, Qiu B, Daisak JI, Worth AJ, Lin N, Lee P, Xie H, et al. 2018. Arginase 2 suppresses renal carcinoma progression via biosynthetic cofactor pyridoxal phosphate depletion and increased polyamine toxicity. *Cell Metab* **27**: 1263–1280.e6. doi:10.1016/j.cmet.2018.04.009

Ogando DG, Choi M, Shyam R, Li S, Bonanno JA. 2019. Ammonia sensitive SLC4A11 mitochondrial uncoupling reduces glutamine induced oxidative stress. *Redox Biol* **26**: 101260. doi:10.1016/j.redox.2019.101260

Ohshima K, Nojima S, Tahara S, Kurashige M, Hori Y, Hagiwara K, Okuzaki D, Oki S, Wada N, Ikeda JI, et al. 2017. Argininosuccinate synthase 1-deficiency enhances the cell sensitivity to arginine through decreased DEPTOR expression in endometrial cancer. *Sci Rep* **7**: 1–14. doi:10.1038/srep4550

Passarelli A, Tucci M, Mannavola F, Felici C, Silvestris F. 2019. The metabolic milieu in melanoma: role of immune suppression by CD73/adenosine. *Tumour Biol* **41**: 101042831983713. doi:10.1177/1010428319837138

Pavlova NN, Hui S, Ghergurovich JM, Fan J, Intlekofer AM, White RM, Rabinowitz JD, Thompson CB, Zhang J. 2018. As extracellular glutamine levels decline, asparagine becomes an essential amino acid. *Cell Metab* **27**: 428–438.e5. doi:10.1016/j.cmet.2017.12.006

Rabinovich S, Adler L, Yizhak K, Sarver A, Silberman A, Agron S, Stettner N, Sun Q, Brandis A, Helbling D, et al. 2015. Diversion of aspartate in ASS1-deficient tumours fosters de novo pyrimidine synthesis. *Nature* **527**: 379–383. doi:10.1038/nature15529

Rabinovich S, Silberman A, Adler L, Agron S, Levin-Zaidman S, Bahat A, Porat Z, Ben-Zeev E, Geva I, Itkin M, et al. 2020. The mitochondrial carrier citrin plays a role in regulating cellular energy during carcinogenesis. *Oncogene* **39**: 164–175. doi:10.1038/s41388-019-0976-2

Raskovalova T, Huang X, Sitkovsky M, Zacharia LC, Jackson EK, Gorelik E. 2005. Gs protein-coupled adenosine receptor signaling and lytic function of activated NK cells. *J Immunol* **175**: 4383–4391. doi:10.4049/jimmunol.175.7.4383

Ridder DA, Schindeldecker M, Weinmann A, Berndt K, Urbansky L, Witzel HR, Heinrich S, Roth W, Straub BK. 2021. Key enzymes in pyrimidine synthesis, CAD and CPS1, predict prognosis in hepatocellular carcinoma. *Cancers (Basel)* **13**: 744. doi:10.3390/cancers13040744

Roci I, Watrous JD, Lagerborg KA, Lafranchi L, Lindqvist A, Jain M, Nilsson R. 2019. Mapping metabolic events in the cancer cell cycle reveals arginine catabolism in the committed SG2M phase. *Cell Rep* **26**: 1691–1700.e5. doi:10.1016/j.celrep.2019.01.059

Rodriguez PC, Quiceno DG, Zabaleta J, Ortiz B, Zea AH, Piazuelo MB, Delgado A, Correa P, Brayer J, Sotomayor EM, et al. 2004. Arginase I production in the tumor microenvironment by mature myeloid cells inhibits T-cell receptor expression and antigen-specific T-cell responses. *Cancer Res* **64**: 5839–5849. doi:10.1158/0008-5472.CAN-04-0465

Rodriguez PC, Ernstoff MS, Hernandez C, Atkins M, Zabaleta J, Sierra R, Ochoa AC. 2009. Arginase I–producing myeloid-derived suppressor cells in renal cell carcinoma are a subpopulation of activated granulocytes. *Cancer Res* **69**: 1553–1560. doi:10.1158/0008-5472.CAN-08-1921

Rotondo R, Barisione G, Mastracci L, Grossi F, Orengo AM, Costa R, Truini M, Fabbi M, Ferrini S, Barbieri O. 2009. IL-8 induces exocytosis of arginase 1 by neutrophil polymorphonuclears in nonsmall cell lung cancer. *Int J Cancer* **125**: 887–893. doi:10.1002/ijc.24448

Serafini P, Mgebroff S, Noonan K, Borrello I. 2008. Myeloid-derived suppressor cells promote cross-tolerance in B-cell lymphoma by expanding regulatory T cells. *Cancer Res* **68**: 5439–5449. doi:10.1158/0008-5472.CAN-07-6621

Shan YS, Hsu HP, Lai MD, Yen MC, Chen WC, Fang JH, Weng TY, Chen YL. 2015. Argininosuccinate synthetase 1 suppression and arginine restriction inhibit cell migration in gastric cancer cell lines. *Sci Rep* **5**: 9783. doi:10.1038/srep09783

Silberman A, Goldman O, Boukobza Assayag O, Jacob A, Rabinovich S, Adler L, Lee JS, Keshet R, Sarver A, Frug J, et al. 2019. Acid-induced downregulation of ASS1 contributes to the maintenance of intracellular pH in cancer. *Cancer Res* **79**: 518–533. doi:10.1158/0008-5472.CAN-18-1062

Sousa CM, Biancur DE, Wang X, Halbrook CJ, Sherman MH, Zhang L, Kremer D, Hwang RF, Witkiewicz AK, Ying H, et al. 2016. Pancreatic stellate cells support tumour metabolism through autophagic alanine secretion. *Nature* **536**: 479–483. doi:10.1038/nature19084

Spinelli JB, Yoon H, Ringel AE, Jeanfavre S, Clish CB, Haigis MC. 2017. Metabolic recycling of ammonia via glutamate

dehydrogenase supports breast cancer biomass. *Science* **358**: 941–946. doi:10.1126/science.aam9305

Syed N, Langer J, Janczar K, Singh P, Lo Nigro C, Lattanzio L, Coley HM, Hatzimichael E, Bomalaski J, Szlosarek P, et al. 2013. Epigenetic status of argininosuccinate synthetase and argininosuccinate lyase modulates autophagy and cell death in glioblastoma. *Cell Death Dis* **4**: e458–e458. doi:10.1038/cddis.2012.197

Szlosarek PW, Grimshaw MJ, Wilbanks GD, Hagemann T, Wilson JL, Burke F, Stamp G, Balkwill FR. 2007. Aberrant regulation of argininosuccinate synthetase by TNF-α in human epithelial ovarian cancer. *Int J Cancer* **121**: 6–11. doi:10.1002/ijc.22666

Szlosarek PW, Phillips MM, Pavlyk I, Steele J, Shamash J, Spicer J, Kumar S, Pacey S, Feng X, Johnston A, et al. 2020. Expansion phase 1 study of pegargiminase plus pemetrexed and cisplatin in patients with argininosuccinate synthetase 1–deficient mesothelioma: safety, efficacy, and resistance mechanisms. *JTO Clin Res Rep* **1**: 100093.

Tajan M, Hock AK, Blagih J, Robertson NA, Labuschagne CF, Kruiswijk F, Humpton TJ, Adams PD, Vousden KH. 2018. A role for p53 in the adaptation to glutamine starvation through the expression of SLC1A3. *Cell Metab* **28**: 721–736.e6. doi:10.1016/j.cmet.2018.07.005

Takenawa H, Kurosaki M, Enomoto N, Miyasaka Y, Kanazawa N, Sakamoto N, Ikeda T, Izumi N, Sato C, Watanabe M. 2004. Differential gene-expression profiles associated with gastric adenoma. *Br J Cancer* **90**: 216–223. doi:10.1038/sj.bjc.6601399

Takeuchi Y, Nakayama Y, Fukusaki E, Irino Y. 2018. Glutamate production from ammonia via glutamate dehydrogenase 2 activity supports cancer cell proliferation under glutamine depletion. *Biochem Biophys Res Commun* **495**: 761–767. doi:10.1016/j.bbrc.2017.11.088

Tan GS, Lim KH, Tan HT, Khoo ML, Tan SH, Toh HC, Ching Ming Chung M. 2014. Novel proteomic biomarker panel for prediction of aggressive metastatic hepatocellular carcinoma relapse in surgically resectable patients. *J Proteome Res* **13**: 4833–4846. doi:10.1021/pr500229n

Tao X, Zuo Q, Ruan H, Wang H, Jin H, Cheng Z, Lv Y, Qin W, Wang C. 2019. Argininosuccinate synthase 1 suppresses cancer cell invasion by inhibiting STAT3 pathway in hepatocellular carcinoma. *Acta Biochem Biophys Sin (Shanghai)* **51**: 263–276. doi:10.1093/abbs/gmz005

Tardito S, Oudin A, Ahmed SU, Fack F, Keunen O, Zheng L, Miletic H, Sakariassen PØ, Weinstock A, Wagner A, et al. 2015. Glutamine synthetase activity fuels nucleotide biosynthesis and supports growth of glutamine-restricted glioblastoma. *Nat Cell Biol* **17**: 1556–1568. doi:10.1038/ncb3272

Thevenot PT, Sierra RA, Raber PL, Al-Khami AA, Trillo-Tinoco J, Zarreii P, Ochoa AC, Cui Y, Del Valle L, Rodriguez PC. 2014. The stress–response sensor chop regulates the function and accumulation of myeloid-derived suppressor cells in tumors. *Immunity* **41**: 389–401. doi:10.1016/j.immuni.2014.08.015

Thongkum A, Wu C, Li YY, Wangpaichitr M, Navasumrit P, Parnlob V, Sricharunrat T, Bhudhisawasdi V, Ruchirawat M, Savaraj N. 2017. The combination of arginine deprivation and 5-fluorouracil improves therapeutic efficacy in argininosuccinate synthetase negative hepatocellular carcinoma. *Int J Mol Sci* **18**: 1175. doi:10.3390/ijms18061175

Tsai CY, Chi HC, Chi LM, Yang HY, Tsai MM, Lee KF, Huang HW, Chou LF, Cheng AJ, Yang CW, et al. 2018. Argininosuccinate synthetase 1 contributes to gastric cancer invasion and progression by modulating autophagy. *FASEB J* **32:** 2601–2614. doi:10.1096/fj.201700094r

van de Poll MC, Siroen MP, van Leeuwen PA, Soeters PB, Melis GC, Boelens PG, Deutz NE, Dejong CH. 2007. Interorgan amino acid exchange in humans: consequences for arginine and citrulline metabolism. *Am J Clin Nutr* **85:** 167–172. doi:10.1093/ajcn/85.1.167

von Stechow L, Ruiz-Aracama A, van de Water B, Peijnenburg A, Danen E, Lommen A. 2013. Identification of cisplatin-regulated metabolic pathways in pluripotent stem cells. *PLoS ONE* **8:** e76476. doi:10.1371/journal.pone.0076476

Wang X, Xiang H, Toyoshima Y, Shen W, Shichi S, Nakamoto H, Kimura S, Sugiyama K, Homma S, Miyagi Y, et al. 2023. Arginase-1 inhibition reduces migration ability and metastatic colonization of colon cancer cells. *Cancer Metab* **11:** 1–14. doi:10.1186/s40170-022-00301-z

Watford M. 2003. The urea cycle: teaching intermediary metabolism in a physiological setting. *Biochem Mol Biol Educ* **31:** 289–297. doi:10.1002/bmb.2003.494031050249

Weis-Banke SE, Hübbe ML, Holmström MO, Jørgensen MA, Bendtsen SK, Martinenaite E, Carretta M, Svane IM, Ødum N, Pedersen AW, et al. 2020. The metabolic enzyme arginase-2 is a potential target for novel immune modulatory vaccines. *Oncoimmunology* **9:** 1771142. doi:10.1080/2162402X.2020.1771142

Yan W, Wu X, Zhou W, Fong MY, Cao M, Liu J, Liu X, Chen CH, Fadare O, Pizzo DP, et al. 2018. Cancer-cell-secreted exosomal miR-105 promotes tumour growth through the MYC-dependent metabolic reprogramming of stromal cells. *Nat Cell Biol* **20:** 597–609. doi:10.1038/s41556-018-0083-6

Yang L, Achreja A, Yeung TL, Mangala LS, Jiang D, Han C, Baddour J, Marini JC, Ni J, Nakahara R, et al. 2016. Targeting stromal glutamine synthetase in tumors disrupts tumor microenvironment-regulated cancer cell growth. *Cell Metab* **24:** 685–700. doi:10.1016/j.cmet.2016.10.011

Yao S, Nguyen TV, Rolfe A, Agrawal AA, Ke J, Peng S, Colombo F, Yu S, Bouchard P, Wu J. 2020. Small molecule inhibition of CPS1 activity through an allosteric pocket. *Cell Chem Biol* **27:** 259–268. doi:10.1016/j.chembiol.2020.01.009

Yau T, Cheng PN, Chiu J, Kwok GGW, Leung R, Liu AM, Cheung TT, Ng CT. 2022. A phase 1 study of pegylated recombinant arginase (PEG-BCT-100) in combination with systemic chemotherapy (capecitabine and oxaliplatin) [PACOX] in advanced hepatocellular carcinoma patients. *Invest New Drugs* **40:** 1–8. doi:10.1007/s10637-021-01178-3

You J, Chen W, Chen J, Zheng Q, Dong J, Zhu Y. 2018. The oncogenic role of ARG1 in progression and metastasis of hepatocellular carcinoma. *BioMed Res Int* **2018:** 2109865. doi:10.1155/2018/2109865

Zeng W, Zhang Y, Zheng W, Luo Q, Han J, Liu JA, Zhao Y, Jia F, Wu K, Wang F. 2019. Discovery of cisplatin binding to thymine and cytosine on a single-stranded oligodeoxynucleotide by high resolution FT-ICR mass spectrometry. *Molecules* **24:** 1852. doi:10.3390/molecules24101852

Zhang L, Zou Y, Lu Y, Li Z, Gao F. 2023a. Unraveling the therapeutic potential of carbamoyl phosphate synthetase 1 (CPS1) in human diseases. *Bioorg Chem* **130:** 106253. doi:10.1016/j.bioorg.2022.106253

Zhang S, Hu Y, Wu Z, Zhou X, Wu T, Li P, Lian Q, Xu S, Gu J, Chen L, et al. 2023b. Deficiency of carbamoyl phosphate synthetase 1 engenders radioresistance in hepatocellular carcinoma via deubiquitinating c-Myc. *Int J Radiat Oncol Biol Phys* **115:** 1244–1256. doi:10.1016/j.ijrobp.2022.11.022

Zhao Z, Liu H, Fang D, Zhou X, Zhao S, Zhang C, Ye J, Xu J. 2022. Patient stratification based on urea cycle metabolism for exploration of combination immunotherapy in colon cancer. *BMC Cancer* **22:** 883. doi:10.1186/s12885-022-09958-7

Tracing the Diverse Paths of One-Carbon Metabolism in Cancer and Beyond

Esther W. Lim[1,2] and Christian M. Metallo[1,2]

[1]Department of Molecular and Cell Biology, Salk Institute for Biological Studies, La Jolla, California 92037, USA

[2]Department of Bioengineering, University of California, San Diego, La Jolla, California 92093, USA

Correspondence: metallo@salk.edu

One-carbon (1C) metabolism is a network of biochemical reactions distributed across organelles that delivers folate-activated 1C units to support macromolecule synthesis, methylation, and reductive homeostasis. Fluxes through these pathways are up-regulated in highly proliferative cancer cells, and anti-folates, which target enzymes within the 1C pathway, have long been used in the treatment of cancer. In this work, we review fundamental aspects of 1C metabolism and place it in context with other biosynthetic and redox pathways, such that 1C metabolism acts to bridge pathways across compartments. We further discuss the importance of stable-isotope-tracing techniques combined with mass spectrometry analysis to study 1C metabolism and conclude by highlighting therapeutic approaches that could exploit cancer cells' dependency on 1C metabolism.

Metabolic reprogramming is essential for tumorigenesis (Pavlova and Thompson 2016; Faubert et al. 2020). The altered metabolic state of glycolysis and mitochondrial metabolism tumors and proliferating cells was first described almost a century ago by Warburg et al. (1927). Since then, many new biochemical mechanisms that drive the growth and survival of tumors have been discovered (DeBerardinis and Chandel 2020). Many of these alterations are needed to support the increased bioenergetic and biosynthetic demand for survival and proliferation. As such, these metabolic alterations often include up-regulated nutrient acquisition (e.g., glucose, lactate, amino acids), increased need for electron acceptors, expanded biosynthesis pathways, and changes in gene regulation (Pavlova and Thompson 2016). One such metabolic pathway that supports many of these needs is one-carbon (1C) metabolism.

1C metabolism consists of a broad range of biochemical reactions that are essential for maintaining cellular homeostasis. In cancer, genes in this pathway are often transcriptionally up-regulated. These include dihydrofolate reductase (DHFR) (Guo et al. 1999; Yang et al. 2003), thymidylate synthase (TYMS) (Burdelski et al. 2015; Sun et al. 2015; Fu et al. 2019), mitochondrial serine hydroxymethyl transferase (SHMT2) (Jain et al. 2012; Lee et al. 2014), and mitochondrial methylenetetrahydrofolate dehydrogenase (MTHFD2) (Fig. 1; Nilsson et al. 2014). In fact, patients with high expression of these genes such as *SHMT2*, *MTHFD2*, and *ALDH1L2* have a

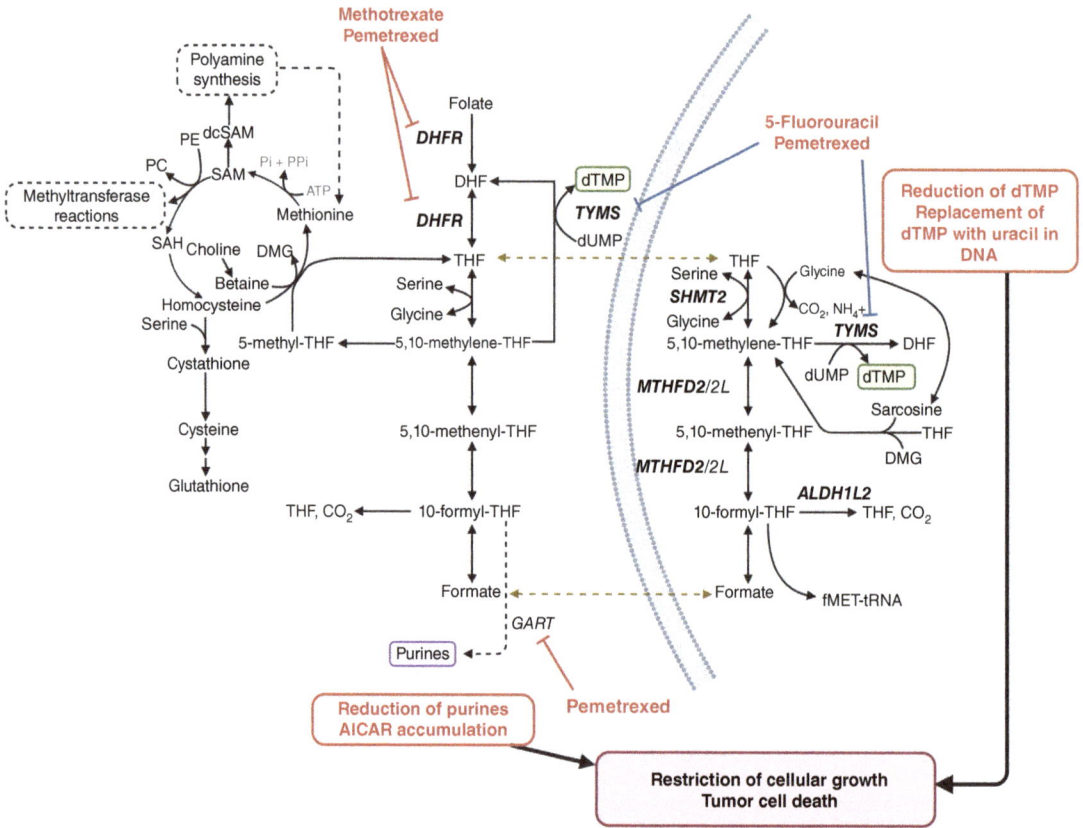

Figure 1. Overview of 1C metabolism and established therapeutics that target this pathway and their effects on cancer. Genes in bold encode enzymes in the 1C metabolic pathway that are transcriptionally up-regulated in some cancers. These include dihydrofolate reductase (DHFR), thymidylate synthase (TYMS), mitochondrial serine hydroxymethyl transferase (SHMT2), and mitochondrial methylenetetrahydrofolate dehydrogenase (MTHFD2). Chemotherapeutics such as methotrexate, pemetrexed, and 5-Fluorouracil inhibit annotated enzymes in the pathway. (Figure generated with BioRender; https://biorender.com.)

shorter survival rate compared to patients with low expression of these genes (Koseki et al. 2018). The gene for the first enzyme for serine synthesis, phosphoglycerate dehydrogenase (PHGDH), is often up-regulated in cancer as well (Locasale et al. 2011; Possemato et al. 2011) and this is important because serine is one of the inputs for 1C metabolism. The reliance on 1C metabolism in cancer cells is also reflected in the use of antifolates for the treatment of cancer (Fig. 1), although these therapies have harmful side effects due to the importance of 1C metabolism in nontransformed cells as well.

Here, we review 1C metabolism in the context of other biosynthetic and redox pathways and discuss how this reaction network acts as a dynamic system to bridge pathways across compartments such as the nucleus, cytosol, and mitochondria. Additionally, we highlight the utility of stable-isotope tracing techniques combined with mass spectrometry measurement to study 1C metabolism and then discuss therapeutic approaches that could exploit cancer cells' dependency on 1C metabolism.

1C METABOLISM IN RELATION TO THE TRICARBOXYLIC ACID CYCLE

The Warburg effect, which describes the high rate of glucose uptake and lactate secretion even in the presence of oxygen, is well known. The observation that cancer cells actively take up

Cite this article as *Cold Spring Harb Perspect Med* doi: 10.1101/cshperspect.a041533

glucose has led to the routine use of 2-[18F]-fluor-2-deoxy-D-glucose position emission tomography/computed tomography (FDG-PET/CT) to diagnose many different cancers in the clinic (Otsuka et al. 2004; Rohren et al. 2004). Although Warburg postulated that cancer cells have defective mitochondria, many cancer cells use these glucose-derived carbons to feed into the Krebs or tricarboxylic acid (TCA) cycle in the mitochondria to support multiple metabolic processes. The TCA cycle produces reducing equivalents in the form of NADH and $FADH_2$, which are used to generate ATP though oxidative phosphorylation. Additionally, the TCA cycle provides precursors for fatty acid and steroid biosynthesis and fuels other anabolic pathways including amino acid biosynthesis and gluconeogenesis. Beyond these anabolic pathways, TCA cycle intermediates can act as effector molecules to modulate signaling pathways and gene expression (Martínez-Reyes and Chandel 2020).

In many ways, 1C metabolism is like the TCA cycle (Fig. 2), where both pathways include a cyclic network of reactions to generate precursors for the synthesis of other metabolites. Additionally, both 1C and TCA cycles consume and regenerate re-

ducing equivalents as cofactors to support bioenergetics and maintain redox homeostasis (with production of reducing equivalents favored in the matrix). Like the TCA cycle, several enzymatic reactions of 1C metabolism such as MTHFD2/2L and ALDH1L2 produce NAD(P)H in the mitochondrial matrix. As such, many of the reactions in 1C metabolism are linked to changes in redox status. For example, metastatic melanoma cells reversibly increase the expression of NADPH-regenerating enzyme ALDH1L2 to increase their capacity to withstand oxidative stress (Piskounova et al. 2015). Notably, folate-dependent serine catabolism within mitochondria can generate NADPH under hypoxia (Ye et al. 2014) and NADH when respiration is impaired (Yang et al. 2020), indicating the critical role of 1C metabolism in regulating redox homeostasis. On the other hand, both pathways are fueled by substrates carried by vitamin cofactors in the form of tetrahydrofolate and coenzyme A.

1C metabolism encompasses a complex metabolic network that supports multiple biological processes through the generation of 1C units. These pathways include the interconversion of serine to glycine and 1C units, the glycine cleav-

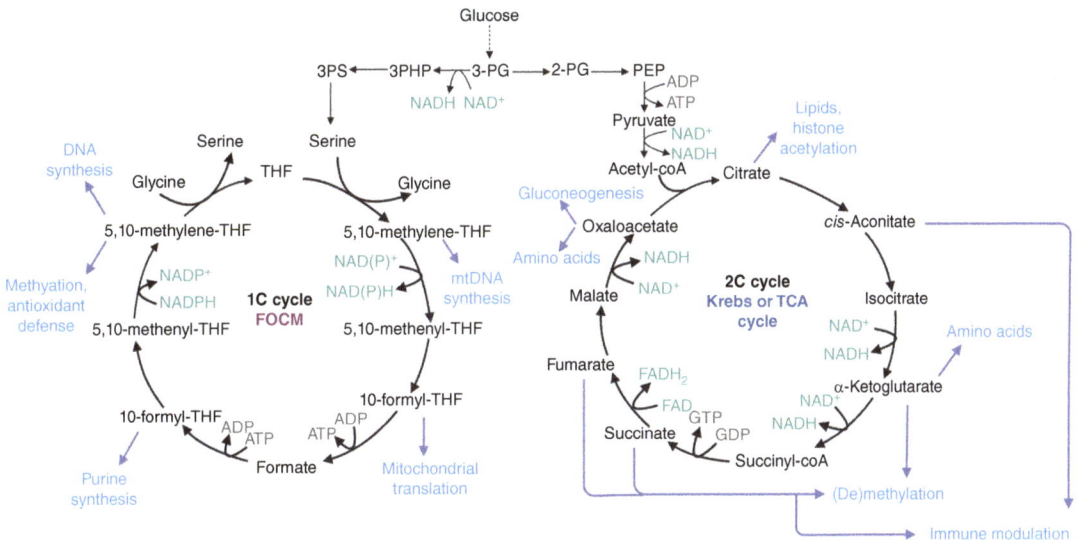

Figure 2. Comparison between 1C and 2C cycle. It can be helpful to think of 1C metabolism in the context of the Krebs or tricarboxylic acid (TCA) cycle. (2-PG) 2-phosphoglycerate, (3-PG) 3-phosphoglycerate, (PEP) phosphoenolpyruvate, (3PHP) 3-phosphohydroxypyruvate, (3PS) 3-phosphoserine, (THF) tetrahydrofolate. (Figure generated with BioRender; https://biorender.com.)

age system (GCS), betaine and choline metabolism, and the catabolism of histidine as well as other amino acids. Among these inputs, serine is a major source of 1C units (Labuschagne et al. 2014; Maddocks et al. 2016). Serine is metabolized to/from formate by two complementary pathways in the cytosol and mitochondria (Fig. 3), which consist of similar biochemical reactions: (1) transfer of 1C unit to tetrahydrofolate (THF) by forming 5,10-methylene-THF and glycine, and (2) oxidation of 5,10-methylene-THF to 10-formyl-THF. In the cytosol, these steps are

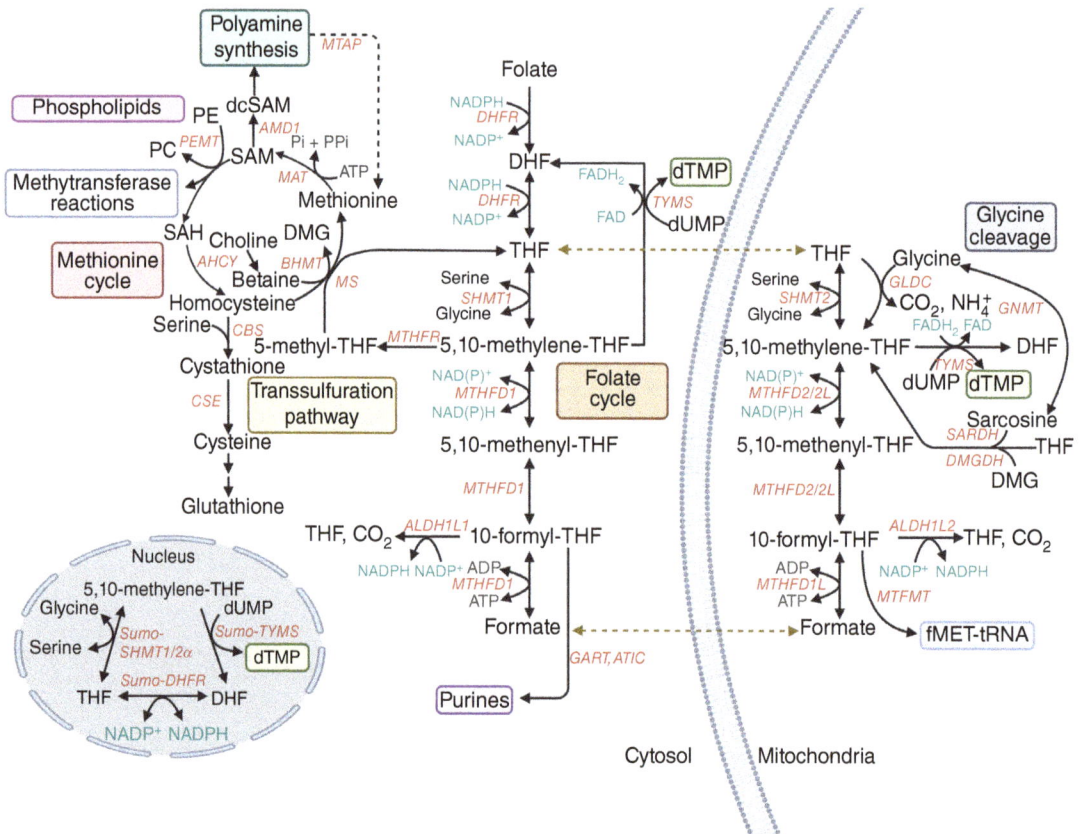

Figure 3. 1C metabolism network across organelles. 1C pathways are distributed across the cytosol, mitochondria, and nucleus. (DHF) Dihydrofolate, (THF) tetrahydrofolate, (DMG) dimethylglycine, (SAM) S-adenosylmethionine, (SAH) S-adenosylhomocysteine, (dcSAM) decarboxylated SAM, (AMD1) S-adenosylmethionine decarboxylase, (MTAP) methylthioadenosine phosphorylase, (PE) phosphatidylethanolamine, (PC) phosphatidylcholine, (PEMT) phosphatidylethanolamine N-methyltransferase, (DHFR) dihydrofolate reductase, (SHMT1/2) serine hydroxymethyl transferase, cytosolic(1)/mitochondrial(2), (MTHFD1) methylenetetrahydrofolate dehydrogenase, cyclohydrolase, and formyltetrahydrofolate synthetase 1, (MTHFD2/2L) methylenetetrahydrofolate dehydrogenase 2/2-like, (MTHFD1L) monofunctional tetrahydrofolate synthase, (ALDH1L1/2) cytosolic(1)/ mitochondrial (2) 10-formyltetrahydrofolate dehydrogenase, (GLDC) glycine decarboxylase, (TYMS) thymidylate synthase, (GNMT) glycine N-methyltransferase, (SARDH) sarcosine dehydrogenase, (DMGDH) dimethylglycine dehydrogenase, (MTFMT) mitochondrial methionyl-tRNA formyltransferase, (MTHFR) methylenetetrahydrofolate reductase, (MS) methionine synthase, (BHMT) betaine-homocysteine S-methyltransferase, (MAT) methionine adenosyltransferase, (AHCY) S-adenosyl-L-homocysteine hydrolase, (CBS) cystathionine beta synthase, (CSE) cystathionine γ lyase, (GART) phosphoribosylglycinamide formyltransferase, (ATIC) 5-aminoimidazole-4-carboxamideribonucleotide formyltransferase/IMP cyclohydrolase. (Figure generated with BioRender; https://biorender.com.)

catalyzed by SHMT1 and MTHFD1, whereas in the mitochondrial matrix these steps are catalyzed by SHMT2, MTHFD2 or MTHFD2L, and MTHFD1L. In the cytosol, CH_2-THF is also reduced to 5-methyl-THF to support methyl group synthesis. Through these intermediates, the 1C metabolism is associated and interlinked with other metabolic pathways such as the folate cycle, methionine cycle, and indirectly the TCA cycle through redox status (Fig. 2). Folate molecules chemically activate 1C units and must first be reduced from folic acid to dihydrofolate (DHF) by DHF reductase and subsequently to tetrahydrofolate (THF). Once bound to a folate molecule, 1C units exist at different oxidation states: 5, 10-methylene THF, 5-methyl-THF, and 10-formyl-THF with each supporting a different biosynthetic function.

1C metabolism contributes to the methionine cycle by reduction of CH_2-THF to 5-methyl-THF. The methionine cycle produces S-adenosylmethionine (SAM), a ubiquitous methyl group donor that is used by SAM-dependent methyltransferases for the methylation of DNA, RNA, proteins, and lipids. 5,10-methylene-THF derived from the folate cycle is irreversibly converted to 5-methyl-THF by MTHFR. 5-methyl-THF then donates its methyl group to homocysteine in a B12-dependent reaction catalyzed by methionine synthase to produce methionine and THF. THF can then reenter the folate cycle. The remethylation of homocysteine to form methionine is also driven by choline through the generation of betaine via betaine-homocysteine S-methyltransferase (BHMT). A product of that reaction, dimethylglycine (DMG) can further contribute 1C units to the mitochondrial folate cycle. Methionine is then converted into SAM by S-adenosylmethionine synthase in an ATP-dependent process. The folate cycle helps contribute to this reaction as well by maintaining ATP levels through de novo purine synthesis in cancer cells (Maddocks et al. 2016). SAM can also be diverted to the polyamine synthesis pathway after decarboxylation by adenosylmethionine decarboxylase 1 (AMD1). Decarboxylated SAM along with putrescine are precursors for polyamines, spermidine, and spermine, and generate 5-methylthioadenosine as a byproduct that can be recycled back to me-

thionine by 5-methylthioadenosine phosphorylase (MTAP).

The methionine cycle is also involved in the biosynthesis of phospholipids such as phosphatidylcholine through SAM (Zatz et al. 1981). The head group of phosphatidylcholines is synthesized from choline through the adenylation of methionine to SAM, such that alterations in 1C metabolism may influence the balance of phosphatidylcholine and phosphoethanolamine. These glycerophospholipids are abundant in tissues and are important components of the plasma membrane that facilitate transport and signaling across cells (Szlasa et al. 2020; Saito et al. 2022).

Besides choline, glycine is another potential source of 1C units through the GCS, which catalyzes the breakdown of glycine to CO_2, ammonia, and a 1C unit in the form of 5,10-methylene-THF. As such, the GCS is coupled to 1C metabolism via the activity of MTHFD2/2L and MTHFD1L. Glycine is subsequently catabolized or converted to serine by SHMT1, as patients lacking GCS function accumulate glycine (Kralik et al. 2023). While highly active in liver, kidney, and select cell types (Handzlik and Metallo 2023), immortalized cancer cell lines lack a significant contribution of GCS activity to the 1C pool (Labuschagne et al. 2014; Meiser et al. 2016).

The 1C cycle is also influenced by redox homeostasis. Tetrahydrofolate reductase reduces THF, which enters the folate-mediated 1C cycle, and this reaction consumes one molecule of NADPH for each turn of the cycle. The reactions catalyzed by MTHFD1 or MTHFD2/L either consume or produce NAD(P)H depending on the direction of the reaction. While many of these reactions are reversible, the oxidation of 10-formyl-THF to CO_2 is not and generates NADPH in the mitochondrial matrix. In addition to supporting redox maintenance, NAPDH also supports lipid synthesis and NADPH oxidase (NOX) signaling to support cancer cell proliferation. In some cancers, the mitochondrial 1C pathway is a contributor to the NADPH pool (Fan et al. 2014; Ye et al. 2014; Piskounova et al. 2015). Finally, the transsulfuration pathway connects to the methionine and folate cycle through homocysteine, such that the condensation of serine and homocysteine yields cystathionine and subsequently cysteine, a precursor for glutathione. Glutathione is an important antioxidant that helps maintain redox homeostasis as levels are maintained at mM concentrations in cells and tissues.

Overall, 1C metabolism is highly interconnected and dependent on multiple inputs that fuel the folate-mediated 1C cycle. It may therefore be helpful to think about the 1C cycle in relation to the 2-carbon TCA cycle. Both pathways are amphibolic in that they are involved in catabolic and anabolic processes, they are both linked directly by electron flow to/from reducing equivalents, and they also influence epigenetic regulation. In the same way, reactions in both of these pathways occur in the cytosol, mitochondrial matrix, and nucleus.

COMPARTMENTALIZATION OF 1C METABOLISM

The wide network of metabolic reactions in 1C metabolism and associated pathways occur in various organelles, such that specific reactions are compartmentalized across the cytoplasm, mitochondria, and nucleus (Fig. 3; Tibbetts and Appling 2010). While MTHFD1 catalyzes the conversion of formate to 10-formyl-THF, 5,10-methenyl-THF, and 5,10-methylene-THF in the cytosol, these reactions are catalyzed separately by MTHFD2/2L and MTHFD1L in the mitochondria. 1C-activated folates are not known to travel across intracellular membranes, so to enable the transfer of 1C units between compartments, 10-formyl-THF is converted to formate. The hydrolysis of 10-formyl-THF is coupled to ATP production and is reversible. Transport of 1C units between organelles can also occur through serine and glycine. In the mitochondria, dimethylglycine and sarcosine can also serve as 1C donors via dimethylglycine and sarcosine dehydrogenase reactions, highlighting the fact that different sources exist for 1C units in distinct organelles.

The reversibility and compartmentation of enzymes in the cytosol and mitochondria allow pathway flexibility. In most cells, serine is catabolized in the mitochondria (Lewis et al. 2014) to generate 1C units in the cytosol, which end up on thymidylate, formate (Meiser et al. 2016), or methionine (Maddocks et al. 2016). This unidirectional flow of 1C units is thermodynamically driven by the higher NADPH/NADP$^+$ ratio in the cytosol through MTHFD1 reaction (Yang and MacKenzie 1993). In contrast, there is more oxidative redox potential in the mitochondria, which would favor the MTHFD2/2L reaction to use NAD(P)$^+$ as a cofactor to drive the reaction. These redox-dependent reactions in the 1C cycle can influence the mitochondrial state through redox homeostasis. Mitochondrial enzymes, ALDH1L2 and MTHFD2/2L can produce NADPH through their reactions and the NADPH/NADP$^+$ ratio can help maintain the flux of 1C units through the cytosol. Although mitochondrial serine catabolism dominates in most cells, there are cells that show mixed cytosolic and mitochondrial 1C generation since some of these enzymes are differentially expressed across tissues (Girgis et al. 1998). Furthermore, reversal of the MTHFD1 reaction can occur when formyl-THF is depleted (Ducker et al. 2016).

The connection between mitochondrial function and 1C metabolism is further supported by studies that show the remodeling of 1C metabolism upon mitochondrial respiratory chain deficiency. Disruption of the electron transport chain reduces mitochondrial formate production, although the expression of serine synthesis genes is increased through ATF4 (Bao et al. 2016). Similarly, mtDNA replication dysfunction reduces formate and 10-formyl-THF levels while increasing flux to through the de novo serine synthesis pathway in mitochondrial myopathy mice (Nikkanen et al. 2016). The 1C pool can also impact mitochondrial function through production of SAM. While SAM is synthesized in the cytosol, it is transported into the matrix through the mitochondrial SAM carrier (Agrimi et al. 2004) and influences mitochondrial energy metabolism though protein methylation in complex I and iron–sulfur cluster biosynthesis (Schober et al. 2021), highlighting other biosynthetic fates for 1C metabolites.

1C metabolic reactions also exist in the nucleus (Anderson et al. 2007; Woeller et al. 2007). Nuclear folate metabolism occurs through the small ubiquitin-related modifier (SUMO)-dependent import of the enzymes that support de novo thymidylate synthesis from the cytosol to the nucleus (Anderson et al. 2007; Woeller et al. 2007). Upon sumoylation, SHMT, thymidylate synthase, and DHFR can be translocated to the nucleus during the S and G_2/M phase of cell replication (Anderson et al. 2007; Woeller et al. 2007). Using 5,10-methylene-THF as a 1C donor, thymidylate synthase catalyzes the methylation of deoxyuridylate (dUMP) to form thymidylate (dTMP). To reenter the 1C pool, DHF is reduced back to THF and eventually back to 5,10-methylene-THF through Sumo-SHMT1. Other subnetworks in this pathway are localized to distinct organelles as well. While the GCS occurs only in mitochondria (Kikuchi and Hiraga 1982), thymidylate synthesis takes place in the cytosol, mitochondria, and nucleus to support DNA synthesis (MacFarlane et al. 2011). On the other hand, purine synthesis occurs in the cytosol (An et al. 2008). Similarly, the methionine cycle operates in the cytosol although its downstream products are transported into mitochondria (Schober et al. 2021).

In addition to being highly compartmentalized intracellularly, 1C metabolism is differentially active across tissues and cell types. While many nonproliferative adult tissues express 1C enzymes such as SHMT1 and SHMT2, they are highly expressed in the liver and kidney (Girgis et al. 1998). On the other hand, the expression of SHMT2 is greater than that of SHMT1 in tissues like the brain, skeletal muscle, and heart (Girgis et al. 1998). As SHMT1 and SHMT2 operate in different directions and support distinct metabolic pathways, this specification suggests that different functions exist for 1C metabolism across tissues. For example, SHMT1 in mammalian cells has been shown to behave like a switch diverting 1C units for SAM or dTMP synthesis (Herbig et al. 2002). Perturbing 1C metabolism in the liver usually results in a fatty liver phenotype and is thought to be associated with impaired phosphatidylcholine synthesis (Pogribny et al. 2013). Furthermore, the knockout of me-

thionine adenosyltransferase has been shown to induce a fatty liver phenotype, reduce 1C-related metabolites, and lead to hepatocellular carcinoma (Lu et al. 2001). Beyond 1C enzymes, genes encoding enzymes in the GCS are also distinctly expressed in the liver (Yoshida and Kikuchi 1973), which suggests a differential preference for sources of 1C units across tissues. Similarly, transporters for serine and choline, inputs to the 1C cycle, vary according to tissue type (Hediger et al. 2013).

QUANTIFYING 1C METABOLISM FLUX AND METABOLITE LEVELS

The interconnected pathways and compartmentalization of these reactions make studying 1C metabolism challenging. However, by combining stable isotope tracers with mass spectrometry analysis researchers have made great insights into the topology of this pathway. Serine contributes to the 1C pool and stable isotope tracers such as $[2,3,3-^2H]$serine and $[3,3-^2H]$serine will generate ^2H-labeled 1C folate intermediates downstream of SHMT (Gregory et al. 2000; Herbig et al. 2002). Tracing with $[2,3,3-^2H]$serine, however, provides compartment-specific information on this pathway (detailed in Fig. 4A). If serine is metabolized in the mitochondria, one deuterium on the third carbon eventually ends up on NADPH and the other on formate. The incorporation of this 1C unit from formate into DNA will result in formation of a singly deuterated thymidine monophosphate (TMP M + 1). In contrast, if serine is metabolized in the cytosol by SHMT1, both deuterons on serine will be transferred to 5,10-methylene THF that will eventually result in doubly labeled TMP M + 2 (Fig. 4A). In most cells and tissues analyzed, TMP M + 1 is the predominant product from this tracer, suggesting that mitochondrial serine catabolism occurs along with cytosolic reduction of formate by MTHFD1.

Another serine tracer that may effectively be used to investigate 1C metabolism is $[3-^{13}C]$serine (Fig. 4B). This serine tracer enables one to exclude the carbon contribution from glycine cleavage because the ^{13}C carbon on serine transfers to 5,10-methylene-THF only via SHMT (Fig. 4B). This

A

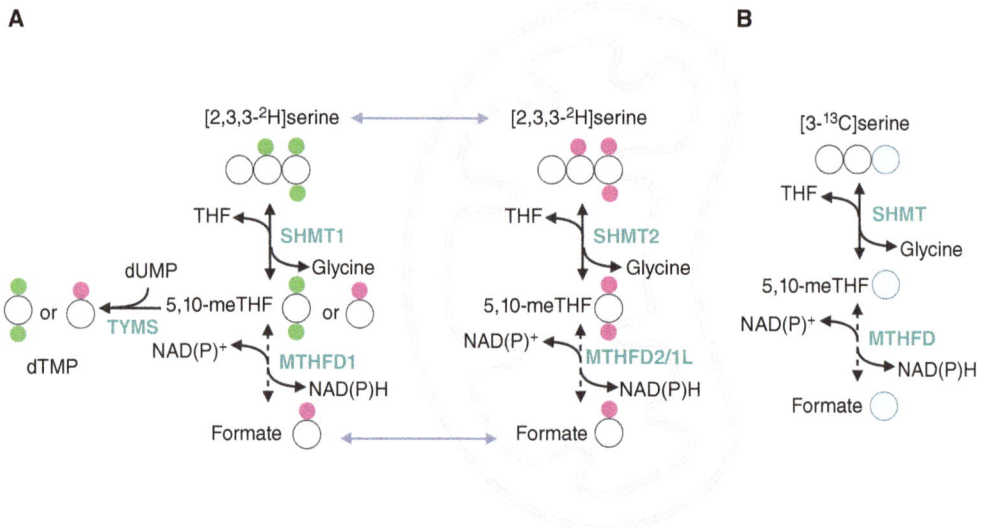

B

Figure 4. Tracing 1C metabolism. (*A*) [2,3,3-^{2}H]serine can be used to distinguish compartment-specific metabolism of serine since ^{2}H from serine is incorporated differently into 1C intermediates and dTMP. (*B*) [3-^{13}C] serine allows us to exclude the carbon contribution from glycine cleavage because only the ^{13}C carbon on serine transfers to 5,10-me-THF (5,10-methylene-THF) via SHMT. (THF) Tetrahydrofolate, (SHMT1/2) serine hydroxymethyl transferase, cytosolic(1)/mitochondrial(2), (MTHFD1) methylenetetrahydrofolate dehydrogenase, cyclohydrolase, and formyltetrahydrofolate synthetase 1, (MTHFD2/2L), methylenetetrahydrofolate dehydrogenase 2/2-like, (MTHFD1L) monofunctional tetrahydrofolate synthase, (TYMS) thymidylate synthase. (Figure generated with BioRender; https://biorender.com.)

tracer has been used to observe serine catabolism to formate in vivo (Meiser et al. 2016). Similarly, ^{13}C-MeOH may be employed to quantify serine catabolism to formate in vivo because methanol is metabolized to formate in the liver (Meiser et al. 2018). Fully ^{13}C- and ^{15}N-labeled serine or methionine can track flux into intermediates of the methionine cycle and methylation of DNA and RNA, which is helpful to study methylation dynamics (Newman et al. 2019). Multiple stable-isotope tracers can also be used in parallel to perform dynamic flux analysis. For example, parallel use of [4-^{2}H]glucose and [^{2}H]formate was performed to demonstrate that MTHFD2 has a noncanonical oxidative function to provide mitochondrial NAD$^+$ (Achreja et al. 2022). This experiment is possible because [4-^{2}H]glucose labels NADH and if the MTHFD2 reaction operates oxidatively rather than reductively, the ^{2}H label appears on serine. Isotope from [^{2}H]formate appears on serine through the folate cycle, and this helped Achreja et al. to deconvolute the noncanonical mitochondrial MTHFD2 activity.

As our knowledge of 1C metabolism advances, alternative sources for 1C units in specific cell and tissue contexts are being discovered. One example of a nontraditional source for 1C units is tryptophan in pancreatic ductal adenocarcinoma (PDAC) (Newman et al. 2021). Indoleamine 2,3-dioxygenase (IDO) expression in cancer cells promotes the generation of 1C units from tryptophan to support de novo purine synthesis, observed using ^{13}C-tryptophan (Newman et al. 2021). Similarly, ^{13}C-formaldehyde was used to show that formaldehyde detoxification by alcohol dehydrogenase 5 supplies 1C units for nucleotide synthesis in cells (Burgos-Barragan et al. 2017). Overall, these examples show the utility of stable isotope tracing in exploring the many pathways fueling 1C metabolism.

To better characterize organelle-specific directionality of 1C metabolism, Lewis et al. (2014) leveraged [2,3,3-^{2}H]serine labeling of NAD(P)H and a compartment-specific reporter system. Specifically, cells were engineered to inducibly express either cytosolic IDH1 or mitochondrial

IDH2 harboring neomorphic mutations that result in production of (D)2-hydroxyglutarate (2-HG) from α-ketoglutarate (Lewis et al. 2014). As this reaction reduces αKG by transferring a hydride from NADPH to form 2HG, the label on NADPH is transferred to 2HG. 2HG is typically present at low levels (Matsunaga et al. 2012) and the labeled 2HG can be used as a readout of NADPH metabolism. By using [2,3,3-^{2}H]serine or other tracers in this reporter system, the authors have characterized redox reaction directionality of 1C (Lewis et al. 2014) and TCA cycle (Jiang et al. 2016; Badur et al. 2018) reactions in both the cytosol and mitochondria.

Quantitation of metabolites over time is the most direct approach to measure flux. Absolute quantification of formate by GC-MS has enabled measurements of key exchange fluxes between formate, serine, and glycine (Meiser et al. 2016). Quantifying rates of purine synthesis and formate release revealed the latter as the dominant fate of 1C metabolites (Meiser et al. 2016, 2018). These results when paired with metabolic flux analysis indicate that formate efflux exceeds anabolic 1C demands (Meiser et al. 2016, 2018). Similarly, measuring the flux of CO_2 released from [1-^{13}C] glycine has demonstrated that the GCS is a major contributor for entry of 5,10-methylene-THF into 1C metabolism at a rate that exceeds the demand for methyl groups (Lamers et al. 2009). The ability to quantitatively assess and model these reactions greatly improves our ability to target 1C metabolism in specific tissues or contexts.

DYNAMIC REGULATION OF 1C METABOLISM

As described above, 1C metabolism functions as a central metabolic hub that connects metabolites and reactions across organelles to not only produce critical macromolecules but also for maintenance of redox homeostasis and epigenetic status. The many inputs into the cycle make it a dynamic system that is responsive to multiple perturbations and regulation. In fact, many of the reactions in the 1C cycle are reversible, highlighting the flexibility ingrained in the system (Ducker et al. 2016). The existence of multiple isoforms for most of the 1C enzymes

enables such specialization and redundancy such that different isoforms to compensate for one if the other is comprised (Ducker et al. 2016). Again, this metabolic architecture and behavior are manifested in the TCA cycle, where NADP$^+$-dependent isocitrate dehydrogenases afford flexibility under hypoxic or lipid stress. Although mitochondrial 1C metabolism is dominant in most cells, reversal of cytosolic 1C reactions can compensate for the loss of the mitochondrial folate pathway (Ducker et al. 2016). Additionally, when the cytosolic pathway is compromised, alternative sources of 1C units such as endogenous formaldehyde feeds the cycle, further emphasizing the adaptability of this critical pathway (Burgos-Barragan et al. 2017).

At the same time, the demand and role for 1C metabolism may be different across developmental stages. For example, consumption rates for 1C units are highest during fetal development, and folate deficiency is a known driver of neural tube and congenital heart defects (Bailey and Berry 2005; Beaudin et al. 2011). Additionally, genes encoding 1C enzymes are differentially expressed during embryonic development in the liver and brain, highlighting the dynamic regulation of this pathway as tissue morphogenesis and specialization occur (Imbard et al. 2021). Highly proliferative cells such as hematopoietic, immune, and gastrointestinal lineages are highly dependent on 1C metabolism (Ponziani et al. 2012; Henry et al. 2017; Kurniawan et al. 2021). Activated T cells, which likely exhibit the highest rates of nucleotide synthesis in the body, up-regulate 1C metabolism in the mitochondria to promote thymidylate and purine synthesis, while genetic targeting of mitochondrial 1C metabolism enzymes impairs T-cell survival (Ron-Harel et al. 2016). Recent research also suggests that MTHFD2 regulates both effector and regulatory T-cell fate and function through various mechanisms (Sugiura et al. 2022).

Given its contributions to diverse proliferating (and nonproliferating) normal cell types, it is not surprising that expression of 1C enzymes is altered in the context of cancer. MTHFD2 is mostly absent in healthy adult tissues, yet its expression is frequently up-regulated in many cancer types (Nilsson et al. 2014) and is associated with a poor prognosis in breast cancer (Liu et al. 2014). Other 1C enzymes that are highly expressed in various cancer types are TYMS (Burdelski et al. 2015; Sun et al. 2015; Fu et al. 2019), SHMT (Jain et al. 2012; Lee et al. 2014), and DHFR (Guo et al. 1999; Yang et al. 2003). In addition, the robust up-regulation of 1C metabolic enzymes has been observed in response to cancers associated with cancers associated with viral infection (Wang et al. 2019; Zhang et al. 2021). Epstein–Barr virus (EBV) is a driver of B-cell lymphomas (Epstein et al. 1964). Upon infection, EBV remodels B-cell mitochondrial 1C metabolism along with serine uptake and catabolism, and these were among the most highly induced pathways (Wang et al. 2019). Functionally, EBV-induced mitochondrial 1C metabolism generates NADPH, fuels nucleotide synthesis through formate, and generates glutathione (Wang et al. 2019). Outside of cancer, the 1C metabolism pathway is remodeled by viruses such as severe acute respiratory syndrome coronavirus 2 (SARS-CoV-2) (Zhang et al. 2021). These findings also highlight the potential for inhibition of 1C metabolism as a therapeutic for viral infections, as practiced in cancer therapy.

1C metabolism is also responsive to perturbations in redox homeostasis. Formate production and efflux are sensitive to cellular redox state (Meiser et al. 2018). Specifically, shifting cells toward a more oxidative state induces increased formate efflux and vice versa (Meiser et al. 2018). During hypoxia, MYC-transformed cells induce the expression of SHMT2 to maintain mitochondrial redox balance, specifically cellular NADPH: NADP$^+$ ratio (Ye et al. 2014). This is clinically relevant as hypoxia develops during tumor progression when there is insufficient vasculature to supply oxygen to tumor cells. During metastasis, some melanoma cells reversibly increase their expression of ALDH1L2, an NAPDH-regenerating enzyme, and knockdown of MTHFD1 or ALDH1L2 inhibits metastasis to distant organs (Piskounova et al. 2015). As discussed previously, 1C metabolism is linked to mitochondrial function through cofactors and intermediates such as NAD(P)H and SAM, providing various mechanisms for cross-regulation upon perturbation (Schober et al. 2021). Additionally, mitochondrial 10-formyl-THF is

used for N-formylation of the initiator methionine in mitochondrial methionyl-tRNA^{met}, which is important for translation of mitochondrial-encoded proteins (Tucker et al. 2011).

Evidence indicates that 1C metabolism is tightly regulated by mammalian target of rapamycin (mTORC1), a critical nutrient sensor (Ben-Sahra et al. 2016; Rathore et al. 2021). A known downstream target of mTOR is ATF4, which regulates the expression of serine biosynthesis enzymes including PHGDH (Ye et al. 2012). When serine levels are low, ATF4 is activated to sustain glucose uptake, serine synthesis, and flux through the 1C pathway, as ATF4 also regulates expression of MTHFD2 (Ben-Sahra et al. 2016). mTORC1 also regulates the expression of other 1C enzymes, including SHMT2 and MTHFD1L through FOXK1 (He et al. 2018). Unsurprisingly, mTORC1 signaling is often hyperactivated in various cancers (Zhang et al. 2017). An upstream effector of mTORC1, LKB1, is a known tumor suppressor (Hemminki et al. 1998; Sanchez-Cespedes 2007). LKB1 loss results in up-regulation of enzymes involved in 1C metabolism and SAM biosynthesis, further connecting mTOR signaling to changes in DNA methylation and tumorigenesis (Kottakis et al. 2016). The activation of the energy sensor and LKB1 targeted AMP-activated kinase (AMPK), also down-regulates MTHFD1, MTHFD1L, and MTHFD2 expression through the PGC1a/ERRa axis (Audet-Walsh et al. 2016). Notably, expression of PGC1a is reduced in some cancers relative to healthy tissue (Deblois et al. 2013). Overall, these observations suggest that cells tune 1C pathway flux based on their energetic status and biosynthetic demands such that they can respond to perturbations to support the dynamic metabolic needs associated with tumor cell growth and survival. Redundancy and parallelization across compartments in enzymes within this pathway highlight the metabolic flexibility necessary to respond to the stresses, which is critical for embryonic cells and tumors.

TARGETING 1C METABOLISM

As tumor cells commonly overexpress key 1C enzymes, numerous therapeutics direct targeted key critical nodes in the pathway (Fig. 1). For example, methotrexate, pemetrexed, and 5-Fluoruoacil are commonly used chemotherapeutics approved for treatment of lymphomas, osteosarcomas, breast cancer, and lung cancer (Huennekens 1994; Longley et al. 2003; Vander Heiden 2011). Both methotrexate and pemetrexed target dihydrofolate reductase (DHFR), with pemetrexed targeting thymidylate synthase (TYMS) and serine hydroxymethyltransferases (SHMTs) as well (Shih et al. 1997; Goodsell 1999). While these drugs are effective against tumors, the benefits of these drugs are hampered due to toxicities caused by inhibition of 1C metabolism in nontransformed cells, including those in the bone marrow and intestinal epithelium resulting in various complications.

The challenge with targeting components of 1C metabolism more specifically is that tumors may rewire their metabolism to compensate for the intervention and eventually resist treatment. As such, combination therapies to target 1C metabolism have been explored in preclinical models. Combination treatment with SHMT1/2 inhibitor (e.g., SHIN2) and methotrexate showed a synergistic response in a patient-derived xenograft (PDX) T-cell acute lymphoblastic leukemia mouse model (García-Cañaveras et al. 2021). This result is likely due to methotrexate-induced depletion of cellular THF, resulting in decreased competition for SHIN2 that effectively inhibits SHMT. An alternate strategy is to design multitargeted inhibitors of 1C cycle enzymes, as they are traditionally targeted using antimetabolites (García-Cañaveras et al. 2021). Small molecules that possess structural features to inhibit de novo purine biosynthesis, SHMT1, and SHMT2 demonstrated significant in vivo antitumor efficacy in early- and late-stage pancreatic adenocarcinoma xenografts in mice (Dekhne et al. 2019).

Recent efforts to uncover collateral deletion of essential genes in chromosomal proximity during inactivation of tumor suppressor genes can provide potential targets for combination therapies. For example, MTHFD2 has recently been identified as a collateral gene in UQCR11-deleted ovarian tumors, and inhibiting MTHFD2 in UQCR11-null cancers dramatically decreased xenograft tumor growth, showing the essentiality of MTHFD2 in these cancers (Achreja et al. 2022). Inhibitors against 1C metabolism combined with inhibitors of other targets such as PHGDH or mTOR could be effective in such cases. Indeed, the rewiring of the serine synthesis pathway has been identified as a mechanism for resistance in certain cancer cells (Ross et al. 2017; Rathore et al. 2021).

Nutrient availability has a significant impact on the progression of some tumors. Special diets such as the ketogenic diet can sensitize some cancers to standard treatment by exploiting the reprogrammed metabolism of cancer cells (Hopkins et al. 2018; Tajan and Vousden 2020; Ferrere et al. 2021). Studies have shown that dietary removal of amino acids including serine/glycine (Maddocks et al. 2013; Muthusamy et al. 2020), methionine (Gao et al. 2019), and asparagine (Krall et al. 2016) can modulate cancer growth in animal models. In some tumors, this effect was further improved when combining serine restriction with biguanides (i.e., metformin) that disrupt mitochondrial oxidative phosphorylation (Maddocks et al. 2017). The response to dietary serine/glycine restriction, however, is limited in tumors that can effectively up-regulate expression of PHGDH or serine transporters, which can occur downstream of activated KRAS (Maddocks et al. 2017). To address this issue, a combination of dietary serine restriction with PHGDH or PSAT inhibitors has been tested in animal models and demonstrated some effect against tumors that are resistant to diet or inhibitor alone (Méndez-Lucas et al. 2020; Tajan et al. 2021). Similarly, dietary methionine restriction has been shown to have anticancer effects mediated through changes to 1C metabolism (Gao et al. 2019). In addition to reducing tumor growth in colorectal PDX models, methionine restriction also sensitized these models to chemotherapy 5-FU and radiation, providing evidence that targeted dietary manipulation can affect specific tumor metabolism and impact cancer progression in mice (Gao et al. 2019). On the other hand, dietary supplementation of histidine enhances the sensitivity of cancer cells to methotrexate by up-regulating the histidine degradation pathway to deplete THF (Kanarek et al. 2018), highlighting the interconnected nature and complexity of targeting 1C metabolism.

BYSTANDER EFFECTS

Antifolates have been the standard of care for cancer patients since the 1950s, and yet patients still must endure the deleterious side effects during treatment due to the importance of 1C metabolism in healthy proliferating, nontransformed cells. Toxicities caused by these drugs tend to cause anemia, gastric complications, and immune deficiency. In fact, the immunosuppressant impact from methotrexate has made it useful to treat chronic inflammatory conditions such as rheumatoid arthritis, psoriasis, and Crohn's disease (Willkens et al. 1984; Weinblatt et al. 1985; Kozarek et al. 1989; Feagan et al. 1995; Esteitie et al. 2005). However, immunosuppression can be devastating to cancer patients as the protective role of immune cells such as T-cell lymphocytes are instrumental in the body's defense against tumors. The efficacy of cell-based therapies and vaccinations are dependent on the generation of robust and stable populations of antigen-specific T-cell populations (Waldman et al. 2020). As such, the disruption of T-cell metabolism through cancer therapy is deleterious to immune function and patient outcomes in the long run.

CONCLUDING REMARKS

Advances in analytical chemistry, molecular biology techniques, and genetically engineered mouse models have improved our understanding of 1C metabolism in various contexts relevant to cancer. Nonetheless, the complexity and compartmentalization of 1C cycle reactions across organelles are yet to be fully deciphered. While some mitochondrial transporters for 1C metabolites have been identified (Porter et al. 1992; Titus and Moran 2000; Agrimi et al. 2004; Kory et al. 2018), genes encoding other transporters remain unknown. Additionally, metabolic cross talk between organelles such as the mitochondria and nucleus is not well understood, yet this communication between organelles is likely to have important implications for

tumor growth and metastasis. New disciplines such as functional genomics and organelle-specific biology are rapidly enabling discoveries in this area. The challenge then remains to translate such mechanistic and biological insights into physiologically relevant therapies that have improved precision or efficacy in cancer patients.

ACKNOWLEDGMENTS

We thank all members of the Metallo Laboratory for helpful discussions, and we apologize to those researchers whose work we were unable to cite. This work was supported by the NIH (R01CA234245 to C.M.M.).

REFERENCES

Achreja A, Yu T, Mittal A, Choppara S, Animasahun O, Nenwani M, Wuchu F, Meurs N, Mohan A, Jeon JH, et al. 2022. Metabolic collateral lethal target identification reveals MTHFD2 paralogue dependency in ovarian cancer. Nat Metab 4: 1119–1137. doi:10.1038/s42255-022-00636-3

Agrimi G, Di Noia MA, Marobbio CMT, Fiermonte G, Lasorsa FM, Palmieri F. 2004. Identification of the human mitochondrial S-adenosylmethionine transporter: bacterial expression, reconstitution, functional characterization and tissue distribution. Biochem J 379: 183–190. doi:10.1042/bj20031664

An S, Kumar R, Sheets ED, Benkovic SJ. 2008. Reversible compartmentalization of de novo purine biosynthetic complexes in living cells. Science 320: 103–106. doi:10.1126/science.1152241

Anderson DD, Woeller CF, Stover PJ. 2007. Small ubiquitin-like modifier-1 (SUMO-1) modification of thymidylate synthase and dihydrofolate reductase. Clin Chem Lab Med 45: 1760–1763. doi:10.1515/CCLM.2007.355

Audet-Walsh É, Papadopoli DJ, Gravel SP, Yee T, Bridon G, Caron M, Bourque G, Giguère V, St-Pierre J. 2016. The PGC-1α/ERRα axis represses one-carbon metabolism and promotes sensitivity to anti-folate therapy in breast cancer. Cell Rep 14: 920–931. doi:10.1016/j.celrep.2015.12.086

Badur MG, Muthusamy T, Parker SJ, Ma S, McBrayer SK, Cordes T, Magana JH, Guan KL, Metallo CM. 2018. Oncogenic R132 IDH1 mutations limit NADPH for de novo lipogenesis through (D)2-hydroxyglutarate production in fibrosarcoma cells. Cell Rep 25: 1018–1026.e4. doi:10.1016/j.celrep.2018.09.074

Bailey LB, Berry RJ. 2005. Folic acid supplementation and the occurrence of congenital heart defects, orofacial clefts, multiple births, and miscarriage. Am J Clin Nutr 81: 1213S–1217S. doi:10.1093/ajcn/81.5.1213

Bao XR, Ong SE, Goldberger O, Peng J, Sharma R, Thompson DA, Vafai SB, Cox AG, Marutani E, Ichinose F, et al. 2016. Mitochondrial dysfunction remodels one-carbon metabolism in human cells. eLife 5: e10575.

Cite this article as Cold Spring Harb Perspect Med doi: 10.1101/cshperspect.a041533

Beaudin AE, Abarinov EV, Noden DM, Perry CA, Chu S, Stabler SP, Allen RH, Stover PJ. 2011. Shmt1 and de novo thymidylate biosynthesis underlie folate-responsive neural tube defects in mice. *Am J Clin Nutr* **93:** 789–798. doi:10.3945/ajcn.110.002766

Ben-Sahra I, Hoxhaj G, Ricoult SJH, Asara JM, Manning BD. 2016. mTORC1 induces purine synthesis through control of the mitochondrial tetrahydrofolate cycle. *Science* **351:** 728–733. doi:10.1126/science.aad0489

Burdelski C, Strauss C, Tsourlakis MC, Kluth M, Hube-Magg C, Melling N, Lebok P, Minner S, Koop C, Graefen M, et al. 2015. Overexpression of thymidylate synthase (TYMS) is associated with aggressive tumor features and early PSA recurrence in prostate cancer. *Oncotarget* **6:** 8377. doi:10.18632/oncotarget.3107

Burgos-Barragan G, Wit N, Meiser J, Dingler FA, Pietzke M, Mulderrig L, Pontel LB, Rosado IV, Brewer TF, Cordell RL, et al. 2017. Mammals divert endogenous genotoxic formaldehyde into one-carbon metabolism. *Nature* **548:** 549. doi:10.1038/nature23481

DeBerardinis RJ, Chandel NS. 2020. We need to talk about the Warburg effect. *Nat Metab* **2:** 127–129. doi:10.1038/s42255-020-0172-2

Deblois G, St-Pierre J, Giguère V. 2013. The PGC-1/ERR signaling axis in cancer. *Oncogene* **32:** 3483–3490. doi:10.1038/onc.2012.529

Dekhne AS, Shah K, Ducker GS, Katinas JM, Wong-Roushar J, Junayed Nayeen M, Doshi A, Ning C, Bao X, Frühauf J, et al. 2019. Novel Pyrrolo[3,2-d]pyrimidine compounds target mitochondrial and cytosolic one-carbon metabolism with broad-spectrum antitumor efficacy. *Mol Cancer Ther* **18:** 1787–1799. doi:10.1158/1535-7163.MCT-19-0037

Ducker GS, Chen L, Morscher RJ, Gherurovich JM, Esposito M, Teng X, Kang Y, Rabinowitz JD. 2016. Reversal of cytosolic one-carbon flux compensates for loss of the mitochondrial folate pathway. *Cell Metab* **23:** 1140–1153. doi:10.1016/j.cmet.2016.04.016

Epstein MA, Achong BG, Barr YM. 1964. Virus particles in cultured lymphoblasts from Burkitt's lymphoma. *Lancet* **1:** 702–703. doi:10.1016/S0140-6736(64)91524-7

Esteitie N, Hinttala R, Wibom R, Nilsson H, Hance N, Naess K, Teär-Fahnehjelm K, Von Döbeln U, Majamaa K, Larsson NG. 2005. Secondary metabolic effects in complex I deficiency. *Ann Neurol* **58:** 544–552. doi:10.1002/ana.20570

Fan J, Ye J, Kamphorst JJ, Shlomi T, Thompson CB, Rabinowitz JD. 2014. Quantitative flux analysis reveals folate-dependent NADPH production. *Nature* **510:** 298–302. doi:10.1038/nature13236

Faubert B, Solmonson A, DeBerardinis RJ. 2020. Metabolic reprogramming and cancer progression. *Science* **368:** eaaw5473. doi:10.1126/science.aaw5473

Feagan BG, Rochon J, Fedorak RN, Irvine EJ, Wild G, Sutherland L, Steinhart AH, Greenberg GR, Gillies R, Hopkins M. 1995. Methotrexate for the treatment of Crohn's disease. The North American Crohn's Study Group Investigators. *N Engl J Med* **332:** 292–297. doi:10.1056/NEJM199502023320503

Ferrere G, Alou MT, Liu P, Goubet AG, Fidelle M, Kepp O, Durand S, Iebba V, Fluckiger A, Daillère R, et al. 2021. Ketogenic diet and ketone bodies enhance the anticancer effects of PD-1 blockade. *JCI Insight* **6:** e145207. doi:10.1172/jci.insight.145207

Fu Z, Jiao Y, Li Y, Ji B, Jia B, Liu B. 2019. TYMS presents a novel biomarker for diagnosis and prognosis in patients with pancreatic cancer. *Medicine (Baltimore)* **98:** e18487. doi:10.1097/MD.0000000000018487

Gao X, Sanderson SM, Dai Z, Reid MA, Cooper DE, Lu M, Richie JP, Ciccarella A, Calcagnotto A, Mikhael PG, et al. 2019. Dietary methionine links nutrition and metabolism to the efficacy of cancer therapies. *Nature* **572:** 397–401. doi:10.1038/s41586-019-1437-3

García-Cañaveras JC, Lancho O, Ducker GS, Ghergurovich JM, Xu X, da Silva-Diz V, Minuzzo S, Indraccolo S, Kim H, Herranz D, et al. 2021. SHMT inhibition is effective and synergizes with methotrexate in T-cell acute lymphoblastic leukemia. *Leukemia* **35:** 377–388. doi:10.1038/s41375-020-0845-6

Girgis S, Nasrallah IM, Suh JR, Oppenheim E, Zanetti KA, Mastri MG, Stover PJ. 1998. Molecular cloning, characterization and alternative splicing of the human cytoplasmic serine hydroxymethyltransferase gene. *Gene* **210:** 315–324. doi:10.1016/S0378-1119(98)00085-7

Goodsell DS. 1999. The molecular perspective: methotrexate. *Stem Cells* **17:** 314–315. doi:10.1002/stem.170314

Gregory JF, Cuskelly GJ, Shane B, Toth JP, Baumgartner TG, Stacpoole PW. 2000. Primed, constant infusion with [^{2}H$_3$] serine allows in vivo kinetic measurement of serine turnover, homocysteine remethylation, and transsulfuration processes in human one-carbon metabolism. *Am J Clin Nutr* **72:** 1535–1541. doi:10.1093/ajcn/72.6.1535

Guo W, Healey JH, Meyers PA, Ladanyi M, Huvos AG, Bertino JR, Gorlick R. 1999. Mechanisms of methotrexate resistance in osteosarcoma. *Clin Cancer Res* **5:** 621–627.

Handzlik MK, Metallo CM. 2023. Sources and sinks of serine in nutrition, health, and disease. *Annu Rev Nutr* **43:** 123–151. doi:10.1146/annurev-nutr-061021-022648

He L, Gomes AP, Wang X, Yoon SO, Lee G, Nagiec MJ, Cho S, Chavez A, Islam T, Yu Y, et al. 2018. mTORC1 promotes metabolic reprogramming by the suppression of GSK3-dependent Foxk1 phosphorylation. *Mol Cell* **70:** 949–960.e4. doi:10.1016/j.molcel.2018.04.024

Hediger MA, Clémençon B, Burrier RE, Bruford EA. 2013. The ABCs of membrane transporters in health and disease (SLC series): introduction. *Mol Aspects Med* **34:** 95–107. doi:10.1016/j.mam.2012.12.009

Hemminki A, Markie D, Tomlinson I, Avizienyte E, Roth S, Loukola A, Bignell G, Warren W, Aminoff M, Höglund P, et al. 1998. A serine/threonine kinase gene defective in Peutz–Jeghers syndrome. *Nature* **391:** 184–187. doi:10.1038/34432

Henry CJ, Nemkov T, Casás-Selves M, Bilousova G, Zaberezhnyy V, Higa KC, Serkova NJ, Hansen KC, D'Alessandro A, DeGregori J. 2017. Folate dietary insufficiency and folic acid supplementation similarly impair metabolism and compromise hematopoiesis. *Haematologica* **102:** 1985–1994. doi:10.3324/haematol.2017.171074

Herbig K, Chiang EP, Lee LR, Hills J, Shane B, Stover PJ. 2002. Cytoplasmic serine hydroxymethyltransferase mediates competition between folate-dependent deoxyribonucleotide and S-adenosylmethionine biosyntheses. *J Biol Chem* **277:** 38381–38389. doi:10.1074/jbc.M205000200

Hopkins BD, Pauli C, Xing D, Wang DG, Li X, Wu D, Amadiume SC, Goncalves MD, Hodakoski C, Lundquist MR, et al. 2018. Suppression of insulin feedback enhances the efficacy of PI3K inhibitors. *Nature* **560:** 499–503. doi:10.1038/s41586-018-0343-4

Huennekens FM. 1994. The methotrexate story: a paradigm for development of cancer chemotherapeutic agents. *Adv Enzyme Regul* **34:** 397–419. doi:10.1016/0065-2571(94)90025-6

Imbard A, Schwendimann L, Lebon S, Gressens P, Blom HJ, Benoist JF. 2021. Liver and brain differential expression of one-carbon metabolism genes during ontogenesis. *Sci Reports* **11:** 1–9. doi:10.1038/s41598-021-00311-9

Jain M, Nilsson R, Sharma S, Madhusudhan N, Kitami T, Souza AL, Kafri R, Kirschner MW, Clish CB, Mootha VK. 2012. Metabolite profiling identifies a key role for glycine in rapid cancer cell proliferation. *Science* **336:** 1040–1044. doi:10.1126/science.1218595

Jiang L, Shestov AA, Swain P, Yang C, Parker SJ, Wang QA, Terada LS, Adams ND, McCabe MT, Pietrak B, et al. 2016. Reductive carboxylation supports redox homeostasis during anchorage-independent growth. *Nature* **532:** 255–258. doi:10.1038/nature17393

Kanarek N, Keys HR, Cantor JR, Lewis CA, Chan SH, Kunchok T, Abu-Remaileh M, Freinkman E, Schweitzer LD, Sabatini DM. 2018. Histidine catabolism is a major determinant of methotrexate sensitivity. *Nature* **559:** 632–636. doi:10.1038/s41586-018-0316-7

Kikuchi G, Hiraga K. 1982. The mitochondrial glycine cleavage system. Unique features of the glycine decarboxylation. *Mol Cell Biochem* **45:** 137–149. doi:10.1007/BF00230082

Kory N, Wyant GA, Prakash G, Uit de Bos J, Bottanelli F, Pacold ME, Chan SH, Lewis CA, Wang T, Keys HR, et al. 2018. SFXN1 is a mitochondrial serine transporter required for one-carbon metabolism. *Science* **362:** eaat9528. doi:10.1126/science.aat9528

Koseki J, Konno M, Asai A, Colvin H, Kawamoto K, Nishida N, Sakai D, Kudo T, Satoh T, Doki Y, et al. 2018. Enzymes of the one-carbon folate metabolism as anticancer targets predicted by survival rate analysis. *Sci Reports* **8:** 303. doi:10.1038/s41598-017-18456-x

Kottakis F, Nicolay BN, Roumane A, Karnik R, Gu H, Nagle JM, Boukhali M, Hayward MC, Li YY, Chen T, et al. 2016. LKB1 loss links serine metabolism to DNA methylation and tumorigenesis. *Nature* **539:** 390–395. doi:10.1038/nature20132

Kozarek RA, Patterson DJ, Gelfand MD, Botoman VA, Ball TJ, Wilske KR. 1989. Methotrexate induces clinical and histologic remission in patients with refractory inflammatory bowel disease. *Ann Intern Med* **110:** 353–356. doi:10.7326/0003-4819-110-5-353

Kralik S, Desai N, Meoded A, Huisman T. 2023. Inherited and acquired metabolic disorders. In *Fetal, neonatal and pediatric neuroradiology* (ed. Kralik S, Desai N, Meoded A, Huisman T), pp. 225–286. Elsevier, St. Louis, MO.

Krall AS, Xu S, Graeber TG, Braas D, Christofk HR. 2016. Asparagine promotes cancer cell proliferation through use as an amino acid exchange factor. *Nat Commun* **7:** 11457. doi:10.1038/ncomms11457

Kurniawan H, Kobayashi T, Brenner D. 2021. The emerging role of one-carbon metabolism in T cells. *Curr Opin Biotechnol* **68:** 193–201. doi:10.1016/j.copbio.2020.12.001

Labuschagne CF, van den Broek NJF, Mackay GM, Vousden KH, Maddocks ODK. 2014. Serine, but not glycine, supports one-carbon metabolism and proliferation of cancer cells. *Cell Rep* **7:** 1248–1258. doi:10.1016/j.celrep.2014.04.045

Lamers Y, Williamson J, Theriaque DW, Shuster JJ, Gilbert LR, Keeling C, Stacpoole PW, Gregory JF. 2009. Production of 1-carbon units from glycine is extensive in healthy men and women. *J Nutr* **139:** 666–671. doi:10.3945/jn.108.103580

Lee GY, Haverty PM, Li L, Kljavin NM, Bourgon R, Lee J, Stern H, Modrusan Z, Seshagiri S, Zhang Z, et al. 2014. Comparative oncogenomics identifies PSMB4 and SHMT2 as potential cancer driver genes. *Cancer Res* **74:** 3114–3126. doi:10.1158/0008-5472.CAN-13-2683

Lewis CA, Parker SJ, Fiske BP, McCloskey D, Gui DY, Green CR, Vokes NI, Feist AM, Vander Heiden MG, Metallo CM. 2014. Tracing compartmentalized NADPH metabolism in the cytosol and mitochondria of mammalian cells. *Mol Cell* **55:** 253–263. doi:10.1016/j.molcel.2014.05.008

Liu F, Liu Y, He C, Tao L, He X, Song H, Zhang G. 2014. Increased MTHFD2 expression is associated with poor prognosis in breast cancer. *Tumour Biol* **35:** 8685–8690. doi:10.1007/s13277-014-2111-x

Locasale JW, Grassian AR, Melman T, Lyssiotis CA, Mattaini KR, Bass AJ, Heffron G, Metallo CM, Muranen T, Sharfi H, et al. 2011. Phosphoglycerate dehydrogenase diverts glycolytic flux and contributes to oncogenesis. *Nat Genet* **43:** 869–874. doi:10.1038/ng.890

Longley DB, Harkin DP, Johnston PG. 2003. 5-Fluorouracil: mechanisms of action and clinical strategies. *Nat Rev Cancer* **3:** 330–338. doi:10.1038/nrc1074

Lu SC, Alvarez L, Huang ZZ, Chen L, An W, Corrales FJ, Avila MA, Kanel G, Mato JM. 2001. Methionine adenosyltransferase 1A knockout mice are predisposed to liver injury and exhibit increased expression of genes involved in proliferation. *Proc Natl Acad Sci* **98:** 5560–5565. doi:10.1073/pnas.091016398

MacFarlane AJ, Anderson DD, Flodby P, Perry CA, Allen RH, Stabler SP, Stover PJ. 2011. Nuclear localization of de novo thymidylate biosynthesis pathway is required to prevent uracil accumulation in DNA. *J Biol Chem* **286:** 44015–44022. doi:10.1074/jbc.M111.307629

Maddocks ODK, Berkers CR, Mason SM, Zheng L, Blyth K, Gottlieb E, Vousden KH. 2013. Serine starvation induces stress and p53-dependent metabolic remodelling in cancer cells. *Nature* **493:** 542–546. doi:10.1038/nature11743

Maddocks ODK, Labuschagne CF, Adams PD, Vousden KH. 2016. Serine metabolism supports the methionine cycle and DNA/RNA methylation through de novo ATP synthesis in cancer cells. *Mol Cell* **61:** 210–221. doi:10.1016/j.molcel.2015.12.014

Maddocks ODK, Athineos D, Cheung EC, Lee P, Zhang T, Van Den Broek NJF, Mackay GM, Labuschagne CF, Gay D, Kruiswijk F, et al. 2017. Modulating the therapeutic response of tumours to dietary serine and glycine starvation. *Nature* **544:** 372–376. doi:10.1038/nature22056

Cite this article as *Cold Spring Harb Perspect Med* doi: 10.1101/cshperspect.a041533

Martínez-Reyes I, Chandel NS. 2020. Mitochondrial TCA cycle metabolites control physiology and disease. *Nat Commun* **11**: 102. doi:10.1038/s41467-019-13668-3

Matsunaga H, Futakuchi-Tsuchida A, Takahashi M, Ishikawa T, Tsuji M, Ando O. 2012. IDH1 and IDH2 have critical roles in 2-hydroxyglutarate production in D-2-hydroxyglutarate dehydrogenase depleted cells. *Biochem Biophys Res Commun* **423**: 553–556. doi:10.1016/j.bbrc.2012.06.002

Meiser J, Tumanov S, Maddocks O, Labuschagne CF, Athineos D, Van Den Broek N, Mackay GM, Gottlieb E, Blyth K, Vousden K, et al. 2016. Serine one-carbon catabolism with formate overflow. *Sci Adv* **2**: e1601273. doi:10.1126/sciadv.1601273

Meiser J, Schuster A, Pietzke M, Vande Voorde J, Athineos D, Oizel K, Burgos-Barragan G, Wit N, Dhayade S, Morton JP, et al. 2018. Increased formate overflow is a hallmark of oxidative cancer. *Nat Commun* **9**: 368. doi:10.1038/s41467-018-03777-w

Méndez-Lucas A, Lin W, Driscoll PC, Legrave N, Novellasdemunt L, Xie C, Charles M, Wilson Z, Jones NP, Rayport S, et al. 2020. Identifying strategies to target the metabolic flexibility of tumours. *Nat Metab* **2**: 335–350. doi:10.1038/s42255-020-0195-8

Muthusamy T, Cordes T, Handzlik MK, You L, Lim EW, Gengatharan J, Pinto AFM, Badur MG, Kolar MJ, Wallace M, et al. 2020. Serine restriction alters sphingolipid diversity to constrain tumour growth. *Nature* **586**: 790–795. doi:10.1038/s41586-020-2609-x

Newman AC, Labuschagne CF, Vousden KH, Maddocks ODK. 2019. Use of 13C315N1-serine or 13C515N1-methionine for studying methylation dynamics in cancer cell metabolism and epigenetics. *Methods Mol Biol* **1928**: 55–67. doi:10.1007/978-1-4939-9027-6_4

Newman AC, Falcone M, Huerta Uribe A, Zhang T, Athineos D, Pietzke M, Vazquez A, Blyth K, Maddocks ODK. 2021. Immune-regulated IDO1-dependent tryptophan metabolism is source of one-carbon units for pancreatic cancer and stellate cells. *Mol Cell* **81**: 2290–2302.e7. doi:10.1016/j.molcel.2021.03.019

Nikkanen J, Forsström S, Euro L, Paetau I, Kohnz RA, Wang L, Chilov D, Viinamäki J, Roivainen A, Marjamäki P, et al. 2016. Mitochondrial DNA replication defects disturb cellular dNTP pools and remodel one-carbon metabolism. *Cell Metab* **23**: 635–648. doi:10.1016/j.cmet.2016.01.019

Nilsson R, Jain M, Madhusudhan N, Sheppard NG, Strittmatter L, Kampf C, Huang J, Asplund A, Mootha VK. 2014. Metabolic enzyme expression highlights a key role for MTHFD2 and the mitochondrial folate pathway in cancer. *Nat Commun* **5**: 1–10. doi:10.1038/ncomms4128

Otsuka H, Graham M, Kubo A, Nishitani H. 2004. Clinical utility of FDG PET. *J Med Invest* **51**: 14–19. doi:10.2152/jmi.51.14

Pavlova NN, Thompson CB. 2016. The emerging hallmarks of cancer metabolism. *Cell Metab* **23**: 27–47. doi:10.1016/j.cmet.2015.12.006

Piskounova E, Agathocleous M, Murphy MM, Hu Z, Huddlestun SE, Zhao Z, Leitch AM, Johnson TM, DeBerardinis RJ, Morrison SJ. 2015. Oxidative stress inhibits distant metastasis by human melanoma cells. *Nature* **527**: 186–191. doi:10.1038/nature15726

Pogribny IP, Kutanzi K, Melnyk S, de Conti A, Tryndyak V, Montgomery B, Pogribna M, Muskhelishvili L, Latendresse JR, James SJ, et al. 2013. Strain-dependent dysregulation of one-carbon metabolism in male mice is associated with choline- and folate-deficient diet-induced liver injury. *FASEB J* **27**: 2233–2243. doi:10.1096/fj.12-227116

Ponziani FR, Cazzato IA, Danese S, Fagiuoli S, Gionchetti P, Annicchiarico BE, D'Aversa F, Gasbarrini A. 2012. Folate in gastrointestinal health and disease. *Eur Rev Med Pharmacol Sci* **16**: 376–385.

Porter RK, Scott JM, Brand MD. 1992. Choline transport into rat liver mitochondria. Characterization and kinetics of a specific transporter. *J Biol Chem* **267**: 14637–14646. doi:10.1016/S0021-9258(18)42089-3

Possemato R, Marks KM, Shaul YD, Pacold ME, Kim D, Birsoy K, Sethumadhavan S, Woo HK, Jang HG, Jha AK, et al. 2011. Functional genomics reveal that the serine synthesis pathway is essential in breast cancer. *Nature* **476**: 346–350. doi:10.1038/nature10350

Rathore R, Caldwell KE, Schutt C, Brashears CB, Prudner BC, Ehrhardt WR, Leung CH, Lin H, Daw NC, Beird HC, et al. 2021. Metabolic compensation activates pro-survival mTORC1 signaling upon 3-phosphoglycerate dehydrogenase inhibition in osteosarcoma. *Cell Rep* **34**: 108678. doi:10.1016/j.celrep.2020.108678

Rohren EM, Turkington TG, Coleman RE. 2004. Clinical applications of PET in oncology. *Radiology* **231**: 305–332. doi:10.1148/radiol.2312021185

Ron-Harel N, Santos D, Ghergurovich JM, Sage PT, Reddy A, Lovitch SB, Dephoure N, Satterstrom FK, Sheffer M, Spinelli JB, et al. 2016. Mitochondrial biogenesis and proteome remodeling promote one-carbon metabolism for T cell activation. *Cell Metab* **24**: 104–117. doi:10.1016/j.cmet.2016.06.007

Ross KC, Andrews AJ, Marion CD, Yen TJ, Bhattacharjee V. 2017. Identification of the serine biosynthesis pathway as a critical component of BRAF inhibitor resistance of melanoma, pancreatic, and non-small cell lung cancer cells. *Mol Cancer Ther* **16**: 1596–1609. doi:10.1158/1535-7163.MCT-16-0798

Saito RF, Andrade LNS, Bustos SO, Chammas R. 2022. Phosphatidylcholine-derived lipid mediators: the crosstalk between cancer cells and immune cells. *Front Immunol* **13**: 215. doi:10.3389/fimmu.2022.768606

Sanchez-Cespedes M. 2007. A role for LKB1 gene in human cancer beyond the Peutz–Jeghers syndrome. *Oncogene* **26**: 7825–7832. doi:10.1038/sj.onc.1210594

Schober FA, Moore D, Atanassov I, Moedas MF, Clemente P, Végvári Á, El FN, Filograna R, Bucher AL, Hinze Y, et al. 2021. The one-carbon pool controls mitochondrial energy metabolism via complex I and iron–sulfur clusters. *Sci Adv* **7**. doi:10.1126/sciadv.abf0717

Shih C, Chen VJ, Gossett LS, Gates SB, MacKellar WC, Habeck LL, Shackelford KA, Mendelsohn LG, Soose DJ, Patel VF, et al. 1997. LY231514, a pyrrolo[2,3-d]pyrimidine-based antifolate that inhibits multiple folate-requiring enzymes. *Cancer Res* **57**: 1116–1123.

Sugiura A, Andrejeva G, Voss K, Heintzman DR, Xu X, Madden MZ, Ye X, Beier KL, Chowdhury NU, Wolf MM, et al. 2022. MTHFD2 is a metabolic checkpoint controlling effector and regulatory T cell fate and function. *Immunity* **55**: 65–81.e9. doi:10.1016/j.immuni.2021.10.011

Sun S, Shi W, Wu Z, Zhang G, Yang B, Jiao S. 2015. Prognostic significance of the mRNA expression of ERCC1, RRM1, TUBB3 and TYMS genes in patients with non-small cell lung cancer. *Exp Ther Med* **10:** 937–941. doi:10.3892/etm .2015.2636

Szlasa W, Zendran I, Zalesińska A, Tarek M, Kulbacka J. 2020. Lipid composition of the cancer cell membrane. *J Bioenerg Biomembr* **52:** 321–342. doi:10.1007/s10863-020-09846-4

Tajan M, Vousden KH. 2020. Dietary approaches to cancer therapy. *Cancer Cell* **37:** 767–785. doi:10.1016/j.ccell.2020 .04.005

Tajan M, Hennequart M, Cheung EC, Zani F, Hock AK, Legrave N, Maddocks ODK, Ridgway RA, Athineos D, Suárez-Bonnet A, et al. 2021. Serine synthesis pathway inhibition cooperates with dietary serine and glycine limitation for cancer therapy. *Nat Commun* **12:** 366. doi:10 .1038/s41467-020-20223-y

Tibbetts AS, Appling DR. 2010. Compartmentalization of mammalian folate-mediated one-carbon metabolism. *Annu Rev Nutr* **30:** 57–81. doi:10.1146/annurev.nutr .012809.104810

Titus SA, Moran RG. 2000. Retrovirally mediated complementation of the glyB phenotype. *J Biol Chem* **275:** 36811–36817. doi:10.1074/jbc.M005163200

Tucker EJ, Hershman SG, Köhrer C, Belcher-Timme CA, Patel J, Goldberger OA, Christodoulou J, Silberstein JM, McKenzie M, Ryan MT, et al. 2011. Mutations in MTFMT underlie a human disorder of formylation causing impaired mitochondrial translation. *Cell Metab* **14:** 428–434. doi:10.1016/j.cmet.2011.07.010

Vander Heiden MG. 2011. Targeting cancer metabolism: a therapeutic window opens. *Nat Rev Drug Discov* **10:** 671–684. doi:10.1038/nrd3504

Waldman AD, Fritz JM, Lenardo MJ. 2020. A guide to cancer immunotherapy: from T cell basic science to clinical practice. *Nat Rev Immunol* **20:** 651–668. doi:10.1038/s41577-020-0306-5

Wang LW, Shen H, Nobre L, Ersing I, Paulo JA, Trudeau S, Wang Z, Smith NA, Ma Y, Reinstadler B, et al. 2019. Epstein–Barr-Virus-induced one-carbon metabolism drives B cell transformation. *Cell Metab* **30:** 539–555.e11. doi:10 .1016/j.cmet.2019.06.003

Warburg O, Wind F, Negelein E. 1927. The metabolism of tumors in the body. *J Gen Physiol* **8:** 519–530. doi:10.1085/ jgp.8.6.519

Weinblatt ME, Coblyn JS, Fox DA, Fraser PA, Holdsworth DE, Glass DN, Trentham DE. 1985. Efficacy of low-dose methotrexate in rheumatoid arthritis. *N Engl J Med* **312:** 818–822. doi:10.1056/NEJM198503283121303

Willkens RF, Williams HJ, Ward JR, Egger MJ, Reading JC, Clements PJ, Cathcart ES, Samuelson COJ, Solsky MA, Kaplan SB, et al. 1984. Randomized, double-blind, placebo controlled trial of low-dose pulse methotrexate in psoriatic arthritis. *Arthritis Rheum* **27:** 376–381. doi:10.1002/art .1780270403

Woeller CF, Anderson DD, Szebenyi DME, Stover PJ. 2007. Evidence for small ubiquitin-like modifier-dependent nuclear import of the thymidylate biosynthesis pathway. *J Biol Chem* **282:** 17623–17631. doi:10.1074/jbc .M702526200

Yang XM, MacKenzie RE. 1993. NAD-Dependent methylenetetrahydrofolate dehydrogenase-methenyltetrahydrofolate cyclohydrolase is the mammalian homolog of the mitochondrial enzyme encoded by the yeast MIS1 gene. *Biochemistry* **32:** 11118–11123. doi:10.1021/bi00092a022

Yang R, Sowers R, Mazza B, Healey JH, Huvos A, Grier H, Bernstein M, Beardsley GP, Krailo MD, Devidas M, et al. 2003. Sequence alterations in the reduced folate carrier are observed in osteosarcoma tumor samples. *Clin Cancer Res* **9:** 837–844.

Yang L, Garcia Canaveras JC, Chen Z, Wang L, Liang L, Jang C, Mayr JA, Zhang Z, Ghergurovich JM, Zhan L, et al. 2020. Serine catabolism feeds NADH when respiration is impaired. *Cell Metab* **31:** 809–821.e6. doi:10.1016/j.cmet .2020.02.017

Ye J, Mancuso A, Tong X, Ward PS, Fan J, Rabinowitz JD, Thompson CB. 2012. Pyruvate kinase M2 promotes de novo serine synthesis to sustain mTORC1 activity and cell proliferation. *Proc Natl Acad Sci* **109:** 6904–6909. doi:10.1073/pnas.1204176109

Ye J, Fan J, Venneti S, Wan YW, Pawel BR, Zhang J, Finley LWS, Lu C, Lindsten T, Cross JR, et al. 2014. Serine catabolism regulates mitochondrial redox control during hypoxia. *Cancer Discov* **4:** 1406–1417. doi:10.1158/2159-8290.CD-14-0250

Yoshida T, Kikuchi G. 1973. Major pathways of serine and glycine catabolism in various organs of the rat and cock. *J Biochem* **73:** 1013–1022. doi:10.1093/oxfordjournals .jbchem.a130155

Zatz M, Dudley PA, Kloog Y, Markey SP. 1981. Nonpolar lipid methylation. Biosynthesis of fatty acid methyl esters by rat lung membranes using *S*-adenosylmethionine. *J Biol Chem* **256:** 10028–10032. doi:10.1016/S0021-9258(19) 68735-1

Zhang Y, Kwok-Shing Ng P, Kucherlapati M, Chen F, Liu Y, Tsang YH, de Velasco G, Jeong KJ, Akbani R, Hadjipanayis A, et al. 2017. A pan-cancer proteogenomic atlas of PI3K/AKT/mTOR pathway alterations. *Cancer Cell* **31:** 820–832.e3. doi:10.1016/j.ccell.2017.04.013

Zhang Y, Guo R, Kim SH, Shah H, Zhang S, Liang JH, Fang Y, Gentili M, Leary CNO, Elledge SJ, et al. 2021. SARS-CoV-2 hijacks folate and one-carbon metabolism for viral replication. *Nat Commun* **12:** 1676. doi:10.1038/s41467-020-20314-w

Cite this article as *Cold Spring Harb Perspect Med* doi: 10.1101/cshperspect.a041533

Iron, Copper, and Selenium: Cancer's Thing for Redox Bling

Erdem M. Terzi[1,2] and Richard Possemato[1,2]

[1]Department of Pathology, New York University Grossman School of Medicine, New York, New York 10016, USA

[2]Laura and Isaac Perlmutter Cancer Center, New York, New York 10016, USA

Correspondence: Richard.Possemato@nyulangone.org; Erdem.Terzi@nyulangone.org

Cells require micronutrients for numerous basic functions. Among these, iron, copper, and selenium are particularly critical for redox metabolism, and their importance is heightened during oncogene-driven perturbations in cancer. In this review, which particularly focuses on iron, we describe how these micronutrients are carefully chaperoned about the body and made available to tissues, a process that is designed to limit the toxicity of free iron and copper or by-products of selenium metabolism. We delineate perturbations in iron metabolism and iron-dependent proteins that are observed in cancer, and describe the current approaches being used to target iron metabolism and iron-dependent processes.

IRON

Iron is essential for living organisms and is used in a variety of different functions including oxidative phosphorylation, oxygen transport, and DNA synthesis and maintenance. Many of these cellular processes are dependent on iron-containing proteins, which either directly bind to iron molecules or to iron-containing cofactors, namely, heme and iron–sulfur clusters (Sviderskiy et al. 2019). As such, iron is required at a minimum level to maintain viability in almost all living cells.

One of the primary reasons that cells use iron abundantly is its high potential to accept or donate electrons. Although this redox potential is useful in various cellular processes (for example, the electron transport chain) excess iron can enhance the production of reactive oxygen species (ROS), mainly via a process called the Fenton reactions (Winterbourn 1995). During this process, iron catalyzes the conversion of hydrogen peroxide to highly reactive hydroxyl radical species. Excessive iron-catalyzed ROS production can lead to protein and lipid oxidation and ROS-dependent cell death.

As insufficient or excessive iron is harmful for cell viability, iron regulation pathways have evolved to maintain an optimal iron concentration. In mammals, iron is regulated at the systemic level to control iron intake to the body as well as at the cellular level to regulate cellular iron concentration (Hentze et al. 2010). Misregulation in either of these iron regulatory pathways can contribute to various diseases and disorders, including cancer.

Systemic Iron Regulation

Systemic iron levels are sensed in the liver, resulting in modulation of expression of the hormone hepcidin, which regulates iron mainly by controlling dietary iron absorption and iron release from macrophages (Fig. 1; Ganz 2011; Ward and Kaplan 2012). Briefly, hepcidin triggers the internalization and subsequent degradation of iron exporter ferroportin (Nemeth et al. 2004b). The duodenum, the first part of small intestine where iron is primarily absorbed, as well as macro-phages, which recycle iron from red blood cells, express high levels of ferroportin to control the release of iron into the blood (Ganz 2013). Upon transport into the blood, ferrous iron (Fe^{2+}) is oxidized to ferric iron (Fe^{3+}) by two main oxidases, hephaestin and ceruloplasmin, whereupon Fe^{3+} binds to serum transferrin, the main iron carrier protein in the circulation (Osaki et al. 1966; Vulpe et al. 1999). Iron absorbed in this way is not excreted—blood loss or sloughing of endothelial cells are the primary mechanisms of body iron loss and are not regulated by iron. Di-

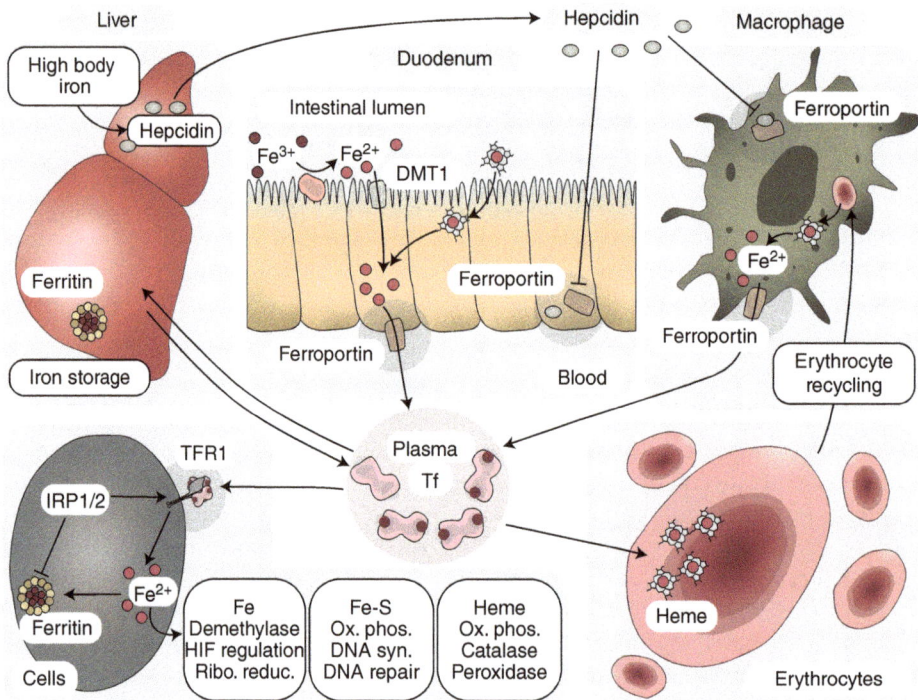

Figure 1. Systemic iron handling. Iron intake in intestine: Dietary iron is primarily absorbed in the duodenum in Fe^{2+} or heme form. Iron can be released to the plasma via iron exporter ferroportin and bind to transferrin in plasma to be transported across the body. Erythrocytes and iron recycling by macrophages: Most iron in the body is used by erythrocytes in the form of heme in hemoglobin. Old and damaged erythrocytes are cleared by macrophages in the spleen, and iron is released from the macrophages back to plasma via the iron exporter ferroportin. Liver and hepcidin: Excess iron in the body is stored in ferritin in the liver. When systemic iron levels are too high, the liver secretes the hormone hepcidin to inhibit iron release into the plasma. Hepcidin binds and internalizes ferroportin, mainly in the intestines and macrophages. Without this iron exporter, iron is not released into the plasma, lowering systemic iron availability. Cellular iron handling: Cells express transferrin receptor 1 (TFR1) to facilitate iron intake and store excess iron in ferritin. Iron regulatory protein 1 (IRP1) and 2 (IRP2) maintain cellular iron homeostasis, facilitating various cell essential functions like oxidative phosphorylation (Ox. phos.) and DNA synthesis (syn.) and repair, while ensuring that excess reactive iron does not accumulate. (Ribo. reduc.) Ribonucleotide reductase.

Cite this article as *Cold Spring Harb Perspect Med* doi: 10.1101/cshperspect.a041545

etary iron intake, on the other hand, compensates the daily loss of iron and maintains body iron levels (Korolnek and Hamza 2015). Thus, by excluding iron from the body via duodenal enterocytes and trapping iron in macrophages, hepcidin alters the total iron intake of the body and regulates systemic iron levels. Of note, the contribution of dietary iron intake to the overall organismal iron pool is dwarfed by the recycling of erythrocyte iron by macrophages.

Regulation of Hepcidin

Hepcidin is a 25-amino-acid hormone expressed predominantly in the liver (Park et al. 2001). Lower expression of hepcidin is observed in other tissues as well, which might contribute to local iron regulation. Hepatic hepcidin levels are mainly regulated by systemic iron levels, erythropoiesis, hypoxia, and inflammation, as outlined below and reviewed in detail in Rishi et al. (2015).

Iron-dependent regulation of hepcidin levels is conferred by a signaling pathway involving transferrin receptors 1 and 2 (TFR1 and TFR2), homeostatic iron regulator (HFE), bone morphogenetic protein (BMP), and the SMA and mother against decapentaplegic (SMAD) pathway (Andriopoulos et al. 2009; Rishi et al. 2015). High iron saturation of circulating transferrin promotes hepcidin production and inhibits further iron uptake (Kautz et al. 2008).

Most iron in the body is used by erythrocytes as heme in hemoglobin to transport oxygen in the blood (Kohgo et al. 2008). As such, erythropoiesis factors and hypoxia regulate hepcidin levels to ensure sufficient iron intake for new red blood cell production, and red blood cell loss is a major cause of low organismal iron levels (Pak et al. 2006). Specifically, peritubular fibroblasts in the renal cortex sense blood oxygen levels via hypoxia-inducible factor 2α (HIF-2α) (Kapitsinou et al. 2010). Hypoxia stimulates expression of the HIF-2α target and erythropoiesis hormone erythropoietin within the kidney, triggering erythroid expansion and expression of the hormone erythroferrone within erythroblasts (Rankin et al. 2007). Erythroferrone directly suppresses hepatic hepcidin expression,

increasing iron availability (Kautz et al. 2014). Conversely, inhibition of erythropoiesis significantly increases hepcidin expression indirectly, via elevated systemic iron levels.

As almost all organisms require iron to proliferate, iron restriction is hypothesized to have evolved as an innate defense against infection. Inflammation is a major regulator of hepcidin mainly through inflammatory cytokines, especially IL-6, which limits iron availability locally and systemically (Nemeth et al. 2004a; Lee et al. 2005). IL-6 triggers hepatic hepcidin expression dependent upon classical JAK/STAT3 signaling (Wrighting and Andrews 2006). In chronic diseases, hepcidin induced by persistent inflammation can limit dietary iron uptake, resulting in anemia due to subsequent lack of iron for erythropoiesis (Weinstein et al. 2002). Moreover, innate immune cells release iron-binding proteins (e.g., lactoferrin and lipocalin-2) to locally limit iron available for invading microbes (Ganz 2009).

Anemia of Cancer

Anemia is a common condition in cancer patients either due to the disease itself or due to cancer treatment. Tumor-associated bleeding and subsequent red blood cell loss, malabsorption or malnutrition, and myeloablative chemotherapy can result in iron deficiency and decreased red blood cell production, negatively affecting the quality of life and prognosis of cancer patients (Gilreath et al. 2014).

Chronic inflammation is a hallmark of some cancer subtypes, and inflammatory cytokines are elevated in serum and tumor tissues of patients with various cancers (Kumari et al. 2016). In mouse cancer models that exhibit anemia of cancer, chronic inflammation and iron deficiency anemia can be accompanied by hepcidin up-regulation, although anemia can occur independently of hepcidin as well (Kim et al. 2014). Recent studies suggest that ectopic expression of hepcidin in colorectal cancer cells themselves can support tumor growth. In these models, hepcidin is thought to act in an autocrine/paracrine fashion to block ferroportin-mediated iron export, sequestering iron in cancer cells for important cellular functions such as mitochondrial oxidative phosphorylation and nucleotide metabolism (Schwartz et al. 2021). Of note, iron deficiency–dependent anemia is more common in colorectal cancer, where intestinal bleeding, malabsorption, and inflammation-associated hepcidin up-regulation are all major factors (Bhurosy et al. 2022).

Dietary Iron Overload and Cancer

Epidemiological studies investigating the relationship between iron uptake and cancer incidence suggest a potential positive correlation between high heme-bound iron intake and the incidence of certain cancer types, including colorectal, lung, pancreas, and breast (Fonseca-Nunes et al. 2014). In colorectal cancer, a comprehensive analysis of several studies revealed a strong association with red meat consumption, which is abundant in heme-bound iron (Torti et al. 2018). This increase in colorectal cancer incidence is attributed to overload of heme oxygenase (HMOX), an enzyme that degrades heme, and the subsequent damage to the colonic epithelium of excess heme, a highly oxidative molecule in its free form (Fiorito et al. 2019). Dietary heme also increases systemic iron availability and heme-dependent formation of N-nitroso compounds, which are associated with cancer risk (Lunn et al. 2007).

Hereditary hemochromatosis is a relatively common disorder (1:200 persons of Northern European ancestry), and is caused by mutations in genes involved in the hepcidin pathway, with mutations in *HFE* representing the vast majority of cases. These mutations lead to excess iron absorption and consequent iron overload specifically in the liver, heart, and endocrine glands. This excess iron can be stored safely in cellular iron storage protein ferritin, yet consistently high iron uptake can saturate cellular and serum ferritin, leading to iron toxicity. Depending on the specific gene mutated and disease severity, patients can experience early or late onset of symptoms related to iron overload, including liver cirrhosis (Pietrangelo 2010). In accordance with the positive cancer correlation with iron intake, liver cancer risk is 20-fold higher in patients with hereditary hemochromatosis (Elmberg et al. 2003).

Iron Chelators and Cancer Therapy

As cancer cells display an enhanced requirement for iron, iron chelation was suggested as a potential method to target cancer cells (Yu et al. 2012). Deferoxamine (DFO) and related compounds are siderophores with high affinity to Fe^{3+} that are commonly used clinically as iron chelators for the treatment of hemochromatosis (Ibrahim and O'Sullivan 2020). Although DFO treatment can decrease the proliferation of cancer cells in neonatal acute leukemia and moderately decrease bone marrow infiltration in neuroblastoma patients, it had no effect on hormone-refractory metastatic prostate cancer, among other tumor subtypes, and is not currently used clinically for cancer treatment (Estrov et al. 1987; Donfrancesco et al. 1990; Dreicer et al. 1997).

Deferasirox is an orally bioavailable iron chelator with a longer half-life compared to DFO, and as such has been proposed as a superior iron chelator option in cancer clinical trials (Ibrahim and O'Sullivan 2020). Deferasirox suppressed tumor xenografts in mice, yet in a small clinical trial failed to show a significant difference in tumor response (Lui et al. 2013; Saeki et al. 2016).

Ribonucleotide reductase (RNR) has a di-iron center that is required for its catalytic function to convert ribonucleotides to deoxyribonucleotides, required for DNA synthesis and repair. This iron group is targeted by the small molecule inhibitor triapine (Popović-Bijelić et al. 2011). Unlike other iron chelators, triapine is suggested to act primarily via a radical tyrosyl-based mechanism instead of direct iron chelation to selectively inhibit RNR activity (Aye et al. 2012). Similar to other iron chelators, triapine had a limited response in clinical trials, in this case in renal cell carcinoma and head and neck squamous cell carcinoma patients (Knox et al. 2007; Nutting et al. 2009).

In general, iron chelation presents a potential method to target cancer cells; however, the toxicity of iron chelation at the doses required to inhibit cancer cell function is the most significant roadblock to clinical translation. Future studies may find specific contexts in which iron chelation therapy is efficacious or targets specific downstream processes that use iron.

Cellular Iron Regulation and Cancer-Relevant Alterations

In mammals, a complex array of iron sensing, import, and storage proteins regulate cellular iron trafficking and homeostasis (Fig. 2). Cellular iron levels are mainly regulated by iron regulatory proteins 1 and 2 (IRP1, IRP2). IRPs sense both iron and iron–sulfur cluster levels in the cell to regulate iron import, export, storage, and utilization (Hentze et al. 2010). Aside from IRPs, iron storage is directly regulated by cytoplasmic iron levels via controlling degradation of iron storage protein ferritin. In a process called ferritinophagy, cargo receptor NCOA4 delivers ferritin to the cellular autophagy machinery where it is released into the lysosome (Mancias et al. 2014). As iron metabolism is intricately connected to ROS

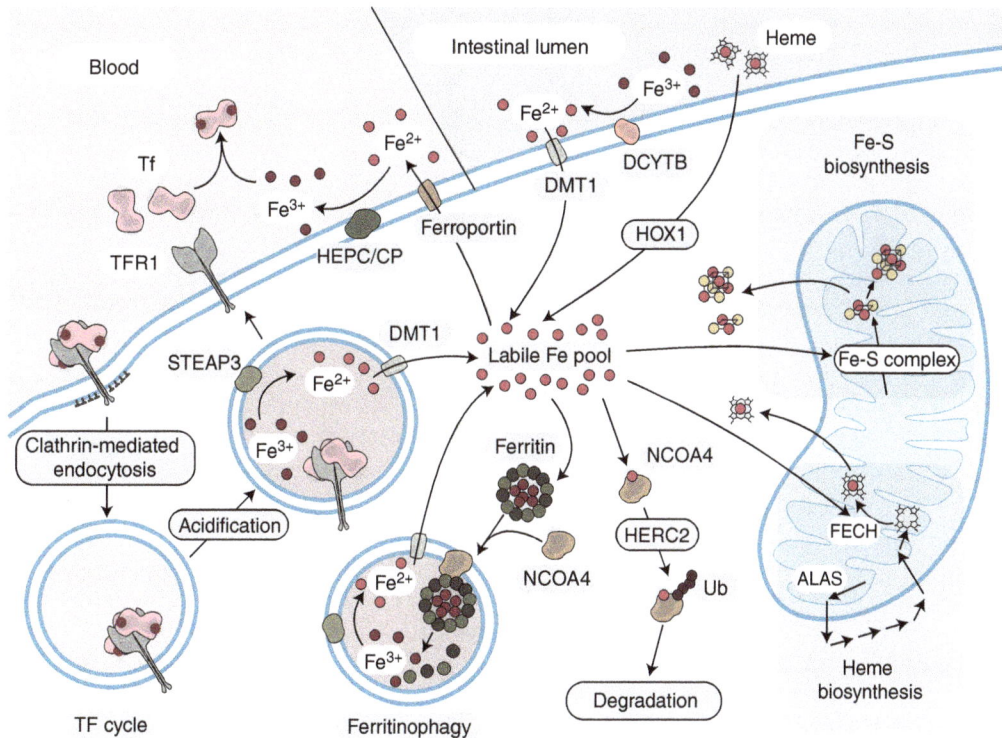

Figure 2. Cellular iron management and utilization. Iron intake in intestine: In the intestinal lumen, Fe^{3+} can be reduced to Fe^{2+} by duodenal cytochrome B (DCYTB), and Fe^{2+} can be taken into the cell via divalent metal transporter 1 (DMT1). Heme can be also absorbed in the intestine and subsequently degraded by heme oxygenase 1 (HMOX1) to release iron. Transferrin cycle: Transferrin receptor 1 (TFR1) binds Fe^{3+}-bound transferrin and is internalized via clathrin-mediated endocytosis. Endosomes are subsequently acidified and Fe^{3+} is released from transferrin in this lower pH. Fe^{3+} is reduced by metalloreductases such as STEAP3 and released into the cytosol via transporters including DMT1. TFR1 is recycled back to the cell membrane, and apotransferrin released back into the plasma, as it has low affinity to TFR1 when not bound to iron in neutral pH. Ferritin and ferritinophagy: Excess iron is stored in a 24-unit ferritin complex formed by ferritin heavy and light chains. Ferritin heavy chain can oxidase Fe^{2+} to Fe^{3+}, which is subsequently stored within the core of ferritin complex. In an iron-replete condition, iron-bound NCOA4 is degraded via HERC2. In iron-depleted conditions, NCOA4 can bind and target ferritin for degradation in a process called ferritinophagy. Iron utilization: Iron can either be used as a cofactor directly or used to synthesize iron-containing cofactors, iron–sulfur clusters, and heme. Different steps of heme biosynthesis occur in mitochondria and cytosol, with the last step of iron incorporation occurring in the mitochondria. Iron sulfur cluster biosynthesis occurs within the mitochondria, emphasizing the key role of mitochondria in cellular iron metabolism.

metabolism, oxygen and ROS have important roles in regulating cellular iron metabolism via both IRPs and the key transcriptional regulator of antioxidant defense, NRF2 (Meyron-Holtz et al. 2004; Kerins and Ooi 2018; Wang et al. 2020; Terzi et al. 2021). Oxidative stress in the cytoplasm triggers NRF2 stabilization and nuclear translocation, where ferritin heavy and light chains and HMOX are among its canonical targets.

To maintain optimal available iron concentration in cells, iron import, storage, and export is controlled by different layers of regulation (Sviderskiy et al. 2019). Iron import is primarily accomplished by TFR-dependent uptake of transferrin, although non-transferrin-bound iron can be obtained via other transporters like divalent metal transporter 1 ([DMT1] gene symbol *SLC11A2*). Ferritin is the main storage protein in the cell, regulating the available iron levels by oxidizing labile ferrous iron (Fe^{2+}) and storing iron within its core in the ferric (Fe^{3+}) form. Ferroportin is the primary iron exporter and plays an important role in systemic iron regulation together with hepcidin, as explained above. Here, we discuss each of these major players in iron trafficking and regulation in turn, along with their cancer relevance (Table 1).

Transferrin-Dependent Iron Uptake

The transferrin cycle is the main iron import pathway for most mammalian cells and is essential for the regulation of iron homeostasis. Since free iron can be highly reactive, iron is preferentially transported in the blood by iron-binding proteins. Transferrin is a 76-kD glycoprotein and main iron transporter in blood serum in vertebrates (Lambert 2012). One transferrin molecule can bind to two Fe^{3+} atoms (Aisen et al. 1978), enabling this less soluble and less active form to be transported across the body. While TFR1 is ubiquitously expressed, it can be further induced in normally proliferative cells, and is particularly up-regulated during erythroid differentiation, owing to the massive amount of iron required for hemoglobin synthesis (Sieff et al. 1982). TFR1 binds to iron-bound transferrin with high affinity to initiate the transferrin cycle

(Kleven et al. 2018). Transferrin-bound TFR1 is internalized via clathrin-mediated endocytosis and enters acidified endosomes, reducing the affinity of Fe^{3+} to transferrin (Aisen et al. 1978; Lakadamyali et al. 2006). Apotransferrin has a low affinity for the transferrin receptor, thus upon returning back to the plasma membrane, transferrin is released to the extracellular space (Dautry-Varsat et al. 1983). Internalized Fe^{3+} is reduced to Fe^{2+} by metalloreductases such as STEAP3 in acidified endosomes, and transported to the cytosol via transporters like DMT1 (Tabuchi et al. 2000; Ohgami et al. 2005), although iron reduction and export processes are very likely supported by other, redundant proteins.

TFR2 is expressed primarily in liver tissues, where it is involved in systemic iron regulation (Nemeth et al. 2005). TFR2 has different iron binding dynamics and lower binding affinity compared to TFR1 (Kleven et al. 2018), and as such TFR2 is suggested to detect transferrin saturation and initiate signaling cascades that regulate hepcidin expression. TFR2 also has functions in modulating erythropoiesis by interacting with the erythropoietin receptor in erythroblasts, and TFR2 expression is reported in several cancer cell lines (Calzolari et al. 2007; Forejtnikovà et al. 2010). However, unlike TFR1, TFR2 has not been reported to have a significant role in tumorigenesis.

Transferrin-Independent Iron Uptake and Transport

When released into the blood, iron is oxidized to Fe^{3+} and bound to transferrin and (to a much smaller degree) serum ferritin (Soldin et al. 2004). In chronic iron overload disorders or upon cytotoxic chemotherapy (Belotti et al. 2015), serum transferrin can become saturated, leading to increased levels of non-transferrin-bound iron (NTBI) (Brissot et al. 2012). NTBI is suggested to loosely bind other serum proteins such as albumin. Unlike transferrin-bound iron, NTBI can more easily catalyze unwanted ROS production (Silva and Hider 2009). As NTBI is not bound to transferrin, other transporters like Zip14 are suggested to facilitate NTBI intake,

Cite this article as *Cold Spring Harb Perspect Med* doi: 10.1101/cshperspect.a041545

Table 1. Cancer relevance of key iron-, copper-, and selenium-regulated proteins and processes

Gene	Ion-relevant function	Cancer relevance	References
Iron			
NRF2	Activates ferritin expression, stabilizes Bach1 via HMOX1	NRF2 activation in lung and esophageal cancers	Sporn and Liby 2012; Kerins and Ooi 2018; Wu and Papagiannakopoulos 2020
NFS1	Fe-S synthesis	Higher NFS1 expression/ requirement in lung cancer	Alvarez et al. 2017
HQ/ lysosome inhibitor	Blocks iron intake via TFR1; blocks ferritinophagy	Clinical trials in various solid tumors	Yambire et al. 2019; Weber et al. 2020; Mukhopadhyay et al. 2023
NCOA4	Ferritinophagy cargo receptor	Pancreatic cancer dependence (mouse models)	Hasan et al. 2020; Santana-Codina et al. 2021, 2022
TFR1 (CD71)	Iron uptake	Up-regulated in many tumors and proliferating cells	Habashy et al. 2010; Chan et al. 2014; Shen et al. 2018
HFE	Systemic iron regulation	Mutation causes hereditary hemochromatosis (HH), which promotes liver cancer	Elmberg et al. 2003
HMOX1	Heme degradation	Expressed in cancer and stroma, regulates BACH1 via NRF2	Nitti et al. 2017; Fiorito et al. 2019; Unlu et al. 2022
TET2	DNA demethylation function is iron-dependent	TET2 is mutated in myeloid malignancies	Ko et al. 2010; López-Cimmino et al. 2017; Moyado et al. 2019
HIF-1α	HIF stabilization is iron-dependent	HIF-1α is activated in cancer, enhances glycolysis	Masoud and Li 2015; Hirota 2019
HIF-2α	HIF stabilization is iron-dependent	HIF-2α is activated in clear cell renal cell carcinoma (VHL-mut)	Anderson et al. 2013; Chen et al. 2016; Cho et al. 2016
Copper			
MEK1/2	Copper regulates MEK1/2 phosphorylation of ERK	MAP kinase pathway is commonly activated in cancer	Turski et al. 2012; Brady et al. 2014
ULK1/2	Copper is required for ULK1/2 activity, autophagy stimulation	Autophagy is activated in specific cancer (e.g., pancreas)	Tsang et al. 2020
Selenium			
GPX4	GPX4 has a catalytic active site selenocysteine	GPX4 may protect cancer cells from ferroptosis	Yang et al. 2014; Chen et al. 2021

primarily by hepatic clearance (Liuzzi et al. 2006).

Several other pathways independent of transferrin exist to transport iron such as DMT1. DMT1 is the main transferrin-independent iron import pathway and is expressed highly in the apical membrane of duodenum cells for the systemic uptake of iron into the body (Shawki et al. 2015). DMT1 mainly transports Fe^{2+} from the intestinal lumen, which is subsequently released into blood via ferroportin (Donovan et al. 2005). Aside from its systemic role in intestinal cells, DMT1 is localized to the endosomal membrane, contributing to iron transport within the cells (Tabuchi et al. 2000).

Transferrin-Dependent Iron Uptake and Cancer

Cancer cells have a higher iron requirement due to their high proliferation rate. TFR1—also named CD71—is commonly up-regulated in cancer cells and has been suggested as a prognostic marker and target for cancer therapy (Habashy et al. 2010; Chan et al. 2014; Shen et al. 2018). Accordingly, TFR1 is also a proliferation marker in other contexts such as immune cell expansion, which would limit its specificity as a target (Dinh et al. 2020). As cancer therapy often targets proliferative cells, recurrence can be driven by the persistence of dormant or low-cycling populations. In these contexts, down-regulation of TFR1 is observed in such dormant cells, and re-expression of TFR1 is a hallmark of recurrent disease (Brown et al. 2017).

Since the transferrin cycle requires endosomal acidification to release Fe^{3+} from transferrin, maintaining the transferrin cycle is one of the primary functions of endosomal acidification, especially in proliferating cells (Weber et al. 2020). The inability to maintain acidification can impair iron metabolism and mitochondrial function, leading to cell death (Yambire et al. 2019). As such, alteration in endosomal acidification, either due to cancer progression or via cancer treatment, inevitably affects iron metabolism via the transferrin pathway as well. In particular, the autophagy inhibitor hydroxychloroquine is currently being tested in pancreas cancer clinical trials, and can limit iron availability to pancreas cancer cells, suppressing tumor growth (Mukhopadhyay et al. 2023).

Blocking antibodies can limit TFR1 function or potentially promote antibody-dependent cellular cytotoxicity (ADCC) (Candelaria et al. 2021). For example, anti-TFR1 antibodies can inhibit the growth of leukemia xenografts by disturbing iron homeostasis (Callens et al. 2010; Daniels et al. 2011). Moreover, certain viruses use TFR1 to enter the cell, such as New World hemorrhagic fever arenaviruses or hepatitis C virus (Radoshitzky et al. 2007; Martin and Uprichard 2013). Viral carriers similar to these viruses, or nanomolecular carriers, can be used to deliver cytotoxic molecules to the cancer cells. (Daniels et al. 2012).

Ferritin

Iron is essential for various cellular functions, yet cells need to control the available iron pool to avoid excessive ROS production. Only a small portion of iron in the cell exists in a readily bioaccessible state bound transiently to chaperones, known as the labile iron pool (LIP). In contrast, iron is predominantly stored by iron storage protein ferritin (Arosio et al. 2017). In animals, ferritin heavy- and light-chain subunits (FTH1/FTL) form a 24-subunit hollow spherical complex, which can contain up to 4000 iron molecules within its core (Harrison and Arosio 1996). FTH1 has a ferroxidase activity and oxidizes Fe^{2+} to Fe^{3+}, storing excess iron in this less reactive form (Levi et al. 1988).

Ferritin is mainly found in the cytosol, although nuclear and mitochondrial ferritin is described in specific tissues. (Santambrogio et al. 2007; Alkhateeb and Connor 2010) Ferritin can be also secreted into the blood as serum ferritin, which is relatively iron poor (Worwood et al. 1976). Although serum ferritin has limited functional utility as an iron-transport system, its levels correlate positively with systemic iron overload (Harrison and Arosio 1996) or independently with inflammation (Alkhateeb and Connor 2013). Compared to cellular ferritin, the physiological role of serum ferritin is not well understood. Functions independent of iron metabolism have been suggested, such as triggering inflammatory signaling pathways in the liver (Ruddell et al. 2009).

Ferritin transcription, translation, and degradation is regulated by different pathways to control iron availability. High ROS levels oxidize redox-active cysteine residues in the E3-ligase component KEAP1, resulting in its inactivation and the accumulation of its target, NRF2 (Deshmukh et al. 2017). As such, the KEAP1/NRF2 pathway constitutes the major cellular redox sensor, a principle function of which is to activate transcription of both FTH1 and FTL when cytoplasmic oxidative potential is high (Kerins and Ooi 2018). Additionally, low-iron or iron-sulfur cluster levels can inhibit translation of ferritin mRNAs via activation of IRP1 and IRP2 (Sviderskiy et al. 2019). Finally, ferritin degradation is actively regulated via NCOA4 in an iron-dependent manner (Mancias et al. 2014). Thus, ferritin is an integral part of iron homeostasis and an important factor to sustain sufficient iron for cancer growth while protecting cells from excessive ROS production.

Ferritin is targeted to autophagic degradation upon iron starvation in a process called ferritinophagy. Ferritinophagy is mediated through NCOA4-FTH1 binding, which targets ferritin to autophagosomes and lysosomes (Mancias et al. 2015). NCOA4 is itself targeted to degradation by E3 ligase component HERC2 in an iron-dependent manner, regulating ferritin degradation based on cellular iron concentration (Mancias et al. 2015). Activation of ferritinophagy can increase the LIP by releasing stored iron, increasing iron availability but potentially enhancing ROS production (Ajoolabady et al. 2021).

Ferritin and Cancer

Cancer cells need to acquire sufficient iron to sustain their proliferation, while avoiding excessive ROS production. By storing excess iron and releasing it when required, ferritin can maintain iron homeostasis efficiently. Ferritinophagy regulates the degradation of ferritin, and as such plays a role in iron maintenance in cancer cells (Santana-Codina et al. 2021). In particular, pancreatic ductal adenocarcinomas have very high levels of basal autophagy, and ferritinophagy supports pancreatic tumor growth by sustaining iron availability and enabling iron–sulfur cluster synthesis (Santana-Codina et al. 2022). In contrast, NCOA4 deletion has limited effect on pancreas cancer cell growth in vitro in 10% serum (Hasan et al. 2020), but a vulnerability is revealed upon serum limitation, suggesting that ferritinophagy can compensate for low extracellular levels of transferrin/TFR1 (Santana-Codina et al. 2022). Future work will be needed to determine whether ferritinophagy can be targeted in other tumor types, including those with low basal autophagy rates. Ferritinophagy also is a key factor in ferroptosis and released iron via ferritinophagy can sensitize cells to ferroptosis (Gao et al. 2016; Hou et al. 2016).

NRF2 is the main antioxidant defense pathway in the cell and can be up-regulated in cancer to enhance antioxidant defense (Sporn and Liby 2012). In particular, loss-of-function mutations in *KEAP1* activate NRF2 in a substantial proportion of lung and esophageal cancers, and these tumors have poor clinical outcomes (Wu and Papagiannakopoulos 2020). As an NRF2 target, ferritin expression can be up-regulated in KEAP1 mutant cells or those experiencing oxidative stress to restrict iron availability and avoid excessive ROS production (Pietsch et al. 2003). Cells can express different basal levels of ferritin (Shpyleva et al. 2011), and the degree of NRF2 activation can be a determinant of these levels. Since down-regulation of ferritin can alter sensitivity of cells to drugs such as doxorubicin (Buranrat and Connor 2015) and promote cell death by ferroptosis, ferritin may influence the effectiveness of cancer treatments via controlling iron availability and ROS balance.

Aside from the role of cytosolic ferritin in cancer, serum ferritin is commonly elevated in cancer and proposed as a prognostic cancer biomarker, albeit one that is relatively nonspecific (Hazard and Drysdale 1977; Ramírez-Carmona et al. 2022). Serum ferritin is not appreciated to have a role in tumor iron metabolism.

Ferroportin

Ferroportin (SLC40A1) is the only known cellular iron exporter in mammals, and in conjunction with hepcidin, has an important role in systemic iron regulation (Drakesmith et al. 2015). Ferroportin controls the efflux of iron from duodenal enterocytes, macrophages, and the liver. Hepcidin can bind ferroportin and initiate its internalization to inhibit iron efflux into the blood (Nemeth et al. 2004b). Ferroportin deficiency causes accumulation of iron in enterocytes, hepatocytes, and macrophages, as iron is unable to exit these cells and leads to iron deficiency anemia (Donovan et al. 2005).

Ferroportin and Cancer

Although ferroportin expression is high in the duodenum to support systemic iron regulation, ferroportin is still expressed in some other tissues, albeit to much lower levels, including the breast ductal epithelium (Pinnix et al. 2010). Hepcidin is suggested to regulate iron efflux in these cancer cells via ferroportin inhibition, similar to its role in systemic iron regulation and as described above in colorectal cancer (Schwartz et al. 2021). Ferroportin levels are reduced upon transformation, which would serve to maintain intracellular iron levels and support cancer cell function. One interesting question is therefore whether ferroportin inhibition or down-regulation can promote biologically meaningful iron retention outside of colorectal cancer, perhaps in transformed cells that normally express ferroportin highly.

Iron Regulatory Proteins

Levels of primary iron import protein TFR1, iron storage protein ferritin, iron transporter DMT1, and iron exporter ferroportin, control the LIP in the cell (Sviderskiy et al. 2019). IRP1 (gene symbol *ACO1*) and IRP2 (*IREB2*) regulate iron metabolism genes directly and maintain iron homeostasis in mammalian cells (Fig. 3; Hentze et al. 2010).

Both IRP1 and IRP2 bind hairpin-like structures called iron response elements (IREs) within $3'$ or $5'$ untranslated regions (UTRs) of their target mRNAs (Addess et al. 1997). When bound to the $5'$UTR, IRPs inhibit the translation of target mRNAs, including ferritin subunits FTH1 and FTL, ferroportin, heme synthesis enzyme ALAS2, and hypoxia-inducible factor 2α (HIF-2α) (Aziz and Munro 1987; Hentze et al. 1987; Cox et al. 1991; Dandekar et al. 1991; Liu et al. 2002; Sanchez et al. 2007). On the other hand, IRPs stabilize target mRNAs upon binding to the $3'$UTR, increasing the levels of proteins such as TFR1 and DMT1 (Koeller et al. 1989; Gunshin et al. 2001). As such, IRP activation during periods of low iron down-regulates iron storage, export, and utilization and up-regulates iron intake to increase iron availability in the cell. We term this process of IRP activation the iron-starvation response.

Although IRP1 and IRP2 have similar targets, they are activated in a different manner. IRP1 has an iron–sulfur cluster binding site and acts as cytosolic aconitase when it is bound to this iron–sulfur cluster. Upon losing its cluster, an mRNA binding site becomes exposed and IRP1 can bind to its target mRNA (Volz 2008). The iron–sulfur cluster in IRP1 is sensitive to the O_2 level and cytosolic redox potential, and can be absent in chronic iron limiting conditions

(Meyron-Holtz et al. 2004). Unlike IRP1, IRP2 is acutely regulated both by cytosolic iron concentration and iron–sulfur cluster availability. FBXL5 is an E3 ubiquitin ligase component that can target IRP2 for degradation in an iron, oxygen, and iron–sulfur cluster–dependent manner (Salahudeen et al. 2009; Vashisht et al. 2009), while iron sulfur cluster deficiency can also activate IRP2 independent of FBXL5 (Terzi et al. 2021). Together, IRP1 and IRP2 integrate iron, iron–sulfur clusters, redox, and O_2 inputs to modulate iron availability.

Although having a similar role in regulating IRE-containing genes, IRP1 and IRP2 are appreciated to have tissue-specific and context-dependent roles in iron homeostasis. Thus, IRP1 and IRP2 can only functionally compensate for each other to an extent, whereas deletion of both IRPs is embryonic lethal in mice (Smith et al. 2006). Single ACO1 or IREB2 knockout mice are viable, but with distinct dysregulation of erythropoiesis as well as neurological phenotypes and altered glucose homeostasis specifically in IREB2 knockout mice (Wilkinson and Pantopoulos 2014; Sviderskiy et al. 2019; Santos et al. 2020). Nevertheless, activation of either IRP is sufficient to induce the iron-starvation response, iron loading, and ferroptosis sensitivity in cellular models (Terzi et al. 2021).

Iron Regulatory Proteins and Cancer

Although both IRPs regulate cellular iron metabolism, IRP2 specifically is essential to maintain basal iron levels in most tissues (Meyron-Holtz et al. 2004). Deletion of IRP2 reduces basal TFR1 and increases basal ferritin levels, decreasing overall iron availability in the cell (Terzi et al. 2021). Accordingly, IRP2 deletion in breast cancer xenografts decreases the LIP and drastically decreases tumor growth and increases survival (Wang et al. 2014). In contrast, overexpression of IRP2 increases tumor growth in xenografts by increasing iron availability (Maffettone et al. 2010). Similar to IRP2, activation of IRP1 is suggested to increase tumor growth as well. These data support the notion that iron availability is a common bottleneck for tumor growth (Jeong et al. 2015).

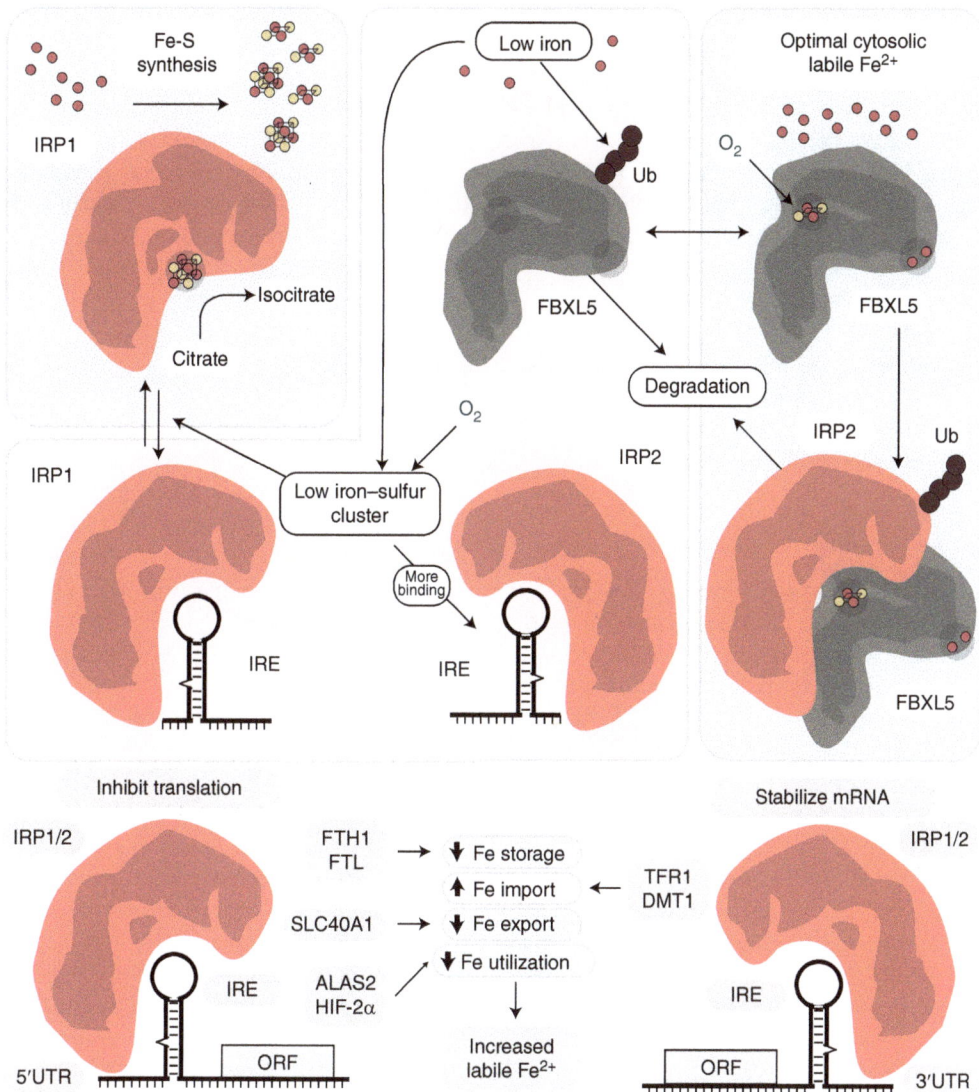

Figure 3. Iron sensing by iron regulatory proteins. Regulation of iron regulatory protein 1 (IRP1) activity: In an iron-replete condition, IRP1 is mostly bound to [4Fe-4S] clusters and acts as a cytosolic aconitase. In an iron-depleted condition, iron sulfur cluster synthesis is inhibited and IRP1 loses its cluster leading to a conformational change. In this state, IRP1 can bind to hairpin-like structures in target mRNAs, called iron response elements (IREs). Regulation of IRP2 activity: IRP2 does not bind to iron–sulfur clusters. Instead its activity is regulated by a complex interplay between iron–sulfur clusters and protein levels. In an iron-replete condition, FBXL5 binds and targets IRP2 for ubiquitination and subsequent degradation. In iron-depleted conditions, FXBL5 no longer binds to iron and is degraded, leading to increased IRP2 protein levels. FXBL5 has a binding site for a [2Fe-2S] cluster, and oxidation of the cluster is necessary for FBXL5-IRP2 binding. Independent of FXBL5-dependent regulation, low iron–sulfur cluster levels can increase IRP2-IRE binding without altering protein level. IRP targets: IRP1 and IRP2 can bind to IREs in the 5′ or 3′ untranslated region (UTR) of the target mRNA. If bound to an IRE in the 5′ UTR, IRPs inhibit the translation of the target mRNA (e.g., FTH1, FTL, SLC40A1, ALAS2, HIF-2α). If bound to an IRE in the 3′UTR, IRPs stabilize the target mRNA and increase protein levels (e.g., TFR1, DMT1). Through regulation of iron storage, import, export and utilization, the activation of IRPs increases the LIP and restores iron homeostasis.

Although IRPs maintain iron homeostasis to promote tumor growth, aberrant activation of either IRP increases the LIP significantly and enhances ROS production. Iron–sulfur cluster deficiency can activate IRPs, sensitizing cells to ferroptosis (Alvarez et al. 2017; Terzi et al. 2021). Because of their redundant function, deleting both IRPs is necessary to block ferroptosis, and demonstrates the role of iron regulation in ferroptotic cell death (Terzi et al. 2021). As such, IRP activation can have antitumor effects when coupled with excessive ROS production (Alvarez et al. 2017). Future work will be needed to determine whether IRP activation can cooperate with ROS-promoting anticancer therapies.

Iron–Sulfur Clusters

Iron–sulfur clusters are formed by a complex assembly mechanism, ultimately producing mainly [2Fe-2S], [3Fe-4S], and [4Fe-4S] clusters that serve as cofactors in multiple essential cellular functions, including the electron transport chain, and DNA synthesis, and repair (Sviderskiy et al. 2019). Iron–sulfur cluster synthesis begins in the mitochondria with the abstraction of an atom of sulfur from the amino acid cysteine by the enzyme NFS1, in association with other key assembly factors FXN, ISD11, and ACP (Rouault 2015; Braymer and Lill 2017). The nascent cluster is assembled on scaffold protein ISCU, after which a complex array of chaperones and assembly proteins are involved in targeting iron–sulfur clusters to resident proteins in the mitochondria, cytosol, and the nucleus (Braymer and Lill 2017).

Similar to iron deficiency, iron–sulfur cluster deficiency is detected by IRPs, increasing the LIP to restore iron–sulfur cluster biosynthesis (Hentze et al. 2010; Terzi et al. 2021). In addition to iron levels, iron–sulfur cluster availability is also determined by oxygen and ROS, which directly destabilizes exposed iron–sulfur clusters and increases their degradation rate (Imlay 2006). Indeed, cells in which iron–sulfur cluster synthesis is partially inhibited fail to grow in ambient oxygen concentrations ($[O_2]$), but are rescued by culture in reduced $[O_2]$ (Alvarez et al. 2017). Moreover, increasing $[O_2]$ selectively degrades the iron–sulfur clusters in specific proteins, including IRP1

and FBXL5, increasing IRP activation and iron loading (Alvarez et al. 2017; Wang et al. 2020). In contrast, while ROS levels can directly damage iron–sulfur clusters, antioxidant systems typically act to neutralize moderate levels of ROS in the cellular environment without substantial effects on iron–sulfur cluster proteins (Alvarez et al. 2017). Due to this interaction, iron–sulfur clusters create a strong link between $[O_2]$, oxidative stress, and iron metabolism.

Iron–Sulfur Clusters and Cancer

Unlike ambient oxygen levels (21% $[O_2]$), most tissues experience 3%–8% $[O_2]$, while cancer cells within a tumor can experience even lower $[O_2]$ due to poor vasculature (McKeown 2014). During metastasis, cancer cells migrating via the blood or lymphatic vessels can experience higher $[O_2]$—as high as 14% $[O_2]$ in the lung microenvironment (McKeown 2014). This change in $[O_2]$ is especially important for the maintenance of iron–sulfur clusters. For example, NFS1 is positively selected at the genomic level in lung tumors, and lung metastases exhibit higher NFS1 levels than primary tumors from which they are derived in breast cancer xenograft models (Alvarez et al. 2017). This observation indicates that iron–sulfur cluster biosynthesis can be limiting for tumorigenesis, particularly in high $[O_2]$. Accordingly, partial inhibition of NFS1 drastically decreases lung metastatic spread from primary mammary tumor or intravenous injection models of metastasis, but does not affect the growth of primary mammary or subcutaneous tumors (Alvarez et al. 2017), indicating that the metastatic process or the lung microenvironment provides a barrier for cancer cells with low iron–sulfur cluster synthesis.

The requirement for iron-sulfur cluster synthesis also varies across tumor types, and breast cancer cells in particular exhibit subtype-specific differences in the response to NFS1 inhibition (Sviderskiy et al. 2020). This difference in sensitivity has been attributed to a selective requirement for iron–sulfur cluster protein DNA polymerase ε (POLE) in triple-negative breast cancer (Sviderskiy et al. 2020). POLE performs leading strand replication, whose suppression may selec-

Cite this article as *Cold Spring Harb Perspect Med* doi: 10.1101/cshperspect.a041545

tively affect triple-negative breast cancer due to genomic instability and abrogation of cell-cycle checkpoints specific to this disease. Surprisingly, the other replicative polymerases, iron–sulfur cluster proteins POLA and POLD, are not selectively required in triple-negative breast cancer, indicating a specific liability related to leading strand replication (Sviderskiy et al. 2020). Taken together, these data suggest that alterations in iron metabolism can influence cancer cells selectively based on both their genetic background and microenvironment.

Iron–sulfur cluster deficiency activates both IRP1 and IRP2 and increases the labile iron concentration, sensitizing cells to ferroptosis through the iron-starvation response mechanism described above (Terzi et al. 2021). Enhanced ferroptosis sensitivity may especially alter cancer progression in tissues with high oxygen exposure due to the higher turnover of iron–sulfur clusters and basal activation of IRPs. Indeed, NRF2 activation, which suppresses ferroptosis, is most commonly activated in lung and esophageal cancers through mutation of *KEAP1*, as described above (Sporn and Liby 2012).

Heme

Iron is a component of heme, which acts as an important cofactor in essential functions such as the electron transport chain (complexes II, III, and IV) or oxygen transport and storage (hemoglobin and myoglobin) (Kim et al. 2012; Poulos 2014). The enzyme catalase uses a heme cofactor to catabolize hydrogen peroxide to water and oxygen using a heme cofactor (Alfonso-Prieto et al. 2009). Heme peroxidases use hydrogen peroxide as an electron acceptor for oxidation of other substrates as well (Poulos 2014).

Heme synthesis starts at the mitochondria with ALA-synthetase. Subsequent steps of heme synthesis take place in the cytosol, finally returning to the mitochondria for the final steps, which includes the ultimate incorporation of iron into protoporphyrin IX by ferrochelatase, forming heme (Ajioka et al. 2006). Ferrochelatase requires an iron–sulfur cluster for its activity and stability, linking heme and iron–sulfur cluster metabolism (Dailey et al. 1994). Heme biosynthesis is also regulated during erythropoiesis by iron availability, as the erythroid ALA-synthase isoform, ALAS2, is inhibited by IRPs when iron levels are low (Cox et al. 1991; Dandekar et al. 1991).

HMOX1 and HMOX2 can facilitate degradation of heme to biliverdin, Fe^{2+}, and CO. HMOX2 is constitutively expressed, while HMOX1 is induced in response to various cellular stresses and stimuli such as hypoxia via HIF-1α and oxidative stress via NRF2, thereby limiting the levels of free heme, which are highly oxidative (Kikuchi et al. 2005; Chiabrando et al. 2014).

Heme and Cancer

As described above, high dietary iron and heme intake is correlated strongly with colorectal, lung, pancreas, and breast cancers (Rishi et al. 2015). Similar to their higher iron requirement, cancer cells can also display a higher heme requirement and enhanced heme biosynthesis, including non-small-cell lung cancer (Fiorito et al. 2019; Sohoni et al. 2019). As a highly reactive molecule, free heme is unlikely to exist in appreciable quantities in the circulation, and is therefore unlikely to be a major contributor to intracellular heme levels in cancer and normal tissues. However, microglia-restricted transporter SLCO2B1 and heme carrier protein HCP1 (SLC46A1) have been reported to import heme, and have been hypothesized to clear extracellular heme present during tissue damage (Unlu et al. 2022).

HMOX1, the inducible heme degradation enzyme, is expressed by various cancer types as well as tumor-associated macrophages. HMOX1 is suggested to influence proliferation, differentiation, angiogenesis, metastasis, and cell death, and suppress immune responses (Nitti et al. 2017; Fiorito et al. 2019). NFR2 can increase HMOX1 and subsequently stabilize Bach1 in lung cancer, promoting metastasis (Lignitto et al. 2019). Interestingly, nuclear localization of enzymatically inactive HMOX1 can activate oxidant-responsive transcription factors, indicating a heme-independent role in some of these processes (Lin et al. 2007).

Non-Heme Iron Proteins

In addition to iron-sulfur clusters or heme-bound iron, proteins can directly bind iron molecules, primarily in the Fe^{2+} form. Non-heme iron protein contains either one or two iron molecules, and includes α-ketoglutarate (αKG)-dependent dioxygenases, which bind a single iron atom, or RNR, which has a di-iron center (Ryle and Hausinger 2002).

αKG-Dependent Dioxygenases

αKG-dependent dioxygenases are the major class of non-heme proteins that require Fe^{2+} as cofactor and use αKG decarboxylation for oxidizing C-H bonds into C-OH bonds (Fletcher and Coleman 2020; Baksh and Finley 2021). αKG-dependent dioxygenases can catalyze the hydroxylation of proteins, such as the hydroxylation of HIF-1/2α proteins by prolyl hydroxylases (PHDs). In addition to the well-known sensitivity of PHDs to $[O_2]$, these proteins can be sensitive to changes in iron levels or can be inhibited by metals that compete with iron, such as cobalt (Hewitson et al. 2002; Salnikow et al. 2004).

αKG-dependent dioxygenases can also target nucleotides for hydroxylation catalyzed by ten-eleven translocation (TET) enzymes (Kohli and Zhang 2013). Histone demethylation can also be catalyzed by αKG-dependent dioxygenases like Jumonji C (JmJC) domain-containing demethylases. (Fletcher and Coleman 2020).

αKG-Dependent Dioxygenases and Cancer

As αKG-dependent dioxygenases require iron and αKG, lack of either can inhibit their activity. Accumulation of metabolites or specific transition metals can compete with αKG or iron to block this activity, and is a common mechanism in transformation (Chen and Costa 2009; Xiao et al. 2012). For example, accumulation of fumarate and succinate underlies the tumor suppressive function of succinate dehydrogenase and fumarate hydratase in clear cell renal cell carcinoma (ccRCC), and fumarate accumulation promotes epithelial-to-mesenchymal transition (Xiao et al. 2012; Sciacovelli et al. 2016).

Epigenetic regulation via histone and DNA demethylation are also important factors in cancer progression. For example, TET enzymes catalyze the hydroxylation of 5-methylcystosine, ultimately resulting in demethylation. This function is frequently lost in cancers, as TET2 is commonly mutated in many myeloid malignancies (An et al. 2017). These TET2 mutations impair catalytic activity, potentially via disturbing TET2 binding to Fe^{2+} and αKG (Ko et al. 2010). Counterintuitively, recent evidence demonstrates that TET2 loss-of-function mutations, while increasing methylation in euchromatic regions, actually induce demethylation of heterochromatic regions, leading to the expression of normally silenced Alu retroviral elements and induction of inflammatory responses (López-Moyado et al. 2019). Iron availability can influence DNA methylation by regulating TET activity and altering epigenetic regulation in normal and malignant cells. Interestingly, treatment of AML cells with Vitamin C, a TET2 cofactor and electron donor that increases recycling of Fe^{3+} to Fe^{2+}, can restore TET2 activity in TET2-deficient leukemia models (Cimmino et al. 2017). Moreover, neomorphic mutations in genes encoding TCA enzymes IDH1 and IDH2 enhance the production of the oncometabolite 2-hydroxyglutarate, which inhibits αKG-dependent dioxygenases, including TET enzymes (Xu et al. 2011). Indeed, TET2 mutations and IDH1/2 mutations are mutually exclusive in AML, supporting their common function in transformation of myeloid cells (Figueroa et al. 2010).

Aside from DNA demethylation, histone demethylases regulate gene expression epigenetically and are mutated in various cancers (D'Oto et al. 2016). JmJC histone demethylases, such as JMJD2C, are implicated in oncogenic transformation in breast cancer (Cloos et al. 2006; Liu et al. 2009), while JMJD3 controls oncogenic genes and promotes initiation and maintenance of T-cell acute lymphoblastic leukemia (Ntziachristos et al. 2014).

HIF-1α activation is correlated strongly with metastasis, angiogenesis, and poor prognosis, and is a potential target in cancer therapy (Masoud and Li 2015). PHDs and factor-inhibiting HIF (FIH) require iron to regulate the activity of

HIF-1α and HIF-2α, in addition to being sensitive to oxygen concentration, which underlies their role as oxygen sensors (Hirota 2019). As such, iron deprivation or inhibition of PHDs (e.g., by cobalt) can induce HIF-1α stabilization and "pseudo-hypoxia." HIF-2α stabilization is commonly observed in ccRCC due to mutation of the von Hippel–Lindau (*VHL*) tumor suppressor, an E3 ligase subunit that normally targets HIFs for proteasomal degradation. Inhibitors of HIF-2α have recently been developed and have advanced to clinical trials in ccRCC (Chen et al. 2016; Cho et al. 2016). Coincidentally, HIF-2α is also regulated primarily by IRP1 in vivo, one example of the differential roles of IRPs (Anderson et al. 2013). This function of IRP1 enables iron levels to regulate erythropoiesis, as HIF-2α translational control by IRP1 in the kidney affects the expression of its target, erythropoietin.

Ribonucleotide Reductase and Cancer

RNR converts ribonucleotides to deoxyribonucleotides, substrates required for DNA synthesis and repair. The β-subunit of the RNR complex contains a di-iron binding site required to activate the α-subunit, which contains the catalytic site to reduce ribonucleotides (Gaur et al. 2021). Due to the iron dependency of the β-subunit, iron chelation can inhibit RNR activity (Sanvisens et al. 2011). Inhibition of RNR or replicative DNA polymerases, which contain iron–sulfur clusters, can explain why iron chelation blocks replication and S-phase progression (Sviderskiy et al. 2020).

Because proliferating cells require deoxyribonucleotides, RNR expression is essential for tumor growth and can be targeted for cancer treatment. The pyrimidine analog gemcitabine, widely used in treatment of ovarian, breast, lung, and pancreatic cancer, is converted intracellularly into gemcitabine diphosphate and triphosphate and incorporated into DNA to terminate DNA synthesis. Gemcitabine triphosphate is also a potent inhibitor of the RNR α-subunit (Mini et al. 2006). Clofarabine, a purine analog approved for acute lymphoblastic leukemia, also inhibits the RNR α-subunit as well as DNA polymerases (Aye et al. 2015). Hydroxyurea, a classic RNR inhibitor, targets the RNR β-subunit as a promiscuous metal chelator. Hydroxyurea historically has been used in treatment of chronic myelogenous leukemia and head and neck cancer, although its current clinical use in cancer is limited. (Akerblom et al. 1981).

COPPER

Copper is an essential cofactor in copper-dependent enzymes such as cytochrome *c* oxidase, the cytoplasmic superoxide dismutase (SOD1), and other oxygenase/oxidase enzymes. Similar to iron, the high redox potential of copper enables it to catalyze these reactions (Ge et al. 2022). Intracellular free copper is almost undetectable, and is estimated to be ~9 orders of magnitude lower than iron (Foster et al. 2014; Kaplan and Maryon 2016). As such, copper binding proteins and chaperones have exquisitely high affinity for copper, and proteins that bind iron intracellularly often have higher affinity for copper than iron. Like iron, copper is highly reactive and can be toxic in supraphysiological concentrations; however, this effect is likely due to mismetallation driven by Irving Williams series properties of copper (substitution of copper for other metals, like iron) resulting in the inhibition of iron-dependent processes, such as iron–sulfur cluster biosynthesis (Macomber and Imlay 2009; Garcia-Santamarina et al. 2017; Tan et al. 2017), although induction of ROS via the Fenton-like copper reactions has also been proposed as a mode of copper toxicity (Pham et al. 2013; Ge et al. 2022). Accordingly, copper availability is regulated at both the cellular and systemic level to maintain homeostasis.

Dietary copper is bound to intestinal mucin, which prevents copper toxicity and enables copper absorption mainly in the small intestines via copper transporter 1 (CTR1) (Nose et al. 2006; Reznik et al. 2022). Aside from its function in iron metabolism, DMT1 is recently reported to act as a Cu^{2+} importer as well (Pezacki et al. 2022). Absorbed copper is released to the bloodstream via ATP7A, and excess copper is stored in the liver by metallothioneins MT1 and MT2 (Luza and Speisky 1996; Kaler 2011). Copper in the liver can be released into the blood via ATP7B and binds to ceruloplasmin (Huster et al. 2006). Ceruloplasmin is a secreted oxidase protein that serves as the dedicated Cu delivery protein and transports it around the body (Linder 2016). Aside from ceruloplasmin, other proteins in the blood such as albumin can bind to copper to a lesser degree (Linder 2016). Excess copper can be excreted from the body via ATP7B to control systemic copper levels (Polishchuk et al. 2014). Most tissues uptake copper in reduced Cu^{1+} form via CTR1 potentially with metalloreductases like STEAP or in complex with glutathione (Kuo et al. 2001; Lee et al. 2002; Ge et al. 2022). Within the cell, metallochaperones facilitate transport of copper to target proteins (Ge et al. 2022). Together, these proteins maintain the optimal copper availability by regulating influx, efflux, and storage.

Copper and Cancer

Demand for copper is higher in cancer cells due to increased proliferation, and elevated serum copper levels are reported in people harboring breast, lung, gastrointestinal, prostate, thyroid, gallbladder, and oral cancer tumors (Ge et al. 2022). Although correlation exists between circulating copper levels and cancer occurrence, it is not clear whether tumors stimulate serum copper levels indirectly or directly, or whether elevated serum copper levels contribute to tumor initiation, growth, or metastasis. Wilson's disease patients accumulate copper primarily in the liver and brain due to mutations in *ATP7B*, where progressive tissue damage is observed (Tanzi et al. 1993). Although a high incidence of hepatocellular carcinoma is reported in animal models of Wilson's disease, the occurrence rate of hepatic cancer in a Wilson's disease patient is not elevated compared to the general population, suggesting that copper accumulation might not directly increase tumor formation in humans (Pfeiffenberger et al. 2015; Reed et al. 2018).

Copper metabolism alters various important processes in the cell and can promote tumor growth either directly or indirectly. Aside from its role in oxidative respiration, copper is involved in the activation of known oncogenic pathways such as the MAP kinase pathway via modulating MEK1/2 activity toward ERK (Tur-

ski et al. 2012; Brady et al. 2014). This activity has been best studied in *BRAF* mutation–driven melanoma and lung adenocarcinoma models where inhibition of MEK1/2 via copper chelation limits tumor growth and counters resistance to MEK or BRAF inhibitors (Brady et al. 2014). AKT, a commonly activated protein kinase in cancer, is reported to be activated via direct copper binding to PDK1 (Guo et al. 2021). Copper also regulates autophagic flux via its interaction with autophagic kinases ULK1 and ULK2, and thus can promote tumor growth in lung adenocarcinoma (Tsang et al. 2020). In orthotopic breast cancer models in mice, loss of ATP7A inhibited the activity of copper-dependent LOX and LOXL enzymes and inhibited tumor growth and metastasis (Shanbhag et al. 2019). Angiogenesis is an important factor in tumor progression, and copper promotes angiogenesis potentially via activation of angiogenic factors such as vascular endothelial growth factor (VEGF) (Xie and Kang 2009).

Tetrathiomolybdate, a copper chelator, progressed to a phase I trial due to its potential antiangiogenic activity (Brewer et al. 2000). A separate phase II trial in triple-negative breast cancer patients observed that copper depletion can alter the tumor microenvironment and decrease metastasis to the lung (Chan et al. 2017). These data suggest that copper depletion can indirectly influence metastasis by promoting a less receptive environment, in addition to its potential roles in modulating oxidative respiration, signaling, and autophagy in cancer cells themselves.

Similar to iron, induction of copper overload has been proposed as an anticancer strategy. Indeed, deletion of copper exporter *ATP7A* results in aberrant copper retention and is suggested as a potential vulnerability in *KRAS*-mutated colorectal cancer, which exhibits elevated autophagy and therefore increased acquisition of copper from extracellular protein (Aubert et al. 2020). Disulfiram, originally used as an alcohol aversion agent, has recently been repurposed to deliver copper to cancer cells. Disulfiram forms a complex with copper and is efficiently internalized, exerting an antitumorigenic effect (Lu et al. 2021). Disulfiram–copper complexes are well-tolerated and have antitumor effects in combination with other treatments in clinical trials (Nechushtan et al. 2015; Huang et al. 2016). Another copper-binding molecule, elesclomol, promotes a copper-dependent cell death in cells that exhibit increased dependence on oxidative phosphorylation (Tsvetkov et al. 2019). Elesclomol promotes intake of excess copper, which binds to lipoylated proteins leading to protein aggregation and cell death (Tsvetkov et al. 2022). The antitumor effect of elesclomol has been investigated in advanced-stage melanoma in combination with paclitaxel. Although well-tolerated, this combination therapy did not improve progression-free survival in a phase III study (O'Day et al. 2013).

SELENIUM

The metalloid selenium is an essential micronutrient used forming selenocysteine residues of at least 25 proteins in humans, called selenoproteins. Among selenoproteins, those with a known function have important roles in redox and thyroid metabolism, including five of the eight known glutathione peroxidases, thioredoxin reductases, methionine-R-sulfoxide reductase 1, and iodothyronine deodinases (Gladyshev et al. 2016).

Selenium is absorbed from the diet mainly in the form of selenomethionine that is randomly present in protein in place of methionine. Selenium levels in the body are mainly regulated via excretion of excess selenium (Hadrup and Ravn-Haren 2021). The liver acts as a selenium storage depot and regulates delivery of selenium to the rest of the body via secretion of selenium transport protein SELENOP (SEPP1) (Hill et al. 2012; Burk and Hill 2015). Selenomethionine or selenoproteins, such as Gpx1, can function as a reserve for selenium in the body. The selenocysteine residues of selenoproteins cannot be directly recycled to load tRNAs. They must first be converted to the intermediate selenide, which is incorporated in the selenocysteine biosynthesis pathway where selenocysteine-tRNA is synthesized from a specialized serine-tRNA precursor. Selenium either in selenomethionine form or in inorganic forms such as selenite must also first be converted to selenide then processed in the same manner. Selenocysteine is structurally similar to cysteine, replacing sulfur with selenium, with significantly different biochemical properties (Nauser et al. 2012).

Selenocysteine is incorporated into target selenoproteins by a complex co-translational machinery (Labunskyy et al. 2014). Briefly, mRNAs encoding selenoproteins contain a stem-loop structure in the 3′UTR, called a selenocysteine insertion sequence (SECIS), and an internal UGA codon at the selenocystine insertion site (UGA codons normally terminate translation) (Berry et al. 1993). Upon reaching the internal UGA codon, the selenocysteine tRNA inserts selenocysteine into the nascent protein via SECIS-binding protein 2 (SBP2) and selenocysteine-specific eukaryotic elongation factor (eEFSec) (Copeland and Driscoll 1999; Low et al. 2000).

Selenium and Cancer

Due to its role in redox metabolism, selenium may play a role in cancer progression via regulating ROS. Indeed, initial studies have shown a negative correlation between selenium exposure and risk of some cancer types, suggesting dietary selenium intake may have preventative effects on cancer (Whanger 2004). However, selenium supplementation failed to show any preventative effect against cancer risk in several randomized controlled trials, with potential negative side effects including a nonsignificant increased risk of type 2 diabetes mellitus (Lippman et al. 2009; Vinceti et al. 2018) The relationship between selenium exposure and cancer risk is ambiguous, as contradicting results from these studies can be interpreted differently based on cancer type, source of the selenium supplement, and study design (Radomska et al. 2021).

Nevertheless, increased selenium uptake was recognized decades ago as a tumor-specific feature (Cavalieri et al. 1966). Cancer cells can indirectly promote selenium uptake via the system xCT cystine–glutamate antiporter SLC7A11 (Carlisle et al. 2020). In this model, cystine imported by SLC7A11 is reduced to cysteine intracellularly and effluxed from the cell, where it can promote the reduction of extracellular selenite to selenide, a cell-permeable form of selenium. Increased selenium uptake and the subsequent increase in selenocysteine biosynthesis creates a cancer-specific requirement to detoxify products of selenium metabolism, such as selenide, dependent upon the selenophosphate synthetase 2 (SEPHS2) (Carlisle et al. 2020). Targeting this vulnerability has shown promise in preclinical breast cancer mouse models.

One of the most relevant selenoproteins to redox homeostasis is GPX4, which inhibits ferroptosis by selectively reducing phospholipid hydroperoxides (Friedmann Angeli et al. 2014; Yang et al. 2014). GPX4 is highly sensitive to selenium depletion, and modulation of dietary selenium levels are capable of modulating GPX4 protein levels in vivo (Lei et al. 1998). As there is evidence that ferroptosis is a barrier to transformation, identifying methods to target selenium metabolism or GPX4 might be directly beneficial for future cancer therapy (Chen et al. 2021).

CONCLUSION

Oncogenic transformation places a number of demands on metabolic and biosynthetic processes that are the object of multiple ongoing approaches to target cancer cells. Of these, altered redox homeostasis is a hallmark of cancer metabolism that is intimately linked to the cellular functions of iron, copper, and selenium. Approaches to target cancer by broadly eliminating these micronutrients from the diet or circulation have largely been unsuccessful due to a poor therapeutic window. However, a more sophisticated understanding of specific cancer-relevant processes that depend on these nutrients is beginning to come into view. Apart from direct targeting of proteins that contain iron, copper, and selenium such as RNR, MEK1/2, and GPX4, work to induce ferroptosis in cancer cells, or protect antitumor immune cells from oxidative damage, are among the most promising avenues of ongoing research. These future discoveries will be built on the understanding of the fundamental sensing, regulatory, and transport processes described here and amassed over decades.

ACKNOWLEDGMENTS

We thank Dohoon Kim and Donita Brady for their critical reading of this manuscript.

REFERENCES

Addess KJ, Basilion JP, Klausner RD, Rouault TA, Pardi A. 1997. Structure and dynamics of the iron responsive element RNA: implications for binding of the RNA by iron regulatory binding proteins. *J Mol Biol* 274: 72–83. doi:10.1006/jmbi.1997.1377

Aisen P, Leibman A, Zweier J. 1978. Stoichiometric and site characteristics of the binding of iron to human transferrin. *J Biol Chem* 253: 1930–1937. doi:10.1016/S0021-9258(19)62337-9

Ajioka RS, Phillips JD, Kushner JP. 2006. Biosynthesis of heme in mammals. *Biochim Biophys Acta* 1763: 723–736. doi:10.1016/j.bbamcr.2006.05.005

Ajoolabady A, Aslkhodapasandhokmabad H, Libby P, Tuomilehto J, Lip GYH, Penninger JM, Richardson DR, Tang D, Zhou H, Wang S, et al. 2021. Ferritinophagy and ferroptosis in the management of metabolic diseases. *Trends Endocrinol Metab* 32: 444–462. doi:10.1016/j.tem.2021.04.010

Akerblom L, Ehrenberg A, Gräslund A, Lankinen H, Reichard P, Thelander L. 1981. Overproduction of the free radical of ribonucleotide reductase in hydroxyurea-resistant mouse fibroblast 3T6 cells. *Proc Natl Acad Sci* 78: 2159–2163. doi:10.1073/pnas.78.4.2159

Alfonso-Prieto M, Biarnés X, Vidossich P, Rovira C. 2009. The molecular mechanism of the catalase reaction. *J Am Chen Soc* 131: 11751–11761. doi:10.1021/ja9018572

Alkhateeb AA, Connor JR. 2010. Nuclear ferritin: a new role for ferritin in cell biology. *Biochim Biophys Acta* 1800: 793–797. doi:10.1016/j.bbagen.2010.03.017

Alkhateeb AA, Connor JR. 2013. The significance of ferritin in cancer: anti-oxidation, inflammation and tumorigenesis. *Biochim Biophys Acta* 1836: 245–254.

Alvarez SW, Sviderskiy VO, Terzi EM, Papagiannakopoulos T, Moreira AL, Adams S, Sabatini DM, Birsoy K, Possemato R. 2017. NFS1 undergoes positive selection in lung tumours and protects cells from ferroptosis. *Nature* 551: 639–643. doi:10.1038/nature24637

An J, Rao A, Ko M. 2017. TET family dioxygenases and DNA demethylation in stem cells and cancers. *Exp Mol Med* 49: e323. doi:10.1038/emm.2017.5

Anderson SA, Nizzi CP, Chang YI, Deck KM, Schmidt PJ, Galy B, Damnernsawad A, Broman AT, Kendziorski C, Hentze MW, et al. 2013. The IRP1-HIF-2α axis coordinates iron and oxygen sensing with erythropoiesis and iron absorption. *Cell Metab* 17: 282–290. doi:10.1016/j.cmet.2013.01.007

Andriopoulos B, Corradini E, Xia Y, Faasse SA, Chen S, Grgurevic L, Knutson MD, Pietrangelo A, Vukicevic S, Lin HY, et al. 2009. BMP6 is a key endogenous regulator of hepcidin expression and iron metabolism. *Nat Genet* 41: 482–487. doi:10.1038/ng.335

Arosio P, Elia L, Poli M. 2017. Ferritin, cellular iron storage and regulation. *IUBMB Life* 69: 414–422. doi:10.1002/iub.1621

Aubert L, Nandagopal N, Steinhart Z, Lavoie G, Nourreddine S, Berman J, Saba-El-Leil MK, Papadopoli D, Lin S, Hart T, et al. 2020. Copper bioavailability is a KRAS-specific vulnerability in colorectal cancer. *Nat Commun* 11: 3701. doi:10.1038/s41467-020-17549-y

Cite this article as *Cold Spring Harb Perspect Med* doi: 10.1101/cshperspect.a041545

Aye Y, Long MJC, Stubbe J. 2012. Mechanistic studies of semicarbazone triapine targeting human ribonucleotide reductase in vitro and in mammalian cells: tyrosyl radical quenching not involving reactive oxygen species. *J Biol Chem* **287:** 35768–35778. doi:10.1074/jbc.M112.396911

Aye Y, Li M, Long MJC, Weiss RS. 2015. Ribonucleotide reductase and cancer: biological mechanisms and targeted therapies. *Oncogene* **34:** 2011–2021. doi:10.1038/onc.2014.155

Aziz N, Munro HN. 1987. Iron regulates ferritin mRNA translation through a segment of its 5′ untranslated region. *Proc Natl Acad Sci* **84:** 8478–8482. doi:10.1073/pnas.84.23.8478

Baksh SC, Finley LWS. 2021. Metabolic coordination of cell fate by α-ketoglutarate-dependent dioxygenases. *Trends Cell Biol* **31:** 24–36. doi:10.1016/j.tcb.2020.09.010

Belotti A, Duca L, Borin L, Realini S, Renso R, Parma M, Pioltelli P, Pogliani E, Cappellini MD. 2015. Non transferrin bound iron (NTBI) in acute leukemias throughout conventional intensive chemotherapy: kinetics of its appearance and potential predictive role in infectious complications. *Leuk Res* **39:** 88–91. doi:10.1016/j.leukres.2014.11.003

Berry MJ, Banu L, Harney JW, Larsen PR. 1993. Functional characterization of the eukaryotic SECIS elements which direct selenocysteine insertion at UGA codons. *EMBO J* **12:** 3315–3322. doi:10.1002/j.1460-2075.1993.tb06001.x

Bhurosy T, Jishan A, Boland PM, Lee YH, Heckman CJ. 2022. Underdiagnosis of iron deficiency anemia among patients with colorectal cancer: an examination of electronic medical records. *BMC Cancer* **22:** 435. doi:10.1186/s12885-022-09542-z

Brady DC, Crowe MS, Turski ML, Hobbs GA, Yao X, Chaikuad A, Knapp S, Xiao K, Campbell SL, Thiele DJ, et al. 2014. Copper is required for oncogenic BRAF signalling and tumorigenesis. *Nature* **509:** 492–496. doi:10.1038/nature13180

Braymer JJ, Lill R. 2017. Iron–sulfur cluster biogenesis and trafficking in mitochondria. *J Biol Chem* **292:** 12754–12763. doi:10.1074/jbc.R117.787101

Brewer GJ, Dick RD, Grover DK, LeClaire V, Tseng M, Wicha M, Pienta K, Redman BG, Jahan T, Sondak VK, et al. 2000. Treatment of metastatic cancer with tetrathiomolybdate, an anticopper, antiangiogenic agent: phase I study. *Clin Cancer Res* **6:** 1–10.

Brissot P, Ropert M, Le Lan C, Loréal O. 2012. Non-transferrin bound iron: a key role in iron overload and iron toxicity. *Biochim Biophys Acta* **1820:** 403–410. doi:10.1016/j.bbagen.2011.07.014

Brown JA, Yonekubo Y, Hanson N, Sastre-Perona A, Basin A, Rytlewski JA, Dolgalev I, Meehan S, Tsirigos A, Beronja S, et al. 2017. TGF-β-induced quiescence mediates chemoresistance of tumor-propagating cells in squamous cell carcinoma. *Cell Stem Cell* **21:** 650–664.e8. doi:10.1016/j.stem.2017.10.001

Buranrat B, Connor JR. 2015. Cytoprotective effects of ferritin on doxorubicin-induced breast cancer cell death. *Oncol Rep* **34:** 2790–2796. doi:10.3892/or.2015.4250

Burk RF, Hill KE. 2015. Regulation of selenium metabolism and transport. *Annu Rev Nutr* **35:** 109–134. doi:10.1146/annurev-nutr-071714-034250

Callens C, Coulon S, Naudin J, Radford-Weiss I, Boissel N, Raffoux E, Wang PHM, Agarwal S, Tamouza H, Paubelle E, et al. 2010. Targeting iron homeostasis induces cellular differentiation and synergizes with differentiating agents in acute myeloid leukemia. *J Exp Med* **207:** 731–750. doi:10.1084/jem.20091488

Calzolari A, Oliviero I, Deaglio S, Mariani G, Biffoni M, Sposi NM, Malavasi F, Peschle C, Testa U. 2007. Transferrin receptor 2 is frequently expressed in human cancer cell lines. *Blood Cells Mol Dis* **39:** 82–91. doi:10.1016/j.bcmd.2007.02.003

Candelaria PV, Leoh LS, Penichet ML, Daniels-Wells TR. 2021. Antibodies targeting the transferrin receptor 1 (TfR1) as direct anti-cancer agents. *Front Immunol* **12:** 607692. doi:10.3389/fimmu.2021.607692

Carlisle AE, Lee N, Matthew-Onabanjo AN, Spears ME, Park SJ, Youkana D, Doshi MB, Peppers A, Li R, Joseph AB, et al. 2020. Selenium detoxification is required for cancer-cell survival. *Nat Metab* **2:** 603–611. doi:10.1038/s42255-020-0224-7

Cavalieri RR, Scott KG, Sairenji E. 1966. Selenite (75Se) as a tumor-localizing agent in man. *J Nucl Med* **7:** 197–208.

Chan KT, Choi MY, Lai KK, Tan W, Tung LN, Lam HY, Tong DK, Lee NP, Law S. 2014. Overexpression of transferrin receptor CD71 and its tumorigenic properties in esophageal squamous cell carcinoma. *Oncol Rep* **31:** 1296–1304. doi:10.3892/or.2014.2981

Chan N, Willis A, Kornhauser N, Ward MM, Lee SB, Nackos E, Seo BR, Chuang E, Cigler T, Moore A, et al. 2017. Influencing the tumor microenvironment: a phase II study of copper depletion using tetrathiomolybdate in patients with breast cancer at high risk for recurrence and in preclinical models of lung metastases. *Clin Cancer Res* **23:** 666–676. doi:10.1158/1078-0432.CCR-16-1326

Chen H, Costa M. 2009. Iron- and 2-oxoglutarate-dependent dioxygenases: an emerging group of molecular targets for nickel toxicity and carcinogenicity. *Biometals* **22:** 191–196. doi:10.1007/s10534-008-9190-3

Chen W, Hill H, Christie A, Kim MS, Holloman E, Pavia-Jimenez A, Homayoun F, Ma Y, Patel N, Yell P, et al. 2016. Targeting renal cell carcinoma with a HIF-2 antagonist. *Nature* **539:** 112–117. doi:10.1038/nature19796

Chen X, Kang R, Kroemer G, Tang D. 2021. Broadening horizons: the role of ferroptosis in cancer. *Nat Rev Clin Oncol* **18:** 280–296. doi:10.1038/s41571-020-00462-0

Chiabrando D, Vinchi F, Fiorito V, Mercurio S, Tolosano E. 2014. Heme in pathophysiology: a matter of scavenging, metabolism and trafficking across cell membranes. *Front Pharmacol* **5:** 61. doi:10.3389/fphar.2014.00061

Cho H, Du X, Rizzi JP, Liberzon E, Chakraborty AA, Gao W, Carvo I, Signoretti S, Bruick RK, Josey JA, et al. 2016. On-target efficacy of a HIF-2α antagonist in preclinical kidney cancer models. *Nature* **539:** 107–111. doi:10.1038/nature19795

Cimmino L, Dolgalev I, Wang Y, Yoshimi A, Martin GH, Wang J, Ng V, Xia B, Witkowski MT, Mitchell-Flack M, et al. 2017. Restoration of TET2 function blocks aberrant self-renewal and leukemia progression. *Cell* **170:** 1079–1095.e20. doi:10.1016/j.cell.2017.07.032

Cloos PAC, Christensen J, Agger K, Maiolica A, Rappsilber J, Antal T, Hansen KH, Helin K. 2006. The putative oncogene GASC1 demethylates tri- and dimethylated lysine 9

on histone H3. *Nature* **442:** 307–311. doi:10.1038/na
ture04837

Copeland PR, Driscoll DM. 1999. Purification, redox sensitivity, and RNA binding properties of SECIS-binding protein 2, a protein involved in selenoprotein biosynthesis. *J
Biol Chem* **274:** 25447–25454. doi:10.1074/jbc.274.36
.25447

Cox TC, Bawden MJ, Martin A, May BK. 1991. Human
erythroid 5-aminolevulinate synthase: promoter analysis and identification of an iron-responsive element in
the mRNA. *EMBO J* **10:** 1891–1902. doi:10.1002/j.1460-
2075.1991.tb07715.x

Dailey HA, Finnegan MG, Johnson MK. 1994. Human ferrochelatase is an iron-sulfur protein. *Biochemistry* **33:**
403–407. doi:10.1021/bi00168a003

Dandekar T, Stripecke R, Gray NK, Goossen B, Constable A,
Johansson HE, Hentze MW. 1991. Identification of a novel iron-responsive element in murine and human erythroid δ-aminolevulinic acid synthase mRNA. *EMBO J*
10: 1903–1909. doi:10.1002/j.1460-2075.1991.tb07716.x

Daniels TR, Ortiz-Sánchez E, Luria-Pérez R, Quintero R,
Helguera G, Bonavida B, Martínez-Maza O, Penichet
ML. 2011. An antibody-based multifaceted approach tar-
geting the human transferrin receptor for the treatment of
B-cell malignancies. *J Immunother* **34:** 500–508. doi:10
.1097/CJI.0b013e318222ffc8

Daniels TR, Bernabeu E, Rodríguez JA, Patel S, Kozman M,
Chiappetta DA, Holler E, Ljubimova JY, Helguera G,
Penichet ML. 2012. The transferrin receptor and the targeted delivery of therapeutic agents against cancer. *Biochim Biophys Acta* **1820:** 291–317. doi:10.1016/j.bbagen
.2011.07.016

Dautry-Varsat A, Ciechanover A, Lodish HF. 1983. pH and
the recycling of transferrin during receptor-mediated endocytosis. *Proc Natl Acad Sci* **80:** 2258–2262. doi:10.1073/
pnas.80.8.2258

Deshmukh P, Unni S, Krishnappa G, Padmanabhan B. 2017.
The Keap1-Nrf2 pathway: promising therapeutic target to
counteract ROS-mediated damage in cancers and neuro-
degenerative diseases. *Biophys Rev* **9:** 41–56. doi:10.1007/
s12551-016-0244-4

Dinh HQ, Eggert T, Meyer MA, Zhu YP, Olingy CE, Llewel-
lyn R, Wu R, Hedrick CC. 2020. Coexpression of CD71
and CD117 identifies an early unipotent neutrophil progenitor population in human bone marrow. *Immunity* **53:**
319–334.e6. doi:10.1016/j.immuni.2020.07.017

Donfrancesco A, Deb G, Dominici C, Pileggi D, Castello
MA, Helson L. 1990. Effects of a single course of deferoxamine in neuroblastoma patients. *Cancer Res* **50:** 4929–
4930.

Donovan A, Lima CA, Pinkus JL, Pinkus GS, Zon LI, Robine
S, Andrews NC. 2005. The iron exporter ferroportin/
Slc40a1 is essential for iron homeostasis. *Cell Metab* **1:**
191–200. doi:10.1016/j.cmet.2005.01.003

D'Oto A, Tian QW, Davidoff AM, Yang J. 2016. Histone
demethylases and their roles in cancer epigenetics. *J
Med Oncol Ther* **1:** 34–40.

Drakesmith H, Nemeth E, Ganz T. 2015. Ironing out ferroportin. *Cell Metab* **22:** 777–787. doi:10.1016/j.cmet.2015
.09.006

Dreicer R, Kemp JD, Stegink LD, Cardillo T, Davis CS, Forest
PK, See WA. 1997. A phase II trial of deferoxamine in

patients with hormone-refractory metastatic prostate cancer. *Cancer Invest* **15:** 311–317. doi:10.3109/0735790970
9039731

Elmberg M, Hultcrantz R, Ekbom A, Brandt L, Olsson S,
Olsson R, Lindgren S, Lööf L, Stål P, Wallerstedt S, et al.
2003. Cancer risk in patients with hereditary hemochromatosis and in their first-degree relatives. *Gastroenterology* **125:** 1733–1741. doi:10.1053/j.gastro.2003.09.035

Estrov Z, Tawa A, Wang XH, Dubé ID, Sulh H, Cohen A,
Gelfand EW, Freedman MH. 1987. In vitro and in vivo
effects of deferoxamine in neonatal acute leukemia. *Blood*
69: 757–761. doi:10.1182/blood.V69.3.757.757

Figueroa ME, Abdel-Wahab O, Lu C, Ward PS, Patel J, Shih
A, Li Y, Bhagwat N, Vasanthakumar A, Fernandez HF, et
al. 2010. Leukemic IDH1 and IDH2 mutations result in a
hypermethylation phenotype, disrupt TET2 function,
and impair hematopoietic differentiation. *Cancer Cell*
18: 553–567. doi:10.1016/j.ccr.2010.11.015

Fiorito V, Chiabrando D, Petrillo S, Bertino F, Tolosano E.
2020. The multifaceted role of heme in cancer. *Front Oncol* **9:** 1540. doi:10.3389/fonc.2019.01540

Fletcher SC, Coleman ML. 2020. Human 2-oxoglutarate-de-
pendent oxygenases: nutrient sensors, stress responders,
and disease mediators. *Biochem Soc Trans* **48:** 1843–1858.
doi:10.1042/BST20190333

Fonseca-Nunes A, Jakszyn P, Agudo A. 2014. Iron and cancer risk—a systematic review and meta-analysis of the
epidemiological evidence. *Cancer Epidemiol Biomarkers
Prev* **23:** 12–31. doi:10.1158/1055-9965.EPI-13-0733

Forejtniková H, Vieillevoye M, Zermati Y, Lambert M, Pelle-
grino RM, Guihard S, Gaudry M, Camaschella C, La-
combe C, Roetto A, et al. 2010. Transferrin receptor 2 is
a component of the erythropoietin receptor complex and
is required for efficient erythropoiesis. *Blood* **116:** 5357–
5367. doi:10.1182/blood-2010-04-281360

Foster AW, Osman D, Robinson NJ. 2014. Metal preferences
and metallation. *J Biol Chem* **289:** 28095–28103. doi:10
.1074/jbc.R114.588145

Friedmann Angeli JP, Schneider M, Proneth B, Tyurina YY,
Tyurin VA, Hammond VJ, Herbach N, Aichler M, Walch
A, Eggenhofer E, et al. 2014. Inactivation of the ferropto-
sis regulator Gpx4 triggers acute renal failure in mice. *Nat
Cell Biol* **16:** 1180–1191. doi:10.1038/ncb3064

Ganz T. 2009. Iron in innate immunity: starve the invaders.
Curr Opin Immunol **21:** 63–67. doi:10.1016/j.coi.2009.01
.011

Ganz T. 2011. Hepcidin and iron regulation, 10 years
later. *Blood* **117:** 4425–4433. doi:10.1182/blood-2011-
01-258467

Ganz T. 2013. Systemic iron homeostasis. *Physiol Rev* **93:**
1721–1741. doi:10.1152/physrev.00008.2013

Gao M, Monian P, Pan Q, Zhang W, Xiang J, Jiang X. 2016.
Ferroptosis is an autophagic cell death process. *Cell Res*
26: 1021–1032. doi:10.1038/cr.2016.95

Garcia-Santamarina S, Uzarska MA, Festa RA, Lill R, Thiele
DJ. 2017. Cryptococcus neoformans iron-sulfur protein
biogenesis machinery is a novel layer of protection against
Cu stress. *MBio* **8:** e01742-17. doi:10.1128/mBio.01742-
17

Gaur K, Pérez Otero SC, Benjamín-Rivera JA, Rodríguez I,
Loza-Rosas SA, Vázquez Salgado AM, Akam EA, Her-

nández-Matias L, Sharma RK, Alicea N, et al. 2021. Iron chelator transmetalative approach to inhibit human ribonucleotide reductase. *JACS Au* **1**: 865–878. doi:10.1021/jacsau.1c00078

Ge EJ, Bush AI, Casini A, Cobine PA, Cross JR, DeNicola GM, Dou QP, Franz KJ, Gohil VM, Gupta S, et al. 2022. Connecting copper and cancer: from transition metal signalling to metalloplasia. *Nat Rev Cancer* **22**: 102–113. doi:10.1038/s41568-021-00417-2

Gilreath JA, Stenehjem DD, Rodgers GM. 2014. Diagnosis and treatment of cancer-related anemia. *Am J Hematol* **89**: 203–212. doi:10.1002/ajh.23628

Gladyshev VN, Arnér ES, Berry MJ, Brigelius-Flohé R, Bruford EA, Burk RF, Carlson BA, Castellano S, Chavatte L, Conrad M, et al. 2016. Selenoprotein gene nomenclature. *J Biol Chem* **291**: 24036–24040. doi:10.1074/jbc.M116.756155

Gunshin H, Allerson CR, Polycarpou-Schwarz M, Rofts A, Rogers JT, Kishi F, Hentze MW, Rouault TA, Andrews NC, Hediger MA. 2001. Iron-dependent regulation of the divalent metal ion transporter. *FEBS Lett* **509**: 309–316. doi:10.1016/S0014-5793(01)03189-1

Guo J, Cheng J, Zheng N, Zhang X, Dai X, Zhang L, Hu C, Wu X, Jiang Q, Wu D, et al. 2021. Copper promotes tumorigenesis by activating the PDK1-AKT oncogenic pathway in a copper transporter 1 dependent manner. *Adv Sci (Weinh)* **8**: e2004303. doi:10.1002/advs.202004303

Habashy HO, Powe DG, Staka CM, Rakha EA, Ball G, Green AR, Aleskandarany M, Paish EC, Douglas Macmillan R, Nicholson RI, et al. 2010. Transferrin receptor (CD71) is a marker of poor prognosis in breast cancer and can predict response to tamoxifen. *Breast Cancer Res Treat* **119**: 283–293. doi:10.1007/s10549-009-0345-x

Hadrup N, Ravn-Haren G. 2021. Absorption, distribution, metabolism and excretion (ADME) of oral selenium from organic and inorganic sources: a review. *J Trace Elem Med Biol* **67**: 126801. doi:10.1016/j.jtemb.2021.126801

Harrison PM, Arosio P. 1996. The ferritins: molecular properties, iron storage function and cellular regulation. *Biochim Biophys Acta* **1275**: 161–203. doi:10.1016/0005-2728(96)00022-9

Hasan M, Reddy SM, Das NK. 2020. Ferritinophagy is not required for colon cancer cell growth. *Cell Biol Int* **44**: 2307–2314. doi:10.1002/cbin.11439

Hazard JT, Drysdale JW. 1977. Ferritinaemia in cancer. *Nature* **265**: 755–756. doi:10.1038/265755a0

Hentze MW, Caughman SW, Rouault TA, Barriocanal JG, Dancis A, Harford JB, Klausner RD. 1987. Identification of the iron-responsive element for the translational regulation of human ferritin mRNA. *Science* **238**: 1570–1573. doi:10.1126/science.3685996

Hentze MW, Muckenthaler MU, Galy B, Camaschella C. 2010. Two to tango: regulation of mammalian iron metabolism. *Cell* **142**: 24–38. doi:10.1016/j.cell.2010.06.028

Hewitson KS, McNeill LA, Riordan MV, Tian YM, Bullock AN, Welford RW, Elkins JM, Oldham NJ, Bhattacharya S, Gleadle JM, et al. 2002. Hypoxia-inducible factor (HIF) asparagine hydroxylase is identical to factor inhibiting HIF (FIH) and is related to the cupin structural family. *J Biol Chem* **277**: 26351–26355. doi:10.1074/jbc.C200273200

Hill KE, Wu S, Motley AK, Stevenson TD, Winfrey VP, Capecchi MR, Atkins JF, Burk RF. 2012. Production of selenoprotein P (Sepp1) by hepatocytes is central to selenium homeostasis. *J Biol Chem* **287**: 40414–40424. doi:10.1074/jbc.M112.421404

Hirota K. 2019. An intimate crosstalk between iron homeostasis and oxygen metabolism regulated by the hypoxia-inducible factors (HIFs). *Free Radic Biol Med* **133**: 118–129. doi:10.1016/j.freeradbiomed.2018.07.018

Hou W, Xie Y, Song X, Sun X, Lotze MT, Zeh HJ III, Kang R, Tang D. 2016. Autophagy promotes ferroptosis by degradation of ferritin. *Autophagy* **12**: 1425–1428. doi:10.1080/15548627.2016.1187366

Huang J, Campian JL, Gujar AD, Tran DD, Lockhart AC, DeWees TA, Tsien CI, Kim AH. 2016. A phase I study to repurpose disulfiram in combination with temozolomide to treat newly diagnosed glioblastoma after chemoradiotherapy. *J Neurooncol* **128**: 259–266. doi:10.1007/s11060-016-2104-2

Huster D, Finegold MJ, Morgan CT, Burkhead JL, Nixon R, Vanderwerf SM, Gilliam CT, Lutsenko S. 2006. Consequences of copper accumulation in the livers of the *Atp7b⁻/⁻* (Wilson disease gene) knockout mice. *Am J Pathol* **168**: 423–434. doi:10.2353/ajpath.2006.050312

Ibrahim O, O'Sullivan J. 2020. Iron chelators in cancer therapy. *Biometals* **33**: 201–215. doi:10.1007/s10534-020-00243-3

Imlay JA. 2006. Iron–sulphur clusters and the problem with oxygen. *Mol Microbiol* **59**: 1073–1082. doi:10.1111/j.1365-2958.2006.05028.x

Jeong SM, Lee J, Finley LWS, Schmidt PJ, Fleming MD, Haigis MC. 2015. SIRT3 regulates cellular iron metabolism and cancer growth by repressing iron regulatory protein 1. *Oncogene* **34**: 2115–2124. doi:10.1038/onc.2014.124

Kaler SG. 2011. ATP7A-related copper transport diseases—emerging concepts and future trends. *Nat Rev Neurol* **7**: 15–29. doi:10.1038/nrneurol.2010.180

Kapitsinou PP, Liu Q, Unger TL, Rha J, Davidoff O, Keith B, Epstein JA, Moores SL, Erickson-Miller CL, Haase VH. 2010. Hepatic HIF-2 regulates erythropoietic responses to hypoxia in renal anemia. *Blood* **116**: 3039–3048. doi:10.1182/blood-2010-02-270322

Kaplan JH, Maryon EB. 2016. How mammalian cells acquire copper: an essential but potentially toxic metal. *Biophys J* **110**: 7–13. doi:10.1016/j.bpj.2015.11.025

Kautz L, Meynard D, Monnier A, Darnaud V, Bouvet R, Wang RH, Deng C, Vaulont S, Mosser J, Coppin H, et al. 2008. Iron regulates phosphorylation of Smad1/5/8 and gene expression of Bmp6, Smad7, Id1, and Atoh8 in the mouse liver. *Blood* **112**: 1503–1509. doi:10.1182/blood-2008-03-143354

Kautz L, Jung G, Valore EV, Rivella S, Nemeth E, Ganz T. 2014. Identification of erythroferrone as an erythroid regulator of iron metabolism. *Nat Genet* **46**: 678–684. doi:10.1038/ng.2996

Kerins MJ, Ooi A. 2018. The roles of NRF2 in modulating cellular iron homeostasis. *Antioxid Redox Signal* **29**: 1756–1773. doi:10.1089/ars.2017.7176

Kikuchi G, Yoshida T, Noguchi M. 2005. Heme oxygenase and heme degradation. *Biochem Biophys Res Commun* **338**: 558–567. doi:10.1016/j.bbrc.2005.08.020

Kim HJ, Khalimonchuk O, Smith PM, Winge DR. 2012. Structure, function, and assembly of heme centers in mitochondrial respiratory complexes. *Biochim BIophys Acta* **1823:** 1604–1616. doi:10.1016/j.bbamcr.2012.04.008

Kim A, Rivera S, Shprung D, Limbrick D, Gabayan V, Nemeth E, Ganz T. 2014. Mouse models of anemia of cancer. *PLoS ONE* **9:** e93283. doi:10.1371/journal.pone.0093283

Kleven MD, Jue S, Enns CA. 2018. Transferrin receptors TfR1 and TfR2 bind transferrin through differing mechanisms. *Biochemistry* **57:** 1552–1559. doi:10.1021/acs.biochem.8b00006

Knox JJ, Hotte SJ, Kollmannsberger C, Winquist E, Fisher B, Eisenhauer EA. 2007. Phase II study of Triapine in patients with metastatic renal cell carcinoma: a trial of the national cancer institute of Canada clinical trials group (NCIC IND.161). *Invest New Drugs* **25:** 471–477. doi:10.1007/s10637-007-9044-9

Ko M, Huang Y, Jankowska AM, Pape UJ, Tahiliani M, Bandukwala HS, An J, Lamperti ED, Koh KP, Ganetzky R, et al. 2010. Impaired hydroxylation of 5-methylcytosine in myeloid cancers with mutant TET2. *Nature* **468:** 839–843. doi:10.1038/nature09586

Koeller DM, Casey JL, Hentze MW, Gerhardt EM, Chan LN, Klausner RD, Harford JB. 1989. A cytosolic protein binds to structural elements within the iron regulatory region of the transferrin receptor mRNA. *Proc Natl Acad Sci* **86:** 3574–3578. doi:10.1073/pnas.86.10.3574

Kohgo Y, Ikuta K, Ohtake T, Torimoto Y, Kato J. 2008. Body iron metabolism and pathophysiology of iron overload. *Int J Hematol* **88:** 7–15. doi:10.1007/s12185-008-0120-5

Kohli RM, Zhang Y. 2013. TET enzymes, TDG and the dynamics of DNA demethylation. *Nature* **502:** 472–479. doi:10.1038/nature12750

Korolnek T, Hamza I. 2015. Macrophages and iron trafficking at the birth and death of red cells. *Blood* **125:** 2893–2897. doi:10.1182/blood-2014-12-567776

Kumari N, Dwarakanath BS, Das A, Bhatt AN. 2016. Role of interleukin-6 in cancer progression and therapeutic resistance. *Tumor Biol* **37:** 11553–11572. doi:10.1007/s13277-016-5098-7

Kuo YM, Zhou B, Cosco D, Gitschier J. 2001. The copper transporter CTR1 provides an essential function in mammalian embryonic development. *Proc Natl Acad Sci* **98:** 6836–6841. doi:10.1073/pnas.111057298

Labunskyy VM, Hatfield DL, Gladyshev VN. 2014. Selenoproteins: molecular pathways and physiological roles. *Physiol Rev* **94:** 739–777. doi:10.1152/physrev.00039.2013

Lakadamyali M, Rust MJ, Zhuang X. 2006. Ligands for clathrin-mediated endocytosis are differentially sorted into distinct populations of early endosomes. *Cell* **124:** 997–1009. doi:10.1016/j.cell.2005.12.038

Lambert LA. 2012. Molecular evolution of the transferrin family and associated receptors. *Biochim Biophys Acta Gen Subj* **1820:** 244–255. doi:10.1016/j.bbagen.2011.06.002

Lee J, Peña MM, Nose Y, Thiele DJ. 2002. Biochemical characterization of the human copper transporter Ctr1. *J Biol Chem* **277:** 4380–4387. doi:10.1074/jbc.M104728200

Lee P, Peng H, Gelbart T, Wang L, Beutler E. 2005. Regulation of hepcidin transcription by interleukin-1 and interleukin-6. *Proc Natl Acad Sci* **102:** 1906–1910. doi:10.1073/pnas.0409808102

Lei XG, Dann HM, Ross DA, Cheng WH, Combs GF Jr, Roneker KR. 1998. Dietary selenium supplementation is required to support full expression of three selenium-dependent glutathione peroxidases in various tissues of weanling pigs. *J Nutr* **128:** 130–135. doi:10.1093/jn/128.1.130

Levi S, Luzzago A, Cesareni G, Cozzi A, Franceschinelli F, Albertini A, Arosio P. 1988. Mechanism of ferritin iron uptake: activity of the H-chain and deletion mapping of the ferro-oxidase site. A study of iron uptake and ferro-oxidase activity of human liver, recombinant H-chain ferritins, and of two H-chain deletion mutants. *J Biol Chem* **263:** 18086–18092. doi:10.1016/S0021-9258(19)81326-1

Lignitto L, LeBoeuf SE, Homer H, Jiang S, Askenazi M, Karakousi TR, Pass HI, Bhutkar AJ, Tsirigos A, Ueberheide B, et al. 2019. Nrf2 activation promotes lung cancer metastasis by inhibiting the degradation of Bach1. *Cell* **178:** 316–329.e18. doi:10.1016/j.cell.2019.06.003

Lin Q, Weis S, Yang G, Weng YH, Helston R, Rish K, Smith A, Bordner J, Polte T, Gaunitz F, et al. 2007. Heme oxygenase-1 protein localizes to the nucleus and activates transcription factors important in oxidative stress. *J Biol Chem* **282:** 20621–20633. doi:10.1074/jbc.M607954200

Linder MC. 2016. Ceruloplasmin and other copper binding components of blood plasma and their functions: an update. *Metallomics* **8:** 887–905. doi:10.1039/C6MT00103C

Lippman SM, Klein EA, Goodman PJ, Lucia MS, Thompson IM, Ford LG, Parnes HL, Minasian LM, Gaziano JM, Hartline JA, et al. 2009. Effect of selenium and vitamin E on risk of prostate cancer and other cancers: the selenium and vitamin E cancer prevention trial (SELECT). *J Am Med Assoc* **301:** 39–51. doi:10.1001/jama.2008.864

Liu XB, Hill P, Haile DJ. 2002. Role of the ferroportin iron-responsive element in iron and nitric oxide dependent gene regulation. *Blood Cells Mol Dis* **29:** 315–326. doi:10.1006/bcmd.2002.0572

Liu G, Bollig-Fischer A, Kreike B, van de Vijver MJ, Abrams J, Ethier SP, Yang ZQ. 2009. Genomic amplification and oncogenic properties of the GASC1 histone demethylase gene in breast cancer. *Oncogene* **28:** 4491–4500. doi:10.1038/onc.2009.297

Liuzzi JP, Aydemir F, Nam H, Knutson MD, Cousins RJ. 2006. Zip14 (Slc39a14) mediates non-transferrin-bound iron uptake into cells. *Proc Natl Acad Sci* **103:** 13612–13617. doi:10.1073/pnas.0606424103

López-Moyado IF, Tsagaratou A, Yuita H, Seo H, Delatte B, Heinz S, Benner C, Rao A. 2019. Paradoxical association of TET loss of function with genome-wide DNA hypomethylation. *Proc Natl Acad Sci* **116:** 16933–16942. doi:10.1073/pnas.1903059116

Low SC, Grundner-Culemann E, Harney JW, Berry MJ. 2000. SECIS–SBP2 interactions dictate selenocysteine incorporation efficiency and selenoprotein hierarchy. *EMBO J* **19:** 6882–6890. doi:10.1093/emboj/19.24.6882

Lu C, Li X, Ren Y, Zhang X. 2021. Disulfiram: a novel repurposed drug for cancer therapy. *Cancer Chemother Pharmacol* **87:** 159–172. doi:10.1007/s00280-020-04216-8

Lui GY, Obeidy P, Ford SJ, Tselepis C, Sharp DM, Jansson PJ, Kalinowski DS, Kovacevic Z, Lovejoy DB, Richardson

DR. 2013. The iron chelator, deferasirox, as a novel strategy for cancer treatment: oral activity against human lung tumor xenografts and molecular mechanism of action. *Mol Pharmacol* **83**: 179–190. doi:10.1124/mol.112.081893

Lunn JC, Kuhnle G, Mai V, Frankenfeld C, Shuker DE, Glen RC, Goodman JM, Pollock JR, Bingham SA. 2006. The effect of haem in red and processed meat on the endogenous formation of N-nitroso compounds in the upper gastrointestinal tract. *Carcinogenesis* **28**: 685–690. doi:10.1093/carcin/bgl192

Luza SC, Speisky HC. 1996. Liver copper storage and transport during development: implications for cytotoxicity. *Am J Clin Nutr* **63**: 812S–820S. doi:10.1093/ajcn/63.5.812

Macomber L, Imlay JA. 2009. The iron-sulfur clusters of dehydratases are primary intracellular targets of copper toxicity. *Proc Natl Acad Sci* **106**: 8344–8349. doi:10.1073/pnas.0812808106

Maffettone C, Chen G, Drozdov I, Ouzounis C, Pantopoulos K. 2010. Tumorigenic properties of iron regulatory protein 2 (IRP2) mediated by its specific 73-amino acids insert. *PLoS ONE* **5**: e10163. doi:10.1371/journal.pone.0010163

Mancias JD, Wang X, Gygi SP, Harper JW, Kimmelman AC. 2014. Quantitative proteomics identifies NCOA4 as the cargo receptor mediating ferritinophagy. *Nature* **509**: 105–109. doi:10.1038/nature13148

Mancias JD, Pontano Vaites L, Nissim S, Biancur DE, Kim AJ, Wang X, Liu Y, Goessling W, Kimmelman AC, Harper JW. 2015. Ferritinophagy via NCOA4 is required for erythropoiesis and is regulated by iron dependent HERC2-mediated proteolysis. *eLife* **4**: e10308. doi:10.7554/eLife.10308

Martin DN, Uprichard SL. 2013. Identification of transferrin receptor 1 as a hepatitis C virus entry factor. *Proc Natl Acad Sci* **110**: 10777–10782. doi:10.1073/pnas.1301764110

Masoud GN, Li W. 2015. HIF-1α pathway: role, regulation and intervention for cancer therapy. *Acta Pharm Sin B* **5**: 378–389. doi:10.1016/j.apsb.2015.05.007

McKeown SR. 2014. Defining normoxia, physoxia and hypoxia in tumours—implications for treatment response. *Br J Radiol* **87**: 20130676. doi:10.1259/bjr.20130676

Meyron-Holtz EG, Ghosh MC, Rouault TA. 2004. Mammalian tissue oxygen levels modulate iron-regulatory protein activities in vivo. *Science* **306**: 2087–2090. doi:10.1126/science.1103786

Mini E, Nobili S, Caciagli B, Landini I, Mazzei T. 2006. Cellular pharmacology of gemcitabine. *Ann Oncol* **17**: v7–v12. doi:10.1093/annonc/mdj941

Mukhopadhyay S, Encarnación-Rosado J, Lin EY, Sohn ASW, Zhang H, Mancias JD, Kimmelman AC. 2023. Autophagy supports mitochondrial metabolism through the regulation of iron homeostasis in pancreatic cancer. *Sci Adv* **9**: eadf9284. doi:10.1126/sciadv.adf9284

Nauser T, Steinmann D, Koppenol WH. 2012. Why do proteins use selenocysteine instead of cysteine? *Amino Acids* **42**: 39–44. doi:10.1007/s00726-010-0602-7

Nechushtan H, Hamamreh Y, Nidal S, Gotfried M, Baron A, Shalev YI, Nisman B, Peretz T, Peylan-Ramu N. 2015. A phase IIb trial assessing the addition of disulfiram to chemotherapy for the treatment of metastatic non-small cell lung cancer. *Oncologist* **20**: 366–367. doi:10.1634/theoncologist.2014-0424

Nemeth E, Rivera S, Gabayan V, Keller C, Taudorf S, Pedersen BK, Ganz T. 2004a. IL-6 mediates hypoferremia of inflammation by inducing the synthesis of the iron regulatory hormone hepcidin. *J Clin Invest* **113**: 1271–1276. doi:10.1172/JCI200420945

Nemeth E, Tuttle MS, Powelson J, Vaughn MB, Donovan A, Ward DM, Ganz T, Kaplan J. 2004b. Hepcidin regulates cellular iron efflux by binding to ferroportin and inducing its internalization. *Science* **306**: 2090–2093. doi:10.1126/science.1104742

Nemeth E, Roetto A, Garozzo G, Ganz T, Camaschella C. 2005. Hepcidin is decreased in TFR2 hemochromatosis. *Blood* **105**: 1803–1806. doi:10.1182/blood-2004-08-3042

Nitti M, Piras S, Marinari UM, Moretta L, Pronzato MA, Furfaro AL. 2017. HO-1 induction in cancer progression: a matter of cell adaptation. *Antioxidants (Basel)* **6**: 29. doi:10.3390/antiox6020029

Nose Y, Kim BE, Thiele DJ. 2006. Ctr1 drives intestinal copper absorption and is essential for growth, iron metabolism, and neonatal cardiac function. *Cell Metab* **4**: 235–244. doi:10.1016/j.cmet.2006.08.009

Ntziachristos P, Tsirigos A, Welstead GG, Trimarchi T, Bakogianni S, Xu L, Loizou E, Holmfeldt L, Strikoudis A, King B, et al. 2014. Contrasting roles of histone 3 lysine 27 demethylases in acute lymphoblastic leukaemia. *Nature* **514**: 513–517. doi:10.1038/nature13605

Nutting CM, van Herpen CM, Miah AB, Bhide SA, Machiels JP, Buter J, Kelly C, de Raucourt D, Harrington KJ. 2009. Phase II study of 3-AP Triapine in patients with recurrent or metastatic head and neck squamous cell carcinoma. *Ann Oncol* **20**: 1275–1279. doi:10.1093/annonc/mdn775

O'Day SJ, Eggermont AM, Chiarion-Sileni V, Kefford R, Grob JJ, Mortier L, Robert C, Schachter J, Testori A, Mackiewicz J, et al. 2013. Final results of phase III SYMMETRY study: randomized, double-blind trial of elesclomol plus paclitaxel versus paclitaxel alone as treatment for chemotherapy-naive patients with advanced melanoma. *J Clin Oncol* **31**: 1211–1218. doi:10.1200/JCO.2012.44.5585

Ohgami RS, Campagna DR, Greer EL, Antiochos B, McDonald A, Chen J, Sharp JJ, Fujiwara Y, Barker JE, Fleming MD. 2005. Identification of a ferrireductase required for efficient transferrin-dependent iron uptake in erythroid cells. *Nat Genet* **37**: 1264–1269. doi:10.1038/ng1658

Osaki S, Johnson DA, Frieden E. 1966. The possible significance of the ferrous oxidase activity of ceruloplasmin in normal human serum. *J Biol Chem* **241**: 2746–2751. doi:10.1016/S0021-9258(18)96527-0

Pak M, Lopez MA, Gabayan V, Ganz T, Rivera S. 2006. Suppression of hepcidin during anemia requires erythropoietic activity. *Blood* **108**: 3730–3735. doi:10.1182/blood-2006-06-028787

Park CH, Valore EV, Waring AJ, Ganz T. 2001. Hepcidin, a urinary antimicrobial peptide synthesized in the liver. *J Biol Chem* **276**: 7806–7810. doi:10.1074/jbc.M008922200

Pezacki AT, Matier CD, Gu X, Kummelstedt E, Bond SE, Torrente L, Jordan-Sciutto KL, DeNicola GM, Su TA, Brady DC, et al. 2022. Oxidation state-specific fluorescent copper sensors reveal oncogene-driven redox changes that regulate labile copper(II) pools. *Proc Natl Acad Sci* 119: e2202736119. doi:10.1073/pnas.2202736119

Pfeiffenberger J, Mogler C, Gotthardt DN, Schulze-Bergkamen H, Litwin T, Reuner U, Hefter H, Huster D, Schemmer P, Członkowska A, et al. 2015. Hepatobiliary malignancies in Wilson disease. *Liver Int* 35: 1615–1622. doi:10.1111/liv.12727

Pham AN, Xing G, Miller CJ, Waite TD. 2013. Fenton-like copper redox chemistry revisited: hydrogen peroxide and superoxide mediation of copper-catalyzed oxidant production. *J Catal* 301: 54–64. doi:10.1016/j.jcat.2013.01.025

Pietrangelo A. 2010. Hereditary hemochromatosis: pathogenesis, diagnosis, and treatment. *Gastroenterology* 139: 393–408.e2. doi:10.1053/j.gastro.2010.06.013

Pietsch EC, Chan JY, Torti FM, Torti SV. 2003. Nrf2 mediates the induction of ferritin H in response to xenobiotics and cancer chemopreventive dithiolethiones. *J Biol Chem* 278: 2361–2369. doi:10.1074/jbc.M210664200

Pinnix ZK, Miller LD, Wang W, D'Agostino R, Kute T, Willingham MC, Hatcher H, Tesfay L, Sui G, Di X, et al. 2010. Ferroportin and iron regulation in breast cancer progression and prognosis. *Sci Transl Med* 2: 43ra56. doi:10.1126/scitranslmed.3001127

Polishchuk EV, Concilli M, Iacobacci S, Chesi G, Pastore N, Piccolo P, Paladino S, Baldantoni D, van ISC, Chan J, et al. 2014. Wilson disease protein ATP7B utilizes lysosomal exocytosis to maintain copper homeostasis. *Dev Cell* 29: 686–700. doi:10.1016/j.devcel.2014.04.033

Popović-Bijelić A, Kowol CR, Lind ME, Luo J, Himo F, Enyedy EA, Arion VB, Gräslund A. 2011. Ribonucleotide reductase inhibition by metal complexes of Triapine (3-aminopyridine-2-carboxaldehyde thiosemicarbazone): a combined experimental and theoretical study. *J Inorg Biochem* 105: 1422–1431. doi:10.1016/j.jinorgbio.2011.07.003

Poulos TL. 2014. Heme enzyme structure and function. *Chem Rev* 114: 3919–3962. doi:10.1021/cr400415k

Radomska D, Czarnomysy R, Radomski D, Bielawska A, Bielawski K. 2021. Selenium as a bioactive micronutrient in the human diet and its cancer chemopreventive activity. *Nutrients* 13: 1649. doi:10.3390/nu13051649

Radoshitzky SR, Abraham J, Spiropoulou CF, Kuhn JH, Nguyen D, Li W, Nagel J, Schmidt PJ, Nunberg JH, Andrews NC, et al. 2007. Transferrin receptor 1 is a cellular receptor for new world haemorrhagic fever arenaviruses. *Nature* 446: 92–96. doi:10.1038/nature05539

Ramírez-Carmona W, Díaz-Fabregat B, Yuri Yoshigae A, Musa de Aquino A, Scarano WR, de Souza Castilho AC, Avansini Marsicano J, Leal do Prado R, Pessan JP, de Oliveira Mendes L. 2022. Are serum ferritin levels a reliable cancer biomarker? A systematic review and meta-analysis. *Nutr Cancer* 74: 1917–1926. doi:10.1080/01635581.2021.1982996

Rankin EB, Biju MP, Liu Q, Unger TL, Rha J, Johnson RS, Simon MC, Keith B, Haase VH. 2007. Hypoxia-inducible factor-2 (HIF-2) regulates hepatic erythropoietin in vivo. *J Clin Invest* 117: 1068–1077. doi:10.1172/JCI30117

Reed E, Lutsenko S, Bandmann O. 2018. Animal models of Wilson disease. *J Neurochem* 146: 356–373. doi:10.1111/jnc.14323

Reznik N, Gallo AD, Rush KW, Javitt G, Fridmann-Sirkis Y, Ilani T, Nairner NA, Fishilevich S, Gokhman D, Chacón KN, et al. 2022. Intestinal mucin is a chaperone of multivalent copper. *Cell* 185: 4206–4215.e11. doi:10.1016/j.cell.2022.09.021

Rishi G, Wallace DF, Subramaniam VN. 2015. Hepcidin: regulation of the master iron regulator. *Biosci Rep* 35. doi:10.1042/BSR20150014

Rouault TA. 2015. Mammalian iron–sulphur proteins: novel insights into biogenesis and function. *Nat Rev Mol Cell Biol* 16: 45–55. doi:10.1038/nrm3909

Ruddell RG, Hoang-Le D, Barwood JM, Rutherford PS, Piva TJ, Watters DJ, Santambrogio P, Arosio P, Ramm GA. 2009. Ferritin functions as a proinflammatory cytokine via iron-independent protein kinase C zeta/nuclear factor κB-regulated signaling in rat hepatic stellate cells. *Hepatology* 49: 887–900. doi:10.1002/hep.22716

Ryle MJ, Hausinger RP. 2002. Non-heme iron oxygenases. *Curr Opin Chem Biol* 6: 193–201. doi:10.1016/S1367-5931(02)00302-2

Saeki I, Yamamoto N, Yamasaki T, Takami T, Maeda M, Fujisawa K, Iwamoto T, Matsumoto T, Hidaka I, Ishikawa T, et al. 2016. Effects of an oral iron chelator, deferasirox, on advanced hepatocellular carcinoma. *World J Gastroenterol* 22: 8967–8977. doi:10.3748/wjg.v22.i40.8967

Salahudeen AA, Thompson JW, Ruiz JC, Ma HW, Kinch LN, Li Q, Grishin NV, Bruick RK. 2009. An E3 ligase possessing an iron-responsive hemerythrin domain is a regulator of iron homeostasis. *Science* 326: 722–726. doi:10.1126/science.1176326

Salnikow K, Donald SP, Bruick RK, Zhitkovich A, Phang JM, Kasprzak KS. 2004. Depletion of intracellular ascorbate by the carcinogenic metals nickel and cobalt results in the induction of hypoxic stress. *J Biol Chem* 279: 40337–40344. doi:10.1074/jbc.M403057200

Sanchez M, Galy B, Muckenthaler MU, Hentze MW. 2007. Iron-regulatory proteins limit hypoxia-inducible factor-2α expression in iron deficiency. *Nat Struct Mol Biol* 14: 420–426. doi:10.1038/nsmb1222

Santambrogio P, Biasiotto G, Sanvito F, Olivieri S, Arosio P, Levi S. 2007. Mitochondrial ferritin expression in adult mouse tissues. *J Histochem Cytochem* 55: 1129–1137. doi:10.1369/jhc.7A7273.2007

Santana-Codina N, Gikandi A, Mancias JD. 2021. The role of NCOA4-mediated ferritinophagyferritinophagy in ferroptosisferroptosis. In *Ferroptosis: mechanism and diseases* (ed. Florez AF, Alborzinia H), pp. 41–57. Springer, New York.

Santana-Codina N, Del Rey MQ, Kapner KS, Zhang H, Gikandi A, Malcolm C, Poupault C, Kuljanin M, John KM, Biancur DE, et al. 2022. NCOA4-mediated ferritinophagy is a pancreatic cancer dependency via maintenance of iron bioavailability for iron-sulfur cluster proteins. *Cancer Discov* 12: 2180–2197. doi:10.1158/2159-8290.CD-22-0043

Santos M, Anderson CP, Neschen S, Zumbrennen-Bullough KB, Romney SJ, Kahle-Stephan M, Rathkolb B, Gailus-Durner V, Fuchs H, Wolf E, et al. 2020. Irp2 regulates insulin production through iron-mediated Cdkal1-catalyzed tRNA modification. *Nat Commun* 11: 296. doi:10.1038/s41467-019-14004-5

Sanvisens N, Bañó MC, Huang M, Puig S. 2011. Regulation of ribonucleotide reductase in response to iron deficiency. *Mol Cell* **44:** 759–769. doi:10.1016/j.molcel.2011.09.021

Schwartz AJ, Goyert JW, Solanki S, Kerk SA, Chen B, Castillo C, Hsu PP, Do BT, Singhal R, Dame MK, et al. 2021. Hepcidin sequesters iron to sustain nucleotide metabolism and mitochondrial function in colorectal cancer epithelial cells. *Nat Metab* **3:** 969–982. doi:10.1038/s42255-021-00406-7

Sciacovelli M, Gonçalves E, Johnson TI, Zecchini VR, da Costa AS, Gaude E, Drubbel AV, Theobald SJ, Abbo SR, Tran MG, et al. 2016. Fumarate is an epigenetic modifier that elicits epithelial-to-mesenchymal transition. *Nature* **537:** 544–547. doi:10.1038/nature19353

Shanbhag V, Jasmer-McDonald K, Zhu S, Martin AL, Gudekar N, Khan A, Ladomersky E, Singh K, Weisman GA, Petris MJ. 2019. ATP7A delivers copper to the lysyl oxidase family of enzymes and promotes tumorigenesis and metastasis. *Proc Natl Acad Sci* **116:** 6836–6841. doi:10.1073/pnas.1817473116

Shawki A, Anthony SR, Nose Y, Engevik MA, Niespodzany EJ, Barrientos T, Öhrvik H, Worrell RT, Thiele DJ, Mackenzie B. 2015. Intestinal DMT1 is critical for iron absorption in the mouse but is not required for the absorption of copper or manganese. *Am J Physiol Gastrointest Liver Physiol* **309:** G635–G647. doi:10.1152/ajpgi.00160.2015

Shen Y, Li X, Dong D, Zhang B, Xue Y, Shang P. 2018. Transferrin receptor 1 in cancer: a new sight for cancer therapy. *Am J Cancer Res* **8:** 916–931.

Shpyleva SI, Tryndyak VP, Kovalchuk O, Starlard-Davenport A, Chekhun VF, Beland FA, Pogribny IP. 2011. Role of ferritin alterations in human breast cancer cells. *Breast Cancer Res Treat* **126:** 63–71. doi:10.1007/s10549-010-0849-4

Sieff C, Bicknell D, Caine G, Robinson J, Lam G, Greaves MF. 1982. Changes in cell surface antigen expression during hemopoietic differentiation. *Blood* **60:** 703–713. doi:10.1182/blood.V60.3.703.703

Silva AM, Hider RC. 2009. Influence of non-enzymatic post-translation modifications on the ability of human serum albumin to bind iron. Implications for non-transferrin-bound iron speciation. *Biochim Biophys Acta* **1794:** 1449–1458. doi:10.1016/j.bbapap.2009.06.003

Smith SR, Ghosh MC, Ollivierre-Wilson H, Hang Tong W, Rouault TA. 2006. Complete loss of iron regulatory proteins 1 and 2 prevents viability of murine zygotes beyond the blastocyst stage of embryonic development. *Blood Cells Mol Dis* **36:** 283–287. doi:10.1016/j.bcmd.2005.12.006

Sohoni S, Ghosh P, Wang T, Kalainayakan SP, Vidal C, Dey S, Konduri PC, Zhang L. 2019. Elevated heme synthesis and uptake underpin intensified oxidative metabolism and tumorigenic functions in non-small cell lung cancer cells. *Cancer Res* **79:** 2511–2525. doi:10.1158/0008-5472.CAN-18-2156

Soldin OP, Bierbower LH, Choi JJ, Choi JJ, Thompson-Hoffman S, Soldin SJ. 2004. Serum iron, ferritin, transferrin, total iron binding capacity, hs-CRP, LDL cholesterol and magnesium in children; new reference intervals using the Dade Dimension Clinical Chemistry System. *Clin Chim Acta* **342:** 211–217. doi:10.1016/j.cccn.2004.01.002

Sporn MB, Liby KT. 2012. NRF2 and cancer: the good, the bad and the importance of context. *Nat Rev Cancer* **12:** 564–571. doi:10.1038/nrc3278

Sviderskiy VO, Terzi EM, Possemato R. 2019. Iron–sulfur cluster metabolism impacts iron homeostasis, ferroptosis sensitivity, and human disease. In *Ferroptosis in health and disease* (ed. Tang D), pp. 215–237. Springer, New York.

Sviderskiy VO, Blumenberg L, Gorodetsky E, Karakousi TR, Hirsh N, Alvarez SW, Terzi EM, Kaparos E, Whiten GC, Ssebyala S, et al. 2020. Hyperactive CDK2 activity in basal-like breast cancer imposes a genome integrity liability that can be exploited by targeting DNA polymerase ε. *Mol Cell* **80:** 682–698.e7. doi:10.1016/j.molcel.2020.10.016

Tabuchi M, Yoshimori T, Yamaguchi K, Yoshida T, Kishi F. 2000. Human NRAMP2/DMT1, which mediates iron transport across endosomal membranes, is localized to late endosomes and lysosomes in HEp-2 cells. *J Biol Chem* **275:** 22220–22228. doi:10.1074/jbc.M001478200

Tan G, Yang J, Li T, Zhao J, Sun S, Li X, Lin C, Li J, Zhou H, Lyu J, et al. 2017. Anaerobic copper toxicity and iron-sulfur cluster biogenesis in *Escherichia coli*. *Appl Environ Microbiol* **83:** e00867-17. doi:10.1128/AEM.00867-17

Tanzi RE, Petrukhin K, Chernov I, Pellequer JL, Wasco W, Ross B, Romano DM, Parano E, Pavone L, Brzustowicz LM, et al. 1993. The Wilson disease gene is a copper transporting ATPase with homology to the Menkes disease gene. *Nat Genet* **5:** 344–350. doi:10.1038/ng1293-344

Terzi EM, Sviderskiy VO, Alvarez SW, Whiten GC, Possemato R. 2021. Iron-sulfur cluster deficiency can be sensed by IRP2 and regulates iron homeostasis and sensitivity to ferroptosis independent of IRP1 and FBXL5. *Sci Adv* **7:** eabg4302. doi:10.1126/sciadv.abg4302

Torti SV, Manz DH, Paul BT, Blanchette-Farra N, Torti FM. 2018. Iron and cancer. *Annu Rev Nutr* **38:** 97–125. doi:10.1146/annurev-nutr-082117-051732

Tsang T, Posimo JM, Gudiel AA, Cicchini M, Feldser DM, Brady DC. 2020. Copper is an essential regulator of the autophagic kinases ULK1/2 to drive lung adenocarcinoma. *Nat Cell Biol* **22:** 412–424. doi:10.1038/s41556-020-0481-4

Tsvetkov P, Detappe A, Cai K, Keys HR, Brune Z, Ying W, Thiru P, Reidy M, Kugener G, Rossen J, et al. 2019. Mitochondrial metabolism promotes adaptation to proteotoxic stress. *Nat Chem Biol* **15:** 681–689. doi:10.1038/s41589-019-0291-9

Tsvetkov P, Coy S, Petrova B, Dreishpoon M, Verma A, Abdusamad M, Rossen J, Joesch-Cohen L, Humeidi R, Spangler RD, et al. 2022. Copper induces cell death by targeting lipoylated TCA cycle proteins. *Science* **375:** 1254–1261. doi:10.1126/science.abf0529

Turski ML, Brady DC, Kim HJ, Kim BE, Nose Y, Counter CM, Winge DR, Thiele DJ. 2012. A novel role for copper in Ras/mitogen-activated protein kinase signaling. *Mol Cell Biol* **32:** 1284–1295. doi:10.1128/MCB.05722-11

Unlu G, Prizer B, Erdal R, Yeh HW, Bayraktar EC, Birsoy K. 2022. Metabolic-scale gene activation screens identify SLCO2B1 as a heme transporter that enhances cellular iron availability. *Mol Cell* **82:** 2832–2843.e7. doi:10.1016/j.molcel.2022.05.024

Vashisht AA, Zumbrennen KB, Huang X, Powers DN, Durazo A, Sun D, Bhaskaran N, Persson A, Uhlen M, Sangfelt O, et al. 2009. Control of iron homeostasis by an iron-regulated ubiquitin ligase. *Science* **326:** 718–721. doi:10.1126/science.1176333

Vinceti M, Filippini T, Del Giovane C, Dennert G, Zwahlen M, Brinkman M, Zeegers MP, Horneber M, D'Amico R, Crespi CM. 2018. Selenium for preventing cancer. *Cochrane Database Syst Rev* **1:** Cd005195.

Volz K. 2008. The functional duality of iron regulatory protein 1. *Curr Opin Struct Biol* **18:** 106–111. doi:10.1016/j.sbi.2007.12.010

Vulpe CD, Kuo YM, Murphy TL, Cowley L, Askwith C, Libina N, Gitschier J, Anderson GJ. 1999. Hephaestin, a ceruloplasmin homologue implicated in intestinal iron transport, is defective in the *sla* mouse. *Nat Genet* **21:** 195–199. doi:10.1038/5979

Wang W, Deng Z, Hatcher H, Miller LD, Di X, Tesfay L, Sui G, D'Agostino RB Jr, Torti FM, Torti SV. 2014. IRP2 regulates breast tumor growth. *Cancer Res* **74:** 497–507. doi:10.1158/0008-5472.CAN-13-1224

Wang H, Shi H, Rajan M, Canarie ER, Hong S, Simoneschi D, Pagano M, Bush MF, Stoll S, Leibold EA, et al. 2020. FBXL5 regulates IRP2 stability in iron homeostasis via an oxygen-responsive [2Fe2S] cluster. *Mol Cell* **78:** 31–41.e5. doi:10.1016/j.molcel.2020.02.011

Ward DM, Kaplan J. 2012. Ferroportin-mediated iron transport: expression and regulation. *Biochim BIophys Acta* **1823:** 1426–1433. doi:10.1016/j.bbamcr.2012.03.004

Weber RA, Yen FS, Nicholson SPV, Alwaseem H, Bayraktar EC, Alam M, Timson RC, La K, Abu-Remaileh M, Molina H, et al. 2020. Maintaining iron homeostasis is the key role of lysosomal acidity for cell proliferation. *Mol Cell* **77:** 645–655.e7. doi:10.1016/j.molcel.2020.01.003

Weinstein DA, Roy CN, Fleming MD, Loda MF, Wolfsdorf JI, Andrews NC. 2002. Inappropriate expression of hepcidin is associated with iron refractory anemia: implications for the anemia of chronic disease. *Blood* **100:** 3776–3781. doi:10.1182/blood-2002-04-1260

Whanger PD. 2004. Selenium and its relationship to cancer: an update. *Br J Nutr* **91:** 11–28. doi:10.1079/BJN20031015

Wilkinson N, Pantopoulos K. 2014. The IRP/IRE system in vivo: insights from mouse models. *Front Pharmacol* **5:** 176. doi:10.3389/fphar.2014.00176

Winterbourn CC. 1995. Toxicity of iron and hydrogen peroxide: the Fenton reaction. *Toxicol Lett* **82-83:** 969–974. doi:10.1016/0378-4274(95)03532-X

Worwood M, Dawkins S, Wagstaff M, Jacobs A. 1976. The purification and properties of ferritin from human serum. *Biochem J* **157:** 97–103. doi:10.1042/bj1570097

Wrighting DM, Andrews NC. 2006. Interleukin-6 induces hepcidin expression through STAT3. *Blood* **108:** 3204–3209. doi:10.1182/blood-2006-06-027631

Wu WL, Papagiannakopoulos T. 2020. The pleiotropic role of the KEAP1/NRF2 pathway in cancer. *Ann Rev Cancer Biol* **4:** 413–435. doi:10.1146/annurev-cancerbio-030518-055627

Xiao M, Yang H, Xu W, Ma S, Lin H, Zhu H, Liu L, Liu Y, Yang C, Xu Y, et al. 2012. Inhibition of α-KG-dependent histone and DNA demethylases by fumarate and succinate that are accumulated in mutations of FH and SDH tumor suppressors. *Genes Dev* **26:** 1326–1338. doi:10.1101/gad.191056.112

Xie H, Kang YJ. 2009. Role of copper in angiogenesis and its medicinal implications. *Curr Med Chem* **16:** 1304–1314. doi:10.2174/092986709787846622

Xu W, Yang H, Liu Y, Yang Y, Wang P, Kim SH, Ito S, Yang C, Wang P, Xiao MT, et al. 2011. Oncometabolite 2-hydroxyglutarate is a competitive inhibitor of α-ketoglutarate-dependent dioxygenases. *Cancer Cell* **19:** 17–30. doi:10.1016/j.ccr.2010.12.014

Yambire KF, Rostosky C, Watanabe T, Pacheu-Grau D, Torres-Odio S, Sanchez-Guerrero A, Senderovich O, Meyron-Holtz EG, Milosevic I, Frahm J, et al. 2019. Impaired lysosomal acidification triggers iron deficiency and inflammation in vivo. *eLife* **8:** e51031. doi:10.7554/eLife.51031

Yang WS, SriRamaratnam R, Welsch ME, Shimada K, Skouta R, Viswanathan VS, Cheah JH, Clemons PA, Shamji AF, Clish CB, et al. 2014. Regulation of ferroptotic cancer cell death by GPX4. *Cell* **156:** 317–331. doi:10.1016/j.cell.2013.12.010

Yu Y, Gutierrez E, Kovacevic Z, Saletta F, Obeidy P, Suryo Rahmanto Y, Richardson DR. 2012. Iron chelators for the treatment of cancer. *Curr Med Chem* **19:** 2689–2702. doi:10.2174/092986712800609706

The Complex Roles of Redox and Antioxidant Biology in Cancer

Makiko Hayashi,[1,3] Keito Okazaki,[2,3] Thales Papgiannakopoulos,[1] and Hozumi Motohashi[2]

[1]Department of Pathology, New York University School of Medicine, New York, New York 10016, USA

[2]Department of Gene Expression Regulation, Institute of Development, Aging and Cancer, Tohoku University, Sendai 980-8575, Japan

Correspondence: hozumim@med.tohoku.ac.jp; papagt01@nyumc.org

Redox reactions control fundamental biochemical processes, including energy production, metabolism, respiration, detoxification, and signal transduction. Cancer cells, due to their generally active metabolism for sustained proliferation, produce high levels of reactive oxygen species (ROS) compared to normal cells and are equipped with antioxidant defense systems to counteract the detrimental effects of ROS to maintain redox homeostasis. The KEAP1-NRF2 system plays a major role in sensing and regulating endogenous antioxidant defenses in both normal and cancer cells, creating a bivalent contribution of NRF2 to cancer prevention and therapy. Cancer cells hijack the NRF2-dependent antioxidant program and exploit a very unique metabolism as a trade-off for enhanced antioxidant capacity. This work provides an overview of redox metabolism in cancer cells, highlighting the role of the KEAP1-NRF2 system, selenoproteins, sulfur metabolism, heme/iron metabolism, and antioxidants. Finally, we describe therapeutic approaches that can be leveraged to target redox metabolism in cancer.

Redox reactions are fundamental chemical reactions in life and play a central role in the acquisition of energy to sustain life. Among the various chemical reactions that support life, redox reactions play an extremely important role in energy production in mitochondria, intracellular signal transduction, quality control through proper folding of proteins, bactericidal action by leukocytes, and detoxification of environmental chemicals present in food and air. Biomolecules responsible for these fundamental chemical reactions in biological contexts include electron donors such as NADH and $FADH_2$, iron–sulfur clusters, heme, metal ions such as iron and copper, selenocysteine in selenoproteins, and a whole variety of reactive molecules, such as reactive oxygen species (ROS), reactive nitrogen species (Cronin et al. 2018), and reactive sulfur species (Sayin et al. 2014). Given their importance, a plethora of studies have been investigating the role of redox molecules in normal physiology and disease.

While many aerobic organisms utilize oxygen for more efficient energy metabolism, they

[3]These authors contributed equally to this work.

Copyright © 2025 Cold Spring Harbor Laboratory Press; all rights reserved
Cite this article as *Cold Spring Harb Perspect Med* doi: 10.1101/cshperspect.a041546

are also exposed to oxygen toxicity and must constantly cope with oxidative stress. Although cancer cells reside in a relatively hypoxic environment in tumor tissues, increased proliferation in cancer cells is accompanied by increased production of ROS (Harris and DeNicola 2020). To detoxify ROS, cancer cells often activate a battery of antioxidants machinery to maintain homeostasis in response to the ROS associated with proliferation, inflammation or acquired resistance to anticancer drugs and radiation therapy (Motohashi and Yamamoto 2004; Perillo et al. 2020). Inhibition of such antioxidant functions is expected to have tumor suppressive effects (Harder et al. 2017; Tsuchida et al. 2017). While this is a therapeutic idea to tilt the redox balance toward oxidation, tilting the balance toward reduction is also an effective way to inhibit a certain battery of cancers (Kong et al. 2020; Weiss-Sadan et al. 2023). Recent studies further revealed more dynamic ROS controls depending on different stages of cancer development (Cheung et al. 2020; He et al. 2022), making us recognize the need to understand the multifaceted roles of redox balance control. Therefore, understanding redox reactions and oxidative stress and their contributions to the hallmarks of carcinogenesis is fundamental to cancer cell biology. Furthermore, elucidating the regulatory mechanisms governing the redox state in cancer cells provides powerful insights into potential therapeutic strategies. In this review, we outline the factors that can disturb the redox balance in cancer cells and their microenvironment, discuss how cancer cells utilize redox regulation for malignant transformation, and how this can potentially be leveraged to develop novel therapeutic strategies aimed at targeting redox pathways.

REDOX IMBALANCE IN CANCER INITIATION AND PROGRESSION

Reactive Species Involved in Determination of Cellular Redox Status

The cellular redox environment, or the balance between oxidizing and reducing molecules in a cell, is influenced by various reactive species. The production of ROS in cells primarily origi-

nates from mitochondria and various enzymatic reactions in the cell (Murphy 2009; Cheung and Vousden 2022). Mitochondrial electron transport chain (Chafe et al. 2021) generates the majority of ROS in the form of superoxide anion (O_2^-). Outside the mitochondria, O_2^- is produced by enzymes such as nicotinamide adenine dinucleotide phosphate (NADPH) oxidase (NOX) family proteins (Moghadam et al. 2021). O_2^- is converted to hydrogen peroxide (H_2O_2) by SOD (superoxide dismutase), SOD2 in mitochondria, SOD1 in cytoplasm, and SOD3 in the extracellular space, leading to induction of the localized signaling by H_2O_2, as H_2O_2 is the most stable form of ROS and plays an important role as a signaling molecule (Glasauer and Chandel 2014). Peroxisomal oxidases, cytochrome P-450, and oxidative protein folding also contribute to H_2O_2 production. H_2O_2 is neutralized by enzymes such as catalase and peroxiredoxin. Cytosolic H_2O_2 leads to the formation of highly potent hydroxyl radicals through the Fenton reaction in the presence of ferrous or cuprous ions. H_2O_2 is also sensed by cysteine residues on KEAP1 that lead to the stabilization of the antioxidant transcription factor NRF2 (Suzuki et al. 2019). Nitrogen-containing reactive molecules such as nitric oxide (NO) and peroxynitrite ($ONOO^-$) are called RNS. Peroxynitrite undergoes protonation and homolytic scission to form $NO_2^{\cdot}$, which, as well as NO, readily reacts with polyunsaturated fatty acids with conjugated dienes and produces electrophilic nitro-fatty acids (Schopfer et al. 2011). RSS include thiyl radicals, sulfenic acids, disulfide-S-oxide, and persulfides/polysulfides (Ida et al. 2014; Giles and Jacob 2022). Because perthiyl radicals are relatively stable but sufficiently reactive, hydropersulfides serve as efficient radical trapping antioxidants, being able to antagonize ferroptotic cell death (Chauvin et al. 2019; Barayeu et al. 2023).

Early Stage of Carcinogenesis

Environmental chemicals, including ones in food ingredients and additives, often have electrophilic properties or are converted to electrophilic substances through metabolism in the body (Talalay 1989; Talalay and Fahey 2001). They form adducts in nucleic acids, proteins, lip-

Cite this article as *Cold Spring Harb Perspect Med* doi: 10.1101/cshperspect.a041546

ids, and other biomolecules, thereby altering their functions, which can ultimately generate cellular diversity and contribute to the process of cellular transformation (Jacobs and Marnett 2010). Subsequently, the emergence of cells that have a proliferative advantage over normal cells, evade cell death and immune cell surveillance, can give rise to a cancerous state and tumor formation. Redox disruption is thought to be one of the important steps in the early stage of chemical carcinogenesis (Trush and Kensler 1991).

Interestingly, several oncogenes have been shown to increase mitochondrial ROS production (Vafa et al. 2002; Weinberg et al. 2010). Mitochondrial ROS activates PI3K-AKT pathway and hypoxia inducible factors (HIF), promoting cell proliferation (Sullivan and Chandel 2014). An active site cysteine on PTEN, a negative regulator of PI3K pathway, inactivates PTEN and consequent activation of the PI3K-AKT pathway (Cully et al. 2006; Badr et al. 2017). Phosphatases, PP2A and PTP1B, both of which inactivate AKT, are also inhibited by ROS. PHD2 is another target suppressed by mitochondrial ROS, resulting in the activation of HIF (Tojo et al. 2015; Lee et al. 2016). As such, once a cell acquires an oncogenic mutation, the increased mitochondrial ROS can stimulate its proliferation. However, this can be a turnaround situation when cancers are treated with anticancer therapies, which increase ROS and induce oxidative damage in cancer cells. Mitochondrial translation for the maintenance of mitochondrial activity has been shown critical for cancer cells to be sensitive to the ROS-inducing chemotherapeutic reagents (Zhang et al. 2023).

From the viewpoint of cell competition and cancer evolution (Morata and Calleja 2020; Maruyama and Fujita 2022), cells that have undergone oncogenic changes are often eliminated as losers exhibiting increased intracellular ROS (Kucinski et al. 2017). In contrast, cells that acquire genetic or epigenetic changes that enable them to produce endogenous antioxidants and detoxify ROS can remain protected from excess macromolecule damage (e.g., genomic DNA damage, lipid peroxidation) and gain a competitive advantage (Hirose et al. 2022). Dissecting how redox regulation influences the destiny of cells undergoing oncogenic changes, escaping cell competition and surviving, awaits further investigation.

Cancer Malignancy and Redox Dysregulation

Oxidative stress is a condition that arises when there is an imbalance between the production of ROS and the ability of cells to detoxify these potentially harmful molecules. Proliferative signals can increase the levels of ROS in cancer cells, which can cause damage to cellular components and promote tumor growth (Jackson and Loeb 2001; Tubbs and Nussenzweig 2017). Therefore, tight regulation of oxidative stress is essential for cancer cells and can be accomplished by diverse genetic or epigenetic changes in cancer cells (Kreuz and Fischle 2016; Reczek and Chandel 2017). For example, in cancer cells in which NRF2, a key factor in the oxidative stress response, is constitutively activated by somatic loss-of-function (LOF) mutations in the KEAP1 or gain-of-function (GOF) mutations in NFE2L2 (encoding NRF2), strong activation of NRF2 target genes results in increased glutathione (GSH) synthesis, increased NADPH production, increased expression of various detoxifying enzymes and antioxidant proteins, leading to the enhancement of antioxidant capacity (Singh et al. 2006; Shibata et al. 2008a; Suzuki et al. 2016). On the other hand, there is a metabolic trade-off to support such strong antioxidant capacity, which can lead to reductive stress and metabolic vulnerabilities (Romero et al. 2017). For example, some many cancers are dependent on mitochondrial function and inhibition of NADH oxidation by suppression of the mitochondrial electron transfer system has been shown to result in reductive stress and growth inhibition (Morita et al. 2018; Weiss-Sadan et al. 2023).

Metastatic process is accompanied by a unique redox balance tilted toward oxidation. In KRAS-mutant pancreatic cancers, increased ROS contributes to the acquisition of the invasive phenotype of the cancer cells. Inhibition of TI-GAR or NRF2 leading to the ROS increase delays initial tumor development but accelerates metastatic progression at later stages (Cheung et al. 2020). Furthermore, there is evidence that host tissues with ROS accumulation due to genetic knockout of *Nrf2* are more receptive to metastatic colonization (Satoh et al. 2010), and bone marrow–derived myeloid cells may play a role in this process (Hiramoto et al. 2014). Reduced expression of methionine sulfoxide reductase A (MSRA) increases protein methionine oxidation resulting in the enhanced metastasis (He et al. 2022). Oxidative proteome appears to be advantageous for cancer cells to be metastatic.

REGULATORS INVOLVED IN CANCER REDOX METABOLISM

1. KEAP1-NRF2 SYSTEM

The KEAP1-NRF2 system plays a central role the defense mechanism against oxidative and electrophilic stress (Fig. 1; Yamamoto et al. 2018). NRF2 is a potent transcription activator, heterodimerizing with small Maf proteins (Motohashi et al. 2004) and binding to antioxidant response elements (AREs) (Rushmore et al. 1991), CNC-sMaf-binding element (CsMBE) (Otsuki et al. 2016) or electrophile response element (EpRE) (Friling et al. 1990) for activation of its target genes. As part of a larger transcriptional complex, NRF2 can interact with histone acetyltransferases

(Katoh et al. 2001), SWI/SNF chromatin remodeling complex (Zhang 2006; Ogiwara et al. 2019), mediator complex (Sekine et al. 2016), and specific transcription factors (Alam et al. 2017; Okazaki et al. 2020, 2022). KEAP1 is a substrate recognizing subunit of CUL3-based ubiquitin E3 ligase for ubiquitination of NRF2, serving as a negative regulator of NRF2 in unstressed conditions (Kobayashi et al. 2004; Zhang et al. 2004; Furukawa and Xiong 2005). Electrophiles and ROS directly modify reactive cysteine residues of KEAP1 and suppress the ubiquitination of NRF2, which makes KEAP1 a major biosensor of oxidative stress. Neddylation of CUL3 forms another regulatory layer of NRF2 activity (Lo and Hannink 2006), and its inhibition was shown to promote activation of NRF2 (Mehine et al. 2022). KEAP1-independent regulation of NRF2 is mediated by b-TrCP-CUL1 ubiquitin E3 ligase after being phosphorylated by GSK3 (Chowdhry et al. 2013; Taguchi et al. 2014; Kuga et al. 2022). The physiological relevance of NRF2 has been shown by using both NRF2-deficient mice (Enomoto et al. 2001; Shah et al. 2007) and analysis of human single-nucleotide polymorphisms (SNPs) in the *NRF2* gene locus (Suzuki et al. 2013; Honkura et al. 2016). Although NRF2 activation contributes to maintenance of

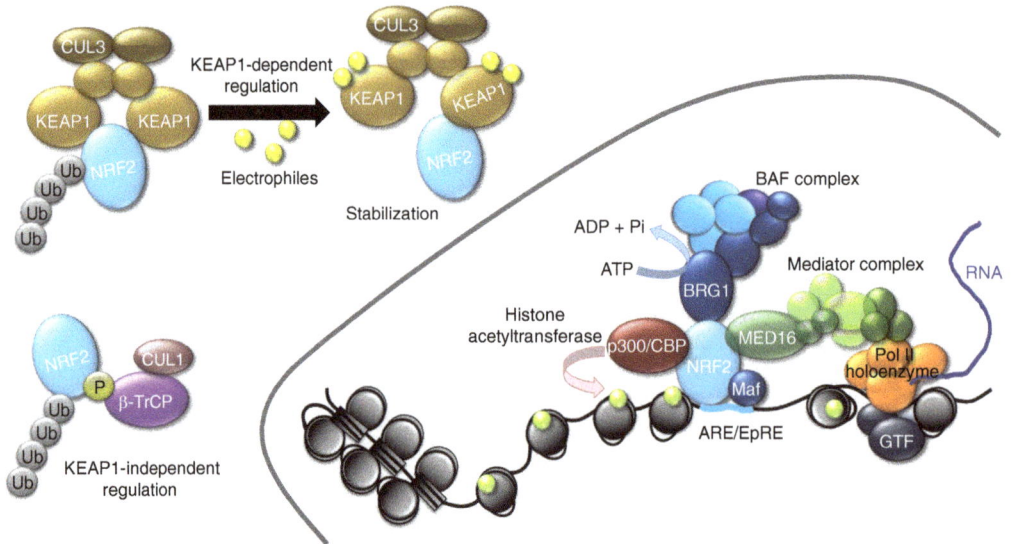

Figure 1. KEAP1-NRF2 system. NRF2 is an antioxidant transcriptional factor interacting with multiple coactivators. KEAP1-dependent and -independent degradation mechanisms of NRF2 are known to regulate NRF2 at the posttranslational level.

health in the setting for various pathological conditions, excessive activation of NRF2 in normal cells sometimes results in deleterious effects (Wakabayashi et al. 2003; Yoshida et al. 2018; Kuga et al. 2022). Systemic loss of KEAP1 leads to NRF2-dependent hyperkeratosis of the esophagus and forestomach that causes gastric obstruction and death (Wakabayashi et al. 2003). Moreover, constitutive NRF2 activation in hematopoietic stem cells leads to failure in bone marrow reconstitution due to stem cell exhaustion (Murakami et al. 2017). Consistently, high levels of NRF2 activation in adult flies leads to accelerated aging, while mild NRF2 activation extends life span, suggesting that homeostatic regulation of NRF2 by KEAP1 and redox-dependent cellular mechanisms is required for organismal health (Tsakiri et al. 2019).

Molecular Mechanisms Leading to NRF2-Activated Cancers

Hyperactivation of NRF2 occurs in many tumor types, including lung, esophagus, bladder, ovar-

ian, and colorectal cancers (Kandoth et al. 2013). As NRF2 primarily serves as a defense system against xenobiotics as well as oxidative and electrophilic stress (Kobayashi et al. 2006; Yamamoto et al. 2018), cancers within tissues that are highly exposed to such stressors are more likely to acquire hyperactivation of NRF2 to endure and survive, leading to NRF2 addiction (Kitamura and Motohashi 2018; Wu and Papagiannakopoulos 2020; Kitamura et al. 2022; Pillai et al. 2022). In this section, we discuss the molecular mechanisms of regulation of the KEAP1-NRF2 system in cancer cells (Fig. 2).

Genetic Alterations in NRF2-Activated Cancer Cells

Among all cancers, non-small-cell lung cancer (NSCLC), such as lung squamous cell carcinoma (LUSC) and lung adenocarcinoma (LUAD), most frequently harbor mutations in the *NRF2* or *KEAP1* loci, which result in NRF2 hyperactivation (Ohta et al. 2008; The Cancer Genome Atlas Research Network 2012; Marinelli et al.

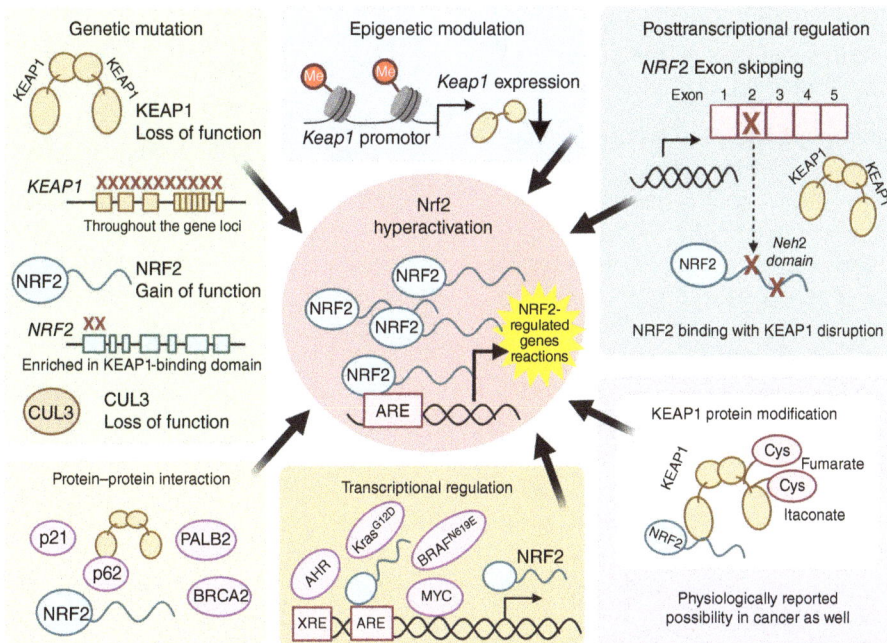

Figure 2. Mechanisms of NRF2 activation in cancer. KEAP1-mediated degradation of NRF2 is often impaired in NRF2-activated cancers, resulting in the persistent stabilization and hyperactivation of NRF2. Additional mechanisms of increased NRF2 production include the transcriptional up-regulation of NRF2.

2020). Somatic LOF (Stafford et al. 2018) mutations of *KEAP1* occur throughout the gene (Hast et al. 2013), whereas somatic GOF mutations of *NRF2* are enriched in its ETGE and DLG domain (Shibata et al. 2011; Fukutomi et al. 2014), leading to conformational changes that prevent NRF2 degradation by disrupting its interaction with KEAP1. Paradoxically, some mutations in *KEAP1* were reported to increase binding to NRF2 but blocked its degradation (Hast et al. 2014). *KEAP1* LOF mutations and *NRF2* GOF mutations are mutually exclusive, suggesting that hyperactivation of NRF2 by either mechanism is sufficient for cancer progression. From the perspective of cancer evolution, *KEAP1* mutations typically occur in early tumorigenesis alongside oncogenic *KRAS* mutations, which are frequent driver mutations in LUAD (Jamal-Hanjani et al. 2017). Additionally, since CUL3 is a major component of the complex targeting NRF2 for degradation, *CUL3* somatic LOF mutations are also detected in multiple cancer types, including LUSC and papillary renal cell carcinoma (The Cancer Genome Atlas Research Network 2012; Kandoth et al. 2013).

Protein–Protein Interaction (PPI) and Inhibition of NRF2–KEAP1 Complex

The interaction of KEAP1 and NRF2 is thought to be a hinge and latch mechanism (Tong et al. 2006, 2007; Horie et al. 2021). Unlike the mechanism by which modification of the cysteine residue in KEAP1 changes the conformation of KEAP1 and prevents it from capturing NRF2, the binding of these proteins is inhibited by getting stuck in the pocket at the point of contact between NRF2 and KEAP1. p62 (SQSTM1), a transcriptional target of NRF2 that functions as an anchor for the autophagosome membrane and targets proteins for ubiquitination, was reported to competitively bind KEAP1 at the same site as the ETGE motif of NRF2 (Komatsu et al. 2010; Ichimura et al. 2013; Katsuragi et al. 2016), thereby disruption KEAP1-NRF2 PPI, which is often observed in hepatocellular carcinoma (Saito et al. 2016). Similarly, other competitive proteins, such as PALB2 (Ma et al. 2012), BRCA2 (Gorrini et al. 2013), and DPP3 (Hast et al. 2013)

are also reported to block KEAP1–NRF2 interaction without modification of cysteine residues of KEAP1.

Cysteine Modification by Oncometabolites Inducing NRF2 Stabilization

KEAP1 functions as a major sensor of ROS and electrophiles (Saito et al. 2016), so its subsequent cytoprotective function of NRF2 induction needs to be sensitive and quick. Hence, multiple sensory cysteine residues in KEAP1 can directly react with xenobiotics and oxidative stressors (Suzuki et al. 2019). Some of the endogenous factors, such as the tricarboxylic acid (Chafe et al. 2021) cycle metabolites itaconate (Mills et al. 2018) and fumarate (Sullivan et al. 2013), glycolytic intermediate methylglyoxal (Bollong et al. 2018), threonine catabolism and acetoacetate oxidation (Kold-Christensen and Johannsen 2020), and the lipid mediators 15-deoxy PGJ2 (Mochizuki et al. 2005), react with these sensory cysteines to alter the conformation of the KEAP1 dimer and drive NRF2 activation. In the fumarate, its accumulation occurs in response to LOF mutations in fumarate hydratase (*FH*) gene, which are observed in multiple cancers (Kinch et al. 2011; Schmidt et al. 2020).

Transcriptional Up-Regulation of NRF2

In physiological conditions, the promotor of the *NRF2 (NFE2L2)* gene contains xenobiotic response elements where aryl hydrocarbon receptor (Adam et al. 2011) directly binds, which enables AhR to regulate Nrf2 transcriptionally (Kensler et al. 2007). The *NFE2L2* promotor also contains ARE sequence, and it has been suggested that NRF2 activates its own transcription (Kwak et al. 2002). Interestingly, Notch family proteins seem to have both up- and downstream roles in NRF2 transcriptional regulation. While NOTCH signaling directly activates NRF2 expression, specifically in the physiological liver development (Wakabayashi et al. 2014), *NOTCH3* is a target gene of NRF2 in NRF2-hyperactivated cancers (Okazaki et al. 2020). In the context of cancers, transcriptional up-regulation of *NFE2L2* gene has been reported. For example, major oncogenes like

KRAS, BRAF, and *MYC* have been found to drive transcriptional NRF2 expression to mitigate the increase of excessive ROS (DeNicola et al. 2011; Gorrini et al. 2013).

Posttranscriptional Regulation of NRF2

In addition to the transcriptional regulation, posttranscriptional changes can cause persistent activation of NRF2 (Wu and Papagiannakopoulos 2020; Pillai et al. 2022). For example, aberrant splicing of *NFE2L2* gene leading to skipping of exon 2, which contains the Neh2 domain that mediates interaction with KEAP1, leads to KEAP1-mediated ubiquitination and degradation and consequently exhibits NRF2 hyperactivation (Goldstein et al. 2016).

Epigenetic Suppression of *KEAP1* Gene

Epigenetic regulation of *KEAP1* has been proposed as another mechanism of NRF2 induction. Hypermethylation of the *KEAP1* promotor region is observed in multiple cancer types, including brain, lung, breast, colorectal, and prostate cancer (Wang et al. 2008; Zhang 2010; Hanada et al. 2012; Barbano et al. 2013). In fact, epigenetic profiling of 47 NSCLC patient samples revealed methylation of the *KEAP1* promoter region in half of the tumor tissues, suggesting that epigenetic suppression of *KEAP1* expression may also contribute to NRF2 deregulation in lung cancer (Muscarella et al. 2011). Triple-negative breast cancers with KEAP1 promoter hypermethylation were associated with worse prognosis (Barbano et al. 2013).

Metabolic Characteristics of NRF2-Activated Cancer Cells

NRF2 is a transcription factor that regulates redox balance by driving robust expression of molecules responsible for scavenging ROS and mitigating oxidative stress (Singh et al. 2006; Shibata et al. 2008a). Since the antioxidant function of NRF2 is based primarily on functions of redox-regulating enzymes induced by NRF2, in this section we discuss how NRF2 target genes control multiple aspects of cellular metabolism involved in anabolic processes and redox biology.

One of the most important modulators of redox balance is GSH (Fig. 3). The synthesis of GSH involves the conjugation of glutamate, cysteine, and glycine (Lu 2009). Upon exposure to ROS, GSH is oxidized to glutathione sulfenic acid (GSOH), which rapidly reacts with GSH to form oxidized glutathione (GSSG) and water. Physiologically, GSH is maintained in the reduced state by the NRF2 target glutathione disulfide reductase (GSR) (Harris et al. 2015), in a reaction that requires NADPH, a reducing equivalent also under the regulation of NRF2. GSH biosynthesis is highly dependent on the system xC (xCT), which is an antiporter of cystine and glutamate. Cystine pumped in via xCT is converted intracellularly to cysteine by the thioredoxin system (see the section Selenoproteins). Cysteine is conjugated with glutamate to form γ-glutamyl cysteine, which is catalyzed by γ-glutamyl cysteine ligase (GCL), a rate-limiting enzyme of the glutathione synthesis pathway. GCL is composed of two subunits, catalytic subunit (GCLC) (Nguyen et al. 2003; McWalter et al. 2004) and modulatory subunit (GCLM) (Jyrkkänen et al. 2008). γ-Glutamyl cysteine is ultimately conjugated with glycine to form GSH. *SLC7A11* encoding the cystine transporter xCT, *GCLC*, and *GCLM* are all bona fide target genes of NRF2. A large pool of GSH is advantageous for cancer cells as it leads to multidrug and radiation resistance, protection against mutagenesis, or against ROS produced along with growth, resulting in survival (Wu and Papagiannakopoulos 2020; Pillai et al. 2022).

NADPH serves as an important reducing equivalent in the biological redox reactions. NRF2 coordinately regulates NADPH synthesizing enzymes, such as the first two enzymes on the pentose phosphate pathway (PPP), glucose-6-phosphate dehydrogenase (G6PD), and 6-phosphogluconate dehydrogenase (PGD), and the central carbon metabolism enzymes, malic enzyme 1 (ME1) and isocitrate dehydrogenase 1 (IDH1) (Mitsuishi et al. 2012). NADPH has two important roles in metabolism. First, NADPH works as a source of synthesis of nucleotide (Tong et al. 2009), cholesterols (Porter 2015), and fatty acids (Wakil 1989). Second,

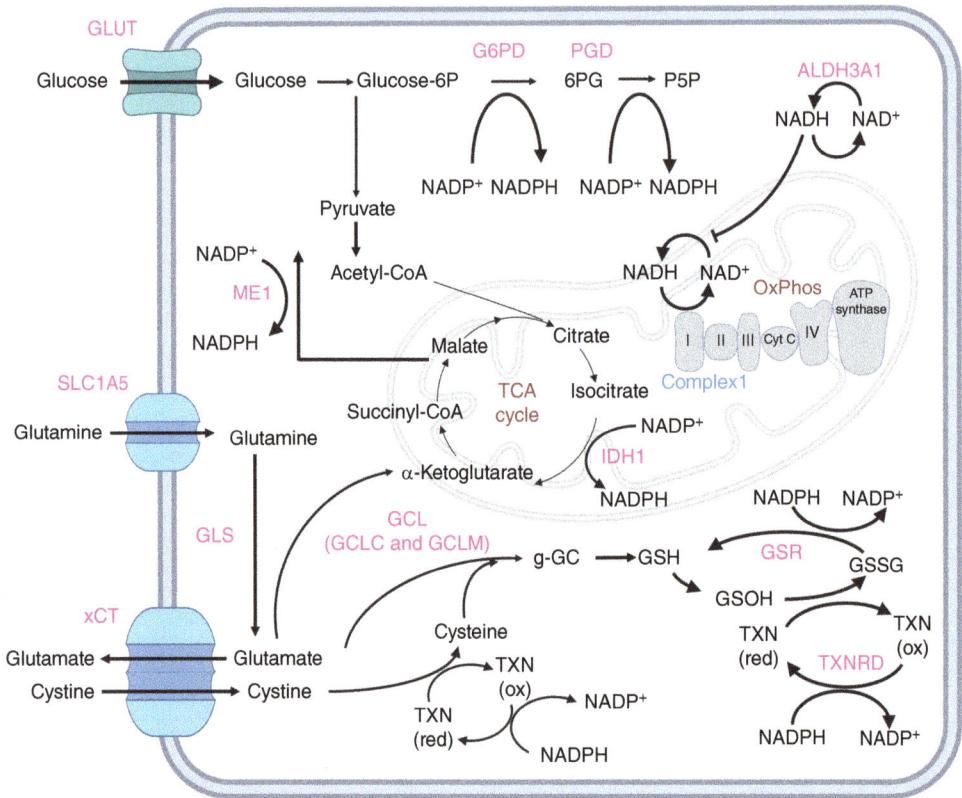

Figure 3. Metabolic characteristics of NRF2-activated cancer cells. One of the most prominent characteristics of NRF2-activated cancer cells is the extensive metabolic rewiring of multiple redox pathways, including glutathione synthesis. Due to the increased consumption of glutamate, NRF2-activated cancer cells are heavily dependent on glutamine uptake and utilization.

NADPH is used to reduce oxidized glutathione (GSSH) into GSH and to reduce thioredoxin (TXN). As NRF2 induces GSR and thioredoxin reductase 1 (TXNRD1) (Stafford et al. 2018), Nrf2-activated cancer continuously consumes NADPH as compensation of its large production of GSH and reduced TXN.

However, NRF2 activation is a double-edged sword, because at the cost of increased antioxidant production and the high reductive potential, chronic NRF2 activation can lead to reductive stress and metabolic vulnerabilities (Fig. 3; Wu and Papagiannakopoulos 2020; Pillai et al. 2022). Because xCT is an antiporter of cystine and glutamate, increased cystine uptake due to highly expressed xCT is inevitably accompanied by increased export of glutamate. Moreover, high GSH production requires glutamate in addition to

cysteine, which ultimately leads to reduction of intracellular glutamate and decreased glutamate availability for fueling the TCA cycle and nonessential amino acid (NEAA) synthesis in NRF2-activated cancer cells (Sayin et al. 2017; LeBoeuf et al. 2020). Therefore, NRF2-activated cancers are heavily dependent on glutamine uptake and glutaminase (GLS1), which converts glutamine to glutamate (Romero et al. 2017; Sayin et al. 2017; Galan-Cobo et al. 2019; Fox et al. 2020). Furthermore, NRF2-activated cells are highly dependent on the PPP (Mitsuishi et al. 2012; Best et al. 2019; Ding et al. 2021) and recent research demonstrated that this dependence is due to compensatory up-regulation of NADPH-producing enzymes ME1 and IDH1, which consume malate and isocitrate away from the TCA cycle (Ding et al. 2021). Intriguingly the G6PD inhibition synergizes with glutaminase inhibition because both independently deplete TCA intermediates, resulting in the efficient suppression of NRF2-activated tumor growth (Ding et al. 2021).

Finally, a recent study demonstrated that NRF2 activation leads to NADH accumulation, an overall reduction of the NAD^+/NADH ratio and reductive stress (Weiss-Sadan et al. 2023). While NADH is a major electron donor to the complex I of the mitochondrial electron transport chain (Chafe et al. 2021), alcohol dehydrogenases, such as *ALDH3A1*, utilize NAD^+ as a cofactor for electron acceptance and generate NADH. Thus, NRF2-activated cancers are selectively vulnerable to complex I inhibition, which impairs oxidation of NADH and exacerbates NADH-mediated reductive stress (Weiss-Sadan et al. 2023).

NRF2 Activation and Its Role in Different Stages of Tumorigenesis

Over the last decade, multiple studies have dissected the role of NRF2 in the various stages of cancer progression. These studies have demonstrated a clear role of NRF2 in tumor initiation, progression, and immune evasion.

NRF2 in Tumor Initiation and Progression

DeNicola et al. (2011) were the first to demonstrate that *Nrf2* is required for *Kras*-driven lung and pancreas tumorigenesis. Using patient-derived organoid models, Chio et al. (2016) demonstrated that *Nrf2* knockdown suppressed tumor initiation and maintenance. These studies support the idea that NRF2 is necessary for tumorigenesis in tumors with known oncogenic drivers such as *KRAS*. Genomic studies suggest that activation of the NRF2 pathway by genetic alterations in KEAP1/NRF2 play an important role in cancer development (Shibata et al. 2008b, 2011; Kim et al. 2010; Solis et al. 2010; Zhang et al. 2010; Konstantinopoulos et al. 2011), including lung adenocarcinoma (Satoh et al. 2013; Romero et al. 2017), papillary lung adenomas (Best et al. 2018), and squamous cell carcinomas (Jeong et al. 2017). In addition to the importance of the KEAP1/NRF2-pathway in tumor initiation

and maintenance, NRF2 has been to shown to also promote metastases (Lignitto et al. 2019). Overall, NRF2 activation by any number of mechanisms including somatic mutations, transcriptional regulation, or metabolic reprogramming-triggered modifications of KEAP1 promotes tumorigenesis.

Tumor Microenvironment (TME) of NRF2-Activated Cancers

NRF2 activation in immune cells has been reported to enhance the antitumor immunity. NRF2-deficient mice exhibit increased cancer cell colonization in lung (Satoh et al. 2010), and this phenotype was recapitulated in myeloid cell–specific NRF2-deficient mice (Hiramoto et al. 2014), suggesting that NRF2 in myeloid cells is responsible for the suppressed colonization of cancer cells in lung tissues. Conversely, NRF2 activation in cancer-bearing hosts attenuates tumor growth (Hayashi et al. 2020), supporting the idea that NRF2 activation in the tumor microenvironment (TME) enhances antitumor immunity. NRF2 pathway activation in regulatory T cells were shown to limit their suppressive activity, enhancing the antitumor immunity (Maj et al. 2017).

NRF2 in cancer cells has been implicated to suppress antitumor immunity in a mouse model (Fig. 4; Kitamura et al. 2017). Recent clinical data consistently suggest that hyperactivation of the NRF2 pathway in cancer cells modulates or remodels the TME and promotes immune evasion, leading to immunotherapy inactivation. NRF2-hyperactive cancers respond poorly to immune checkpoint inhibitor (The Cancer Genome Atlas Research Network 2012) treatment (Arbour et al. 2018; Brogden et al. 2018; Cristescu et al. 2018; Marinelli et al. 2020). In fact, studies have reported that patients harboring *KEAP1* LOF mutations or *NRF2* GOF mutations exhibit worse survival after immunotherapy (Arbour et al. 2018; Hellmann et al. 2018). Pancancer analysis revealed immune evasive characteristics in NRF2-activated cancers, especially NRF2-activated squamous cell carcinoma (Härkönen et al. 2023). As for the mechanism of how NRF2-activated cancers evade antitumor immunity,

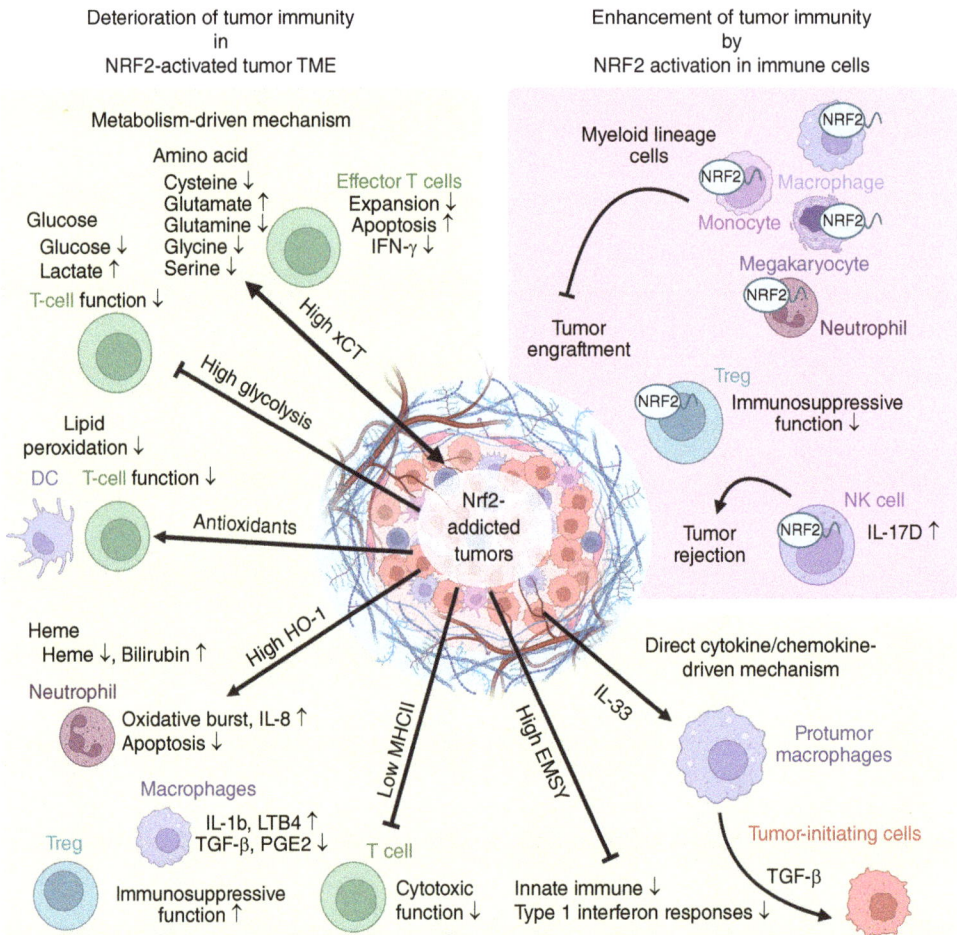

Figure 4. Tumor microenvironment of NRF2-activated cancer. Effects of *Keap1/Nrf2* mutated tumor on tumor microenvironment and antitumor immune responses. Nrf2-activated tumors display increase of glutamate and depletion of cystine, glycine, glutamine, and serine. This imbalance affects T-cell function. Increased glucose consumption and lactate secretion also impacts T-cell function. Accumulation of antioxidants decreases reactive oxygen species (ROS) and lipid peroxides, which can affect dendritic cells, T-cell effector cells, and Treg cells. Remodeled heme metabolism by NRF2-activation drives by-products, which can affect other immune cells infiltrating TME.

newly identified KEAP1 substrates in addition to NRF2 may also play a role (Marzio et al. 2022).

2. SELENOPROTEINS

Proteins with selenocysteine, the 2I amino acid (Fig. 5A), are collectively called selenoproteins, and 25 selenoproteins are known in humans. Selenocysteine tRNA (Trsp) is a single-copy gene and essential for the selenoprotein synthesis

mediating selenocysteine incorporation into the growing polypeptides (Tsuji et al. 2021). Trsp deficiency inhibits production of whole selenoproteins, leading to remarkable increase of oxidative stress, which implies critical contributions of selenoproteins to antioxidant function (Suzuki et al. 2008; Kawatani et al. 2011). The selenoproteins play important roles in the removal of ROS and in redox regulation, the major ones being glutathione peroxidase family and thiore-

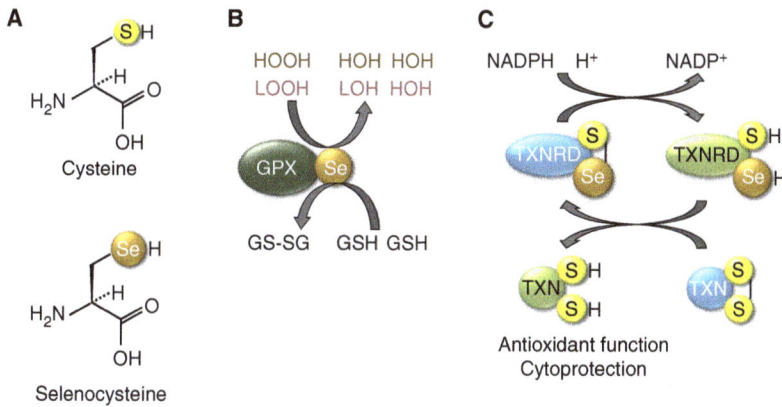

Figure 5. Redox regulation by selenoproteins. (*A*) Comparison of cysteine and selenocysteine. (*B*) GPX enzymes use glutathione (GSH) as a cosubstrate to catalyze the reduction of lipid hydroperoxides to their corresponding alcohols. (*C*) Thioredoxin system is composed of thioredoxin (TXN) and thioredoxin reductase (TXNRD) using NADPH as a reducing equivalent.

doxin reductase family. As selenium is more re-active than sulfur, selenocysteine is used as the active center of the redox reaction in these en-zymes.

There are four family members of glutathi-one peroxidase (Fig. 5B). GPX1 reduces hydro-gen peroxide to water using reduced glutathione (Lubos et al. 2011). GPX4, which has recently attracted attention as a suppressor of ferroptosis, plays a particularly important function in cancer cells (Seiler et al. 2008; Yang et al. 2014). GPX4 uses reduced glutathione to reduce lipid peroxide in biological membranes to alcohol, thereby sup-pressing lipid peroxide accumulation (Yoo et al. 2010). In cancer cells, lipid peroxide tends to accumulate due to the generation of reactive ox-ygen species. GPX4 reduces lipid peroxide, thereby imparting resistance to ferroptosis in cancer cells (Wu et al. 2019).

There are three family members of thiore-doxin reductase (Fig. 5C). Of particular impor-tance for oxidative stress tolerance in cancer cells is TXNRD1. Specific inhibition of the cytoplas-mic thioredoxin reductase, TXNRD1, was effec-tive in producing specific cytotoxicity in cancer cells (Stafford et al. 2018). Furthermore, inhibi-tion of TXNRD1 has been reported to induce cancer cell death (Busker et al. 2020) and sensi-tize NRF2-activated cancer cells to an anticancer drug (Torrente and DeNicola 2022). Under

physiological conditions, the thioredoxin system is an important antioxidant system regulated by NRF2 along with the glutathione system. Thio-redoxin (TXN) and TXNRD1 are both canonical NRF2 target genes.

3. SULFUR METABOLISM

Sulfur is an essential element for life and plays a central role in redox reactions in the body. Cys-teine/cystine and methionine are the main sources of sulfur for living organisms, and both are closely linked to the redox balance of cancer cells. Com-prehensive metabolic tracing revealed that activity of cysteine synthesis from methionine via a *trans*-sulfuration pathway varies from tissue to tissue and is generally down-regulated during tumori-genesis (Yoon et al. 2023). Consistently, many cancer cells appear to save cysteine and activate cystine uptake from outside of cells. For example, CDO1, which reduces cysteine availability by feeding cysteine into the taurine synthesis path-way (Fig. 6A), is frequently silenced cancer cells (Kang et al. 2019). Pancreatic cancers with higher expression of mitochondrial calcium uniporter have higher activity of NRF2 and heavily rely on cystine transporter xCT (Wang et al. 2022). In contrast, lung cancer cells, especially those with NRF2 activation, are resistant to xCT inhibition despite the remarkable up-regulation of xCT and

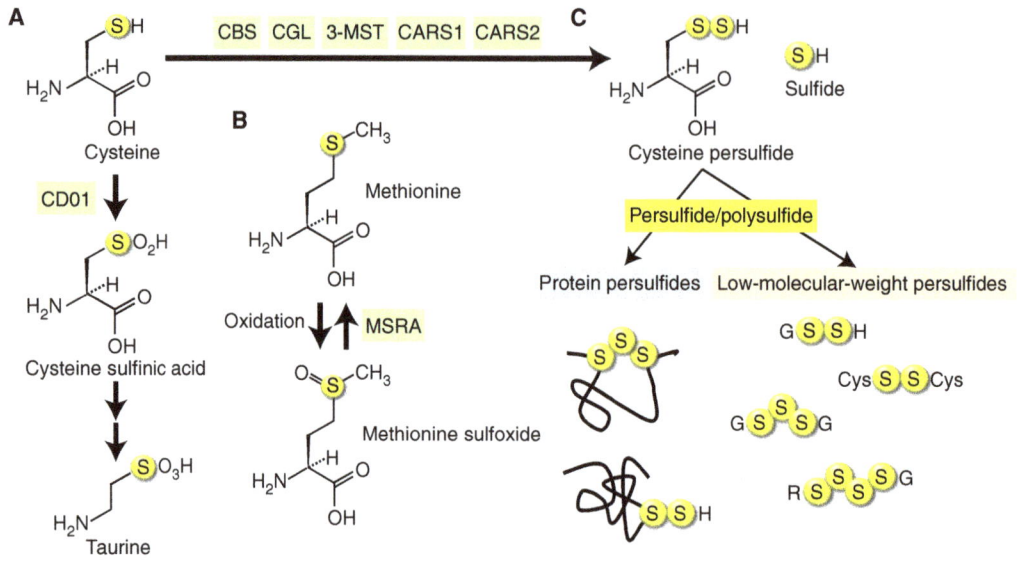

Figure 6. Sulfur metabolism regulating cellular redox homeostasis. (*A*) Cysteine is oxidized by CDO1 and eventually converted to taurine. (*B*) Methionine oxidation is reversed by methionine sulfoxide reductase A (MSRA). (*C*) Cysteine persulfide synthesis is catalyzed by several enzymes including CBS, CGL, 3-MST, CARS1, and CARS2. Persulfides and polysulfides are present in the form of low molecular weight metabolites and in the side chains of proteins.

increased uptake of cystine, which is explained by a novel regulation of ferroptosis by glutamate sequestration (Kang et al. 2021).

While cysteine thiols are sensitive to oxidation, alkylation and other redox-mediated modification, methionine is also sensitive to oxidation especially in cancer cells that tend to generate high levels of ROS. MSRA, which protects proteins from oxidation of methionine residues (Fig. 6B), is down-regulated in breast cancers especially of advanced stage (De Luca et al. 2010). Similar tendencies are observed in metastatic pancreatic cancers, in which oxidation of methionine residue in pyruvate kinase M2 plays a role in the promotion of migration and metastasis (He et al. 2022).

Enzymes involved in the *trans*-sulfuration pathway, CBS and CGL, are regarded to catalyze hydrogen sulfide production, which has been reported to exhibit a variety of physiological activities as an intracellular signaling molecule. For example, it has been reported that the life span extension conferred by caloric restriction is dependent on hydrogen sulfide produced by CGL in the liver (Hine et al. 2015) and that CGL expres-

sion in the liver is regulated by the hypothalamic–pituitary axis (Hine et al. 2017). One of the biological actions of hydrogen sulfide is to promote angiogenesis (Coletta et al. 2012), which is observed as a downstream event of GCN2-ATF4 pathway activation as an amino acid starvation response (Longchamp et al. 2018). Coordinated action of hydrogen sulfide with the anti-aging effect of the NAD$^+$–Sirt1 axis is responsible for the maintenance of peripheral capillaries and consequent good peripheral tissue circulation (Das et al. 2018). CBS and CGL are expressed in cancer cells and promote their energy metabolism and cell proliferation, as well as angiogenesis and metastasis (Szabo et al. 2013; Wang et al. 2019; Ascenção and Szabo 2022). Hydrogen sulfide also affects antitumor immunity based on experiments in mouse models, showing that hydrogen sulfide suppression improves the efficacy of immune checkpoint inhibitors (Yue et al. 2023).

On the other hand, recent improvements in analytical techniques have revealed that many of the biological phenomena previously understood as hydrogen sulfide effects are persulfide/polysulfide effects (Ida et al. 2014; Akaike et al.

2017; Zivanovic et al. 2019). One of the characteristics of sulfur atoms is that they can form catenation on their own. That is, in addition to small molecule metabolites such as cysteine and glutathione, sulfur atoms are present in the side chains of cysteine residues in proteins in the form of catenation. Such persulfide/polysulfide can now be detected in biological samples, and it is assumed that most of what has been considered hydrogen sulfide is produced secondary to the degradation of persulfide/polysulfide during the preparation of biological samples. Persulfides/polysulfides are present in the form of low-molecular weight metabolites as well as in side chains of cysteine residues of proteins (Fig. 6C). Several enzymes involved in the production of persulfide/polysulfide have been described. CBS and CGL, which are considered hydrogen sulfide-producing enzymes, produce persulfide/polysulfide (Yadav et al. 2013, 2016; Ida et al. 2014). Cysteinyl-tRNA synthetases CARS1 and CARS2, which are localized in cytoplasm and mitochondria, respectively, possess cysteine persulfide synthesizing activity as a moonlighting function (Akaike et al. 2017). 3-Mercaptopyruvate sulfur transferase (Zhu et al. 2019) has been identified as a protein persulfidating enzyme (Pedre et al. 2023). Persulfide/polysulfide has an antioxidant function (Ida et al. 2014) and an anti-inflammatory function (Zhang et al. 2019), and is involved in protein quality control (Doka et al. 2020) and mediates mitochondrial activation (Akaike et al. 2017; Alam et al. 2023). Decrease in protein persulfide/polysulfide has been observed during the organismal aging process (Zivanovic et al. 2019). The role of persulfide/polysulfide in cancer includes supporting cell survival by inhibiting ferroptosis (Erdélyi et al. 2021; Wu et al. 2022; Barayeu et al. 2023) and promoting metastasis by activating EMT (Czikora et al. 2022). In addition, CBS promotes persulfidation of PHD2, resulting in the suppression of PHD2 and consequent activation of the HIF pathway (Dey et al. 2020). This may be one of the mechanisms by which cancer cells use the HIF pathway to achieve malignant transformation. NRF2 activates the cystine transporter to increase cystine uptake into the cell, thus increasing cysteine persulfide production (Alam et al. 2023).

Persulfide/polysulfide may be one of the mediators enhancing malignant attitudes of cancer.

4. HEME AND IRON METABOLISM

Heme and iron metabolism play important roles in both normal cellular functions and cancer development. Heme consists of a porphyrin ring coordinated with an iron atom at its center and serves as a critical vehicle for iron incorporation and utilization in various biological processes, being one of the major ways in which life utilizes iron. Although iron is an essential element for life, it needs to be tightly regulated because free iron is rather dangerous causing Fenton reaction, which occurs when free iron reacts with hydrogen peroxide (H_2O_2) or other ROS in cells and generates highly reactive hydroxy radicals, resulting in the lipid peroxidation and ferroptosis. Cancer cells, especially NRF2-activated cancers, are resistance to ferroptosis due to the NRF2-regulated iron metabolism, which can be regarded as a part of NRF2-mediated antioxidant function (Kerins and Ooi 2017).

Heme Metabolism in Cancer

Heme serves as a cofactor for various proteins involved in oxygen transport, energy production, and drug metabolism. Cellular heme levels are tightly regulated by synthesis and degradation. A rate limiting enzyme for the heme synthesis is δ-aminolevulinic acid synthase 1 (ALAS1), whereas a key enzyme for heme degradation is heme oxygenase 1 (HO-1). HO-1 expression is transcriptionally controlled under various stressed conditions including oxidative stress, inflammation, and hypoxia (Campbell et al. 2021). Among them, NRF2 and BACH1 play major roles in the regulation of HO-1: transcriptional activation by the former and transcriptional repression by the latter. An interesting twist is that BACH1 protein stability and nuclear translocation is regulated by HO-1 via heme availability as BACH1 is a heme-binding protein (Suzuki et al. 2004; Hira et al. 2007; Zenke-Kawasaki et al. 2007). FBXO22 turned out to mediate the heme-induced degradation of BACH1 by interacting with heme-loaded BACH1 (Lignitto et al. 2019).

BACH1 has been shown to enhance metastasis of lung cancers (Wiel et al. 2019) and pancreatic cancers by repressing epithelial gene expression and promoting epithelial–mesenchymal transition (Sato et al. 2020). In NRF2-activated NSCLC, HO-1 is up-regulated, resulting in the heme degradation, consequent decline of FBXO22-mediated BACH1 degradation, and enhanced metastasis by the stabilized BACH1 (Lignitto et al. 2019). Although BACH1 is stabilized, which is expected to shut off HO-1 expression in normal conditions, HO-1 expression remains high enough to maintain the low levels of heme in NRF2-activated cancer cells, suggesting that transcriptional activation of HO-1 by constitutively activated NRF2 dominates over the BACH1-mediated repression of HO-1. The persistent activation of NRF2 creates a unique coexistence of NRF2 and BACH1 via heme metabolism, which drives metastasis, the most serious fatal event for cancer patients.

Iron Metabolism and Ferroptosis in Cancer

Iron metabolism and the process of ferroptosis are closely related to each other, and how they are regulated has a significant impact on the biological characteristics of cancer. Dysregulation of iron metabolism and alterations in the ferroptosis pathway play important roles in cancer development, progression, and therapeutic response.

Cancer cells often exhibit increased iron uptake to support their high metabolic demands for cell proliferation and growth and an enhanced dependence on iron, being dramatically more susceptible to iron depletion than noncancer cells, a phenomenon termed "iron addiction" (Manz et al. 2016). Up-regulation of iron transporters, such as transferrin receptor 1 (TFR1) is often observed in various cancers, and increased expression of TFR1 is associated with poor prognosis (Shen et al. 2018). At the same time, cancer cells are equipped with protective systems against iron-induced oxidative stress. For example, iron storage proteins, such as ferritin, to sequester excess iron and iron exporter, ferroportin, to transport iron from the inside of a cell to the outside of the cell are frequently up-regulated in cancer cells (Manz et al. 2016). NRF2 directly activates FTH and FTL genes encoding ferritin

heavy chain and ferritin light chain, respectively, and SLC40A1 encoding ferropotin is also a direct target gene of NRF2 (Kerins and Ooi 2017), suggesting that the regulation of iron metabolism by NRF2 is a part of the NRF2-mediated antioxidant cytoprotective system.

Homeostatic iron levels are maintained by the function of iron regulatory proteins (IRPs) that recognize iron-responsive elements (IREs) in the mRNA sequence of iron regulatory proteins such as ferritin and transferrin receptor (Rouault 2006). IRP1 is a functional aconitase that interconverts citrate and isocitrate in the cytosol of iron-sufficient cells, whereas IRP1 acquires IRE-binding activity in iron-depleted cells enhancing iron uptake. The mechanistic basis of the "iron-sulfur cluster switch" performed by IRP1 is based on the ability of IRP1 to alternate between two major forms: the cytosolic aconitase form, which contains a [4Fe-4S] cluster bound to the enzymatic active site and does not bind IREs, and the apoprotein form, which lacks an iron–sulfur cluster and binds IREs. The cysteine desulfurase NFS1, which is an essential enzyme in eukaryotes that harvests sulfur from cysteine for the biosynthesis of iron–sulfur clusters, was shown to protect cancer cells from ferroptosis (Alvarez et al. 2017). Inhibition of NFS1 decreases the iron–sulfur cluster and consequently enhances IRP-meditated increase of iron uptake, which sensitizes ferroptosis induction. NFS1 inhibition shows synthetic lethality with inhibition of CA9, which is one of the carbonic anhydrases responsible for buffering pH through cooperation with bicarbonate transporters to avoid intracellular acidification of tumor cells (Chafe et al. 2021). CA9 inhibition acidifies intracellularly and promotes ROS accumulation, leading to the susceptibility to ferroptosis, which synergizes with NFS1 inhibition.

5. ANTIOXIDANTS

Antioxidants play complex roles in the context of cancer. Antioxidants are known for their ability to counteract oxidative stress and protect cells from damage caused by ROS, preventing carcinogenesis. On the other hand, high-dose antioxidant supplementation has been reported to promote tumor growth and interfere with anticancer therapy. This is a similar scenario to the bivalent effects of NRF2 activation, which exerts antioxidant function, on cancer prevention and cancer promotion. Of note, NRF2 activation is suppressed by antioxidants in cells with an intact KEAP1-NRF2 system because NRF2 is activated in response to electrophiles and ROS, which is quenched by antioxidants.

Antioxidants for Cancer Prevention and Therapeutics

ROS functions as both a carcinogenic and mutagenic agent against DNA, and the formation of ROS-induced DNA adducts, particularly 8-hydroxydeoxy guanine (8-OHdG), are a representative biomarker of oxidative DNA damage (Valko et al. 2007; Shigenaga et al. 1989). 8-OHdG leads to base mispairing from G:C to T:A, which can induce mutations by conversion of guanine to thymine (Moriya 1993) and underlie LOF mutations in tumor suppressor genes (Harris and Hollstein 1993; Hainaut and Pfeifer 2001) or GOF mutations in oncogenes (Hruban et al. 1993; Madison et al. 2022). In addition, cancer cells produce abundant ROS, which is beneficial to some extent for tumor expansion and growth (Perillo et al. 2020). Antioxidants, such as vitamins C and E, β-carotene, and selenium, can scavenge ROS and neutralize their harmful effects, thus potentially reducing DNA damage and protecting against cancer initiation as well as limiting tumor growth facilitated by optimal levels of ROS. Observational studies showed that diets rich in fruits, vegetables, and other antioxidant-rich foods are associated with a lower risk of cancers (Weisburger 1991). These foods naturally contain a variety of antioxidants, along with other phytochemicals, which may serve as NRF2 inducers. Thus, it is not easy to separate the specific effects of antioxidants on cancer pretension from those of other components in these foods.

While the antioxidant effects in cancer prevention are still inconclusive, mitochondria-targeted antioxidants, such as mito-vitamin E and MitoTEMPO, in combination with mitochondrial complex I inhibitors are likely to induce reductive stress in cancer cells, providing an effective therapeutic strategy (Kong et al. 2020). Because mito-vitamin E reduces superoxide production in mitochondria and because Mito-TEMPO promotes superoxide quenching as a mitochondria-targeted SOD (SOD2) mimetics, superoxide elimination in mitochondria may mainly account for the therapeutic effect. Inhibition of mitochondrial complex I increases NADH/NAD ratio and is effective for the induction of reductive stress. KEAP1-mutant cancers in which NRF2 is constitutively activated are especially vulnerable to the mitochondrial complex I inhibition (Weiss-Sadan et al. 2023).

Antioxidants for Cancer Promotion

Some studies suggest that supplementation of high-dose antioxidants during cancer treatment, such as radiation therapy or chemotherapy, interferes with the effectiveness of these treatments (Wang et al. 2011; Kashif et al. 2023). This is because cancer therapies often exert their effects by generating ROS to induce tumor cell death. Antioxidants quench ROS and consequently decrease the efficacy of the treatments. In addition to affecting the treatment efficacy, mouse cancer models have been used to demonstrate protumorigenic effects of antioxidants. Supplementation of antioxidants N-acetylcysteine (NAC) and vitamin E to the diet markedly increases tumor progression and reduces survival in mouse models of BRAF- and KRAS-induced lung cancer. Both antioxidants reduced expression of endogenous antioxidant genes (Sayin et al. 2014). In the case of an endogenous mouse model of malignant melanoma, NAC supplementation increases lymph node metastases. Importantly, NAC and the soluble vitamin E analog Trolox markedly increased the migration and invasive properties of human malignant melanoma cells. These results suggest that antioxidants are involved in the malignant melanoma progression (Le Gal et al. 2015).

THERAPEUTICS STRATEGIES TARGETING REDOX METABOLISM

Given the importance of redox biology in cancer, there are many therapeutic strategies being developed to target redox metabolism. As we have highlighted throughout this paper, cancer cells build up their antioxidant capacity to buffer against ROS-dependent toxicity, which can often lead to reductive stress. Thus, many emerging anticancer therapeutic agents today aim to disrupt ROS homeostasis by modulating cellular metabolism (Table 1).

Therapeutic strategies that promote ROS production have been shown to suppress growth and promote cell death. Targeting antioxidant pathways directly responsible for ROS scavenging, such as TXN and GSH metabolism, is being explored by many groups. The GCL inhibitor, buthionine sulfoximine (Cronin et al. 2018), is well-tolerated compound that has shown some efficacy in several cancer models (Tagde et al. 2014; Villablanca et al. 2016). Furthermore, blocking cystine uptake by inhibiting xCT (sulfasalazine and erastin) or degradation of exogenous cystine by cyste(i)nase has shown therapeutic efficacy in several cancers (Cramer et al. 2017; Badgley et al. 2020; Joly et al. 2020; Xia et al. 2021). Inhibitors of glutamine uptake (V-9302) and glutaminase (CB-839) can block glutamine-derived glutamate use for GSH synthesis (Li et al. 2014; Romero et al. 2017; Jin et al. 2020; Xia et al. 2021). In addition, small molecules inhibitors of the TXN system (auranofin, Tri-1/2) have shown antitumor activity in preclinical models (Chaffman et al. 1984; Gromer et al. 1998; Sobhakumari et al. 2012; Stafford et al. 2018).

As discussed extensively in this paper, a major form of redox-dependent cell death resulting from excessive lipid peroxidation and loss of membrane integrity in cancer cells is ferroptosis. Therefore, drugs directly targeting the enzymes that prevent lipid peroxidation, Gpx4 (RSL3; ML210; DPIs) and Fsp1 (iFSP1, icFSP1), are being developed (Stockwell et al. 2017; Doll et al. 2019; Nakamura et al. 2023). Inhibition of cysteine metabolism with sulfasalazine, erastin, and cyste(i)nase may be able to effectively defeat cancer by inducing ferroptosis (Cramer et al. 2017; Badgley et al. 2020; Joly et al. 2020; Xia et al. 2021).

Several clinical trials have been recently conducted in patients with LOF mutations in *KEAP1* or GOF mutations in *NRF2* that have putative activation in NRF2, high antioxidant capacity.

Table 1. Summary of metabolic therapies targeting redox metabolism

Drug name	Target	Pathway	Clinical trial
BSO	GCL inhibitor	GSH metabolism	NCT00002730
CB-839	Inhibition of GLS	GSH/Glutamine metabolism	NCT03875313, NCT04265534 NCT03872427
V-9302	Inhibition of SLC1A5	GSH/Glutamine metabolism	
Sulfasalazine Erastin	Inhibition of xCT	GSH/Glutamine/Cysteine metabolism Ferroptosis induction	NCT04205357 and NCT03847311
DRP-104 (Sirpiglenastat) DON	Glutamine antagonism	Glutamine metabolism	NCT04471415
Auranofin Tri1 Tri2	Inhibition of TXNRD1	Thioredoxin pathway	NCT01747798, NCT01419691, and NCT01737502
Cysteinase	Depletion of cysteine	Ferroptosis induction	
RSL3 ML210 DPIs	Inhibition of Gpx4	Ferroptosis induction	
iFSP1 icFSP1	Inhibition of Fsp1	Ferroptosis induction	

Cite this article as *Cold Spring Harb Perspect Med* doi: 10.1101/cshperspect.a041546

The majority of these trials targeted metabolic liabilities that result from the constitutive activation of NRF2, including glutamine addiction, which has been shown to be a major metabolic vulnerability in multiple preclinical studies (Romero et al. 2017; Sayin et al. 2017; Galan-Cobo et al. 2019; Fox et al. 2020). Specifically, one of the approaches combined standard of care immunotherapy/chemotherapy with the glutaminase inhibitor CB-839 (telaglenastat). This phase 2 clinical trial (KEAPSAKE, NCT04265534) targeted cancer patients with LOF mutations in *KEAP1*. This combination therapy was based on preclinical studies demonstrating that CB-839 promotes antitumor immune responses (Zavitsanou et al. 2023). Unfortunately, this study was terminated early because of no added benefit when CB-839 was added to standard of care. Glutaminase inhibition only blocks one of the many glutamine-dependent reactions, which may explain the limited therapeutic efficacy.

More recently, a phase 1/2 clinical trial (NCT04471415) focused on patients with advanced NSCLC harboring mutations in *KEAP1*, *NRF2*, or *STK11* tested the efficacy of single-agent therapy of a prodrug DRP-104 (Sirpiglenastat) or in combination with immune checkpoint inhibition. DRP-104 is prodrug of the glutamine antagonist 6-dizao-5-oxo-L-norleucine (DON) (Rais et al. 2022). As DON can be toxic, the DRP-104 prodrug is selectively converted to DON in the tumor microenvironment (Tenora et al. 2019; Rais et al. 2022). Interestingly, multiple preclinical studies have shown that administration of DRP-104, or earlier versions of this prodrug, results in higher infiltration of cytotoxic T cells and increased response to immunotherapy (Leone et al. 2019; Rais et al. 2022; Yokoyama et al. 2022; Pillai et al. 2023). It remains to be seen whether DRP-104 will display greater therapeutic efficacy compared to CB-839 by suppressing tumor growth and boosting antitumor immune responses.

A variety of approaches have been used to treat NRF2-addicted cancers, including inhibition of the NRF2 protein itself, or inhibition of downstream genes, and targeting the characteristic amino acid or redox metabolism. However, no highly effective therapy has yet been identified. Future studies will likely need to combine therapies that target cancer cell redox regulation and those that promote antitumor immune responses by altering immune cell landscapes.

CONCLUSION

Redox reactions play an extremely important role in the acquisition of life function. Cancer cells, being highly proliferative, generate higher levels of ROS compared to normal cells. To counteract the detrimental effects of ROS and promote their survival and growth, cancer cells are often equipped with potent antioxidant mechanisms, which allows them to evade the damaging effects of ROS, contributing to their ability to resist radiotherapy and chemotherapy. Understanding how cancer cells utilize redox regulation in tumor progression has powerful implications for the development of effective therapeutic strategies, leading to novel therapies for cancer cases refractory to ordinary and standard treatments due to highly enhanced antioxidant capacities of cancer cells.

ACKNOWLEDGMENTS

We thank all the members in the Papagiannakopoulos laboratory and Motohashi laboratory for their daily efforts and achievements in establishing a new landscape of redox metabolism in cancer. T.P. is supported by NIH grants (R37CA222504 and R01CA227649) and an American Cancer Society Research Scholar grant (RSG-17-200-01–TBE). M.H. is supported by a JSPS Overseas Research Fellowship, K.O. is supported by a JSPS grant (22K15504), and H.M. is supported by JSPS grants 21H05258, 21H05264, and 21H04799. We thank K. Wu for their critical reading of this review.

REFERENCES

Adam J, Hatipoglu E, O'Flaherty L, Ternette N, Sahgal N, Lockstone H, Baban D, Nye E, Stamp GW, Wolhuter K, et al. 2011. Renal cyst formation in Fh1-deficient mice is independent of the Hif/Phd pathway: roles for fumarate in KEAP1 succination and Nrf2 signaling. *Cancer Cell* **20**: 524–537. doi:10.1016/j.ccr.2011.09.006

Akaike T, Ida T, Wei FY, Nishida M, Kumagai Y, Alam MM, Ihara H, Sawa T, Matsunaga T, Kasamatsu S, et al. 2017. Cysteinyl-tRNA synthetase governs cysteine polysulfidation and mitochondrial bioenergetics. *Nat Commun* **8:** 1177. doi:10.1038/s41467-017-01311-y

Alam MM, Okazaki K, Nguyen LTT, Ota N, Kitamura H, Murakami S, Shima H, Igarashi K, Sekine H, Motohashi H. 2017. Glucocorticoid receptor signaling represses the antioxidant response by inhibiting histone acetylation mediated by the transcriptional activator NRF2. *J Biol Chem* **292:** 7519–7530. doi:10.1074/jbc.M116.773960

Alam MM, Kishino A, Sung E, Sekine H, Abe T, Murakami S, Akaike T, Motohashi H. 2023. Contribution of NRF2 to sulfur metabolism and mitochondrial activity. *Redox Biol* **60:** 102624. doi:10.1016/j.redox.2023.102624

Alvarez SW, Sviderskiy VO, Terzi EM, Papagiannakopoulos T, Moreira AL, Adams S, Sabatini DM, Birsoy K, Possemato R. 2017. NFS1 undergoes positive selection in lung tumours and protects cells from ferroptosis. *Nature* **551:** 639–643. doi:10.1038/nature24637

Arbour KC, Jordan E, Kim HR, Dienstag J, Yu HA, Sanchez-Vega F, Lito P, Berger M, Solit DB, Hellmann M, et al. 2018. Effects of co-occurring genomic alterations on outcomes in patients with *KRAS*-mutant non-small cell lung cancer. *Clin Cancer Res* **24:** 334–340. doi:10.1158/1078-0432 .CCR-17-1841

Ascenção K, Szabo C. 2022. Emerging roles of cystathionine β-synthase in various forms of cancer. *Redox Biol* **53:** 102331. doi:10.1016/j.redox.2022.102331

Badgley MA, Kremer DM, Maurer HC, DelGiorno KE, Lee HJ, Purohit V, Sagalovskiy IR, Ma A, Kapilian J, Firl CEM, et al. 2020. Cysteine depletion induces pancreatic tumor ferroptosis in mice. *Science* **368:** 85–89. doi:10.1126/sci ence.aaw9872

Badr H, Federman AD, Wolf M, Revenson TA, Wisnivesky JP. 2017. Depression in individuals with chronic obstructive pulmonary disease and their informal caregivers. *Aging Ment Health* **21:** 975–982. doi:10.1080/13607863.2016 .1186153

Barayeu U, Schilling D, Eid M, Xavier da Silva TN, Schlicker L, Mitreska N, Zapp C, Gräter F, Miller AK, Kappl R, et al. 2023. Hydropersulfides inhibit lipid peroxidation and ferroptosis by scavenging radicals. *Nat Chem Biol* **19:** 28–37. doi:10.1038/s41589-022-01145-w

Barbano R, Muscarella LA, Pasculli B, Valori VM, Fontana A, Coco M, la Torre A, Balsamo T, Poeta ML, Marangi GF, et al. 2013. Aberrant *Keap1* methylation in breast cancer and association with clinicopathological features. *Epigenetics* **8:** 105–112. doi:10.4161/epi.23319

Best SA, De Souza DP, Kersbergen A, Policheni AN, Dayalan S, Tull D, Rathi V, Gray DH, Ritchie ME, McConville MJ, et al. 2018. Synergy between the KEAP1/NRF2 and PI3K pathways drives non-small-cell lung cancer with an altered immune microenvironment. *Cell Metab* **27:** 935–943.e4. doi:10.1016/j.cmet.2018.02.006

Best SA, Ding S, Kersbergen A, Dong X, Song JY, Xie Y, Reljic B, Li K, Vince JE, Rathi V, et al. 2019. Distinct initiating events underpin the immune and metabolic heterogeneity of KRAS-mutant lung adenocarcinoma. *Nat Commun* **10:** 4190. doi:10.1038/s41467-019-12164-y

Bollong MJ, Lee G, Coukos JS, Yun H, Zambaldo C, Chang JW, Chin EN, Ahmad I, Chatterjee AK, Lairson LL, et al.

2018. A metabolite-derived protein modification integrates glycolysis with KEAP1-NRF2 signalling. *Nature* **562:** 600–604. doi:10.1038/s41586-018-0622-0

Brogden KA, Parashar D, Hallier AR, Braun T, Qian F, Rizvi NA, Bossler AD, Milhem MM, Chan TA, Abbasi T, et al. 2018. Genomics of NSCLC patients both affirm PD-L1 expression and predict their clinical responses to anti-PD-1 immunotherapy. *BMC Cancer* **18:** 225. doi:10 .1186/s12885-018-4134-y

Busker S, Qian W, Haraldsson M, Espinosa B, Johansson L, Attarha S, Kolosenko I, Liu J, Dagnell M, Grandér D, et al. 2020. Irreversible TrxR1 inhibitors block STAT3 activity and induce cancer cell death. *Sci Adv* **6:** eaax7945. doi:10 .1126/sciadv.aax7945

Campbell NK, Fitzgerald HK, Dunne A. 2021. Regulation of inflammation by the antioxidant haem oxygenase 1. *Nat Rev Immunol* **21:** 411–425. doi:10.1038/s41577-020-00491-x

Chafe SC, Vizeacoumar FS, Venkateswaran G, Nemirovsky O, Awrey S, Brown WS, McDonald PC, Carta F, Metcalfe A, Karasinska JM, et al. 2021. Genome-wide synthetic lethal screen unveils novel CAIX-NFS1/xCT axis as a targetable vulnerability in hypoxic solid tumors. *Sci Adv* **7:** eabj0364. doi:10.1126/sciadv.abj0364

Chaffman M, Brogden RN, Heel RC, Speight TM, Avery GS. 1984. Auranofin. A preliminary review of its pharmacological properties and therapeutic use in rheumatoid arthritis. *Drugs* **27:** 378–424. doi:10.2165/00003495-198427050-00002

Chauvin JR, Griesser M, Pratt DA. 2019. The antioxidant activity of polysulfides: It's radical!. *Chem Sci* **10:** 4999–5010. doi:10.1039/C9SC00276F

Cheung EC, Vousden KH. 2022. The role of ROS in tumour development and progression. *Nat Rev Cancer* **22:** 280–297. doi:10.1038/s41568-021-00435-0

Cheung EC, DeNicola GM, Nixon C, Blyth K, Labuschagne CF, Tuveson DA, Vousden KH. 2020. Dynamic ROS control by TIGAR regulates the initiation and progression of pancreatic cancer. *Cancer Cell* **37:** 168–182.e4. doi:10 .1016/j.ccell.2019.12.012

Chio IIC, Jafarnejad SM, Ponz-Sarvise M, Park Y, Rivera K, Palm W, Wilson J, Sangar V, Hao Y, Öhlund D, et al. 2016. NRF2 promotes tumor maintenance by modulating mRNA translation in pancreatic cancer. *Cell* **166:** 963–976. doi:10.1016/j.cell.2016.06.056

Chowdhry S, Zhang Y, McMahon M, Sutherland C, Cuadrado A, Hayes JD. 2013. Nrf2 is controlled by two distinct β-TrCP recognition motifs in its Neh6 domain, one of which can be modulated by GSK-3 activity. *Oncogene* **32:** 3765–3781. doi:10.1038/onc.2012.388

Coletta C, Papapetropoulos A, Erdelyi K, Olah G, Módis K, Panopoulos P, Asimakopoulou A, Gerö D, Sharina I, Martin E, et al. 2012. Hydrogen sulfide and nitric oxide are mutually dependent in the regulation of angiogenesis and endothelium-dependent vasorelaxation. *Proc Natl Acad Sci* **109:** 9161–9166. doi:10.1073/pnas.1202916109

Cramer SL, Saha A, Liu J, Tadi S, Tiziani S, Yan W, Triplett K, Lamb C, Alters SE, Rowlinson S, et al. 2017. Systemic depletion of L-cyst(e)ine with cyst(e)inase increases reactive oxygen species and suppresses tumor growth. *Nat Med* **23:** 120–127. doi:10.1038/nm.4232

Cristescu R, Mogg R, Ayers M, Albright A, Murphy E, Yearley J, Sher X, Liu XQ, Lu H, Nebozhyn M, et al. 2018. Pantumor genomic biomarkers for PD-1 checkpoint blockade-based immunotherapy. *Science* **362**: eaar3593. doi:10.1126/science.aar3593

Cronin SJF, Seehus C, Weidinger A, Talbot S, Reissig S, Seifert M, Pierson Y, McNeill E, Longhi MS, Turnes BL, et al. 2018. The metabolite BH4 controls T cell proliferation in autoimmunity and cancer. *Nature* **563**: 564–568. doi:10.1038/s41586-018-0701-2

Cully M, You H, Levine AJ, Mak TW. 2006. Beyond PTEN mutations: the PI3K pathway as an integrator of multiple inputs during tumorigenesis. *Nat Rev Cancer* **6**: 184–192. doi:10.1038/nrc1819

Czikora Á, Erdélyi K, Ditrói T, Szántó N, Jurányi EP, Szanyi S, Tóvári J, Strausz T, Nagy P. 2022. Cystathionine β-synthase overexpression drives metastatic dissemination in pancreatic ductal adenocarcinoma via inducing epithelial-to-mesenchymal transformation of cancer cells. *Redox Biol* **57**: 102505. doi:10.1016/j.redox.2022.102505

Das A, Huang GX, Bonkowski MS, Longchamp A, Li C, Schultz MB, Kim LJ, Osborne B, Joshi S, Lu Y, et al. 2018. Impairment of an endothelial NAD^+-H_2S signaling network is a reversible cause of vascular aging. *Cell* **173**: 74–89.e20. doi:10.1016/j.cell.2018.02.008

De Luca A, Sanna F, Sallese M, Ruggiero C, Grossi M, Sacchetta P, Rossi C, De Laurenzi V, Di Ilio C, Favaloro B. 2010. Methionine sulfoxide reductase a down-regulation in human breast cancer cells results in a more aggressive phenotype. *Proc Natl Acad Sci* **107**: 18628–18633. doi:10.1073/pnas.1010171107

DeNicola GM, Karreth FA, Humpton TJ, Gopinathan A, Wei C, Frese K, Mangal D, Yu KH, Yeo CJ, Calhoun ES, et al. 2011. Oncogene-induced Nrf2 transcription promotes ROS detoxification and tumorigenesis. *Nature* **475**: 106–109. doi:10.1038/nature10189

Dey A, Prabhudesai S, Zhang Y, Rao G, Thirugnanam K, Hossen MN, Dwivedi SKD, Ramchandran R, Mukherjee P, Bhattacharya R. 2020. Cystathione β-synthase regulates HIF-1α stability through persulfidation of PHD2. *Sci Adv* **6**: eaaz8534. doi:10.1126/sciadv.aaz8534

Ding H, Chen Z, Wu K, Huang SM, Wu WL, LeBoeuf SE, Pillai RG, Rabinowitz JD, Papagiannakopoulos T. 2021. Activation of the NRF2 antioxidant program sensitizes tumors to G6PD inhibition. *Sci Adv* **7**: eabk1023. doi:10.1126/sciadv.abk1023

Dóka É, Ida T, Dagnell M, Abiko Y, Luong NC, Balog N, Takata T, Espinosa B, Nishimura A, Cheng Q, et al. 2020. Control of protein function through oxidation and reduction of persulfidated states. *Sci Adv* **6**: eaax8358. doi:10.1126/sciadv.aax8358

Doll S, Freitas FP, Shah R, Aldrovandi M, da Silva MC, Ingold I, Goya Grocin A, Xavier da Silva TN, Panzilius E, Scheel CH, et al. 2019. FSP1 is a glutathione-independent ferroptosis suppressor. *Nature* **575**: 693–698. doi:10.1038/s41586-019-1707-0

Enomoto A, Itoh K, Nagayoshi E, Haruta J, Kimura T, O'Connor T, Harada T, Yamamoto M. 2001. High sensitivity of Nrf2 knockout mice to acetaminophen hepatotoxicity associated with decreased expression of ARE-regulated drug metabolizing enzymes and antioxidant genes. *Toxicol Sci* **59**: 169–177. doi:10.1093/toxsci/59.1.169

Erdélyi K, Ditrói T, Johansson HJ, Czikora Á, Balog N, Silwal-Pandit L, Ida T, Olasz J, Hajdú D, Mátrai Z, et al. 2021. Reprogrammed transsulfuration promotes basal-like breast tumor progression via realigning cellular cysteine persulfidation. *Proc Natl Acad Sci* **118**: e2100050118. doi:10.1073/pnas.2100050118

Fox DB, Garcia NMG, McKinney BJ, Lupo R, Noteware LC, Newcomb R, Liu J, Locasale JW, Hirschey MD, Alvarez JV. 2020. NRF2 activation promotes the recurrence of dormant tumour cells through regulation of redox and nucleotide metabolism. *Nat Metab* **2**: 318–334. doi:10.1038/s42255-020-0191-z

Friling RS, Bensimon A, Tichauer Y, Daniel V. 1990. Xenobiotic-inducible expression of murine glutathione S-transferase Ya subunit gene is controlled by an electrophile-responsive element. *Proc Natl Acad Sci* **87**: 6258–6262. doi:10.1073/pnas.87.16.6258

Fukutomi T, Takagi K, Mizushima T, Ohuchi N, Yamamoto M. 2014. Kinetic, thermodynamic, and structural characterizations of the association between Nrf2-DLGex degron and Keap1. *Mol Cell Biol* **34**: 832–846. doi:10.1128/MCB.01191-13

Furukawa M, Xiong Y. 2005. BTB protein Keap1 targets antioxidant transcription factor Nrf2 for ubiquitination by the cullin 3-Roc1 ligase. *Mol Cell Biol* **25**: 162–171. doi:10.1128/MCB.25.1.162-171.2005

Galan-Cobo A, Sitthideatphaiboon P, Qu X, Poteete A, Pisegna MA, Tong P, Chen PH, Boroughs LK, Rodriguez MLM, Zhang W, et al. 2019. LKB1 and KEAP1/NRF2 pathways cooperatively promote metabolic reprogramming with enhanced glutamine dependence in *KRAS*-mutant lung adenocarcinoma. *Cancer Res* **79**: 3251–3267. doi:10.1158/0008-5472.CAN-18-3527

Giles GI, Jacob C. 2002. Reactive sulfur species: an emerging concept in oxidative stress. *Biol Chem* **383**: 375–388. doi:10.1515/BC.2002.042

Glasauer A, Chandel NS. 2014. Targeting antioxidants for cancer therapy. *Biochem Pharmacol* **92**: 90–101. doi:10.1016/j.bcp.2014.07.017

Goldstein LD, Lee J, Gnad F, Klijn C, Schaub A, Reeder J, Daemen A, Bakalarski CE, Holcomb T, Shames DS, et al. 2016. Recurrent loss of NFE2L2 exon 2 is a mechanism for Nrf2 pathway activation in human cancers. *Cell Rep* **16**: 2605–2617. doi:10.1016/j.celrep.2016.08.010

Gorrini C, Baniasadi PS, Harris IS, Silvester J, Inoue S, Snow B, Joshi PA, Wakeham A, Molyneux SD, Martin B, et al. 2013. BRCA1 interacts with Nrf2 to regulate antioxidant signaling and cell survival. *J Exp Med* **210**: 1529–1544. doi:10.1084/jem.20121337

Gromer S, Arscott LD, Williams CH Jr, Schirmer RH, Becker K. 1998. Human placenta thioredoxin reductase: isolation of the selenoenzyme, steady state kinetics, and inhibition by therapeutic gold compounds. *J Biol Chem* **273**: 20096–20101. doi:10.1074/jbc.273.32.20096

Hainaut P, Pfeifer GP. 2001. Patterns of p53 G->T transversions in lung cancers reflect the primary mutagenic signature of DNA-damage by tobacco smoke. *Carcinogenesis* **22**: 367–374. doi:10.1093/carcin/22.3.367

Hanada N, Takahata T, Zhou Q, Ye X, Sun R, Itoh J, Ishiguro A, Kijima H, Mimura J, Itoh K, et al. 2012. Methylation of the KEAP1 gene promoter region in human colorectal cancer. *BMC Cancer* **12**: 66. doi:10.1186/1471-2407-12-66

Harder B, Tian W, La Clair JJ, Tan AC, Ooi A, Chapman E, Zhang DD. 2017. Brusatol overcomes chemoresistance through inhibition of protein translation. *Mol Carcinog* **56:** 1493–1500. doi:10.1002/mc.22609

Härkönen J, Pölönen P, Deen AJ, Selvarajan I, Teppo HR, Dimova EY, Kietzmann T, Ahtiainen M, Väyrynen JP, Väyrynen SA, et al. 2023. A pan-cancer analysis shows immunoevasive characteristics in NRF2 hyperactive squamous malignancies. *Redox Biol* **61:** 102644. doi:10.1016/j.redox.2023.102644

Harris IS, DeNicola GM. 2020. The complex interplay between antioxidants and ROS in cancer. *Trends Cell Biol* **30:** 440–451. doi:10.1016/j.tcb.2020.03.002

Harris IS, Treloar AE, Inoue S, Sasaki M, Gorrini C, Lee KC, Yung KY, Brenner D, Knobbe-Thomsen CB, Cox MA, et al. 2015. Glutathione and thioredoxin antioxidant pathways synergize to drive cancer initiation and progression. *Cancer Cell* **27:** 211–222. doi:10.1016/j.ccell.2014.11.019

Hast BE, Goldfarb D, Mulvaney KM, Hast MA, Siesser PF, Yan F, Hayes DN, Major MB. 2013. Proteomic analysis of ubiquitin ligase KEAP1 reveals associated proteins that inhibit NRF2 ubiquitination. *Cancer Res* **73:** 2199–2210. doi:10.1158/0008-5472.CAN-12-4400

Hast BE, Cloer EW, Goldfarb D, Li H, Siesser PF, Yan F, Walter V, Zheng N, Hayes DN, Major MB. 2014. Cancer-derived mutations in KEAP1 impair NRF2 degradation but not ubiquitination. *Cancer Res* **74:** 808–817. doi:10.1158/0008-5472.CAN-13-1655

Hayashi M, Kuga A, Suzuki M, Panda H, Kitamura H, Motohashi H, Yamamoto M. 2020. Microenvironmental activation of Nrf2 restricts the progression of Nrf2-activated malignant tumors. *Cancer Res* **80:** 3331–3344. doi:10.1158/0008-5472.CAN-19-2888

He D, Feng H, Sundberg B, Yang J, Powers J, Christian AH, Wilkinson JE, Monnin C, Avizonis D, Thomas CJ, et al. 2022. Methionine oxidation activates pyruvate kinase M2 to promote pancreatic cancer metastasis. *Mol Cell* **82:** 3045–3060.e11. doi:10.1016/j.molcel.2022.06.005

Hellmann MD, Nathanson T, Rizvi H, Creelan BC, Sanchez-Vega F, Ahuja A, Ni A, Novik JB, Mangarin LMB, Abu-Akeel M, et al. 2018. Genomic features of response to combination immunotherapy in patients with advanced non-small-cell lung cancer. *Cancer Cell* **33:** 843–852.e4. doi:10.1016/j.ccell.2018.03.018

Hine C, Harputlugil E, Zhang Y, Ruckenstuhl C, Lee BC, Brace L, Longchamp A, Treviño-Villarreal JH, Mejia P, Ozaki CK, et al. 2015. Endogenous hydrogen sulfide production is essential for dietary restriction benefits. *Cell* **160:** 132–144. doi:10.1016/j.cell.2014.11.048

Hine C, Kim HJ, Zhu Y, Harputlugil E, Longchamp A, Matos MS, Ramadoss P, Bauerle K, Brace L, Asara JM, et al. 2017. Hypothalamic-pituitary axis regulates hydrogen sulfide production. *Cell Metab* **25:** 1320–1333.e5. doi:10.1016/j.cmet.2017.05.003

Hira S, Tomita T, Matsui T, Igarashi K, Ikeda-Saito M. 2007. Bach1, a heme-dependent transcription factor, reveals presence of multiple heme binding sites with distinct coordination structure. *IUBMB Life* **59:** 542–551. doi:10.1080/15216540701225941

Hiramoto K, Satoh H, Suzuki T, Moriguchi T, Pi J, Shimosegawa T, Yamamoto M. 2014. Myeloid lineage-specific deletion of antioxidant system enhances tumor metastasis.

Cancer Prev Res **7:** 835–844. doi:10.1158/1940-6207.CAPR-14-0094

Hirose W, Oshikiri H, Taguchi K, Yamamoto M. 2022. The KEAP1-NRF2 system and esophageal cancer. *Cancers (Basel)* **14:** 4702. doi:10.3390/cancers14194702

Honkura Y, Matsuo H, Murakami S, Sakiyama M, Mizutari K, Shiotani A, Yamamoto M, Morita I, Shinomiya N, Kawase T, et al. 2016. NRF2 is a key target for prevention of noise-induced hearing loss by reducing oxidative damage of cochlea. *Sci Rep* **6:** 19329. doi:10.1038/srep19329

Horie Y, Suzuki T, Inoue J, Iso T, Wells G, Moore TW, Mizushima T, Dinkova-Kostova AT, Kasai T, Kamei T, et al. 2021. Molecular basis for the disruption of Keap1-Nrf2 interaction via hinge & latch mechanism. *Commun Biol* **4:** 576. doi:10.1038/s42003-021-02100-6

Hruban RH, van Mansfeld AD, Offerhaus GJ, van Weering DH, Allison DC, Goodman SN, Kensler TW, Bose KK, Cameron JL, Bos JL. 1993. K-ras oncogene activation in adenocarcinoma of the human pancreas. A study of 82 carcinomas using a combination of mutant-enriched polymerase chain reaction analysis and allele-specific oligonucleotide hybridization. *Am J Pathol* **143:** 545–554.

Ichimura Y, Waguri S, Sou YS, Kageyama S, Hasegawa J, Ishimura R, Saito T, Yang Y, Kouno T, Fukutomi T, et al. 2013. Phosphorylation of p62 activates the Keap1-Nrf2 pathway during selective autophagy. *Mol Cell* **51:** 618–631. doi:10.1016/j.molcel.2013.08.003

Ida T, Sawa T, Ihara H, Tsuchiya Y, Watanabe Y, Kumagai Y, Suematsu M, Motohashi H, Fujii S, Matsunaga T, et al. 2014. Reactive cysteine persulfides and S-polythiolation regulate oxidative stress and redox signaling. *Proc Natl Acad Sci* **111:** 7606–7611. doi:10.1073/pnas.1321232111

Jackson AL, Loeb LA. 2001. The contribution of endogenous sources of DNA damage to the multiple mutations in cancer. *Mutat Res* **477:** 7–21. doi:10.1016/S0027-5107(01)00091-4

Jacobs AT, Marnett LJ. 2010. Systems analysis of protein modification and cellular responses induced by electrophile stress. *Acc Chem Res* **43:** 673–683. doi:10.1021/ar900286y

Jamal-Hanjani M, Wilson GA, McGranahan N, Birkbak NJ, Watkins TBK, Veeriah S, Shafi S, Johnson DH, Mitter R, Rosenthal R, et al. 2017. Tracking the evolution of non-small-cell lung cancer. *N Engl J Med* **376:** 2109–2121. doi:10.1056/NEJMoa1616288

Jeong Y, Hoang NT, Lovejoy A, Stehr H, Newman AM, Gentles AJ, Kong W, Truong D, Martin S, Chaudhuri A, et al. 2017. Role of *KEAP1/NRF2* and *TP53* mutations in lung squamous cell carcinoma development and radiation resistance. *Cancer Discov* **7:** 86. doi:10.1158/2159-8290.CD-16-0127

Jin H, Wang S, Zaal EA, Wang C, Wu H, Bosma A, Jochems F, Isima N, Jin G, Lieftink C, et al. 2020. A powerful drug combination strategy targeting glutamine addiction for the treatment of human liver cancer. *eLife* **9:** e56749. doi:10.7554/eLife.56749

Joly JH, Delfarah A, Phung PS, Parrish S, Graham NA. 2020. A synthetic lethal drug combination mimics glucose deprivation–induced cancer cell death in the presence of glucose. *J Biol Chem* **295:** 1350–1365. doi:10.1074/jbc.RA119.011471

Cite this article as *Cold Spring Harb Perspect Med* doi: 10.1101/cshperspect.a041546

Jyrkkänen HK, Kansanen E, Inkala M, Kivelä AM, Hurttila H, Heinonen SE, Goldsteins G, Jauhiainen S, Tiainen S, Makkonen H, et al. 2008. Nrf2 regulates antioxidant gene expression evoked by oxidized phospholipids in endothelial cells and murine arteries in vivo. *Circ Res* **103**: e1–e9. doi:10.1161/CIRCRESAHA.108.176883

Kandoth C, McLellan MD, Vandin F, Ye K, Niu B, Lu C, Xie M, Zhang Q, McMichael JF, Wyczalkowski MA, et al. 2013. Mutational landscape and significance across 12 major cancer types. *Nature* **502**: 333–339. doi:10.1038/nature12634

Kang YP, Torrente L, Falzone A, Elkins CM, Liu M, Asara JM, Dibble CC, DeNicola GM. 2019. Cysteine dioxygenase 1 is a metabolic liability for non-small cell lung cancer. *eLife* **8**: e45572. doi:10.7554/eLife.45572

Kang YP, Mockabee-Macias A, Jiang C, Falzone A, Prieto-Farigua N, Stone E, Harris IS, DeNicola GM. 2021. Non-canonical glutamate-cysteine ligase activity protects against ferroptosis. *Cell Metab* **33**: 174–189.e7. doi:10.1016/j.cmet.2020.12.007

Kashif M, Yao H, Schmidt S, Chen X, Truong M, Tüksammel E, Liu Y, Bergo MO. 2023. ROS-lowering doses of vitamins C and A accelerate malignant melanoma metastasis. *Redox Biol* **60**: 102619. doi:10.1016/j.redox.2023.102619

Katoh Y, Itoh K, Yoshida E, Miyagishi M, Fukamizu A, Yamamoto M. 2001. Two domains of Nrf2 cooperatively bind CBP, a CREB binding protein, and synergistically activate transcription. *Genes Cells* **6**: 857–868. doi:10.1046/j.1365-2443.2001.00469.x

Katsuragi Y, Ichimura Y, Komatsu M. 2016. Regulation of the Keap1–Nrf2 pathway by p62/SQSTM1. *Curr Opin Toxicol* **1**: 54–61. doi:10.1016/j.cotox.2016.09.005

Kawatani Y, Suzuki T, Shimizu R, Kelly VP, Yamamoto M. 2011. Nrf2 and selenoproteins are essential for maintaining oxidative homeostasis in erythrocytes and protecting against hemolytic anemia. *Blood* **117**: 986–996. doi:10.1182/blood-2010-05-285817

Kensler TW, Wakabayashi N, Biswal S. 2007. Cell survival responses to environmental stresses via the Keap1-Nrf2-ARE pathway. *Annu Rev Pharmacol Toxicol* **47**: 89–116. doi:10.1146/annurev.pharmtox.46.120604.141046

Kerins MJ, Ooi A. 2017. The roles of NRF2 in modulating cellular iron homeostasis. *Antioxid Redox Signal* **29**: 1756–1773. doi:10.1089/ars.2017.7176

Kim YR, Oh JE, Kim MS, Kang MR, Park SW, Han JY, Eom HS, Yoo NJ, Lee SH. 2010. Oncogenic *NRF2* mutations in squamous cell carcinomas of oesophagus and skin. *J Pathol* **220**: 446–451. doi:10.1002/path.2653

Kinch L, Grishin NV, Brugarolas J. 2011. Succination of Keap1 and activation of Nrf2-dependent antioxidant pathways in FH-deficient papillary renal cell carcinoma type 2. *Cancer Cell* **20**: 418–420. doi:10.1016/j.ccr.2011.10.005

Kitamura H, Motohashi H. 2018. NRF2 addiction in cancer cells. *Cancer Sci* **109**: 900–911. doi:10.1111/cas.13537

Kitamura H, Onodera Y, Murakami S, Suzuki T, Motohashi H. 2017. IL-11 contribution to tumorigenesis in an NRF2 addiction cancer model. *Oncogene* **36**: 6315–6324. doi:10.1038/onc.2017.236

Kitamura H, Takeda H, Motohashi H. 2022. Genetic, metabolic and immunological features of cancers with NRF2

addiction. *FEBS Lett* **596**: 1981–1993. doi:10.1002/1873-3468.14458

Kobayashi A, Kang MI, Okawa H, Ohtsuji M, Zenke Y, Chiba T, Igarashi K, Yamamoto M. 2004. Oxidative stress sensor Keap1 functions as an adaptor for Cul3-based E3 ligase to regulate proteasomal degradation of Nrf2. *Mol Cell Biol* **24**: 7130–7139. doi:10.1128/MCB.24.16.7130-7139.2004

Kobayashi A, Kang MI, Watai Y, Tong KI, Shibata T, Uchida K, Yamamoto M. 2006. Oxidative and electrophilic stresses activate Nrf2 through inhibition of ubiquitination activity of Keap1. *Mol Cell Biol* **26**: 221–229. doi:10.1128/MCB.26.1.221-229.2006

Kold-Christensen R, Johannsen M. 2020. Methylglyoxal metabolism and aging-related disease: Moving from correlation toward causation. *Trends Endocrinol Metab* **31**: 81–92. doi:10.1016/j.tem.2019.10.003

Komatsu M, Kurokawa H, Waguri S, Taguchi K, Kobayashi A, Ichimura Y, Sou YS, Ueno I, Sakamoto A, Tong KI, et al. 2010. The selective autophagy substrate p62 activates the stress responsive transcription factor Nrf2 through inactivation of Keap1. *Nat Cell Biol* **12**: 213–223. doi:10.1038/ncb2021

Kong H, Reczek CR, McElroy GS, Steinert EM, Wang T, Sabatini DM, Chandel NS. 2020. Metabolic determinants of cellular fitness dependent on mitochondrial reactive oxygen species. *Sci Adv* **6**: eabb7272. doi:10.1126/sciadv.abb7272

Konstantinopoulos PA, Spentzos D, Fountzilas E, Francoeur N, Sanisetty S, Grammatikos AP, Hecht JL, Cannistra SA. 2011. Keap1 mutations and Nrf2 pathway activation in epithelial ovarian cancer. *Cancer Res* **71**: 5081–5089. doi:10.1158/0008-5472.CAN-10-4668

Kreuz S, Fischle W. 2016. Oxidative stress signaling to chromatin in health and disease. *Epigenomics* **8**: 843–862. doi:10.2217/epi-2016-0002

Kucinski I, Dinan M, Kolahgar G, Piddini E. 2017. Chronic activation of JNK JAK/STAT and oxidative stress signalling causes the loser cell status. *Nat Commun* **8**: 136. doi:10.1038/s41467-017-00145-y

Kuga A, Tsuchida K, Panda H, Horiuchi M, Otsuki A, Taguchi K, Katsuoka F, Suzuki M, Yamamoto M. 2022. The β-TrCP-mediated pathway cooperates with the keap1-mediated pathway in Nrf2 degradation in vivo. *Mol Cell Biol* **42**: e0056321. doi:10.1128/mcb.00563-21

Kwak MK, Itoh K, Yamamoto M, Kensler TW. 2002. Enhanced expression of the transcription factor Nrf2 by cancer chemopreventive agents: role of antioxidant response element-like sequences in the *nrf2* promoter. *Mol Cell Biol* **22**: 2883–2892. doi:10.1128/MCB.22.9.2883-2892.2002

LeBoeuf SE, Wu WL, Karakousi TR, Karadal B, Jackson SR, Davidson SM, Wong KK, Koralov SB, Sayin VI, Papagiannakopoulos T. 2020. Activation of oxidative stress response in cancer generates a druggable dependency on exogenous non-essential amino acids. *Cell Metab* **31**: 339–350.e4. doi:10.1016/j.cmet.2019.11.01

Lee G, Won HS, Lee YM, Choi JW, Oh TI, Jang JH, Choi DK, Lim BO, Kim YJ, Park JW, et al. 2016. Oxidative dimerization of PHD2 is responsible for its inactivation and contributes to metabolic reprogramming via HIF-1α activation. *Sci Rep* **6**: 18928. doi:10.1038/srep18928

Le Gal K, Ibrahim MX, Wiel C, Sayin VI, Akula MK, Karlsson C, Dalin MG, Akyürek LM, Lindahl P, Nilsson J, et al. 2015.

Antioxidants can increase melanoma metastasis in mice. *Sci Transl Med* **7**: 308re8. doi:10.1126/scitranslmed.aad3740

Leone RD, Zhao L, Englert JM, Sun IM, Oh MH, Sun IH, Arwood ML, Bettencourt IA, Patel CH, Wen J, et al. 2019. Glutamine blockade induces divergent metabolic programs to overcome tumor immune evasion. *Science* **366**: 1013–1021. doi:10.1126/science.aav2588

Li M, Zhang Z, Yuan J, Zhang Y, Jin X. 2014. Altered glutamate cysteine ligase expression and activity in renal cell carcinoma. *Biomed Rep* **2**: 831–834. doi:10.3892/br.2014.359

Lignitto L, LeBoeuf SE, Homer H, Jiang S, Askenazi M, Karakousi TR, Pass HI, Bhutkar AJ, Tsirigos A, Ueberheide B, et al. 2019. Nrf2 activation promotes lung cancer metastasis by inhibiting the degradation of Bach1. *Cell* **178**: 316–329.e18. doi:10.1016/j.cell.2019.06.003

Lo SC, Hannink M. 2006. PGAM5, a Bcl-XL-interacting protein, is a novel substrate for the redox-regulated Keap1-dependent ubiquitin ligase complex. *J Biol Chem* **281**: 37893–37903. doi:10.1074/jbc.M606539200

Longchamp A, Mirabella T, Arduini A, MacArthur MR, Das A, Treviño-Villarreal JH, Hine C, Ben-Sahra I, Knudsen NH, Brace LE, et al. 2018. Amino acid restriction triggers angiogenesis via GCN2/ATF4 regulation of VEGF and H_2S production. *Cell* **173**: 117–129.e14. doi:10.1016/j.cell.2018.03.001

Lu SC. 2009. Regulation of glutathione synthesis. *Mol Aspects Med* **30**: 42–59. doi:10.1016/j.mam.2008.05.005

Lubos E, Loscalzo J, Handy DE. 2011. Glutathione peroxidase-1 in health and disease: from molecular mechanisms to therapeutic opportunities. *Antioxid Redox Signal* **15**: 1957–1997. doi:10.1089/ars.2010.3586

Ma J, Cai H, Wu T, Sobhian B, Huo Y, Alcivar A, Mehta M, Cheung KL, Ganesan S, Kong AN, et al. 2012. PALB2 interacts with KEAP1 to promote NRF2 nuclear accumulation and function. *Mol Cell Biol* **32**: 1506–1517. doi:10.1128/MCB.06271-11

Madison RW, Hu X, Ramanan V, Xu Z, Huang RSP, Sokol ES, Frampton GM, Schrock AB, Ali SM, Ganesan S, et al. 2022. Clustered 8-oxo-guanine mutations and oncogenic gene fusions in microsatellite-unstable colorectal cancer. *JCO Precis Oncol* **6**: e2100477. doi:10.1200/PO.21.00477

Maj T, Wang W, Crespo J, Zhang H, Wang W, Wei S, Zhao L, Vatan L, Shao I, Szeliga W, et al. 2017. Oxidative stress controls regulatory T cell apoptosis and suppressor activity and PD-L1-blockade resistance in tumor. *Nat Immunol* **18**: 1332–1341. doi:10.1038/ni.3868

Manz DH, Blanchette NL, Paul BT, Torti FM, Torti SV. 2016. Iron and cancer: recent insights. *Ann NY Acad Sci* **1368**: 149–161. doi:10.1111/nyas.13008

Marinelli D, Mazzotta M, Scalera S, Terrenato I, Sperati F, D'Ambrosio L, Pallocca M, Corleone G, Krasniqi E, Pizzuti L, et al. 2020. KEAP1-driven co-mutations in lung adenocarcinoma unresponsive to immunotherapy despite high tumor mutational burden. *Ann Oncol* **31**: 1746–1754. doi:10.1016/j.annonc.2020.08.2105

Maruyama T, Fujita Y. 2022. Cell competition in vertebrates —a key machinery for tissue homeostasis. *Curr Opin Genet Dev* **72**: 15–21. doi:10.1016/j.gde.2021.09.006

Marzio A, Kurz E, Sahni JM, Di Feo G, Puccini J, Jiang S, Hirsch CA, Arbini AA, Wu WL, Pass HI, et al. 2022. EMSY

inhibits homologous recombination repair and the interferon response, promoting lung cancer immune evasion. *Cell* **185**: 169–183.e19. doi:10.1016/j.cell.2021.12.005

McWalter GK, Higgins LG, McLellan LI, Henderson CJ, Song L, Thornalley PJ, Itoh K, Yamamoto M, Hayes JD. 2004. Transcription factor Nrf2 is essential for induction of NAD(P)H:Quinone oxidoreductase 1, glutathione S-transferases, and glutamate cysteine ligase by broccoli seeds and isothiocyanates. *J Nutr* **134**: 3499S–3506S. doi:10.1093/jn/134.12.3499S

Mehine M, Ahvenainen T, Khamaiseh S, Härkönen J, Reinikka S, Heikkinen T, Äyräväinen A, Pakarinen P, Härkki P, Pasanen A, et al. 2022. A novel uterine leiomyoma subtype exhibits NRF2 activation and mutations in genes associated with neddylation of the cullin 3-RING E3 ligase. *Oncogenesis* **11**: 52. doi:10.1038/s41389-022-00425-3

Mills EL, Ryan DG, Prag HA, Dikovskaya D, Menon D, Zaslona Z, Jedrychowski MP, Costa ASH, Higgins M, Hams E, et al. 2018. Itaconate is an anti-inflammatory metabolite that activates Nrf2 via alkylation of KEAP1. *Nature* **556**: 113–117. doi:10.1038/nature25986

Mitsuishi Y, Taguchi K, Kawatani Y, Shibata T, Nukiwa T, Aburatani H, Yamamoto M, Motohashi H. 2012. Nrf2 redirects glucose and glutamine into anabolic pathways in metabolic reprogramming. *Cancer Cell* **22**: 66–79. doi:10.1016/j.ccr.2012.05.016

Mochizuki M, Ishii Y, Itoh K, Iizuka T, Morishima Y, Kimura T, Kiwamoto T, Matsuno Y, Hegab AE, Nomura A, et al. 2005. Role of 15-deoxy $\Delta^{12,14}$ prostaglandin J_2 and Nrf2 pathways in protection against acute lung injury. *Am J Respir Crit Care Med* **171**: 1260–1266. doi:10.1164/rccm.200406-755OC

Moghadam ZM, Henneke P, Kolter J. 2021. From flies to men: ROS and the NADPH oxidase in phagocytes. *Front Cell Dev Biol* **9**: 628991. doi:10.3389/fcell.2021.628991

Morata G, Calleja M. 2020. Cell competition and tumorigenesis in the imaginal discs of *Drosophila*. *Semin Cancer Biol* **63**: 19–26. doi:10.1016/j.semcancer.2019.06.010

Morita M, Sato T, Nomura M, Sakamoto Y, Inoue Y, Tanaka R, Ito S, Kurosawa K, Yamaguchi K, Sugiura Y, et al. 2018. PKM1 confers metabolic advantages and promotes cell-autonomous tumor cell growth. *Cancer Cell* **33**: 355–367.e7. doi:10.1016/j.ccell.2018.02.004

Moriya M. 1993. Single-stranded shuttle phagemid for mutagenesis studies in mammalian cells: 8-oxoguanine in DNA induces targeted GC-> TA transversions in simian kidney cells. *Proc Natl Acad Sci* **90**: 1122–1126. doi:10.1073/pnas.90.3.1122

Motohashi H, Yamamoto M. 2004. Nrf2-Keap1 defines a physiologically important stress response mechanism. *Trends Mol Med* **10**: 549–557. doi:10.1016/j.molmed.2004.09.003

Motohashi H, Katsuoka F, Engel JD, Yamamoto M. 2004. Small Maf proteins serve as transcriptional cofactors for keratinocyte differentiation in the Keap1-Nrf2 regulatory pathway. *Proc Natl Acad Sci* **101**: 6379–6384. doi:10.1073/pnas.0305902101

Murakami S, Suzuki T, Harigae H, Romeo PH, Yamamoto M, Motohashi H. 2017. NRF2 activation impairs quiescence and bone marrow reconstitution capacity of hematopoietic stem cells. *Mol Cell Biol* **37**: e00086-17. doi:10.1128/MCB.00086-17

Murphy MP. 2009. How mitochondria produce reactive oxygen species. *Biochem J* **417**: 1–13. doi:10.1042/BJ20081386

Muscarella LA, Parrella P, D'Alessandro V, la Torre A, Barbano R, Fontana A, Tancredi A, Guarnieri V, Balsamo T, Coco M, et al. 2011. Frequent epigenetics inactivation of KEAP1 gene in non-small cell lung cancer. *Epigenetics* **6**: 710–719. doi:10.4161/epi.6.6.15773

Nakamura T, Hipp C, Santos Dias Mourão A, Borggräfe J, Aldrovandi M, Henkelmann B, Wanninger J, Mishima E, Lytton E, Emler D, et al. 2023. Phase separation of FSP1 promotes ferroptosis. *Nature* **619**: 371–377. doi:10.1038/s41586-023-06255-6

Nguyen T, Sherratt PJ, Pickett CB. 2003. Regulatory mechanisms controlling gene expression mediated by the antioxidant response element. *Annu Rev Pharmacol Toxicol* **43**: 233–260. doi:10.1146/annurev.pharmtox.43.100901.140229

Ogiwara H, Takahashi K, Sasaki M, Kuroda T, Yoshida H, Watanabe R, Maruyama A, Makinoshima H, Chiwaki F, Sasaki H, et al. 2019. Targeting the vulnerability of glutathione metabolism in ARID1A-deficient cancers. *Cancer Cell* **35**: 177–190.e8. doi:10.1016/j.ccell.2018.12.009

Ohta T, Iijima K, Miyamoto M, Nakahara I, Tanaka H, Ohtsuji M, Suzuki T, Kobayashi A, Yokota J, Sakiyama T, et al. 2008. Loss of Keap1 function activates Nrf2 and provides advantages for lung cancer cell growth. *Cancer Res* **68**: 1303–1309. doi:10.1158/0008-5472.CAN-07-5003

Okazaki K, Anzawa H, Liu Z, Ota N, Kitamura H, Onodera Y, Alam MM, Matsumaru D, Suzuki T, Katsuoka F, et al. 2020. Enhancer remodeling promotes tumor-initiating activity in NRF2-activated non-small cell lung cancers. *Nat Commun* **11**: 5911. doi:10.1038/s41467-020-19593-0

Okazaki K, Anzawa H, Katsuoka F, Kinoshita K, Sekine H, Motohashi H. 2022. CEBPB is required for NRF2-mediated drug resistance in NRF2-activated non-small cell lung cancer cells. *J Biochem* **171**: 567–578. doi:10.1093/jb/mvac013

Otsuki A, Suzuki M, Katsuoka F, Tsuchida K, Suda H, Morita M, Shimizu M, Yamamoto M. 2016. Unique cistrome defined as CsMBE is strictly required for Nrf2-sMaf heterodimer function in cytoprotection. *Free Radic Biol Med* **91**: 45–57. doi:10.1016/j.freeradbiomed.2015.12.005

Pedre B, Talwar D, Barayeu U, Schilling D, Luzarowski M, Sokolowski M, Glatt S, Dick TP. 2023. 3-Mercaptopyruvate sulfur transferase is a protein persulfidase. *Nat Chem Biol* **19**: 507–517. doi:10.1038/s41589-022-01244-8

Perillo B, Di Donato M, Pezone A, Di Zazzo E, Giovannelli P, Galasso G, Castoria G, Migliaccio A. 2020. ROS in cancer therapy: the bright side of the moon. *Exp Mol Med* **52**: 192–203. doi:10.1038/s12276-020-0384-2

Pillai R, Hayashi M, Zavitsanou AM, Papagiannakopoulos T. 2022. NRF2: KEAPing tumors protected. *Cancer Discov* **12**: 625–643. doi:10.1158/2159-8290.CD-21-0922

Pillai R, LeBoeuf SE, Hao Y, New C, Blum JLE, Rashidfarrokhi A, Huang SM, Bahamon C, Wu WL, Karadal-Ferrena B, et al. 2023. Glutamine antagonist DRP-104 suppresses tumor growth and enhances response to checkpoint blockade in *KEAP1* mutant lung cancer. bioRxiv doi:10.1101/2023.06.27.546750

Porter TD. 2015. Electron transfer pathways in cholesterol synthesis. *Lipids* **50**: 927–936. doi:10.1007/s11745-015-4065-1

Rais R, Lemberg KM, Tenora L, Arwood ML, Pal A, Alt J, Wu Y, Lam J, Aguilar JMH, Zhao L, et al. 2022. Discovery of DRP-104, a tumor-targeted metabolic inhibitor prodrug. *Sci Adv* **8**: eabq5925. doi:10.1126/sciadv.abq5925

Reczek CR, Chandel NS. 2017. The two faces of reactive oxygen species in cancer. *Annu Rev Cancer Biol* **1**: 79–98. doi:10.1146/annurev-cancerbio-041916-065808

Romero R, Sayin VI, Davidson SM, Bauer MR, Singh SX, LeBoeuf SE, Karakousi TR, Ellis DC, Bhutkar A, Sánchez-Rivera FJ, et al. 2017. Keap1 loss promotes kras-driven lung cancer and results in dependence on glutaminolysis. *Nat Med* **23**: 1362–1368. doi:10.1038/nm.4407

Rouault TA. 2006. The role of iron regulatory proteins in mammalian iron homeostasis and disease. *Nature Chem Biol* **2**: 406–414. doi:10.1038/nchembio807

Rushmore TH, Morton MR, Pickett CB. 1991. The antioxidant responsive element. Activation by oxidative stress and identification of the DNA consensus sequence required for functional activity. *J Biol Chem* **266**: 11632–11639. doi:10.1016/S0021-9258(18)99004-6

Saito R, Suzuki T, Hiramoto K, Asami S, Naganuma E, Suda H, Iso T, Yamamoto H, Morita M, Baird L, et al. 2016. Characterizations of three major cysteine sensors of Keap1 in stress response. *Mol Cell Biol* **36**: 271–284. doi:10.1128/MCB.00868-15

Sato M, Matsumoto M, Saiki Y, Alam M, Nishizawa H, Rokugo M, Brydun A, Yamada S, Kaneko MK, Funayama R, et al. 2020. BACH1 promotes pancreatic cancer metastasis by repressing epithelial genes and enhancing epithelial-mesenchymal transition. *Cancer Res* **80**: 1279–1292. doi:10.1158/0008-5472.CAN-18-4099

Satoh H, Moriguchi T, Taguchi K, Takai J, Maher JM, Suzuki T, Winnard PT, Raman V, Ebina M, Nukiwa T, et al. 2010. Nrf2-deficiency creates a responsive microenvironment for metastasis to the lung. *Carcinogenesis* **31**: 1833–1843. doi:10.1093/carcin/bgq105

Satoh H, Moriguchi T, Takai J, Ebina M, Yamamoto M. 2013. Nrf2 prevents initiation but accelerates progression through the kras signaling pathway during lung carcinogenesis. *Cancer Res* **73**: 4158–4168. doi:10.1158/0008-5472.CAN-12-4499

Sayin VI, Ibrahim MX, Larsson E, Nilsson JA, Lindahl P, Bergo MO. 2014. Antioxidants accelerate lung cancer progression in mice. *Sci Transl Med* **6**: 221ra15. doi:10.1126/scitranslmed.3007653

Sayin VI, LeBoeuf SE, Singh SX, Davidson SM, Biancur D, Guzelhan BS, Alvarez SW, Wu WL, Karakousi TR, Zavitsanou AM, et al. 2017. Activation of the NRF2 antioxidant program generates an imbalance in central carbon metabolism in cancer. *eLife* **6**: e28083. doi:10.7554/eLife.28083

Schmidt C, Sciacovelli M, Frezza C. 2020. Fumarate hydratase in cancer: a multifaceted tumour suppressor. *Semin Cell Dev Biol* **98**: 15–25. doi:10.1016/j.semcdb.2019.05.002

Schopfer FJ, Cipollina C, Freeman BA. 2011. Formation and signaling actions of electrophilic lipids. *Chem Rev* **111**: 5997–6021. doi:10.1021/cr200131e

Seiler A, Schneider M, Förster H, Roth S, Wirth EK, Culmsee C, Plesnila N, Kremmer E, Rådmark O, Wurst W, et al. 2008. Glutathione peroxidase 4 senses and translates oxidative stress into 12/15-lipoxygenase dependent- and AIF-mediated cell death. *Cell Metab* **8**: 237–248. doi:10.1016/j.cmet.2008.07.005

Sekine H, Okazaki K, Ota N, Shima H, Katoh Y, Suzuki N, Igarashi K, Ito M, Motohashi H, Yamamoto M. 2016. The mediator subunit MED16 transduces NRF2-activating signals into antioxidant gene expression. *Mol Cell Biol* **36**: 407–420. doi:10.1128/MCB.00785-15

Shah ZA, Li RC, Thimmulappa RK, Kensler TW, Yamamoto M, Biswal S, Doré S. 2007. Role of reactive oxygen species in modulation of Nrf2 following ischemic reperfusion injury. *Neuroscience* **147**: 53–59. doi:10.1016/j.neuroscience.2007.02.066

Shen Y, Li X, Dong D, Zhang B, Xue Y, Shang P. 2018. Transferrin receptor 1 in cancer: a new sight for cancer therapy. *Am J Cancer Res* **8**: 916–931.

Shibata T, Kokubu A, Gotoh M, Ojima H, Ohta T, Yamamoto M, Hirohashi S. 2008a. Genetic alteration of Keap1 confers constitutive Nrf2 activation and resistance to chemotherapy in gallbladder cancer. *Gastroenterology* **135**: 1358–1368.e4. doi:10.1053/j.gastro.2008.06.082

Shibata T, Ishimaru K, Kawaguchi S, Yoshikawa H, Hama Y. 2008b. Antioxidant activities of phlorotannins isolated from japanese laminariaceae. *J App Phycol* **20**: 705–711. doi:10.1007/s10811-007-9254-8

Shibata T, Kokubu A, Saito S, Narisawa-Saito M, Sasaki H, Aoyagi K, Yoshimatsu Y, Tachimori Y, Kushima R, Kiyono T, et al. 2011. NRF2 mutation confers malignant potential and resistance to chemoradiation therapy in advanced esophageal squamous cancer. *Neoplasia* **13**: 864–873. doi:10.1593/neo.11750

Shigenaga MK, Gimeno CJ, Ames BN. 1989. Urinary 8-hydroxy-2′-deoxyguanosine as a biological marker of in vivo oxidative DNA damage. *Proc Natl Acad Sci* **86**: 9697–9701. doi:10.1073/pnas.86.24.9697

Singh M, Govindarajan R, Nath V, Rawat AK, Mehrotra S. 2006. Antimicrobial, wound healing and antioxidant activity of plagiochasma appendiculatum lehm. et lind. *J Ethnopharmacol* **107**: 67–72. doi:10.1016/j.jep.2006.02.007

Sobhakumari A, Love-Homan L, Fletcher EV, Martin SM, Parsons AD, Spitz DR, Knudson CM, Simons AL. 2012. Susceptibility of human head and neck cancer cells to combined inhibition of glutathione and thioredoxin metabolism. *PLoS ONE* **7**: e48175. doi:10.1371/journal.pone.0048175

Solis LM, Behavrens C, Dong W, Suraokar M, Ozburn NC, Moran CA, Corvalan AH, Biswal S, Swisher SG, Bekele BN. 2010. Nrf2 and Keap1 abnormalities in non–small cell lung carcinoma and association with clinicopathologic features. *Clin Cancer Res* **16**: 3743. doi:10.1158/1078-0432.CCR-09-3352

Stafford WC, Peng X, Olofsson MH, Zhang X, Luci DK, Lu L, Cheng Q, Trésaugues L, Dexheimer TS, Coussens NP, et al. 2018. Irreversible inhibition of cytosolic thioredoxin reductase 1 as a mechanistic basis for anticancer therapy. *Sci Transl Med* **10**: eaaf7444. doi:10.1126/scitranslmed.aaf7444

Stockwell BR, Friedmann Angeli JP, Bayir H, Bush AI, Conrad M, Dixon SJ, Fulda S, Gascón S, Hatzios SK, Kagan VE, et al. 2017. Ferroptosis: a regulated cell death nexus linking metabolism, redox biology, and disease. *Cell* **171**: 273–285. doi:10.1016/j.cell.2017.09.021

Sullivan LB, Chandel NS. 2014. Mitochondrial reactive oxygen species and cancer. *Cancer Metab* **2**: 17. doi:10.1186/2049-3002-2-17

Sullivan LB, Martinez-Garcia E, Nguyen H, Mullen AR, Dufour E, Sudarshan S, Licht JD, Deberardinis RJ, Chandel NS. 2013. The proto-oncometabolite fumarate binds glutathione to amplify ROS-dependent signaling. *Mol Cell* **51**: 236–248. doi:10.1016/j.molcel.2013.05.003

Suzuki H, Tashiro S, Hira S, Sun J, Yamazaki C, Zenke Y, Ikeda-Saito M, Yoshida M, Igarashi K. 2004. Heme regulates gene expression by triggering Crm1-dependent nuclear export of Bach1. *EMBO J* **23**: 2544–2553. doi:10.1038/sj.emboj.7600248

Suzuki T, Kelly VP, Motohashi H, Nakajima O, Takahashi S, Nishimura S, Yamamoto M. 2008. Deletion of the selenocysteine tRNA gene in macrophages and liver results in compensatory gene induction of cytoprotective enzymes by Nrf2. *J Biol Chem* **283**: 2021–2030. doi:10.1074/jbc.M708352200

Suzuki T, Shibata T, Takaya K, Shiraishi K, Kohno T, Kunitoh H, Tsuta K, Furuta K, Goto K, Hosoda F, et al. 2013. Regulatory nexus of synthesis and degradation deciphers cellular Nrf2 expression levels. *Mol Cell Biol* **33**: 2402–2412. doi:10.1128/MCB.00065-13

Suzuki M, Otsuki A, Keleku-Lukwete N, Yamamoto M. 2016. Overview of redox regulation by Keap1–Nrf2 system in toxicology and cancer. *Curr Opin Toxicol* **1**: 29–36. doi:10.1016/j.cotox.2016.10.001

Suzuki T, Muramatsu A, Saito R, Iso T, Shibata T, Kuwata K, Kawaguchi SI, Iwawaki T, Adachi S, Suda H, et al. 2019. Molecular mechanism of cellular oxidative stress sensing by Keap1. *Cell Rep* **28**: 746–758.e4. doi:10.1016/j.celrep.2019.06.047

Szabo C, Coletta C, Chao C, Módis K, Szczesny B, Papapetropoulos A, Hellmich MR. 2013. Tumor-derived hydrogen sulfide, produced by cystathionine-β-synthase, stimulates bioenergetics, cell proliferation, and angiogenesis in colon cancer. *Proc Natl Acad Sci* **110**: 12474–12479. doi:10.1073/pnas.1306241110

Tagde A, Singh H, Kang MH, Reynolds CP. 2014. The glutathione synthesis inhibitor buthionine sulfoximine synergistically enhanced melphalan activity against preclinical models of multiple myeloma. *Blood Cancer J* **4**: e229. doi:10.1038/bcj.2014.45

Taguchi K, Hirano I, Itoh T, Tanaka M, Miyajima A, Suzuki A, Motohashi H, Yamamoto M. 2014. Nrf2 enhances cholangiocyte expansion in pten-deficient livers. *Mol Cell Biol* **34**: 900–913. doi:10.1128/MCB.01384-13

Talalay P. 1989. Mechanisms of induction of enzymes that protect against chemical carcinogenesis. *Adv Enzyme Regul* **28**: 237–250. doi:10.1016/0065-2571(89)90074-5

Talalay P, Fahey JW. 2001. Phytochemicals from cruciferous plants protect against cancer by modulating carcinogen metabolism. *J Nutr* **131**: 3027s–3033s. doi:10.1093/jn/131.11.3027S

Tenora L, Alt J, Dash RP, Gadiano AJ, Novotná K, Veeravalli V, Lam J, Kirkpatrick QR, Lemberg KM, Majer P, et al. 2019. Tumor-targeted delivery of 6-diazo-5-oxo-l-norleucine (DON) using substituted acetylated lysine prodrugs. *J Med Chem* **62**: 3524–3538. doi:10.1021/acs.jmedchem.8b02009

Cite this article as *Cold Spring Harb Perspect Med* doi: 10.1101/cshperspect.a041546

The Cancer Genome Atlas Research Network. 2012. Comprehensive genomic characterization of squamous cell lung cancers. *Nature* **489:** 519–525. doi:10.1038/nature 11404

Tojo Y, Sekine H, Hirano I, Pan X, Souma T, Tsujita T, Kawaguchi S, Takeda N, Takeda K, Fong GH, et al. 2015. Hypoxia signaling cascade for erythropoietin production in hepatocytes. *Mol Cell Biol* **35:** 2658–2672. doi:10.1128/MCB.00161-15

Tong KI, Kobayashi A, Katsuoka F, Yamamoto M. 2006. Two-site substrate recognition model for the Keap1-Nrf2 system: a hinge and latch mechanism. *Biol Chem* **387:** 1311–1320. doi:10.1515/BC.2006.164

Tong KI, Padmanabhan B, Kobayashi A, Shang C, Hirotsu Y, Yokoyama S, Yamamoto M. 2007. Different electrostatic potentials define ETGE and DLG motifs as hinge and latch in oxidative stress response. *Mol Cell Biol* **27:** 7511–7521. doi:10.1128/MCB.00753-07

Tong X, Zhao F, Thompson CB. 2009. The molecular determinants of de novo nucleotide biosynthesis in cancer cells. *Curr Opin Genet Dev* **19:** 32–37. doi:10.1016/j.gde.2009.01 .002

Torrente L, DeNicola GM. 2022. Targeting NRF2 and its downstream processes: opportunities and challenges. *Annu Rev Pharmacol Toxicol* **62:** 279–300. doi:10.1146/ annurev-pharmtox-052220-104025

Trush MA, Kensler TW. 1991. An overview of the relationship between oxidative stress and chemical carcinogenesis. *Free Radic Biol Med* **10:** 201–209. doi:10.1016/0891-5849 (91)90077-G

Tsakiri EN, Gumeni S, Iliaki KK, Benaki D, Vougas K, Sykiotis GP, Gorgoulis VG, Mikros E, Scorrano L, Trougakos IP. 2019. Hyperactivation of Nrf2 increases stress tolerance at the cost of aging acceleration due to metabolic deregulation. *Aging Cell* **18:** e12845. doi:10.1111/acel.12845

Tsuchida K, Tsujita T, Hayashi M, Ojima A, Keleku-Lukwete N, Katsuoka F, Otsuki A, Kikuchi H, Oshima Y, Suzuki M, et al. 2017. Halofuginone enhances the chemo-sensitivity of cancer cells by suppressing NRF2 accumulation. *Free Radic Biol Med* **103:** 236–247. doi:10.1016/j.freeradbiomed.2016 .12.041

Tsuji PA, Santesmasses D, Lee BJ, Gladyshev VN, Hatfield DL. 2021. Historical roles of selenium and selenoproteins in health and development: the good, the bad and the ugly. *Int J Mol Sci* **23:** 5. doi:10.3390/ijms23010005

Tubbs A, Nussenzweig A. 2017. Endogenous DNA damage as a source of genomic instability in cancer. *Cell* **168:** 644–656. doi:10.1016/j.cell.2017.01.002

Vafa O, Wade M, Kern S, Beeche M, Pandita TK, Hampton GM, Wahl GM. 2002. c-Myc can induce DNA damage, increase reactive oxygen species, and mitigate p53 function: a mechanism for oncogene-induced genetic instability. *Mol Cell* **9:** 1031–1044. doi:10.1016/s1097-2765(02) 00520-8

Valko M, Leibfritz D, Moncol J, Cronin MT, Mazur M, Telser J. 2007. Free radicals and antioxidants in normal physiological functions and human disease. *Int J Biochem Cell Biol* **39:** 44–84. doi:10.1016/j.biocel.2006.07.001

Villablanca JG, Volchenboum SL, Cho H, Kang MH, Cohn SL, Anderson CP, Marachelian A, Groshen S, Tsao-Wei D, Matthay KK, et al. 2016. A phase I new approaches to neuroblastoma therapy study of buthionine sulfoximine and melphalan with autologous stem cells for recurrent/refractory high-risk neuroblastoma. *Pediatr Blood Cancer* **63:** 1349–1356. doi:10.1002/pbc.25994

Wakabayashi N, Itoh K, Wakabayashi J, Motohashi H, Noda S, Takahashi S, Imakado S, Kotsuji T, Otsuka F, Roop DR, et al. 2003. Keap1-null mutation leads to postnatal lethality due to constitutive Nrf2 activation. *Nat Genet* **35:** 238–245. doi:10.1038/ng1248

Wakabayashi N, Skoko JJ, Chartoumpekis DV, Kimura S, Slocum SL, Noda K, Palliyaguru DL, Fujimuro M, Boley PA, Tanaka Y, et al. 2014. Notch-Nrf2 axis: regulation of *Nrf2* gene expression and cytoprotection by notch signaling. *Mol Cell Biol* **34:** 653–663. doi:10.1128/MCB.01408-13

Wakil SJ. 1989. Fatty acid synthase, a proficient multifunctional enzyme. *Biochemistry* **28:** 4523–4530. doi:10.1021/ bi00437a001

Wang R, An J, Ji F, Jiao H, Sun H, Zhou D. 2008. Hypermethylation of the Keap1 gene in human lung cancer cell lines and lung cancer tissues. *Biochem Biophys Res Commun* **373:** 151–154. doi:10.1016/j.bbrc.2008.06.004

Wang H, Liu F, Yang L, Zu Y, Wang H, Qu S, Zhang Y. 2011. Oxidative stability of fish oil supplemented with carnosic acid compared with synthetic antioxidants during long-term storage. *Food Chem* **128:** 93–99. doi:10.1016/j .foodchem.2011.02.082

Wang YH, Huang JT, Chen WL, Wang RH, Kao MC, Pan YR, Chan SH, Tsai KW, Kung HJ, Lin KT, et al. 2019. Dysregulation of cystathionine γ-lyase promotes prostate cancer progression and metastasis. *EMBO Rep* **20:** e45986. doi:10.15252/embr.201845986

Wang X, Li Y, Li Z, Lin S, Wang H, Sun J, Lan C, Wu L, Sun D, Huang C, et al. 2022. Mitochondrial calcium uniporter drives metastasis and confers a targetable cystine dependency in pancreatic cancer. *Cancer Res* **82:** 2254–2268. doi:10.1158/0008-5472.CAN-21-3230

Weinberg F, Hamanaka R, Wheaton WW, Weinberg S, Joseph J, Lopez M, Kalyanaraman B, Mutlu GM, Budinger GR, Chandel NS. 2010. Mitochondrial metabolism and ROS generation are essential for kras-mediated tumorigenicity. *Proc Natl Acad Sci* **107:** 8788–8793. doi:10.1073/ pnas.1003428107

Weisburger JH. 1991. Nutritional approach to cancer prevention with emphasis on vitamins, antioxidants, and carotenoids. *Am J Clin Nutr* **53:** 226S–237S. doi:10.1093/ajcn/ 53.1.226S

Weiss-Sadan T, Ge M, Hayashi M, Gohar M, Yao CH, de Groot A, Harry S, Carlin A, Fischer H, Shi L, et al. 2023. NRF2 activation induces NADH-reductive stress, providing a metabolic vulnerability in lung cancer. *Cell Metab* **35:** 487–503.e7. doi:10.1016/j.cmet.2023.01.012

Wiel C, Le Gal K, Ibrahim MX, Jahangir CA, Kashif M, Yao H, Ziegler DV, Xu X, Ghosh T, Mondal T, et al. 2019. BACH1 stabilization by antioxidants stimulates lung cancer metastasis. *Cell* **178:** 330–345.e22. doi:10.1016/j.cell.2019.06 .005

Wu WL, Papagiannakopoulos T. 2020. The pleiotropic role of the KEAP1/NRF2 pathway in cancer. *Annu Rev Cancer Biol* **4:** 413–435. doi:10.1146/annurev-cancerbio-030518-055627

Wu J, Minikes AM, Gao M, Bian H, Li Y, Stockwell BR, Chen ZN, Jiang X. 2019. Intercellular interaction dictates cancer cell ferroptosis via NF2-YAP signalling. *Nature* **572**: 402–406. doi:10.1038/s41586-019-1426-6

Wu Z, Khodade VS, Chauvin JR, Rodriguez D, Toscano JP, Pratt DA. 2022. Hydropersulfides inhibit lipid peroxidation and protect cells from ferroptosis. *J Am Chem Soc* **144**: 15825–15837. doi:10.1021/jacs.2c06804

Xia M, Li X, Diao Y, Du B, Li Y. 2021. Targeted inhibition of glutamine metabolism enhances the antitumor effect of selumetinib in KRAS-mutant NSCLC. *Transl Oncol* **14**: 100920. doi:10.1016/j.tranon.2020.100920

Yadav PK, Yamada K, Chiku T, Koutmos M, Banerjee R. 2013. Structure and kinetic analysis of H2S production by human mercaptopyruvate sulfurtransferase. *J Biol Chem* **288**: 20002–20013. doi:10.1074/jbc.M113.466177

Yadav PK, Martinov M, Vitvitsky V, Seravalli J, Wedmann R, Filipovic MR, Banerjee R. 2016. Biosynthesis and reactivity of cysteine persulfides in signaling. *J Am Chem Soc* **138**: 289–299. doi:10.1021/jacs.5b10494

Yamamoto M, Kensler TW, Motohashi H. 2018. The KEAP1-NRF2 system: a thiol-based sensor-effector apparatus for maintaining redox homeostasis. *Physiol Rev* **98**: 1169–1203. doi:10.1152/physrev.00023.2017

Yang WS, SriRamaratnam R, Welsch ME, Shimada K, Skouta R, Viswanathan VS, Cheah JH, Clemons PA, Shamji AF, Clish CB, et al. 2014. Regulation of ferroptotic cancer cell death by GPX4. *Cell* **156**: 317–331. doi:10.1016/j.cell.2013.12.010

Yokoyama Y, Estok TM, Wild R. 2022. Sirpiglenastat (DRP-104) induces antitumor efficacy through direct, broad antagonism of glutamine metabolism and stimulation of the innate and adaptive immune systems. *Mol Cancer Ther* **21**: 1561–1572. doi:10.1158/1535-7163.MCT-22-0282

Yoo MH, Gu X, Xu XM, Kim JY, Carlson BA, Patterson AD, Cai H, Gladyshev VN, Hatfield DL. 2010. Delineating the role of glutathione peroxidase 4 in protecting cells against lipid hydroperoxide damage and in Alzheimer's disease. *Antioxid Redox Signal* **12**: 819–827. doi:10.1089/ars.2009.2891

Yoon SJ, Combs JA, Falzone A, Prieto-Farigua N, Caldwell S, Ackerman HD, Flores ER, DeNicola GM. 2023. Comprehensive metabolic tracing reveals the origin and catabolism of cysteine in mammalian tissues and tumors. *Cancer Res* **83**: 1426–1442. doi:10.1158/0008-5472.CAN-22-3000

Yoshida E, Suzuki T, Morita M, Taguchi K, Tsuchida K, Motohashi H, Doita M, Yamamoto M. 2018. Hyperactivation of Nrf2 leads to hypoplasia of bone in vivo. *Genes Cells* **23**: 386–392. doi:10.1111/gtc.12579

Yue T, Li J, Zhu J, Zuo S, Wang X, Liu Y, Liu J, Liu X, Wang P, Chen S. 2023. Hydrogen sulfide creates a favorable immune microenvironment for colon cancer. *Cancer Res* **83**: 595–612. doi:10.1158/0008-5472.CAN-22-1837

Zavitsanou AM, Pillai R, Hao Y, Wu WL, Bartnicki E, Karakousi T, Rajalingam S, Herrera A, Karatza A, Rashidfarrokhi A, et al. 2023. KEAP1 mutation in lung adenocarcinoma promotes immune evasion and immunotherapy resistance. *Cell Rep* **42**: 113295. doi:10.1016/j.celrep.2023.113295

Zenke-Kawasaki Y, Dohi Y, Katoh Y, Ikura T, Ikura M, Asahara T, Tokunaga F, Iwai K, Igarashi K. 2007. Heme induces ubiquitination and degradation of the transcription factor Bach1. *Mol Cell Biol* **27**: 6962–6971. doi:10.1128/MCB.02415-06

Zhang DD. 2006. Mechanistic studies of the Nrf2-Keap1 signaling pathway. *Drug Metab Rev* **38**: 769–789. doi:10.1080/03602530600971974

Zhang DD. 2010. The Nrf2-Keap1-ARE signaling pathway: the regulation and dual function of Nrf2 in cancer. *Antioxid Redox Signal* **13**: 1623–1626. doi:10.1089/ars.2010.3301

Zhang DD, Lo SC, Cross JV, Templeton DJ, Hannink M. 2004. Keap1 is a redox-regulated substrate adaptor protein for a Cul3-dependent ubiquitin ligase complex. *Mol Cell Biol* **24**: 10941–10953. doi:10.1128/MCB.24.24.10941-10953.2004

Zhang P, Singh A, Yegnasubramanian S, Esopi D, Kombairaju P, Bodas M, Wu H, Bova SG, Biswal S. 2010. Loss of kelch-like ECH-associated protein 1 function in prostate cancer cells causes chemoresistance and radioresistance and promotes tumor growth. *Mol Cancer Ther* **9**: 336–346. doi:10.1158/1535-7163.MCT-09-0589

Zhang T, Ono K, Tsutsuki H, Ihara H, Islam W, Akaike T, Sawa T. 2019. Enhanced cellular polysulfides negatively regulate TLR4 signaling and mitigate lethal endotoxin shock. *Cell Chem Biol* **26**: 686–698.e4. doi:10.1016/j.chembiol.2019.02.003

Zhang J, Simpson CM, Berner J, Chong HB, Fang J, Ordulu Z, Weiss-Sadan T, Possemato AP, Harry S, Takahashi M, et al. 2023. Systematic identification of anticancer drug targets reveals a nucleus-to-mitochondria ROS-sensing pathway. *Cell* **186**: 2361–2379.e25. doi:10.1016/j.cell.2023.04.026

Zhu XG, Nicholson Puthenveedu S, Shen Y, La K, Ozlu C, Wang T, Klompstra D, Gultekin Y, Chi J, Fidelin J, et al. 2019. CHP1 regulates compartmentalized glycerolipid synthesis by activating GPAT4. *Mol Cell* **74**: 45–58.e7. doi:10.1016/j.molcel.2019.01.037

Zivanovic J, Kouroussis E, Kohl JB, Adhikari B, Bursac B, Schott-Roux S, Petrovic D, Miljkovic JL, Thomas-Lopez D, Jung Y, et al. 2019. Selective persulfide detection reveals evolutionarily conserved antiaging effects of *S*-sulfhydration. *Cell Metab* **30**: 1152–1170.e13. doi:10.1016/j.cmet.2019.10.007

Cite this article as *Cold Spring Harb Perspect Med* doi: 10.1101/cshperspect.a041546

The Role of Stroma in Cancer Metabolism

Alec C. Kimmelman[1,2] and Mara H. Sherman[3]

[1]Perlmutter Cancer Center, New York University Grossman School of Medicine, New York, New York 10016, USA

[2]Department of Radiation Oncology, New York University Grossman School of Medicine, New York, New York 10016, USA

[3]Cancer Biology & Genetics Program, Memorial Sloan Kettering Cancer Center, New York, New York 10065, USA

Correspondence: shermam1@mskcc.org; alec.kimmelman@nyulangone.org

The altered metabolism of tumor cells is a well-known hallmark of cancer and is driven by multiple factors such as mutations in oncogenes and tumor suppressor genes, the origin of the tissue where the tumor arises, and the microenvironment of the tumor. These metabolic changes support the growth of cancer cells by providing energy and the necessary building blocks to sustain proliferation. Targeting these metabolic alterations therapeutically is a potential strategy to treat cancer, but it is challenging due to the metabolic plasticity of tumors. Cancer cells have developed ways to scavenge nutrients through autophagy and macropinocytosis and can also form metabolic networks with stromal cells in the tumor microenvironment. Understanding the role of the tumor microenvironment in tumor metabolism is crucial for effective therapeutic targeting. This review will discuss tumor metabolism and the contribution of the stroma in supporting tumor growth through metabolic interactions.

It is well established that altered tumor cell metabolism is a hallmark of cellular transformation and a characteristic of the malignant state (Hanahan 2022). These changes are driven by a combination of factors including the mutational spectrum of the tumor (including oncogenes and tumor suppressor genes), the tissue of origin of the tumor, and the tumor microenvironment (TME) (DeBerardinis and Chandel 2016). Such metabolic alterations serve to support the unconstrained growth of cancer cells, providing the bioenergetic and anabolic needs for the developing tumor (Zhu and Thompson 2019). Causal roles for these metabolic alterations in tumor progression have motivated extensive effort to target these metabolic changes therapeutically as they represent potential therapeutic vulnerabilities. While some of these have shown promise and have moved forward into the clinic with mixed results (Luengo et al. 2017), a common theme is that there is metabolic plasticity of tumors that is difficult to overcome (Biancur and Kimmelman 2018). Indeed, inhibition of single metabolic pathways in various tumor models often results in rapid metabolic rewiring to bypass the inhibited pathway (Biancur et al. 2017). Additionally, cancer cells have developed various mechanisms of "metabolic scavenging." These include catabolic processes such as autophagy and macropinocytosis whereby intracellular (autophagy) and extracellular (macropinocytosis) cargo are degraded by the lysosome and the resultant degraded products can fuel cellular metabolism (Encarnación-Rosado and Kimmelman 2021). Tumor cells can also form heterocellular metabolic networks with stromal cells in the TME that can support various aspects of cancer growth (Lyssiotis and Kimmelman 2017). This review discusses tumor metabolism with a particular focus on the various roles of the stroma in supporting tumor growth through metabolic contributions. We contend that to effectively target metabolism in the cancer cells themselves, one must also understand the contributions of the TME to these processes.

METABOLIC FEATURES OF NONMALIGNANT CELL TYPES IN THE TUMOR STROMA

Metabolic Milieu of the TME Is a Critical Determinant of Tumor Biology

During tumorigenesis, the evolution of a unique TME imparts a set of selection pressures on the epithelial tumor cells that influences the fundamental biology of the cancer. The TME consists of a multitude of cell types, including fibroblasts, immune cells, neurons, and an abundant stromal matrix. The specific composition of TME cellular and acellular components are determined in part by the mutational landscape of the developing tumor, and reflect a perturbed wound-healing response. Recruitment, activation, and expansion of these TME components can lead to heterogeneous alterations in tissue oxygen (hypoxia) and nutrient content depending on stromal contexture, with profound consequences for the metabolic state of the tumor. The metabolic composition of the TME has gained attention in recent years and a great deal of effort has gone into trying to assess the altered nutrient levels in various tumor types. Among solid tumors, pancreatic ductal adenocarcinoma (PDA) has particularly complex and abundant stroma, and is poorly perfused and extremely hypoxic (Halbrook et al. 2023). Because of this, there have

been substantial efforts to understand the nutrient content of its TME and the impact of this on its metabolic dependencies. Based on the seminal findings that PDA can use extracellular protein to fuel metabolism via a process of bulk uptake and lysosomal degradation, termed macropinocytosis (Commisso et al. 2013), several groups have attempted to compare the nutrient content of freshly resected human PDA tumors compared to the adjacent normal pancreas (Kamphorst et al. 2015). This work demonstrated that tumors had reduced levels of glucose (including upper glycolytic intermediates), glutamine, and serine. It was also noted that amino acids used primarily for protein synthesis were enriched, which was consistent with increased protein scavenging via macropinocytosis. In an attempt to further refine the PDA nutrient content, Sullivan and colleagues performed metabolomics on tumor interstitial fluid (TIF) from mouse PDA models, as well as lung cancer models (Sullivan et al. 2019a). Interestingly, they showed that the nutrient content differed between lung and PDA, even when driven by the same oncogenic driver and tumor-suppressor gene loss. Factors such as tumor location, type of tumors cells, and diet also influenced TIF metabolite concentrations. Other groups have confirmed the altered nutrient content is affected by diet in head and neck cancer patients (Schroeder et al. 2013). Similar microdialysis studies in high grade astrocytoma patients showed decreased glucose in tumor compared to adjacent tissue (Roslin et al. 2003).

In addition to defining the altered nutrient content of the TME, several groups have explored how these nutrient differences impact aspects of tumor metabolism and biology. Using experimental models, Sullivan et al. (2019b) showed that expression of PHGDH, the first rate-limiting step of serine biosynthesis, benefits tumors specifically in tissues where serine is limited. The Pacold and Cantley laboratories demonstrated that the ability of tumor cells to metastasize to the brain, an environment where serine is present at low levels, requires an intact serine synthesis pathway (Ngo et al. 2020). Indeed, inhibition of PHGDH selectively attenuated brain metastasis growth, while extracranial growth was largely unaffected. Similarly, Ferraro et al. show that the brain is low in lipid availability and this causes breast cancer cells that metastasize to the brain to up-regulate fatty acid synthesis (Ferraro et al. 2021). Given the impact of the nutrient content of the TME on the tumor, there are significant efforts to use this information for the purposes of understanding the metabolic dependencies of cancer cells. These include developing modified media formulations to better reflect the metabolic content of the TME and enable more meaningful cell culture studies (Cantor et al. 2017), as well as performing functional genomic screens in the in vivo setting where cells are in the appropriate TME (Biancur et al. 2021; Zhu et al. 2021). Both approaches have yielded potential novel metabolic targets, but more work is needed in these areas.

As mentioned previously, there are a multitude of cell types within the TME, making it likely that a competition for nutrient availability exists. Indeed, several groups have demonstrated that infiltrating immune cells compete with tumor cells for critical nutrients. The Pearce and Kaech groups showed that there is intense competition between tumor-infiltrating T cells and the highly glycolytic tumor cells in sarcoma and melanoma models, respectively (Chang et al. 2015; Ho et al. 2015). Limiting glucose to the effector T cells can impair their function and dampen antitumor immunity. Treatment with anti-PD-L1 blocking antibodies can decrease tumor cell glycolytic activity, improve T-cell access to glucose, and enhance T-cell activation. Alternatively, T cells can up-regulate phosphoenolpyruvate (PEP) production (a glycolytic intermediate) through overexpression of phosphoenolpyruvate carboxykinase 1 (PCK1), which leads to improved antitumor functions. Similarly, it was shown that the hypoxic and glucose-deprived melanoma TME causes an increased utilization of fatty acids by the effector T cells, thereby improving their antitumor response. Reinfeld and colleagues used positron emission tomography (PET) tracers to show that there was preferential uptake of glutamine by the tumor cells, with myeloid cells and T cells showing the highest avidity for glucose (Reinfeld et al. 2021). Interestingly, they demonstrated that

this nutrient partitioning was cell intrinsic and not due to glucose being limiting in the TME. Thus, it appears that there are multiple mechanisms that govern nutrient competition in the TME that can include limiting concentrations in the tumor- or cell-intrinsic properties of particular cell types. Understanding these factors will be critical to optimize therapeutic efficacy.

Metabolic Features and Consequences of the Tumor Vasculature

Solid tumors require a vascular supply to enable progression. Sufficient vascularization results from one of two general mechanisms: induction of angiogenesis or the formation of new blood vessels by reprogramming of quiescent endothelial cells, known as the angiogenic switch; or vessel co-option, whereby cancer cells migrate along or infiltrate between preexisting vessels in benign tumor-adjacent tissue, ultimately leading to the incorporation of these vessels into the tumor (Kuczynski et al. 2019; Hanahan 2022). This requirement reflects the dependence of cancer cells on oxygen and nutrients delivered by the circulatory system, such that tumor-associated vasculature provides critical metabolic inputs once the limits of oxygen diffusion are exceeded. This need for the vasculature to provide metabolites is overcome to some extent by metabolic reprogramming of other nonmalignant cell types in the TME, discussed in detail in the sections below. However, the association between microvessel density and tumor grade in multiple tumor types (Weidner et al. 1991, 1993; Macchiarini et al. 1992; Benckert et al. 2012) as well as the pervasive use of hematogenous or lymphatic dissemination as a route of metastasis (Lambert et al. 2017; Follain et al. 2020; Reticker-Flynn et al. 2022) underscore the significance of endothelial cells in cancer. While the mechanisms underlying vessel co-option remain poorly understood, tumor angiogenesis is known to require extensive metabolic adaptation among endothelial cells (Zecchin et al. 2017). Quiescent endothelial cells switch to migratory tip cell or proliferative stalk cell fates and sprout into poorly vascularized tissues including hypoxic tumors to form new blood vessels during angiogenesis, a process featuring activation of glycolysis in both migratory tip cells and proliferative stalk cells by 6-phosphofructo-2-kinase/fructose-2,6-bisphosphate 3 (PFKFB3) (De Bock et al. 2013; Li et al. 2019). Tracing studies of tumor endothelial cells in culture using ^{14}C-glucose and ^{13}C-glucose showed use of glucose carbons for nucleotide synthesis (Cantelmo et al. 2016), linking the hyperglycolytic metabolism of tumor endothelial cells to biomass production. Loss of a single allele of *Pfkfb3* in endothelial cells did not impact tumor size, but reduced cancer cell intravasation and metastasis together with reduced vessel tortuosity and improved perfusion dynamics (Cantelmo et al. 2016). These structural features of a normalized vasculature are typically associated with intact adherens junctions and vascular barriers that limit cancer cell spread, suggesting endothelial cell metabolism as a potential target to normalize tumor vasculature and limit metastasis.

Blood vessels in tumors are structurally abnormal or tortuous and typically hyperpermeable, together causing fluid leakage, compromising blood perfusion, and exacerbating hypoxia and acidity (Jain 2005). Vessel dysfunction results in part from mechanical forces within the tumor stroma (Provenzano et al. 2012; Stylianopoulos et al. 2012), and necessitates adaptive mechanisms in the neoplastic compartment to maintain viability and proliferative capacity in the context of relatively low oxygen, serum nutrients, and pH. These adaptive mechanisms include hypoxia-driven enhancement of macropinocytosis to obtain amino acids and other nutrients from the extracellular space, mediated by hypoxia-inducible factor 1α (HIF-1α) as well as mutant KRAS (Commisso et al. 2013; Garcia-Bermudez et al. 2022). Metabolic heterogeneity among poorly perfused versus relatively well-perfused regions of human lung cancer have been reported, highlighting potentially limited nutrient availability in poorly perfused tissue areas reflected by increased contribution of glucose—as opposed to other available metabolites—to the tricarboxylic acid (TCA) cycle (Hensley et al. 2016). Important adaptations to tumor acidification include use of lactate as a carbon source (Faubert et al. 2017; Hui et al. 2017),

while adaptations to low oxygen include increased uptake and use of unsaturated fatty acids that do not require oxygen-dependent desaturation (Ackerman and Simon 2014). While these and other adaptations to metabolic stress enable cancer cell proliferation and survival, they may also represent vulnerabilities for therapeutic intervention.

STROMAL CATABOLIC PROCESSES SUPPORTING CANCER CELL METABOLIC FITNESS

Significance of Stromal Autophagy and Macropinocytosis for Cancer Cell Viability

While the importance of nutrient scavenging and catabolism in the tumor epithelium has been recognized for over a decade, the significance of these processes in the adjacent stroma has more recently come to light. In an effort to explore additional nutrient sources for pancreatic cancer cells, Sousa et al. (2016) identified a novel metabolic cross talk between the cancer-associated fibroblasts (CAFs) and the pancreatic cancer epithelial tumor cells. The CAFs were secreting high levels of the amino acid alanine, which the tumor cells could use to fuel metabolic processes under nutrient-limiting conditions. Interestingly, the secretion of alanine was dependent on the autophagy/lysosome system (Fig. 1). Consistent with this, inhibition of autophagy in the CAFs decreased alanine secretion and impaired tumor take in coinjection studies. Other studies have also confirmed the importance of autophagy in the stroma in promoting pancreatic cancer growth (Endo et al. 2017). In a follow-up study, the nutrient transporter required for alanine uptake in pancreatic cancer cells, SLC38A2, was identified. SLC38A2 was shown to be critical for metabolic homeostasis in these cells and was required for tumor growth (Parker et al. 2020). In a related manner, Zhang et al. (2021) demonstrated that pancreatic CAFs use macropinocytosis under nutrient-limited conditions to support their own metabolism, but also to allow the secretion of amino acids to fuel the metabolism of pancreatic cancer cells. Studies in prostate cancer showed similar find-

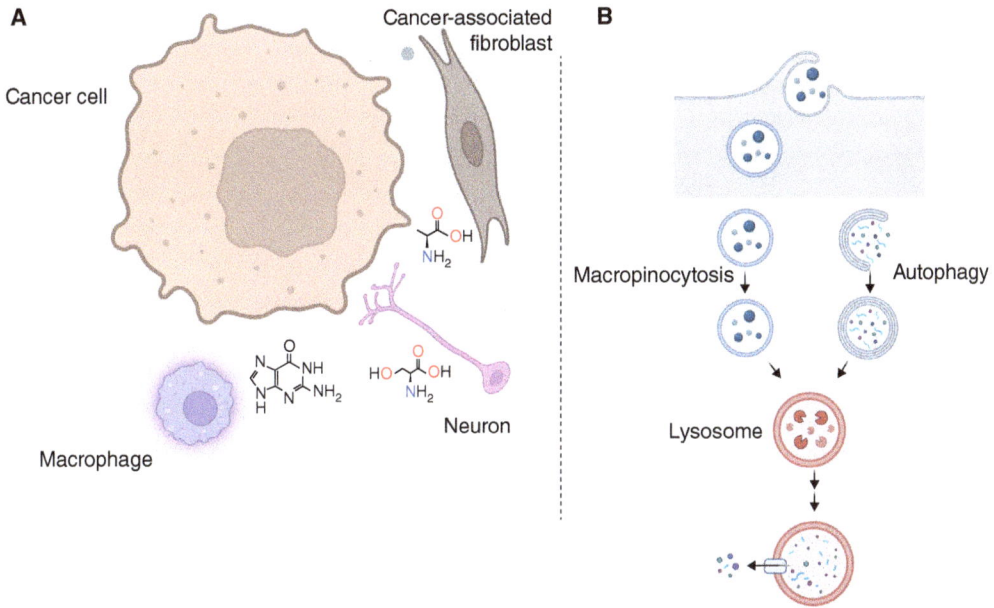

Figure 1. Catabolic processes in the neoplastic and surrounding stromal compartments cooperate to enable tumor progression. (*A*) Cancer cells obtain nutrients from surrounding immune and nonimmune stromal cells to support proliferation, viability, and resistance to therapy. This paracrine metabolic support includes alanine and specific lysolipid species from cancer-associated fibroblasts, which support mitochondrial metabolism and membrane synthesis, respectively: serine from peripheral axons to regulate mRNA translation and pyrimidines from macrophages, which promote resistance to standard-of-care chemotherapeutic agent gemcitabine. (*B*) Both cancer cells and nontransformed stromal cells take up nutrients from the extracellular space via macropinocytosis, and degrade intracellular cargo by autophagy. These processes converge at the lysosome, enabling recycling of nutrients that may be secreted and used by neighboring cells to support metabolic processes in a paracrine manner.

ings, whereby Ras activity is up-regulated in prostate CAFs through the epigenetic silencing of a negative Ras regulator (Mishra et al. 2018). This increases macropinocytosis and allows the CAFs to supply glutamine to the cancer cells to fuel metabolic processes, but also promotes neuroendocrine differentiation.

Paracrine Regulation of Lipid Metabolism

Co-option of nonmalignant cell types in the TME for metabolic support extends to cancer-associated adipocytes in several tissue contexts where tumors or metastases grow in the vicinity of adipose tissue. Multiple tumor types, including prostate, breast, lung, colon, and ovarian cancer, melanoma, and hematologic malignancies, stimulate lipolysis in nearby adipocytes and take up adipocyte-derived fatty acids to support tu-

mor growth and metastasis (Mukherjee et al. 2022). For example, advanced melanoma grows past the dermis into adipocyte-rich subcutaneous tissue, with the potential to metastasize to secondary subcutaneous tissues. Melanoma cells have long been known to harbor lipolytic activity (Hollander et al. 1986), and a recent study demonstrated that adipocytes increase melanoma cell proliferation and invasion (Zhang et al. 2018). Melanoma cells stimulate fatty acid release by adipocytes, which are in turn taken up by melanoma cells in part via FATP1 to contribute to melanoma cell lipid pools. Inhibition of FATP proteins with the small molecule inhibitor lipofermata blocked lipid transfer into melanoma cells, and this suppression of adipocyte-melanoma cross talk reduced paracrine induction of proliferation and invasion. The mechanistic links between fatty acid uptake and cancer cell invasiveness remain unclear and warrant further investigation. Functional, bidirectional interactions between adipocytes and cancer cells were also reported in ovarian cancer, which frequently metastasizes to the adipocyte-rich omentum. Ovarian cancer cells induce lipolysis in adipocytes, which in turn provide lipids to cancer cells, induce β-oxidation, and promote tumor growth (Nieman et al. 2011). The tumor-promoting effects of adipocytes were also mediated by adipokines including IL-8, which promote ovarian cancer cell homing, migration, and invasion in the omentum. Adipocytes were later shown to induce expression of lipid chaperone protein FABP4 in ovarian cancer cells, which critically regulates adipocyte-driven alterations to ovarian cancer cell lipid metabolism and ultimately supports both tumor growth and, somewhat surprisingly, resistance to the chemotherapeutic agent carboplatin (Mukherjee et al. 2020). Additional mechanisms by which stromal metabolism promotes chemoresistance are discussed in the next section.

Breast cancer is somewhat unique in that primary breast tumors develop within the adipose-dominated mammary TME. Recent transcriptomic analysis of both breast cancer cells and adjacent mammary adipose tissue identified critical roles for glycine amidinotransferase (GATM) in adipocytes and acyl-CoA synthetase bubblegum family member 1 (ACSBG1) in cancer cells for breast tumor progression (Maguire et al. 2021). Linking these pathways is creatine, which is released by adipocytes and taken up by breast cancer cells to promote proliferation. Breast cancer–associated adipocytes also express extracellular matrix remodeling enzymes such as MMP-11 and proinflammatory cytokines such as IL-6 and IL-1β, together supporting breast cancer cell invasiveness (Dirat et al. 2011). Further highlighting the metastasis-promoting potential of local adipose tissue, expression of the fatty acid translocase CD36, a transmembrane glycoprotein receptor with a high affinity for long-chain fatty acids, is high on metastasis-initiating cells and associates with a poor prognosis among breast cancer patients (Pascual et al. 2017). These tumor-promoting functions of local adipose tissue and adipose-derived fatty acids

may explain in part the epidemiologic evidence supporting an association of obesity with breast cancer (Lauby-Secretan et al. 2016).

Stromal Supply of Nucleic and Branched-Chain Amino Acids to Cancer Cells

Tumor cells stimulate catabolic processes in surrounding stromal cells beyond lipolysis and autophagy as described above, which make distinct contributions to tumor cell metabolic fitness. One such process was recently demonstrated in the context of pancreatic cancer. PDA cells take up and use glutamine as a TCA carbon source (Son et al. 2013), such that environmental glutamine levels in the PDA microenvironment are low compared to benign pancreas tissue (Kamphorst et al. 2015; Lee et al. 2019). A recent study demonstrated that conditions of low glutamine stimulate the accumulation of nuclear fragile X mental retardation–interacting protein 1 (NUFIP1) in the cytoplasm of pancreatic CAFs, where NUFIP1 degrades ribosomal RNAs (rRNAs) (Yuan et al. 2022). These NUFIP1-generated nucleosides are then secreted and taken up by PDA cells, resulting in stabilization of oncogenic transcription factor MYC, elevated expression of MYC target SLC2A1, and increased glucose uptake to promote tumor growth. While CAFs provide secreted factors that enable PDA cell proliferation under low-glutamine conditions, loss of NUFIP1 expression by CAFs abolished this effect. CAFs also support PDA cell proliferation by providing substrates for de novo protein synthesis (Zhu et al. 2020). CAFs express high levels of branched-chain amino acid transaminase 1 (BCAT1), far exceeding BCAT1 expression in tumor cells. BCAT1 induction in CAFs results from TGF-β signaling, originating from cancer cells and perhaps additional cellular sources, via SMAD5. Stromal BCAT1 in turn catabolizes extracellular matrix proteins and potentially other substrates to generate branched-chain ketoacids, which are taken up by PDA cells and used for protein synthesis. In addition to supporting proliferation under conditions of nutrient challenge, CAFs also support PDA cell resistance to chemotherapy and viability in the context of gemcitabine treatment. PDA CAFs secrete sufficiently high levels of deoxycytidine through equilibrative nucleoside transporters, to inhibit the processing and cytotoxic activity of gemcitabine in PDA cells (Dalin et al. 2019). Tumor-associated macrophages in PDA were similarly shown to secrete deoxycytidine and promote gemcitabine resistance (Halbrook et al. 2019), further linking stromal metabolism to therapeutic resistance.

Role of p62 in the Stroma for Metabolic Reprogramming and Tumor Progression

P62 (SQSTM1) is a multifunctional signaling hub that has been most well studied as an autophagy adaptor (Moscat and Diaz-Meco 2011). Interestingly, while p62 up-regulation in the tumor epithelium has been shown in several cancers to be oncogenic in nature (Reina-Campos et al. 2018), its loss in the stroma of certain tumor types has been shown to support cancer growth through a number of mechanisms including altering cellular metabolism. In prostate cancer CAFs, loss of P62 causes a series of metabolic effects that ultimately supports prostate cancer growth. For example, in a low glutamine environment, CAFs lacking p62 increase expression of asparagine synthetase (ASNS), which leads to increased secretion of asparagine. This asparagine can be used by the tumor cells as a fuel source. These CAFs also up-regulate pyruvate carboxylase (PC) that can help compensate for decreased α-ketoglutarate from a low glutamine environment and allow the CAFs to thrive. Consistent with the importance of stromal P62 in supporting tumor growth, knockout of P62 in fibroblasts induced premalignant prostate lesions (Valencia et al. 2014). Loss of p62 expression in adjacent fibroblasts is driven by malignant epithelial cells via secreted lactate, which suppresses activity of AP-1 transcription factors in CAFs leading to transcriptional down-regulation of *Sqstm1* (encoding p62) (Linares et al. 2022). Tumor-restraining potential of stromal p62 extends to adipose tissue as well, where p62 loss results in osteopontin release from adipocytes and consequent increases in cancer cell CPT1 expression, fatty acid oxidation, and tumor progression (Huang et al. 2018). While these context-dependent roles for p62 have mostly been studied in prostate cancer, these roles may extend to other tumor types, and opposing roles of metabolic signaling hubs in tumor cells versus surrounding stroma may also be more broadly relevant.

PARACRINE REGULATION OF CANCER CELL METABOLIC SIGNALING NETWORKS

Activation of Mitogenic and Metabolic Signaling Nodes by Stromal Cues

The studies discussed above provide evidence that stromal cells secrete metabolites through diverse mechanisms that can be taken up by cancer cells to contribute to their metabolite pools and reduce the need for de novo synthesis reactions. However, these stroma-derived metabolites also serve as functional mediators of paracrine signaling, which can further impact cancer cell-intrinsic metabolic processes via metabolite-responsive signaling pathways (Fig. 2). This basis for coupling of stromal and epithelial metabolic processes was recently demonstrated in PDA. Normal pancreas tissue harbors a population of tissue-resident mesenchymal cells called stellate cells, which regulate tissue homeostasis including baseline production and recycling of extracellular matrix and basement membrane components (Sherman 2018). Pancreatic stellate cells (PSCs) are characterized in part by abundant, cytoplasmic lipid droplets that store vitamin A as retinyl esters and give PSCs a blue-green autofluorescence that facilitates visualization and analysis. In the context of tissue damage or during pancreatic tumorigenesis, PSCs become activated, and differentiate from their quiescent state to a myofibroblastic phenotype. In the activation process, PSCs lose their lipid droplets and down-regulate a transcriptional program associated with lipid storage, coincident with up-regulation of genes associated with CAF functions (Sherman et al. 2014). As this stromal lipid metabolic switch accompanies pancreatic tumor progression, lipidomic analyses of PSC-intrinsic and secreted lipid species were performed and revealed that PSCs undergo extensive lipidomic remodeling upon activation

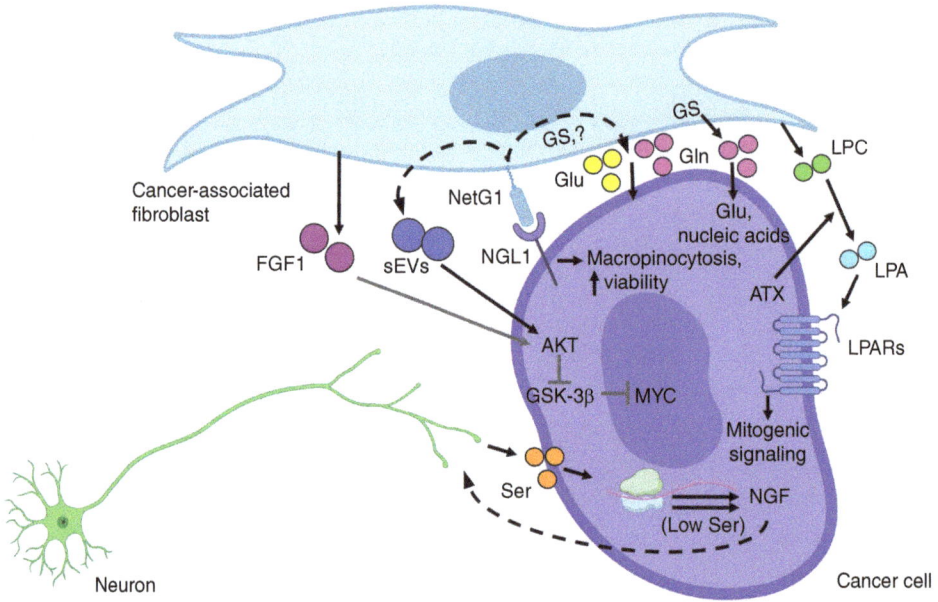

Figure 2. Signaling mediators from stromal cells, including cancer-associated fibroblasts and neurons, regulate cancer cell metabolic and mitogenic pathways in a paracrine manner. (ATX) Autotaxin, (FGF1) acidic fibroblast growth factor, (Gln) glutamine, (Glu) glutamate, (GS) glutamine synthetase, (LPA) lysophosphatidic acid, (LPAR) LPA receptor, (LPC) lysophosphatidylcholine, (NetG1) Netrin G1, (NGF) nerve growth factor, (NGL1) NetG1 ligand 1, (Ser) serine, (sEVs) small extracellular vesicles.

(Auciello et al. 2019). Activated PSCs secrete abundant lysophosphatidylcholines (LPCs), the preferred fatty acid–scavenging substrate for RAS-transformed cells, including PDA cells (Kamphorst et al. 2013). In addition to their utility for uptake and nutrient scavenging, though, LPCs can also regulate cancer cell metabolism via signaling. LPCs are hydrolyzed by the secreted enzyme autotaxin, with lysophospholipase D activity, to yield lysophosphatidic acid (LPA) species (Perrakis and Moolenaar 2014). PDA cells express and secrete high levels of autotaxin, which hydrolyzes stroma-derived LPC to yield LPA in the pancreatic TME (Auciello et al. 2019). LPA in turn signals through G-protein-coupled LPA receptors (LPARs) on PDA cells to activate mitogenic signaling pathways including the PI-3 kinase (PI3K)/AKT pathway, significant in the context of PDA as PI3K mutations are exceedingly rare in this disease setting. Genetic or pharmacologic inhibition of autotaxin reduces both AKT activation and PDA growth in vivo, and may also impact additional

metabolic signaling pathways downstream of LPARs (Mills and Moolenaar 2003).

An unexpected signaling mechanism was recently shown to coregulate AKT signaling in both tumor cells and stromal cells. Compared to normal tissue fibroblasts, CAFs express high levels of presynaptic protein Netrin G1 (NetG1), which signals through NetG1 ligand 1 (NGL1) or NGL1-independent mechanisms on neighboring cells (Francescone et al. 2021). NetG1 expression on CAFs positively regulates AKT activation in a cell-intrinsic manner, but also activates AKT in PDA cells in a paracrine manner mediated by NetG1-dependent small extracellular vesicle production (Raghavan et al. 2022). Stromal NetG1 and consequent paracrine activation of AKT helps PDA cells survive under relevant conditions of nutrient challenge. NetG1 on CAFs further regulates PDA cell metabolism by interacting with NGL1 on the PDA cell surface and inducing macropinocytosis, although the precise signaling pathway linking NetG1-NGL1 engagement to induction of macropino-

Cite this article as *Cold Spring Harb Perspect Med* doi: 10.1101/cshperspect.a041540

cytosis remains to be determined. The relevance of stromal NetG1 for cancer cell metabolic signaling in other tumor settings has not been assessed and warrants investigation.

Neuron-Derived Serine in Cancer Cell mRNA Translation

Pancreatic cancers are among the most highly innervated of human tumors that can lead to an intractable pain syndrome in patients (Lohse and Brothers 2020). While it has been well known that neurons can support the growth of cancers, including pancreatic cancer, most of this work has focused on the secretion of growth factors by the neurons that are used by cancer cells (Renz et al. 2018). Recently, it was shown that nerves also play a critical metabolic role in pancreatic tumors through the secretion of metabolites (Banh et al. 2020). Conceptually, neurons are ideally suited to be a nutritional conduit to the nutrient-deprived areas of the tumor. While the axons are in the TME, the cell body is actually in the ganglion, bathed by the nutrient-rich systemic circulation. Using a microfluidic chamber, Banh et al. showed that rat dorsal root ganglion neurons were capable of secreting amino acids from their axons (Banh et al. 2020). They went on to show that neuronal secretion of serine and glycine could support the growth of a large subset of pancreatic cancer cells that are unable to biosynthesize serine due to loss of PHGDH. Interestingly, they identified that the cancer cells required serine and glycine for proper RNA translation and that pancreatic cancer cells deficient in serine synthesis showed differential translation of particular serine codons, resulting in an adaptive biological program that slows proliferation, but increased secretion of nerve growth factor (NGF). Thus, serine deprivation resulted in increased innervation of the pancreatic tumors to support tumor growth by providing serine. Combining a serine/glycine-free diet with an NGF receptor inhibitor significantly decreased the growth of serine-dependent pancreatic cancer cells. Further efforts are underway to determine whether this biological adaptation can be exploited for therapeutic purposes and warrants investigation

in other tumor types featuring peripheral innervation.

Cross Talk between Fibroblasts and Cancer Cells to Support Oncogene Signaling

Examples of stroma-derived metabolites supporting cancer cell proliferation and survival call into question how stromal cells can bioenergetically "afford" to spare metabolites for the purpose of cancer cell fitness, as these stromal cells (with the exception of nerves, as described above) reside in the same inhospitable microenvironment as the tumor cells they functionally feed. These interactions may reflect an evolutionarily conserved relationship for stromal cells in the context of wound-healing reactions, where professional fibroinflammatory cells secrete diverse factors to enable epithelial cell proliferation and tissue repair. Stromal cell proliferation rates are lower than those of regenerating epithelium in wounds, and lower than cancer cells in tumors, consistent with coevolution of epithelial and stromal compartments such that stromal cells secrete metabolites that help tumor cells proliferate and survive. Even with a relatively low proliferation rate to limit biomass demand among stromal cells, these cells must adapt to their surroundings in the context of a tumor to produce and secrete molecules that facilitate growth in a paracrine manner. An important adaptation enabling metabolic cross talk between stromal and cancer cells was identified by comparing normal ovarian fibroblasts to ovarian CAFs (Yang et al. 2016). Transcriptional profiling of high-grade serous ovarian CAFs compared to normal fibroblasts revealed strikingly higher expression of genes involved in glutamine anabolic pathways in CAFs. Further, CAFs had far greater metabolic flexibility than normal fibroblasts, including adaptive mechanisms for harnessing carbon and nitrogen from atypical sources to enable glutamine synthesis in environments where glutamine is scarce. High expression of glutamine synthetase by CAFs was crucial for efficient stromal glutamine production, and combined inhibition of stromal glutamine synthetase, and glutaminase within tumor cells served as a synthetic lethal approach leading to reduced tumor growth and metastasis. In-depth analyses of coevolving metabolic adaptations in tumor and stroma may point to additional avenues for combined targeting to suppress tumor progression.

While cancer cells undergo cell-intrinsic metabolic reprogramming over the course of tumor initiation and progression mediated by core oncogenic signaling pathways, stromal components further influence cancer cell metabolism by cooperatively activating oncogenic signaling nodes to augment metabolic transcriptional outputs. In the pancreas, oncogenic KRAS and its gene-regulatory effector MYC drive an anabolic transcriptional program including components of the hexosamine biosynthesis and pentose phosphate pathways (Ying et al. 2012). Despite pervasive regulation of oncogenic transcription by mutant KRAS and MYC, expression of KRAS G12D throughout the pancreatic epithelium is insufficient to drive tumorigenesis in adult mice (Guerra et al. 2007). A fibroinflammatory reaction cooperated with oncogenic KRAS to promote pancreatic tumorigenesis, implicating this stromal reaction as a permissive context for tumor initiation and early progression. While inflammation limits barriers to tumor formation in place under homeostatic conditions, stromal cues also promote KRAS-driven tumorigenesis by cooperating with cancer cell–intrinsic KRAS signaling to promote expression of genes involved in metabolic reprogramming and immune suppression (Sherman et al. 2017; Alonso-Curbelo et al. 2021). Gene-expression programs and many gene identities were co-regulated by KRAS and stromal cues, with highest expression of these genes in the context of both cell-intrinsic and microenvironmental inputs. These findings suggest gene-regulatory points of convergence for oncogenic and stromal signaling pathways that together enable metabolic reprogramming to support tumor growth.

WOUND-HEALING MEDIATORS AS METABOLIC REGULATORS

The dense extracellular matrix associated with many solid tumors has long been implicated in mechanosignaling and tumor progression, but recently has been reported as a metabolic signaling mediator and a potential fuel source. Collagen is particularly abundant in solid TMEs, and dynamic matrix remodeling yields collagen fragments that may be taken up by cancer cells via macropinocytosis or other mechanisms (Olivares et al. 2017). As proline comprises 25% of the total amino acid composition of collagen, these collagen fragments serve as a proline reservoir that can promote cancer cell viability under nutrient-limited conditions. Collagen-derived proline contributes to PDA cell metabolism, and proline oxidase is required for PDA cell proliferation both in vitro and in vivo (Olivares et al. 2017). Proline oxidase is similarly needed to support colorectal cancer cell survival, yielding ATP in the setting of nutrient restriction and inducing autophagy under hypoxic conditions (Liu et al. 2012). Collagen is mostly produced by CAFs, and the metabolic state of CAFs dictates their capacity for matrix production. The cystine transporter SLC7A11, previously implicated as a therapeutic target on PDA cells (Badgley et al. 2020), also promotes tumor growth through its functions in the stroma (Sharbeen et al. 2021). SLC7A11 promotes cystine uptake and glutathione synthesis by CAFs, and stromal SLC7A11 inhibition reduces CAF proliferation as well as their ability to produce and remodel collagen and to support tumor growth. Protumorigenic collagen production by CAFs also requires proline synthesis from glutamine by PYCR1 (Kay et al. 2022), such that PYCR1 inhibition in breast CAFs is sufficient to reduce collagen production, tumor growth, and metastatic spread. The master fibrogenic signaling mediator TGF-β promotes collagen production by CAFs, and was recently shown to support the bioenergetic cost of matrix protein synthesis in part by increasing mitochondrial oxidation of glucose and glutamine (Schwörer et al. 2020). TGF-β signaling also stimulates proline biosynthesis from glutamine in a SMAD4-dependent manner. To reconcile collagen production with the glutamine- and glucose-low environments in which CAFs often function, a recent study demonstrated that PC-mediated anaplerosis within CAFs supports use of extracellular lactate to fuel the TCA cycle, nonessential amino acid biosynthesis, and collagen synthesis (Schwörer et al. 2021). Like collagen, hyaluronic acid (HA) is an abundant component of TMEs, and can also be used as a fuel source. HA consists of repeating N-acetylglucosamine (GlcNAc) and glucuronic acid sugars, and can contribute to the hexosamine biosynthesis pathway via GlcNAc salvage (Kim et al. 2021). Consistent with these findings, GlcNAc salvage via N-acetylglucosamine kinase (NAGK) promotes protein glycosylation and tumor growth in vivo (Campbell et al. 2021). HA remodeling and fragmentation further impacts cancer cell metabolism by negatively regulating TXNIP, increasing GLUT1 abundance at the plasma membrane, and increasing glucose uptake and glycolysis (Sullivan et al. 2018). Together, these studies highlight the significance of the extracellular matrix for cancer metabolism and, in turn, the importance of fibroblast metabolism for matrix production in tumors.

In addition to matrix components, soluble mediators of wound-healing reactions have also been implicated in the regulation of cancer cell metabolism. As described above, cancer cell–intrinsic KRAS signaling cooperates with stromal cues to promote expression of an anabolic transcriptional program, including many MYC target genes. Mechanistically, CAFs secrete high levels of acidic fibroblast growth factor (FGF1), which signals to cancer cells in a paracrine manner to activate AKT, negatively regulate GSK-3β, and elevate MYC stability and expression in the context of mutant KRAS (Bhattacharyya et al. 2020). CAF-derived cytokines and chemokines may also indirectly impact cancer cell metabolism by regulating the abundance and phenotypes of tumor-infiltrating immune cells. CAF secretion of CXCL12/SDF1, M-CSF/CSF1, IL-6, and CCL2/MCP1 can all contribute to the recruitment of tumor-associated macrophages as well as their arginase-expressing, immunosuppressive phenotype (Sanford-Crane et al. 2019). Arginine-metabolizing myeloid cells create a growth-permissive niche for lung cancer (Fu et al. 2022), neuroblastoma (Van de Velde et al. 2021), and other tumor types (Grzywa et al. 2020), perhaps reflecting the role of arginine metabolism in the resolution of tissue injury (Yurdagul et al. 2020).

TARGETING STROMAL METABOLISM FOR CANCER THERAPY

While the wound-like microenvironments associated with many solid tumors permits or supports progression, these niches also establish growth requirements distinct from healthy tissue, which may be targetable for therapeutic benefit. Targeting tumor cells as well as their niche may overcome cancer cell–intrinsic metabolic plasticity that has limited the efficacy of therapeutic agents targeting metabolic pathways. For example, Ras-transformed cancer cells as well as cancer cells under hypoxia take up lipids from the extracellular space and scavenge fatty acids from these lipids to limit the need for de novo lipid synthesis and oxygen-dependent desaturation reactions (Kamphorst et al. 2013). As stromal cells provide specific lipid species to tumor cells to support their proliferative capacity (Zhang et al. 2018; Auciello et al. 2019), particularly within poorly perfused contexts, combination therapies targeting stromal lipid metabolism as well as adaptation mechanisms in tumor cells may meaningfully limit cancer cell viability within an intact TME. Evidence in melanoma suggests that targeting stromal lipid metabolism may also foster the efficacy of targeted therapies (Alicea et al. 2020). Along a similar vein, recent work demonstrated the tumor-promoting roles for catabolic processes including autophagy and macropinocytosis in the stroma associated with cancer cells (Yang et al. 2018; Zhang et al. 2021). These findings in PDA complement recent work in lung cancer, indicating the potential to foster antitumor immunity by inhibiting autophagy systemically (Poillet-Perez et al. 2020; Khayati et al. 2022) via cancer cell-non-autonomous mechanisms that may include stromal cells in the TME as well as distant organs. These studies highlight the potential for inhibitors of these mechanisms to perturb stromal metabolic support to tumor cells, as well as growth-permissive cross talk with the immune system. While the antitumor potential of autophagy inhibitor hydroxychloroquine is already under investigation in clinical trials in combination with cytotoxic chemotherapy (Zeh et al. 2020) and other agents, a deeper understanding of the consequences of stromal catabolic processes may point to new, rationally designed combination therapy studies.

CONCLUSIONS AND FUTURE DIRECTIONS

Over the course of this review, we have described diverse modes of tumor-stroma cross talk that impact cancer cell metabolism and tumor progression. Some of these cross-talk mechanisms may reflect the metabolic reprogramming associated with productive wound-healing reactions (Shyh-Chang et al. 2013), highjacked in the context of cancer. Others may be tumor-specific. Given the increasingly appreciated role of stromal metabolism in both tumor progression and therapeutic resistance, our evolving understanding of metabolic support functions in intact TMEs may point to critical pathways to target for combination therapy. While the heterogeneity and plasticity of tumor cells with respect to their metabolism creates a challenge for productive therapeutic targeting of metabolic pathways, further study of cancer metabolism in the proper tissue setting has the potential to identify contextual dependencies that may be exploited effectively. To this end, important goals of future investigation include a deeper understanding of intratumor metabolic heterogeneity as well as the mechanisms enabling metabolic plasticity. State-of-the-art metabolomic technologies increasingly enable analysis of metabolic processes within heterocellular tumor tissues (Nascentes Melo et al. 2022), and their continued development will serve the field well in striving to understand relationships between tumor cell and stromal cell metabolism within relevant anatomic contexts.

COMPETING INTEREST STATEMENT

A.C.K. has financial interests in Vescor Therapeutics and is an inventor on patents pertaining to KRAS-regulated metabolic pathways and redox control pathways in pancreatic cancer, targeting GOT1 as a therapeutic approach, targeting alanine transport, and the autophagic control of iron metabolism. A.C.K. is on the scientific advisory board of Rafael/Cornerstone Pharmaceuticals, OcoRev, and has been a con-

sultant for Deciphera and Abbvie. M.H.S. declares no competing interests.

ACKNOWLEDGMENTS

The authors apologize for the omission of any primary references. This work was supported by NCI Grants P01CA117969, R35CA232124, P30CA016087-38, and 1R01CA251726-01A1; the Lustgarten Foundation, and SU2C to A.C.K. M.H.S. is supported by MSK Cancer Center Support Grant/Core Grant (P30 CA008748).

REFERENCES

Ackerman D, Simon MC. 2014. Hypoxia, lipids, and cancer: surviving the harsh tumor microenvironment. *Trends Cell Biol* **24:** 472–478. doi:10.1016/j.tcb.2014.06.001

Alicea GM, Rebecca VW, Goldman AR, Fane ME, Douglass SM, Behera R, Webster MR, Kugel CH III, Ecker BL, Caino MC, et al. 2020. Changes in aged fibroblast lipid metabolism induce age-dependent melanoma cell resistance to targeted therapy via the fatty acid transporter FATP2. *Cancer Discov* **10:** 1282–1295. doi:10.1158/2159-8290.CD-20-0329

Alonso-Curbelo D, Ho YJ, Burdziak C, Maag JLV, Morris JP IV, Chandwani R, Chen HA, Tsanov KM, Barriga FM, Luan W, et al. 2021. A gene-environment-induced epigenetic program initiates tumorigenesis. *Nature* **590:** 642–648. doi:10.1038/s41586-020-03147-x

Auciello FR, Bulusu V, Oon C, Tait-Mulder J, Berry M, Bhattacharyya S, Tumanov S, Allen-Petersen BL, Link J, Kendsersky ND, et al. 2019. A stromal lysolipid-autotaxin signaling axis promotes pancreatic tumor progression. *Cancer Discov* **9:** 617–627. doi:10.1158/2159-8290.CD-18-1212

Badgley MA, Kremer DM, Maurer HC, DelGiorno KE, Lee HJ, Purohit V, Sagalovskiy IR, Ma A, Kapilian J, Firl CEM, et al. 2020. Cysteine depletion induces pancreatic tumor ferroptosis in mice. *Science* **368:** 85–89. doi:10.1126/science.aaw9872

Banh RS, Biancur DE, Yamamoto K, Sohn ASW, Walters B, Kuljanin M, Gikandi A, Wang H, Mancias JD, Schneider RJ, et al. 2020. Neurons release serine to support mRNA translation in pancreatic cancer. *Cell* **183:** 1202–1218.e25. doi:10.1016/j.cell.2020.10.016

Benckert C, Thelen A, Cramer T, Weichert W, Gaebelein G, Gessner R, Jonas S. 2012. Impact of microvessel density on lymph node metastasis and survival after curative resection of pancreatic cancer. *Surg Today* **42:** 169–176. doi:10.1007/s00595-011-0045-0

Bhattacharyya S, Oon C, Kothari A, Horton W, Link J, Sears RC, Sherman MH. 2020. Acidic fibroblast growth factor underlies microenvironmental regulation of MYC in pancreatic cancer. *J Exp Med* **217:** e20191805. doi:10.1084/jem.20191805

Biancur DE, Kimmelman AC. 2018. The plasticity of pancreatic cancer metabolism in tumor progression and therapeutic resistance. *Biochim Biophys Acta Rev Cancer* **1870**: 67–75. doi:10.1016/j.bbcan.2018.04.011

Biancur DE, Paulo JA, Małachowska B, Quiles Del Rey M, Sousa CM, Wang X, Sohn ASW, Chu GC, Gygi SP, Harper JW, et al. 2017. Compensatory metabolic networks in pancreatic cancers upon perturbation of glutamine metabolism. *Nat Commun* **8**: 15965. doi:10.1038/ncomms15965

Biancur DE, Kapner KS, Yamamoto K, Banh RS, Neggers JE, Sohn ASW, Wu W, Manguso RT, Brown A, Root DE, et al. 2021. Functional genomics identifies metabolic vulnerabilities in pancreatic cancer. *Cell Metab* **33**: 199–210.e8. doi:10.1016/j.cmet.2020.10.018

Campbell S, Mesaros C, Izzo L, Affronti H, Noji M, Schaffer BE, Tsang T, Sun K, Trefely S, Kruijning S, et al. 2021. Glutamine deprivation triggers NAGK-dependent hexosamine salvage. *eLife* **10**: e62644. doi:10.7554/eLife.62644

Cantelmo AR, Conradi LC, Brajic A, Goveia J, Kalucka J, Pircher A, Chaturvedi P, Hol J, Thienpont B, Teuwen LA, et al. 2016. Inhibition of the glycolytic activator PFKFB3 in endothelium induces tumor vessel normalization, impairs metastasis, and improves chemotherapy. *Cancer Cell* **30**: 968–985. doi:10.1016/j.ccell.2016.10.006

Cantor JR, Abu-Remaileh M, Kanarek N, Freinkman E, Gao X, Louissaint A Jr, Lewis CA, Sabatini DM. 2017. Physiologic medium rewires cellular metabolism and reveals uric acid as an endogenous inhibitor of UMP synthase. *Cell* **169**: 258–272.e17. doi:10.1016/j.cell.2017.03.023

Chang CH, Qiu J, O'Sullivan D, Buck MD, Noguchi T, Curtis JD, Chen Q, Gindin M, Gubin MM, van der Windt GJ, et al. 2015. Metabolic competition in the tumor microenvironment is a driver of cancer progression. *Cell* **162**: 1229–1241. doi:10.1016/j.cell.2015.08.016

Commisso C, Davidson SM, Soydaner-Azeloglu RG, Parker SJ, Kamphorst JJ, Hackett S, Grabocka E, Nofal M, Drebin JA, Thompson CB, et al. 2013. Macropinocytosis of protein is an amino acid supply route in Ras-transformed cells. *Nature* **497**: 633–637. doi:10.1038/nature12138

Dalin S, Sullivan MR, Lau AN, Grauman-Boss B, Mueller HS, Kreidl E, Fenoglio S, Luengo A, Lees JA, Vander Heiden MG, et al. 2019. Deoxycytidine release from pancreatic stellate cells promotes gemcitabine resistance. *Cancer Res* **79**: 5723–5733. doi:10.1158/0008-5472.CAN-19-0960

DeBerardinis RJ, Chandel NS. 2016. Fundamentals of cancer metabolism. *Sci Adv* **2**: e1600200. doi:10.1126/sciadv.1600200

De Bock K, Georgiadou M, Schoors S, Kuchnio A, Wong BW, Cantelmo AR, Quaegebeur A, Ghesquière B, Cauwenberghs S, Eelen G, et al. 2013. Role of PFKFB3-driven glycolysis in vessel sprouting. *Cell* **154**: 651–663. doi:10.1016/j.cell.2013.06.037

Dirat B, Bochet L, Dabek M, Daviaud D, Dauvillier S, Majed B, Wang YY, Meulle A, Salles B, Le Gonidec S, et al. 2011. Cancer-associated adipocytes exhibit an activated phenotype and contribute to breast cancer invasion. *Cancer Res* **71**: 2455–2465. doi:10.1158/0008-5472.CAN-10-3323

Encarnación-Rosado J, Kimmelman AC. 2021. Harnessing metabolic dependencies in pancreatic cancers. *Nat Rev Gastroenterol Hepatol* **18**: 482–492. doi:10.1038/s41575-021-00431-7

Endo S, Nakata K, Ohuchida K, Takesue S, Nakayama H, Abe T, Koikawa K, Okumura T, Sada M, Horioka K, et al. 2017. Autophagy is required for activation of pancreatic stellate cells, associated with pancreatic cancer progression and promotes growth of pancreatic tumors in mice. *Gastroenterology* **152**: 1492–1506.e24. doi:10.1053/j.gastro.2017.01.010

Faubert B, Li KY, Cai L, Hensley CT, Kim J, Zacharias LG, Yang C, Do QN, Doucette S, Burguete D, et al. 2017. Lactate metabolism in human lung tumors. *Cell* **171**: 358–371.e9. doi:10.1016/j.cell.2017.09.019

Ferraro GB, Ali A, Luengo A, Kodack DP, Deik A, Abbott KL, Bezwada D, Blanc L, Prideaux B, Jin X, et al. 2021. Fatty acid synthesis is required for breast cancer brain metastasis. *Nat Cancer* **2**: 414–428. doi:10.1038/s43018-021-00183-y

Follain G, Herrmann D, Harlepp S, Hyenne V, Osmani N, Warren SC, Timpson P, Goetz JG. 2020. Fluids and their mechanics in tumour transit: shaping metastasis. *Nat Rev Cancer* **20**: 107–124. doi:10.1038/s41568-019-0221-x

Francescone R, Barbosa Vendramini-Costa D, Franco-Barraza J, Wagner J, Muir A, Lau AN, Gabitova L, Pazina T, Gupta S, Luong T, et al. 2021. Netrin G1 promotes pancreatic tumorigenesis through cancer-associated fibroblast-driven nutritional support and immunosuppression. *Cancer Discov* **11**: 446–479. doi:10.1158/2159-8290.CD-20-0775

Fu Y, Pajulas A, Wang J, Zhou B, Cannon A, Cheung CCL, Zhang J, Zhou H, Fisher AJ, Omstead DT, et al. 2022. Mouse pulmonary interstitial macrophages mediate the pro-tumorigenic effects of IL-9. *Nat Commun* **13**: 3811. doi:10.1038/s41467-022-31596-7

Garcia-Bermudez J, Badgley MA, Prasad S, Baudrier L, Liu Y, La K, Soula M, Williams RT, Yamaguchi N, Hwang RF, et al. 2022. Adaptive stimulation of macropinocytosis overcomes aspartate limitation in cancer cells under hypoxia. *Nat Metab* **4**: 724–738. doi:10.1038/s42255-022-00583-z

Grzywa TM, Sosnowska A, Matryba P, Rydzynska Z, Jasinski M, Nowis D, Golab J. 2020. Myeloid cell-derived arginase in cancer immune response. *Front Immunol* **11**: 938. doi:10.3389/fimmu.2020.00938

Guerra C, Schuhmacher AJ, Cañamero M, Grippo PJ, Verdaguer L, Pérez-Gallego L, Dubus P, Sandgren EP, Barbacid M. 2007. Chronic pancreatitis is essential for induction of pancreatic ductal adenocarcinoma by K-Ras oncogenes in adult mice. *Cancer Cell* **11**: 291–302. doi:10.1016/j.ccr.2007.01.012

Halbrook CJ, Pontious C, Kovalenko I, Lapienyte L, Dreyer S, Lee HJ, Thurston G, Zhang Y, Lazarus J, Sajjakulnukit P, et al. 2019. Macrophage-released pyrimidines inhibit gemcitabine therapy in pancreatic cancer. *Cell Metab* **29**: 1390–1399.e6. doi:10.1016/j.cmet.2019.02.001

Halbrook CJ, Lyssiotis CA, Pasca di Magliano M, Maitra A. 2023. Pancreatic cancer: advances and challenges. *Cell* **186**: 1729–1754. doi:10.1016/j.cell.2023.02.014

Hanahan D. 2022. Hallmarks of cancer: new dimensions. *Cancer Discov* **12**: 31–46. doi:10.1158/2159-8290.CD-21-1059

Hensley CT, Faubert B, Yuan Q, Lev-Cohain N, Jin E, Kim J, Jiang L, Ko B, Skelton R, Loudat L, et al. 2016. Metabolic heterogeneity in human lung tumors. *Cell* **164**: 681–694. doi:10.1016/j.cell.2015.12.034

Ho PC, Bihuniak JD, Macintyre AN, Staron M, Liu X, Amezquita R, Tsui YC, Cui G, Micevic G, Perales JC, et al. 2015. Phosphoenolpyruvate is a metabolic checkpoint of antitumor T cell responses. *Cell* 162: 1217–1228. doi:10.1016/j.cell.2015.08.012

Hollander DM, Devereux DF, Taylor CG, Taylor DD. 1986. Demonstration of lipolytic activity from cultured human melanoma cells. *J Surg Res* 40: 445–449. doi:10.1016/0022-4804(86)90213-1

Huang J, Duran A, Reina-Campos M, Valencia T, Castilla EA, Müller TD, Tschöp MH, Moscat J, Diaz-Meco MT. 2018. Adipocyte p62/SQSTM1 suppresses tumorigenesis through opposite regulations of metabolism in adipose tissue and tumor. *Cancer Cell* 33: 770–784.e6. doi:10.1016/j.ccell.2018.03.001

Hui S, Ghergurovich JM, Morscher RJ, Jang C, Teng X, Lu W, Esparza LA, Reya T, Le Z, Yanxiang Guo J, et al. 2017. Glucose feeds the TCA cycle via circulating lactate. *Nature* 551: 115–118. doi:10.1038/nature24057

Jain RK. 2005. Normalization of tumor vasculature: an emerging concept in antiangiogenic therapy. *Science* 307: 58–62. doi:10.1126/science.1104819

Kamphorst JJ, Cross JR, Fan J, de Stanchina E, Mathew R, White EP, Thompson CB, Rabinowitz JD. 2013. Hypoxic and Ras-transformed cells support growth by scavenging unsaturated fatty acids from lysophospholipids. *Proc Natl Acad Sci* 110: 8882–8887. doi:10.1073/pnas.1307237110

Kamphorst JJ, Nofal M, Commisso C, Hackett SR, Lu W, Grabocka E, Vander Heiden MG, Miller G, Drebin JA, Bar-Sagi D, et al. 2015. Human pancreatic cancer tumors are nutrient poor and tumor cells actively scavenge extracellular protein. *Cancer Res* 75: 544–553. doi:10.1158/0008-5472.CAN-14-2211

Kay EJ, Paterson K, Riera-Domingo C, Sumpton D, Däbritz JHM, Tardito S, Boldrini C, Hernandez-Fenaud JR, Athineos D, Dhayade S, et al. 2022. Cancer-associated fibroblasts require proline synthesis by PYCR1 for the deposition of pro-tumorigenic extracellular matrix. *Nat Metab* 4: 693–710. doi:10.1038/s42255-022-00582-0

Khayati K, Bhatt V, Lan T, Alogaili F, Wang W, Lopez E, Hu ZS, Gokhale S, Cassidy L, Narita M, et al. 2022. Transient systemic autophagy inhibition is selectively and irreversibly deleterious to lung cancer. *Cancer Res* 82: 4429–4443. doi:10.1158/0008-5472.CAN-22-1039

Kim PK, Halbrook CJ, Kerk SA, Radyk M, Wisner S, Kremer DM, Sajjakulnukit P, Andren A, Hou SW, Trivedi A, et al. 2021. Hyaluronic acid fuels pancreatic cancer cell growth. *eLife* 10: e62645. doi:10.7554/eLife.62645

Kuczynski EA, Vermeulen PB, Pezzella F, Kerbel RS, Reynolds AR. 2019. Vessel co-option in cancer. *Nat Rev Clin Oncol* 16: 469–493. doi:10.1038/s41571-019-0181-9

Lambert AW, Pattabiraman DR, Weinberg RA. 2017. Emerging biological principles of metastasis. *Cell* 168: 670–691. doi:10.1016/j.cell.2016.11.037

Lauby-Secretan B, Scoccianti C, Loomis D, Grosse Y, Bianchini F, Straif K; International Agency for Research on Cancer Handbook Working Group. 2016. Body fatness and cancer—viewpoint of the IARC Working Group. *N Engl J Med* 375: 794–798. doi:10.1056/NEJMsr1606602

Lee SW, Zhang Y, Jung M, Cruz N, Alas B, Commisso C. 2019. EGFR-Pak signaling selectively regulates glutamine deprivation-induced macropinocytosis. *Dev Cell* 50: 381–392.e5. doi:10.1016/j.devcel.2019.05.043

Li X, Kumar A, Carmeliet P. 2019. Metabolic pathways fueling the endothelial cell drive. *Annu Rev Physiol* 81: 483–503. doi:10.1146/annurev-physiol-020518-114731

Linares JF, Cid-Diaz T, Duran A, Osrodek M, Martinez-Ordoñez A, Reina-Campos M, Kuo HH, Elemento O, Martin ML, Cordes T, et al. 2022. The lactate-NAD$^+$ axis activates cancer-associated fibroblasts by downregulating p62. *Cell Rep* 39: 110792. doi:10.1016/j.celrep.2022.110792

Liu W, Glunde K, Bhujwalla ZM, Raman V, Sharma A, Phang JM. 2012. Proline oxidase promotes tumor cell survival in hypoxic tumor microenvironments. *Cancer Res* 72: 3677–3686. doi:10.1158/0008-5472.CAN-12-0080

Lohse I, Brothers SP. 2020. Pathogenesis and treatment of pancreatic cancer related pain. *Anticancer Res* 40: 1789–1796. doi:10.21873/anticanres.14133

Luengo A, Gui DY, Vander Heiden MG. 2017. Targeting metabolism for cancer therapy. *Cell Chem Biol* 24: 1161–1180. doi:10.1016/j.chembiol.2017.08.028

Lyssiotis CA, Kimmelman AC. 2017. Metabolic interactions in the tumor microenvironment. *Trends Cell Biol* 27: 863–875. doi:10.1016/j.tcb.2017.06.003

Macchiarini P, Fontanini G, Hardin MJ, Squartini F, Angeletti CA. 1992. Relation of neovascularisation to metastasis of non-small-cell lung cancer. *Lancet* 340: 145–146. doi:10.1016/0140-6736(92)93217-B

Maguire OA, Ackerman SE, Szwed SK, Maganti AV, Marchildon F, Huang X, Kramer DJ, Rosas-Villegas A, Gelfer RG, Turner LE, et al. 2021. Creatine-mediated crosstalk between adipocytes and cancer cells regulates obesity-driven breast cancer. *Cell Metab* 33: 499–512.e6. doi:10.1016/j.cmet.2021.01.018

Mills GB, Moolenaar WH. 2003. The emerging role of lysophosphatidic acid in cancer. *Nat Rev Cancer* 3: 582–591. doi:10.1038/nrc1143

Mishra R, Haldar S, Placencio V, Madhav A, Rohena-Rivera K, Agarwal P, Duong F, Angara B, Tripathi M, Liu Z, et al. 2018. Stromal epigenetic alterations drive metabolic and neuroendocrine prostate cancer reprogramming. *J Clin Invest* 128: 4472–4484. doi:10.1172/JCI99397

Moscat J, Diaz-Meco MT. 2011. Feedback on fat: p62-mTORC1-autophagy connections. *Cell* 147: 724–727. doi:10.1016/j.cell.2011.10.021

Mukherjee A, Chiang CY, Daifotis HA, Nieman KM, Fahrmann JF, Lastra RR, Romero IL, Fiehn O, Lengyel E. 2020. Adipocyte-induced FABP4 expression in ovarian cancer cells promotes metastasis and mediates carboplatin resistance. *Cancer Res* 80: 1748–1761. doi:10.1158/0008-5472.CAN-19-1999

Mukherjee A, Bilecz AJ, Lengyel E. 2022. The adipocyte microenvironment and cancer. *Cancer Metastasis Rev* 41: 575–587. doi:10.1007/s10555-022-10059-x

Nascentes Melo LM, Lesner NP, Sabatier M, Ubellacker JM, Tasdogan A. 2022. Emerging metabolomic tools to study cancer metastasis. *Trends Cancer* 8: 988–1001. doi:10.1016/j.trecan.2022.07.003

Ngo B, Kim E, Osorio-Vasquez V, Doll S, Bustraan S, Liang RJ, Luengo A, Davidson SM, Ali A, Ferraro GB, et al. 2020.

Limited environmental serine and glycine confer brain metastasis sensitivity to PHGDH inhibition. *Cancer Discov* 10: 1352–1373. doi:10.1158/2159-8290.CD-19-1228

Nieman KM, Kenny HA, Penicka CV, Ladanyi A, Buell-Gutbrod R, Zillhardt MR, Romero IL, Carey MS, Mills GB, Hotamisligil GS, et al. 2011. Adipocytes promote ovarian cancer metastasis and provide energy for rapid tumor growth. *Nat Med* 17: 1498–1503. doi:10.1038/nm.2492

Olivares O, Mayers JR, Gouirand V, Torrence ME, Gicquel T, Borge L, Lac S, Roques J, Lavaut MN, Berthezene P, et al. 2017. Collagen-derived proline promotes pancreatic ductal adenocarcinoma cell survival under nutrient limited conditions. *Nat Commun* 8: 16031. doi:10.1038/ncomms16031

Parker SJ, Amendola CR, Hollinshead KER, Yu Q, Yamamoto K, Encarnación-Rosado J, Rose RE, LaRue MM, Sohn ASW, Biancur DE, et al. 2020. Selective alanine transporter utilization creates a targetable metabolic niche in pancreatic cancer. *Cancer Discov* 10: 1018–1037. doi:10.1158/2159-8290.CD-19-0959

Pascual G, Avgustinova A, Mejetta S, Martín M, Castellanos A, Attolini CS, Berenguer A, Prats N, Toll A, Hueto JA, et al. 2017. Targeting metastasis-initiating cells through the fatty acid receptor CD36. *Nature* 541: 41–45. doi:10.1038/nature20791

Perrakis A, Moolenaar WH. 2014. Autotaxin: structure-function and signaling. *J Lipid Res* 55: 1010–1018. doi:10.1194/jlr.R046391

Poillet-Perez L, Sharp DW, Yang Y, Laddha SV, Ibrahim M, Bommareddy PK, Hu ZS, Vieth J, Haas M, Bosenberg MW, et al. 2020. Autophagy promotes growth of tumors with high mutational burden by inhibiting a T-cell immune response. *Nat Cancer* 1: 923–934. doi:10.1038/s43018-020-00110-7

Provenzano PP, Cuevas C, Chang AE, Goel VK, Von Hoff DD, Hingorani SR. 2012. Enzymatic targeting of the stroma ablates physical barriers to treatment of pancreatic ductal adenocarcinoma. *Cancer Cell* 21: 418–429. doi:10.1016/j.ccr.2012.01.007

Raghavan KS, Francescone R, Franco-Barraza J, Gardiner JC, Vendramini-Costa DB, Luong T, Pourmandi N, Andren A, Kurimchak A, Ogier C, et al. 2022. Netrin g1+ cancer-associated fibroblasts generate unique extracellular vesicles that support the survival of pancreatic cancer cells under nutritional stress. *Cancer Res Commun* 2: 1017–1036. doi:10.1158/2767-9764.CRC-21-0147

Reina-Campos M, Shelton PM, Diaz-Meco MT, Moscat J. 2018. Metabolic reprogramming of the tumor microenvironment by p62 and its partners. *Biochim Biophys Acta Rev Cancer* 1870: 88–95. doi:10.1016/j.bbcan.2018.04.010

Reinfeld BI, Madden MZ, Wolf MM, Chytil A, Bader JE, Patterson AR, Sugiura A, Cohen AS, Ali A, Do BT, et al. 2021. Cell-programmed nutrient partitioning in the tumour microenvironment. *Nature* 593: 282–288. doi:10.1038/s41586-021-03442-1

Renz BW, Takahashi R, Tanaka T, Macchini M, Hayakawa Y, Dantes Z, Maurer HC, Chen X, Jiang Z, Westphalen CB, et al. 2018. β2 adrenergic-neurotrophin feedforward loop promotes pancreatic cancer. *Cancer Cell* 33: 75–90.e7. doi:10.1016/j.ccell.2017.11.007

Reticker-Flynn NE, Zhang W, Belk JA, Basto PA, Escalante NK, Pilarowski GOW, Bejnood A, Martins MM, Kenkel JA, Linde IL, et al. 2022. Lymph node colonization induces tumor-immune tolerance to promote distant metastasis. *Cell* 185: 1924–1942.e23. doi:10.1016/j.cell.2022.04.019

Roslin M, Henriksson R, Bergström P, Ungerstedt U, Bergenheim AT. 2003. Baseline levels of glucose metabolites, glutamate and glycerol in malignant glioma assessed by stereotactic microdialysis. *J Neurooncol* 61: 151–160. doi:10.1023/A:1022106910017

Sanford-Crane H, Abrego J, Sherman MH. 2019. Fibroblasts as modulators of local and systemic cancer metabolism. *Cancers (Basel)* 11: 619. doi:10.3390/cancers11050619

Schroeder U, Himpe B, Pries R, Vonthein R, Nitsch S, Wollenberg B. 2013. Decline of lactate in tumor tissue after ketogenic diet: in vivo microdialysis study in patients with head and neck cancer. *Nutr Cancer* 65: 843–849. doi:10.1080/01635581.2013.804579

Schwörer S, Berisa M, Violante S, Qin W, Zhu J, Hendrickson RC, Cross JR, Thompson CB. 2020. Proline biosynthesis is a vent for TGFβ-induced mitochondrial redox stress. *EMBO J* 39: e103334. doi:10.15252/embj.2019103334

Schwörer S, Pavlova NN, Cimino FV, King B, Cai X, Sizemore GM, Thompson CB. 2021. Fibroblast pyruvate carboxylase is required for collagen production in the tumour microenvironment. *Nat Metab* 3: 1484–1499. doi:10.1038/s42255-021-00480-x

Sharbeen G, McCarroll JA, Akerman A, Kopecky C, Youkhana J, Kokkinos J, Holst J, Boyer C, Erkan M, Goldstein D, et al. 2021. Cancer-associated fibroblasts in pancreatic ductal adenocarcinoma determine response to SLC7A11 inhibition. *Cancer Res* 81: 3461–3479. doi:10.1158/0008-5472.CAN-20-2496

Sherman MH. 2018. Stellate cells in tissue repair, inflammation, and cancer. *Annu Rev Cell Dev Biol* 34: 333–355. doi:10.1146/annurev-cellbio-100617-062855

Sherman MH, Yu RT, Engle DD, Ding N, Atkins AR, Tiriac H, Collisson EA, Connor F, Van Dyke T, Kozlov S, et al. 2014. Vitamin D receptor-mediated stromal reprogramming suppresses pancreatitis and enhances pancreatic cancer therapy. *Cell* 159: 80–93. doi:10.1016/j.cell.2014.08.007

Sherman MH, Yu RT, Tseng TW, Sousa CM, Liu S, Truitt ML, He N, Ding N, Liddle C, Atkins AR, et al. 2017. Stromal cues regulate the pancreatic cancer epigenome and metabolome. *Proc Natl Acad Sci* 114: 1129–1134. doi:10.1073/pnas.1620164114

Shyh-Chang N, Zhu H, Yvanka de Soysa T, Shinoda G, Seligson MT, Tsanov KM, Nguyen L, Asara JM, Cantley LC, Daley GQ. 2013. Lin28 enhances tissue repair by reprogramming cellular metabolism. *Cell* 155: 778–792. doi:10.1016/j.cell.2013.09.059

Son J, Lyssiotis CA, Ying H, Wang X, Hua S, Ligorio M, Perera RM, Ferrone CR, Mullarky E, Shyh-Chang N, et al. 2013. Glutamine supports pancreatic cancer growth through a KRAS-regulated metabolic pathway. *Nature* 496: 101–105. doi:10.1038/nature12040

Sousa CM, Biancur DE, Wang X, Halbrook CJ, Sherman MH, Zhang L, Kremer D, Hwang RF, Witkiewicz AK, Ying H, et al. 2016. Pancreatic stellate cells support tumour metabolism through autophagic alanine secretion. *Nature* **536:** 479–483. doi:10.1038/nature19084

Stylianopoulos T, Martin JD, Chauhan VP, Jain SR, Diop-Frimpong B, Bardeesy N, Smith BL, Ferrone CR, Hornicek FJ, Boucher Y, et al. 2012. Causes, consequences, and remedies for growth-induced solid stress in murine and human tumors. *Proc Natl Acad Sci* **109:** 15101–15108. doi:10.1073/pnas.1213353109

Sullivan WJ, Mullen PJ, Schmid EW, Flores A, Momcilovic M, Sharpley MS, Jelinek D, Whiteley AE, Maxwell MB, Wilde BR, et al. 2018. Extracellular matrix remodeling regulates glucose metabolism through TXNIP destabilization. *Cell* **175:** 117–132.e21. doi:10.1016/j.cell.2018.08.017

Sullivan MR, Danai LV, Lewis CA, Chan SH, Gui DY, Kunchok T, Dennstedt EA, Vander Heiden MG, Muir A. 2019a. Quantification of microenvironmental metabolites in murine cancers reveals determinants of tumor nutrient availability. *eLife* **8:** e44235. doi:10.7554/eLife.44235

Sullivan MR, Mattaini KR, Dennstedt EA, Nguyen AA, Sivanand S, Reilly MF, Meeth K, Muir A, Darnell AM, Bosenberg MW, et al. 2019b. Increased serine synthesis provides an advantage for tumors arising in tissues where serine levels are limiting. *Cell Metab* **29:** 1410–1421.e4. doi:10.1016/j.cmet.2019.02.015

Valencia T, Kim JY, Abu-Baker S, Moscat-Pardos J, Ahn CS, Reina-Campos M, Duran A, Castilla EA, Metallo CM, Diaz-Meco MT, et al. 2014. Metabolic reprogramming of stromal fibroblasts through p62-mTORC1 signaling promotes inflammation and tumorigenesis. *Cancer Cell* **26:** 121–135. doi:10.1016/j.ccr.2014.05.004

Van de Velde LA, Allen EK, Crawford JC, Wilson TL, Guy CS, Russier M, Zeitler L, Bahrami A, Finkelstein D, Pelletier S, et al. 2021. Neuroblastoma formation requires unconventional CD4 T cells and arginase-1-dependent myeloid cells. *Cancer Res* **81:** 5047–5059. doi:10.1158/0008-5472.CAN-21-0691

Weidner N, Semple JP, Welch WR, Folkman J. 1991. Tumor angiogenesis and metastasis—correlation in invasive breast carcinoma. *N Engl J Med* **324:** 1–8. doi:10.1056/NEJM199101033240101

Weidner N, Carroll PR, Flax J, Blumenfeld W, Folkman J. 1993. Tumor angiogenesis correlates with metastasis in invasive prostate carcinoma. *Am J Pathol* **143:** 401–409.

Yang L, Achreja A, Yeung TL, Mangala LS, Jiang D, Han C, Baddour J, Marini JC, Ni J, Nakahara R, et al. 2016. Targeting stromal glutamine synthetase in tumors disrupts tumor microenvironment-regulated cancer cell growth. *Cell Metab* **24:** 685–700. doi:10.1016/j.cmet.2016.10.011

Yang A, Herter-Sprie G, Zhang H, Lin EY, Biancur D, Wang X, Deng J, Hai J, Yang S, Wong KK, et al. 2018. Autophagy sustains pancreatic cancer growth through both cell-autonomous and nonautonomous mechanisms. *Cancer Discov* **8:** 276–287. doi:10.1158/2159-8290.CD-17-0952

Ying H, Kimmelman AC, Lyssiotis CA, Hua S, Chu GC, Fletcher-Sananikone E, Locasale JW, Son J, Zhang H, Coloff JL, et al. 2012. Oncogenic Kras maintains pancreatic tumors through regulation of anabolic glucose metabolism. *Cell* **149:** 656–670. doi:10.1016/j.cell.2012.01.058

Yuan M, Tu B, Li H, Pang H, Zhang N, Fan M, Bai J, Wang W, Shu Z, DuFort CC, et al. 2022. Cancer-associated fibroblasts employ NUFIP1-dependent autophagy to secrete nucleosides and support pancreatic tumor growth. *Nat Cancer* **3:** 945–960. doi:10.1038/s43018-022-00426-6

Yurdagul A Jr, Subramanian M, Wang X, Crown SB, Ilkayeva OR, Darville L, Kolluru GK, Rymond CC, Gerlach BD, Zheng Z, et al. 2020. Macrophage metabolism of apoptotic cell-derived arginine promotes continual efferocytosis and resolution of injury. *Cell Metab* **31:** 518–533. e10. doi:10.1016/j.cmet.2020.01.001

Zecchin A, Kalucka J, Dubois C, Carmeliet P. 2017. How endothelial cells adapt their metabolism to form vessels in tumors. *Front Immunol* **8:** 1750. doi:10.3389/fimmu.2017.01750

Zeh HJ, Bahary N, Boone BA, Singhi AD, Miller-Ocuin JL, Normolle DP, Zureikat AH, Hogg ME, Bartlett DL, Lee KK, et al. 2020. A randomized phase II preoperative study of autophagy inhibition with high-dose hydroxychloroquine and gemcitabine/nab-paclitaxel in pancreatic cancer patients. *Clin Cancer Res* **26:** 3126–3134. doi:10.1158/1078-0432.CCR-19-4042

Zhang M, Di Martino JS, Bowman RL, Campbell NR, Baksh SC, Simon-Vermot T, Kim IS, Haldeman P, Mondal C, Yong-Gonzales V, et al. 2018. Adipocyte-derived lipids mediate melanoma progression via FATP proteins. *Cancer Discov* **8:** 1006–1025. doi:10.1158/2159-8290.CD-17-1371

Zhang Y, Recouvreux MV, Jung M, Galenkamp KMO, Li Y, Zagnitko O, Scott DA, Lowy AM, Commisso C. 2021. Macropinocytosis in cancer-associated fibroblasts is dependent on CaMKK2/ARHGEF2 signaling and functions to support tumor and stromal cell fitness. *Cancer Discov* **11:** 1808–1825. doi:10.1158/2159-8290.CD-20-0119

Zhu J, Thompson CB. 2019. Metabolic regulation of cell growth and proliferation. *Nat Rev Mol Cell Biol* **20:** 436–450. doi:10.1038/s41580-019-0123-5

Zhu Z, Achreja A, Meurs N, Animasahun O, Owen S, Mittal A, Parikh P, Lo TW, Franco-Barraza J, Shi J, et al. 2020. Tumour-reprogrammed stromal BCAT1 fuels branched-chain ketoacid dependency in stromal-rich PDAC tumours. *Nat Metab* **2:** 775–792. doi:10.1038/s42255-020-0226-5

Zhu XG, Chudnovskiy A, Baudrier L, Prizer B, Liu Y, Ostendorf BN, Yamaguchi N, Arab A, Tavora B, Timson R, et al. 2021. Functional genomics in vivo reveal metabolic dependencies of pancreatic cancer cells. *Cell Metab* **33:** 211–221.e6. doi:10.1016/j.cmet.2020.10.017

Cancer Metabolism under Limiting Oxygen Conditions

Laura C. Kim,[1,2,3] Nicholas P. Lesner,[1,2,3] and M. Celeste Simon[1,2]

[1]Abramson Family Cancer Research Institute, Perelman School of Medicine; [2]Department of Cell and Developmental Biology, University of Pennsylvania, Philadelphia, Pennsylvania 19104, USA

Correspondence: celeste2@pennmedicine.upenn.edu

Molecular oxygen (O_2) is essential for cellular bioenergetics and numerous biochemical reactions necessary for life. Solid tumors outgrow the native blood supply and diffusion limits of O_2, and therefore must engage hypoxia response pathways that evolved to withstand acute periods of low O_2. Hypoxia activates coordinated gene expression programs, primarily through hypoxia inducible factors (HIFs), to support survival. Many of these changes involve metabolic rewiring such as increasing glycolysis to support ATP generation while suppressing mitochondrial metabolism. Since low O_2 is often coupled with nutrient stress in the tumor microenvironment, other responses to hypoxia include activation of nutrient uptake pathways, metabolite scavenging, and regulation of stress and growth signaling cascades. Continued development of models that better recapitulate tumors and their microenvironments will lead to greater understanding of oxygen-dependent metabolic reprogramming and lead to more effective cancer therapies.

Molecular oxygen (O_2) is required for life-sustaining biological processes, and this extends to tumor cell survival as well. Despite this, the relatively rapid proliferation rate of cells within solid tumors causes them to outgrow their native blood supply and diffusion limits of oxygen resulting in hypoxic stress. Cancer cells have therefore evolved to overcome these harsh conditions by co-opting pathways used by healthy cells to resist transient periods of hypoxia.

The best studied oxygen-sensing pathway is the hypoxia inducible factor (HIF)/prolyl hydroxylase (PHD)/von Hippel–Lindau tumor suppressor (pVHL) axis (Fig. 1; Lee et al. 2020a). Briefly, HIFs are transcription factors that form heterodimers and bind to hypoxia response elements (HREs) in the regulatory regions of target genes under low oxygen conditions. While the aryl hydrocarbon receptor nuclear translocator (ARNT) subunit (also known as HIF-1β) is constitutively expressed, expression of HIF-α subunits (HIF-1α or HIF-2α) is tightly regulated and dependent on oxygen levels. At ambient oxygen, the "VHL" complex, including pVHL, elongins B/C, and Cullin 2, polyubiquitylates HIFα, leading to its proteasomal degradation.

[3]These authors contributed equally to this work.

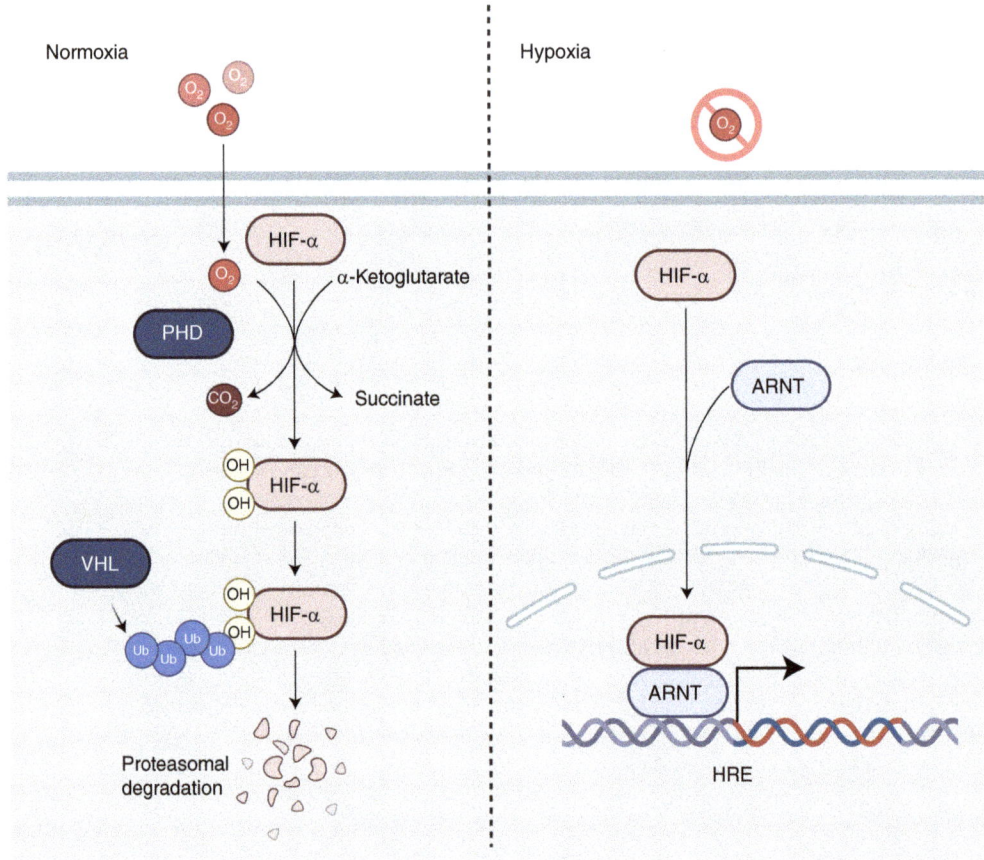

Figure 1. Hypoxia inducible factor (HIF) pathway. Under normoxia, HIF-α is degraded upon hydroxylation by prolyl hydroxylases (PHDs) and ubiquitylation by von Hippel–Lindau complex (VHL). When O_2 is low, stable HIF-α can dimerize with aryl hydrocarbon receptor nuclear translocator (ARNT) to initiate transcription of target genes. (HIF-α) Hypoxia-inducible factor α, (HRE) hypoxia response element. (Figure generated with BioRender, biorender.com.)

To be recognized by VHL for ubiquitylation, two proline residues in the HIF-α oxygen-dependent domain must be hydroxylated via PHD1-3, which require oxygen, iron, and α-ketoglutarate (αKG). When oxygen is limited, the PHDs cannot hydroxylate HIF-α, preventing its degradation. HIF-α therefore dimerizes with ARNT, binds to HREs of target genes, and promotes transcription. Some examples of well-characterized HIF targets include the angiogenic factor VEGF, red blood cell growth factor EPO, and glycolytic enzymes like LDHA and GLUT1. In tumors, increased expression of HIF targets can relieve hypoxic stress by increasing the local blood supply through tumor angiogenesis and rewiring cellular metabolism to continue producing ATP in an anaerobic environment.

Interestingly, in clear cell renal cell carcinoma (ccRCC) ~90% of cases arise from pVHL loss, leading to constitutive HIF-α stabilization and mimicking a hypoxic state (hereafter "pseudohypoxic"). The significance of the HIF pathway's role in renal cancer progression is further supported by the recent approval of Belzutifan, an HIF-2α inhibitor, as a first-line treatment for ccRCC patients with VHL disease (Choueiri and Kaelin 2020). Considering the tumor-promoting roles of HIF-mediated gene expression, it is unsurprising that many other cancer types also exhibit increased expression of HIF-1α and HIF-2α (Wicks and Semenza 2022).

Beyond the HIF pathway, many other cellular biochemical reactions are oxygen sensitive. Several examples include oxidases located in the electron transport chain (ETC) required for ATP generation during aerobic respiration (Ashton et al. 2018), cyclooxygenases that catalyze prostaglandin synthesis and inflammation (Menter et al. 2010), the heme dioxygenases responsible for tryptophan and kynurenine regulation (Zhai et al. 2015), TET methylcytosine dioxygenases responsible for DNA demethylation (Losman et al. 2020), and lysine-specific demethylases that regulate histone methylation (Kooistra and Helin 2012).

In this work, we will focus on the impact of low oxygen conditions on tumor metabolism.

MITOCHONDRIAL METABOLISM

Mitochondrial metabolite oxidation requires an electron acceptor: typically, oxidized nicotinamide adenine dinucleotide (NAD$^+$) or flavin adenine dinucleotide (FAD)-generating reduced nicotinamide adenine dinucleotide (NADH) and flavin adenine dinucleotide (FADH$_2$), respectively. These molecules can then be used to fuel the ETC, where O$_2$ serves as the terminal electron acceptor. The ETC is the primary consumer of cellular oxygen for ATP generation through oxidative phosphorylation (OXPHOS). Therefore, hypoxic conditions result in decreased ETC activity and increased reactive oxygen species (ROS), whereby cells must adapt their metabolism to maintain ATP, mitochondrial membrane potential (ΔΨm), and prevent uncontrolled ROS production. The role of mitochondrial function in cancer has been extensively reviewed (Vyas et al. 2016; Zong et al. 2016). Here, we will summarize the literature describing hypoxia-mediated changes to mitochondrial metabolism and their implications in cancer.

THE ETC AND TCA CYCLE

An intracellular oxygen tension of 0.3% is rate-limiting for ETC function (Wilson et al. 1988).

The ETC is composed of four complexes with the terminal step cytochrome c oxidase (complex IV or COX). Complex IV (cIV) donates four electrons (originating from either NADH or FADH$_2$) to O$_2$ to generate two water molecules. Interestingly, under chronic hypoxia and subsequent HIF activation, decreased ETC function is independent of oxygen's role as a substrate for cIV (Wheaton and Chandel 2011). Hypoxia and HIF-1α activation induce a switch in cIV subunits (Fukuda et al. 2007). Canonically, cIV contains a total of 13 subunits: 10 encoded by nuclear DNA and three encoded by mitochondrial DNA, along with >30 associated assembly factors (Schon et al. 2012). HIF-1α activation induces expression of COX4 isoform 2 (COX4I2) and mitochondrial LON protease (LONP1), resulting in the degradation of COX4 isoform 1 (COX4I1) (Fig. 2). Replacement with COX4I2 results in increased cIV activity under hypoxic conditions (Fukuda et al. 2007).

Low oxygen results in decreased ETC flux and a subsequent buildup of reduced to oxidized NADH:NAD$^+$ and FADH$_2$:FAD$^+$ ratios (Donnelly et al. 2012; Eales et al. 2016). NADH buildup inhibits NADH-producing enzymes in the tricarboxylic acid (TCA) cycle, thereby decreasing TCA cycle activity (Martínez-Reyes and Chandel 2020). In addition to decreased flux, hypoxia influences the TCA cycle by reducing pyruvate entry into the mitochondria. This is achieved via HIF-1α-induced expression of pyruvate dehydrogenase kinase 1 (PDK1) and lactate dehydrogenase A (LDHA). PDK1 phosphorylates the active site of pyruvate dehydrogenase (PDH), reducing its activity and subsequently limiting the generation of mitochondrial acetyl-CoA (AcCoA) from pyruvate (Kim et al. 2006; Papandreou et al. 2006). LDHA induction also affects TCA activity through consumption of pyruvate and regeneration of cytosolic NAD$^+$, thereby reinforcing glycolysis (Fig. 2). This may partially explain why Kras- and p53-mutant pancreatic mouse tumors, which are extremely hypoxic, show reduced contribution from glucose into the TCA cycle and a concomitant increased contribution from lactate (Hui et al. 2017; McGinn et al. 2017). However, this also occurs in more aerobic environments (lung tumors), suggesting this result is not exclu-

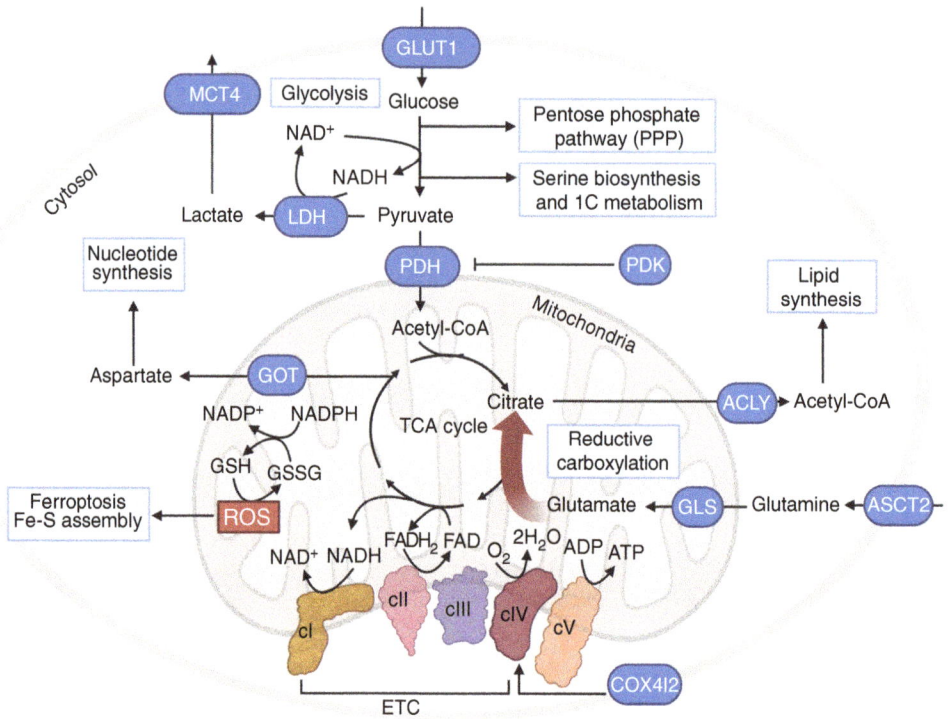

Figure 2. Metabolic pathway adaptations in response to low oxygen. Hypoxia results in up-regulation of glycolytic metabolism with some glucose being used in the pentose phosphate pathway (PPP) and for one carbon (1C) metabolism. Due to limited pyruvate entry into mitochondria, glutamine-derived carbons undergo reductive carboxylation to generate citrate and cytosolic acetyl-CoA for lipid synthesis. Decreased tricarboxylic acid (TCA) cycle flux results in a dependency for aspartate for nucleotide synthesis, and subsequently changes in electron transport chain (ETC) activity result in reactive oxygen species (ROS) accumulation and dysregulated iron metabolism. (ACLY) ATP citrate lyase, (ASCT2) alanine, serine, cysteine transporter 2, (COX4I2) cytochrome *c* oxidase subunit 4I2, (GLS) glutaminase, (*Glut1*) glucose transporter 1, (GOT) glutamatic-oxaloacetic transaminase, (LDH) lactate dehydrogenase, (MCT4) monocarboxylate transporter 4, (PDK) pyruvate dehydrogenase, (PDK) pyruvate dehydrogenase kinase. (Figure generated with BioRender, biorender.com.)

sive to hypoxic environments (Faubert et al. 2017; Hui et al. 2017).

Aspartate, generated from TCA cycle intermediate oxaloacetate via glutamic-oxaloacetic transamination (GOT1 or GOT2), is required for nucleotide synthesis and cell proliferation (Fig. 2; Birsoy et al. 2015; Sullivan et al. 2015). Under hypoxia (0.5% O_2), proliferation and aspartate abundance are significantly decreased in pancreatic cancer cells and are rescued by exogenous aspartate supplementation (Garcia-Bermudez et al. 2018). Furthermore, primary solid tumors with high VEGFA levels (suggestive of HIF-1α activity and hypoxia) display decreased steady-state aspartate levels (Garcia-Bermudez

et al. 2018). This correlation suggests aspartate restriction may be beneficial for treatment of hypoxic tumors by eliminating a necessary and already limiting nutrient.

Typically, the TCA cycle operates in the oxidative direction (i.e., production of NADH and CO_2); however, under hypoxia or impaired ETC function, isocitrate dehydrogenase 2 (IDH2) operates in the reductive direction generating citrate from glutamine-derived αKG (Metallo et al. 2011; Mullen et al. 2011; Wise et al. 2011). This reductive carboxylation (RC) is critical to maintain lipogenesis from citrate via ATP citrate lyase (ACLY) (Figs. 2 and 3; Sun and Denko 2014). RC has been extensively confirmed in vitro, but evi-

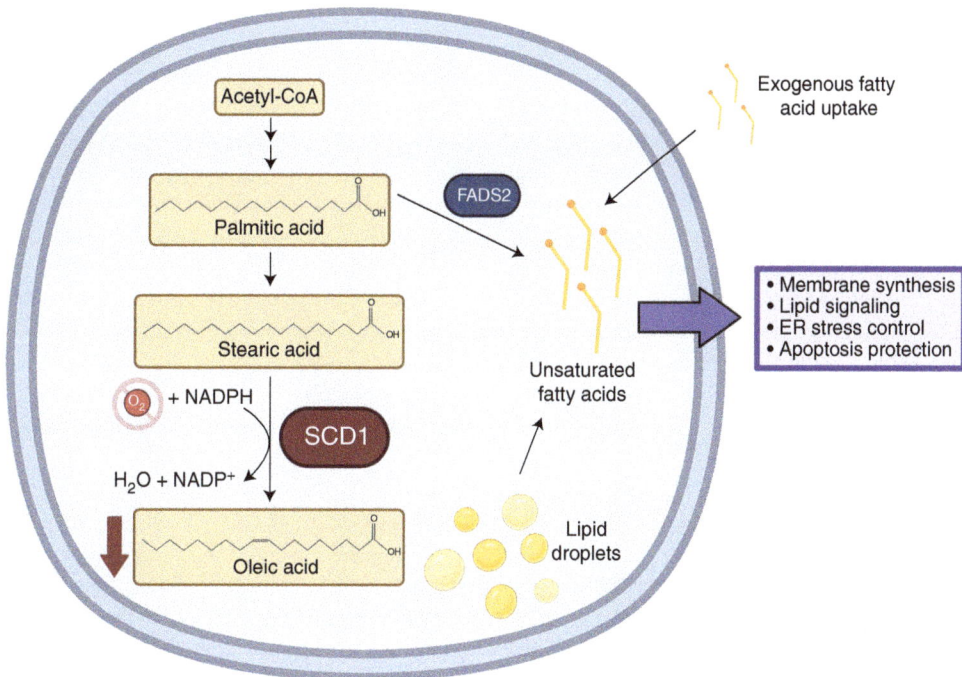

Figure 3. Response to hypoxia-mediated stearoyl-coA desaturase (SCD) inhibition. SCD1 requires O$_2$ to desaturate fatty acids. Buildup of saturated fatty acids under hypoxia can be stressful to cancer cells. Mechanisms to protect against this stress include exogenous fatty acid uptake, breakdown of lipid droplets, and activation of alternative desaturase enzymes. (FADS2) Fatty acid desaturase 2. (Figure generated with BioRender, biorender.com.)

dence in in vivo models is limited. Patient-derived xenografts (PDXs) of "pseudohypoxic" ccRCC tumors also display a significant increase in RC compared to normal kidney tissue, suggesting this adaptive pathway is critical for tumor proliferation (Kaushik et al. 2022). Due to the glutamine requirement of hypoxic cancer cells, there has been significant interest in targeting glutamine metabolism as a cancer therapy (DeBerardinis et al. 2007; Altman et al. 2016; Leone et al. 2019; Lee et al. 2020b; Oh et al. 2020; Tao et al. 2021; Jin et al. 2023; Park et al. 2023). Recently, the glutaminase inhibitor CB-839 (telaglenastat) was tested in a clinical trial against metastatic renal cell carcinoma (RCC); however, no changes in progression-free survival were observed (Lee et al. 2022; Tannir et al. 2022). Clinical trials of the panglutamine antagonist 6-diazo-5-oxo-L-norleucine (DON) suggested modest antitumor activity, but trials were halted

due to dosing and toxicity issues (Lemberg et al. 2018). Currently, less toxic prodrugs (e.g., JHU083) are under investigation to inhibit tumor metabolic processes and promote immune responses (Leone et al. 2019; Oh et al. 2020).

Metabolic flux analysis has recently demonstrated that murine pancreatic ductal adenocarcinoma (PDAC) tumors exhibit lower TCA cycle flux and an overall lower rate of ATP synthesis relative to normal tissue (Bartman et al. 2023). Interestingly, these results suggest that tumor cells are not hypermetabolic, as often assumed, and lose tissue-specific functions to grow despite reduced ATP availability.

MITOCHONDRIAL QUALITY CONTROL

As part of the overall shift away from mitochondrial metabolism, hypoxia also affects mitochondrial quality control processes by suppressing mitochondrial biogenesis and activating mitophagy, the selective degradation of damaged mitochondria through autophagy. Hypoxia can block biogenesis through inhibition of lysine demethylase 3A (KDM3A), which requires oxygen for enzymatic activity. Reduced KDM3A output enhances methylation of lysine 2224 on peroxisome proliferator-activated receptor γ coactivator-1α (PGC-1α), suppressing transactivation of mitochondrial genes (Qian et al. 2019). Along these lines, constitutive PGC-1α activation increased mitochondrial content and inhibited growth of brain tumors in mice (Qian et al. 2019). In ccRCC, PGC-1α and mitochondrial biogenesis are also suppressed, although suppression is regulated by HIF stabilization in this case (LaGory et al. 2015). Additionally, in primary HCC patient cell lines, HIF activation induces the transcriptional repressor HEY1 to prevent transcription of PTEN-induced kinase 1 (PINK1), a gene critical for mitochondrial biogenesis and mitophagy (Kung-Chun Chiu et al. 2019). However, under some contexts, hypoxia may induce mitochondrial biogenesis. Hypoxic HCC cells were found to activate PGC-1α via high mobility group box 1 (HMGB1) protein, leading to increased mitochondria and promotion of tumor survival and proliferation (Tohme et al. 2017). These results suggest that mitochondrial biogenesis is important to tumor proliferation; however, this role is likely both cancer- and genotype-dependent.

Mitophagy is an important mechanism by which cells maintain mitochondrial homeostasis. In mammalian cells, mitophagy is triggered through ubiquitylation or receptor-mediated pathways that engage the cellular autophagy machinery for selective mitochondrial degradation (Youle and Narendra 2010). Cancer cells have been shown to engage the pathway in response to different environmental stimuli, including in response to hypoxia. Hypoxia can activate mitophagy through multiple mechanisms, but the consequences of hypoxia-induced mitophagy on tumor growth are context-dependent (Chang et al. 2017).

In healthy mitochondria, the ubiquitin-mediated mitophagy pathway is regulated through PINK1 and PARKIN. PINK1 is continuously im-ported into mitochondria through the translocase inner membrane and translocase outer membrane (TIM/TOM) complex, where its mitochondrial targeting sequence is cleaved by proteases, ubiquitinated, and degraded by the proteasome. However, in damaged mitochondria (no ΔΨm or blocked import), PINK1 accumulates on the mitochondria and phosphorylates Serine 65 on PARKIN, an E3-ubitquitin ligase. Phosphorylated PARKIN binds LC3 and recruits autophagosomes to be degraded by lysosomes (Pickrell and Youle 2015). In HCC cells, HIF-1α targets miR-210-5P, which suppresses the transcription of AAA domain-containing 3A protein (ATAD3A), a mitophagy regulatory protein that prevents PINK1 accumulation (Wu et al. 2020). ATAD3A depletion results in PINK1 stabilization on the outer mitochondrial membrane, facilitating binding of PARKIN to trigger the mitophagy cascade (Jin et al. 2017). Moreover, this hypoxia-induced mitophagy activation drives HCC resistance to multikinase inhibitor sorafenib (Wu et al. 2020).

Hypoxia can also affect the stability of FUN14 domain-containing 1 (FUNDC1), a mitophagy receptor that interacts with LC3 to induce autophagosome formation (Liu et al. 2012). Mechanistically, hypoxia can affect the function of various kinases and phosphatases that alter the phosphorylation status and subsequently, the activity, of FUNDC1. For example, hypoxia suppresses Src kinase activity, preventing FUNDC1 phosphorylation at Tyr18, which increases FUNDC1-LC3 binding (Liu et al. 2012). Alternatively, HIF-target LONP1 binds the Na^+/Ca^{2+} exchanger (NCLX) and prevents Ca^{2+}-dependent phosphorylation of FUNDC1 (Ser17). Loss of phosphorylation stabilizes the FUNDC1-ULK1 (Unc-51-like autophagy-activating kinase) complex at endoplasmic reticulum (ER)–mitochondrial contact sites, where FUNDC1 binds LC3 (Ponneri Babuharisankar et al. 2023). Additional studies suggest FUNDC1 stability may be further regulated by a feedback mechanism, as prolonged hypoxia can induce FUNDC1 degradation, preventing hypoxia-induced mitophagy (Chen et al. 2017).

Hypoxia can also regulate receptor-mediated mitophagy in an HIF-dependent manner

Cite this article as *Cold Spring Harb Perspect Med* doi: 10.1101/cshperspect.a041542

through activation of BCL2/adenovirus E1B 19-kDa protein-interacting protein 3 (BNIP3) and NIX (Fu et al. 2020; Sulkshane et al. 2021). BNIP3/NIX homo- and heterodimers more robustly recruit autophagosomes through recognition of LC3 (Marinković et al. 2021). BNIP3 also has roles in global autophagy, a process discussed later in the article. The role of hypoxia-induced BNIP-mediated mitophagy in tumor promotion is unclear. In the MMTV-PyMT mouse model of breast cancer, loss of BNIP3 and mitophagy accelerates progression to carcinoma, increases metastasis, and increases dysfunctional mitochondria (Chourasia et al. 2015). Conversely, in melanoma, BNIP3 loss impairs mitophagy but delays tumor growth (Vara-Pérez et al. 2021). Regulation of mitochondrial quality control has many implications in disease including cancer progression and drug resistance. Therefore, it will be important to clarify the contexts in which tumor hypoxia mediates these processes across cancer subtypes.

GLUCOSE METABOLISM

Cancer cells were commonly believed to up-regulate glycolytic activity at the expense of mitochondrial metabolism (i.e., the "Warburg effect"); however, many recent studies suggest that this may be an oversimplification of tumor metabolic rewiring and does not take into account the heterogeneity of cancers and their microenvironments (Heiden et al. 2009; DeBerardinis and Chandel 2020). While likely a generalization overall, it is well understood that under hypoxic conditions, tumor cells shift their metabolism from mitochondrial-mediated ATP generation to glycolysis-driven ATP production. HIF-1α-mediated up-regulation of glycolysis (Semenza 2017; Kierans and Taylor 2021; Missiaen et al. 2023) and glycolysis in cancer (Lunt and Vander Heiden 2011; Liberti and Locasale 2016; DeBerardinis and Chandel 2016, 2020) have been extensively reviewed elsewhere, so we will only highlight a few important studies here. Generally, glycolytic genes, including glucose transporter 1 (GLUT1) and LDHA, are major targets of HIF-1α-mediated transcription. Furthermore, HIF induces expression of PDK1,

which inhibits PDH activity to promote glycolytic utilization (Fig. 2). The relevance of hypoxic regulation of glycolysis was confirmed in vivo in ccRCC patients who underwent intraoperative infusions of [U-^{13}C] glucose. These tumors, the majority of which harbor VHL mutations and subsequently constitutive HIF stabilization, displayed increased glycolytic intermediates and decreased TCA cycle labeling, consistent with the Warburg effect (Courtney et al. 2018). Hypoxic zones of PDAC tumors or PDAC cells cultured under hypoxia also showed increased glucose uptake and lactate secretion (Guillaumond et al. 2013; Hao et al. 2021). Slight increases in glucose utilization flux in PDAC tumors further confirmed these results (Bartman et al. 2023). Interestingly, while PDAC cells had significantly decreased rates of ATP synthesis overall, these cells derived more of their ATP from glycolysis relative to healthy tissue. As the importance of glycolytic metabolism in hypoxic cells is evident, targeting glycolysis has been a fundamental notion in cancer therapy (Abdel-Wahab et al. 2019).

The pentose phosphate pathway (PPP) is a parallel, branched (oxidative and nonoxidative) pathway to glycolysis that generates NADPH and five-carbon sugars necessary for nucleotide synthesis. The PPP is also regulated by hypoxia and has implications in cancer. Following glucose phosphorylation via hexokinase, glucose 6-phosphate (G6P) can proceed through glycolysis or enter the PPP. The first step in the PPP is the conversion of G6P and NADP$^+$ to 6-phosphogluconate and NADPH through glucose 6-phosphate dehydrogenase (G6PD), which is transactivated by HIF-1α (Gao et al. 2004). Therefore, G6PD activity is critical for redox homeostasis and regeneration of the antioxidant reduced glutathione (GSH), which requires NADPH (Fig. 2). When subjected to hypoxia, breast cancer cells displayed an increased steady-state concentration of glycolytic and PPP intermediates, which could be partially ameliorated by NRF2 (a transcription factor controlling genes related to oxidative stress) knockdown and downstream inhibition of HIF-1α (Lee et al. 2019). Although the nonoxidative branch of the PPP can regenerate glycolytic in-

---

termediates (glyceraldehyde 6-phosphate and fructose 6-phosphate), cancer cells need to balance their energetic needs between glycolysis and PPP for proliferation (Ros et al. 2012).

Excess glucose is stored as glycogen and, under fasting conditions, glycogen is broken down to release glucose. During periods of hypoxia, glycogen synthesis enzymes, including glycogen synthase 1, are up-regulated by HIF-1α signaling (Pescador et al. 2010). Intriguingly, ccRCC tumors are characterized by high glycogen content. Glycogen accumulation, however, seems to be a byproduct of constitutive HIF-1α signaling rather than a requirement for tumor progression, as disruption of glycogen synthesis or breakdown did not influence xenograft tumor growth (Xie et al. 2021). This contrasts with breast cancer cells that also exhibit increased glycogen stores. Inhibition of glycogen utilization in MCF7 and MDA-MB-231 breast cancer cell lines reduced their invasive capacity (Altemus et al. 2019). This result suggests a potential link between glycogen metabolism and metastasis, although this has yet to be confirmed in an in vivo setting. This result suggests a potential link between glycogen metabolism and metastasis and highlights the unique cancer subtype dependencies in response to hypoxia.

ROS AND IRON

ROS are a broad class of molecules with varying activities sometimes difficult to distinguish; however, the principal ROS in biology are hydrogen peroxide (H_2O_2) and superoxide ($O_2^{\bullet-}$) (Sies and Jones 2020). As the major cellular O_2 consumer, the ETC generates mitochondrial ROS through electron leakage at multiple sites. Levels of ROS generation are related to the concentration of electron donors, oxygen concentrations, and the reaction rate between them (Murphy 2009). Hypoxic conditions result in increased ROS production, primarily through complex III activity (cIII, coenzyme Q—cytochrome c reductase) (Chandel et al. 2000; Guzy et al. 2005; Waypa et al. 2013; Orr et al. 2015). In cancer, ROS is required for cell proliferation, but depending on the form and context, ROS can be damaging and cause cell death (Fig. 2; Cheung and Vous-

den 2022). Thus, ROS levels and redox state must be carefully managed by hypoxic cancer cells.

Most cells possess multiple mechanisms to control ROS levels primarily through GSH, the most abundant antioxidant cofactor. NADPH is required as an electron donor for reduction of oxidized glutathione (GSSG). Although NADPH can be formed through multiple pathways, cancer cells have been shown to rely primarily on NADPH generated from PPP or one carbon metabolism (Fan et al. 2014). Hypoxia regulates NADPH generation through HIF-mediated induction of mitochondrial serine metabolism via the reversible enzyme serine hydroxymethyltransferase (SHMT2) (Ye et al. 2014). Serine can be locally produced in tumors through metabolism of the glycolytic intermediate, 3-phosphoglycerate, via phosphoglycerate dehydrogenase (PHGDH). After generation of glycine from SHMT2, methylenetetrahydrofolate dehydrogenase 2 (MTHFD2) produces NADPH and 10-formyl-tetrahydrofolate. In neuroblastoma, SHMT2 and HIF-1α expression levels are positively correlated, with higher expression of both correlating with worse prognosis (Ye et al. 2014). Breast cancer cells also up-regulate expression of serine biosynthesis and one carbon metabolism enzyme in response to hypoxia to produce NADPH, moderate ROS levels, and maintain stemness features (Samanta et al. 2016). Conversely, hypoxia has also been shown to suppress GSH in an HIF-independent manner (Mansfield et al. 2004). As such, careful interrogation of the contexts in which hypoxia stimulates or inhibits GSH generation is warranted.

Abundant ROS can also trigger lipid peroxidation that occurs when free radicals, with the help of metal ions, take electrons from and damage polyunsaturated fatty acids in cell membranes. Accumulation of intracellular iron and lipid peroxidation leads to ferroptosis, a form of nonapoptotic, programmed cell death (Dixon et al. 2012). Ferroptosis is limited by glutathione peroxidase 4 (GPX4), an isoform of GPX that can reduce peroxidation on lipid membranes. ccRCC cells that have high ROS levels due to stabilized HIF, also rely heavily on GSH and GPX activity for ROS maintenance and ferroptosis inhibition (Miess et al. 2018; Bansal et al. 2019; Zou et al.

2019). HIF activation mediates this protective response as well, through induction of cystine-glutamate antiporter, xCT, to import cysteine (the limiting metabolite) for GSH synthesis (Miess et al. 2018). Interestingly, mechanisms of hypoxia-mediated resistance to ferroptosis do not seem to be universal, rendering some cell types more sensitive to ferroptosis induction than others (Fuhrmann et al. 2020).

In addition to ferroptosis, iron is required for many fundamental biological processes related to oxygen levels. Perhaps most well-characterized is the role of iron in hemoglobin as carrier of O$_2$ throughout the body. Iron is also important for formation of iron-sulfur (Fe-S) clusters, which are present in various electron transfer proteins involved in the ETC and redox homeostasis (Read et al. 2021). Moreover, iron preferentially accumulates in cancer cells compared to normal cells, and Fe-S clusters are required for many cancer cell growth pathways (Petronek et al. 2019). Although yet to be investigated in the tumor context, 1% O$_2$ levels restored Fe-S clusters and viability in cells lacking mitochondrial protein frataxin, a chaperone protein involved in Fe-S biosynthesis, whose mutation is typically lethal (Ast et al. 2019). Interestingly, this Fe-S restoration occurs via an HIF-independent mechanism, potentially through the cytosolic Fe-S cluster assembly (CIA) pathway. Low oxygen tension strengthens the association between cytosolic Fe-S assembly component 3 (CIAO3) and the rest of the CIA scaffold, suggesting a mechanism of Fe-S cluster preservation that functions independently of HIF (Fan et al. 2022). Conversely, hyperoxia results in destabilization of specific Fe-S cluster-containing proteins suggesting that oxygen tension must be maintained for proper function (Baik et al. 2023). Future studies investigating the mechanisms of hypoxic regulation of Fe-S clusters and their role in cancer will be important, as there is mounting interest in targeting iron metabolism for cancer therapy.

LIPIDS

Lipids are necessary for tumors for a multitude of reasons including generation of the phospho-lipid bilayer, organelle membranes, and signaling molecules. Thus, tumors must rewire their lipid metabolism pathways to meet these demands. Canonical lipid synthesis begins with AcCoA generated in the cytosol by ACLY cleavage activity on citrate transported from the mitochondria. AcCoA is then used by acetyl-CoA carboxylase (ACC) and fatty acid synthase (FASN) to produce free fatty acids or by acetyl-CoA acetyltransferase (ACAT) and hydroxymethylglutaryl-CoA synthase (HMGCS) to feed the mevalonate pathway and produce sterols and isoprenoids (Guertin and Wellen 2023).

As described previously, the increased conversion of glucose to lactate under hypoxic conditions is an active process that requires HIF activation of *PDK1*, the kinase responsible for inhibition of PDH, resulting in suppression of TCA activity (Kim et al. 2006). Another consequence of reduced PDH activity is reduced AcCoA levels generated from pyruvate. Therefore, tumor cells must use alternative ways to produce AcCoA for lipogenesis. Low oxygen or oncogenic HIF stabilization can drive RC of glutamine-derived αKG by IDH to sustain citrate pools (Metallo et al. 2011; Mullen et al. 2011; Wise et al. 2011). HIF further promotes this process through Siah E3 ubiquitin protein ligase 2-mediated ubiquitination and subsequent proteolysis of αKG dehydrogenase, a subunit of the αKG dehydrogenase complex and the fourth step of the oxidative TCA cycle (Sun and Denko 2014). Alternatively, cells can generate AcCoA from acetate pools under hypoxia through the activity of acyl-coenzyme A synthetase short-chain family member 2 (ACSS2), which has been shown to be up-regulated in hypoxic regions of tumors (Kamphorst et al. 2014; Schug et al. 2015).

In addition to alternative pathways of de novo fatty acid synthesis, hypoxic tumor cells also block fatty acid oxidation and increase lipid droplet formation. HIF-1α suppresses expression of acyl-CoA dehydrogenases, repressing fatty acid oxidation when oxygen levels are low (Huang et al. 2014). *FABP3*, *FABP7*, and *ADRP* (also called *PLIN2*), all genes involved in lipid droplet formation, are induced by low oxygen in an HIF-dependent manner (Bensaad et al. 2014). The importance of cellular lipid droplets is supported in pseudohypoxic ccRCC, where *PLIN2* expression and lipid droplet formation are regulated by HIF-2α (Qiu et al. 2015). CPT1a, a mitochondrial lipid transporter, is repressed by HIF-1α and HIF-2α, forcing fatty acids into lipid droplets in ccRCC (Du et al. 2017). Lipid droplets are also maintained in hypoxia through inhibition of lipid droplet catabolism. HIG2 is an HIF-1α target that inhibits adipose triglyceride lipase (ATGL), blocking intracellular lipolysis in hypoxic colorectal cancer and ccRCC cell lines (Zhang et al. 2017).

Interestingly, stearoyl-coA desaturase (SCD1), an enzyme responsible for production of monounsaturated fatty acids, requires oxygen for the desaturation reaction; therefore, under hypoxic conditions, SCD1 activity becomes compromised (Fig. 3; Kamphorst et al. 2013; Young et al. 2013). This results in accumulation of saturated fatty acid precursors, which can disrupt ER membranes and trigger apoptosis (Kamphorst et al. 2013; Young et al. 2013). Cancer cells relieve this stress through uptake of exogenous unsaturated fatty acids (Kamphorst et al. 2013) and through selective release of unsaturated lipids from lipid droplets to "buffer" against saturated lipid accumulations (Ackerman et al. 2018). Tumor cells can also use an alternative fatty acid desaturation pathway, via the enzyme FADS2 to synthesize sapienate (Vriens et al. 2019), suggesting additional ways cancer cells may cope with lipotoxic stress. A recent study has shown that hypoxic inhibition of the ETC results in poor NAD^+ regeneration and inability to synthesize lipids de novo as NAD^+ is a critical cofactor for this process (Li et al. 2022). Therefore, uptake of exogenous lipids under hypoxia may relieve stress from NAD^+ deficiency as well as from accumulation of saturated lipids.

ER STRESS CONTROL

Nutrient stressed and hypoxic conditions can impair the protein folding process and cause accumulation of unfolded proteins at the ER. Specifically, hypoxia limits disulfide bond formation during posttranslational protein folding (May et al. 2005; Koritzinsky et al. 2013). Additionally, hypoxia hinders desaturated lipid syn-

thesis, which limits ER membrane expansion and triggers ER stress (Young et al. 2013). To combat this ER stress, cells respond to hypoxia by activating the unfolded protein response (UPR), which includes inhibition of translation and increased protein degradation through ER-associated degradation and autophagy (Lee et al. 2020a). Three sensors regulate activation of the UPR: protein kinase R (PKR)-like ER kinase (PERK), inositol-requiring transmembrane kinase/endoribonuclease 1α (IRE1α), and activating transcription factor 6 (ATF6) (Chen and Brandizzi 2013). During hypoxia, PERK phosphorylates eukaryotic translation initiation factor 2A (eIF2α) to halt translation initiation and conserve energy and decrease ER protein load (Brewer and Diehl 2000; Harding et al. 2000b). Interestingly, this inhibition of protein synthesis increases available ribosomes for translation of specific transcripts, such as *ATF4* and *CHOP*, which have important downstream UPR functions (Harding et al. 2000a, 2003).

The second branch of the UPR is activated by IRE1α, which has endoribonuclease activity to splice x-box-binding protein 1 (*XBP1*) mRNA, generating a functional, spliced form (*sXBP1*) that functions as a transcription factor regulating expression of numerous ER and metabolic genes (Calfon et al. 2002; Liu et al. 2009, 2016; Bouchecareilh et al. 2011; Zhou et al. 2011; So et al. 2012; Xie et al. 2018). Hypoxia induces XBP1 expression and splicing in an HIF-independent manner resulting in an increased expression of sXBP1 protein (Romero-Ramirez et al. 2004). Interestingly, sXBP1 interacts with many transcription factors including HIF-1α. By recruiting RNA polymerase II to HIF-1α, sXBP1 can coordinate transcriptional programs important for combatting hypoxic and ER stress (Chen et al. 2014).

Upon ER stress, ATF6 translocates to the Golgi and is subsequently activated via cleavage by two proteases (Haze et al. 1999; Ye et al. 2000). Activated ATF6 then translocates to the nucleus to induce UPR gene expression to increase ER folding capacity, including XBP1 and C/EBP homologous protein (CHOP), which plays an important role in UPR-induced apoptosis (Fawcett et al. 1999; Yoshida et al. 2001;

Shen et al. 2002; Yamamoto et al. 2007). UPR activation further protects tumor cells under hypoxia by regulating autophagy genes to promote survival (Rouschop et al. 2010a). Cells with a compromised UPR, from either disrupted PERK or eIF2α signaling, are more sensitive to ER-induced cell death (Harding et al. 2000b).

UPR engagement can be protective during hypoxic stress and promote tumor growth. For example, in hypoxic breast cancers, loss of XBP1 inhibited tumor growth, suggesting the UPR is important for protecting tumor cells from hypoxia and ER stress (Chen et al. 2014). These data have prompted interest in targeting ER stress-response pathways for cancer therapy. However, chronic, high levels of ER stress can instead induce apoptosis, suggesting deletion of UPR pathways might be cytoprotective in certain contexts (Chen and Cubillos-Ruiz 2021). Unresolved ER stress promotes immune evasion in disseminated cancer cells thereby promoting latent metastasis (Pommier et al. 2018). It will be important to distinguish the contexts in which the UPR is engaged in tumors, and when its inhibition will be beneficial, as ER stress therapies continue to be developed.

AUTOPHAGY AND NUTRIENT SCAVENGING

Cancer cells must find ways to acquire high levels of macromolecules required for rapid proliferation, particularly in the nutrient limited tumor microenvironment (TME). Two mechanisms used by cancer cells to fulfill nutrient needs are autophagy and macropinocytosis. Since nutrient scarcity and hypoxia are often paired, both processes are directly regulated by oxygen levels.

Macropinocytosis, the nonselective endocytic process for uptake of extracellular fluid and macromolecules via generation of large, uncoated vesicles, can be used to import extracellular protein, exosomes, and necrotic cell debris (Finicle et al. 2018). These vesicles will then empty their contents into the cytoplasm or fuse with lysosomes for degradation into metabolites that become available to the cell. Several oncogenic alterations including *RAS* mutations and *PTEN* loss have been shown to induce macropinosome

formation as a means of replenishing nutrient pools under nutrient-starved conditions (Commisso et al. 2013; Kim et al. 2018).

Cancer cells also employ macropinocytosis to adapt to metabolic stresses that occur during hypoxia. ETC inhibition caused by low oxygen levels results in reduced synthesis of the amino acid aspartate, which becomes limiting for cancer cell proliferation (Garcia-Bermudez et al. 2018). Albumin supplementation restored aspartate to normoxic levels in pancreatic cancer cells, suggesting macropinocytosis could provide sufficient aspartate to support tumor growth (Garcia-Bermudez et al. 2022). Further, macropinocytosis was up-regulated under hypoxic conditions in an HIF-1α-dependent manner via HIF-1α target CA9 and its product bicarbonate (Garcia-Bermudez et al. 2022). Bicarbonate has previously been shown to stimulate V-ATPase and Rac1 plasma membrane association, a prerequisite for membrane ruffling and macropinocytosis (Ramirez et al. 2019). Studies in hepatocellular carcinoma suggest that HIF-1α may also activate macropinocytosis directly through transcriptional up-regulation of *EHD2*, a dynamin-related ATPase that plays important roles in membrane fission and vesicle formation (Zhang et al. 2022).

In addition to scavenging nutrients from the extracellular environment, cancer cells use autophagy to acquire key macromolecules through degradation of their own proteins and organelles (Kimmelman and White 2017). In healthy cells, autophagy is maintained at a basal level as a quality-control mechanism to clear damaged proteins and organelles. Cancer cells, however, have been shown to rely on up-regulated autophagy to recycle nutrients for pathways important for growth and survival (Frezza et al. 2011). Autophagy is also responsive to stress signals in the TME including low oxygen conditions. Initial studies showed that autophagosomes were localized to hypoxic regions in tumors, suggesting oxygen levels regulated the autophagic response (Degenhardt et al. 2006). Subsequent studies have since shown that hypoxia does indeed regulate autophagy in tumors through multiple mechanisms. First, HIF is directly involved in the transcription of *BNIP3* and *BNIP3L*, genes involved in the formation of the autophagosome to degrade mitochondria and ER (Bellot et al. 2009). Second, hypoxia can trigger the UPR, leading to activation of the PERK-signaling cascade and its downstream effectors ATF4 and CHOP (Rouschop et al. 2010b). Targets of these transcription factors include autophagy genes *MAP1LC3B* and *ATG5*, leading to increased autophagosome formation and tumor cell survival (Rouschop et al. 2010b). Finally, low oxygen levels regulate autophagy through major metabolic signaling nodes AMP-activated protein kinase (AMPK) and mechanistic target of rapamycin (mTOR) (discussed in detail later). Both kinases can phosphorylate autophagy activator ULK1, although at unique sites that differentially regulate autophagy (Kim et al. 2011). Phosphorylation of ULK by mTOR negatively regulates autophagy (Ganley et al. 2009; Jung et al. 2009), while phosphorylation by AMPK results in autophagy activation (Egan et al. 2011). Further, AMPK is a negative regulator of mTOR; thus, AMPK can activate autophagy through multiple mechanisms.

NUTRIENT SENSING

Hypoxia is often accompanied by low nutrient conditions; therefore, it is unsurprising that nutrient sensing and growth control signaling pathways are also regulated by oxygen levels.

AMPK is a trimeric complex that regulates cellular energy homeostasis (Garcia and Shaw 2017). AMPK stimulation is mediated by phosphorylation of its activation loop through two mechanisms: canonically by LKB1 and increased AMP:ATP ratios and noncanonically through increased Ca^{2+} and calcium/calmodulin-dependent protein kinase kinase 2 (CaMKK2) activity. Of note, AMPK is activated under hypoxic conditions. Under low oxygen conditions, AMP:ATP ratios are unchanged (Emerling et al. 2009), but Ca^{2+} levels are increased, suggesting hypoxia stimulates AMPK through CaMKK2 phosphorylation (Gusarova et al. 2011; Mungai et al. 2011).

In contrast to AMPK, the mTOR and its functional complexes (mTORC1 and mTORC2) are activated by high cellular energy and abundant nutrients to coordinate numerous growth-promoting processes including, but not limited to, translation, nucleotide synthesis, lipid metabolism, and autophagy (Liu and Sabatini 2020). Hypoxia has been shown to inhibit mTOR signaling and its downstream anabolic programs via multiple mechanisms (Arsham et al. 2003; Wouters and Koritzinsky 2008). Acute hypoxia activates AMPK, an upstream regulator of mTOR. AMPK phosphorylates and inhibits tuberous sclerosis complex 2 (TSC2), a GTPase-activating protein for Rheb GTPase. Inactive Rheb leads to loss of mTORC1 activation signals (Liu et al. 2006). HIF-1α target BNIP3 also interacts with Rheb to prevent mTOR activation (Li et al. 2007). Chronic hypoxia mediates mTORC1 independently of AMPK instead by up-regulation of *REDD1* (Brugarolas et al. 2004; Sofer et al. 2005). *REDD1* expression is normally curtailed by miR-7 (Seong et al. 2019), but hypoxia suppresses miR-7, allowing REDD1 to release TSC2 from inhibitory 14-3-3 proteins and inhibit mTORC1 (Deyoung et al. 2008). REDD1 up-regulation also requires HIF-1α phosphorylation by ataxia-telangiectasia mutated kinase, a stress-response protein activated by DNA double-strand breaks, further underlining the connections between stress, hypoxia, and growth signaling (Cam et al. 2010).

Hypoxic AMPK activation and mTOR suppression can be beneficial to cancer cells through promotion of autophagy and macropinocytosis nutrient scavenging pathways, particularly under nutrient stressed conditions (described previously). However, to maintain high levels of macromolecule biosynthesis required for rapid tumor cell proliferation, constitutive mTOR signaling can also be beneficial. For example, some tumors exhibit loss of TSC2, a major point for hypoxic regulation of mTOR, allowing growth-promoting processes such translation to persist despite low oxygen levels (Mieulet and Lamb 2010). Furthermore, HIF-1α translation is promoted by mTORC1 (Hudson et al. 2002; Düvel et al. 2010), suggesting oncogenic alterations that activate the mTOR pathway may lead to preemptive HIF stabilization, preventing hypoxia-induced inhibition of the mTOR node.

METABOLIC REWIRING OF THE TUMOR STROMA BY HYPOXIA

Cancer cells can induce broad changes in the TME, including metabolite availability in the tumor interstitial fluid (Sullivan et al. 2019) and reprogramming of nutrient uptake programs in other cell types (Reinfeld et al. 2021). Tumor hypoxia, therefore, can have significant consequences beyond tumor-intrinsic metabolic rewiring, affecting other cell types in the TME.

Hypoxia is a well-known modulator of immune responses (Taylor and Colgan 2017); however, the role of tumor hypoxia in metabolic rewiring of cells involved in the tumor immune response continues to be explored. Moreover, hypoxia seems to have both tumor promoting and suppressing effects on the immune compartment. In CD8 T cells, hypoxia improves antitumor cytotoxic responses in part through HIF-1α-mediated promotion of glycolysis (Gropper et al. 2017; Palazon et al. 2017). In contrast, hypoxia rewires Treg metabolism to support protumorigenic functions. HIF-1α induction in Tregs shunts glucose away from the mitochondria, forcing Tregs to depend on extracellular fatty acids for fuel (Miska et al. 2019). In glioblastoma models, reliance on extracellular fatty acids promoted immune suppression and Treg-specific HIF-1α knockout improved mouse survival (Miska et al. 2019). Tregs also support their function in hypoxic, lactate-rich environments by increasing reliance on OXPHOS through a FoxP3-dependent mechanism (Angelin et al. 2017). Beyond T cells, tumor hypoxia also influences functional macrophage polarization: specifically "M2" or alternative activation, which is characterized by tumor-promoting, immunosuppressive phenotypes and metabolism of arginine by Arginase 1 (Arg 1). Macrophage HIF-1α regulates "M2" gene expression signatures and HIF-1α can be stabilized by hypoxia and lactate secreted from highly glycolytic tumors (Colegio et al. 2014).

Cancer-associated fibroblasts (CAFs) are also a major component of tumor stroma with important roles in regulating extracellular matrix deposition, cancer cell signaling cascades, and modulation of the immune response (Sahai et al. 2020). CAFs also secrete metabolites to support nearby cancer cells (Sanford-Crane et al. 2019). Interestingly, chronic hypoxia in the TME can epigenetically alter *HIF1A* expression and glycolytic enzymes in normal fibroblasts, pushing them toward a proglycolytic, CAF-like phenotype that supports cancer progression (Becker et al. 2020). Like cancer cells, hypoxia also induces autophagy in CAFs (Chiavarina et al. 2010; Martinez-Outschoorn et al. 2010), leading to generation of metabolites including alanine, which has been shown to fuel the TCA cycle in neighboring pancreatic cancer cells (Sousa et al. 2016).

CONCLUSIONS

Reprogrammed cellular metabolism is a well-recognized hallmark of cancer (Hanahan 2022). Moreover, we now understand that metabolic reprogramming is not permanent, but can change dynamically depending on the tumor context. O$_2$ levels are an important factor that regulates tumor metabolic changes, particularly because of its role as a substrate for metabolic enzymes and as a cofactor for the HIF transcriptional network.

In this review, we have covered many aspects of tumor metabolism that are affected by hypoxia and how this metabolic rewiring can impact tumor growth. Looking forward, we expect many studies to investigate the impact of hypoxia in in vivo tumor models, as much of the work presented herein has been conducted in in vitro cell culture systems that are important, but do not always accurately recapitulate the TME. Better in vivo model systems may also uncover novel impacts of hypoxia on the cross talk between tumor and stromal cells. Additionally, we are excited about the availability of new techniques that can capture both metabolic and spatial information. Since hypoxia can be hyperlocalized to specific avascular tumor regions, these techniques may provide greater insight into hypoxia's role on metabolic rewiring at the tumor neighborhood and cell-type-specific level. Overall, we anticipate that better understanding of oxygen-dependent tumor metabolic rewiring will lead to development of more effective cancer therapies.

AUTHOR CONTRIBUTIONS

L.C.K., N.P.L., and M.C.S. wrote and reviewed the manuscript.

ACKNOWLEDGMENTS

The authors thank the entire Simon laboratory for comments and discussion on the manuscript. We apologize to any colleagues whose work we failed to cite owing to space and reference constraints. This work was supported by the American Cancer Society Postdoctoral Fellowship PF-23-1034739-01-TBE to L.C.K., Damon Runyon postdoctoral fellowship DRG2497-23 to N.P.L., and the National Cancer Institute (NCI) grants 5T32CA009140 to L.C.K. and N.P.L, and P01 CA104838 and R35 CA197602 to M.C.S.

REFERENCES

Abdel-Wahab AF, Mahmoud W, Al-Harizy RM. 2019. Targeting glucose metabolism to suppress cancer progression: prospective of anti-glycolytic cancer therapy. *Pharmacol Res* **150:** 104511. doi:10.1016/j.phrs.2019.104511

Ackerman D, Tumanov S, Qiu B, Michalopoulou E, Spata M, Azzam A, Xie H, Simon MC, Kamphorst JJ. 2018. Triglycerides promote lipid homeostasis during hypoxic stress by balancing fatty acid saturation. *Cell Rep* **24:** 2596–2605.e5. doi:10.1016/j.celrep.2018.08.015

Altemus MA, Goo LE, Little AC, Yates JA, Cheriyan HG, Wu ZF, Merajver SD. 2019. Breast cancers utilize hypoxic glycogen stores via PYGB, the brain isoform of glycogen phosphorylase, to promote metastatic phenotypes. *PLoS ONE* **14:** e0220973. doi:10.1371/journal.pone.0220973

Altman BJ, Stine ZE, Dang CV. 2016. From Krebs to clinic: glutamine metabolism to cancer therapy. *Nat Rev Cancer* **16:** 619–634. doi:10.1038/nrc.2016.71

Angelin A, Gil-de-Gómez L, Dahiya S, Jiao J, Guo L, Levine MH, Wang Z, Quinn WJ, Kopinski PK, Wang L, et al. 2017. Foxp3 reprograms T cell metabolism to function in low-glucose, high-lactate environments. *Cell Metab* **25:** 1293.e7. doi:10.1016/j.cmet.2016.12.018

Arsham AM, Howell JJ, Simon MC. 2003. A novel hypoxia-inducible factor-independent hypoxic response regulating mammalian target of rapamycin and its targets. *J Biol Chem* **278:** 29655–29660. doi:10.1074/jbc.M212770200

Ashton TM, Gillies McKenna W, Kunz-Schughart LA, Higgins GS. 2018. Oxidative phosphorylation as an emerging target in cancer therapy. *Clin Cancer Res* **24:** 2482–2490. doi:10.1158/1078-0432.CCR-17-3070

Ast T, Meisel JD, Patra S, Wang H, Grange RMH, Kim SH, Calvo SE, Orefice LL, Nagashima F, Ichinose F, et al. 2019. Hypoxia rescues frataxin loss by restoring iron sulfur cluster biogenesis. *Cell* **177:** 1507–1521.e16. doi:10.1016/j.cell.2019.03.045

Baik AH, Haribowo AG, Chen X, Queliconi BB, Barrios AM, Garg A, Maishan M, Campos AR, Matthay MA, Jain IH. 2023. Oxygen toxicity causes cyclic damage by destabilizing specific Fe-S cluster-containing protein complexes. *Mol Cell* **83:** 942–960.e9. doi:10.1016/j.molcel.2023.02.013

Bansal A, Sanchez DJ, Nimgaonkar V, Sanchez D, Riscal R, Skuli N, Simon MC. 2019. γ-Glutamyltransferase 1 promotes clear cell renal cell carcinoma initiation and progression. *Mol Cancer Res* **17:** 1881–1892. doi:10.1158/1541-7786.MCR-18-1204

Bartman CR, Weilandt DR, Shen Y, Lee WD, Han Y, TeSlaa T, Jankowski CSR, Samarah L, Park NR, da Silva-Diz V, et al. 2023. Slow TCA flux and ATP production in primary solid tumours but not metastases. *Nature* **614:** 349–357. doi:10.1038/s41586-022-05661-6

Becker LM, O'Connell JT, Vo AP, Cain MP, Tampe D, Bizarro L, Sugimoto H, McGow AK, Asara JM, Lovisa S, et al. 2020. Epigenetic reprogramming of cancer-associated fibroblasts deregulates glucose metabolism and facilitates progression of breast cancer. *Cell Rep* **31:** 107701. doi:10.1016/j.celrep.2020.107701

Bellot G, Garcia-Medina R, Gounon P, Chiche J, Roux D, Pouysségur J, Mazure NM. 2009. Hypoxia-induced autophagy is mediated through hypoxia-inducible factor induction of BNIP3 and BNIP3L via their BH3 domains. *Mol Cell Biol* **29:** 2570–2581. doi:10.1128/MCB.00166-09

Bensaad K, Favaro E, Lewis CA, Peck B, Lord S, Collins JM, Pinnick KE, Wigfield S, Buffa FM, Li JL, et al. 2014. Fatty acid uptake and lipid storage induced by HIF-1α contribute to cell growth and survival after hypoxia-reoxygenation. *Cell Rep* **9:** 349–365. doi:10.1016/j.celrep.2014.08.056

Birsoy K, Wang T, Chen WW, Freinkman E, Abu-Remaileh M, Sabatini DM. 2015. An essential role of the mitochondrial electron transport chain in cell proliferation is to enable aspartate synthesis. *Cell* **162:** 540–551. doi:10.1016/j.cell.2015.07.016

Bouchecareilh M, Higa A, Fribourg S, Moenner M, Chevet E. 2011. Peptides derived from the bifunctional kinase/RNase enzyme IRE1α modulate IRE1α activity and protect cells from endoplasmic reticulum stress. *FASEB J* **25:** 3115–3129. doi:10.1096/fj.11-182931

Brewer JW, Diehl JA. 2000. PERK mediates cell-cycle exit during the mammalian unfolded protein response. *Proc Natl Acad Sci* **97:** 12625–12630. doi:10.1073/pnas.220247197

Brugarolas J, Lei K, Hurley RL, Manning BD, Reiling JH, Hafen E, Witters LA, Ellisen LW, Kaelin WG. 2004. Regulation of mTOR function in response to hypoxia by REDD1 and the TSC1/TSC2 tumor suppressor complex. *Genes Dev* **18:** 2893–2904. doi:10.1101/gad.1256804

Calfon M, Zeng H, Urano F, Till JH, Hubbard SR, Harding HP, Clark SG, Ron D. 2002. IRE1 couples endoplasmic reticulum load to secretory capacity by processing the XBP-1 mRNA. *Nature* **415:** 92–96. doi:10.1038/415092a

Cam H, Easton JB, High A, Houghton PJ. 2010. mTORC1 signaling under hypoxic conditions is controlled by ATM-dependent phosphorylation of HIF-1α. *Mol Cell* **40:** 509–520. doi:10.1016/j.molcel.2010.10.030

Chandel NS, McClintock DS, Feliciano CE, Wood TM, Melendez JA, Rodriguez AM, Schumacker PT. 2000. Reactive oxygen species generated at mitochondrial complex III stabilize hypoxia-inducible factor-1α during hypoxia: a mechanism of O$_2$ sensing. *J Biol Chem* **275:** 25130–25138. doi:10.1074/jbc.M001914200

Chang JY, Yi HS, Kim HW, Shong M. 2017. Dysregulation of mitophagy in carcinogenesis and tumor progression. *Biochim Biophys Acta* **1858:** 633–640. doi:10.1016/j.bbabio .2016.12.008

Chen Y, Brandizzi F. 2013. IRE1: ER stress sensor and cell fate executor. *Trends Cell Biol* **23:** 547–555. doi:10.1016/j .tcb.2013.06.005

Chen X, Cubillos-Ruiz JR. 2021. Endoplasmic reticulum stress signals in the tumour and its microenvironment. *Nat Rev Cancer* **21:** 71–88. doi:10.1038/s41568-020-00312-2

Chen X, Iliopoulos D, Zhang Q, Tang Q, Greenblatt MB, Hatziapostolou M, Lim E, Tam WL, Ni M, Chen Y, et al. 2014. XBP1 promotes triple-negative breast cancer by controlling the HIF1α pathway. *Nature* **508:** 103–107. doi:10.1038/nature13119

Chen Z, Liu L, Cheng Q, Li Y, Wu H, Zhang W, Wang Y, Sehgal SA, Siraj S, Wang X, et al. 2017. Mitochondrial E3 ligase MARCH5 regulates FUNDC1 to fine-tune hypoxic mitophagy. *EMBO Rep* **18:** 495–509. doi:10.15252/embr .201643309

Cheung EC, Vousden KH. 2022. The role of ROS in tumour development and progression. *Nat Rev Cancer* **22:** 280–297. doi:10.1038/s41568-021-00435-0

Chiavarina B, Whitaker-Menezes D, Migneco G, Martinez-Outschoorn UE, Pavlides S, Howell A, Tanowitz HB, Casimiro MC, Wang C, Pestell RG, et al. 2010. HIF1-α functions as a tumor promoter in cancer associated fibroblasts, and as a tumor suppressor in breast cancer cells: autophagy drives compartment-specific oncogenesis. *Cell Cycle* **9:** 3534–3551. doi:10.4161/cc.9.17.12908

Choueiri TK, Kaelin WG. 2020. Targeting the HIF2–VEGF axis in renal cell carcinoma. *Nat Med* **26:** 1519–1530. doi:10.1038/s41591-020-1093-z

Chourasia AH, Tracy K, Frankenberger C, Boland ML, Sharifi MN, Drake LE, Sachleben JR, Asara JM, Locasale JW, Karczmar GS, et al. 2015. Mitophagy defects arising from BNip3 loss promote mammary tumor progression to metastasis. *EMBO Rep* **16:** 1145–1163. doi:10.15252/embr .201540759

Colegio OR, Chu NQ, Szabo AL, Chu T, Rhebergen AM, Jairam V, Cyrus N, Brokowski CE, Eisenbarth SC, Phillips GM, et al. 2014. Functional polarization of tumour-associated macrophages by tumour-derived lactic acid. *Nature* **513:** 559–563. doi:10.1038/nature13490

Commisso C, Davidson SM, Soydaner-Azeloglu RG, Parker SJ, Kamphorst JJ, Hackett S, Grabocka E, Nofal M, Drebin JA, Thompson CB, et al. 2013. Macropinocytosis of protein is an amino acid supply route in Ras-transformed cells. *Nature* **497:** 633–637. doi:10.1038/nature12138

Courtney KD, Bezwada D, Mashimo T, Pichumani K, Vemireddy V, Funk AM, Wimberly J, McNeil SS, Kapur P, Lotan Y, et al. 2018. Isotope tracing of human clear cell renal cell carcinomas demonstrates suppressed glucose oxidation in vivo. *Cell Metab* **28:** 793–800.e2. doi:10 .1016/j.cmet.2018.07.020

DeBerardinis RJ, Chandel NS. 2016. Fundamentals of cancer metabolism. *Sci Adv* **2:** e1600200. doi:10.1126/sciadv .1600200

DeBerardinis RJ, Chandel NS. 2020. We need to talk about the Warburg effect. *Nat Metab* **2:** 127–129. doi:10.1038/ s42255-020-0172-2

DeBerardinis RJ, Mancuso A, Daikhin E, Nissim I, Yudkoff M, Wehrli S, Thompson CB. 2007. Beyond aerobic glycolysis: transformed cells can engage in glutamine metabolism that exceeds the requirement for protein and nucleotide synthesis. *Proc Natl Acad Sci* **104:** 19345–19350. doi:10.1073/pnas.0709747104

Degenhardt K, Mathew R, Beaudoin B, Bray K, Anderson D, Chen G, Mukherjee C, Shi Y, Gélinas C, Fan Y, et al. 2006. Autophagy promotes tumor cell survival and restricts necrosis, inflammation, and tumorigenesis. *Cancer Cell* **10:** 51–64. doi:10.1016/j.ccr.2006.06.001

Deyoung MP, Horak P, Sofer A, Sgroi D, Ellisen LW. 2008. Hypoxia regulates TSC1/2-mTOR signaling and tumor suppression through REDD1-mediated 14-3-3 shuttling. *Genes Dev* **22:** 239–251. doi:10.1101/gad.1617608

Dixon SJ, Lemberg KM, Lamprecht MR, Skouta R, Zaitsev EM, Gleason CE, Patel DN, Bauer AJ, Cantley AM, Yang WS, et al. 2012. Ferroptosis: an iron-dependent form of nonapoptotic cell death. *Cell* **149:** 1060–1072. doi:10 .1016/j.cell.2012.03.042

Donnelly PS, Liddell JR, Lim SC, Paterson BM, Cater MA, Savva MS, Mot AI, James JL, Trounce IA, White AR, et al. 2012. An impaired mitochondrial electron transport chain increases retention of the hypoxia imaging agent diacetylbis(4-methylthiosemicarbazonato)copper[II]. *Proc Natl Acad Sci* **109:** 47–52. doi:10.1073/pnas .1116227108

Du W, Zhang L, Brett-Morris A, Aguila B, Kerner J, Hoppel CL, Puchowicz M, Serra D, Herrero L, Rini BI, et al. 2017. HIF drives lipid deposition and cancer in ccRCC via repression of fatty acid metabolism. *Nat Commun* **8:** 1769. doi:10.1038/s41467-017-01965-8

Düvel K, Yecies JL, Menon S, Raman P, Lipovsky AI, Souza AL, Triantafellow E, Ma Q, Gorski R, Cleaver S, et al. 2010. Activation of a metabolic gene regulatory network downstream of mTOR complex 1. *Mol Cell* **39:** 171–183. doi:10.1016/j.molcel.2010.06.022

Eales KL, Hollinshead KER, Tennant DA. 2016. Hypoxia and metabolic adaptation of cancer cells. *Oncogenesis* **5:** e190–e190. doi:10.1038/oncsis.2015.50

Egan DF, Shackelford DB, Mihaylova MM, Gelino S, Kohnz RA, Mair W, Vasquez DS, Joshi A, Gwinn DM, Taylor R, et al. 2011. Phosphorylation of ULK1 (hATG1) by AMP-activated protein kinase connects energy sensing to mitophagy. *Science* **331:** 456–461. doi:10.1126/science .1196371

Emerling BM, Weinberg F, Snyder C, Burgess Z, Mutlu GM, Viollet B, Budinger GRS, Chandel NS. 2009. Hypoxic activation of AMPK is dependent on mitochondrial ROS but independent of an increase in AMP/ATP ratio. *Free Radic Biol Med* **46:** 1386–1391. doi:10.1016/j .freeradbiomed.2009.02.019

Fan J, Ye J, Kamphorst JJ, Shlomi T, Thompson CB, Rabinowitz JD. 2014. Quantitative flux analysis reveals folate-dependent NADPH production. *Nature* **510:** 298–302. doi:10.1038/nature13236

Fan X, Barshop WD, Vashisht AA, Pandey V, Leal S, Rayat-pisheh S, Jami-Alahmadi Y, Sha J, Wohlschlegel JA. 2022. Iron-regulated assembly of the cytosolic iron–sulfur cluster biogenesis machinery. *J Biol Chem* **298:** 102094. doi:10.1016/j.jbc.2022.102094

Faubert B, Li KY, Cai L, Hensley CT, Kim J, Zacharias LG, Yang C, Do QN, Doucette S, Burguete D, et al. 2017. Lactate metabolism in human lung tumors. *Cell* **171:** 358–371.e9. doi:10.1016/j.cell.2017.09.019

Fawcett TW, Martindale JL, Guyton KZ, Hai T, Holbrook NJ. 1999. Complexes containing activating transcription factor (ATF)/cAMP-responsive-element-binding protein (CREB) interact with the CCAAT/enhancer-binding protein (C/EBP)-ATF composite site to regulate Gadd153 expression during the stress response. *Biochem J* **339:** 135–141. doi:10.1042/bj3390135

Finicle BT, Jayashankar V, Edinger AL. 2018. Nutrient scavenging in cancer. *Nat Rev Cancer* **18:** 619–633. doi:10.1038/s41568-018-0048-x

Frezza C, Zheng L, Tennant DA, Papkovsky DB, Hedley BA, Kalna G, Watson DG, Gottlieb E. 2011. Metabolic profiling of hypoxic cells revealed a catabolic signature required for cell survival. *PLoS ONE* **6:** e24411. doi:10.1371/journal.pone.0024411

Fu ZJ, Wang ZY, Xu L, Chen XH, Li XX, Liao WT, Ma HK, Di JM, Xu TT, Xu J, et al. 2020. HIF-1α-BNIP3-mediated mitophagy in tubular cells protects against renal ischemia/reperfusion injury. *Redox Biol* **36:** 101671. doi:10.1016/j.redox.2020.101671

Fuhrmann DC, Mondorf A, Beifuß J, Jung M, Brüne B. 2020. Hypoxia inhibits ferritinophagy, increases mitochondrial ferritin, and protects from ferroptosis. *Redox Biol* **36:** 101670. doi:10.1016/j.redox.2020.101670

Fukuda R, Zhang H, Kim JW, Shimoda L, Dang CV, Semenza GLL. 2007. HIF-1 regulates cytochrome oxidase subunits to optimize efficiency of respiration in hypoxic cells. *Cell* **129:** 111–122. doi:10.1016/j.cell.2007.01.047

Ganley IG, Lam DH, Wang J, Ding X, Chen S, Jiang X. 2009. ULK1-ATG13-FIP200 complex mediates mTOR signaling and is essential for autophagy. *J Biol Chem* **284:** 12297–12305. doi:10.1074/jbc.M900573200

Gao L, Mejías R, Echevarría M, López-Barneo J. 2004. Induction of the glucose-6-phosphate dehydrogenase gene expression by chronic hypoxia in PC12 cells. *FEBS Lett* **569:** 256–260. doi:10.1016/j.febslet.2004.06.004

Garcia D, Shaw RJ. 2017. AMPK: mechanisms of cellular energy sensing and restoration of metabolic balance. *Mol Cell* **66:** 789–800. doi:10.1016/j.molcel.2017.05.032

Garcia-Bermudez J, Baudrier L, La K, Zhu XG, Fidelin J, Sviderskiy VO, Papagiannakopoulos T, Molina H, Snuderl M, Lewis CA, et al. 2018. Aspartate is a limiting metabolite for cancer cell proliferation under hypoxia and in tumours. *Nat Cell Biol* **20:** 775–781. doi:10.1038/s41556-018-0118-z

Garcia-Bermudez J, Badgley MA, Prasad S, Baudrier L, Liu Y, La K, Soula M, Williams RT, Yamaguchi N, Hwang RF, et al. 2022. Adaptive stimulation of macropinocytosis overcomes aspartate limitation in cancer cells under hypoxia. *Nat Metab* **4:** 724–738. doi:10.1038/s42255-022-00583-z

Gropper Y, Feferman T, Shalit T, Salame TM, Porat Z, Shakhar G. 2017. Culturing CTLs under hypoxic conditions enhances their cytolysis and improves their anti-

tumor function. *Cell Rep* **20:** 2547–2555. doi:10.1016/j.celrep.2017.08.071

Guertin DA, Wellen KE. 2023. Acetyl-CoA metabolism in cancer. *Nat Rev Cancer* **23:** 156–172. doi:10.1038/s41568-022-00543-5

Guillaumond F, Leca J, Olivares O, Lavaut MN, Vidal N, Berthezène P, Dusetti NJ, Loncle C, Calvo E, Turrini O, et al. 2013. Strengthened glycolysis under hypoxia supports tumor symbiosis and hexosamine biosynthesis in pancreatic adenocarcinoma. *Proc Natl Acad Sci* **110:** 3919–3924. doi:10.1073/pnas.1219555110

Gusarova GA, Trejo HE, Dada LA, Briva A, Welch LC, Hamanaka RB, Mutlu GM, Chandel NS, Prakriya M, Sznajder JI. 2011. Hypoxia leads to Na,K-ATPase downregulation via Ca²⁺ release-activated Ca²⁺ channels and AMPK activation. *Mol Cell Biol* **31:** 3546–3556. doi:10.1128/MCB.05114-11

Guzy RD, Hoyos B, Robin E, Chen H, Liu L, Mansfield KD, Simon MC, Hammerling U, Schumacker PT. 2005. Mitochondrial complex III is required for hypoxia-induced ROS production and cellular oxygen sensing. *Cell Metab* **1:** 401–408. doi:10.1016/j.cmet.2005.05.001

Hanahan D. 2022. Hallmarks of cancer: new dimensions. *Cancer Discov* **12:** 31–46. doi:10.1158/2159-8290.CD-21-1059

Hao X, Ren Y, Feng M, Wang Q, Wang Y. 2021. Metabolic reprogramming due to hypoxia in pancreatic cancer: implications for tumor formation, immunity, and more. *Biomed Pharmacother* **141:** 111798. doi:10.1016/j.biopha.2021.111798

Harding HP, Novoa I, Zhang Y, Zeng H, Wek R, Schapira M, Ron D. 2000a. Regulated translation initiation controls stress-induced gene expression in mammalian cells. *Mol Cell* **6:** 1099–1108. doi:10.1016/S1097-2765(00)00108-8

Harding HP, Zhang Y, Bertolotti A, Zeng H, Ron D. 2000b. Perk is essential for translational regulation and cell survival during the unfolded protein response. *Mol Cell* **5:** 897–904. doi:10.1016/S1097-2765(00)80330-5

Harding HP, Zhang Y, Zeng H, Novoa I, Lu PD, Calfon M, Sadri N, Yun C, Popko B, Paules R, et al. 2003. An integrated stress response regulates amino acid metabolism and resistance to oxidative stress. *Mol Cell* **11:** 619–633. doi:10.1016/S1097-2765(03)00105-9

Haze K, Yoshida H, Yanagi H, Yura T, Mori K. 1999. Mammalian transcription factor ATF6 is synthesized as a transmembrane protein and activated by proteolysis in response to endoplasmic reticulum stress. *Mol Biol Cell* **10:** 3787–3799. doi:10.1091/mbc.10.11.3787

Heiden MGV, Cantley LC, Thompson CB. 2009. Understanding the Warburg effect: the metabolic requirements of cell proliferation. *Science* **324:** 1029–1033. doi:10.1126/science.1160809

Huang D, Li T, Li X, Zhang L, Sun L, He X, Zhong X, Jia D, Song L, Semenza GL, et al. 2014. HIF-1-mediated suppression of acyl-CoA dehydrogenases and fatty acid oxidation is critical for cancer progression. *Cell Rep* **8:** 1930–1942. doi:10.1016/j.celrep.2014.08.028

Hudson CC, Liu M, Chiang GG, Otterness DM, Loomis DC, Kaper F, Giaccia AJ, Abraham RT. 2002. Regulation of hypoxia-inducible factor 1α expression and function by the mammalian target of rapamycin. *Mol Cell Biol* **22:** 7004–7014. doi:10.1128/MCB.22.20.7004-7014.2002

Hui S, Ghergurovich JM, Morscher RJ, Jang C, Teng X, Lu W, Esparza LA, Reya T, Zhan L, Yanxiang Guo J, et al. 2017. Glucose feeds the TCA cycle via circulating lactate. *Nature* 551: 115–118. doi:10.1038/nature24057

Jin G, Xu C, Zhang X, Long J, Rezaeian AH, Liu C, Furth ME, Kridel S, Pasche B, Bian XW, et al. 2017. Atad3a suppresses Pink1-dependent mitophagy to maintain homeostasis of hematopoietic progenitor cells. *Nat Immunol* 19: 29–40. doi:10.1038/s41590-017-0002-1

Jin J, Byun JK, Choi YK, Park KG. 2023. Targeting glutamine metabolism as a therapeutic strategy for cancer. *Exp Mol Med* 55: 706–715. doi:10.1038/s12276-023-00971-9

Jung CH, Jun CB, Ro SH, Kim YM, Otto NM, Cao J, Kundu M, Kim DH. 2009. ULK-Atg13-FIP200 complexes mediate mTOR signaling to the autophagy machinery. *Mol Biol Cell* 20: 1992–2003. doi:10.1091/mbc.e08-12-1249

Kamphorst JJ, Cross JR, Fan J, De Stanchina E, Mathew R, White EP, Thompson CB, Rabinowitz JD. 2013. Hypoxic and Ras-transformed cells support growth by scavenging unsaturated fatty acids from lysophospholipids. *Proc Natl Acad Sci* 110: 8882–8887. doi:10.1073/pnas.1307237110

Kamphorst JJ, Chung MK, Fan J, Rabinowitz JD. 2014. Quantitative analysis of acetyl-CoA production in hypoxic cancer cells reveals substantial contribution from acetate. *Cancer Metab* 2: 23. doi:10.1186/2049-3002-2-23

Kaushik AK, Tarangelo A, Boroughs LK, Ragavan M, Zhang Y, Wu CY, Li X, Ahumada K, Chiang JC, Tcheuyap VT, et al. 2022. In vivo characterization of glutamine metabolism identifies therapeutic targets in clear cell renal cell carcinoma. *Sci Adv* 8: eabp8293. doi:10.1126/sciadv.abp8293

Kierans SJ, Taylor CT. 2021. Regulation of glycolysis by the hypoxia-inducible factor (HIF): implications for cellular physiology. *J Physiol* 599: 23–37. doi:10.1113/JP280572

Kim JW, Tchernyshyov I, Semenza GL, Dang CV. 2006. HIF-1-mediated expression of pyruvate dehydrogenase kinase: a metabolic switch required for cellular adaptation to hypoxia. *Cell Metab* 3: 177–185. doi:10.1016/j.cmet.2006.02.002

Kim J, Kundu M, Viollet B, Guan KL. 2011. AMPK and mTOR regulate autophagy through direct phosphorylation of Ulk1. *Nat Cell Biol* 13: 132–141. doi:10.1038/ncb2152

Kim SM, Nguyen TT, Ravi A, Kubiniok P, Finicle BT, Jayashankar V, Malacrida L, Hou J, Robertson J, Gao D, et al. 2018. PTEN deficiency and AMPK activation promote nutrient scavenging and anabolism in prostate cancer cells. *Cancer Discov* 8: 866–883. doi:10.1158/2159-8290.CD-17-1215

Kimmelman AC, White E. 2017. Autophagy and tumor metabolism. *Cell Metab* 25: 1037–1043. doi:10.1016/j.cmet.2017.04.004

Kooistra SM, Helin K. 2012. Molecular mechanisms and potential functions of histone demethylases. *Nat Rev Mol Cell Biol* 13: 297–311. doi:10.1038/nrm3327

Koritzinsky M, Levitin F, Van Den Beucken T, Rumantir RA, Harding NJ, Chu KC, Boutros PC, Braakman I, Wouters BG. 2013. Two phases of disulfide bond formation have differing requirements for oxygen. *J Cell Biol* 203: 615–627. doi:10.1083/jcb.201307185

Kung-Chun Chiu D, Pui-Wah Tse A, Law CT, Ming-Jing Xu I, Lee D, Chen M, Kit-Ho Lai R, Wai-Hin Yuen V, Wing-

Sum Cheu J, Wai-Hung Ho D, et al. 2019. Hypoxia regulates the mitochondrial activity of hepatocellular carcinoma cells through HIF/HEY1/PINK1 pathway. *Cell Death Dis* 10: 934. doi:10.1038/s41419-019-2155-3

LaGory EL, Wu C, Taniguchi CM, Ding CKC, Chi JT, von Eyben R, Scott DA, Richardson AD, Giaccia AJ. 2015. Suppression of PGC-1α is critical for reprogramming oxidative metabolism in renal cell carcinoma. *Cell Rep* 12: 116–127. doi:10.1016/j.celrep.2015.06.006

Lee S, Hallis SP, Jung KA, Ryu D, Kwak MK. 2019. Impairment of HIF-1α-mediated metabolic adaption by NRF2-silencing in breast cancer cells. *Redox Biol* 24: 101210. doi:10.1016/j.redox.2019.101210

Lee P, Chandel NS, Simon MC. 2020a. Cellular adaptation to hypoxia through hypoxia inducible factors and beyond. *Nat Rev Mol Cell Biol* 21: 268–283. doi:10.1038/s41580-020-0227-y

Lee P, Malik D, Perkons N, Huangyang P, Khare S, Rhoades S, Gong YY, Burrows M, Finan JM, Nissim I, et al. 2020b. Targeting glutamine metabolism slows soft tissue sarcoma growth. *Nat Commun* 11: 498. doi:10.1038/s41467-020-14374-1

Lee CH, Motzer R, Emamekhoo H, Matrana M, Percent I, Hsieh JJ, Hussain A, Vaishampayan U, Liu S, McCune S, et al. 2022. Telaglenastat plus everolimus in advanced renal cell carcinoma: a randomized, double-blinded, placebo-controlled, phase II ENTRATA trial. *Clin Cancer Res* 28: 3248–3255. doi:10.1158/1078-0432.CCR-22-0061

Lemberg KM, Vornov JJ, Rais R, Slusher BS. 2018. We're not "DON" yet: optimal dosing and prodrug delivery of 6-Diazo-5-oxo-L-norleucine. *Mol Cancer Ther* 17: 1824–1832. doi:10.1158/1535-7163.MCT-17-1148

Leone RD, Zhao L, Englert JM, Sun IM, Oh MH, Sun IH, Arwood ML, Bettencourt IA, Patel CH, Wen J, et al. 2019. Glutamine blockade induces divergent metabolic programs to overcome tumor immune evasion. *Science* 366: 1013–1021. doi:10.1126/science.aav2588

Li Y, Wang Y, Kim E, Beemiller P, Wang CY, Swanson J, You M, Guan KL. 2007. Bnip3 mediates the hypoxia-induced inhibition on mammalian target of rapamycin by interacting with Rheb. *J Biol Chem* 282: 35803–35813. doi:10.1074/jbc.M705231200

Li Z, Ji BW, Dixit PD, Tchourine K, Lien EC, Hosios AM, Abbott KL, Rutter JC, Westermark AM, Gorodetsky EF, et al. 2022. Cancer cells depend on environmental lipids for proliferation when electron acceptors are limited. *Nat Metab* 4: 711–723. doi:10.1038/s42255-022-00588-8

Liberti MV, Locasale JW. 2016. The Warburg effect: how does it benefit cancer cells? *Trends Biochem Sci* 41: 211–218. doi:10.1016/j.tibs.2015.12.001

Liu GY, Sabatini DM. 2020. mTOR at the nexus of nutrition, growth, ageing and disease. *Nat Rev Mol Cell Biol* 21: 183–203. doi:10.1038/s41580-019-0199-y

Liu L, Cash TP, Jones RG, Keith B, Thompson CB, Simon MC. 2006. Hypoxia-induced energy stress regulates mRNA translation and cell growth. *Mol Cell* 21: 521–531. doi:10.1016/j.molcel.2006.01.010

Liu Y, Adachi M, Zhao S, Hareyama M, Koong AC, Luo D, Rando TA, Imai K, Shinomura Y. 2009. Preventing oxidative stress: a new role for XBP1. *Cell Death Differ* 16: 847–857. doi:10.1038/cdd.2009.14

Liu L, Feng D, Chen G, Chen M, Zheng Q, Song P, Ma Q, Zhu C, Wang R, Qi W, et al. 2012. Mitochondrial outer-membrane protein FUNDC1 mediates hypoxia-induced mitophagy in mammalian cells. *Nat Cell Biol* **14:** 177–185. doi:10.1038/ncb2422

Liu J, Ibi D, Taniguchi K, Lee J, Herrema H, Akosman B, Mucka P, Salazar Hernandez MA, Uyar MF, Park SW, et al. 2016. Inflammation improves glucose homeostasis through IKKβ-XBP1s interaction. *Cell* **167:** 1052–1066. e18. doi:10.1016/j.cell.2016.10.015

Losman JA, Koivunen P, Kaelin WG. 2020. 2-Oxoglutarate-dependent dioxygenases in cancer. *Nat Rev Cancer* **20:** 710–726. doi:10.1038/s41568-020-00303-3

Lunt SY, Vander Heiden MG. 2011. Aerobic glycolysis: meeting the metabolic requirements of cell proliferation. *Annu Rev Cell Dev Biol* **27:** 441–464. doi:10.1146/annurev-cellbio-092910-154237

Mansfield KD, Simon MC, Keith B. 2004. Hypoxic reduction in cellular glutathione levels requires mitochondrial reactive oxygen species. *J Appl Physiol* **97:** 1358–1366. doi:10.1152/japplphysiol.00449.2004

Marinković M, Šprung M, Novak I. 2021. Dimerization of mitophagy receptor BNIP3L/NIX is essential for recruitment of autophagic machinery. *Autophagy* **17:** 1232–1243. doi:10.1080/15548627.2020.1755120

Martinez-Outschoorn UE, Trimmer C, Lin Z, Whitaker-Menezes D, Chiavarina B, Zhou J, Wang C, Pavlides S, Martinez-Cantarin MP, Capozza F, et al. 2010. Autophagy in cancer associated fibroblasts promotes tumor cell survival: role of hypoxia, HIF1 induction and NFκB activation in the tumor stromal microenvironment. *Cell Cycle* **9:** 3515–3533. doi:10.4161/cc.9.17.12928

Martínez-Reyes I, Chandel NS. 2020. Mitochondrial TCA cycle metabolites control physiology and disease. *Nat Commun* **11:** 1–11. doi:10.1038/s41467-019-13668-3

May D, Itin A, Gal O, Kalinski H, Feinstein E, Keshet E. 2005. Ero1-Lα plays a key role in a HIF-1-mediated pathway to improve disulfide bond formation and VEGF secretion under hypoxia: implication for cancer. *Oncogene* **24:** 1011–1020. doi:10.1038/sj.onc.1208325

McGinn O, Gupta VK, Dauer P, Arora N, Sharma N, Nomura A, Dudeja V, Saluja A, Banerjee S. 2017. Inhibition of hypoxic response decreases stemness and reduces tumorigenic signaling due to impaired assembly of HIF1 transcription complex in pancreatic cancer. *Sci Rep* **7:** 7872. doi:10.1038/s41598-017-08447-3

Menter DG, Schilsky RL, DuBois RN. 2010. Cyclooxygenase-2 and cancer treatment: understanding the risk should be worth the reward. *Clin Cancer Res* **16:** 1384–1390. doi:10.1158/1078-0432.CCR-09-0788

Metallo CM, Gameiro PA, Bell EL, Mattaini KR, Yang J, Hiller K, Jewell CM, Johnson ZR, Irvine DJ, Guarente L, et al. 2011. Reductive glutamine metabolism by IDH1 mediates lipogenesis under hypoxia. *Nature* **481:** 380–384. doi:10.1038/nature10602

Miess H, Dankworth B, Gouw AM, Rosenfeldt M, Schmitz W, Jiang M, Saunders B, Howell M, Downward J, Felsher DW, et al. 2018. The glutathione redox system is essential to prevent ferroptosis caused by impaired lipid metabolism in clear cell renal cell carcinoma. *Oncogene* **37:** 5435–5450. doi:10.1038/s41388-018-0315-z

Mieulet V, Lamb RF. 2010. Tuberous sclerosis complex: linking cancer to metabolism. *Trends Mol Med* **16:** 329–335. doi:10.1016/j.molmed.2010.05.001

Miska J, Lee-Chang C, Rashidi A, Muroski ME, Chang AL, Lopez-Rosas A, Zhang P, Panek WK, Cordero A, Han Y, et al. 2019. HIF-1α is a metabolic switch between glycolytic-driven migration and oxidative phosphorylation-driven immunosuppression of Tregs in glioblastoma. *Cell Rep* **27:** 226–237.e4. doi:10.1016/j.celrep.2019.03.029

Missiaen R, Lesner NP, Simon MC. 2023. HIF: a master regulator of nutrient availability and metabolic crosstalk in the tumor microenvironment. *EMBO J* **42:** e112067. doi:10.15252/embj.2022112067

Mullen AR, Wheaton WW, Jin ES, Chen PH, Sullivan LB, Cheng T, Yang Y, Linehan WM, Chandel NS, Deberardinis RJ. 2011. Reductive carboxylation supports growth in tumour cells with defective mitochondria. *Nature* **481:** 385–388. doi:10.1038/nature10642

Mungai PT, Waypa GB, Jairaman A, Prakriya M, Dokic D, Ball MK, Schumacker PT. 2011. Hypoxia triggers AMPK activation through reactive oxygen species-mediated activation of calcium release-activated calcium channels. *Mol Cell Biol* **31:** 3531–3545. doi:10.1128/MCB.05124-11

Murphy MP. 2009. How mitochondria produce reactive oxygen species. *Biochem J* **417:** 1–13. doi:10.1042/BJ20081386

Oh MH, Sun IH, Zhao L, Leone RD, Sun IM, Xu W, Collins SL, Tam AJ, Blosser RL, Patel CH, et al. 2020. Targeting glutamine metabolism enhances tumor-specific immunity by modulating suppressive myeloid cells. *J Clin Invest* **130:** 3865–3884. doi:10.1172/JCI131859

Orr AL, Vargas L, Turk CN, Baaten JE, Matzen JT, Dardov VJ, Attle SJ, Li J, Quackenbush DC, Goncalves RLS, et al. 2015. Suppressors of superoxide production from mitochondrial complex III. *Nat Chem Biol* **11:** 834–836. doi:10.1038/nchembio.1910

Palazon A, Tyrakis PA, Macias D, Veliça P, Rundqvist H, Fitzpatrick S, Vojnovic N, Phan AT, Loman N, Hedenfalk I, et al. 2017. An HIF-1α/VEGF-A axis in cytotoxic T cells regulates tumor progression. *Cancer Cell* **32:** 669–683.e5. doi:10.1016/j.ccell.2017.10.003

Papandreou I, Cairns RA, Fontana L, Lim AL, Denko NC. 2006. HIF-1 mediates adaptation to hypoxia by actively downregulating mitochondrial oxygen consumption. *Cell Metab* **3:** 187–197. doi:10.1016/j.cmet.2006.01.012

Park SJ, Yoo HC, Ahn E, Luo E, Kim Y, Sung Y, Yu YC, Kim K, Min DS, Lee HS, et al. 2023. Enhanced glutaminolysis drives hypoxia-induced chemoresistance in pancreatic cancer. *Cancer Res* **83:** 735–752. doi:10.1158/0008-5472.CAN-22-2045

Pescador N, Villar D, Cifuentes D, Garcia-Rocha M, Ortiz-Barahona A, Vazquez S, Ordoñez A, Cuevas Y, Saez-Morales D, Garcia-Bermejo ML, et al. 2010. Hypoxia promotes glycogen accumulation through hypoxia inducible factor (HIF)-mediated induction of glycogen synthase 1. *PLoS ONE* **5:** e9644. doi:10.1371/journal.pone.0009644

Petronek MS, Spitz DR, Buettner GR, Allen BG. 2019. Linking cancer metabolic dysfunction and genetic instability through the lens of iron metabolism. *Cancers (Basel)* **11:** 1077. doi:10.3390/cancers11081077

Cite this article as *Cold Spring Harb Perspect Med* doi: 10.1101/cshperspect.a041542

Pickrell AM, Youle RJ. 2015. The roles of PINK1, parkin and mitochondrial fidelity in Parkinson's disease. *Neuron* 85: 257–273. doi:10.1016/j.neuron.2014.12.007

Pommier A, Anaparthy N, Memos N, Larkin Kelley Z, Gouronnec A, Yan R, Auffray C, Albrengues J, Egeblad M, Iacobuzio-Donahue CA, et al. 2018. Unresolved endoplasmic reticulum stress engenders immune-resistant, latent pancreatic cancer metastases. *Science* 360: eaao4908. doi:10.1126/science.aao4908

Ponneri Babuharisankar A, Kuo CL, Chou HY, Tangeda V, Fan CC, Chen CH, Kao YH, Lee AYL. 2023. Mitochondrial Ion-induced mitophagy benefits hypoxic cancer resistance via Ca^{2+}-dependent FUNDC1 phosphorylation at the ER-mitochondria interface. *Cell Death Dis* 14: 1–17. doi:10.1038/s41419-023-05723-1

Qian X, Li X, Shi Z, Bai X, Xia Y, Zheng Y, Xu D, Chen F, You Y, Fang J, et al. 2019. KDM3A senses oxygen availability to regulate PGC-1α-mediated mitochondrial biogenesis. *Mol Cell* 76: 885–895.e7. doi:10.1016/j.molcel.2019.09.019

Qiu B, Ackerman D, Sanchez DJ, Li B, Ochocki JD, Grazioli A, Bobrovnikova-Marjon E, Alan Diehl J, Keith B, Celeste Simon M. 2015. HIF2α-dependent lipid storage promotes endoplasmic reticulum homeostasis in clear-cell renal cell carcinoma. *Cancer Discov* 5: 653–667.

Ramirez C, Hauser AD, Vucic EA, Bar-Sagi D. 2019. Plasma membrane V-ATPase controls oncogenic RAS-induced macropinocytosis. *Nature* 576: 477–481. doi:10.1038/s41586-019-1831-x

Read AD, Bentley RE, Archer SL, Dunham-Snary KJ. 2021. Mitochondrial iron–sulfur clusters: structure, function, and an emerging role in vascular biology. *Redox Biol* 47: 102164. doi:10.1016/j.redox.2021.102164

Reinfeld BI, Madden MZ, Wolf MM, Chytil A, Bader JE, Patterson AR, Sugiura A, Cohen AS, Ali A, Do BT, et al. 2021. Cell-programmed nutrient partitioning in the tumour microenvironment. *Nature* 593: 282–288 doi:10.1038/s41586-021-03442-1

Romero-Ramirez L, Cao H, Nelson D, Hammond E, Lee AH, Yoshida H, Mori K, Glimcher LH, Denko NC, Giaccia AJ, et al. 2004. XBP1 is essential for survival under hypoxic conditions and is required for tumor growth. *Cancer Res* 64: 5943–5947. doi:10.1158/0008-5472.CAN-04-1606

Ros S, Santos CR, Moco S, Baenke F, Kelly G, Howell M, Zamboni N, Schulze A. 2012. Functional metabolic screen identifies 6-phosphofructo-2-kinase/fructose-2,6-biphosphatase 4 as an important regulator of prostate cancer cell survival. *Cancer Discov* 2: 328–343. doi:10.1158/2159-8290.CD-11-0234

Rouschop KMA, Van Den Beucken T, Dubois L, Niessen H, Bussink J, Savelkouls K, Keulers T, Mujcic H, Landuyt W, Voncken JW, et al. 2010a. The unfolded protein response protects human tumor cells during hypoxia through regulation of the autophagy genes MAP1LC3B and ATG5. *J Clin Invest* 120: 127–141. doi:10.1172/JCI40027

Rouschop KMA, Van Den Beucken T, Dubois L, Niessen H, Bussink J, Savelkouls K, Keulers T, Mujcic H, Landuyt W, Voncken JW, et al. 2010b. The unfolded protein response protects human tumor cells during hypoxia through regulation of the autophagy genes MAP1LC3B and ATG5. *J Clin Invest* 120: 127–141. doi:10.1172/JCI40027

Sahai E, Astsaturov I, Cukierman E, DeNardo DG, Egeblad M, Evans RM, Fearon D, Greten FR, Hingorani SR, Hunter T, et al. 2020. A framework for advancing our understanding of cancer-associated fibroblasts. *Nat Rev Cancer* 20: 174–186. doi:10.1038/s41568-019-0238-1

Samanta D, Park Y, Andrabi SA, Shelton LM, Gilkes DM, Semenza GL. 2016. PHGDH expression is required for mitochondrial redox homeostasis, breast cancer stem cell maintenance, and lung metastasis. *Cancer Res* 76: 4430–4442. doi:10.1158/0008-5472.CAN-16-0530

Sanford-Crane H, Abrego J, Sherman MH. 2019. Fibroblasts as modulators of local and systemic cancer metabolism. *Cancers (Basel)* 11: 619. doi:10.3390/cancers11050619

Schon EA, Dimauro S, Hirano M. 2012. Human mitochondrial DNA: roles of inherited and somatic mutations. *Nat Rev Genet* 13: 878–890. doi:10.1038/nrg3275

Schug ZT, Peck B, Jones DT, Zhang Q, Grosskurth S, Alam IS, Goodwin LM, Smethurst E, Mason S, Blyth K, et al. 2015. Acetyl-CoA synthetase 2 promotes acetate utilization and maintains cancer cell growth under metabolic stress. *Cancer Cell* 27: 57–71. doi:10.1016/j.ccell.2014.12.002

Semenza GL. 2017. Hypoxia-inducible factors: coupling glucose metabolism and redox regulation with induction of the breast cancer stem cell phenotype. *EMBO J* 36: 252–259. doi:10.15252/embj.201695204

Seong M, Lee J, Kang H. 2019. Hypoxia-induced regulation of mTOR signaling by miR-7 targeting REDD1. *J Cell Biochem* 120: 4523–4532. doi:10.1002/jcb.27740

Shen J, Chen X, Hendershot L, Prywes R. 2002. ER stress regulation of ATF6 localization by dissociation of BiP/GRP78 binding and unmasking of Golgi localization signals. *Dev Cell* 3: 99–111. doi:10.1016/S1534-5807(02)00203-4

Sies H, Jones DP. 2020. Reactive oxygen species (ROS) as pleiotropic physiological signalling agents. *Nat Rev Mol Cell Biol* 21: 363–383. doi:10.1038/s41580-020-0230-3

So JS, Hur KY, Tarrio M, Ruda V, Frank-Kamenetsky M, Fitzgerald K, Koteliansky V, Lichtman AH, Iwawaki T, Glimcher LH, et al. 2012. Silencing of lipid metabolism genes through IRE1α-mediated mRNA decay lowers plasma lipids in mice. *Cell Metab* 16: 487–499. doi:10.1016/j.cmet.2012.09.004

Sofer A, Lei K, Johannessen CM, Ellisen LW. 2005. Regulation of mTOR and cell growth in response to energy stress by REDD1. *Mol Cell Biol* 25: 5834–5845. doi:10.1128/MCB.25.14.5834-5845.2005

Sousa CM, Biancur DE, Wang X, Halbrook CJ, Sherman MH, Zhang L, Kremer D, Hwang RF, Witkiewicz AK, Ying H, et al. 2016. Pancreatic stellate cells support tumour metabolism through autophagic alanine secretion. *Nature* 536: 479–483. doi:10.1038/nature19084

Sulkshane P, Ram J, Thakur A, Reis N, Kleifeld O, Glickman MH. 2021. Ubiquitination and receptor-mediated mitophagy converge to eliminate oxidation-damaged mitochondria during hypoxia. *Redox Biol* 45: 102047. doi:10.1016/j.redox.2021.102047

Sullivan LB, Gui DY, Hosios AM, Bush LN, Freinkman E, Vander Heiden MG. 2015. Supporting aspartate biosynthesis is an essential function of respiration in proliferating cells. *Cell* 162: 552–563. doi:10.1016/j.cell.2015.07.017

Sullivan MR, Danai LV., Lewis CA, Chan SH, Gui DY, Kunchok T, Dennstedt EA, Heiden MGV, Muir A. 2019. Quantification of microenvironmental metabolites in murine cancers reveals determinants of tumor nutrient availability. *eLife* **8**: e44235. doi:10.7554/eLife .44235

Sun RC, Denko NC. 2014. Hypoxic regulation of glutamine metabolism through HIF1 and SIAH2 supports lipid synthesis that is necessary for tumor growth. *Cell Metab* **19**: 285–292. doi:10.1016/j.cmet.2013.11.022

Tannir NM, Agarwal N, Porta C, Lawrence NJ, Motzer R, McGregor B, Lee RJ, Jain RK, Davis N, Appleman LJ, et al. 2022. Efficacy and safety of telaglenastat plus cabozantinib vs placebo plus cabozantinib in patients with advanced renal cell carcinoma: the CANTATA randomized clinical trial. *JAMA Oncol* **8**: 1411–1418. doi:10.1001/ja maoncol.2022.3511

Tao J, Yang G, Zhou W, Qiu J, Chen G, Luo W, Zhao F, You L, Zheng L, Zhang T, et al. 2021. Targeting hypoxic tumor microenvironment in pancreatic cancer. *J Hematol Oncol* **14**: 1–25. doi:10.1186/s13045-020-01030-w

Taylor CT, Colgan SP. 2017. Regulation of immunity and inflammation by hypoxia in immunological niches. *Nat Rev Immunol* **17**: 774–785. doi:10.1038/nri.2017.103

Tohme S, Yazdani HO, Liu Y, Loughran P, van der Windt DJ, Huang H, Simmons RL, Shiva S, Tai S, Tsung A. 2017. Hypoxia mediates mitochondrial biogenesis in hepatocellular carcinoma to promote tumor growth through HMGB1 and TLR9 interaction. *Hepatology* **66**: 182–197. doi:10.1002/hep.29184

Vara-Pérez M, Rossi M, Van den Haute C, Maes H, Sassano ML, Venkataramani V, Michalke B, Romano E, Rillaerts K, Garg AD, et al. 2021. BNIP3 promotes HIF-1α-driven melanoma growth by curbing intracellular iron homeostasis. *EMBO J* **40**: e106214. doi:10 .15252/embj.2020106214

Vriens K, Christen S, Parik S, Broekaert D, Yoshinaga K, Talebi A, Dehairs J, Escalona-Noguero C, Schmieder R, Cornfield T, et al. 2019. Evidence for an alternative fatty acid desaturation pathway increasing cancer plasticity. *Nature* **566**: 403–406. doi:10.1038/s41586-019-0904-1

Vyas S, Zaganjor E, Haigis MC. 2016. Mitochondria and cancer. *Cell* **166**: 555–566. doi:10.1016/j.cell.2016.07.002

Waypa GB, Marks JD, Guzy RD, Mungai PT, Schriewer JM, Dokic D, Ball MK, Schumacker PT. 2013. Superoxide generated at mitochondrial complex III triggers acute responses to hypoxia in the pulmonary circulation. *Am J Respir Crit Care Med* **187**: 424–432. doi:10.1164/rccm .201207-1294OC

Wheaton WW, Chandel NS. 2011. Hypoxia. 2. Hypoxia regulates cellular metabolism. *Am J Physiol Cell Physiol* **300**: C385–C393. doi:10.1152/ajpcell.00485.2010

Wicks EE, Semenza GL. 2022. Hypoxia-inducible factors: cancer progression and clinical translation. *J Clin Invest* **132**: e159839. doi:10.1172/JCI159839

Wilson DF, Rumsey WL, Green TJ, Vanderkooi JM. 1988. The oxygen dependence of mitochondrial oxidative phosphorylation measured by a new optical method for measuring oxygen concentration. *J Biol Chem* **263**: 2712–2718. doi:10.1016/S0021-9258(18)69126-4

Wise DR, Ward PS, Shay JES, Cross JR, Gruber JJ, Sachdeva UM, Platt JM, DeMatteo RG, Simon MC, Thompson CB.

2011. Hypoxia promotes isocitrate dehydrogenase-dependent carboxylation of α-ketoglutarate to citrate to support cell growth and viability. *Proc Natl Acad Sci* **108**: 19611–19616. doi:10.1073/pnas.1117773108

Wouters BG, Koritzinsky M. 2008. Hypoxia signalling through mTOR and the unfolded protein response in cancer. *Nat Rev Cancer* **8**: 851–864. doi:10.1038/ nrc2501

Wu H, Wang T, Liu Y, Li X, Xu S, Wu C, Zou H, Cao M, Jin G, Lang J, et al. 2020. Mitophagy promotes sorafenib resistance through hypoxia-inducible ATAD3A dependent axis. *J Exp Clin Cancer Res* **39**: 1–16. doi:10.1186/ s13046-020-01768-8

Xie H, Tang CHA, Song JH, Mancuso A, Del Valle JR, Cao J, Xiang Y, Dang CV., Lan R, Sanchez DJ, et al. 2018. IRE1α RNase–dependent lipid homeostasis promotes survival in Myc-transformed cancers. *J Clin Invest* **128**: 1300–1316. doi:10.1172/JCI95864

Xie H, Song J, Godfrey J, Riscal R, Skuli N, Nissim I, Simon MC. 2021. Glycogen metabolism is dispensable for tumour progression in clear cell renal cell carcinoma. *Nat Metab* **3**: 327–336. doi:10.1038/s42255-021-00367-x

Yamamoto K, Sato T, Matsui T, Sato M, Okada T, Yoshida H, Harada A, Mori K. 2007. Transcriptional induction of mammalian ER quality control proteins is mediated by single or combined action of ATF6α and XBP1. *Dev Cell* **13**: 365–376. doi:10.1016/j.devcel.2007 .07.018

Ye J, Rawson RB, Komuro R, Chen X, Davé UP, Prywes R, Brown MS, Goldstein JL. 2000. ER stress induces cleavage of membrane-bound ATF6 by the same proteases that process SREBPs. *Mol Cell* **6**: 1355–1364. doi:10.1016/ S1097-2765(00)00133-7

Ye J, Fan J, Venneti S, Wan YW, Pawel BR, Zhang J, Finley LWS, Lu C, Lindsten T, Cross JR, et al. 2014. Serine catabolism regulates mitochondrial redox control during hypoxia. *Cancer Discov* **4**: 1406–1417. doi:10.1158/2159-8290.CD-14-0250

Yoshida H, Matsui T, Yamamoto A, Okada T, Mori K. 2001. XBP1 mRNA is induced by ATF6 and spliced by IRE1 in response to ER stress to produce a highly active transcription factor. *Cell* **107**: 881–891. doi:10.1016/S0092-8674 (01)00611-0

Youle RJ, Narendra DP. 2010. Mechanisms of mitophagy. *Nat Rev Mol Cell Biol* **12**: 9–14. doi:10.1038/nrm3028

Young RM, Ackerman D, Quinn ZL, Mancuso A, Gruber M, Liu L, Giannoukos DN, Bobrovnikova-Marjon E, Diehl JA, Keith B, et al. 2013. Dysregulated mTORC1 renders cells critically dependent on desaturated lipids for survival under tumor-like stress. *Genes Dev* **27**: 1115–1131. doi:10.1101/gad.198630.112

Zhai L, Spranger S, Binder DC, Gritsina G, Lauing KL, Giles FJ, Wainwright DA. 2015. Molecular pathways: targeting IDO1 and other tryptophan dioxygenases for cancer immunotherapy. *Clin Cancer Res* **21**: 5427–5433. doi:10 .1158/1078-0432.CCR-15-0420

Zhang X, Saarinen AM, Hitosugi T, Wang Z, Wang L, Ho TH, Liu J. 2017. Inhibition of intracellular lipolysis promotes human cancer cell adaptation to hypoxia. *eLife* **6**: e31132. doi:10.7554/eLife.31132

Zhang MS, Di CJ, Lee D, Yuen VWH, Chiu DKC, Goh CC, Cheu JWS, Tse APW, Bao MHR, Wong BPY, et al. 2022.

Hypoxia-induced macropinocytosis represents a metabolic route for liver cancer. *Nat Commun* **13:** 954. doi:10.1038/s41467-022-28618-9

Zhou Y, Lee J, Reno CM, Sun C, Park SW, Chung J, Lee J, Fisher SJ, White MF, Biddinger SB, et al. 2011. Regulation of glucose homeostasis through a XBP-1–FOXO1 interaction. *Nat Med* **17:** 356–365. doi:10.1038/nm.2293

Zong WX, Rabinowitz JD, White E. 2016. Mitochondria and cancer. *Mol Cell* **61:** 667–676. doi:10.1016/j.molcel.2016.02.011

Zou Y, Palte MJ, Deik AA, Li H, Eaton JK, Wang W, Tseng YY, Deasy R, Kost-Alimova M, Dančík V, et al. 2019. A GPX4-dependent cancer cell state underlies the clear-cell morphology and confers sensitivity to ferroptosis. *Nat Commun* **10:** 1617. doi:10.1038/s41467-019-09277-9

Role of Tumor Cell Intrinsic and Host Autophagy in Cancer

Jessie Yanxiang Guo[1,2,3] and Eileen White[1,3,4]

[1]Rutgers Cancer Institute of New Jersey, New Brunswick, New Jersey 08903, USA

[2]Department of Chemical Biology, Rutgers Ernest Mario School of Pharmacy, Piscataway, New Jersey 08854, USA

[3]Ludwig Princeton Branch, Ludwig Institute for Cancer Research, Princeton University, Princeton, New Jersey 08544, USA

[4]Department of Molecular Biology and Biochemistry, Rutgers University, Piscataway, New Jersey 08903, USA

Correspondence: epwhite@cinj.rutgers.edu

Macroautophagy (autophagy hereafter) is an intracellular nutrient scavenging pathway induced by starvation and other stressors whereby cellular components such as organelles are captured in double-membrane vesicles (autophagosomes), whereupon their contents are degraded through fusion with lysosomes. Two main purposes of autophagy are to recycle the intracellular breakdown products to sustain metabolism and survival during starvation and to eliminate damaged or excess cellular components to suppress inflammation and maintain homeostasis. In contrast to most normal cells and tissues in the fed state, tumor cells up-regulate autophagy to promote their growth, survival, and malignancy. This tumor-cell-autonomous autophagy supports elevated metabolic demand and suppresses tumoricidal activation of the innate and adaptive immune responses. Tumor-cell-nonautonomous (e.g., host) autophagy also supports tumor growth by maintaining essential tumor nutrients in the circulation and tumor microenvironment and by suppressing an antitumor immune response. In the setting of cancer therapy, autophagy is a resistance mechanism to chemotherapy, targeted therapy, and immunotherapy. Thus, tumor and host autophagy are protumorigenic and autophagy inhibition is being examined as a novel therapeutic approach to treat cancer.

Autophagy captures and degrades intracellular proteins and organelles in lysosomes. The breakdown products from the autophagosome cargo degradation are then recycled into metabolic pathways to maintain a substrate supply when nutrients are scarce (Poillet-Perez and White 2019; White et al. 2021). A core function of this recycling activity of autophagy is to enable survival in starvation, and cells and animals defective for autophagy fail to survive nutrient deprivation (Poillet-Perez and White 2019; White et al. 2021). Autophagic cargo degradation also eliminates damaged cellular components (e.g., garbage) that can trigger activation of the innate immune response, and autophagy thereby suppresses inflammation. Both the pro-metabolic and anti-inflammatory roles of autophagy are essential for homeostasis and survival, and autophagy induction may underly the health benefits of caloric restriction, fasting, and exercise (He et al. 2012; Lashinger et al. 2016; Shabkhizan et al. 2023).

Autophagic activity or flux through the pathway is low in normal cells and tissues and is up-regulated by nutrient and growth factor starvation and other stressors. In contrast to normal cells and tissues, tumor cells up-regulate autophagy even in the fed state where it promotes growth, survival, malignancy, and resistance to therapy (Poillet-Perez and White 2019; White et al. 2021). The underlying mechanisms include sustaining cancer cell metabolism and a supply of essential circulating and tumor microenvironment (TME) nutrients and enabling immune evasion. Herein we provide an overview of the role of both tumor-cell-autonomous and non-autonomous mechanisms by which autophagy promotes cancer.

THE ROLE OF TUMOR-INTRINSIC AUTOPHAGY IN CANCER

Tumor cells use autophagy's two major functions: garbage disposal and intracellular recycling, thereby enabling uncontrolled proliferation and survival in what is often a nutrient-deprived and hypoxic TME. Potential mechanisms mediated by tumor-cell-intrinsic or -autonomous autophagy include provision of subunits to support mitochondrial function for energy generation and maintenance of nucleotide pools, inhibition of oxidative stress, suppression of p53 activation to prevent apoptosis and senescence, prevention of tumor lymphocyte infiltration, and prevention of antigen presentation to escape T-cell-mediated tumor killing (Fig. 1).

Oncogenic Events Up-Regulate Autophagy by Activating Transcription Programs

The target of rapamycin (TOR) and its mammalian homolog (mTOR) are the master regulators

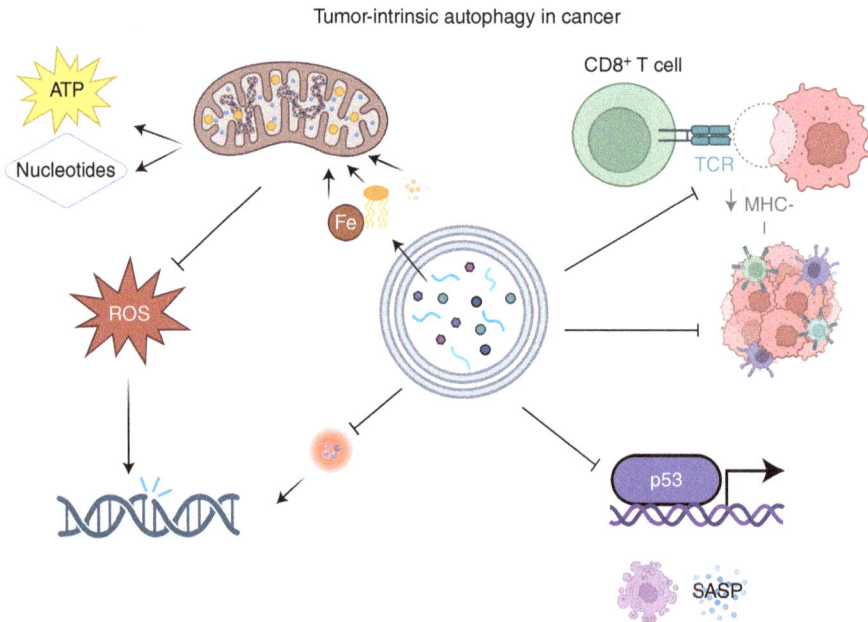

Figure 1. Mechanisms by which tumor-cell-autonomous autophagy supports proliferation and survival. These include recycling of proteins and organelles to provide substrates for macromolecular biosynthesis and iron homeostasis, mitigation of reactive oxygen species (ROS) and cellular damage, suppression of p53 activation, senescence, and inflammation, and inhibition of antigen presentation and killing by T cells. (Figure generated with BioRender, https://biorender.com.)

of cell growth in response to nutrients through kinase signaling that regulates downstream effector pathways (Liu and Sabatini 2020). In the absence of nutrients, the TOR/mTOR pathway is suppressed and autophagy is activated by loss of inhibitory phosphorylation events on proteins controlling initiation of autophagy. mTOR is activated in cancer to promote growth, so autophagy would be expected to be suppressed; however, surprisingly, autophagy is activated even in the context of active mTOR (Poillet-Perez and White 2019; White et al. 2021). This is due to other oncogenic signaling pathways overriding inhibition of autophagy by mTOR (Wong et al. 2013).

Another mechanism by which tumor cells override inhibition of autophagy by mTOR is transcriptional. RAS-driven pancreatic ductal adenocarcinoma (PDAC) requires high levels of autophagy. Oncogenic RAS mutations promote nuclear localization of microphthalmia/transcription factor E (MiT/TFE) family members, leading to activation of expression of genes for the autophagy pathway and for lysosomal biogenesis, which are essential to maintain intracellular amino acid (AA) pools (Perera et al. 2015). Thus, MiT/TFE transcription factors act as master regulators of metabolic reprogramming in PDAC to integrate lysosome with nutrient scavenging pathways, including autophagy and micropinocytosis, to maintain intracellular nutrient availability (Perera et al. 2019).

Tumor-Cell-Autonomous Autophagy Promotes Tumorigenesis

Different types of tumor cells employ cell-autonomous autophagy to maintain their metabolic fitness for survival and proliferation, which has been validated in physiological settings of cancer by conditional deletion of essential autophagy genes in genetically engineered mouse models (GEMMs) for different types of cancer. Deletion of essential autophagy genes (*Atgs*) such as *Atg7* or *Atg5* significantly impairs Kras-driven non-small-cell lung cancer (NSCLC) growth, survival, and malignancy (Guo et al. 2013; Rao et al. 2014; Bhatt et al. 2019). In particular, *Atg7* ablation converts what would be adenocarcinomas to benign oncocytomas, indicating autophagy supports tumor

malignancy (Guo et al. 2013). Deletion of *Atg7* also suppresses Braf^{V600E}-induced lung tumorigenesis (Strohecker et al. 2013). In a PDAC GEMM driven by oncogenic Kras and the stochastic loss of heterozygosity (LOH) of *p53*, *Atg5* ablation in the pancreas leads to increased tumor initiation. However, these premalignant lesions are impaired in their ability to progress to invasive cancer, leading to prolonged survival (Yang et al. 2014). *Atg7* promotes development of Braf^{V600E}-mutant, *Pten*-null melanomas by overcoming senescence (Xie et al. 2015). In a prostate-specific *Pten*-deletion-driven GEMM of prostate cancer, *Atg7* deficiency delayed prostate tumor progression in both castrate-naive and castrate-resistant cancers (Santanam et al. 2016). Deletion of FAK family-interacting protein of 200 kDa (FIP200), which regulates autophagy initiation in mammary epithelial cells (MaECs), suppresses breast cancer initiation, progression, and metastasis in MMTV-PyMT mouse models of breast cancer (Wei et al. 2011). Monoallelic loss of the *Atg* involved in autophagosome maturation and trafficking, *Becn1/Atg6*, reduced *Palb2*-loss-driven mammary tumorigenesis (Huo et al. 2013). In an RCAS/TVA mouse model for gliomagenesis driven by KRAS, inhibition of autophagy via RNAi against *Atg7* (autophagosome assembly), *Atg13*, or Unc-51-like kinase (*Ulk1/Atg1*) (autophagy initiation), strongly reduced glioblastoma development (Gammoh et al. 2016). *Atg7* deficiency in intestinal epithelial cells (IECs) inhibits the formation of precancerous lesions in *Apc$^{+/-}$* mice, leading to a reduction in the number and size of intestinal adenomas (Lévy et al. 2015). These numerous genetic studies indicate that compromising autophagy in cancer cells is specifically detrimental to tumor growth. In the way that normal cells turn on autophagy in response to stress to maintain homeostasis, tumor cells deregulate and activate autophagy to support fitness and tumorigenesis.

Cell-Autonomous Autophagy Promotes Tumorigenesis via Distinct Mechanisms

Autophagy Supports Metabolic Pathways

Autophagy plays an essential role in the removal of damaged organelles and other cellular components and recycles them, which has been usurped by cancer cells to survive and proliferate in the stressed TME. Ras activation up-regulates the autophagy process for cancer cells to maintain mitochondrial metabolism. Autophagy deficiency in cancer cells leads to reduced levels of tricarboxylic acid cycle (TCA) intermediates and impaired tumorigenesis (Guo et al. 2011; Yang et al. 2011). Pulse-chase studies with isotope-labeled nutrients revealed impaired mitochondrial substrate supply during starvation of the autophagy-deficient Ras-driven cancer cells, which is associated with reduced energy charge, increased ROS and caused a dramatic drop of nucleotide pools (Guo et al. 2016). Importantly, nucleotide supplementation in vitro can partly rescue the survival of autophagy-deficient tumor cells demonstrating that the inability to maintain these pools through recycling limits survival in starvation. In a GEMM for Kras-driven NSCLC, accumulation of swollen mitochondria is observed in autophagy-deficient lung tumors. This is aligned with impaired cytochrome *c* oxidase activity (Guo et al. 2013). Autophagy also sustains mitochondrial glutamine metabolism and growth of Braf^{V600E}-driven lung tumors (Strohecker et al. 2013). Autophagy is thus required for proper mitochondrial function and for sustaining tumor cell metabolism, especially under conditions of metabolic stress.

Loss of tumor suppressor liver kinase B1 (*LKB1*) reprograms cancer cell metabolism to efficiently generate energy and biomass components for uncontrolled cell proliferation (Jeon et al. 2012; Parker et al. 2017). However, such alterations in turn cause tumor cells to have less plasticity in dealing with energy crises, creating a metabolic vulnerability. In a study using GEMM of *Lkb1*-deficient Kras-driven (KL) NSCLC, *Atg7* deficiency significantly impaired KL lung tumorigenesis (Bhatt et al. 2019), demonstrating that autophagy compensates for the loss of *Lkb1* in tumorigenesis. Fatty acid oxidation (FAO) plays an important role in KL lung tumor mitochondrial energy production and tumor growth (Svensson et al. 2016; Svensson and Shaw 2016). Autophagy modulates lipid metabolism in KL lung tumorigenesis. In response to nutrient deprivation, autophagy-mediated intracellular recycling is essential for supporting mitochondrial energy production and for maintaining lipid droplet (LD) reserves in KL tumor cells. In the absence of autophagy, KL tumor cells increase their reliance on FAO for energy homeostasis to compensate for defective recycling of TCA cycle intermediates and derivatives, which depletes lipid stores, likely causing an energy crisis (Bhatt et al. 2019). Unlike KL lung tumors, loss of autophagy in KP lung tumors leads to LD accumulation precisely due to defective autophagy and recycling of lipids (lipophagy) and impaired FAO with mitochondrial dysfunction (Guo et al. 2013). Therefore, the type of metabolic liability created by loss of autophagy differs depending on the oncogenic driver mutations.

Besides supplying metabolites to mitochondria, autophagy can regulate mitochondrial function via other ways. Nuclear Receptor Coactivator 4 (NCOA4) is a selective cargo receptor for autophagic turnover of ferritin (ferritinophagy) (Mancias et al. 2014). In PDAC, NCOA4-mediated ferritinophagy is essential for the function of iron–sulfur clusters involved in electron transfer within the mitochondrial respiratory chain (Santana-Codina et al. 2022). Moreover, suppressing iron utilization sensitizes PDAC cells to mitogen-activated extracellular signal-regulated kinase (MEK) inhibition (Ravichandran et al. 2022). Thus, defective mitochondrial metabolism caused by autophagy ablation could be due to impaired iron metabolism. Additionally, oncogenic KRAS in PDAC induces BNIP3L/NIX expression and a selective autophagy of mitochondria (mitophagy) program, which restricts glucose flux to mitochondria and enhances redox capacity (Humpton et al. 2019). Mitophagy also limits ROS that may facilitate survival and metastasis (Labuschagne et al. 2019).

Autophagy Inhibits an Antitumor Immune Response

Immune evasion is one of the hallmarks of cancer and a major obstacle for cancer treatment (Hanahan and Weinberg 2011). One immune escape mechanism in cancer is the loss of antigenicity or immunogenicity, which will lead to a lack of immunogenic peptides presented in the context of a peptide–major histocompatibility complex (MHC). Malignant cells can also gain additional immunosuppressive properties, such as expression of PD-L1 or secretion of suppressive cytokines, which further reduces their immunogenicity. In addition, tumor cells orchestrate an immunosuppressive TME, leading to the recruitment of an immune response that suppresses antitumor immunity (Beatty and Gladney 2015). Cancer cells reprogram metabolism to escape immune surveillance (Villalba et al. 2013). Autophagy activation has been reported to cause the emergence of resistant tumor cells to outmaneuver an effective immune response and escape from immune cell killing (López-Soto et al. 2017; Pietrocola et al. 2017).

Autophagy Inhibits Antigen Presentation

Antigen presentation is responsible for the adaptive immune response against cancer by recognizing foreign protein antigens docked on MHCs on the surface of malignant cells (Schumacher et al. 2019). In addition to proteasome degradation to generate peptides from intracellular antigens (Kloetzel 2001), autophagy-mediated protein degradation is also a route to display antigens on MHC class II molecules to CD4$^+$ T cells, and is implicated in MHC class I cross-presentation of tumor antigens and the activation of CD8$^+$ T cells (Crotzer and Blum 2009). How much this contributes to regulation of tumorigenesis remains to be further elucidated.

PDAC cells display reduced MHC-I cell surface expression and increased localization within autophagosomes and lysosomes. Genetically or pharmaceutically inhibiting autophagy restores surface MHC-I levels, leading to improved antigen presentation, an enhanced antitumor T-cell response, and reduced tumor growth in syngeneic hosts (Yamamoto et al. 2020). Similarly, autophagy inhibits MHC-I presentation in KL lung cancer cells. Upon treatment with autophagy inhibitors, such as chloroquine (CQ) or the ULK1 inhibitor MRT68921, KL cells show restored sensitivity to host immune responses due to enhanced immunoproteasome activity and restoration of antigen processing (Deng et al. 2021).

Thus, MHC-I molecules are selectively targeted for lysosomal degradation through an autophagy-dependent mechanism, which leads to immune evasion. As a result, autophagy inhibition increases the sensitivity of PDAC and KL lung tumors to immune checkpoint blockade (ICB) (Yamamoto et al. 2020; Deng et al. 2021), providing a rationale for the combination of autophagy inhibition and ICB as a therapeutic strategy against cancer.

Autophagy Modulates the TME

Genome-wide CRISPR screens across a panel of genetically diverse mouse cancer cell lines cultured in the presence of cytotoxic T lymphocyte (CTL) revealed that control of interferon responses and tumor necrosis factor α (TNF-α)-induced cytotoxicity are a conserved tumor-cell-autonomous mechanism of CTL evasion. Moreover, tumor-cell-intrinsic autophagy is identified as a conserved mediator of both evasion of CTLs and resistance to cytotoxicity induced by interferon γ (IFN-γ) and TNF-α, which is further validated by an in vivo CRISPR screen in the EMT6 cell model. Such regulation occurs through a hub of autophagy and nuclear factor κB (NF-κβ) signaling (Lawson et al. 2020). Genetic ablation or pharmacological inhibition of autophagy sensitizes cancer cells to TNF-α-induced CTL-mediated cell death (Lawson et al. 2020). In $Apc^{+/-}$ mice, autophagy deficiency in IECs stimulates anticancer adaptive immune responses through the efficient priming and infiltration of antitumoral CD8$^+$ IFN-γ cytotoxic T cells in intestinal mucosa (Lévy and Romagnolo 2015; Lévy et al. 2015). A noncanonical autophagy function of FIP200 is responsible for limiting T-cell recruitment and activation of the TBK1-IFN signaling axis (Okamoto et al. 2020). $Atg5$ knockout significantly increases the accumulation of Tregs in lungs of mice with early autophagy-deficient hyperplastic lesions in a GEMM for Kras-driven NSCLC (Rao et al. 2014). Thus, data from these studies point to the role of autophagy-mediated immune response in the TME, which could be distinct between tumor initiation and tumor growth.

Cite this article as *Cold Spring Harb Perspect Med* doi: 10.1101/cshperspect.a041539

Autophagy Suppresses Oxidative Stress and Maintains Genomic Stability

The role of oxidative stress in tumorigenesis is context dependent. On the one hand, oxidative stress can effectively increase the mutation rates within cells, leading to tumorigenesis. On the other hand, severe oxidative stress can cause cell death that limits cancer. Autophagy mitigates oxidative stress by removing damaged mitochondria, a key source of ROS, thereby maintaining genome integrity to prevent tumor initiation. Autophagy deficiency conferred by either allelic loss of *Becn1* or *Atg5* leads to an enhanced DNA damage response, increased gene amplification, and chromosomal instability, resulting in aneuploidy (Mathew et al. 2007). Autophagy loss decreases levels of checkpoint kinase 1 (Chk1), thereby diminishing DNA repair through error-free homologous recombination (HR), relying instead on the error-prone nonhomologous end joining for repair (Liu et al. 2015). In addition, autophagy deficiency leads to accumulation of p62, which is sufficient to induce ROS, the DNA damage response, and tumorigenesis (Mathew et al. 2009). Mitigation of oxidative stress and preservation of genome stability of autophagy likely enhance the fitness and survival of tumor cells as recurrent mutations in *Atgs* are not seen in human cancers.

Becn1 allelic loss in mouse mammary epithelial cells (MMECs) predisposes to DNA damage and genomic instability through gene amplification, thereby promoting breast cancer progression in a mouse model (Karantza-Wadsworth et al. 2007). However, allelic loss of *Becn1* is not observed in human breast cancers independent of loss of heterozygosity of the well-known tumor suppressor breast cancer gene 1 (*BRCA1*), where it resides next to the genome, indicating that these observations may not be relevant in humans (Laddha et al. 2014).

In cancer cells, persistent autophagy defects may cause elevated ROS and either permanent genomic damage or rapid cell death especially when DNA repair is inhibited. *Atg7* deletion in Braf^{V600E}-induced lung cancer initially induced oxidative stress and accelerated tumor cell proliferation (Guo and White 2016; Guo et al. 2016).

Cysteine plays a critical role in sustaining the antioxidant pool. In PDAC, autophagy regulates SLC7A11 proper membrane localization to maintain cysteine homeostasis via allowing proper cystine transport (Mukhopadhyay et al. 2021). Autophagy inhibition enhances the formation of benign neoplasms in the liver that never progress to hepatocellular carcinoma (HCC) (Takamura et al. 2011). Similarly, in a GEMMs of PDAC, autophagy deficiency promotes the growth of benign Pancreatic intraepithelial neoplasia (PanIN) that do not progress to adenocarcinoma (Yang et al. 2014). These findings suggest that autophagy may have a dual role: blocking tumor initiation and promoting progression to cancer, and while there is evidence for the latter, recurrent mutations in *Atgs* are not found in human cancers. Thus, if autophagy plays a role in prevention of cancer initiation it may be indirect or it may not occur at all as autophagy is required to progress from benign to malignant disease.

Autophagy Inhibits p53-Mediated Tumor Suppression

The *TP53* is the most commonly mutated gene in human cancers. DNA damage and oxidative stress activate p53, leading to cell-cycle arrest, senescence, and apoptosis (Hayes et al. 2020). Overcoming such effects caused by p53 activation is critical for tumorigenesis. p53 is a barrier to *Palb2*-associated mammary tumor growth. Partial autophagy loss due to allelic loss of *Becn1* significantly delays mammary tumor development caused by *Palb2* loss but only when p53 is present, indicating that autophagy suppresses p53 activation to facilitate DNA damage–induced mammary tumorigenesis (Huo et al. 2013). Autophagy supports Kras-driven lung tumorigenesis by inhibiting p53 activation (Guo et al. 2013). However, autophagy also supports lung tumorigenesis independent of p53 suppression (Guo et al. 2013; Strohecker et al. 2013). Autophagy also promotes PDAC independent of p53 status (Yang et al. 2014). These findings suggest that while loss of autophagy can promote p53 activation to suppress tumorigenesis, p53-independent mechanisms also exist.

Cite this article as *Cold Spring Harb Perspect Med* doi: 10.1101/cshperspect.a041539

Autophagy Suppresses Inflammation

The interaction between autophagy, inflammation, and cancer is complex, context-dependent, and mediated by a number of mechanisms (White 2015). A typical inflammatory response in conjunction with the metabolic stress and DNA damage results from production of ROS that occurs in persistent and chronic inflammation contributes to tumorigenesis (Greten et al. 2004; Balkwill et al. 2005; Degenhardt et al. 2006; Mathew et al. 2009; Grivennikov et al. 2010). Autophagy inhibits inflammasome activation and modulates type I interferon responses (White et al. 2010; Deretic et al. 2013). By comparing the global proteome of autophagy-intact and autophagy-deficient Ras-driven cancer cells, autophagy is found to affect levels of the majority of proteins in the proteome. However, the classes of proteins that specifically accumulate when autophagy is defective and that are likely autophagy substrates are not random, indicating that autophagy is selective. Specifically, the proteins involved in the innate immune response preferentially accumulate in autophagy-deficient cells (Mathew et al. 2014). Autophagy also inhibits inflammation through regulation of inflammasome complexes, which are required to process and activate proinflammatory signals such as procaspase 1 or pro-IL-1β (Mathew et al. 2014). Additionally, autophagy is a key regulator of RIP homotypic interaction motif (RHIM) domain proteins, which are molecules important for inflammatory signaling and cell death. Indeed, defective autophagy causes a decrease in turnover in RHIM domain proteins in cells, leading to an increase in necroptosis and inflammatory signaling (Lim et al. 2019). Defective mitochondrial function is associated with accumulation of ROS inside the cell as well as inflammasome activation, suggesting that impaired mitochondrial quality control as a consequence of autophagy inhibition could be another mechanism connecting autophagy and inflammasome activation (Ichinohe et al. 2013).

Autophagy and Metastasis

Unlike its role in supporting primary tumor growth, autophagy plays a complex role in metastases in different types of cancers, which is dependent on the specific metastatic stage (Marsh et al. 2021). Epithelial–mesenchymal transition (EMT) is an important process during tumor metastatic dissemination of solid tumors. Autophagy inhibition suppresses pulmonary metastasis of hepatocellular carcinoma (HCC) in mice via impairing resistance to cell-detachment-induced cell death (anoikis) and colonization of HCC cells (Li et al. 2013; Peng et al. 2013). Autophagy induction impairs migration and invasion by reversing EMT in glioblastoma cells (Catalano et al. 2015). Autophagy in RAS-transformed mammary cancer cells induces tumor cell invasion and lung metastasis through multiple secretory factors including IL-6 (Lock et al. 2014). Inhibition of autophagy promotes metastasis and glycolysis by inducing protective ROS in gastric cancer cells (Qin et al. 2015). ATG4A promotes tumor metastasis by inducing the EMT and stem-like properties in gastric cells (Yang et al. 2016). In breast cancer models, Neighbor to BRCA1 (NBR1), an autophagy cargo receptor, is both necessary and sufficient for pulmonary metastatic colonization and the acquisition of aggressive disease. Genetic ablation of autophagy strongly attenuates primary mammary tumor growth but promotes spontaneous metastasis and enables the outgrowth of disseminated tumor cells into overt macro-metastases. Transcriptomic analysis reveals that accumulation of NBR1 induced by autophagy deficiency potentiates tumor metastasis by potentiating a population of cells with a basal-like state (Marsh et al. 2020). More evidence is needed to establish whether any of these observations are relevant to metastasis of human cancer.

ROLE OF HOST AUTOPHAGY IN CANCER

With an understanding that there are multiple mechanisms by which autophagy promotes cancer growth, survival, and malignancy, this indicates that targeting the autophagy pathway is a novel approach for cancer therapy. Targeting any pathway in cancer requires an understanding that there is a therapeutic window: establishment that cancer cells are preferentially sensitive to pathway inhibition compared to essential normal tissues. It also necessitates developing an understanding of potential toxicities, and if there are any ways to avoid them. To address the role of autophagy in adult mice, GEMMs were developed to delete essential autophagy genes systemically throughout adult mice genetically conditionally to decern the consequences to normal tissues.

Autophagy Is Important for the Function of Some Normal Tissues

Conditional, systemic deletion of the essential autophagy gene, *Atg7*, was surprisingly well tolerated with mice living for several months (Karsli-Uzunbas et al. 2014). An important finding was that not all tissues are equally autophagy dependent. Primarily, there is liver steatosis and neurodegeneration both with associated inflammation. Most remarkably there is depletion of liver glycogen and wasting of fat and muscle that are hallmarks of cachexia (Karsli-Uzunbas et al. 2014), indicative of a systemic metabolic imbalance and inflammatory response to unresolvable damage (Ferrer et al. 2023). In contrast, lung, for example, was largely unaffected. Thus, some tissues are more dependent on autophagy than others, with the hallmarks of autophagy deficiency, inflammation and metabolic impairment including cachexia, being present to varying degrees across the body. Similar findings were made with deletion of other essential autophagy genes (Yang et al. 2020, 2022; White et al. 2021). Interestingly, some of the tissue damage in autophagy-deficient mice is attributed to p53 activation, whereas some protection from damage was provided by *Nrf2* (Yang et al. 2020, 2022; White et al. 2021), the latter of which is also seen as a protective adaptation to loss of autophagy in cancer cell lines in vitro (Towers et al. 2019). LKB1 is also essential for the survival of adult mice and loss of both autophagy and *Lkb1* further diminishes survival. Therefore, autophagy provides some protection in the context of *Lkb1* deficiency to maintain homeostasis and survival in adult mice (Khayati et al. 2020). In conclusion, loss of autophagy at the cellular level in mammals causes a systemic inflammatory and metabolic imbalance that drives cachexia with wasting of the dedicated nutrient stores (liver glycogen, muscle protein, and adipose triglycerides) (Fig. 2).

Autophagy Is Essential for Mice to Survive Fasting

Autophagy recycles intracellular components to sustain survival of cells and animals to nutrient deprivation. A prime example of that is the fasting intolerance of autophagy-deficient adult mice in comparison to wild-type mice with autophagy intact (Karsli-Uzunbas et al. 2014; Yang et al. 2020). Upon fasting, autophagy-deficient mice display accelerated cachexia, fail to maintain circulating glucose levels, and die from hypoglycemia (Karsli-Uzunbas et al. 2014). Interestingly, deletion of p53 protects from this fasting lethality, suggesting that in autophagy-deficient mice, the stress of fasting triggers p53, but the cell types and mechanisms involved are not known (Yang et al. 2020).

Host Autophagy Is Important for Tumor Growth and Survival

Switching autophagy off in mice with Kras-driven lung cancer has pronounced antitumor activity prior to significant damage to normal tissues (Karsli-Uzunbas et al. 2014; Khayati et al. 2022). As there was more antitumor activity with systemic autophagy ablation than with tumor-specific ablation, this suggests that host autophagy also promotes tumor growth. Indeed, half of the tumor cell lines implanted on autophagy-deficient host mice fail to grow, clearly demonstrating a novel role for host autophagy in contributing to tumor growth as well as tumor-cell-autonomous autophagy (Poillet-Perez et al. 2018; Poillet-Perez and White 2019). Similar findings demonstrating that host autophagy promotes tumor growth were also observed in an autochthonous GEMM for PDAC (Yang et al. 2018). The preferential sensitivity of tumors to autophagy inhibition compared with normal tissues is a prerequisite for the use of autophagy inhibitors as cancer therapy. Some tissues, such as the liver, are more dependent on autophagy than others (Karsli-Uzunbas et al. 2014). Toggling Atg5 expression on-off-on in a GEMM

Cite this article as *Cold Spring Harb Perspect Med* doi: 10.1101/cshperspect.a041539

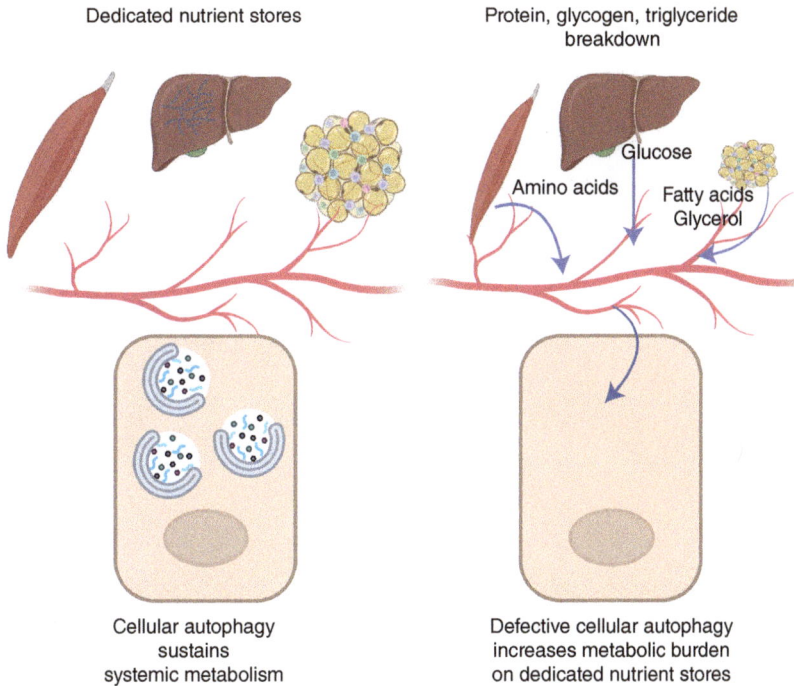

Figure 2. Autophagy in cells in normal tissues preserves dedicated nutrient stores in muscle, liver, and adipose tissue. Systemic conditional autophagy deficiency in adult mice causes a metabolic imbalance that elevates demand for nutrients provided by the dedicated nutrient stores causing cachexia. (Figure generated with BioRender, https://biorender.com.)

for Kras-driven lung cancer revealed that short-term systemic autophagy ablation suppressed tumorigenesis irreversibly, whereas liver injury caused by short-term systemic autophagy inhibition was reversible (Khayati et al. 2022). These findings demonstrate that normal cells and tissues are more tolerant to autophagy inhibition than tumors and that they recover when autophagy is restored, whereas tumors do not.

Host Autophagy Maintains Circulating Arginine Required for Tumor Growth

Since autophagy-deficient mice have a metabolic impairment and inflammation, it was hypothesized that autophagy may promote tumor growth by sustaining essential circulating tumor nutrients or by suppressing inflammation and an antitumor immune response. Both turned out to be true.

Whether a metabolic defect in autophagy-deficient host mice is responsible for defective tumor growth was addressed through serum metabolite profiling, which indicates a striking deficit in circulating arginine (Poillet-Perez et al. 2018). Arginine is an essential tumor nutrient as tumors silence genes for arginine synthesis to devote more carbon to nucleotide synthesis (Poillet-Perez and White 2019). Supplying excess dietary arginine was sufficient to partially rescue tumor growth on autophagy-deficient host mice, demonstrating that a specific metabolic impairment is responsible. The depletion of circulating arginine in autophagy-deficient mice is caused by hepatocytes in the liver secreting Arginase 1 into the circulation, which degrades circulating arginine (Fig. 3; Poillet-Perez et al. 2018). Analogous to immune responses to infection where specific amino acids are depleted as a mechanism to starve pathogens of essential nutrients (e.g., tryptophan) (Zhang and Rubin 2013), similar mechanisms exist and can be used to restrict tumor growth as a novel approach to cancer treatment.

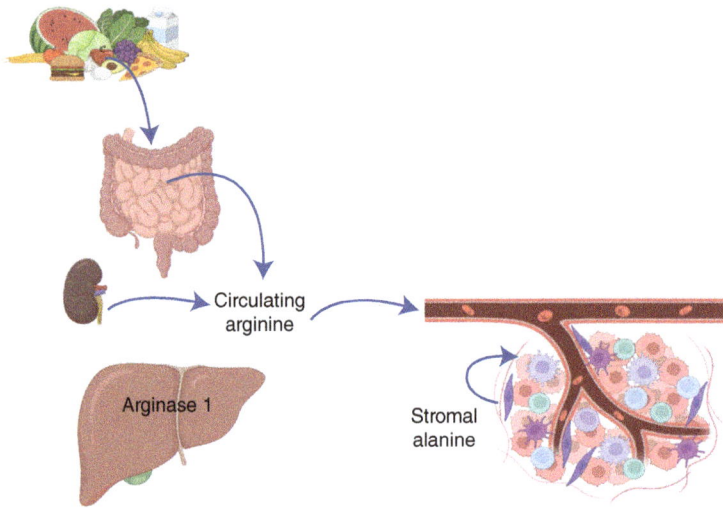

Figure 3. Host autophagy maintains circulating and tumor microenvironment (TME) nutrients essential for tumor growth. Arginine provided by diet and de novo synthesis in the kidney in the host enters the circulation for use by tumors to promote growth and survival. Tumors silence the genes for de novo arginine synthesis and are thereby auxotrophic for arginine and require circulating arginine provided by the host. Autophagy prevents the degradation of circulating arginine and inhibition of tumor growth by inhibiting secretion of Arginase 1 from hepatocytes. Tumor stroma uses autophagy-mediated secretion of alanine to support tumor metabolism and growth. (Figure generated with BioRender, https://biorender.com.)

Autophagy in the Tumor Microenvironment Provides Alanine for Tumor Growth

Provision of essential tumor nutrients through the circulation is not the only mechanism by which host autophagy promotes tumor metabolism and growth. In PDAC, tumor cells make up a minority of the tumor due to tumor cells being surrounded by an expansive desmoplastic stroma that contributes to a hypoxic and nutrient-poor TME. Autophagy in host-derived stromal stellate cells in the TME facilitates secretion of alanine that is used to support tumor metabolism (Fig. 3; Sousa et al. 2016). Tumors use this secreted alanine to fuel TCA cycle metabolism. There is also a similar protumorigenic role for autophagy in stromal fibroblasts in mouse breast cancer models (Rudnick et al. 2021).

Host Autophagy Suppresses Inflammation and an Antitumor T-Cell Response

To test whether inflammation triggered by loss of autophagy in the host suppresses tumor growth, autophagy-competent tumor cells expressing a foreign antigen or with a high mutation burden and high neoantigen load were implanted on wild-type and autophagy-deficient host mice. In contrast to tumors growing on wild-type host mice, those mice deficient for autophagy reject tumors, and eliminating T cells rescues this tumor rejection (Fig. 4; Poillet-Perez et al. 2020). Since autophagy is knocked out in the whole body, this suggests that T cells are functional in the absence of autophagy, at least in the short term of these experiments. Thus, loss of autophagy can stimulate an antitumor T-cell response leading to tumor rejection. This tumor rejection is dependent on stimulator of interferon genes (STING), IFN-γ, and functional antigen presentation (Poillet-Perez et al. 2020). As autophagy eliminates damage-associated molecular patterns (DAMPs) and pathogen-associated molecular patterns (PAMPs) that trigger the innate immune response including activation of interferon α (IFN-α) signaling (Mathew et al. 2014; Yamazaki et al. 2020), loss of autophagy promotes interferon signaling and T-cell activation to eliminate tumors (Fig. 4). Interestingly, the autophagy-driven inflammatory response specifically in the liver is largely respon-

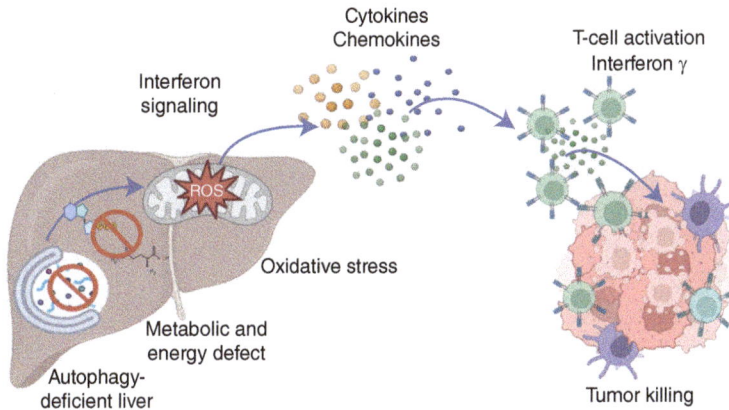

Figure 4. Liver autophagy suppresses inflammation, cytokine production, T-cell activation, and tumor killing by T cells. Inhibition of host and specifically liver autophagy activates interferon signaling and inflammation, which activates T cells and induces tumor killing by T cells. (Figure generated with BioRender, https://biorender.com.)

sible for enhancing tumor immune rejection (Fig. 4; Poillet-Perez et al. 2020). These findings indicate that an antitumor immune response can be elicited by promoting inflammation at a site distant from the tumor.

Host Autophagy Suppresses Effectiveness of Immunotherapy

Autophagy is induced by and is a resistance mechanism to target other forms of cancer therapy (Bryant et al. 2019; Kinsey et al. 2019; Lee et al. 2019; White et al. 2021). Importantly, autophagy is also a resistance mechanism to immunotherapies and autophagy inhibition promotes response to ICB. Autophagy clears MHC class I from the tumor cell surface and autophagy inhibition in PDAC promotes response to ICB (Yamamoto et al. 2020). Pharmacologic inhibition of autophagy also shows promise in enhancing response to ICB through inflammatory mechanisms (Noman et al. 2020; Sharma et al. 2020). The next generation of highly potent and selective small-molecule autophagy inhibitors are in development and are being explored as single agents and in combination to enhance cancer therapy.

CONCLUDING REMARKS

In conclusion, autophagy is a pro-metabolic and anti-inflammatory protective mechanism for normal cells and tissues that tumors usurp to promote their own growth, survival, and malignancy. Autophagy promotes tumorigenesis in the tumor cells themselves, systemically in the host and in the local TME. Tumor cells are more dependent on autophagy than most normal tissues due to a need for metabolic support and immune evasion, and the inability to recover from damage, indicating that there is a therapeutic window. While autophagy is a protective mechanism for normal tissues, if it is tumor suppressive, in this way it may be indirect. Autophagy is a resistance mechanism to cancer therapy including immunotherapy, and harnessing autophagy inhibition for cancer therapy shows great promise. Further determination of the biological role for autophagy in both normal tissues and in tumors that derive from them, and in the context of different driver mutations, will identify how and where deploying this strategy will be most useful.

ACKNOWLEDGMENTS

We thank the Guo and White laboratories for helpful comments and discussions. E.W. is a co-founder of Vescor Therapeutics and receives research funding from Deciphera Pharmaceuticals. Funding sources are R01CA237347, R21CA263136, ACS 134036-RSG-19-165-01-TBG, GO2 Foundation for Lung Cancer, and

Ludwig Princeton Branch of the Ludwig Institute for Cancer Research to J.Y.G. R01CA163591, and Ludwig Princeton Branch of the Ludwig Institute for Cancer Research, NCI 1OT2CA278609-01, and CRUK (CGCATF-2021/100022) to E.W.

REFERENCES

Balkwill F, Charles KA, Mantovani A. 2005. Smoldering and polarized inflammation in the initiation and promotion of malignant disease. *Cancer Cell* **7**: 211–217. doi:10.1016/j.ccr.2005.02.013

Beatty GL, Gladney WL. 2015. Immune escape mechanisms as a guide for cancer immunotherapy. *Clin Cancer Res* **21**: 687–692. doi:10.1158/1078-0432.CCR-14-1860

Bhatt V, Khayati K, Hu ZS, Lee A, Kamran W, Su X, Guo JY. 2019. Autophagy modulates lipid metabolism to maintain metabolic flexibility for *Lkb1*-deficient *Kras*-driven lung tumorigenesis. *Genes Dev* **33**: 150–165. doi:10.1101/gad.320481.118

Bryant KL, Stalnecker CA, Zeitouni D, Klomp JE, Peng S, Tikunov AP, Gunda V, Pierobon M, Waters AM, George SD, et al. 2019. Combination of ERK and autophagy inhibition as a treatment approach for pancreatic cancer. *Nat Med* **25**: 628–640. doi:10.1038/s41591-019-0368-8

Catalano M, D'Alessandro G, Lepore F, Corazzari M, Caldarola S, Valacca C, Faienza F, Esposito V, Limatola C, Cecconi F, et al. 2015. Autophagy induction impairs migration and invasion by reversing EMT in glioblastoma cells. *Mol Oncol* **9**: 1612–1625. doi:10.1016/j.molonc.2015.04.016

Crotzer VL, Blum JS. 2009. Autophagy and its role in MHC-mediated antigen presentation. *J Immunol* **182**: 3335–3341. doi:10.4049/jimmunol.0803458

Degenhardt K, Mathew R, Beaudoin B, Bray K, Anderson D, Chen G, Mukherjee C, Shi Y, Gélinas C, Fan Y, et al. 2006. Autophagy promotes tumor cell survival and restricts necrosis, inflammation, and tumorigenesis. *Cancer Cell* **10**: 51–64. doi:10.1016/j.ccr.2006.06.001

Deng J, Thennavan A, Dolgalev I, Chen T, Li J, Marzio A, Poirier JT, Peng DH, Bulatovic M, Mukhopadhyay S, et al. 2021. ULK1 inhibition overcomes compromised antigen presentation and restores antitumor immunity in LKB1-mutant lung cancer. *Nat Cancer* **2**: 503–514. doi:10.1038/s43018-021-00208-6

Deretic V, Saitoh T, Akira S. 2013. Autophagy in infection, inflammation and immunity. *Nat Rev Immunol* **13**: 722–737. doi:10.1038/nri3532

Ferrer M, Anthony TG, Ayres JS, Biffi G, Brown JC, Caan BJ, Cespedes Feliciano EM, Coll AP, Dunne RF, Goncalves MD, et al. 2023. Cachexia: a systemic consequence of progressive, unresolved disease. *Cell* **186**: 1824–1845. doi:10.1016/j.cell.2023.03.028

Gammoh N, Fraser J, Puente C, Syred HM, Kang H, Ozawa T, Lam D, Acosta JC, Finch AJ, Holland E, et al. 2016. Suppression of autophagy impedes glioblastoma development and induces senescence. *Autophagy* **12**: 1431–1439. doi:10.1080/15548627.2016.1190053

Greten FR, Eckmann L, Greten TF, Park JM, Li ZW, Egan LJ, Kagnoff MF, Karin M. 2004. IKKβ links inflammation and tumorigenesis in a mouse model of colitis-associated cancer. *Cell* **118**: 285–296. doi:10.1016/j.cell.2004.07.013

Grivennikov SI, Greten FR, Karin M. 2010. Immunity, inflammation, and cancer. *Cell* **140**: 883–899. doi:10.1016/j.cell.2010.01.025

Guo JY, White E. 2016. Autophagy, metabolism, and cancer. *Cold Spring Harb Symp Quant Biol* **81**: 73–78. doi:10.1101/sqb.2016.81.030981

Guo JY, Chen HY, Mathew R, Fan J, Strohecker AM, Karsli-Uzunbas G, Kamphorst JJ, Chen G, Lemons JM, Karantza V, et al. 2011. Activated Ras requires autophagy to maintain oxidative metabolism and tumorigenesis. *Genes Dev* **25**: 460–470. doi:10.1101/gad.2016311

Guo JY, Karsli-Uzunbas G, Mathew R, Aisner SC, Kamphorst JJ, Strohecker AM, Chen G, Price S, Lu W, Teng X, et al. 2013. Autophagy suppresses progression of K-ras-induced lung tumors to oncocytomas and maintains lipid homeostasis. *Genes Dev* **27**: 1447–1461. doi:10.1101/gad.219642.113

Guo JY, Teng X, Laddha SV, Ma S, Van Nostrand SC, Yang Y, Khor S, Chan CS, Rabinowitz JD, White E. 2016. Autophagy provides metabolic substrates to maintain energy charge and nucleotide pools in Ras-driven lung cancer cells. *Genes Dev* **30**: 1704–1717. doi:10.1101/gad.283416.116

Hanahan D, Weinberg RA. 2011. Hallmarks of cancer: the next generation. *Cell* **144**: 646–674. doi:10.1016/j.cell.2011.02.013

Hayes JD, Dinkova-Kostova AT, Tew KD. 2020. Oxidative stress in cancer. *Cancer Cell* **38**: 167–197. doi:10.1016/j.ccell.2020.06.001

He C, Bassik MC, Moresi V, Sun K, Wei Y, Zou Z, An Z, Loh J, Fisher J, Sun Q, et al. 2012. Exercise-induced BCL2-regulated autophagy is required for muscle glucose homeostasis. *Nature* **481**: 511–515. doi:10.1038/nature10758

Humpton TJ, Alagesan B, DeNicola GM, Lu D, Yordanov GN, Leonhardt CS, Yao MA, Alagesan P, Zaatari MN, Park Y, et al. 2019. Oncogenic KRAS induces NIX-mediated mitophagy to promote pancreatic cancer. *Cancer Discov* **9**: 1268–1287. doi:10.1158/2159-8290.CD-18-1409

Huo Y, Cai H, Teplova I, Bowman-Colin C, Chen G, Price S, Barnard N, Ganesan S, Karantza V, White E, et al. 2013. Autophagy opposes p53-mediated tumor barrier to facilitate tumorigenesis in a model of *PALB2*-associated hereditary breast cancer. *Cancer Discov* **3**: 894–907. doi:10.1158/2159-8290.CD-13-0011

Ichinohe T, Yamazaki T, Koshiba T, Yanagi Y. 2013. Mitochondrial protein mitofusin 2 is required for NLRP3 inflammasome activation after RNA virus infection. *Proc Natl Acad Sci* **110**: 17963–17968. doi:10.1073/pnas.1312571110

Jeon SM, Chandel NS, Hay N. 2012. AMPK regulates NADPH homeostasis to promote tumour cell survival during energy stress. *Nature* **485**: 661–665. doi:10.1038/nature11066

Karantza-Wadsworth V, Patel S, Kravchuk O, Chen G, Mathew R, Jin S, White E. 2007. Autophagy mitigates metabolic stress and genome damage in mammary tumorigenesis. *Genes Dev* **21**: 1621–1635. doi:10.1101/gad.1565707

Karsli-Uzunbas G, Guo JY, Price S, Teng X, Laddha SV, Khor S, Kalaany NY, Jacks T, Chan CS, Rabinowitz JD, et al.

2014. Autophagy is required for glucose homeostasis and lung tumor maintenance. *Cancer Discov* **4**: 914–927. doi:10.1158/2159-8290.CD-14-0363

Khayati K, Bhatt V, Hu ZS, Fahumy S, Luo X, Guo JY. 2020. Autophagy compensates for Lkb1 loss to maintain adult mice homeostasis and survival. *eLife* **9**: e62377. doi:10.7554/eLife.62377

Khayati K, Bhatt V, Lan T, Alogaili F, Wang W, Lopez E, Hu ZS, Gokhale S, Cassidy L, Narita M, et al. 2022. Transient systemic autophagy inhibition is selectively and irreversibly deleterious to lung cancer. *Cancer Res* **82**: 4429–4443. doi:10.1158/0008-5472.CAN-22-1039

Kinsey CG, Camolotto SA, Boespflug AM, Guillen KP, Foth M, Truong A, Schuman SS, Shea JE, Seipp MT, Yap JT, et al. 2019. Protective autophagy elicited by RAF→MEK→ERK inhibition suggests a treatment strategy for RAS-driven cancers. *Nat Med* **25**: 620–627. doi:10.1038/s41591-019-0367-9

Kloetzel PM. 2001. Antigen processing by the proteasome. *Nat Rev Mol Cell Biol* **2**: 179–187. doi:10.1038/35056572

Labuschagne CF, Cheung EC, Blagih J, Domart MC, Vousden KH. 2019. Cell clustering promotes a metabolic switch that supports metastatic colonization. *Cell Metab* **30**: 720–734.e5. doi:10.1016/j.cmet.2019.07.014

Laddha SV, Ganesan S, Chan CS, White E. 2014. Mutational landscape of the essential autophagy gene *BECN1* in human cancers. *Mol Cancer Res* **12**: 485–490. doi:10.1158/1541-7786.MCR-13-0614

Lashinger LM, O'Flanagan CH, Dunlap SM, Rasmussen AJ, Sweeney S, Guo JY, Lodi A, Tiziani S, White E, Hursting SD. 2016. Starving cancer from the outside and inside: separate and combined effects of calorie restriction and autophagy inhibition on Ras-driven tumors. *Cancer Metab* **4**: 18. doi:10.1186/s40170-016-0158-4

Lawson KA, Sousa CM, Zhang X, Kim E, Akthar R, Caumanns JJ, Yao Y, Mikolajewicz N, Ross C, Brown KR, et al. 2020. Functional genomic landscape of cancer-intrinsic evasion of killing by T cells. *Nature* **586**: 120–126. doi:10.1038/s41586-020-2746-2

Lee CS, Lee LC, Yuan TL, Chakka S, Fellmann C, Lowe SW, Caplen NJ, McCormick F, Luo J. 2019. MAP kinase and autophagy pathways cooperate to maintain RAS mutant cancer cell survival. *Proc Natl Acad Sci* **116**: 4508–4517. doi:10.1073/pnas.1817494116

Lévy J, Romagnolo B. 2015. Autophagy, microbiota and intestinal oncogenesis. *Oncotarget* **6**: 34067–34068. doi:10.18632/oncotarget.5966

Lévy J, Cacheux W, Bara MA, L'Hermitte A, Lepage P, Fraudeau M, Trentesaux C, Lemarchand J, Durand A, Crain AM, et al. 2015. Intestinal inhibition of Atg7 prevents tumour initiation through a microbiome-influenced immune response and suppresses tumour growth. *Nat Cell Biol* **17**: 1062–1073. doi:10.1038/ncb3206

Li J, Yang B, Zhou Q, Wu Y, Shang D, Guo Y, Song Z, Zheng Q, Xiong J. 2013. Autophagy promotes hepatocellular carcinoma cell invasion through activation of epithelial-mesenchymal transition. *Carcinogenesis* **34**: 1343–1351. doi:10.1093/carcin/bgt063

Lim J, Park H, Heisler J, Maculins T, Roose-Girma M, Xu M, McKenzie B, van Lookeren Campagne M, Newton K, Murthy A. 2019. Autophagy regulates inflammatory pro-

grammed cell death via turnover of RHIM-domain proteins. *eLife* **8**: e44452. doi:10.7554/eLife.44452

Liu GY, Sabatini DM. 2020. mTOR at the nexus of nutrition, growth, ageing and disease. *Nat Rev Mol Cell Biol* **21**: 183–203. doi:10.1038/s41580-019-0199-y

Liu EY, Xu N, O'Prey J, Lao LY, Joshi S, Long JS, O'Prey M, Croft DR, Beaumatin F, Baudot AD, et al. 2015. Loss of autophagy causes a synthetic lethal deficiency in DNA repair. *Proc Natl Acad Sci* **112**: 773–778. doi:10.1073/pnas.1409563112

Lock R, Kenific CM, Leidal AM, Salas E, Debnath J. 2014. Autophagy-dependent production of secreted factors facilitates oncogenic RAS-driven invasion. *Cancer Discov* **4**: 466–479. doi:10.1158/2159-8290.CD-13-0841

López-Soto A, Bravo-San Pedro JM, Kroemer G, Galluzzi L, Gonzalez S. 2017. Involvement of autophagy in NK cell development and function. *Autophagy* **13**: 633–636. doi:10.1080/15548627.2016.1274486

Mancias JD, Wang X, Gygi SP, Harper JW, Kimmelman AC. 2014. Quantitative proteomics identifies NCOA4 as the cargo receptor mediating ferritinophagy. *Nature* **509**: 105–109. doi:10.1038/nature13148

Marsh T, Kenific CM, Suresh D, Gonzalez H, Shamir ER, Mei W, Tankka A, Leidal AM, Kalavacherla S, Woo K, et al. 2020. Autophagic degradation of NBR1 restricts metastatic outgrowth during mammary tumor progression. *Dev Cell* **52**: 591–604.e6. doi:10.1016/j.devcel.2020.01.025

Marsh T, Tolani B, Debnath J. 2021. The pleiotropic functions of autophagy in metastasis. *J Cell Sci* **134**: jcs247056. doi:10.1242/jcs.247056

Mathew R, Kongara S, Beaudoin B, Karp CM, Bray K, Degenhardt K, Chen G, Jin S, White E. 2007. Autophagy suppresses tumor progression by limiting chromosomal instability. *Genes Dev* **21**: 1367–1381. doi:10.1101/gad.1545107

Mathew R, Karp CM, Beaudoin B, Vuong N, Chen G, Chen HY, Bray K, Reddy A, Bhanot G, Gelinas C, et al. 2009. Autophagy suppresses tumorigenesis through elimination of p62. *Cell* **137**: 1062–1075. doi:10.1016/j.cell.2009.03.048

Mathew R, Khor S, Hackett SR, Rabinowitz JD, Perlman DH, White E. 2014. Functional role of autophagy-mediated proteome remodeling in cell survival signaling and innate immunity. *Mol Cell* **55**: 916–930. doi:10.1016/j.molcel.2014.07.019

Mukhopadhyay S, Biancur DE, Parker SJ, Yamamoto K, Banh RS, Paulo JA, Mancias JD, Kimmelman AC. 2021. Autophagy is required for proper cysteine homeostasis in pancreatic cancer through regulation of SLC7A11. *Proc Natl Acad Sci* **118**: e2021475118. doi:10.1073/pnas.2021475118

Noman MZ, Parpal S, Van Moer K, Xiao M, Yu Y, Viklund J, De Milito A, Hasmim M, Andersson M, Amaravadi RK, et al. 2020. Inhibition of Vps34 reprograms cold into hot inflamed tumors and improves anti-PD-1/PD-L1 immunotherapy. *Sci Adv* **6**: eaax7881. doi:10.1126/sciadv.aax7881

Okamoto T, Yeo SK, Hao M, Copley MR, Haas MA, Chen S, Guan JL. 2020. FIP200 suppresses immune checkpoint therapy responses in breast cancers by limiting AZI2/TBK1/IRF signaling independent of its canonical autophagy function. *Cancer Res* **80**: 3580–3592. doi:10.1158/0008-5472.CAN-20-0519

Parker SJ, Svensson RU, Divakaruni AS, Lefebvre AE, Murphy AN, Shaw RJ, Metallo CM. 2017. LKB1 promotes metabolic flexibility in response to energy stress. *Metab Eng* **43:** 208–217. doi:10.1016/j.ymben.2016.12.010

Peng YF, Shi YH, Ding ZB, Ke AW, Gu CY, Hui B, Zhou J, Qiu SJ, Dai Z, Fan J. 2013. Autophagy inhibition suppresses pulmonary metastasis of HCC in mice via impairing anoikis resistance and colonization of HCC cells. *Autophagy* **9:** 2056–2068. doi:10.4161/auto.26398

Perera RM, Stoykova S, Nicolay BN, Ross KN, Fitamant J, Boukhali M, Lengrand J, Deshpande V, Selig MK, Ferrone CR, et al. 2015. Transcriptional control of autophagy–lysosome function drives pancreatic cancer metabolism. *Nature* **524:** 361–365. doi:10.1038/nature14587

Perera RM, Di Malta C, Ballabio A. 2019. Mit/TFE family of transcription factors, lysosomes, and cancer. *Annu Rev Cancer Biol* **3:** 203–222. doi:10.1146/annurev-cancerbio-030518-055835

Pietrocola F, Bravo-San Pedro JM, Galluzzi L, Kroemer G. 2017. Autophagy in natural and therapy-driven anticancer immunosurveillance. *Autophagy* **13:** 2163–2170. doi:10.1080/15548627.2017.1310356

Poillet-Perez L, White E. 2019. Role of tumor and host autophagy in cancer metabolism. *Genes Dev* **33:** 610–619. doi:10.1101/gad.325514.119

Poillet-Perez L, Xie X, Zhan L, Yang Y, Sharp DW, Hu ZS, Su X, Maganti A, Jiang C, Lu W, et al. 2018. Autophagy maintains tumour growth through circulating arginine. *Nature* **563:** 569–573. doi:10.1038/s41586-018-0697-7

Poillet-Perez L, Sharp DW, Yang Y, Laddha SV, Ibrahim M, Bommareddy PK, Hu ZS, Vieth J, Haas M, Bosenberg MW, et al. 2020. Autophagy promotes growth of tumors with high mutational burden by inhibiting a T-cell immune response. *Nat Cancer* **1:** 923–934. doi:10.1038/s43018-020-00110-7

Qin W, Li C, Zheng W, Guo Q, Zhang Y, Kang M, Zhang B, Yang B, Li B, Yang H, et al. 2015. Inhibition of autophagy promotes metastasis and glycolysis by inducing ROS in gastric cancer cells. *Oncotarget* **6:** 39839–39854. doi:10.18632/oncotarget.5674

Rao S, Tortola L, Perlot T, Wirnsberger G, Novatchkova M, Nitsch R, Sykacek P, Frank L, Schramek D, Komnenovic V, et al. 2014. A dual role for autophagy in a murine model of lung cancer. *Nat Commun* **5:** 3056. doi:10.1038/ncomms4056

Ravichandran M, Hu J, Cai C, Ward NP, Venida A, Foakes C, Kuljanin M, Yang A, Hennessey CJ, Yang Y, et al. 2022. Coordinated transcriptional and catabolic programs support iron-dependent adaptation to RAS–MAPK pathway inhibition in pancreatic cancer. *Cancer Discov* **12:** 2198–2219. doi:10.1158/2159-8290.CD-22-0044

Rudnick JA, Monkkonen T, Mar FA, Barnes JM, Starobinets H, Goldsmith J, Roy S, Bustamante Eguiguren S, Weaver VM, Debnath J. 2021. Autophagy in stromal fibroblasts promotes tumor desmoplasia and mammary tumorigenesis. *Genes Dev* **35:** 963–975. doi:10.1101/gad.345629.120

Santana-Codina N, Del Rey MQ, Kapner KS, Zhang H, Gikandi A, Malcolm C, Poupault C, Kuljanin M, John KM, Biancur DE, et al. 2022. NCOA4-mediated ferritinophagy is a pancreatic cancer dependency via maintenance of iron bioavailability for iron–sulfur cluster proteins. *Cancer Discov* **12:** 2180–2197. doi:10.1158/2159-8290.CD-22-0043

Santanam U, Banach-Petrosky W, Abate-Shen C, Shen MM, White E, DiPaola RS. 2016. *Atg7* cooperates with *Pten* loss to drive prostate cancer tumor growth. *Genes Dev* **30:** 399–407. doi:10.1101/gad.274134.115

Schumacher TN, Scheper W, Kvistborg P. 2019. Cancer neoantigens. *Annu Rev Immunol* **37:** 173–200. doi:10.1146/annurev-immunol-042617-053402

Shabkhizan R, Haiaty S, Moslehian MS, Bazmani A, Sadeghsoltani F, Saghaei Bagheri H, Rahbarghazi R, Sakhinia E. 2023. The beneficial and adverse effects of autophagic response to caloric restriction and fasting. *Adv Nutr* **14:** 1211–1225. doi:10.1016/j.advnut.2023.07.006

Sharma G, Ojha R, Noguera-Ortega E, Rebecca VW, Attanasio J, Liu S, Piao S, Lee JJ, Nicastri MC, Harper SL, et al. 2020. PPT1 inhibition enhances the antitumor activity of anti-PD-1 antibody in melanoma. *JCI Insight* **5:** e133225. doi:10.1172/jci.insight.133225

Sousa CM, Biancur DE, Wang X, Halbrook CJ, Sherman MH, Zhang L, Kremer D, Hwang RF, Witkiewicz AK, Ying H, et al. 2016. Pancreatic stellate cells support tumour metabolism through autophagic alanine secretion. *Nature* **536:** 479–483. doi:10.1038/nature19084

Strohecker AM, Guo JY, Karsli-Uzunbas G, Price SM, Chen GJ, Mathew R, McMahon M, White E. 2013. Autophagy sustains mitochondrial glutamine metabolism and growth of *Braf*V600E-driven lung tumors. *Cancer Discov* **3:** 1272–1285. doi:10.1158/2159-8290.CD-13-0397

Svensson RU, Shaw RJ. 2016. Lipid synthesis is a metabolic liability of non-small cell lung cancer. *Cold Spring Harb Symp Quant Biol* **81:** 93–103. doi:10.1101/sqb.2016.81.030874

Svensson RU, Parker SJ, Eichner LJ, Kolar MJ, Wallace M, Brun SN, Lombardo PS, Van Nostrand JL, Hutchins A, Vera L, et al. 2016. Inhibition of acetyl-CoA carboxylase suppresses fatty acid synthesis and tumor growth of non-small-cell lung cancer in preclinical models. *Nat Med* **22:** 1108–1119. doi:10.1038/nm.4181

Takamura A, Komatsu M, Hara T, Sakamoto A, Kishi C, Waguri S, Eishi Y, Hino O, Tanaka K, Mizushima N. 2011. Autophagy-deficient mice develop multiple liver tumors. *Genes Dev* **25:** 795–800. doi:10.1101/gad.2016211

Towers CG, Fitzwalter BE, Regan D, Goodspeed A, Morgan MJ, Liu CW, Gustafson DL, Thorburn A. 2019. Cancer cells upregulate NRF2 signaling to adapt to autophagy inhibition. *Dev Cell* **50:** 690–703.e6. doi:10.1016/j.devcel.2019.07.010

Villalba M, Rathore MG, Lopez-Royuela N, Krzywinska E, Garaude J, Allende-Vega N. 2013. From tumor cell metabolism to tumor immune escape. *Int J Biochem Cell Biol* **45:** 106–113. doi:10.1016/j.biocel.2012.04.024

Wei H, Wei S, Gan B, Peng X, Zou W, Guan JL. 2011. Suppression of autophagy by FIP200 deletion inhibits mammary tumorigenesis. *Genes Dev* **25:** 1510–1527. doi:10.1101/gad.2051011

White E. 2015. The role for autophagy in cancer. *J Clin Invest* **125:** 42–46. doi:10.1172/JCI73941

White E, Karp C, Strohecker AM, Guo Y, Mathew R. 2010. Role of autophagy in suppression of inflammation and cancer. *Curr Opin Cell Biol* **22:** 212–217. doi:10.1016/j.ceb.2009.12.008

White E, Lattime EC, Guo JY. 2021. Autophagy regulates stress responses, metabolism, and anticancer immunity.

Trends Cancer **7**: 778–789. doi:10.1016/j.trecan.2021.05
.003

Wong PM, Puente C, Ganley IG, Jiang X. 2013. The ULK1
complex: sensing nutrient signals for autophagy activation. *Autophagy* **9**: 124–137. doi:10.4161/auto.23323

Xie X, Koh JY, Price S, White E, Mehnert JM. 2015. *Atg7*
overcomes senescence and promotes growth of
*Braf*V600E-driven melanoma. *Cancer Discov* **5**: 410–
423. doi:10.1158/2159-8290.CD-14-1473

Yamamoto K, Venida A, Yano J, Biancur DE, Kakiuchi M,
Gupta S, Sohn ASW, Mukhopadhyay S, Lin EY, Parker SJ,
et al. 2020. Autophagy promotes immune evasion of pancreatic cancer by degrading MHC-I. *Nature* **581**: 100–105.
doi:10.1038/s41586-020-2229-5

Yamazaki T, Kirchmair A, Sato A, Buqué A, Rybstein M,
Petroni G, Bloy N, Finotello F, Stafford L, Navarro Manzano E, et al. 2020. Mitochondrial DNA drives abscopal
responses to radiation that are inhibited by autophagy. *Nat
Immunol* **21**: 1160–1171. doi:10.1038/s41590-020-0751-0

Yang S, Wang X, Contino G, Liesa M, Sahin E, Ying H, Bause
A, Li Y, Stommel JM, Dell'antonio G, et al. 2011. Pancreatic
cancers require autophagy for tumor growth. *Genes Dev*
25: 717–729. doi:10.1101/gad.2016111

Yang A, Rajeshkumar NV, Wang X, Yabuuchi S, Alexander
BM, Chu GC, Von Hoff DD, Maitra A, Kimmelman AC.
2014. Autophagy is critical for pancreatic tumor growth

and progression in tumors with p53 alterations. *Cancer
Discov* **4**: 905–913. doi:10.1158/2159-8290.CD-14-0362

Yang SW, Ping YF, Jiang YX, Luo X, Zhang X, Bian XW, Yu
PW. 2016. ATG4A promotes tumor metastasis by inducing the epithelial-mesenchymal transition and stem-like
properties in gastric cells. *Oncotarget* **7**: 39279–39292.
doi:10.18632/oncotarget.9827

Yang A, Herter-Sprie G, Zhang H, Lin EY, Biancur D, Wang
X, Deng J, Hai J, Yang S, Wong KK, et al. 2018. Autophagy
sustains pancreatic cancer growth through both cell-autonomous and nonautonomous mechanisms. *Cancer Discov* **8**: 276–287. doi:10.1158/2159-8290.CD-17-0952

Yang Y, Karsli-Uzunbas G, Poillet-Perez L, Sawant A, Hu ZS,
Zhao Y, Moore D, Hu W, White E. 2020. Autophagy promotes mammalian survival by suppressing oxidative stress
and p53. *Genes Dev* **34**: 688–700. doi:10.1101/gad.335570
.119

Yang Y, Gomez M, Marsh T, Poillet-Perez L, Sawant A, Chen
L, Park NR, Jackson SR, Hu Z, Alon N, et al. 2022. Autophagy in PDGFRα⁺ mesenchymal cells is essential for
intestinal stem cell survival. *Proc Natl Acad Sci* **119**:
e2202016119. doi:10.1073/pnas.2202016119

Zhang YJ, Rubin EJ. 2013. Feast or famine: the host-pathogen
battle over amino acids. *Cell Microbiol* **15**: 1079–1087.
doi:10.1111/cmi.12140

Immunometabolic Maladaptations to the Tumor Microenvironment

Emma S. Hathaway,[1,4] Erin Q. Jennings,[2,4] and Jeffrey C. Rathmell[1,3]

[1]Department of Pathology, Microbiology, and Immunology; [2]Department of Medicine; [3]Vanderbilt Center for Immunobiology, Vanderbilt University Medical Center, Nashville, Tennessee 37232, USA

Correspondence: jeff.rathmell@vumc.org

Tumors consist of cancer cells and a wide range of tissue resident and infiltrating cell types. Tumor metabolism, however, has largely been studied on whole tumors or cancer cells and the metabolism of infiltrating immune cells remains poorly understood. It is now clear from a range of analyses and metabolite rescue studies that metabolic adaptations to the tumor microenvironment (TME) directly impede T-cell and macrophage effector functions. The drivers of metabolic adaptation to the TME and metabolic immune suppression include depletion of essential nutrients, accumulation of waste products or immune suppression metabolites, and metabolic signaling through altered posttranslational modifications. Each infiltrating immune cell subset differs, however, with specific metabolic requirements and adaptations that can be maladaptive for antitumor immunity. Here, we review T-cell and macrophage adaptation and metabolic immune suppression in solid tumors. Ultimately, understanding and addressing these challenges will improve cancer immunotherapy and adoptive chimeric antigen receptor T-cell therapies.

Hanahan and Weinberg first described six hallmarks of cancer in 2000. These have since been expanded to 14, and now include hallmarks for an ability to evade the immune system and deregulation of metabolism (Hanahan 2022). It has become increasingly appreciated that these two new cancer hallmarks are closely linked. While the immune system is designed to recognize foreign or new antigens and damaged tissues, transformation-induced changes to cancer cell metabolism can directly impair this process to contribute to tumor immune evasion. In addition to the disruption of normal tissue structures that ordinarily facilitate immune surveillance for new or mutated antigens in growing tumors, the tumor microenvironment (TME) reflects the metabolic impact of cancer cells. Given the need of activated immune cells for increased nutrient uptake and metabolic reprogramming to support proliferation and effector functions, the TME can offer a hostile environment that prevents metabolic events essential for

---

[4]These authors contributed equally to this work.

immune-mediated tumor killing (Bader et al. 2020). How T cells and macrophages respond to metabolic challenges in the TME and confront metabolic immune suppression can thus place severe limits to antitumor immunity.

While metabolic adaptations of T cells and macrophages to local conditions in the TME may have some benefits to preserve cell viability and avoid processes including activation or restimulation-induced cell death, these adaptations more generally suppress inflammatory immune function and are maladaptive for immune efforts to eliminate cancers (ElTanbouly and Noelle 2021). Both T cells and antigen presenting cells are impaired (McLane et al. 2019; Yang et al. 2023). Given the association of mutational burden with immunotherapy response (Jardim et al. 2021), understanding the nature of metabolic stresses and adaptations of immune cell types in the TME is now critical to improve immune therapies and fully harness the potential of antitumor immunity. These stresses include chronic antigen exposure in large solid tumors that would induce tolerance in normal tissues, tumor-induced changes in tissue architecture, tumor genetics and neoantigen availability, and poor vasculature that cause key nutrients to be depleted and waste products to accumulate. These changes affect signaling, metabolism, and ultimately the antigen presentation and inflammatory functions of tumor-infiltrating immune cells (Fig. 1). Here we review how key immune cell populations adapt and are shaped by stress in the TME in ways that are maladaptive for antitumor immunity.

METABOLIC STRESSES AND MODIFIERS IN THE TME

Nutrient Availability and Competition

The TME presents a complex milieu of many different metabolically active cell types that may compete for limited resources as tumors grow. One hundred years ago, Warburg (1956) proposed cancer cells consume glucose at high rates due to mitochondrial defects. This glycolytic phenotype has provided the rationale for ^{18}F-2-deoxyglucose positron emission tomogra-

phy (PET) for tumor imaging for diagnosis and monitoring. However, Warburg's cancer cell metabolism studies did not consider tumor cell heterogeneity in tumors and PET imaging offers only tissue-level resolution. The contributions of individual cells and various heterogeneous cell types to tumor metabolism have remained largely unclear within the overall TME. Like cancer cells, stimulated immune cells rapidly up-regulate glucose uptake and glycolysis. If vascular exchange in the TME is insufficient to efficiently renew nutrients and remove waste, this may result in an imbalance of glucose consumption and replenishment.

In principle, limited glucose could result in competition between cancer and immune cells for this critical nutrient (Pavlova and Thompson 2016). Indeed, targeted glucose restriction or deletion of the glucose transporter, Glut1, reduces mTORC1 activity and glycolytic capacity in T cells, which blunts interferon γ (IFN-γ) production and effector function (Macintyre et al. 2014; Chang et al. 2015). Decreased glycolysis also reduces availability of the glycolytic metabolite phosphoenolpyruvate (PEP), an important metabolite for sustaining T-cell receptor (TCR)-mediated activation of calcium, nuclear factor of activated T-cell (NFAT) signaling, and ultimately effector function (Ho et al. 2015). In contrast to the Warburg model that presumes cancer cells account for altered metabolism in the tumor as a whole, however, fractionation of cells following infusion of the PET tracer ^{18}F-2-deoxyglucose revealed that tumor-associated macrophages (TAMs), rather than cancer cells, are the predominant consumers of glucose in the TME (Reinfeld et al. 2021). These findings are consistent with proteomics studies showing high expression of glycolytic enzymes in TAMs) (Liu et al. 2017). Importantly, the ability of immune cells to take up glucose was not limited by glucose availability (Reinfeld et al. 2021). Blockade of glutamine uptake within tumors led to increased glucose uptake in all tumor cell types. These data do not preclude locally limiting glucose levels, such as in hypoxic or necrotic tumor regions, but do demonstrate glucose uptake within tumors is not widely capped by availability to glucose itself. Glucose uptake is instead controlled

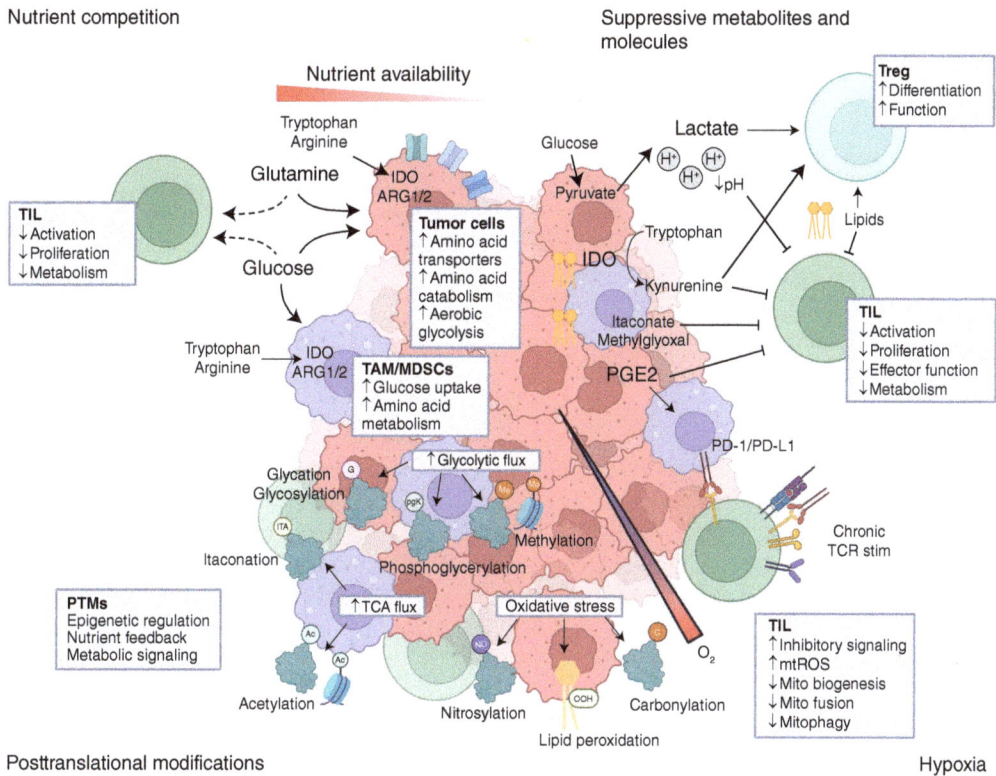

Figure 1. Metabolic stresses in the tumor microenvironment (TME). The TME of solid tumors is characterized by nutrient competition, accumulation of metabolic waste products and immunosuppressive molecules, metabolic feedback by posttranslational modifications (PTMs), and hypoxic regions that contribute to metabolic reprogramming of infiltrating immune cells to both promote tumor progression and suppress antitumor immunity. (ARG1/2) Arginase 1/arginase 2, (IDO) indoleamine 2,3-dioxygenase, (MDSC) myeloid-derived suppressor cell, (Mito) mitochondrial, (mtROS) mitochondrial reactive oxygen species, (PD-1/PD-L1) programmed death 1/programmed death-ligand 1, (PGE2) prostaglandin E2, (TAM) tumor-associated macrophage, (TCR) T-cell receptor, (TIL) tumor-infiltrating lymphocyte, (Treg) regulatory T cell.

by cell-intrinsic metabolic programing within the TME.

Both cancer cells and immune cells rely on amino acid uptake and metabolism. Cancer cells up-regulate multiple transporters to uptake and utilize amino acids, creating potential competition between immune cells for amino acids within the TME (Lieu et al. 2020). In addition to essential amino acids, which must be obtained through diet and transport into cells, amino acids such as glutamine can be conditionally essential and require uptake if synthesis fails to meet demand. Indeed, observations of increased cellular glucose uptake following inhibition of glutamine uptake suggests glutamine uptake in tumors is

limiting in vivo (Reinfeld et al. 2021). Cancer cells avidly consume glutamine to support their bioenergetic and biosynthetic demand, thus potentially depleting available glutamine from the TME (Zhang et al. 2017; Reinfeld et al. 2021). Selectively blocking glutamine metabolism in cancer cells by targeting glutamine uptake or metabolism via glutaminase improved antitumor T-cell function, supporting a model that glutamine accessibility is limiting in the TME (Edwards et al. 2021). Glutamine is a key nutrient for activated effector T cells (Teffs) and insufficient access to glutamine impairs Teff metabolism and function while promoting the development of immune-suppressive regulatory T cells

(Tregs) (Klysz et al. 2015). Glutamine depletion can also induce dysfunction in natural killer (NK) cells, as glutamine is essential to maintain cMyc expression and cytotoxic function (Loftus et al. 2018). Additionally, conventional dendritic cells (cDCs) require glutamine for effective antigen cross-presentation to CD8 T cells; however, cancer cells outcompete cDCs for glutamine by overexpression of the transporter SLC38A2 to impair T-cell priming (Guo et al. 2023). Increased tryptophan uptake and catabolism by cancer cells, certain macrophages, and DCs "starves" T cells of tryptophan, thereby inhibiting antitumor Teff while stimulating suppressive Tregs (Lemos et al. 2019). Cancer cells may also outcompete infiltrating T cells for methionine, resulting in methionine deprivation in T cells and subsequent reductions of intracellular methyl donors and STAT5 signaling, which is important in CD8$^+$ T effector function and regulation of CD4$^+$ T-cell metabolism (Tripathi et al. 2010; Bian et al. 2020; Villarino et al. 2022). Arginine is yet another amino acid important in T-cell activation, effector function, and memory development often depleted in tumors due to high rates of arginine catabolism in tumor cells and myeloid-derived suppressor cells (MDSCs) (Geiger et al. 2016; Lemos et al. 2019).

Hypoxia is a characteristic feature of the solid tumor TME and contributes to an immunosuppressive environment when oxygen is not replenished through the vasculature at the rate it is consumed. Oxygen-dependent prolyl-hydroxylases and the E3 ubiquitin ligase VHL degrade the transcription factor, hypoxia inducible factor 1α (HIF1α) if oxygen is abundant. When limiting HIF1α is stabilized, this leads to transcription of a range of glycolytic genes and immune-suppressive ligands such as programmed death-ligand 1 (PD-L1) (Noman et al. 2014). The combination of hypoxia paired with chronic stimulation of tumor-infiltrating lymphocytes (TILs) inhibits proliferation and drives T-cell exhaustion through repressed mitochondrial biogenesis, function, and heightened reactive oxygen species (ROS) accumulation (Scharping et al. 2016, 2021; Vardhana et al. 2020). Hypoxic conditions can also disturb mitochondrial dynamics and promote the exhausted TIL phenotype

through the repression of Myc-regulated, mitofusin 1 (Mfn1)-mediated mitochondrial fusion (Liu et al. 2020). Hypoxia and chronic TCR signaling also coordinate with programmed death 1 (PD-1) signaling via ligation by PD-L1 on tumor cells or infiltrating myeloid cells, elevating T-cell mitochondrial ROS and inhibiting mitophagy, resulting in the accumulation of depolarized, dysfunctional mitochondria that impair TIL effector function (Yu et al. 2020).

Suppressive Metabolites and Molecules

Cancer cells produce and export metabolites and waste products that directly inhibit immunity. Lactate is produced as a byproduct of aerobic glycolysis, leading to accumulation of lactic acid and creation of an acidic TME. Subsequent lactate and proton uptake by T and NK cells, decrease their intracellular pH, interfering with NFAT translocation to the nucleus and impairing IFN-γ production (Brand et al. 2016). Lactate also suppresses glycolysis in CD4 Teff by inhibiting NAD$^+$ recycling necessary for GAPDH activity and inhibits Teff function by liberating GAPDH from its enzymatic role and facilitating translational repression of IFN-γ (Chang et al. 2013; Haas et al. 2015). Conversely, lactate accumulation promotes Treg function and can drive an immunosuppressive phenotype of DCs within the tumor (Colegio et al. 2014; Angelin et al. 2017; Watson et al. 2021; Møller et al. 2022). Activation of the lactate receptor GPR81 on DCs can disrupt antigen presentation by suppressing MHC class II expression (Brown et al. 2020). Lactate induces polarization of TAMs toward a protumor phenotype and this polarization increases arginine metabolism, to feed back into the cycle of nutrient competition and highlight the metabolic interplay of cells in the TME (Colegio et al. 2014; Zhang et al. 2019).

Lipids are abundant in the TME of many tumors. In addition to promoting tumor growth and metastasis, lipid uptake and storage modulates the metabolism and function of infiltrating immune cells to create an immunosuppressive TME (Prendeville and Lynch 2022). Elevated lipid uptake in Tregs and M2-like TAMs fuels fatty acid oxidation (FAO) to support their immune suppressive functions (Prendeville and Lynch 2022). Conversely, intracellular accumulation of lipid droplets blunts antigen presentation by DCs by preventing the translocation of peptide: MHC complexes to the cell surface (Veglia et al. 2017). Enhanced FAO in DCs has also been shown to promote tolerance in melanoma (Zhao et al. 2018; Giovanelli et al. 2019). In CD8 TILs, the accumulation of very long chain fatty acids or cholesterol induces exhaustion, inhibits cytotoxicity, and production of IFN-γ and TNF-α (Ma et al. 2019; Xu et al. 2021). Uptake of oxidized lipids in the TME via the scavenger receptor and lipid transporter CD36 can impair CD8 T-cell effector function and blocking CD36 can increase antitumor immunity (Xu et al. 2021). Lipid accumulation also interferes with mTOR-mediated glycolysis in NK cells, inhibiting production of IFN-γ and direction of lytic granules to the target cell synapse (Michelet et al. 2018).

In addition to waste products, suppressive cells also actively produce immune inhibitory metabolites. Cancer cells and infiltrating myeloid cells often up-regulate tryptophan catabolism through increased indoleamine 2,3 dioxygenase (IDO). This depletes tryptophan and produces the metabolite kynurenine (Munn and Mellor 2013; Lemos et al. 2019). Kynurenine is exported into the TME where it can activate aryl hydrocarbon receptors (AHRs) on T cells and subsequently inhibit their effector function (Munn and Mellor 2013; Liu et al. 2018). Kynurenine accumulation also promotes the generation of Tregs and Treg-dependent recruitment and activation of MDSCs (Holmgaard et al. 2015; Campesato et al. 2020). MDSCs produce the glycolytic metabolite methylglyoxal, an α-dicarbonyl that can paralyze TILs by cell–cell transfer and subsequent depletion of intracellular L-arginine (Baumann et al. 2020). Methylglyoxal also inhibits TIL metabolism by glycation-induced dysfunction of L-arginine containing proteins imperative for mitochondrial respiration (Baumann et al. 2020). MDSCs also secrete the TCA cycle metabolite itaconate, which is taken up by CD8 TILs and inhibits their activation, proliferation, and cytotoxic function, at least in part,

by disrupting aspartate and serine/glycine biosynthesis (Zhao et al. 2022). The lipid mediator prostaglandin E_2 (PGE₂) is also abundant in the TME. PGE₂ receptor EP1-4 signaling promotes MDSC and TAM recruitment and activation while repressing NK and TIL function, resulting in an immunosuppressive environment (Jin et al. 2023).

An interesting new feature of metabolic suppression may be through the regulation of electron transport and subsequent epigenetic changes. The methylation-controlled J protein (MCJ) can act as an endogenous inhibitor of mitochondrial electron transport complex I and MCJ-deficient T cells had increased respiration, and although proliferation was unchanged secretion of inflammatory cytokines was elevated (Champagne et al. 2016). Ultimately, the greater respiratory capacity through complex I enhanced T-cell survival and memory responses against influenza. This may occur in part because MCJ inhibits complex I, leading to increased glycolysis and cell death through caspase 3 (Secinaro et al. 2019). This pathway has also been shown to affect tumor cells and antigen presentation, with the balance of complex I– and complex II–mediated respiration as key (Mangalhara et al. 2023). In this case, inhibition of complex II–dependent respiration led to elevated succinate and complex I–mediated respiration together with increased expression of MHC-I and antigen presentation. Targeting MCJ in tumor cells had a similar effect and increased both succinate and complex I respiration, leading to greater MHC-I expression and antitumor immunity. Thus, changes that regulate mitochondrial electron transport complex I and II may ultimately shape tumor immunogenicity and the function of antitumor T cells.

Metabolic Signaling and Posttranslational Modifications in the TME

Posttranslational modifications (PTMs) widely influence homeostasis, gene expression, and cell proliferation (Li et al. 2018; Jennings et al. 2022). Importantly, PTMs rely on metabolic intermediates as substrates to modify and influence protein activity, structure, and location (Ducker and Rabinowitz 2017; Li et al. 2018). The availability of these nutrients, therefore, can limit or promote specific PMTs to regulate cell signaling and gene expression. Site specificity and abundance of PTMs is dictated enzymatically through dedicated writer, reader, and eraser enzymes that respond to substrate availability (Jennings et al. 2022). Writer enzymes catalyze the addition of the PTM on amino acid residues, reader enzymes recognize PTMs for downstream signaling, and eraser enzymes catalyze the removal of PTMs. However, not all PTMs require an enzymatic writer and there is growing evidence that eraser enzymes can regulate abundance of nonenzymatic PTMs (Jin et al. 2016; Zheng et al. 2019; Gaffney et al. 2020; Jennings et al. 2021). While listing all PTMs associated with immune cells is beyond the scope here, many reviews have covered PTMs in tumors and the TME (Hitosugi and Chen 2014; Chang and Ding 2018; Chandler et al. 2019; Jennings et al. 2022; Pan and Chen 2022). Less is known, however, on the impact of TME and altered nutrients on PTMs of tumor-infiltrating immune cells (Li et al. 2021; Pan and Chen 2022).

Many immune cells in the TME experience elevated glycolytic flux that can provide glycolytic intermediates for anabolic metabolism and as precursors and substrates for PTMs. Glucose supports a plethora of glycation modifications formed from the nonenzymatic covalent binding of reducing sugars to Arg, Lys, and Cys amino acid residues (Jennings et al. 2022). Fructose-6-phosphate fuels the hexosamine biosynthetic pathway, ultimately leading to the highly studied enzymatic glycosylation PTMs (Palaniappan and Bertozzi 2016; Smith and Bertozzi 2021). 1,3-Bisphosphoglycerate can nonenzymatically modify Lys residues by phosphoglycerylation to regulate glycolytic flux (Moellering and Cravatt 2013). Glycolytic intermediates also support epigenetic modifications on histones. Serine generated by 3-phosphoglycerate through de novo serine metabolism can go through one-carbon metabolism to produce S-adenosylmethionine (SAM), ultimately generating enzymatically driven Lys and Arg methylation of histones (Mentch et al. 2015). While methylation is most known for transcriptional regulation

through epigenetic modifications on histones, methylation is pervasive throughout the cell-regulating cell signaling, cell cycle, and nutrient sensing (Di Blasi et al. 2021). Conversely, TCA intermediates α-ketoglutarate and succinate regulate demethylation reactions.

The TCA cycle is an important supplier of substrates for PTMs. Acetylation is a critical PTM for both epigenetic and nonhistone modifications that is based on cytosolic acetyl-CoA. There are multiple pathways to generate cytosolic acetyl-CoA, including by ATP citrate lyase from mitochondrially derived citrate, by ACSS2 after uptake of acetate, and by nuclear pyruvate dehydrogenase from pyruvate (Sutendra et al. 2014; Zhao et al. 2016; Ali et al. 2018; Guertin and Wellen 2023). In addition to enzymatically generated histone acetylation, acetyl-CoA modifies nonhistone proteins throughout the cell both enzymatically and nonenzymatically on Lys and Cys residues (James et al. 2017). Further, many of the acyl-CoAs generated through the TCA cycle and FAO can enzymatically or nonenzymatically modify proteins throughout the cell, regulating enzyme activity and localization in addition to epigenetic transcriptional regulation (Jennings et al. 2022). Under inflammatory conditions, some cells produce itaconate from cis-aconitate after the induction of IRG1. Itaconate is an α,β-unsaturated electrophile that can nonenzymatically modify proteins (i.e., LDH, ALDOA, KEAP1) through a Michael addition and remodels cells, specifically macrophages, toward an anti-inflammatory phenotype (Mills et al. 2018; Qin et al. 2019, 2020).

Cells within the TME can also experience elevated oxidative stress that leads to protein and lipid modifications (Aboelella et al. 2021). Electron leakage from the mitochondrial electron transport chain is the biggest contributor of oxidative stress and renal carcinoma TILs have increased mitochondrial ROS due in part to reduced mitochondrial superoxide dismutase (Siska et al. 2017). Both ROS and reactive nitrogen species (RNS) can nonenzymatically modify protein Cys residues (Jennings et al. 2022). One such RNS, nitric oxide (NO), can be found within tumor-associated immune cells as a byproduct of elevated arginine metabolism. NO can accumulate and nonenzymatically oxidize Cys residues, generating nitrosylation PTMs (Smith and Marletta 2012). Although NO is a signaling molecule, it can be further metabolized into reactive peroxynitrite and S-nitrosoglutathione in addition to protein S-nitrosylation (Smith and Marletta 2012). Oxidative stress can also lead to secondary metabolites capable of nonenzymatically modifying Cys residues. For example, ROS-generated lipid peroxidation produces α,β-unsaturated alkenals (e.g., 4-hydroxy-2-nonenal, 4-oxo2-nonenal) prone to modifying Cys, His, and Lys residues, resulting in carbonylation PTMs (Yin et al. 2011; Galligan et al. 2014; Chen et al. 2017). Carbonylation modifications can damage proteins and result in protein degradation; additionally, the presence of 4-hydroxy-2-nonenal (HNE) in DCs has been associated with immune suppression in ovarian cancer models (Yin et al. 2011; Galligan et al. 2014; Chen et al. 2017). Last, lipid peroxidation can lead to iron-dependent cell death via ferroptosis (Jiang et al. 2021). Each of these processes are counterbalanced by ROS-modification and KEAP1 to release and stabilize the master redox regulatory transcription factor NRF2, which induces redox neutralization and protective mechanisms (Bellezza et al. 2018).

METABOLISM OF TUMOR-INFILTRATING IMMUNE CELL POPULATIONS

Tumor-Associated Macrophages

Macrophages exist in a wide range of phenotypes and use a metabolic continuum from highly glycolytic to highly lipid oxidative that play roles to promote inflammation or to stimulate tissue repair and inflammatory resolution, respectively (Fig. 2). At the ends of these spectra are proinflammatory, classically activated, M1-like macrophages or anti-inflammatory, alternatively activated, M2-like macrophages. Classically activated macrophages are stimulated by IFN-γ, lipopolysaccharide (LPS) from infection or microbiome, or a combination of both to stimulate IFN-γ receptor (IFNGR) and Toll-like receptors (TLRs) and activate STAT1, NF-κB, and PI3K/AKT/mTORC1 signaling pathways. These sig-

nals induce the proinflammatory M1-associated enzyme, inducible nitric oxide synthase (iNOS) (Liu et al. 2017; Van den Bossche et al. 2017; Kolliniati et al. 2022). In contrast, alternatively activated macrophages are stimulated by interleukin 4, 10, and 13 (IL-4, IL-10, and IL-13), glucocorticoids, and macrophage colony-stimulating factor (M-CSF) (Van den Bossche et al. 2017). The binding of both IL-4 to the IL-4 receptor a (IL-4Ra) and IL-13 to the IL-13 receptor subunit a1 (IL-13Ra1) triggers a dimerization of these two receptors to form a type II cytokine receptor complex (McCormick and Heller 2015). This dimerization leads to downstream anti-inflammatory signaling pathways, including the induction of the M2 anti-inflammatory enzyme arginase-1 (ARG1) (Van den Bossche et al. 2017; Lundahl et al. 2022). Metabolites and danger- or damage-associated molecular patterns (DAMPs) in the TME thus lead to metabolically heterogeneous TAMs (Kolliniati et al. 2022). While TAMs are M2-like for many metabolic pathways, mTORC1-regulated glucose uptake and glycolytic flux are elevated compared to in vitro studied M2 macrophages (Reinfeld et al. 2021; Kolliniati et al. 2022). Despite high metabolic activity, these M2-like TAMs are often regarded as protumorigenic due to their immunosuppressive phenotypes.

HIF1α stabilization induces the expression of Glut1 and glycolytic enzymes that promote elevated glycolytic flux in TAMs. In conjunction with tumor-associated DAMPs, inflammatory cues activate mTORC1 signaling, and increased expression of HIF1α in hypoxic regions of tumors stabilize HIF1α and promote glycolytic flux (Huang et al. 2016; Kolliniati et al. 2022). Exogenous lactate secreted from tumor cells and taken up by TAMs can stabilize HIF1α and induce VEGF expression to drive angiogenesis (Zhang and Li 2020; Kolliniati et al. 2022). In addition to lactate abundance, elevated succinate and low pH in the TME can stabilize HIF1α (Liu et al. 2017; Mehla and Singh 2019). Many TCA intermediates can signal to modify TAM phenotypes and hypoxic responses. For example, itaconate, generated from TCA-derived aconitate after LPS or IFN-γ activation and induction of IRG1, regulates the metabolic switch from proin-

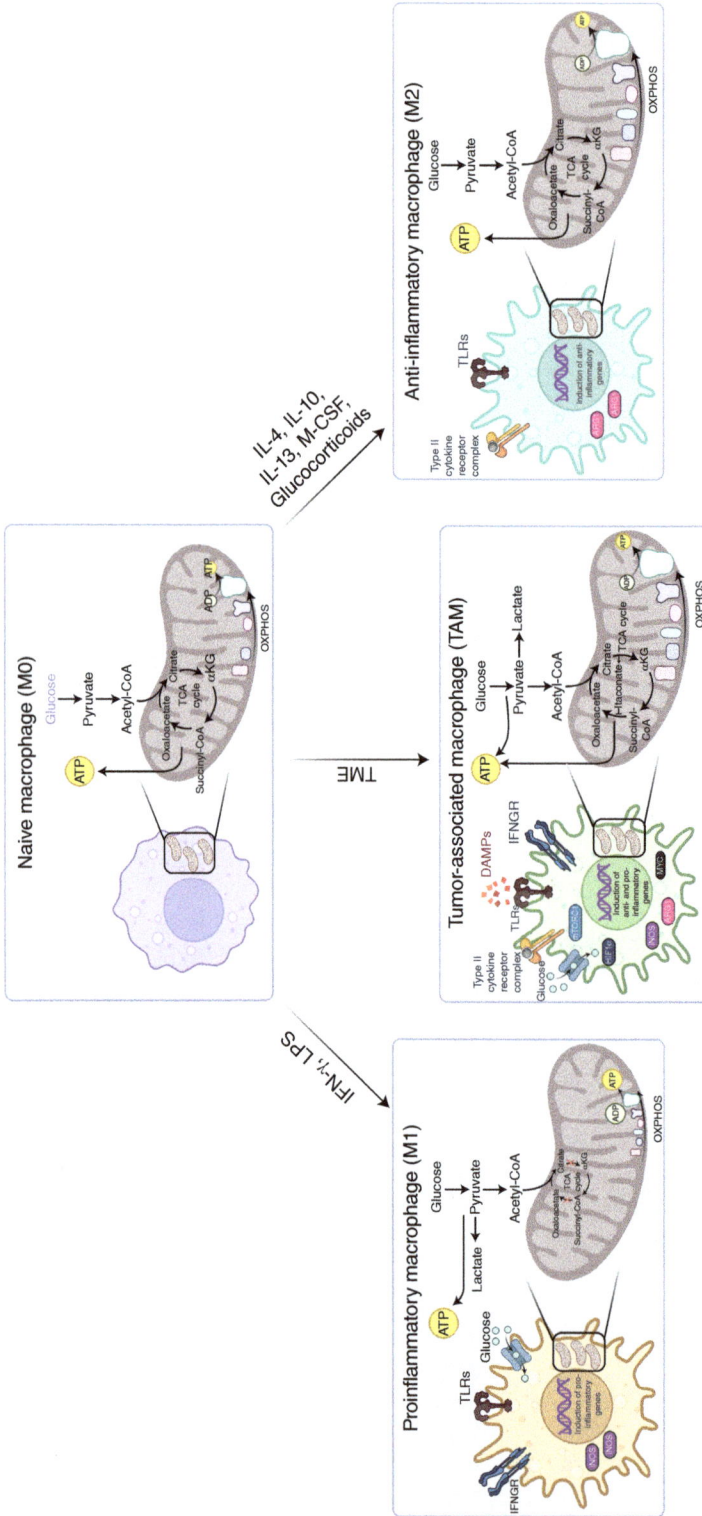

Figure 2. Metabolic reprogramming of macrophages. Naive macrophages undergo context-dependent activation that dictates metabolic programming. M1 macrophages primarily rely on glycolysis for bioenergetic needs and induction of proinflammatory genes, while M2 macrophages use oxidative metabolism and are anti-inflammatory. TAMs are considered M2-like with high mitochondrial metabolism, but also exhibit elevated glycolytic flux. (Acetyl-CoA) Acetyl-coenzyme A, (ADP) adenosine diphosphate, (αKG) α-ketoglutarate, (ARG1) arginase 1, (ATP) adenosine triphosphate, (DAMPs) damage-associated molecular patterns, (HIF1α) hypoxia-inducible factor 1α, (iNOS) inducible nitric oxide synthase, (IFN-γ) interferon γ, (IFNGR) interferon γ receptor, (IL-4) interleukin 4, (IL-10) interleukin 10, (IL-13) interleukin 13, (LPS) lipopolysaccharide, (M-CSF) macrophage colony-stimulating factor, (mTORC1) mammalian target of rapamycin complex 1, (MYC) MYC proto-oncogene, (OXPHOS) oxidative phosphorylation, (succinyl-CoA) succinyl-coenzyme A, (TCA cycle) tricarboxylic acid cycle, (TLRs) Toll-like receptors, (TME) tumor microenvironment.

Cite this article as *Cold Spring Harb Perspect Med* doi: 10.1101/cshperspect.a041547

flammatory to anti-inflammatory phenotypes. Itaconate drives PTMs to reprogram macrophages for OXPHOS and enhanced lactate production through aerobic glycolysis (Lampropoulou et al. 2016; Kolliniati et al. 2022). Inhibition of SDH by itaconate results in succinate accumulation (Lampropoulou et al. 2016; Seim et al. 2019), leading to increased mitochondrial ROS and inhibition of prolyl hydrolases that promote HIF1α degradation and demethylation reactions (Wu et al. 2020). In contrast, α-ketoglutarate provides a substrate for prolyl hydrolases that promote HIF1α degradation, with a high α-ketoglutarate/succinate ratio supporting the anti-inflammatory and protumorigenic phenotype of TAMs (Liu et al. 2017). Glutamine uptake and glutaminolysis can promote this phenotype as a source of α-ketoglutarate for both the replenishment of the TCA cycle and to support α-ketoglutarate-dependent demethylation of histone H3 in promoter regions of anti-inflammatory M2 genes (Mehla and Singh 2019). In hypoxic conditions, or after HIF1α or MYC activation, glutamine supports the TCA cycle through anaplerotic flux and reductive carboxylation (Dubey et al. 2023). MYC-induced glutaminolysis results in the shunting of citrate to cytosolic acetyl-CoA for lipid biogenesis and protein PTMs (Yang et al. 2014). Indeed, blocking glutamine metabolism can enhance the antitumor activity of TAM (Liu et al. 2017; Oh et al. 2020) and regulate antigen presentation by DCs (Guo et al. 2023). Thus, hypoxic TAMs repurpose glutamine for a variety of biosynthetic pathways and immune-suppressive processes rather than for ATP production (Li et al. 2022).

Metabolic changes in M2-like TAMs also augment TME mechanisms that suppress other immune cell types. TAM inhibition of T-cell activity occurs by secreting NOS or ARG1 into the TME that depletes the TME of arginine required for the expression of TCR, proliferation, and memory establishment of T cells (Li et al. 2022). ARG1 is regarded as a universal marker for the M2, anti-inflammatory phenotype. Induction of ARG1 may be perpetuated by IL-4 and acidic pH in the TME (Li et al. 2022). Production of iNOS is supported by T-cell-associated IFN-γ and CD40 (Marigo et al. 2016). While ARG1 and iNOS induction are indicative of distinct polarization states, in vitro evidence has shown iNOS expression in hypoxic states, suggesting the potential for dual expression of iNOS and ARG1 in TAMs of hypoxic TME regions (Carmona-Fontaine et al. 2017; Li et al. 2022). Juxtaposing the M1 antitumor phenotype of iNOS-producing macrophages, inhibition of iNOS in TAMs blocks TAM suppression of T-cell function while inhibition of ARG1 reduces tumor growth (Li et al. 2022). Thus, iNOS expression may regulate the protumorigenic phenotype of TAMs with a higher induction in hypoxic TME regions where ARG1 and iNOS may be coexpressed (Li et al. 2022).

T-Cell Metabolism and Adaptation to Tumor Microenvironments

T cells undergo metabolic reprogramming from catabolism to anabolism upon antigen encounter with appropriate costimulation (Fig. 3). This transition enables T cells to rapidly double cell mass for proliferation while supporting diverse effector functions. While anabolic pathways are broadly elevated, glucose uptake and glycolysis are among the pathways most strikingly increased (Jacobs et al. 2008; Wang et al. 2011; Macintyre et al. 2014). This is initiated in part when the TCR is stimulated by antigen as a first signal and activation of pyruvate dehydrogenase kinase 1 (PDK1), which promotes pyruvate conversion to lactate by preventing pyruvate import into the mitochondria (Menk et al. 2018). Signaling downstream of TCR activation is enhanced by costimulatory signals through CD28 ligation, allowing the T cells to maintain high glycolytic activity (Frauwirth et al. 2002; Jacobs et al. 2008). CD28 stimulation also activates the PI3K/Akt/mTORC1 signaling pathway, leading to Myc-dependent remodeling of the metabolic transcriptome including an increase in genes that regulate glucose uptake and glycolysis (Frauwirth et al. 2002; Jacobs et al. 2008; Wang et al. 2011; Chi 2012). Aerobic glycolysis, while yielding less ATP per cycle than OXPHOS, is important to maintain intracellular redox balance and generate metabolic intermediates for biosynthesis to support rapid cell growth and production of ATP

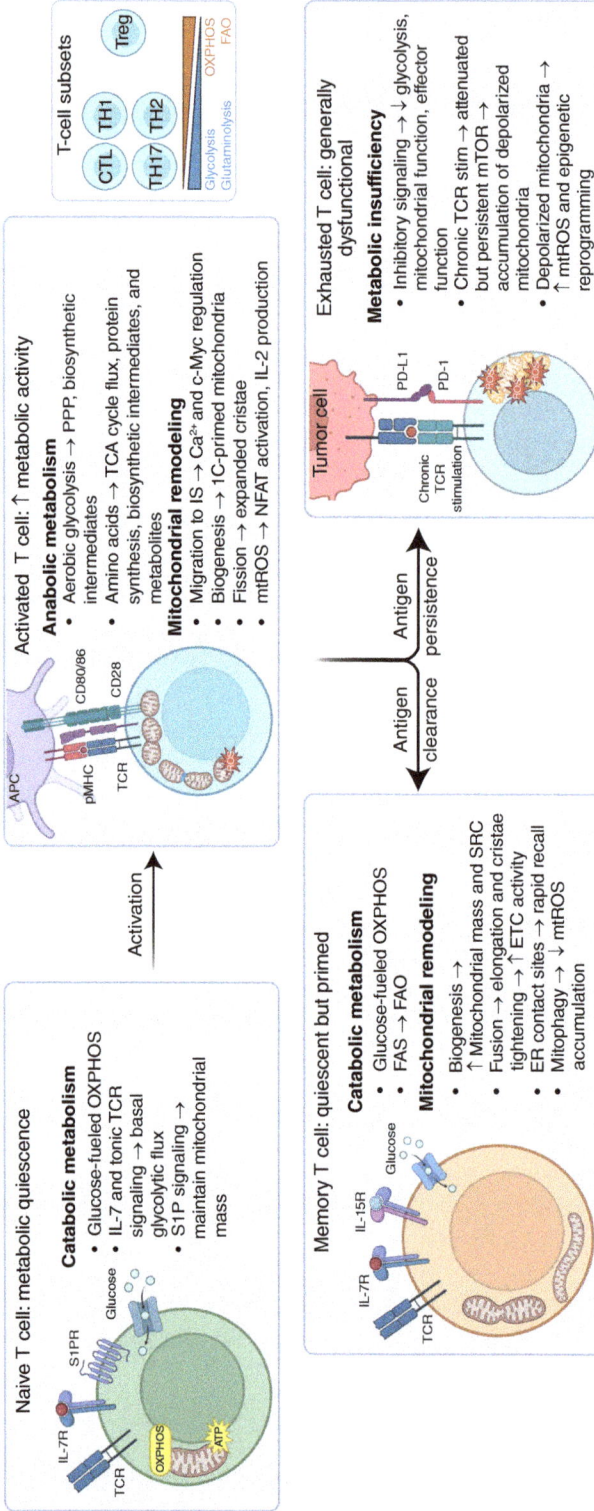

Figure 3. T-cell metabolic programming. Naive T cells are characterized by catabolic metabolism that rapidly switches to anabolism upon activation and costimulation to promote proliferation and effector function. Following antigen clearance, T-cell populations contract to generate a pool of long-lived memory T cells that rely primarily on oxidative metabolism to enable a rapid recall response upon antigen re-encounter. Conversely, antigen persistence promotes differentiation into an exhausted T-cell state characterized by metabolic dysfunction and progressive loss of effector function. (IL-7) Interleukin 7, (IL-7R) interleukin 7 receptor, (S1P) sphingosine-1-phosphate, (S1PRTCR) sphingosine-1-phosphate receptor T-cell receptor.

(Buck et al. 2015; Hosios and Vander Heiden 2018). Glycolytic intermediates enable the shunting of glucose-6-phosphate to the pentose phosphate pathway (PPP) for lipid synthesis, redox balance (Wang et al. 2011; Patra and Hay 2014), and to support the one carbon metabolism pathway that generates nucleotide precursors and SAM for methylation reactions (Ron-Harel et al. 2016; Roy et al. 2020; Sugiura et al. 2022).

Costimulation via the CD28 family plays a central role as a signal two to promote or suppress a productive T-cell response upon TCR stimulation as a signal one. In the absence of CD28-mediated costimulatory activation of the PI3K/Akt/mTORC1 pathway, TCR-stimulated T cells enter an unresponsive state of anergy in which glucose uptake and metabolism are suppressed (Jacobs et al. 2008; Zheng et al. 2009; ElTanbouly and Noelle 2021). Conversely, the inhibitory receptors cytotoxic-T-lymphocyte-associated protein 4 (CTLA4) or PD-1 recruit phosphatases that prevent activation of the PI3K/Akt/mTORC1 pathway and antagonize CD28 costimulation to reduce anabolic metabolism (Frauwirth et al. 2002; Parry et al. 2005). A key mechanism of CTLA4 and PD-1 checkpoint immunotherapies, therefore, is to release this break on T-cell metabolism and enable T-cell anabolism (Bengsch et al. 2016). Indeed, transgenic expression of constitutively active Akt or Glut1 could partially restore T-cell function in models of B-cell leukemia (Siska et al. 2016).

While efficient antigen clearance leads to differentiation of long-lived, protective memory T cells (Tmem), chronic antigen exposure, such as in large solid tumors, promotes restimulation-induced T-cell death or differentiation of dysfunctional, exhausted T cells (Tex) (McLane et al. 2019; ElTanbouly and Noelle 2021). Tex are characterized by loss of effector function and memory recall, sustained expression of inhibitory receptors, and metabolic insufficiency (McLane et al. 2019). Sustained expression and signaling through PD-1 via ligation by PD-L1 expressed on tumor and suppressive myeloid cells reduces glycolysis and mitochondrial function in Tex, partially through inhibition of the master mitochondrial biogenesis and regulatory transcription factor PGC-1α (Bengsch et al.

2016). Additionally, persistent but suboptimal mTORC1 activation during chronic antigen exposure can induce the accumulation of large but dysfunctional, depolarized mitochondria and mtROS production (Bengsch et al. 2016). Accumulation of depolarized mitochondria results in transcriptional and epigenetic changes characteristic of Tex, supporting a link between mitochondrial function and the altered transcriptomic and epigenomic state of exhaustion (Yu et al. 2020).

Among other challenges in tumors, T cells may simultaneously experience chronic TCR stimuli, insufficient costimulation, sustained PD-1 signaling, hypoxia, and altered nutrients. These stresses lead to both functional and metabolic impairments. CD8 T cells isolated from primary patient renal cell carcinoma tumors had accumulated dysfunctional, fragmented mitochondria with elevated production of ROS (Siska et al. 2017). Mitochondrial dysfunction in CD8 T cells is caused by chronic antigen stimulation in hypoxic environments that are frequent in the TME (Scharping et al. 2021). Uptake of oxidized lipids through CD36 in the TME also led to lipid peroxidation and stress response in these CD8 T cells (Xu et al. 2021). While glucose may not be broadly limiting in the TME, TILs also accumulated multiple defects in glycolysis that nonetheless can restrain glucose metabolism. These include deficient Glut1 cell surface trafficking, reduced GAPDH expression, suppression of Enolase 1, and insufficient PEP, which has been reported to signal to drive T-cell calcium responses (Ho et al. 2015; Siska et al. 2017; Gemta et al. 2019). Depletion of amino acids, such as glutamine, in the TME can directly affect T cells and, surprisingly, may promote Teff differentiation and antitumor immunity. Genetically targeting glutaminase (Gls) or broadly inhibiting glutamine metabolism was shown to promote increased glucose metabolism and increased CD4 Th1 and CD8 effector functions (Johnson et al. 2018; Leone et al. 2019; Varghese et al. 2021). However, targeting glutamine metabolism as a whole can also inhibit several essential enzymes (Madden et al. 2023) and promote T-cell exhaustion that may ultimately limit T-cell function (Johnson et al. 2018). In contrast to glutamine depletion, lactate accumulation in the TME may suppress effector functions and both promote Tmem and Treg phenotypes (Angelin et al. 2017; Quinn et al. 2020; Watson et al. 2021; Elia et al. 2022; Feng et al. 2022). Oxidized lipids can also accumulate in the TME, causing stress and impairing T-cell functions, which can be prevented by targeting the lipid transporter CD36 (Xu et al. 2021).

The role of cell metabolism to directly impair or repair T-cell function is evident if metabolic pathways are rescued to restore inflammatory potential, respectively. Consistent with immune checkpoints PD-1 and CTLA4 inhibition of co-stimulatory signals, T-cell function was partially restored in a glycolysis-dependent manner if human kidney tumor T cells were activated with both TCR and CD28-mediated costimulation (Beckermann et al. 2020). Additionally, mito-chondria can be directly rescued by provision of exogenous pyruvate, by neutralizing mito-chondrial ROS (Beckermann et al. 2020), or by overexpression of the mitochondrial biogenesis factor PGC1α (Bengsch et al. 2016; Scharping et al. 2021; Lontos et al. 2023). Each of these metabolic rescue treatments reversed metabolic immune suppression, resulting in improved Teff antitumor function. Metabolic conditioning to enhance mitochondrial quantity and quality prior to T-cell adoptive therapy can also improve antitumor immunity. Stimulation of T cells in low doses of 2-deoxyglucose to suppress glycolysis and effector differentiation increased mito-chondrial capacity in vitro, leading to improved longevity and function upon subsequent transfer in vivo (Sukumar et al. 2013). Similar selection for T cells with highly coupled and efficient mitochondria by selecting T cells with low mitochondrial membrane potential also showed enhanced antitumor activity relative to bulk populations (Sukumar et al. 2016). Other approaches, such as increased temperatures that result in mitochondrial biogenesis, also increased antitumor immunity (O'Sullivan et al. 2021). These findings show that metabolic maladaptations of TIL, and mitochondria in particular, directly contribute to T-cell functional impairments in the TME.

Rewiring T-Cell Metabolism to Improve CAR-T Therapy for Solid Tumors

Adoptive transfer of chimeric antigen receptor–modified T (CAR-T) cells has proven an effective treatment strategy for a variety of hematologic malignancies after FDA approval in 2017 for B-cell acute lymphoblastic leukemia (Schultz and Mackall 2019). Despite success targeting other advanced leukemias, lymphomas, and multiple myeloma, similar clinical efficacy in the solid tumor setting remains elusive. Early clinical trials have demonstrated the feasibility and safety of CAR-T therapy in a variety of solid tumors, but durable responses comparable to those observed in hematologic malignancies have not yet been achieved in solid tumors (Brown et al. 2016; Tchou et al. 2017; Feng et al. 2018; Wang et al. 2018; Adusumilli et al. 2021; Narayan et al. 2022; Qi et al. 2022). A key difference between solid and liquid tumors is the establishment of the TME and the potential for metabolic immune suppression of CAR-T-cell signaling and metabolism (Fig. 4). Challenges faced in developing CAR-T cells for solid tumors include choice of tumor antigen and heterogeneity, tumor bed trafficking, T-cell-intrinsic regulatory programs, and the broadly immunosuppressive TME that limit CAR-T proliferation, function, and persistence (Wagner et al. 2020). It has become increasingly apparent that the metabolic fitness of T cells is a critical determinant of their antitumor function and survival. Components engineered into the CAR can shape CAR-T-cell metabolism. CD3ζ together with CD28 signaling domains yield CAR-T cells with high rates of glycolysis and anabolic metabolism while CD3ζ with 4-1BB signaling domains promote mitochondrial metabolism and CAR-T-cell longevity (Kawalekar et al. 2016; van Bruggen et al. 2019). Thus, there has recently been an intersection between the fields of immunometabolism and CAR-T engineering.

The CAR-T-cell manufacturing process involves cell culture and genetic modification to introduce the CAR, which provides an opportunity to enforce expression of other genes that may improve the metabolism and function of the cells in vivo. The proline metabolism enzyme PRODH2 was identified in a gain-of-function

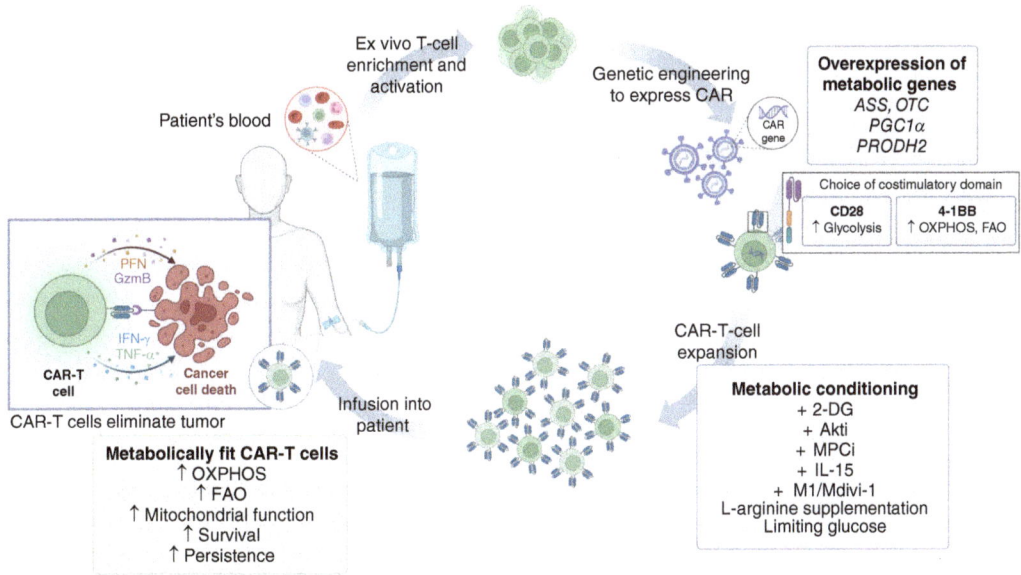

Figure 4. Metabolic reprogramming of chimeric antigen receptor–modified T (CAR-T) cells. CAR design impacts metabolism based on the costimulatory domain used. During manufacturing, CAR-T cells can be induced to overexpress metabolic genes to enable adaptation or resistance to the suppressive tumor microenvironment (TME). Additionally, CAR-T cells may be supplemented with cytokines, nutrients, or metabolic pathway inhibitors to modulate metabolism. Such "metabolically fit" CAR-T cells have improved mitochondrial metabolism, antitumor function, and persistence in vivo.

CRISPR screen as conferring improved effector function and proliferation of CD8 T cells (Ye et al. 2022). Overexpression of this enzyme in CAR-T cells reshaped metabolism to a more memory-like phenotype, including an increase in proline metabolism, mitochondrial mass, and respiration, translating to improved tumor control in both blood and solid tumor models (Ye et al. 2022). Overexpression of the arginine synthesis enzymes argininosuccinate synthase (ASS) or ornithine transcarbamylase (OTC) in CAR-T cells improved proliferation in the arginine-restricted TME, conferring superior tumor control in both acute myeloid leukemia (AML) and solid tumor models (Fultang et al. 2020). Tumor-infiltrating T cells often have dysfunctional mitochondria, but expressing mitochondrial biogenesis transcription factor PGC-1α helped tumor-specific T cells resist mitochondrial deficiency in the TME (Scharping et al. 2016). PGC-1α overexpressing T cells in adoptive cell therapy exhibit increased mitochondrial biogenesis and OXPHOS that enhanced antitumor efficacy in a model of aggressive melanoma

(Scharping et al. 2016) and this translates to CAR-T cells in which PGC-1α has also been reported to have increased antitumor activity (Lontos et al. 2023).

The in vitro CAR-T manufacturing process provides yet another opportunity to modulate metabolism by adjusting culture conditions. This might include the use of pharmacological inhibitors to transiently block certain metabolic pathways. For example, inhibition of glycolysis or Akt signaling can promote a more memory-like phenotype and improves tumor control by tumor-specific T cells and CAR-T cells in models of solid and blood tumors, respectively (Sukumar et al. 2013; Ryan et al. 2017). Additionally, inhibition of the mitochondrial pyruvate carrier (MPC) rewired CAR-T cells to increase glutamine- and lipid-derived acetyl-CoA pools leading to epigenetic reprogramming toward a memory-like CAR-T. This metabolic reprogramming conferred greater antitumor potency and persistence in solid tumor and leukemia models (Wenes et al. 2022). A combination treatment with a mitochondrial fusion promoter (M1) and fission inhibitor (Mdivi-1) generates T cells with memory-like bioenergetic profiles and improved tumor control (Buck et al. 2016). Supplementation of IL-15, a cytokine critical for development and survival of memory T cells, reduces glycolysis and increases FAO in CAR-T cells, conferring superior proliferative capacity, persistence, and tumor control in both lymphoma and glioblastoma models (Alizadeh et al. 2019). L-arginine addition to T-cell cultures promotes a switch to OXPHOS and supplementing TCR transgenic, tumor-specific T cells with L-arginine during in vitro activation leads to improved tumor control in vivo (Geiger et al. 2016).

BARRIERS AND OPPORTUNITIES IN METABOLIC IMMUNOTHERAPY

The TME alters immune cell metabolism in ways maladaptive to antitumor immunity. Models must therefore be refined to better fit the environment of the TME and consider both metabolic and cellular heterogeneity. In addition to altering immune cell metabolism, tumors are spatially heterogeneous, leading to diverse metabolism and methods of regulation across regions of the TME or at different metastatic sites. The tumor is also comprised of a variety of cell types, beyond cancer cells, which all contribute to the metabolic regulation of the TME. Thus, the phenotype of the "tumor" is comprised of many cell types along with a heterogenous metabolic environment. Classically, many cancer studies used bulk tumor processing to provide overarching information on the TME. However, this approach does not provide any nuanced information on what cell types drive the phenotype and differential nutrient uptake and usage between cell subsets (Arner and Rathmell 2023). An additional challenge to model the TME is that in vitro differentiation of immune cells can generate immune cell subtype with metabolic profiles that inherently differ from those seen in vivo (Ma et al. 2019). Another challenge of researching cell types within the TME is that sorting of the tumor into its various cell populations is limited to the abundance of the cell type within the tumor under study.

Although the heterogeneous metabolic character of the TME poses challenges to understand the dynamics of tumor immunobiology, it also offers opportunities to improve tumor immunotherapy. The distinct patterns of nutrient uptake and use by different cell types may be exploited in improved cellular-targeted imaging approaches. This same feature of differential nutrient use may then allow selective molecular targeting of specific cell populations to impair suppressive features of the TME or promote inflammatory functions. The metabolism of tumor-infiltrating immune cells is already being exploited in existing immunotherapies, as PD-1 and CTLA4 blockades appear to act in part by reshaping T-cell metabolism to remove a break on glycolysis and anabolism. Similarly, CAR-T cells with CD28 or 4-1BB costimulatory signaling domains have widely different inflammatory potentials and longevity affecting the tumors being targeted. Many pieces of evidence now point to mitochondrial dysfunction as a weak link in T-cell antitumor immune function (Rostamian et al. 2021). Improved understanding of the maladaptive response of T cells to the TME and how this leads to mitochondrial and general metabolic dysfunction will better identify patients most likely to benefit from immunotherapy and will point to new approaches to increase T-cell longevity and antitumor immunity.

COMPETING INTEREST STATEMENT

Dr. Jeffrey Rathmell is an employee of Vanderbilt University Medical Center and appointed to the Vanderbilt University School of Medicine. He is a founder, scientific advisory board member, and stockholder of Sitryx Therapeutics, a scientific advisory board member and stockholder of Caribou Biosciences and holds stock options for Nirogy Therapeutics. He has consulted and received speaker fees from Merck, Pfizer, and Abbie. He has received research support from Incyte Corp. within the past 3 years.

ACKNOWLEDGMENTS

We thank members of the Jeffrey and W. Kimryn Rathmell laboratories for their input. This work was supported by R01 CA217987 and DOD W81XWH-22-1-0419.

Cite this article as *Cold Spring Harb Perspect Med* doi: 10.1101/cshperspect.a041547

REFERENCES

Aboelella NS, Brandle C, Kim T, Ding ZC, Zhou G. 2021. Oxidative stress in the tumor microenvironment and its relevance to cancer immunotherapy. *Cancers (Basel)* 13: 986. doi:10.3390/cancers13050986

Adusumilli PS, Zauderer MG, Rivière I, Solomon SB, Rusch VW, O'Cearbhaill RE, Zhu A, Cheema W, Chintala NK, Halton E, et al. 2021. A phase I trial of regional mesothelin-targeted CAR T-cell therapy in patients with malignant pleural disease, in combination with the anti–PD-1 agent pembrolizumab. *Cancer Discov* 11: 2748–2763. doi:10.1158/2159-8290.CD-21-0407

Ali I, Conrad RJ, Verdin E, Ott M. 2018. Lysine acetylation goes global: from epigenetics to metabolism and therapeutics. *Chem Rev* 118: 1216–1252. doi:10.1021/acs.chemrev.7b00181

Alizadeh D, Wong RA, Yang X, Wang D, Pecoraro JR, Kuo CF, Aguilar B, Qi Y, Ann DK, Starr R, et al. 2019. IL15 enhances CAR-T cell antitumor activity by reducing mTORC1 activity and preserving their stem cell memory phenotype. *Cancer Immunol Res* 7: 759–772. doi:10.1158/2326-6066.CIR-18-0466

Angelin A, Gil-de-Gómez L, Dahiya S, Jiao J, Guo L, Levine MH, Wang Z, Quinn WJ III, Kopinski PK, Wang L, et al. 2017a. Foxp3 reprograms T cell metabolism to function in low-glucose, high-lactate environments. *Cell Metab* 25: 1282–1293.e7. doi:10.1016/j.cmet.2016.12.018

Arner EN, Rathmell JC. 2023. Metabolic programming and immune suppression in the tumor microenvironment. *Cancer Cell* 41: 421–433. doi:10.1016/j.ccell.2023.01.009

Bader JE, Voss K, Rathmell JC. 2020. Targeting metabolism to improve the tumor microenvironment for cancer immunotherapy. *Mol Cell* 78: 1019–1033. doi:10.1016/j.molcel.2020.05.034

Baumann T, Dunkel A, Schmid C, Schmitt S, Hiltensperger M, Lohr K, Laketa V, Donakonda S, Ahting U, Lorenz-Depiereux B, et al. 2020. Regulatory myeloid cells paralyze T cells through cell–cell transfer of the metabolite methylglyoxal. *Nat Immunol* 21: 555–566. doi:10.1038/s41590-020-0666-9

Beckermann KE, Hongo R, Ye X, Young K, Carbonell K, Healey DCC, Siska PJ, Barone S, Roe CE, Smith CC, et al. 2020. CD28 costimulation drives tumor-infiltrating T cell glycolysis to promote inflammation. *JCI Insight* 5: e138729. doi:10.1172/jci.insight.138729

Bellezza I, Giambanco I, Minelli A, Donato R. 2018. Nrf2-Keap1 signaling in oxidative and reductive stress. *Biochim Biophys Acta Mol Cell Res* 1865: 721–733. doi:10.1016/j.bbamcr.2018.02.010

Bengsch B, Johnson AL, Kurachi M, Odorizzi PM, Pauken KE, Attanasio J, Stelekati E, McLane LM, Paley MA, Delgoffe GM, et al. 2016a. Bioenergetic insufficiencies due to metabolic alterations regulated by the inhibitory receptor PD-1 are an early driver of CD8[+] T cell exhaustion. *Immunity* 45: 358–373. doi:10.1016/j.immuni.2016.07.008

Bian Y, Li W, Kremer DM, Sajjakulnukit P, Li S, Crespo J, Nwosu ZC, Zhang L, Czerwonka A, Pawłowska A, et al. 2020. Cancer SLC43A2 alters T cell methionine metabolism and histone methylation. *Nature* 585: 277–282. doi:10.1038/s41586-020-2682-1

Brand A, Singer K, Koehl Gudrun E, Kolitzus M, Schoenhammer G, Thiel A, Matos C, Bruss C, Klobuch S, Peter K, et al. 2016. LDHA-associated lactic acid production blunts tumor immunosurveillance by T and NK cells. *Cell Metab* 24: 657–671. doi:10.1016/j.cmet.2016.08.011

Brown CE, Alizadeh D, Starr R, Weng L, Wagner JR, Naranjo A, Ostberg JR, Blanchard MS, Kilpatrick J, Simpson J, et al. 2016. Regression of glioblastoma after chimeric antigen receptor T-cell therapy. *N Eng J Med* 375: 2561–2569. doi:10.1056/NEJMoa1610497

Brown TP, Bhattacharjee P, Ramachandran S, Sivaprakasam S, Ristic B, Sikder MOF, Ganapathy V. 2020. The lactate receptor GPR81 promotes breast cancer growth via a paracrine mechanism involving antigen-presenting cells in the tumor microenvironment. *Oncogene* 39: 3292–3304. doi:10.1038/s41388-020-1216-5

Buck MD, O'Sullivan D, Pearce EL. 2015. T cell metabolism drives immunity. *J Exp Med* 212: 1345–1360. doi:10.1084/jem.20151159

Buck MD, O'Sullivan D, Klein Geltink Ramon I, Curtis Jonathan D, Chang CH, Sanin David E, Qiu J, Kretz O, Braas D, van der Windt Gerritje JW, et al. 2016. Mitochondrial dynamics controls T cell fate through metabolic programming. *Cell* 166: 63–76. doi:10.1016/j.cell.2016.05.035

Campesato LF, Budhu S, Tchaicha J, Weng CH, Gigoux M, Cohen IJ, Redmond D, Mangarin L, Pourpe S, Liu C, et al. 2020. Blockade of the AHR restricts a Treg-macrophage suppressive axis induced by L-kynurenine. *Nat Commun* 11: 4011. doi:10.1038/s41467-020-17750-z

Carmona-Fontaine C, Deforet M, Akkari L, Thompson CB, Joyce JA, Xavier JB. 2017. Metabolic origins of spatial organization in the tumor microenvironment. *Proc Natl Acad Sci* 114: 2934–2939. doi:10.1073/pnas.1700600114

Champagne DP, Hatle KM, Fortner KA, D'Alessandro A, Thornton TM, Yang R, Torralba D, Tomás-Cortazar J, Jun YW, Ahn KH, et al. 2016. Fine-Tuning of CD8[+] T cell mitochondrial metabolism by the respiratory chain repressor MCJ dictates protection to influenza virus. *Immunity* 44: 1299–1311. doi:10.1016/j.immuni.2016.02.018

Chandler KB, Costello CE, Rahimi N. 2019. Glycosylation in the tumor microenvironment: implications for tumor angiogenesis and metastasis. *Cells* 8: 544. doi:10.3390/cells8060544

Chang SC, Ding JL. 2018. Ubiquitination and SUMOylation in the chronic inflammatory tumor microenvironment. *Biochim Biophys Acta Rev Cancer* 1870: 165–175. doi:10.1016/j.bbcan.2018.08.002

Chang CH, Curtis Jonathan D, Maggi Leonard B, Faubert B, Villarino Alejandro V, O'Sullivan D, Huang Stanley CC, van der Windt Gerritje JW, Blagih J, Qiu J, et al. 2013. Posttranscriptional control of T cell effector function by aerobic glycolysis. *Cell* 153: 1239–1251. doi:10.1016/j.cell.2013.05.016

Chang CH, Qiu J, O'Sullivan D, Buck Michael D, Noguchi T, Curtis Jonathan D, Chen Q, Gindin M, Gubin Matthew M, van der Windt Gerritje JW, et al. 2015. Metabolic competition in the tumor microenvironment is a driver of cancer progression. *Cell* 162: 1229–1241. doi:10.1016/j.cell.2015.08.016

Chen Y, Cong Y, Quan B, Lan T, Chu X, Ye Z, Hou X, Wang C. 2017. Chemoproteomic profiling of targets of lipid-derived electrophiles by bioorthogonal aminooxy probe. *Redox Biol* 12: 712–718. doi:10.1016/j.redox.2017.04.001

Chi H. 2012. Regulation and function of mTOR signalling in T cell fate decisions. *Nat Rev Immunol* 12: 325–338. doi:10.1038/nri3198

Colegio OR, Chu NQ, Szabo AL, Chu T, Rhebergen AM, Jairam V, Cyrus N, Brokowski CE, Eisenbarth SC, Phillips GM, et al. 2014. Functional polarization of tumour-associated macrophages by tumour-derived lactic acid. *Nature* 513: 559–563. doi:10.1038/nature13490

Di Blasi R, Blyuss O, Timms JF, Conole D, Ceroni F, Whitwell HJ. 2021. Non-histone protein methylation: biological significance and bioengineering potential. *ACS Chem Biol* 16: 238–250. doi:10.1021/acschembio.0c00771

Dubey S, Ghosh S, Goswami D, Ghatak D, De R. 2023. Immunometabolic attributes and mitochondria-associated signaling of tumor-associated macrophages in tumor microenvironment modulate cancer progression. *Biochem Pharmacol* 208: 115369. doi:10.1016/j.bcp.2022.115369

Ducker GS, Rabinowitz JD. 2017. One-carbon metabolism in health and disease. *Cell Metab* 25: 27–42. doi:10.1016/j.cmet.2016.08.009

Edwards DN, Ngwa VM, Raybuck AL, Wang S, Hwang Y, Kim LC, Cho SH, Paik Y, Wang Q, Zhang S, et al. 2021. Selective glutamine metabolism inhibition in tumor cells improves antitumor T lymphocyte activity in triple-negative breast cancer. *J Clin Invest* 131: e140100. doi:10.1172/JCI140100

Elia I, Rowe JH, Johnson S, Joshi S, Notarangelo G, Kurmi K, Weiss S, Freeman GJ, Sharpe AH, Haigis MC. 2022. Tumor cells dictate anti-tumor immune responses by altering pyruvate utilization and succinate signaling in CD8$^+$ T cells. *Cell Metab* 34: 1137–1150.e6. doi:10.1016/j.cmet.2022.06.008

ElTanbouly MA, Noelle RJ. 2021. Rethinking peripheral T cell tolerance: checkpoints across a T cell's journey. *Nat Rev Immunol* 21: 257–267. doi:10.1038/s41577-020-00454-2

Feng K, Liu Y, Guo Y, Qiu J, Wu Z, Dai H, Yang Q, Wang Y, Han W. 2018. Phase I study of chimeric antigen receptor modified T cells in treating HER2-positive advanced biliary tract cancers and pancreatic cancers. *Protein Cell* 9: 838–847. doi:10.1007/s13238-017-0440-4

Feng Q, Liu Z, Yu X, Huang T, Chen J, Wang J, Wilhelm J, Li S, Song J, Li W, et al. 2022. Lactate increases stemness of CD8$^+$ T cells to augment anti-tumor immunity. *Nat Commun* 13: 4981. doi:10.1038/s41467-022-32521-8

Frauwirth KA, Riley JL, Harris MH, Parry RV, Rathmell JC, Plas DR, Elstrom RL, June CH, Thompson CB. 2002a. The CD28 signaling pathway regulates glucose metabolism. *Immunity* 16: 769–777. doi:10.1016/s1074-7613(02)00323-0

Fultang L, Booth S, Yogev O, Martins da Costa B, Tubb V, Panetti S, Stavrou V, Scarpa U, Jankevics A, Lloyd G, et al. 2020. Metabolic engineering against the arginine microenvironment enhances CAR-T cell proliferation and therapeutic activity. *Blood* 136: 1155–1160. doi:10.1182/blood.2019004500

Gaffney DO, Jennings EQ, Anderson CC, Marentette JO, Shi T, Schou Oxvig AM, Streeter MD, Johannsen M, Spiegel DA, Chapman E, et al. 2020. Non-enzymatic lysine lac-

toylation of glycolytic enzymes. *Cell Chem Biol* 27: 206–213.e6. doi:10.1016/j.chembiol.2019.11.005

Galligan JJ, Rose KL, Beavers WN, Hill S, Tallman KA, Tansey WP, Marnett LJ. 2014. Stable histone adduction by 4-oxo-2-nonenal: a potential link between oxidative stress and epigenetics. *J Am Chem Soc* 136: 11864–11866. doi:10.1021/ja503604t

Geiger R, Rieckmann JC, Wolf T, Basso C, Feng Y, Fuhrer T, Kogadeeva M, Picotti P, Meissner F, Mann M, et al. 2016. L-arginine modulates T cell metabolism and enhances survival and anti-tumor activity. *Cell* 167: 829–842.e13. doi:10.1016/j.cell.2016.09.031

Gemta LF, Siska PJ, Nelson ME, Gao X, Liu X, Locasale JW, Yagita H, Slingluff CL Jr, Hoehn KL, Rathmell JC, et al. 2019. Impaired enolase 1 glycolytic activity restrains effector functions of tumor-infiltrating CD8$^+$ T cells. *Sci Immunol* 4: eaap9520. doi:10.1126/sciimmunol.aap9520

Giovanelli P, Sandoval TA, Cubillos-Ruiz JR. 2019. Dendritic cell metabolism and function in tumors. *Trends Immunol* 40: 699–718. doi:10.1016/j.it.2019.06.004

Guertin DA, Wellen KE. 2023. Acetyl-CoA metabolism in cancer. *Nat Rev Cancer* 23: 156–172. doi:10.1038/s41568-022-00543-5

Guo C, You Z, Shi H, Sun Y, Du X, Palacios G, Guy C, Yuan S, Chapman NM, Lim SA, et al. 2023. SLC38A2 and glutamine signalling in cDC1s dictate anti-tumour immunity. *Nature* 620: 200–208. doi:10.1038/s41586-023-06299-8

Haas R, Smith J, Rocher-Ros V, Nadkarni S, Montero-Melendez T, D'Acquisto F, Bland EJ, Bombardieri M, Pitzalis C, Perretti M, et al. 2015. Lactate regulates metabolic and pro-inflammatory circuits in control of T cell migration and effector functions. *PLoS Biol* 13: e1002202. doi:10.1371/journal.pbio.1002202

Hanahan D. 2022. Hallmarks of cancer: new dimensions. *Cancer Discov* 12: 31–46. doi:10.1158/2159-8290.CD-21-1059

Hitosugi T, Chen J. 2014. Post-translational modifications and the Warburg effect. *Oncogene* 33: 4279–4285. doi:10.1038/onc.2013.406

Ho PC, Bihuniak Jessica D, Macintyre Andrew N, Staron M, Liu X, Amezquita R, Tsui YC, Cui G, Micevic G, Perales Jose C, et al. 2015. Phosphoenolpyruvate is a metabolic checkpoint of anti-tumor T cell responses. *Cell* 162: 1217–1228. doi:10.1016/j.cell.2015.08.012

Holmgaard Rikke B, Zamarin D, Li Y, Gasmi B, Munn David H, Allison James P, Merghoub T, Wolchok Jedd D. 2015. Tumor-expressed IDO recruits and activates MDSCs in a Treg-dependent manner. *Cell Rep* 13: 412–424. doi:10.1016/j.celrep.2015.08.077

Hosios AM, Vander Heiden MG. 2018. The redox requirements of proliferating mammalian cells. *J Biol Chem* 293: 7490–7498. doi:10.1074/jbc.TM117.000239

Huang SC, Smith AM, Everts B, Colonna M, Pearce EL, Schilling JD, Pearce EJ. 2016. Metabolic reprogramming mediated by the mTORC2-IRF4 signaling axis is essential for macrophage alternative activation. *Immunity* 45: 817–830. doi:10.1016/j.immuni.2016.09.016

Jacobs SR, Herman CE, Maciver NJ, Wofford JA, Wieman HL, Hammen JJ, Rathmell JC. 2008. Glucose uptake is limiting in T cell activation and requires CD28-mediated Akt-dependent and independent pathways. *J Immunol* 180: 4476–4486. doi:10.4049/jimmunol.180.7.4476

James AM, Hoogewijs K, Logan A, Hall AR, Ding S, Fearnley IM, Murphy MP. 2017. Non-enzymatic N-acetylation of lysine residues by AcetylCoA often occurs via a proximal s-acetylated thiol intermediate sensitive to glyoxalase II. *Cell Rep* 18: 2105–2112. doi:10.1016/j.celrep.2017.02.018

Jardim DL, Goodman A, de Melo Gagliato D, Kurzrock R. 2021. The challenges of tumor mutational burden as an immunotherapy biomarker. *Cancer Cell* 39: 154–173. doi:10.1016/j.ccell.2020.10.001

Jennings EQ, Ray JD, Zerio CJ, Trujillo MN, McDonald DM, Chapman E, Spiegel DA, Galligan J. 2021. Sirtuin 2 regulates protein lactoylLys modifications. *Chembiochem* 22: 2102–2106. doi:10.1002/cbic.202000883

Jennings EQ, Fritz KS, Galligan JJ. 2022. Biochemical genesis of enzymatic and non-enzymatic post-translational modifications. *Mol Aspects Med* 86: 101053. doi:10.1016/j.mam.2021.101053

Jiang X, Stockwell BR, Conrad M. 2021. Ferroptosis: mechanisms, biology and role in disease. *Nat Rev Mol Cell Biol* 22: 266–282. doi:10.1038/s41580-020-00324-8

Jin J, He B, Zhang X, Lin H, Wang Y. 2016. SIRT2 reverses 4-oxononanoyl lysine modification on histones. *J Am Chem Soc* 138: 12304–12307. doi:10.1021/jacs.6b04977

Jin K, Qian C, Lin J, Liu B. 2023. Cyclooxygenase-2-prostaglandin E2 pathway: a key player in tumor-associated immune cells. *Front Oncol* 13: 1099811. doi:10.3389/fonc.2023.1099811

Johnson MO, Wolf MM, Madden MZ, Andrejeva G, Sugiura A, Contreras DC, Maseda D, Liberti MV, Paz K, Kishton RJ, et al. 2018. Distinct regulation of Th17 and Th1 cell differentiation by glutaminase-dependent metabolism. *Cell* 175: 1780–1795.e19. doi:10.1016/j.cell.2018.10.001

Kawalekar OU, O'Connor RS, Fraietta JA, Guo L, McGettigan SE, Posey AD Jr, Patel PR, Guedan S, Scholler J, Keith B, et al. 2016. Distinct signaling of coreceptors regulates specific metabolism pathways and impacts memory development in CAR T cells. *Immunity* 44: 380–390. doi:10.1016/j.immuni.2016.01.021

Klysz D, Tai X, Robert PA, Craveiro M, Cretenet G, Oburoglu L, Mongellaz C, Floess S, Fritz V, Matias MI, et al. 2015. Glutamine-dependent α-ketoglutarate production regulates the balance between T helper 1 cell and regulatory T cell generation. *Sci Signal* 8: ra97. doi:10.1126/scisignal.aab2610

Kolliniati O, Ieronymaki E, Vergadi E, Tsatsanis C. 2022. Metabolic regulation of macrophage activation. *J Innate Immun* 14: 51–68. doi:10.1159/000516780

Lampropoulou V, Sergushichev A, Bambouskova M, Nair S, Vincent EE, Loginicheva E, Cervantes-Barragan L, Ma X, Huang SC, Griss T, et al. 2016. Itaconate links inhibition of succinate dehydrogenase with macrophage metabolic remodeling and regulation of inflammation. *Cell Metab* 24: 158–166. doi:10.1016/j.cmet.2016.06.004

Lemos H, Huang L, Prendergast GC, Mellor AL. 2019. Immune control by amino acid catabolism during tumorigenesis and therapy. *Nat Rev Cancer* 19: 162–175. doi:10.1038/s41568-019-0106-z

Leone RD, Zhao L, Englert JM, Sun IM, Oh MH, Sun IH, Arwood ML, Bettencourt IA, Patel CH, Wen J, et al. 2019. Glutamine blockade induces divergent metabolic programs to overcome tumor immune evasion. *Science* 366: 1013–1021. doi:10.1126/science.aav2588

Li X, Egervari G, Wang Y, Berger SL, Lu Z. 2018. Regulation of chromatin and gene expression by metabolic enzymes and metabolites. *Nat Rev Mol Cell Biol* 19: 563–578. doi:10.1038/s41580-018-0029-7

Li W, Li F, Zhang X, Lin HK, Xu C. 2021. Insights into the post-translational modification and its emerging role in shaping the tumor microenvironment. *Signal Transduct Target Ther* 6: 422. doi:10.1038/s41392-021-00825-8

Li J, DeNicola GM, Ruffell B. 2022. Metabolism in tumor-associated macrophages. *Int Rev Cell Mol Biol* 367: 65–100. doi:10.1016/bs.ircmb.2022.01.004

Lieu EL, Nguyen T, Rhyne S, Kim J. 2020. Amino acids in cancer. *Exp Mol Med* 52: 15–30. doi:10.1038/s12276-020-0375-3

Liu D, Chang C, Lu N, Wang X, Lu Q, Ren X, Ren P, Zhao D, Wang L, Zhu Y, et al. 2017a. Comprehensive proteomics analysis reveals metabolic reprogramming of tumor-associated macrophages stimulated by the tumor microenvironment. *J Proteome Res* 16: 288–297. doi:10.1021/acs.jproteome.6b00604

Liu PS, Wang H, Li X, Chao T, Teav T, Christen S, Di Conza G, Cheng WC, Chou CH, Vavakova M, et al. 2017b. α-ketoglutarate orchestrates macrophage activation through metabolic and epigenetic reprogramming. *Nat Immunol* 18: 985–994. doi:10.1038/ni.3796

Liu T, Zhang L, Joo D, Sun SC. 2017c. NF-κB signaling in inflammation. *Signal Transduct Target Ther* 2: 17023. doi:10.1038/sigtrans.2017.23

Liu Y, Liang X, Dong W, Fang Y, Lv J, Zhang T, Fiskesund R, Xie J, Liu J, Yin X, et al. 2018. Tumor-repopulating cells induce PD-1 expression in CD8+ T cells by transferring kynurenine and AhR activation. *Cancer Cell* 33: 480–494. e7. doi:10.1016/j.ccell.2018.02.005

Liu YN, Yang JF, Huang DJ, Ni HH, Zhang CX, Zhang L, He J, Gu JM, Chen HX, Mai HQ, et al. 2020. Hypoxia induces mitochondrial defect that promotes T cell exhaustion in tumor microenvironment through MYC-regulated pathways. *Front Immunol* 11: 1906. doi:10.3389/fimmu.2020.01906

Loftus RM, Assmann N, Kedia-Mehta N, O'Brien KL, Garcia A, Gillespie C, Hukelmann JL, Oefner PJ, Lamond AI, Gardiner CM, et al. 2018. Amino acid-dependent cMyc expression is essential for NK cell metabolic and functional responses in mice. *Nat Commun* 9: 2341. doi:10.1038/s41467-018-04719-2

Lontos K, Wang Y, Joshi SK, Frisch AT, Watson MJ, Kumar A, Menk AV, Wang Y, Cumberland R, Lohmueller J, et al. 2023. Metabolic reprogramming via an engineered PGC-1α improves human chimeric antigen receptor T-cell therapy against solid tumors. *J Immunother Cancer* 11: e006522. doi:10.1136/jitc-2022-006522

Lundahl MLE, Mitermite M, Ryan DG, Case S, Williams NC, Yang M, Lynch RI, Lagan E, Lebre FM, Gorman AL, et al. 2022. Macrophage innate training induced by IL-4 and IL-13 activation enhances OXPHOS driven anti-mycobacterial responses. *eLife* 11: e74690. doi:10.7554/eLife.74690

Ma EH, Verway MJ, Johnson RM, Roy DG, Steadman M, Hayes S, Williams KS, Sheldon RD, Samborska B, Kosinski PA, et al. 2019a. Metabolic profiling using stable isotope tracing reveals distinct patterns of glucose utilization by physiologically activated CD8+ T cells. *Immunity* 51: 856–870.e5. doi:10.1016/j.immuni.2019.09.003

Ma X, Bi E, Lu Y, Su P, Huang C, Liu L, Wang Q, Yang M, Kalady MF, Qian J, et al. 2019b. Cholesterol induces CD8[+] T cell exhaustion in the tumor microenvironment. *Cell Metab* 30: 143–156.e5. doi:10.1016/j.cmet.2019.04.002

Macintyre AN, Gerriets VA, Nichols AG, Michalek RD, Rudolph MC, Deoliveira D, Anderson SM, Abel ED, Chen BJ, Hale LP, et al. 2014. The glucose transporter Glut1 is selectively essential for CD4 T cell activation and effector function. *Cell Metab* 20: 61–72. doi:10.1016/j.cmet.2014.05.004

Madden MZ, Ye X, Chi C, Fisher EL, Wolf MM, Needle GA, Bader JE, Patterson AR, Reinfeld BI, Landis MD, et al. 2023. Differential effects of glutamine inhibition strategies on antitumor CD8 T cells. *J Immunol* 211: 563–575. doi:10.4049/jimmunol.2200715

Mangalhara KC, Varanasi SK, Johnson MA, Burns MJ, Rojas GR, Esparza Moltó PB, Sainz AG, Tadepalle N, Abbott KL, Mendiratta G, et al. 2023. Manipulating mitochondrial electron flow enhances tumor immunogenicity. *Science* 381: 1316–1323. doi:10.1126/science.abq1053

Marigo I, Zilio S, Desantis G, Mlecnik B, Agnellini AH, Ugel S, Sasso MS, Qualls JE, Kratochvill F, Zanovello P, et al. 2016. T cell cancer therapy requires CD40-CD40L activation of tumor necrosis factor and inducible nitric-oxide-synthase-producing dendritic cells. *Cancer Cell* 30: 377–390. doi:10.1016/j.ccell.2016.08.004

McCormick SM, Heller NM. 2015. Commentary: IL-4 and IL-13 receptors and signaling. *Cytokine* 75: 38–50. doi:10.1016/j.cyto.2015.05.023

McLane LM, Abdel-Hakeem MS, Wherry EJ. 2019. CD8 T cell exhaustion during chronic viral infection and cancer. *Annu Rev Immunol* 37: 457–495. doi:10.1146/annurev-immunol-041015-055318

Mehla K, Singh PK. 2019. Metabolic regulation of macrophage polarization in cancer. *Trends Cancer* 5: 822–834. doi:10.1016/j.trecan.2019.10.007

Menk AV, Scharping NE, Moreci RS, Zeng X, Guy C, Salvatore S, Bae H, Xie J, Young HA, Wendell SG, et al. 2018. Early TCR signaling induces rapid aerobic glycolysis enabling distinct acute T cell effector functions. *Cell Rep* 22: 1509–1521. doi:10.1016/j.celrep.2018.01.040

Mentch SJ, Mehrmohamadi M, Huang L, Liu X, Gupta D, Mattocks D, Gómez Padilla P, Ables G, Bamman MM, Thalacker-Mercer AE, et al. 2015. Histone methylation dynamics and gene regulation occur through the sensing of one-carbon metabolism. *Cell Metab* 22: 861–873. doi:10.1016/j.cmet.2015.08.024

Michelet X, Dyck L, Hogan A, Loftus RM, Duquette D, Wei K, Beyaz S, Tavakkoli A, Foley C, Donnelly R, et al. 2018. Metabolic reprogramming of natural killer cells in obesity limits antitumor responses. *Nat Immunol* 19: 1330–1340. doi:10.1038/s41590-018-0251-7

Mills EL, Ryan DG, Prag HA, Dikovskaya D, Menon D, Zaslona Z, Jedrychowski MP, Costa ASH, Higgins M, Hams E, et al. 2018. Itaconate is an anti-inflammatory metabolite that activates Nrf2 via alkylation of KEAP1. *Nature* 556: 113–117. doi:10.1038/nature25986

Moellering RE, Cravatt BF. 2013. Functional lysine modification by an intrinsically reactive primary glycolytic metabolite. *Science* 341: 549–553. doi:10.1126/science.1238327

Møller SH, Wang L, Ho PC. 2022. Metabolic programming in dendritic cells tailors immune responses and homeostasis.

Cell Mol Immunol 19: 370–383. doi:10.1038/s41423-021-00753-1

Munn DH, Mellor AL. 2013. Indoleamine 2,3 dioxygenase and metabolic control of immune responses. *Trends Immunol* 34: 137–143. doi:10.1016/j.it.2012.10.001

Narayan V, Barber-Rotenberg JS, Jung IY, Lacey SF, Rech AJ, Davis MM, Hwang WT, Lal P, Carpenter EL, Maude SL, et al. 2022. PSMA-targeting TGFβ-insensitive armored CAR T cells in metastatic castration-resistant prostate cancer: a phase 1 trial. *Nat Med* 28: 724–734. doi:10.1038/s41591-022-01726-1

Noman MZ, Desantis G, Janji B, Hasmim M, Karray S, Dessen P, Bronte V, Chouaib S. 2014. PD-L1 is a novel direct target of HIF-1α, and its blockade under hypoxia enhanced MDSC-mediated T cell activation. *J Exp Med* 211: 781–790. doi:10.1084/jem.20131916

Oh MH, Sun IH, Zhao L, Leone RD, Sun IM, Xu W, Collins SL, Tam AJ, Blosser RL, Patel CH, et al. 2020. Targeting glutamine metabolism enhances tumor-specific immunity by modulating suppressive myeloid cells. *J Clin Invest* 130: 3865–3884. doi:10.1172/JCI131859

O'Sullivan D, Stanczak MA, Villa M, Uhl FM, Corrado M, Klein Geltink RI, Sanin DE, Apostolova P, Rana N, Edwards-Hicks J, et al. 2021. Fever supports CD8[+] effector T cell responses by promoting mitochondrial translation. *Proc Natl Acad Sci* 118: e2023752118. doi:10.1073/pnas.2023752118

Palaniappan KK, Bertozzi CR. 2016. Chemical glycoproteomics. *Chem Rev* 116: 14277–14306. doi:10.1021/acs.chemrev.6b00023

Pan S, Chen R. 2022. Pathological implication of protein posttranslational modifications in cancer. *Mol Aspects Med* 86: 101097. doi:10.1016/j.mam.2022.101097

Parry RV, Chemnitz JM, Frauwirth KA, Lanfranco AR, Braunstein I, Kobayashi SV, Linsley PS, Thompson CB, Riley JL. 2005. CTLA-4 and PD-1 receptors inhibit T-cell activation by distinct mechanisms. *Mol Cell Biol* 25: 9543–9553. doi:10.1128/MCB.25.21.9543-9553.2005

Patra KC, Hay N. 2014. The pentose phosphate pathway and cancer. *Trends Biochem Sci* 39: 347–354. doi:10.1016/j.tibs.2014.06.005

Pavlova Natalya N, Thompson Craig B. 2016. The emerging hallmarks of cancer metabolism. *Cell Metab* 23: 27–47. doi:10.1016/j.cmet.2015.12.006

Prendeville H, Lynch L. 2022. Diet, lipids, and antitumor immunity. *Cell Mol Immunol* 19: 432–444. doi:10.1038/s41423-021-00781-x

Qi C, Gong J, Li J, Liu D, Qin Y, Ge S, Zhang M, Peng Z, Zhou J, Cao Y, et al. 2022. Claudin18.2-specific CAR T cells in gastrointestinal cancers: phase 1 trial interim results. *Nat Med* 28: 1189–1198. doi:10.1038/s41591-022-01800-8

Qin W, Qin K, Zhang Y, Jia W, Chen Y, Cheng B, Peng L, Chen N, Liu Y, Zhou W, et al. 2019. S-glycosylation-based cysteine profiling reveals regulation of glycolysis by itaconate. *Nat Chem Biol* 15: 983–991. doi:10.1038/s41589-019-0323-5

Qin W, Zhang Y, Tang H, Liu D, Chen Y, Liu Y, Wang C. 2020. Chemoproteomic profiling of itaconation by bioorthogonal probes in inflammatory macrophages. *J Am Chem Soc* 142: 10894–10898. doi:10.1021/jacs.9b11962

Quinn WJ III, Jiao J, TeSlaa T, Stadanlick J, Wang Z, Wang L, Akimova T, Angelin A, Schäfer PM, Cully MD, et al. 2020. Lactate limits T cell proliferation via the NAD(H) redox state. *Cell Rep* **33:** 108500. doi:10.1016/j.celrep.2020 .108500

Reinfeld BI, Madden MZ, Wolf MM, Chytil A, Bader JE, Patterson AR, Sugiura A, Cohen AS, Ali A, Do BT, et al. 2021. Cell-programmed nutrient partitioning in the tumour microenvironment. *Nature* **593:** 282–288. doi:10 .1038/s41586-021-03442-1

Ron-Harel N, Santos D, Ghergurovich JM, Sage PT, Reddy A, Lovitch SB, Dephoure N, Satterstrom FK, Sheffer M, Spinelli JB, et al. 2016. Mitochondrial biogenesis and proteome remodeling promote one-carbon metabolism for T cell activation. *Cell Metab* **24:** 104–117. doi:10.1016/j.cmet .2016.06.007

Rostamian H, Khakpoor-Koosheh M, Fallah-Mehrjardi K, Mirzaei HR, Brown CE. 2021. Mitochondria as playmakers of CAR T-cell fate and longevity. *Cancer Immunol Res* **9:** 856–861. doi:10.1158/2326-6066.CIR-21-0110

Roy DG, Chen J, Mamane V, Ma EH, Muhire BM, Sheldon RD, Shorstova T, Koning R, Johnson RM, Esaulova E, et al. 2020. Methionine metabolism shapes T helper cell responses through regulation of epigenetic reprogramming. *Cell Metab* **31:** 250–266.e9. doi:10.1016/j.cmet.2020.01 .006

Ryan U, Miriam W, Laura L, ChingLam WW, Lihua EB, Sandra T, Stephen JF, Xiuli W. 2017. Ex vivo Akt inhibition promotes the generation of potent CD19CAR T cells for adoptive immunotherapy. *J ImmunoTher Cancer* **5:** 26. doi:10.1186/s40425-017-0227-4

Scharping NE, Menk AV, Moreci RS, Whetstone RD, Dadey RE, Watkins SC, Ferris RL, Delgoffe GM. 2016. The tumor microenvironment represses T cell mitochondrial biogenesis to drive intratumoral T cell metabolic insufficiency and dysfunction. *Immunity* **45:** 374–388. doi:10.1016/j .immuni.2016.07.009

Scharping NE, Rivadeneira DB, Menk AV, Vignali PDA, Ford BR, Rittenhouse NL, Peralta R, Wang Y, Wang Y, DePeaux K, et al. 2021. Mitochondrial stress induced by continuous stimulation under hypoxia rapidly drives T cell exhaustion. *Nat Immunol* **22:** 205–215. doi:10.1038/s41590-020-00834-9

Schultz L, Mackall C. 2019. Driving CAR T cell translation forward. *Sci Transl Med* **11:** eaaw2127. doi:10.1126/sci translmed.aaw2127

Secinaro MA, Fortner KA, Collins C, Rincón M, Budd RC. 2019. Glycolysis induces MCJ expression that links T cell proliferation with caspase-3 activity and death. *Front Cell Dev Biol* **7:** 28. doi:10.3389/fcell.2019.00028

Seim GL, Britt EC, John SV, Yeo FJ, Johnson AR, Eisenstein RS, Pagliarini DJ, Fan J. 2019. Two-stage metabolic remodelling in macrophages in response to lipopolysaccharide and interferon-γ stimulation. *Nat Metab* **1:** 731–742. doi:10.1038/s42255-019-0083-2

Siska PJ, van der Windt GJ, Kishton RJ, Cohen S, Eisner W, MacIver NJ, Kater AP, Weinberg JB, Rathmell JC. 2016. Suppression of Glut1 and glucose metabolism by decreased Akt/mTORC1 signaling drives T cell impairment in B cell leukemia. *J Immunol* **197:** 2532–2540. doi:10 .4049/jimmunol.1502464

Siska PJ, Beckermann KE, Mason FM, Andrejeva G, Greenplate AR, Sendor AB, Chiang YJ, Corona AL, Gemta LF, Vincent BG, et al. 2017. Mitochondrial dysregulation and glycolytic insufficiency functionally impair CD8 T cells infiltrating human renal cell carcinoma. *JCI Insight* **2:** e93411. doi:10.1172/jci.insight.93411

Smith BAH, Bertozzi CR. 2021. The clinical impact of glycobiology: targeting selectins, siglecs and mammalian glycans. *Nat Rev Drug Discov* **20:** 217–243. doi:10.1038/ s41573-020-00093-1

Smith BC, Marletta MA. 2012. Mechanisms of *S*-nitrosothiol formation and selectivity in nitric oxide signaling. *Curr Opin Chem Biol* **16:** 498–506. doi:10.1016/j.cbpa.2012.10.016

Sugiura A, Andrejeva G, Voss K, Heintzman DR, Xu X, Madden MZ, Ye X, Beier KL, Chowdhury NU, Wolf MM, et al. 2022. MTHFD2 is a metabolic checkpoint controlling effector and regulatory T cell fate and function. *Immunity* **55:** 65–81.e9. doi:10.1016/j.immuni.2021.10.011

Sukumar M, Liu J, Ji Y, Subramanian M, Crompton JG, Yu Z, Roychoudhuri R, Palmer DC, Muranski P, Karoly ED, et al. 2013. Inhibiting glycolytic metabolism enhances CD8[+] T cell memory and antitumor function. *J Clin Invest* **123:** 4479–4488. doi:10.1172/JCI69589

Sukumar M, Liu J, Mehta GU, Patel SJ, Roychoudhuri R, Crompton JG, Klebanoff CA, Ji Y, Li P, Yu Z, et al. 2016. Mitochondrial membrane potential identifies cells with enhanced stemness for cellular therapy. *Cell Metab* **23:** 63–76. doi:10.1016/j.cmet.2015.11.002

Sutendra G, Kinnaird A, Dromparis P, Paulin R, Stenson TH, Haromy A, Hashimoto K, Zhang N, Flaim E, Michelakis ED. 2014. A nuclear pyruvate dehydrogenase complex is important for the generation of acetyl-CoA and histone acetylation. *Cell* **158:** 84–97. doi:10.1016/j.cell.2014.04 .046

Tchou J, Zhao Y, Levine BL, Zhang PJ, Davis MM, Melenhorst JJ, Kulikovskaya I, Brennan AL, Liu X, Lacey SF, et al. 2017. Safety and efficacy of intratumoral injections of chimeric antigen receptor (CAR) T cells in metastatic breast cancer. *Cancer Immunol Res* **5:** 1152–1161. doi:10.1158/ 2326-6066.CIR-17-0189

Tripathi P, Kurtulus S, Wojciechowski S, Sholl A, Hoebe K, Morris SC, Finkelman FD, Grimes HL, Hildeman DA. 2010. STAT5 is critical to maintain effector CD8[+] T cell responses. *J Immunol* **185:** 2116–2124. doi:10.4049/jim munol.1000842

van Bruggen JAC, Martens AWJ, Fraietta JA, Hofland T, Tonino SH, Eldering E, Levin MD, Siska PJ, Endstra S, Rathmell JC, et al. 2019. Chronic lymphocytic leukemia cells impair mitochondrial fitness in CD8[+] T cells and impede CAR T-cell efficacy. *Blood* **134:** 44–58. doi:10.1182/blood .2018885863

Van den Bossche J, O'Neill LA, Menon D. 2017. Macrophage immunometabolism: where are we (going)? *Trends Immunol* **38:** 395–406. doi:10.1016/j.it.2017.03.001

Vardhana SA, Hwee MA, Berisa M, Wells DK, Yost KE, King B, Smith M, Herrera PS, Chang HY, Satpathy AT, et al. 2020. Impaired mitochondrial oxidative phosphorylation limits the self-renewal of T cells exposed to persistent antigen. *Nat Immunol* **21:** 1022–1033. doi:10.1038/s41590-020-0725-2

Varghese S, Pramanik S, Williams LJ, Hodges HR, Hudgens CW, Fischer GM, Luo CK, Knighton B, Tan L, Lorenzi PL, et al. 2021. The glutaminase inhibitor CB-839 (Telaglenastat) enhances the antimelanoma activity of T-cell-mediated immunotherapies. *Mol Cancer Ther* **20**: 500–511. doi:10.1158/1535-7163.MCT-20-0430

Veglia F, Tyurin VA, Mohammadyani D, Blasi M, Duperret EK, Donthireddy L, Hashimoto A, Kapralov A, Amoscato A, Angelini R, et al. 2017. Lipid bodies containing oxidatively truncated lipids block antigen cross-presentation by dendritic cells in cancer. *Nat Commun* **8**: 2122. doi:10.1038/s41467-017-02186-9

Villarino AV, Laurence AD, Davis FP, Nivelo L, Brooks SR, Sun HW, Jiang K, Afzali B, Frasca D, Hennighausen L, et al. 2022. A central role for STAT5 in the transcriptional programing of T helper cell metabolism. *Sci Immunol* **7**: eabl9467. doi:10.1126/sciimmunol.abl9467

Wagner J, Wickman E, DeRenzo C, Gottschalk S. 2020. CAR t cell therapy for solid tumors: bright future or dark reality? *Mol Ther* **28**: 2320–2339. doi:10.1016/j.ymthe.2020.09.015

Wang R, Dillon CP, Shi LZ, Milasta S, Carter R, Finkelstein D, McCormick LL, Fitzgerald P, Chi H, Munger J, et al. 2011. The transcription factor Myc controls metabolic reprogramming upon T lymphocyte activation. *Immunity* **35**: 871–882. doi:10.1016/j.immuni.2011.09.021

Wang Y, Chen M, Wu Z, Tong C, Dai H, Guo Y, Liu Y, Huang J, Lv H, Luo C, et al. 2018. CD133-directed CAR T cells for advanced metastasis malignancies: a phase I trial. *OncoImmunol* **7**: e1440169. doi:10.1080/2162402X.2018.1440169

Warburg O. 1956. On the origin of cancer cells. *Science* **123**: 309–314. doi:10.1126/science.123.3191.309

Watson MJ, Vignali PDA, Mullett SJ, Overacre-Delgoffe AE, Peralta RM, Grebinoski S, Menk AV, Rittenhouse NL, DePeaux K, Whetstone RD, et al. 2021. Metabolic support of tumour-infiltrating regulatory T cells by lactic acid. *Nature* **591**: 645–651. doi:10.1038/s41586-020-03045-2

Wenes M, Jaccard A, Wyss T, Maldonado-Pérez N, Teoh ST, Lepez A, Renaud F, Franco F, Waridel P, Yacoub Maroun C, et al. 2022. The mitochondrial pyruvate carrier regulates memory T cell differentiation and antitumor function. *Cell Metab* **34**: 731–746.e9. doi:10.1016/j.cmet.2022.03.013

Wu JY, Huang TW, Hsieh YT, Wang YF, Yen CC, Lee GL, Yeh CC, Peng YJ, Kuo YY, Wen HT, et al. 2020. Cancer-derived succinate promotes macrophage polarization and cancer metastasis via succinate receptor. *Mol Cell* **77**: 213–227.e5. doi:10.1016/j.molcel.2019.10.023

Xu S, Chaudhary O, Rodríguez-Morales P, Sun X, Chen D, Zappasodi R, Xu Z, Pinto AFM, Williams A, Schulze I, et al. 2021. Uptake of oxidized lipids by the scavenger receptor CD36 promotes lipid peroxidation and dysfunction in CD8$^+$ T cells in tumors. *Immunity* **54**: 1561–1577.e7. doi:10.1016/j.immuni.2021.05.003

Yang C, Ko B, Hensley CT, Jiang L, Wasti AT, Kim J, Sudderth J, Calvaruso MA, Lumata L, Mitsche M, et al. 2014. Glutamine oxidation maintains the TCA cycle and cell survival during impaired mitochondrial pyruvate transport. *Mol Cell* **56**: 414–424. doi:10.1016/j.molcel.2014.09.025

Yang K, Halima A, Chan TA. 2023. Antigen presentation in cancer—mechanisms and clinical implications for immunotherapy. *Nat Rev Clin Oncol* **20**: 604–623. doi:10.1038/s41571-023-00789-4

Ye L, Park JJ, Peng L, Yang Q, Chow RD, Dong MB, Lam SZ, Guo J, Tang E, Zhang Y, et al. 2022. A genome-scale gain-of-function CRISPR screen in CD8 T cells identifies proline metabolism as a means to enhance CAR-T therapy. *Cell Metab* **34**: 595–614.e14. doi:10.1016/j.cmet.2022.02.009

Yin H, Xu L, Porter NA. 2011. Free radical lipid peroxidation: mechanisms and analysis. *Chem Rev* **111**: 5944–5972. doi:10.1021/cr200084z

Yu YR, Imrichova H, Wang H, Chao T, Xiao Z, Gao M, Rincon-Restrepo M, Franco F, Genolet R, Cheng WC, et al. 2020. Disturbed mitochondrial dynamics in CD8$^+$ TILs reinforce T cell exhaustion. *Nat Immunol* **21**: 1540–1551. doi:10.1038/s41590-020-0793-3

Zhang L, Li S. 2020. Lactic acid promotes macrophage polarization through MCT-HIF1α signaling in gastric cancer. *Exp Cell Res* **388**: 111846. doi:10.1016/j.yexcr.2020.111846

Zhang J, Pavlova NN, Thompson CB. 2017. Cancer cell metabolism: the essential role of the nonessential amino acid, glutamine. *EMBO J* **36**: 1302–1315. doi:10.15252/embj.201696151

Zhang D, Tang Z, Huang H, Zhou G, Cui C, Weng Y, Liu W, Kim S, Lee S, Perez-Neut M, et al. 2019. Metabolic regulation of gene expression by histone lactylation. *Nature* **574**: 575–580. doi:10.1038/s41586-019-1678-1

Zhao S, Torres A, Henry RA, Trefely S, Wallace M, Lee JV, Carrer A, Sengupta A, Campbell SL, Kuo YM, et al. 2016. ATP-citrate lyase controls a glucose-to-acetate metabolic switch. *Cell Rep* **17**: 1037–1052. doi:10.1016/j.celrep.2016.09.069

Zhao F, Xiao C, Evans KS, Theivanthiran T, DeVito N, Holtzhausen A, Liu J, Liu X, Boczkowski D, Nair S, et al. 2018. Paracrine Wnt5a-β-catenin signaling triggers a metabolic program that drives dendritic cell tolerization. *Immunity* **48**: 147–160.e7. doi:10.1016/j.immuni.2017.12.004

Zhao H, Teng D, Yang L, Xu X, Chen J, Jiang T, Feng AY, Zhang Y, Frederick DT, Gu L, et al. 2022. Myeloid-derived itaconate suppresses cytotoxic CD8$^+$ T cells and promotes tumour growth. *Nat Metab* **4**: 1660–1673. doi:10.1038/s42255-022-00676-9

Zheng Y, Delgoffe GM, Meyer CF, Chan W, Powell JD. 2009. Anergic T cells are metabolically anergic. *J Immunol* **183**: 6095–6101. doi:10.4049/jimmunol.0803510

Zheng Q, Omans ND, Leicher R, Osunsade A, Agustinus AS, Finkin-Groner E, D'Ambrosio H, Liu B, Chandarlapaty S, Liu S, et al. 2019. Reversible histone glycation is associated with disease-related changes in chromatin architecture. *Nat Commun* **10**: 1289. doi:10.1038/s41467-019-09192-z

Diet and Cancer Metabolism

Jason W. Locasale,[1] Marcus D. Goncalves,[2] Maira Di Tano,[2] and Guillermo Burgos-Barragan[3]

[1]Department of Pharmacology and Cancer Biology, Duke University School of Medicine, 308 Research Drive, Durham, Norh Carolina 27710, USA

[2]Division of Endocrinology, Department of Medicine, Meyer Cancer Center, Weill Cornell Medicine, New York, New York 10065, USA

[3]Department of Pharmacology, Meyer Cancer Center, Weill Cornell Medicine, New York, New York 10056, USA

Correspondence: dr.jason.locasale@gmail.com

Diet and exercise are modifiable lifestyle factors known to have a major influence on metabolism. Clinical practice addresses diseases of altered metabolism such as diabetes or hypertension by altering these factors. Despite enormous public interest, there are limited defined diet and exercise regimens for cancer patients. Nevertheless, the molecular basis of cancer has converged over the past 15 years on an essential role for altered metabolism in cancer. However, our understanding of the molecular mechanisms that underlie the impact of diet and exercise on cancer metabolism is in its very early stages. In this work, we propose conceptual frameworks for understanding the consequences of diet and exercise on cancer cell metabolism and tumor biology and also highlight recent developments. By advancing our mechanistic understanding, we also discuss actionable ways that such interventions could eventually reach the mainstay of both medical oncology and cancer control and prevention.

Nature and nurture are important in shaping the status of a biological system.[4] Both the genetic makeup and the environment that interacts with the living system are highly relevant to all complex diseases and health statuses. For metabolism—broadly defined as the collection of chemical reactions that sustain life—hereditary factors provide the genetic foundation for metabolism, while the environment can modulate the transcription programs, signaling pathways, and chromatin modifying enzymes that regulate metabolic enzymes.

Cancer biology has benefit from the enormous advances in technology over the past 50 years. These advancements have played a crucial role in elucidating the essential genetic characteristics of cancer cells (Ding et al. 2018). For instance, the identification of mutations in oncogenes and tumor suppressor genes has provided valuable insights into the development of tumors, progression of metastasis, and the varying susceptibility to certain therapies. Some of the most common cancer genes, including *KRAS*, *PIK3CA*, *CMYC*, and *TP53*, have substantial im-

---

[4]This is an update to a previous article published in Cancer Discovery [Locasale JW (2022). Diet and exercise in cancer metabolism. *Cancer Discov* **12:** 2249–2257. doi:10.1158/2159-8290.CD-22-0096].

pact on metabolism and these findings have sparked a remarkable surge of interest in cancer metabolism over the last 15 years (Martínez-Reyes and Chandel 2021). As a result, it is now widely recognized that cancer biology is characterized by genetically determined metabolic programs, and the altered metabolism is considered a hallmark of cancer.

The environmental factors that influence cancer metabolism have been far less considered, but numerous studies have shown they are equally, if not more, important (Vander Heiden and DeBerardinis 2017). For example, the composition and quality of the diet can affect cancer cell metabolism directly by providing or removing essential building blocks for tumor growth and survival. Diet can also indirectly influence the local abundance of growth-promoting mitogens, which are substances that bind to cells and stimulate cell division, proliferation, and metabolism. Despite knowledge of these direct and indirect links between diet and cancer, the specific pathways in which diet propagates within the host to influence cancer metabolism remains largely unknown. Further research in these areas is essential for a comprehensive understanding of tumor growth and the development of targeted therapeutic strategies.

PRINCIPLES OF DIET AND MOLECULAR METABOLISM

Diet may impact tumor biology by delivering or restricting specific nutrients to cancer cells or by promoting/reversing a tumorigenic neurohormonal state (Fig. 1). Since both processes are interconnected, it is often difficult to distinguish the specific mediators, which is a limitation of this field.

Dietary nutrients are extracted from food via the process of mastication and digestion, which physically and chemically breaks food into smaller particles that can be absorbed. Digestive enzymes from the salivary glands, stomach, liver, pancreas, and intestine break down proteins into amino acids, complex carbohydrates into simple sugars, and fats into fatty acids and glycerol, which are all transported into the bloodstream or lymphatic system. The absorbed nutrients are then carried to various tissues and organs throughout the body, where they are used for energy production, growth, repair, and various metabolic processes. Any unabsorbed nutrients or indigestible materials accumulate in the large intestine, where they can be metabolized by microbiota or disposed of as waste.

Tumor cells may benefit from direct access to dietary nutrients much like other cells of the body. Studies have demonstrated that plasma metabolite levels can be predicted to some extent by diet, with some nutrients being more heavily modifiable than others. Further, there is also a correlation between nutrient levels and the interstitial tissue fluid where the cancer resides, implying that microenvironmental nutrient availability derives in some or large part from metabolites in blood circulation (Sullivan et al. 2019). Indeed, in cell culture models, such changes are predicted to have a large effect on cancer metabolism in many cases, sometimes larger than the impact of mutating potent oncogenes, which are thought to be the major determinant of altered metabolism.

The processes of ingestion, digestion, and absorption are all under the control of the endocrine system and require the engagement of numerous organs, hormones, and cell signaling pathways that coordinate systemic physiology. Perhaps the best example is that of physiological glucose regulation by insulin. Consumption of dietary carbohydrates results in a systemic rise in insulin levels from the pancreas, which promotes glucose disposal from the blood into tissues. Insulin induces the translocation of the glucose transporter to the plasma membrane in tissues such as skeletal muscle, the phosphorylation of hundreds of metabolic enzymes across all tissues, and the transcriptional regulation of metabolic genes through signaling pathways involving kinases such as AKT and mTOR. Similar nutrient-sensing pathways for protein and lipids influence systemic and cellular metabolism. As additional illustrative examples, there are elevations in growth hormone (GH) and insulin-like growth factor 1 (IGF-1) following ingestion of dietary protein and changes in the levels of circulating lipoproteins following the activation of cholesterol-sensing systems in the liver that are

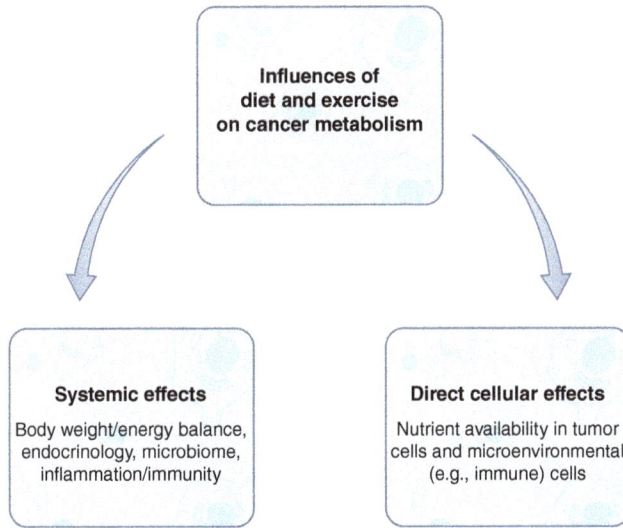

Figure 1. Systemic and direct metabolic influences of diet and exercise on cancer metabolism. Lifestyle factors involving diet and exercise alter tumor metabolism through both systemic influences on organismal physiology (*left*) and direct effects on cellular metabolism through changes in nutrient availability (*right*). (Figure adapted from Locasale 2022, © the authors; Published by the American Association for Cancer Research.)

induced by lipid consumption. This secondary hormonal-metabolic response is an indirect way for diet to impact tumor growth.

Excess consumption of food leads to a disproportionate storage of nutrients in the body, leading to a state of systemic adipocyte expansion called obesity. Currently, over one-third of U.S. adults are obese and this value will rise to one-half by 2030 (Ward et al. 2019). There is sufficient evidence that obesity increases the risk of developing 13 different types of cancer, and the presence of obesity worsens cancer outcomes (Lauby-Secretan et al. 2016; Petrelli et al. 2021). The molecular links between obesity and cancer development and progression are incompletely understood. Obesity increases the abundance of mitogenic hormones like insulin, IGF-1, and leptin, an adipose-secreted hormone that activates proinflammatory signaling in tumor cells (Hopkins et al. 2016). Moreover, obesity promotes low-grade inflammation, which may drive tumor development and perturb antitumor immunity (Iyengar et al. 2016; Ringel et al. 2020). Other recent studies have shown that changes to adipose tissue metabolism can affect tumor growth, which appears to have a mechanism more aligned with nutrient exchange across or-

gans and resulting changes to nutrient uptake in the tumor (Seki et al. 2022). Therefore, weight loss interventions are major avenue for cancer prevention and treatment.

DIET AS CANCER PREVENTION

It has been estimated that about a third of the most common cancers are preventable, in part, through a nutritious diet (Song and Giovannucci 2016). While the specific dietary components driving the risk for cancer have not been fully elucidated, epidemiologic studies have implicated dietary fat. Low fat diets safely promote weight loss, fat loss, lower blood cholesterol, and reduced food intake, suggesting they may be useful as interventions for obese patients with cancer (Hall et al. 2021). The hypothesis that low fat diets reduce cancer incidence was rigorously tested in the Women's Health Initiative Dietary Modification trial, a prospective, randomized, controlled study in postmenopausal women designed to examine the long-term benefits and risks of a low-fat (20% kcal) dietary intervention on the risk of breast and colorectal cancers (Chlebowski et al. 2017, 2018). The low-fat diet arm only missed a significant positive effect to reduce breast cancer incidence (hazard ratio [HR] 0.92, 95% confidence interval [CI] 0.84, 1.01) and it lowered the incidence of deaths after breast cancer diagnosis (Thomson et al. 2014). In the Women's Intervention Nutrition Study and the Women's Healthy Eating and Living studies, women with previously treated, early-stage breast cancer were randomized to a low-fat intervention (Chlebowski et al. 2006; Pierce et al. 2007). Both trials achieved ~9% reduction in dietary fat intake between intervention and control groups, and the data suggests a beneficial effect only in subgroups of patients with breast cancer. For example, there was a diet-induced reduction in recurrences among women who did not experience hot flashes (Gold et al. 2009). To our knowledge, there are no other prospective intervention trials testing the effect of a dietary intervention on the incidence of cancer.

Several medical associations and international guidelines have published dietary guidelines for the prevention of chronic diseases including cancer. The dietary patterns resulting from these guidelines were recently compared using data from more than 205,000 subjects from three prospective, observational studies followed for up to 32 years (Wang et al. 2023). The results demonstrated that adherence to any generally considered healthy diet was associated with a lower risk of major chronic disease, including cancer (HR comparing the 90th with the 10th percentile of dietary pattern scores = 0.58–0.80). However, participants that followed a dietary pattern that suppresses insulin had the largest risk reduction for cancer (HR = 0.58, 95% CI 0.57, 0.60).

Many of the dietary guidelines suggest avoiding alcohol consumption. There is strong evidence to suggest that high alcohol consumption has a significant impact on tumor development, especially those of the breast and organs of the gastrointestinal tract (Cao and Giovannucci 2016). The total amount of alcohol consumed over time, not the type of alcoholic beverage, appears to be the most important factor. Ethanol is metabolized to acetaldehyde, which can promote cancer development through multiple mechanisms, including interference with DNA replication, induction of DNA damage, and for-

mation of DNA adducts (Seitz and Stickel 2007). Moreover, ethanol can fuel central carbon metabolism because it is rapidly metabolized to acetate. The specific mediators that link alcohol to cancer development are still unknown for most cancer types.

Dietary consumption of red and processed meat is an important contributor to the development of certain cancer types. In a comprehensive systematic review and meta-analysis, high red meat intake was positively associated with risk of breast cancer, endometrial cancer, colorectal cancer, colon cancer, rectal cancer, lung cancer, and hepatocellular carcinoma, and high processed meat intake was positively associated with risk of breast, colorectal, colon, rectal, and lung cancers (Farvid et al. 2021). Regarding the mechanistic link between meat and cancer, different hypotheses have been proposed. For example, the lipid peroxidation of heme forms N-nitroso compounds and genotoxic aldehydes, meat contains N-glycolylneuraminic acid and other genotoxic compounds, and the role of the heterocyclic amines and polycyclic aromatic hydrocarbons can promote DNA mutation. A recent study that combined patient diet records with genomic information found an alkylating signature associated with mutagenesis and the acquisition of specific oncogenic mutations in genes such as *KRAS* and *PIK3CA* in subjects consuming higher quantities of red meat (Gurjao et al. 2021); however, it is unknown whether carcinogens and direct mutagenesis are the driver of this alkylating signature or whether the digestion and resulting changes to systemic and cellular metabolism is the cause.

DIETARY INTERVENTIONS AS CANCER THERAPY

In recent years, there has been a surge of interest toward elucidating the mechanisms that link diet to cancer growth and metabolism (Bose et al. 2020; Kanarek et al. 2020; Tajan and Vousden 2020). In preclinical models, dietary interventions synergize with chemo-, radiation, targeted, and immune therapies—all potentially paving the way for dietary interventions as anticancer therapy. Mounting evidence clearly support that diet may impact tumor initiation, progression, and response to therapies, making dietary interventions a potent tool for cancer prevention and treatment. In general, there is a hierarchy of dietary considerations beginning with energy balance, then leading to relative macronutrient intake, and ultimately considering differences in macronutrient consumption (Fig. 2). Here, we

highlight some key and recent findings where new mechanistic insight is emerging.

Dietary interventions can be tailored to address key mediators that support tumor growth. For example, diets that restrict energy intake (hypocaloric) activate a conserved metabolic program that results in weight loss (Ludwig et al. 2021; Hall et al. 2022). For example, an increase

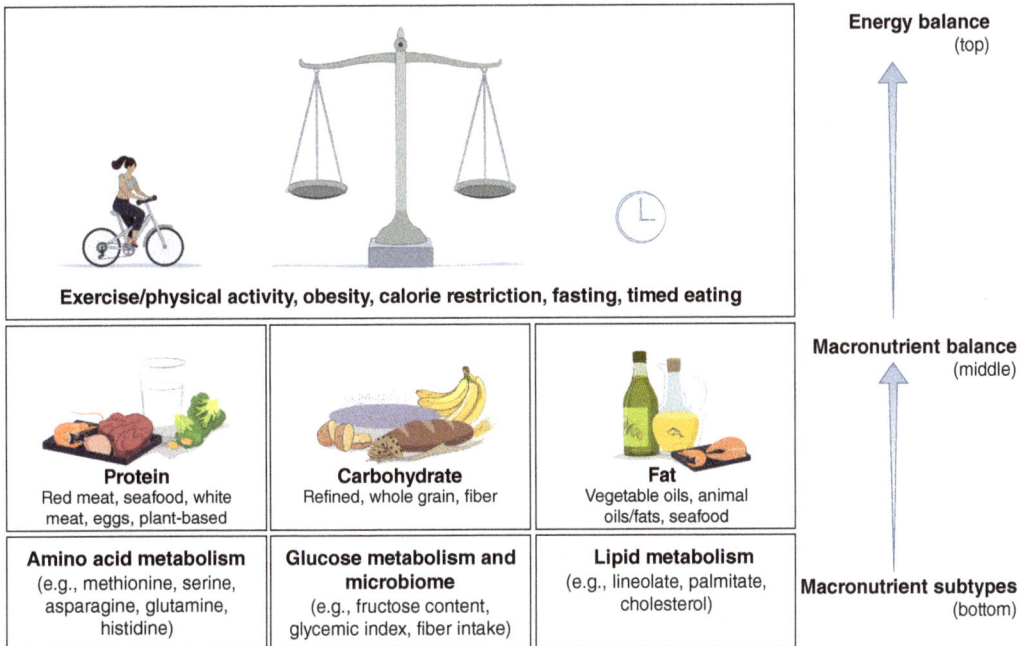

Figure 2. Proposed hierarchical order of influences of diet and exercise on metabolism. A hierarchical view of diet and exercise and its effects on cancer metabolism. Beginning the hierarchy is energy balance (*top*). Energy balance is roughly defined as the total calorie intake from food minus energy expenditure in part through exercise and other energy-dissipating processes such as digestion and thermogenesis. As has been discussed extensively elsewhere and generally speaking, excess energy contributes to obesity. This stage would include obesity, exercise, timed eating, caloric restriction, and fasting. Next in the hierarchy (*middle*) is macronutrient balance. This consideration involves the relative dietary intake of the three caloric sources or macronutrients: protein, carbohydrate, and fat. This would cover diets such ketogenic, paleo, protein restriction, low carbohydrate, vegan, etc. In light of this hierarchical model, these diets of differential macronutrient composition should first be considered relative to their effects on energy balance. For example, low carbohydrate diets are often lower in calories so this should be considered in any conclusions drawn. Finally, the hierarchy considers changes in the dietary intake of macronutrient subtype (*bottom*). These diets involve changes to relative intake of certain types of macronutrients. In lifestyles in the human population, this would involve red meat consumption, veganism, sugary beverage intake, fiber intake, keto, etc. In laboratory studies, this would involve, for example, saturated fat composition and amino acid–depleted diets. In the hierarchical model, the effects these diets have should be considered first in reference to both the over energy balance they alter and next their effects on macronutrient balance. For example, a diet deprived of serine or restricted of methionine should be considered (i.e., these variables should be controlled) in reference to both its total calories and its total protein. Further, a diet high in fructose should also be considered in reference to both its total calories and its total carbohydrate intake. (Figure adapted from Locasale 2022, © the authors; published by the American Association for Cancer Research.)

in adipose tissue lipolysis and hepatic fatty acid oxidation improves obesity, and the resulting reduction in whole-body fat mass lowers the amount of protumorigenic, hormonal mitogens like insulin, IGF-1, and leptin (Hopkins et al. 2016). Hypocaloric diets include portion control or caloric restriction (CR), and those with extended periods of fasting like alternate day fasting (ADF) and fasting-mimicking diets (FMDs). Other dietary interventions that manipulate the macronutrient (carbohydrates, fats, protein) content of the meals can promote satiety and indirectly induce a hypocaloric state, in addition to withholding specific macromolecules. Last, diets can be constructed with nutrients that antagonize tumor metabolism (e.g., antioxidant vitamins) or without nutrients that are required for tumor growth (e.g., nonessential amino acids).

Fasting, Calorie Restriction, and Altering Glucose Metabolism

Extensive research in animal models has shown that diet timing, caloric content, and macronutrient composition impact cancer initiation, progression, and response to therapy (Tajan and Vousden 2020; Longo and Anderson 2022; Taylor et al. 2022).

CR, the oldest dietary intervention, has been described as reduced food intake (15%–30% caloric reduction) without malnutrition, and it has been shown to reduce tumor incidence and retard tumor growth in different animal models (Thompson et al. 2003; Colman et al. 2009; Mercken et al. 2012). Fasting defined as a condition of no or minimal food intake, from 1 d to a wk, represents the most extreme form of CR. CR and fasting have been shown to cause a global decrease of protumorigenic signals, such as insulin, the GH-IGF-1 axis, amino acids, and glucose levels, which are thought to be partially responsible for their antitumor effects (Hofer et al. 2022). However, the benefits of CR are limited by poor adherence and high grades of weight loss. Cycles of fasting have been demonstrated to be more tolerated and to exert a more global action by activating transcriptional programs of protection and regeneration in healthy cells (Raffa-

ghello et al. 2008; Brandhorst et al. 2015; Longo and Anderson 2022). Because of their oncogenes, cancer cells avoid fasting-mediated antigrowth stimuli, and fail to be protected (Raffaghello et al. 2008; Lee et al. 2012). Notably, multiple works in animal models have shown that cycles of fasting sensitize tumor cells to a range of cancer therapies (Lee et al. 2012; Caffa et al. 2020; Di Tano et al. 2020).

Despite the safety and mild side effects, complete fasting may still be challenging, especially for oncological patients. Therefore, FMDs, which consist of a plant-based 5-d regimen characterized by low proteins, sugar, and high unsaturated fats, have been formulated to mimic the effects of fasting. FMD cycles have been shown to be feasible and safe for cancer patients, and to exert a substantial effect on tumor metabolism and antitumor immunity (de Groot et al. 2015, 2020; Wei et al. 2017; Vernieri et al. 2022).

Notably, some metabolic effects induced by CR and FMD, including the beneficial combination with current therapies, can be recapitulated by other dietary interventions that alter macronutrient ratios. For example, a very low carbohydrate diet with high-fat content and low-to-moderate protein also lowers insulin and IGF-1 levels. These diets are also referred to as ketogenic diets because they induce high rates of fatty acid oxidation, which produces large amounts of ketone bodies in the blood. Ketogenic diets enhance the efficacy of PI3K inhibitors (a kinase-directed targeted therapy) by suppressing insulin levels in mice (Hopkins et al. 2018; Lien et al. 2021). Existing data support the feasibility of this approach in patients with cancer (Cohen et al. 2018; Khodabakhshi et al. 2020); however, its efficacy as an anticancer intervention remains unclear.

Restricting sugar may also benefit patients with cancer. Moderate, chronic exposure to fructose in the form of high fructose corn syrup (HFCS) promotes the growth and advances the grade of intestinal adenomas in mice (Goncalves et al. 2019). Fructose metabolites were found to directly promote cell survival through allosteric regulation of cell metabolism (Taylor et al. 2021). These findings suggest that the combination of glucose and fructose in the diet can enhance tumorigenesis. Indeed, early exposure to fructose in sugar-sweetened beverages increases the risk for colorectal adenomas, the precursors to cancer (Hur et al. 2021; Joh et al. 2021).

Despite the progress in understanding the contribution of diets in cancer prevention and treatment, one fundamental question that is still an object of debate is whether the observed beneficial effects are consequences of the reduction in calories or specific macronutrient ratios. Solon-Biet et al. (2014, 2015) showed that macronutrient ratios and not caloric intake dictates the benefits of diets on longevity and health in mice. Notably, they showed that CR achieved by a high protein diet or dietary dilution, fails to improve life span. These data strongly suggest the crucial role of macronutrient ratios as key factors in mediating the prolongevity effect of the diet, without any need to reduce caloric intake (Solon-Biet et al. 2014, 2015).

Lipid Metabolism

Similarly, others have shown that the beneficial effects of CR can be abrogated by altering lipid content (Lien et al. 2021). In this interesting study, the expression of stearoyl-CoA desaturase (SCD) and diets high in palm oil could disrupt the antitumor effects of CR. Several studies have implicated alterations in lipid metabolism in cancer and particularly metastasis through numerous mechanisms including the generation of specific sphingolipids, changes to the activity of acyl carrier proteins, the engagement of an alternative desaturation pathway, and the uptake at lipid-rich environments during metastatic colonization (Broadfield et al. 2021). Saturated fat intake, often modeled in laboratory animals through animal feed containing high palm oil or in cell culture by using palmitate, has been shown to have interesting effects particularly on brain metastasis. One study showed that diets rich in palm oil could promote metastasis through altering epigenetics via the lipid transporter CD36-dependent lipid uptake and histone H3 lysine 4 deposition, which in turn could lead to a neural signature in neighboring cells characterized by altered behavior of intratumoral Schwann cells and innervation (Pascual et al. 2021). Last, studies have shown that excess lipid

intake can impair antitumor immune responses (Michelet et al. 2018). Together, these data highlight the importance of lipid metabolism in cancer, dietary lipid intake, and altered antitumor immunity.

Amino Acid Metabolism

There has been much interest in diets that restrict fat or carbohydrates as an intervention for cancer (Gardner et al. 2018). There are fewer studies investigating diets with altered protein content, possibly due to fears of protein deficiency contributing to catabolic tissue wasting. However, amino acid–metabolizing pathways have been shown to be important for cancer proliferation and have emerged as promising drug targets (Sanderson et al. 2019; Bose et al. 2020; Kanarek et al. 2020; Tajan and Vousden 2020). For example, some tumor cells synthesize increased amounts of the amino acid serine from glucose (Locasale et al. 2011). Serine is biochemically linked to folate and methionine metabolism through the donation of its single carbon side chain to a folate moiety, resulting in the production of glycine. The downstream metabolism is collectively known as one carbon metabolism and serves a plethora of metabolic functions important for cancer such as nucleotide synthesis, maintenance of redox status, and epigenomic status. Consequently, studies in xenografts and later in autochthonous, genetically defined mouse tumors were able to show that removing serine and glycine from the diet could induce substantial antitumor responses and even synergize with inhibition of enzymes that produce serine from glucose (Maddocks et al. 2013, 2017).

The amino acid methionine comprises the other key input to one carbon metabolism (Sanderson et al. 2019). Methionine has been shown in some cohorts to be the most variable amino acid in plasma and estimates using dietary records and quantitative modeling indicated that close to one-half of the variation could be explained by diet (Mentch et al. 2015). In addition, dietary methionine restriction is known to confer anti-aging and anti-obesity properties, while leading to specific changes in one carbon–related metabolism. In several laboratory studies involving patient-derived xenografts and genetically engineered mouse models, this same nutritional intervention could interact with some of the common therapies that are coupled to one carbon metabolism involving radiation and antimetabolite chemotherapy (Gao et al. 2019). The underlying mechanism appeared to be the enhanced dependence on methionine for coupling to and maintenance of the folate cycle downstream effects when methionine was limiting. Other studies have pointed to sphingolipid metabolism as being relevant to the antitumor properties, which could have some effects on metastasis as well (Muthusamy et al. 2020; Rossi et al. 2022). Furthermore, a dietary intervention such as methionine restriction has been shown to achieve a comparable metabolic profile as that in humans eating a plant-based, low-protein diet (Pham et al. 2022).

Additional studies have shown that other amino acids can induce antitumor effects upon removal, restriction, or increasing their dietary intake (Bose et al. 2020; Kanarek et al. 2020; Tajan and Vousden 2020). Dietary asparagine, whose metabolism is only three reaction steps involving glutamate from the TCA cycle, was found to synergize with the anticancer effects of metformin, a drug targeting mitochondrial metabolism (Krall et al. 2021). Dietary supplementation with glutamine, whose metabolism can interact with the TCA cycle via two reaction steps involving glutamate, can also exert anticancer metabolism (Ishak Gabra et al. 2020). Histidine is another example where supplementation can lead to synergy with methotrexate, an antifolate agent, as chemotherapy through its coupling to the folate cycle (Kanarek et al. 2020).

Together, a picture emerges whereby single changes to dietary amino acid content in mice can propagate into the tumor site to influence the metabolic flux related to the amino acid of interest. When that flux is involved in maintaining processes important for cancer proliferation directly or in combination with a therapy of interest, such as its effects on the immune system or on chemo- or radiation therapy, a therapeutic outcome can be achieved. These studies further converge on an important concept that protein content, both in its quantity and quality (i.e., the amino acid content a given type of protein confers), are dietary variables of interest to cancer and more relevant to disease than currently considered (MacArthur et al. 2021). More work is needed however, in relating these laboratory studies to human diet. For example, there is an interesting anticorrelation of serine and methionine (serine is higher in poultry and methionine higher in red meat), but whether this can manifest to specific changes in physiological metabolism is unclear. Applying metabolomics analysis in more controlled studies of human diet will be helpful in parsing these effects. Of course, this is not to say that the better studied macronutrients involving glucose and lipid metabolism are not also important and their relation to cancer and diet are discussed below.

Micronutrients

Micronutrients are the essential vitamins and minerals that our bodies require in small quantities and these too have been shown to impact tumor development and growth. Numerous epidemiological studies have linked the suboptimal consumption of micronutrients with increased cancer risk (Venturelli et al. 2021). Here, we will discuss the complex relationships among micronutrients and cancer, unraveling the multifaceted mechanisms through which these tiny components of our diet exert their influence on cancer. From the paradoxical effects of folate supplementation to the delicate balance of antioxidant vitamins, micronutrients can alter systemic nutrient flux, cancer cell metabolism, and anticancer therapy.

One of the most widely studied micronutrients in cancer is folate, a cofactor required for the synthesis of nucleotides and amino acids. Folate supplementation can promote cancer development, in humans and mice, and the initial observations of this effect inspired the use of antifolates for cancer therapy (Farber et al. 1947; Cole et al. 2007; Deghan Manshadi et al. 2014). While these effects are mostly attributed to the role of folate in anabolic reactions, folate was recently found to spontaneously oxidize in cells generating the mutagen formaldehyde, which suggests folate supplementation might rise mutation rates in cancer cells and fuel tumor evolution (Burgos-Barragan et al. 2017). Paradoxically, while folate deficiency can inhibit growth of established neoplastic lesions in mice, it is associated with an increased risk of many cancer types in humans (Rosen and Nichol 1962; Kotsopoulos 2005; Zhang et al. 2015). Like excess folate, folate deficiency can cause DNA damage by a different mechanism, but its role in cancer development is unclear (Fenech 2001). Folate deficiency can also disrupt methionine metabolism and trigger epigenetic alterations, which have been shown to cause resistance to Myc targeting in mouse models of leukemia (Su et al. 2020).

Folate deficiency can arise from low dietary intake of folate or vitamin B12. Deficiency in vitamin B12 not only impacts folate metabolism but also propionate metabolism, triggering the accumulation of the metabolite methylmalonic acid (MMA). Intriguingly, exposure of cancer cells to high MMA levels induces epithelial-to-mesenchymal transition and promotes metastasis in mouse models (Gomes et al. 2020; Li et al. 2022). Serum MMA levels are found to increase in older people, correlating with a decline B12 levels (Baik and Russell 1999; Gomes et al. 2020). Remarkably, a recent study found that incubation of cancer cells with serum from older people promotes aggressive and metastatic traits, and provided evidence suggesting a role of MMA in this process (Gomes et al. 2020). Thus, it is reasonable to speculate that low B12 levels might contribute to the increased risk of cancer associated with aging. While further investigation is needed, these findings suggest B12 supplementation might be beneficial among the elderly.

Low levels of other vitamins are also associated with increased cancer risk. This observation is true for vitamins E and C, whose potential impact on cancer is generally attributed to their antioxidant properties (Venturelli et al. 2021). Vitamin C deficiency can also support carcinogenesis by altering the activity of α-ketoglutarate-dependent dioxygenases that regulate the epigenome, particularly in leukemias (Agathocleous et al. 2017). Conversely, antioxidants can also promote growth of fully developed tumors and support metastatic colonization, so their supplementation should be carefully assessed (Sayin et al. 2014; Le Gal et al. 2015). On the other hand, high-dose vitamin C has shown anticancer efficacy against several tumor types in preclinical models, and clinical trials are currently assessing its efficacy in humans (Ma et al. 2014; Yun et al. 2015; Schoenfeld et al. 2017; Di Tano et al. 2020). Mechanistically, this therapeutic approach is based on the counterintuitive pro-oxidant effects of vitamin C at high concentrations and requires parenteral administration of the vitamin, since oral supplementation is unable to reach pharmacological concentrations (Ngo et al. 2019).

Low vitamin B6 levels have also been associated with increased cancer risk (Mocellin et al. 2017). Mouse studies have shown a B6-depleted diet can slow down leukemia progression in mice and suggest some leukemias might be particularly dependent on this vitamin (Chen et al. 2020). The inadequate intake of some trace metals, such as iron, zinc, or selenium, has also been implicated in cancer development (Venturelli et al. 2022). Selenium, for instance, is an essential component of several antioxidant enzymes and a low intake of this nutrient is associated with a higher risk of various cancer types (Cai et al. 2016). Iron may have similar roles as well.

In summary, the role of micronutrients in cancer biology is complex and much work is still needed to fully understand the impact of micronutrient intake on cancer development. However, our current knowledge unequivocally underlines the importance of micronutrients in the interaction between diet and cancer.

Fiber, and the Microbiome

Other studies have shown that altering the type of carbohydrate intake can influence tumor growth by altering the microbiota, which responds to diet and especially to carbohydrate intake. This has been shown to be of interest, as one of the emerging areas whereby systemic effects from diet may have relevance to cancer is the microbiota (Park et al. 2022). A series of recent studies are converging on the concept that microbiota can coevolve with tumors, indicating an active role for bacteria in the oncogenic process. The microbiome composition, particularly in the gut, has been implicated in both the efficacy and the toxicity of immune checkpoint inhibitors, currently the most active area of investigation in anticancer therapy (Spencer et al. 2021). In addition, it has been shown that the gut microbiome is highly dynamic and responds to diet (Korem et al. 2017). A controlled trial in humans in Israel, for example, showed that a diet using sourdough-leavened whole-grain bread as opposed to white bread as a carbohydrate source induces widespread changes to the gut microbiome composition in as little as 1 week (Korem et al. 2017). Consistently, observational studies in humans and controlled studies in mice showed that fiber intake, which in large part comes from the carbohydrate source in most diets, was sufficient to alter the microbiota in a manner that could influence the response to immune therapies. Interestingly, probiotic supplementation either abrogated or worsened cancer outcome (Spencer et al. 2021). While these studies provide a convincing link from fiber to cancer, many questions remain as to whether any direct effects on central carbon metabolism via fiber intake or microbiome metabolism might affect therapy outcome or whether the anticancer effects occur predominantly through systemic effects such as what happens to gut inflammation. For example, a change to glycolysis affects both tumor cells and the immune compartment within the tumor, and so it is perhaps reasonable that fiber-mediated changes in glucose metabolism could have a direct role in cancer.

CONCLUDING REMARKS AND FUTURE PERSPECTIVES

Epidemiology, Clinical Investigation, and Mechanistic Biology

Much of nutrition research has historically relied on observational studies rooted in epidemiological frameworks. Epidemiology in general has had an enormous impact in advancing public health. Arguably, the most substantial accomplishments in reducing cancer mortality to date have come from these lines of inquiry. These accomplishments have occurred despite the general belief in the basic sciences that these studies may not provide insight into the mechanism.

Nevertheless, associations between factors such as smoking, exposure to radiation, or human papillomavirus and cancer have led to highly effective mitigation strategies that reduce or sometimes almost eliminate the cancers that may result. In these cases, the effects are so large that confounding factors can be addressed, and long-standing frameworks such as the Bradford–Hill criteria have been developed as evidentiary standards for defining causality. The information one gains from observational studies in a human population is limited by the makeup of that population, but in the case of smoking and cancer, the magnitude of the correlations are so large that they extend beyond any given population and any other possible factors such as germline genetic status. Indeed, in both the public and scientific communities, because the effect size is so large, it is almost universally accepted that smoking causes cancer. This is despite the molecular, mechanistic basis of the connection being very complex and involving a plethora of complicated molecular mechanisms such as direct mutagenesis, inflammation, wound healing, hypoxia adaptation, etc. In stark contrast, the effect sizes in nutritional and exercise epidemiology are much smaller. Common associations with cancer such as calorie intake, sugar intake, red meat consumption, saturated fat intake, coffee consumption, and increased physical activity are much smaller effects. Further, conclusions drawn from the associations depend highly on the nature of the cohort, the confounding variables (age, sex, genetics, other lifestyle factors, etc.) that have been controlled for and the type of statistical model used to assess the correlation strength and effect size. Nevertheless, these studies often garner tremendous public interest and news headlines often occur from analysis that gives rise to relatively small effects.

Compounding these limitations are the challenges of conducting randomized controlled trials in human subjects, which are considered the highest standard in clinical investigation. If the effect sizes are small, larger cohorts are needed, which is usually very difficult if not impossible in oncology, not to mention the compliance-related difficulties in controlling a diet or exercise regimen in humans. Given the challenges of conducting trials and that of epidemiology, scientific advancement into eventual clinical practice requires mechanistic work in this area. Even "N-of-1" studies with firm molecular grounding have yielded important clinical advances despite lacking any statistical information. In the absence of sufficient statistical evidence (from observational studies or controlled trials), mechanistic understanding is the only path forward. Fortunately, in recent years, there has been a surge of interest in this topic, but there is much more to be learned. With this new knowledge, more precisely defined clinical trials could be possible.

Metabolomics as a Path Toward Precision Nutrition in Oncology

Metabolic diseases in general have been diagnosed and treated using measurements of metabolites and metabolic flux (Schmidt et al. 2021). Measures of glucose, cholesterol, and A1C (i.e., a surrogate of glycolysis and glycosylation flux) are standard and widespread clinical mainstays for metabolic disease. These biomarkers are direct measurements of metabolism and do not rely on the underlying complex genetics. They further have mechanistic interpretations about metabolic pathway activity such as increased glucose levels, suggesting lower glucose uptake in muscle or increased cholesterol, possibly implying increased lipid synthesis in liver. In cancer, genetic biomarkers of disease, such as the presence of a certain driver mutations, can inform prognosis as well as the likely response to a therapy targeted toward the mutation. This concept of precision medicine in oncology has been built on genetics. However, it does face challenges. Indeed, a very small portion of cancers responds to targeted therapies, not to mention the resistance that invariably emerges. Thus, genetic biomarkers by themselves are unlikely to have a large role in determining cancer dietary guidelines just as they have proven to be very complex in defining metabolic status (Vander Heiden and DeBerardinis 2017). As the study of diet and exercise in cancer prevention and therapy evolves, new conceptual principles and technological applications are needed to define which cancers might interact with which diet and

exercise regimens. One such technology is metabolomics. Metabolomics provides a methodology for advancing this framework by measuring many aspects of the status of metabolism at once. Metabolomics measurements of metabolites either in plasma or in the fluid at the site of the tumor combined with machine learning approaches and mechanistic understanding may guide the development of the corresponding biomarkers needed to predict what diets might interact with what tumors in the same way that measurements of glucose and cholesterol routinely guide the management of other metabolic diseases. Thus, just as these measurements have proven valuable for other complex metabolic diseases, metabolomics approaches are likely to be fruitful in guiding clinical investigation on the role of diet and exercise in cancer.

ACKNOWLEDGMENTS

J.W.L. thanks Lee Jones for helpful discussions and grants from the National Institutes of Health and American Cancer Society for support. Dr. Locasale receives funding from the National Institutes of Health, the American Cancer Society, the Marc Lustgarten Foundation, and the Swiss Federal Institute of Technology. Dr. Locasale advises Petri Bio, Cornerstone Pharmaceuticals, Nanocare Technologies, and Restoration Foodworks. Dr. Goncalves reports personal fees from Novartis, Pfizer, and Scorpion Therapeutics. He is a cofounder and shareholder of Faeth Therapeutics. We apologize to those authors whose work was omitted in both discussion and citation due to space constraints.

REFERENCES

Agathocleous M, Meacham CE, Burgess RJ, Piskounova E, Zhao Z, Crane GM, Cowin BL, Bruner E, Murphy MM, Chen W, et al. 2017. Ascorbate regulates haematopoietic stem cell function and leukaemogenesis. *Nature* **549**: 476–481. doi:10.1038/nature23876

Baik HW, Russell RM. 1999. Vitamin B$_{12}$ deficiency in the elderly. *Annu Rev Nutr* **19**: 357–377. doi:10.1146/annurev.nutr.19.1.357

Bose S, Allen AE, Locasale JW. 2020. The molecular link from diet to cancer cell metabolism. *Mol Cell* **78**: 1034–1044. doi:10.1016/j.molcel.2020.05.018

Brandhorst S, Choi IY, Wei M, Cheng CW, Sedrakyan S, Navarrete G, Dubeau L, Yap LP, Park R, Vinciguerra M, et al. 2015. A periodic diet that mimics fasting promotes multi-system regeneration, enhanced cognitive performance, and healthspan. *Cell Metab* 22: 86–99. doi:10.1016/j.cmet.2015.05.012

Broadfield LA, Pane AA, Talebi A, Swinnen JV, Fendt SM. 2021. Lipid metabolism in cancer: new perspectives and emerging mechanisms. *Dev Cell* 56: 1363–1393. doi:10.1016/j.devcel.2021.04.013

Burgos-Barragan G, Wit N, Meiser J, Dingler FA, Pietzke M, Mulderrig L, Pontel LB, Rosado IV, Brewer TF, Cordell RL, et al. 2017. Mammals divert endogenous genotoxic formaldehyde into one-carbon metabolism. *Nature* 548: 549–554. doi:10.1038/nature23481

Caffa I, Spagnolo V, Vernieri C, Valdemarin F, Becherini P, Wei M, Brandhorst S, Zucal C, Driehuis E, Ferrando L, et al. 2020. Fasting-mimicking diet and hormone therapy induce breast cancer regression. *Nature* 583: 620–624. doi:10.1038/s41586-020-2502-7

Cai X, Wang C, Yu W, Fan W, Wang S, Shen N, Wu P, Li X, Wang F. 2016. Selenium exposure and cancer risk: an updated meta-analysis and meta-regression. *Sci Rep* 6: 19213. doi:10.1038/srep19213

Cao Y, Giovannucci EL. 2016. Alcohol as a risk factor for cancer. *Semin Oncol Nurs* 32: 325–331. doi:10.1016/j.soncn.2016.05.012

Chen CC, Li B, Millman SE, Chen C, Li X, Morris JP, Mayle A, Ho YJ, Loizou E, Liu H, et al. 2020. Vitamin B6 addiction in acute myeloid leukemia. *Cancer Cell* 37: 71–84.e7. doi:10.1016/j.ccell.2019.12.002

Chlebowski RT, Blackburn GL, Thomson CA, Nixon DW, Shapiro A, Hoy MK, Goodman MT, Giuliano AE, Karanja N, McAndrew P, et al. 2006. Dietary fat reduction and breast cancer outcome: interim efficacy results from the Women's Intervention Nutrition study. *J Natl Cancer Inst* 98: 1767–1776. doi:10.1093/jnci/djj494

Chlebowski RT, Aragaki AK, Anderson GL, Thomson CA, Manson JE, Simon MS, Howard BV, Rohan TE, Snetselar L, Lane D, et al. 2017. Low-fat dietary pattern and breast cancer mortality in the Women's Health Initiative Randomized Controlled trial. *J Clin Oncol* 35: 2919–2926. doi:10.1200/JCO.2016.72.0326

Chlebowski RT, Aragaki AK, Anderson GL, Simon MS, Manson JE, Neuhouser ML, Pan K, Stefanic ML, Rohan TE, Lane D, et al. 2018. Association of low-fat dietary pattern with breast cancer overall survival: a secondary analysis of the Women's Health Initiative Randomized Clinical trial. *JAMA Oncol* 4: e181212. doi:10.1001/jamaoncol.2018.1212

Cohen CW, Fontaine KR, Arend RC, Alvarez RD, Leath CA, Huh WK III, Bevis KS, Kim KH, Straughn JM Jr, Gower BA. 2018. A ketogenic diet reduces central obesity and serum insulin in women with ovarian or endometrial cancer. *J Nutr* 148: 1253–1260. doi:10.1093/jn/nxy119

Cole BF, Baron JA, Sandler RS, Haile RW, Ahnen DJ, Bresalier RS, McKeown-Eyssen G, Summers RW, Rothstein RI, Burke CA, et al. 2007. Folic acid for the prevention of colorectal adenomas: a randomized clinical trial. *JAMA* 297: 2351–2359. doi:10.1001/jama.297.21.2351

Colman RJ, Anderson RM, Johnson SC, Kastman EK, Kosmatka KJ, Beasley TM, Allison DB, Cruzen C, Simmons

HA, Kemnitz JW, et al. 2009. Caloric restriction delays disease onset and mortality in rhesus monkeys. *Science* 325: 201–204. doi:10.1126/science.1173635

Deghan Manshadi S, Ishiguro L, Sohn KJ, Medline A, Renlund R, Croxford R, Kim YI. 2014. Folic acid supplementation promotes mammary tumor progression in a rat model. *PLoS ONE* 9: e84635. doi:10.1371/journal.pone.0084635

de Groot S, Vreeswijk MP, Welters MJ, Gravesteijn G, Boei JJ, Jochems A, Houtsma D, Putter H, van der Hoeven JJ, Nortier JW, et al. 2015. The effects of short-term fasting on tolerance to (neo) adjuvant chemotherapy in HER2-negative breast cancer patients: a randomized pilot study. *BMC Cancer* 15: 652. doi:10.1186/s12885-015-1663-5

de Groot S, Lugtenberg RT, Cohen D, Welters MJP, Ehsan I, Vreeswijk MPG, Smit V, de Graaf H, Heijns JB, Portielje JEA, et al. 2020. Fasting mimicking diet as an adjunct to neoadjuvant chemotherapy for breast cancer in the multicentre randomized phase 2 DIRECT trial. *Nat Commun* 11: 3083. doi:10.1038/s41467-020-16138-3

Ding L, Bailey MH, Porta-Pardo E, Thorsson V, Colaprico A, Bertrand D, Gibbs DL, Weerasinghe A, Huang KL, Tokheim C, et al. 2018. Perspective on oncogenic processes at the end of the beginning of cancer genomics. *Cell* 173: 305–320.e10. doi:10.1016/j.cell.2018.03.033

Di Tano M, Raucci F, Vernieri C, Caffa I, Buono R, Fanti M, Brandhorst S, Curigliano G, Nencioni A, de Braud F, et al. 2020. Synergistic effect of fasting-mimicking diet and vitamin C against KRAS mutated cancers. *Nat Commun* 11: 2332. doi:10.1038/s41467-020-16243-3

Farber S, Cutler EC, Hawkins JW, Harrison JH, Peirce EC 2nd, Lenz GG. 1947. The action of pteroylglutamic conjugates on man. *Science* 106: 619–621. doi:10.1126/science.106.2764.619

Farvid MS, Sidahmed E, Spence ND, Mante Angua K, Rosner BA, Barnett JB. 2021. Consumption of red meat and processed meat and cancer incidence: a systematic review and meta-analysis of prospective studies. *Eur J Epidemiol* 36: 937–951. doi:10.1007/s10654-021-00741-9

Fenech M. 2001. The role of folic acid and vitamin B12 in genomic stability of human cells. *Mutat Res* 475: 57–67. doi:10.1016/s0027-5107(01)00079-3

Gao X, Sanderson SM, Dai Z, Reid MA, Cooper DE, Lu M, Richie JP Jr, Ciccarella A, Calcagnotto A, Mikhael PG, et al. 2019. Dietary methionine influences therapy in mouse cancer models and alters human metabolism. *Nature* 572: 397–401. doi:10.1038/s41586-019-1437-3

Gardner CD, Trepanowski JF, Del Gobbo LC, Hauser ME, Rigdon J, Ioannidis JPA, Desai M, King AC. 2018. Effect of low-fat vs low-carbohydrate diet on 12-month weight loss in overweight adults and the association with genotype pattern or insulin secretion: the DIETFITS randomized clinical trial. *JAMA* 319: 667–679. doi:10.1001/jama.2018.0245

Gold EB, Pierce JP, Natarajan L, Stefanick ML, Laughlin GA, Caan BJ, Flatt SW, Emond JA, Saquib N, Madlensky L, et al. 2009. Dietary pattern influences breast cancer prognosis in women without hot flashes: the women's healthy eating and living trial. *J Clin Oncol* 27: 352–359. doi:10.1200/JCO.2008.16.1067

Gomes AP, Ilter D, Low V, Endress JE, Fernández-García J, Rosenzweig A, Schild T, Broekaert D, Ahmed A, Planque

M, et al. 2020. Age-induced accumulation of methylmalonic acid promotes tumour progression. *Nature* **585:** 283–287. doi:10.1038/s41586-020-2630-0

Gomes AP, Ilter D, Low V, Drapela S, Schild T, Mullarky E, Han J, Elia I, Broekaert D, Rosenzweig A, et al. 2022. Altered propionate metabolism contributes to tumour progression and aggressiveness. *Nat Metab* **4:** 435–443. doi:10.1038/s42255-022-00553-5

Goncalves MD, Lu C, Tutnauer J, Hartman TE, Hwang SK, Murphy CJ, Pauli C, Morris R, Taylor S, Bosch K, et al. 2019. High-fructose corn syrup enhances intestinal tumor growth in mice. *Science* **363:** 1345–1349. doi:10.1126/science.aat8515

Gurjao C, Zhong R, Haruki K, Li YY, Spurr LF, Lee-Six H, Reardon B, Ugai T, Zhang X, Cherniack AD, et al. 2021. Discovery and features of an alkylating signature in colorectal cancer. *Cancer Discov* **11:** 2446–2455. doi:10.1158/2159-8290.CD-20-1656

Hall KD, Guo J, Courville AB, Boring J, Brychta R, Chen KY, Darcey V, Forde CG, Gharib AM, Gallagher I, et al. 2021. Effect of a plant-based, low-fat diet versus an animal-based, ketogenic diet on ad libitum energy intake. *Nat Med* **27:** 344–353. doi:10.1038/s41591-020-01209-1

Hall KD, Farooqi IS, Friedman JM, Klein S, Loos RJF, Mangelsdorf DJ, O'Rahilly S, Ravussin E, Redman LM, Ryan DH, et al. 2022. The energy balance model of obesity: beyond calories in, calories out. *Am J Clin Nutr* **115:** 1243–1254. doi:10.1093/ajcn/nqac031

Hofer SJ, Carmona-Gutierrez D, Mueller MI, Madeo F. 2022. The ups and downs of caloric restriction and fasting: from molecular effects to clinical application. *EMBO Mol Med* **14:** e14418. doi:10.15252/emmm.202114418

Hopkins BD, Goncalves MD, Cantley LC. 2016. Obesity and cancer mechanisms: cancer metabolism. *J Clin Oncol* **34:** 4277–4283. doi:10.1200/JCO.2016.67.9712

Hopkins BD, Pauli C, Du X, Wang DG, Li X, Wu D, Amadiume SC, Goncalves MD, Hodakoski C, Lundquist MR, et al. 2018. Suppression of insulin feedback enhances the efficacy of PI3K inhibitors. *Nature* **560:** 499–503. doi:10.1038/s41586-018-0343-4

Hur J, Otegbeye E, Joh HK, Nimptsch K, Ng K, Ogino S, Meyerhardt JA, Chan AT, Willett WC, Wu K, et al. 2021. Sugar-sweetened beverage intake in adulthood and adolescence and risk of early-onset colorectal cancer among women. *Gut* **70:** 2330–2336. doi:10.1136/gutjnl-2020-323450

Ishak Gabra MB, Yang Y, Li H, Senapati P, Hanse EA, Lowman XH, Tran TQ, Zhang L, Doan LT, Xu X, et al. 2020. Dietary glutamine supplementation suppresses epigenetically-activated oncogenic pathways to inhibit melanoma tumour growth. *Nat Commun* **11:** 3326. doi:10.1038/s41467-020-17181-w

Iyengar NM, Gucalp A, Dannenberg AJ, Hudis CA. 2016. Obesity and cancer mechanisms: tumor microenvironment and inflammation. *J Clin Oncol* **34:** 4270–4276. doi:10.1200/JCO.2016.67.4283

Joh HK, Lee DH, Hur J, Nimptsch K, Chang Y, Joung H, Zhang X, Rezende LFM, Lee JE, Ng K, et al. 2021. Simple sugar and sugar-sweetened beverage intake during adolescence and risk of colorectal cancer precursors. *Gastroenterology* **161:** 128–142.e20. doi:10.1053/j.gastro.2021.03.028

Kanarek N, Petrova B, Sabatini DM. 2020. Dietary modifications for enhanced cancer therapy. *Nature* **579:** 507–517. doi:10.1038/s41586-020-2124-0

Khodabakhshi A, Akbari ME, Mirzaei HR, Mehrad-Majd H, Kalamian M, Davoodi SH. 2020. Feasibility, safety, and beneficial effects of mct-based ketogenic diet for breast cancer treatment: a randomized controlled trial study. *Nutr Cancer* **72:** 627–634. doi:10.1080/01635581.2019.1650942

Korem T, Zeevi D, Zmora N, Weissbrod O, Bar N, Lotan-Pompan M, Avnit-Sagi T, Kosower N, Malka G, Rein M, et al. 2017. Bread affects clinical parameters and induces gut microbiome-associated personal glycemic responses. *Cell Metab* **25:** 1243–1253.e5. doi:10.1016/j.cmet.2017.05.002

Kotsopoulos J. 2005. Effects of dietary folate on the development and progression of mammary tumors in rats. *Carcinogenesis* **26:** 1603–1612. doi:10.1093/carcin/bgi117

Krall AS, Mullen PJ, Surjono F, Momcilovic M, Schmid EW, Halbrook CJ, Thambundit A, Mittelman SD, Lyssiotis CA, Shackelford DB, et al. 2021. Asparagine couples mitochondrial respiration to ATF4 activity and tumor growth. *Cell Metab* **33:** 1013–1026.e6. doi:10.1016/j.cmet.2021.02.001

Lauby-Secretan B, Scoccianti C, Loomis D, Grosse Y, Bianchini F, Straif K. 2016. Body fatness and cancer—viewpoint of the IARC working group. *N Engl J Med* **375:** 794–798. doi:10.1056/NEJMsr1606602

Lee C, Raffaghello L, Brandhorst S, Safdie FM, Bianchi G, Martin-Montalvo A, Pistoia V, Wei M, Hwang S, Merlino A, et al. 2012. Fasting cycles retard growth of tumors and sensitize a range of cancer cell types to chemotherapy. *Sci Transl Med* **4:** 124ra127. doi:10.1126/scitranslmed.3003293

Le Gal K, Ibrahim MX, Wiel C, Sayin VI, Akula MK, Karlsson C, Dalin MG, Akyürek LM, Lindahl P, Nilsson J, et al. 2015. Antioxidants can increase melanoma metastasis in mice. *Sci Transl Med* **7:** 308re308. doi:10.1126/scitranslmed.aad3740

Li Z, Low V, Luga V, Sun J, Earlie E, Parang B, Shobana Ganesh K, Cho S, Endress J, Schild T, et al. 2022. Tumor-produced and aging-associated oncometabolite methylmalonic acid promotes cancer-associated fibroblast activation to drive metastatic progression. *Nat Commun* **13:** 6239. doi:10.1038/s41467-022-33862-0

Lien EC, Westermark AM, Zhang Y, Yuan C, Li Z, Lau AN, Sapp KM, Wolpin BM, Vander Heiden MG. 2021. Low glycaemic diets alter lipid metabolism to influence tumour growth. *Nature* **599:** 302–307. doi:10.1038/s41586-021-04049-2

Locasale JW. 2022. Diet and exercise in cancer metabolism. *Cancer Discov* **12:** 2249–2257. doi:10.1158/2159-8290.CD-22-0096

Locasale JW, Grassian AR, Melman T, Lyssiotis CA, Mattaini KR, Bass AJ, Heffron G, Metallo CM, Muranen T, Sharfi H, et al. 2011. Phosphoglycerate dehydrogenase diverts glycolytic flux and contributes to oncogenesis. *Nat Genet* **43:** 869–874. doi:10.1038/ng.890

Longo VD, Anderson RM. 2022. Nutrition, longevity and disease: from molecular mechanisms to interventions. *Cell* **185:** 1455–1470. doi:10.1016/j.cell.2022.04.002

Ludwig DS, Aronne LJ, Astrup A, de Cabo R, Cantley LC, Friedman MI, Heymsfield SB, Johnson JD, King JC,

Krauss RM, et al. 2021. The carbohydrate-insulin model: a physiological perspective on the obesity pandemic. *Am J Clin Nutr* **114:** 1873–1885. doi:10.1093/ajcn/nqab270

Ma Y, Chapman J, Levine M, Polireddy K, Drisko J, Chen Q. 2014. High-dose parenteral ascorbate enhanced chemosensitivity of ovarian cancer and reduced toxicity of chemotherapy. *Sci Transl Med* **6:** 222ra218. doi:10.1126/scitranslmed.3007154

MacArthur MR, Mitchell SJ, Treviño-Villarreal JH, Grondin Y, Reynolds JS, Kip P, Jung J, Trocha KM, Ozaki CK, Mitchell JR. 2021. Total protein, not amino acid composition, differs in plant-based versus omnivorous dietary patterns and determines metabolic health effects in mice. *Cell Metab* **33:** 1808–1819.e2. doi:10.1016/j.cmet.2021.06.011

Maddocks ODK, Berkers CR, Mason SM, Zheng L, Blyth K, Gottlieb E, Vousden KH. 2013. Serine starvation induces stress and p53-dependent metabolic remodelling in cancer cells. *Nature* **493:** 542–546. doi:10.1038/nature11743

Maddocks ODK, Athineos D, Cheung EC, Lee P, Zhang T, van den Broek NJF, Mackay GM, Labuschagne CF, Gay D, Kruiswijk F, et al. 2017. Modulating the therapeutic response of tumours to dietary serine and glycine starvation. *Nature* **544:** 372–376. doi:10.1038/nature22056

Martínez-Reyes I, Chandel NS. 2021. Cancer metabolism: looking forward. *Nat Rev Cancer* **21:** 669–680. doi:10.1038/s41568-021-00378-6

Mentch SJ, Mehrmohamadi M, Huang L, Liu X, Gupta D, Mattocks D, Gómez Padilla P, Ables G, Bamman MM, Thalacker-Mercer AE, et al. 2015. Histone methylation dynamics and gene regulation occur through the sensing of one-carbon metabolism. *Cell Metab* **22:** 861–873. doi:10.1016/j.cmet.2015.08.024

Mercken EM, Carboneau BA, Krzysik-Walker SM, de Cabo R. 2012. Of mice and men: the benefits of caloric restriction, exercise, and mimetics. *Ageing Res Rev* **11:** 390–398. doi:10.1016/j.arr.2011.11.005

Michelet X, Dyck L, Hogan A, Loftus RM, Duquette D, Wei K, Beyaz S, Tavakkoli A, Foley C, Donnelly R, et al. 2018. Metabolic reprogramming of natural killer cells in obesity limits antitumor responses. *Nat Immunol* **19:** 1330–1340. doi:10.1038/s41590-018-0251-7

Mocellin S, Briarava M, Pilati P. 2017. Vitamin B6 and cancer risk: a field synopsis and meta-analysis. *J Natl Cancer Inst* **109:** djw230. doi:10.1093/jnci/djw230

Muthusamy T, Cordes T, Handzlik MK, You L, Lim EW, Gengatharan J, Pinto AFM, Badur MG, Kolar MJ, Wallace M, et al. 2020. Serine restriction alters sphingolipid diversity to constrain tumour growth. *Nature* **586:** 790–795. doi:10.1038/s41586-020-2609-x

Ngo B, Van Riper JM, Cantley LC, Yun J. 2019. Targeting cancer vulnerabilities with high-dose vitamin C. *Nat Rev Cancer* **19:** 271–282. doi:10.1038/s41568-019-0135-7

Park EM, Chelvanambi M, Bhutiani N, Kroemer G, Zitvogel L, Wargo JA. 2022. Targeting the gut and tumor microbiota in cancer. *Nat Med* **28:** 690–703. doi:10.1038/s41591-022-01779-2

Pascual G, Domínguez D, Elosua-Bayes M, Beckedorff F, Laudanna C, Bigas C, Douillet D, Greco C, Symeonidi A, Hernandez I, et al. 2021. Dietary palmitic acid promotes a prometastatic memory via Schwann cells. *Nature* **599:** 485–490. doi:10.1038/s41586-021-04075-0

Petrelli F, Cortellini A, Indini A, Tomasello G, Ghidini M, Nigro O, Salati M, Dottorini L, Iaculli A, Varricchio A, et al. 2021. Association of obesity with survival outcomes in patients with cancer: a systematic review and meta-analysis. *JAMA Netw Open* **4:** e213520. doi:10.1001/jamanetworkopen.2021.3520

Pham T, Knowles S, Bermingham E, Brown J, Hannaford R, Cameron-Smith D, Braakhuis A. 2022. Plasma amino acid appearance and status of appetite following a single meal of red meat or a plant-based meat analog: a randomized crossover clinical trial. *Curr Dev Nutr* **6:** nzac082. doi:10.1093/cdn/nzac082

Pierce JP, Natarajan L, Caan BJ, Parker BA, Greenberg ER, Flatt SW, Rock CL, Kealey S, Al-Delaimy WK, Bardwell WA, et al. 2007. Influence of a diet very high in vegetables, fruit, and fiber and low in fat on prognosis following treatment for breast cancer: the Women's Healthy Eating and Living (WHEL) randomized trial. *JAMA* **298:** 289–298. doi:10.1001/jama.298.3.289

Raffaghello L, Lee C, Safdie FM, Wei M, Madia F, Bianchi G, Longo VD. 2008. Starvation-dependent differential stress resistance protects normal but not cancer cells against high-dose chemotherapy. *Proc Natl Acad Sci* **105:** 8215–8220. doi:10.1073/pnas.0708100105

Ringel AE, Drijvers JM, Baker GJ, Catozzi A, Garcia-Cañaveras JC, Gassaway BM, Miller BC, Juneja VR, Nguyen TH, Joshi S, et al. 2020. Obesity shapes metabolism in the tumor microenvironment to suppress anti-tumor immunity. *Cell* **183:** 1848–1866.e26. doi:10.1016/j.cell.2020.11.009

Rosen F, Nichol CA. 1962. Inhibition of the growth of an amethopterin-refractory tumor by dietary restriction of folic acid. *Cancer Res* **22:** 495–500.

Rossi M, Altea-Manzano P, Demicco M, Doglioni G, Bornes L, Fukano M, Vandekeere A, Cuadros AM, Fernández-García J, Riera-Domingo C, et al. 2022. PHGDH heterogeneity potentiates cancer cell dissemination and metastasis. *Nature* **605:** 747–753. doi:10.1038/s41586-022-04758-2

Sanderson SM, Gao X, Dai Z, Locasale JW. 2019. Methionine metabolism in health and cancer: a nexus of diet and precision medicine. *Nat Rev Cancer* **19:** 625–637. doi:10.1038/s41568-019-0187-8

Sayin VI, Ibrahim MX, Larsson E, Nilsson JA, Lindahl P, Bergo MO. 2014. Antioxidants accelerate lung cancer progression in mice. *Sci Transl Med* **6:** 221ra215. doi:10.1126/scitranslmed.3007653

Schmidt DR, Patel R, Kirsch DG, Lewis CA, Vander Heiden MG, Locasale JW. 2021. Metabolomics in cancer research and emerging applications in clinical oncology. *CA Cancer J Clin* **71:** 333–358. doi:10.3322/caac.21670

Schoenfeld JD, Sibenaller ZA, Mapuskar KA, Wagner BA, Cramer-Morales KL, Furqan M, Sandhu S, Carlisle TL, Smith MC, Abu Hejleh T, et al. 2017. O_2^- and H_2O_2-mediated disruption of fe metabolism causes the differential susceptibility of NSCLC and GBM cancer cells to pharmacological ascorbate. *Cancer Cell* **32:** 268. doi:10.1016/j.ccell.2017.07.008

Seitz HK, Stickel F. 2007. Molecular mechanisms of alcohol-mediated carcinogenesis. *Nat Rev Cancer* **7:** 599–612. doi:10.1038/nrc2191

Seki T, Yang Y, Sun X, Lim S, Xie S, Guo Z, Xiong W, Kuroda M, Sakaue H, Hosaka K, et al. 2022. Brown-fat-mediated tumour suppression by cold-altered global metabolism. *Nature* **608**: 421–428. doi:10.1038/s41586-022-05030-3

Solon-Biet SM, McMahon AC, Ballard JW, Ruohonen K, Wu LE, Cogger VC, Warren A, Huang X, Pichaud N, Melvin RG, et al. 2014. The ratio of macronutrients, not caloric intake, dictates cardiometabolic health, aging, and longevity in ad libitum-fed mice. *Cell Metab* **19**: 418–430. doi:10.1016/j.cmet.2014.02.009

Solon-Biet SM, Mitchell SJ, Coogan SC, Cogger VC, Gokarn R, McMahon AC, Raubenheimer D, de Cabo R, Simpson SJ, Le Couteur DG. 2015. Dietary protein to carbohydrate ratio and caloric restriction: comparing metabolic outcomes in mice. *Cell Rep* **11**: 1529–1534. doi:10.1016/j.celrep.2015.05.007

Song M, Giovannucci E. 2016. Preventable incidence and mortality of carcinoma associated with lifestyle factors among white adults in the United States. *JAMA Oncol* **2**: 1154–1161. doi:10.1001/jamaoncol.2016.0843

Spencer CN, McQuade JL, Gopalakrishnan V, McCulloch JA, Vetizou M, Cogdill AP, Khan MAW, Zhang X, White MG, Peterson CB, et al. 2021. Dietary fiber and probiotics influence the gut microbiome and melanoma immunotherapy response. *Science* **374**: 1632–1640. doi:10.1126/science.aaz7015

Su A, Ling F, Vaganay C, Sodaro G, Benaksas C, Dal Bello R, Forget A, Pardieu B, Lin KH, Rutter JC, et al. 2020. The folate cycle enzyme MTHFR is a critical regulator of cell response to MYC-targeting therapies. *Cancer Discov* **10**: 1894–1911. doi:10.1158/2159-8290.CD-19-0970

Sullivan MR, Danai LV, Lewis CA, Chan SH, Gui DY, Kunchok T, Dennstedt EA, Vander Heiden MG, Muir A. 2019. Quantification of microenvironmental metabolites in murine cancers reveals determinants of tumor nutrient availability. *eLife* **8**: e44235. doi:10.7554/eLife.44235

Tajan M, Vousden KH. 2020. Dietary approaches to cancer therapy. *Cancer Cell* **37**: 767–785. doi:10.1016/j.ccell.2020.04.005

Taylor SR, Ramsamooj S, Liang RJ, Katti A, Pozovskiy R, Vasan N, Hwang SK, Nahiyaan N, Francoeur NJ, Schatoff EM, et al. 2021. Dietary fructose improves intestinal cell survival and nutrient absorption. *Nature* **597**: 263–267. doi:10.1038/s41586-021-03827-2

Taylor SR, Falcone JN, Cantley LC, Goncalves MD. 2022. Developing dietary interventions as therapy for cancer. *Nat Rev Cancer* **22**: 452–466. doi:10.1038/s41568-022-00485-y

Thompson HJ, Zhu Z, Jiang W. 2003. Dietary energy restriction in breast cancer prevention. *J Mammary Gland Biol Neoplasia* **8**: 133–142. doi:10.1023/a:1025743607445

Thomson CA, Van Horn L, Caan BJ, Aragaki AK, Chlebowski RT, Manson JE, Rohan TE, Tinker LF, Kuller LH, Hou L, et al. 2014. Cancer incidence and mortality during the intervention and postintervention periods of the Women's Health Initiative Dietary Modification trial. *Cancer Epidemiol Biomarkers Prev* **23**: 2924–2935. doi:10.1158/1055-9965.EPI-14-0922

Vander Heiden MG, DeBerardinis RJ. 2017. Understanding the intersections between metabolism and cancer biology. *Cell* **168**: 657–669. doi:10.1016/j.cell.2016.12.039

Venturelli S, Leischner C, Helling T, Burkard M, Marongiu L. 2021. Vitamins as possible cancer biomarkers: significance and limitations. *Nutrients* **13**: 3914. doi:10.3390/nu13113914

Venturelli S, Leischner C, Helling T, Renner O, Burkard M, Marongiu L. 2022. Minerals and cancer: overview of the possible diagnostic value. *Cancers (Basel)* **14**: 1256. doi:10.3390/cancers14051256

Vernieri C, Fucà G, Ligorio F, Huber V, Vingiani A, Iannelli F, Raimondi A, Rinchai D, Frige G, Belfiore A, et al. 2022. Fasting-mimicking diet is safe and reshapes metabolism and antitumor immunity in patients with cancer. *Cancer Discov* **12**: 90–107. doi:10.1158/2159-8290.CD-21-0030

Wang P, Song M, Eliassen AH, Wang M, Fung TT, Clinton SK, Rimm EB, Hu FB, Willett WC, Tabung FK, et al. 2023. Optimal dietary patterns for prevention of chronic disease. *Nat Med* **29**: 719–728. doi:10.1038/s41591-023-02235-5

Ward ZJ, Bleich SN, Cradock AL, Barrett JL, Giles CM, Flax C, Long MW, Gortmaker SL. 2019. Projected U.S. state-level prevalence of adult obesity and severe obesity. *N Engl J Med* **381**: 2440–2450. doi:10.1056/NEJMsa1909301

Wei M, Brandhorst S, Shelehchi M, Mirzaei H, Cheng CW, Budniak J, Groshen S, Mack WJ, Guen E, Di Biase S, et al. 2017. Fasting-mimicking diet and markers/risk factors for aging, diabetes, cancer, and cardiovascular disease. *Sci Transl Med* **9**: eaai8700. doi:10.1126/scitranslmed.aai8700

Yun J, Mullarky E, Lu C, Bosch KN, Kavalier A, Rivera K, Roper J, Chio II, Giannopoulou EG, Rago C, et al. 2015. Vitamin C selectively kills KRAS and BRAF mutant colorectal cancer cells by targeting GAPDH. *Science* **350**: 1391–1396. doi:10.1126/science.aaa5004

Zhang D, Wen X, Wu W, Guo Y, Cui W. 2015. Elevated homocysteine level and folate deficiency associated with increased overall risk of carcinogenesis: meta-analysis of 83 case-control studies involving 35,758 individuals. *PLoS ONE* **10**: e0123423. doi:10.1371/journal.pone.0123423

Metabolic Reprogramming in Human Cancer Patients and Patient-Derived Models

Teresa W.-M. Fan, Richard M. Higashi, and Andrew N. Lane

Center for Environmental and Systems Biochemistry; Markey Cancer Center; Department of Toxicology and Cancer Biology, University of Kentucky, Lexington, Kentucky 40536, USA

Correspondence: twmfan@gmail.com

Stable isotope-resolved metabolomics delineates reprogrammed intersecting metabolic networks in human cancers. Knowledge gained from in vivo patient studies provides the "benchmark" for cancer models to recapitulate. It is particularly difficult to model patients' tumor microenvironment (TME) with its complex cell–cell/cell–matrix interactions, which shapes metabolic reprogramming crucial to cancer development/drug resistance. Patient-derived organotypic tissue cultures (PD-OTCs) represent a unique model that retains an individual patient's TME. PD-OTCs of non-small-cell lung cancer better recapitulated the in vivo metabolic reprogramming of patient tumors than the patient-derived tumor xenograft (PDTX), while enabling interrogation of immunometabolic response to modulators and TME-dependent resistance development. Patient-derived organoids (PDOs) are also good models for reconstituting TME-dependent metabolic reprogramming and for evaluating therapeutic responses. Single-cell based 'omics on combinations of PD-OTC and PDO models will afford an unprecedented understanding on TME dependence of human cancer metabolic reprogramming, which should translate into the identification of novel metabolic targets for regulating TME interactions and drug resistance.

Enhanced lactic fermentation under aerobic conditions (Warburg 1956) was discovered by O. Warburg in the early 1900s to be a distinct trait of cancer. Through subsequent efforts of the cancer community, metabolic reprogramming is now commonly recognized as a hallmark of human cancers that drives cancer development and progression (Hanahan and Weinberg 2011). To support enhanced proliferation and maintain survival, cancer cells must alter their metabolism to produce sufficient metabolic energy and anabolism/survival-requiring substrates. Glycolysis is one such important pathway but not the only one. It is now widely known that oncogenic transformations govern many aspects of central metabolism to support cancer cell proliferation and adaptations to the harsh tumor microenvironment (TME) (Boroughs and DeBerardinis 2015; Hattori et al. 2017). Of note is the consistent reprogramming of glucose and glutamine metabolism by activation of oncogenes such as *MYC* and *KRAS* or inactivation of tumor suppressors such as *TP53* (Boroughs and DeBerardinis 2015). Aberrant metabolism of amino acids other than Gln (e.g., branched-chain amino acids [Mayers et al. 2016; Hattori et al. 2017], arginine, or tryptophan [Mellor and Munn 2008]) has also been implicated in cancer development/progression. Moreover, oncogenic transformations can activate nutrient scavenging to support growth via macropinocytosis (Commisso et al. 2013) or autophagy (Strohecker et al. 2013; White et al. 2021) when cancer cells face nutrient deprivation in the TME (Lane et al. 2020). Thus, the TME can interact with oncogenic transformations to shape cancer cell development and progression via metabolic reprogramming. Reprogrammed metabolism is not only the consequence of but also a driver of carcinogenesis. The latter is exemplified by the ability of mutations in individual enzyme genes such as *FH*, *SDH*, or *IDH1/2* (Toro et al. 2003; King et al. 2006; Thompson 2009) or accumulation of "oncometabolites" such as fumarate, succinate, or 2-hydroxyglutarate (2-HG) (Martínez-Reyes and Chandel 2021) to drive tumorigenesis.

Much of our knowledge of cancer metabolism derives from model studies, most notably 2D cancer cells in vitro (Pavlova and Thompson 2016) and mice in vivo (Martínez-Reyes and Chandel 2021). The information gained has inspired numerous drug discovery efforts (Luengo et al. 2017), which led to large clinical trials (e.g., CB-839, inhibitor of glutaminase 1 or GLS1) and use approval by the U.S. Food and Drug Administration (FDA) (Ivosidenib, inhibitor of isocitrate dehydrogenase 1 [IDH1]) (Dhillon 2018). However, as stated above, the TME is also a key driver of metabolic reprogramming in cancer tissues and it can be highly heterogeneous. Such heterogeneity can lead to the diversity of cancer metabolism, despite sharing the same oncogene such as in the case of mutant *KRAS*-driven non-small-cell lung cancer (NSCLC) and pancreatic ductal adenocarcinoma (PDAC) (Mayers et al. 2016). As the TME is absent in 2D cancer cell cultures, and the mouse TME differs from the human TME, it is of paramount importance to understand how metabolism is reprogrammed in vivo in cancer patients and/or ex vivo in organotypic tissue cultures (OTCs) that retain native

patient TME. This information is needed to guide mechanistic studies on key TME factors that govern metabolic reprogramming and attendant drug resistance in cancer models, whether they be in vitro or in vivo models. Such knowledge not only fulfills a long-standing and major gap in our understanding of cancer biology but will also enable the rational design of therapeutics that target TME-driven drug resistance. In this review, we provide an overview of patient-based metabolic studies with emphasis on the use of stable isotope tracers and the influence of tissue heterogeneity on metabolic reprogramming in cancer tissues. This is not intended to be comprehensive but rather provides examples that demonstrate commonalities and diversities in reprogrammed human cancer metabolism.

IN VIVO CANCER PATIENT STUDIES INFORM COMMON AND DIVERSE TRAITS OF CANCER METABOLISM

Metabolic interrogations in human subjects have been performed for many years in nutritional studies, which benefit greatly from the use of stable isotope tracers including those enriched in ^{2}H, ^{13}C, and ^{15}N (Davies 2020). These studies provided valuable information on energy expenditure, protein turnover (Wagenmakers 1999), and central metabolism such as lipogenesis (Leitch and Jones 1993; Fu et al. 2021) and gluconeogenesis (Landau 1999; Jones et al. 2001). We and others have developed stable isotope tracing in human cancer patients plus a variety of other systems including cells, animal models, and resected tissues (Fan et al. 2005, 2009, 2011; Sellers et al. 2015; Hensley et al. 2016) to broadly define metabolic network activity, which we call stable isotope–resolved metabolomics (SIRM). The use of stable isotope tracers and SIRM application in human cancer patients began with a [U-^{13}C]-glucose study of NSCLC (Fan et al. 2009; Lane et al. 2011), which showed enhanced ^{13}C incorporation into numerous metabolites in cancerous versus benign lung tissues, including those generated by pyruvate carboxylation (Sellers et al. 2015). Subsequently, Maher et al. demonstrated glucose metabolism in glioblastoma

(GBM) where glucose transformations via glycolysis, the Krebs cycle, anaplerosis, and de novo Gln/Gly synthesis were deduced from ^{13}C NMR analysis. Also revealed was a significant contribution of non–blood glucose–derived acetyl CoA to the total pool, and thus tumor bioenergetics (Maher et al. 2012).

Our group then extended the earlier study of reprogrammed cancer metabolism to 34 early-stage NSCLC patients infused with a bolus of [U-^{13}C]-glucose for comparing matched pairs of NSCLC versus benign lung tissues. We again observed consistent activation of anaplerotic pyruvate carboxylation, which was mediated by the overexpression of pyruvate carboxylase (PC). Via PC suppression in NSCLC cells, we demonstrated the importance of this enzyme in supporting lung cancer cell growth both in vitro and in vivo (Sellers et al. 2015). We also revealed enhanced activity of the canonical Krebs cycle in NSCLC tissues, which was contrary to the common thought in the cancer community. Moreover, by tracing the fate of [U-^{13}C,^{15}N]-Gln in 13 ex vivo OTCs of NSCLC and matched benign tissues (see also description below), we saw comparable activities of glutaminase (GLS) in both tissue types, which along with a lack of a consistent trend in GLS1 overexpression, suggest that glutaminolysis is not a key anaplerotic process activated in NSCLC tissues, unlike other types of cancer (Kodama et al. 2020).

Enhanced activities of canonical and PC-mediated anaplerotic Krebs cycle in cancerous versus matched benign tissues were verified by Hensley et al. (2016) in a subsequent in vivo study of nine NSCLC patients with continuous infusion of [U-^{13}C]-glucose. This study also provided evidence for the reutilization of excreted lactate derived from glucose by some tumors, which could be associated with poor survival in adenocarcinoma. Using dynamic contrast-enhanced MRI as a guide for subsampling of resected tumor tissues, the study further demonstrated blood perfusion–driven heterogeneities in fuel oxidation (i.e., glucose being the major fuel in less-perfused regions while alternative fuel sources becoming more significant in regions with higher perfusion). Such TME-imposed metabolic diversities in NSCLC tissues appeared to override intrinsic metabolic phenotypes dictated by oncogenic drivers (Hensley et al. 2016).

The above in-patient metabolic reprogramming was deduced from the analysis of ^{13}C-labeled metabolites in extracts of resected patient tissues using NMR and/or mass spectrometry (MS). Although NMR is capable of in vivo real-time measurement of ^{13}C-metabolites, its relatively low sensitivity of detection, ^{13}C NMR in particular, has been a challenge for such analysis. The advent of hyperpolarized (HP) tracers can enhance sensitivity by more than 10,000-fold, which enables in vivo kinetic analysis of tracer transformation using ^{13}C NMR in a matter of seconds. Nelson et al. (2013) combined HP [1-^{13}C]-pyruvate infusion with ^{13}C-magnetic resonance spectroscopic imaging (MRSI) to show higher fluxes of pyruvate to lactate in biopsy-proven regions of prostate cancer than those in the benign counterparts for 31 patients. In a recent study, Sushentsev et al. (2022) coupled HP ^{13}C-MRI with immunohistochemistry and spatial transcriptomics to detect the emergence of glycolytic conversion of HP [1-^{13}C]-pyruvate to [1-^{13}C]-lactate in the epithelial, rather than the stromal, compartment in intermediate-risk human prostate cancer. In addition to monitoring glycolytic fluxes via [1-^{13}C]-lactate production, HP [1-^{13}C]-pyruvate was found to be converted to HP ^{13}C-bicarbonate in human glioma (Le Page et al. 2020), which was attributed to the activity of pyruvate dehydrogenase as in the brain or a measure of fluxes through anaplerotic PC plus gluconeogenic phosphoenolpyruvate carboxykinase (PCK) in the liver (Merritt et al. 2011). In a healthy human brain, the conversion of HP [2-^{13}C]-pyruvate to [2-^{13}C]-lactate and [5-^{13}C]-glutamate has been observed; the latter can be a measure of the Krebs cycle activity. As such, HP ^{13}C-MRSI is an unparalleled technique for quantifying spatially resolved fluxes through a specific enzyme reaction or a metabolic pathway in situ in human cancer patients. However, it remains a difficult challenge to expand the pathway coverage with this approach due to the very short magnetic half-life and limited choice of HP probes (Fan and Lane 2016).

EX VIVO ORGANOTYPIC TISSUE CULTURES OF CANCER PATIENTS ARE VALUABLE MODELS FOR PROBING HETEROGENEITIES IN METABOLIC REPROGRAMMING IN PATIENTS' TME

It is now generally recognized that many solid tumors including NSCLC and PDAC are highly heterogeneous in their cellular and molecular properties. This is exemplified by the highly variable distribution of cancer cells (panCK⁺ in green), CD8 T cells (CD8⁺ in red), and macrophages (Mϕ, CD68⁺ in yellow) throughout a small and thinly sliced piece of human NSCLC tissue as shown in Figure 1A. Interactions of such variable cell populations with different physicochemical parameters, most notably nutrient availability (Yuneva 2008), extracellular matrix (ECM) (Baghban et al. 2020), pH, and O_2 supply (Zhong et al. 1999), can result in highly complex and distinct TMEs that dictate tumor development/progression and drug resistance (Tredan et al. 2007; Baghban et al. 2020). To recapitulate patients' TME in cancer models has been a major challenge (Baghban et al. 2020), as individual patient's TME can be diverse and a priori un-

known, as well as deviating from that of common in vivo animal models.

To meet this challenge, we were motivated by Warburg's (1924) use of tumor tissue slices for uncovering accelerated aerobic glycolysis. We began by using standard cell culturing techniques to maintain metabolic activity in thinly sliced cancerous (CA) and matched noncancerous (NC) tissues (cf. examples in Fig. 1B) freshly resected from NSCLC patients (Sellers et al. 2015; Fan et al. 2016a). Such ex vivo tissue cultures are also known as OTCs (Humpel 2015) or organotypic multicellular spheres (OMSs) (Barbosa et al. 2021). They offer multiple advantages over other cancer models, including (1) maintenance of the individual patient's TME; (2) interrogation of target tissue responses without systemic influences; (3) matched CA and NC design that circumvents common interferences in functional or drug response studies; (4) flexibility in treatment options, including the use of a full range of tracers; and (5) the ability to acquire the response of the individual patient's target tissue to stressors (Fan et al. 2020).

We found metabolic reprogramming in ex vivo OTCs of CA human lung (blue dash) reca-

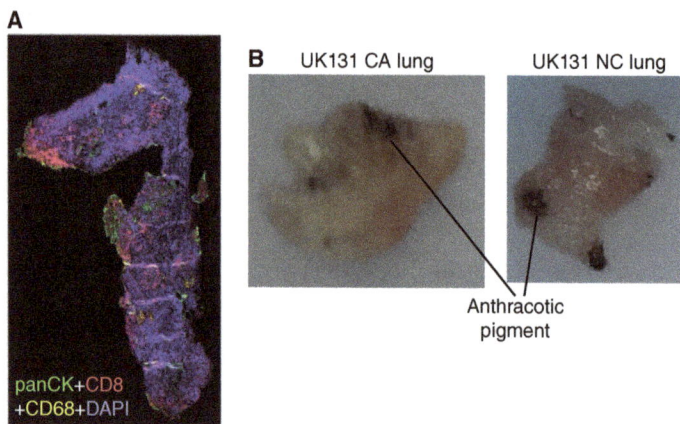

Figure 1. Heterogenous cellular distribution in human non-small-cell lung cancer (NSCLC) tissues. (*A*) The freshly resected NSCLC patient tumor tissues (UK131) were thinly sliced and incubated in $^{13}C_6$-glucose-DMEM medium for 24 hours at 37°C/5% CO_2 before fixing part of the tissues in 4% buffered formalin, embedding in a paraffin block, and sectioning into 4 μm slices for multiplex immunofluorescence (mIF) staining for cancer cells (panCytokeratin or panCK, green), CD8 (cytotoxic T cells, red), and CD68 (Mϕ, yellow) and for nuclei (DAPI, blue). (*A* adapted from Fan et al. 2020; © 2020 by the authors.) (*B*) Example pair of matched cancerous (CA) and noncancerous (NC) organotypic tissue cultures (OTCs), each of 750 μm thickness, prepared from the resected lung of UK131. The yellowish-white tissue in the *left* image is mainly tumor while the pinkish tissue in the *right* image is NC lung tissue. The dark anthracotic pigment denoted is typically found in smoker's lung tissues.

Cite this article as *Cold Spring Harb Perspect Med* doi: 10.1101/cshperspect.a041552

pitulates that in vivo (red dash) from which the OTC was derived (Fig. 2A). For example, compared with the NC counterparts, they exhibit enhanced buildup of ^{13}C-labeled lactate (^{13}C-3-Lac), Ala (^{13}C-3-Ala), Glu (^{13}C-4-Glu), Gln (^{13}C-4-Gln), glycogen (^{13}C-1-glycogen), and nucleotides (^{13}C-1′-UXP, ^{13}C-1′-AXP) but depletion of ^{13}C-labeled glucose and/or glucose-6-phosphate (^{13}C-1-αGlc + G6P) (denoted by dashed lines in Fig. 2A). Such metabolic distinction is common to other matched pairs of CA versus NC OTCs, as shown in Figure 2B, bottom panel. Interestingly, patient-derived subcutaneous xenograft (PDX) of CA lung tissues displayed somewhat different metabolic activities from the corresponding OTCs. Namely, relative to lactate, PDX (red dash) showed enhanced buildup of Ala, Gln, Glu, and glutathiones (reduced GSH

and/or oxidized GSSH) but less buildup of ^{13}C-glucose + G6P and AXP than the OTC counterpart (blue dash) (denoted by dashed lines in Fig. 2B). The different TME in mouse PDX versus human CA OTCs could contribute to these metabolic differences.

Maintaining the viability of ex vivo OTCs is critical to the utility of this model, particularly for investigating long-term responses to therapeutics (e.g., checkpoint inhibitors; see below) and resistance development. We found that thinly sliced (e.g., 750 μm) patient-derived organotypic tissue cultures (PD-OTCs) can remain viable for at least 1 month as measured by metabolic activity and immunohistochemistry (Yan et al. 2023; TWM Fan, T Cassel, RM Higashi, et al., unpubl. results), despite the lack of blood flow. Since the uptake of O_2, nutrients, and treatment agents

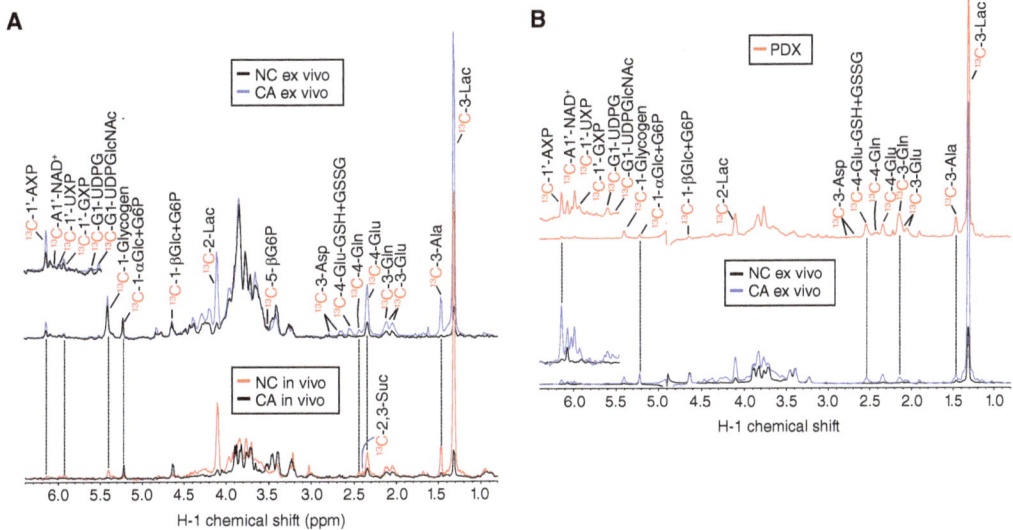

Figure 2. Ex vivo organotypic tissue cultures (OTCs) of human non-small-cell lung cancer (NSCLC) recapitulate in vivo metabolic reprogramming. NSCLC patient UL193 (*A*) was infused with ^{13}C$_6$-glucose for 2 hours before surgery as described previously (Sellers et al. 2015). Cancerous (CA) and surrounding noncancerous (NC) tissues were freshly resected at the operating room, part of which was flash-frozen in liquid N$_2$ (in vivo samples). The rest of the resected tissues were thinly sliced and incubated in ^{13}C$_6$-glucose-DMEM medium for 24 hours at 37°C/5% CO$_2$ (ex vivo OTCs) before flash freezing, pulverization, and extraction for polar metabolites and proteins. ^{1}H{^{13}C} spectra were recorded at 14.1 T and annotated as previously described (Fan et al. 2019). Individual peaks represent protons attached to ^{13}C derived from the metabolic transformation of ^{13}C$_6$-glucose. (*B*) Another patient's (UL025) CA tissues were implanted into the shoulders of NSG mice as patient-derived xenograft (PDX) or prepared for OTCs at the OR, as described previously (Sun et al. 2017). Polar extracts were analyzed by 1D ^{1}H{^{13}C} HSQC as in *A*. (Lac) Lactate, (GSH/GSSH) reduced and oxidized glutathione, (Suc) succinate, (Glc) glucose, (G6P) glucose-6-phosphate, (UDPGlcNAc) N-acetylglucosamine-UDP, (UDPG) UDP-glucose, (GXP/UXP/AXP) guanine/uracil/adenine nucleotides.

relies on diffusion, the thinner the OTC, the lower the diffusion barrier. However, thinner OTCs are more fragile, thereby requiring structural support and the fraction of cells damaged by the cutting process increases with decreasing thickness. To further facilitate the diffusion process, it is important to enable rocking and free medium access from both sides of the OTC.

Although OTCs can be readily treated with inhibitors of protein targets, their genetic manipulations are more difficult presumably due to barriers (e.g., lack of blood delivery, ECM) to the uptake of genetic materials, variable transfection efficiency among different cell types, and slow or no cell growth. Nevertheless, methods are being developed for selective uptake of siRNA or shRNAs (Chastagnier et al. 2023), which can complement studies on small molecule inhibitors. For example, Ruigrok et al. (2017) reported successful transfection of 250–350 μm thick mouse lung and kidney tissue slices using Accell RNA. It is also feasible to deliver target proteins (including antibodies) to cells and potentially tissues using different delivery systems (Oba and Tanaka 2012), although tissue delivery has not been reported. Moreover, mRNA delivery as a result of the development of mRNA-based antiviral therapies (Hou et al. 2021) could be adapted to produce any protein of interest in target cells, either as overexpression of a protein (knockin) or an antibody to the proteins (knockout).

The flexibility of treatments for the OTC model is shown by the following four examples.

1. *Compartmentation of nucleotide biosynthesis was revealed using multiple tracers.* We used [U-^{13}C]-Gly and dual tracers ([U-^{13}C]-Glc in combination with [U-^{2}H]-serine or [U-^{2}H]-glycine) to track simultaneously the transformations of glucose and serine or glycine into purine nucleotides in seven pairs of CA and NC OTCs of NSCLC patients (Fan et al. 2019). Such tracer treatments would be cost-prohibitive for in-patient studies. We were surprised to find that, unlike cultured cancer cells, exogenous glucose was a much-preferred precursor over exogenous serine or glycine for fueling the synthesis of purine nucleotides in CA

OTCs. Based on kinetic modeling of relevant labeled metabolites and protein expression patterns of key enzymes in Ser/Gly synthesis and one-carbon pathways, we attributed this preference to the activation and dynamic compartmentation of de novo serine synthesis pathway in the cytoplasm as well as reversed serine to one-carbon flux in the mitochondrion. It would be difficult to reach such a conclusion without the flexible use of these tracers.

2. *Activation of tumor-associated macrophages (TAM) by β-glucan.* We used [U-^{13}C]-glucose to determine the effect of an experimental immune modulator β-glucan formulated as whole glucan particulates (WGPs) (Fan et al. 2016b) on paired CA and NC lung OTCs. WGP treatment would require clinical trial approval for in-patient studies, which was circumvented for ex vivo OTC studies as OTCs were derived from discarded patient tissues. We have shown that WGPs repolarize anti-inflammatory M2-type macrophages (M2-Mφ) or immunosuppressive TAM to proinflammatory M1-type macrophages (M1-Mφ) in mouse studies. This immunostimulatory response was accompanied by enhanced glycolysis, Krebs cycle activity, and glutamine utilization, as the case for M1 polarization (Liu et al. 2015). However, it was unclear whether TAM in cancer patient tissues similarly respond to WGPs. Patient-derived CA OTCs represent a unique model for addressing this question, as they maintain individual patients' tissue architecture and TME. We found that CA lung OTCs from one NSCLC patient (UK021) with chronic obstructive pulmonary disease (COPD) and abundant TAM responded to WGPs by increasing the expression of inducible nitric oxide synthase (iNOS), reduced mitotic index, and increased necrosis (Fan et al. 2016b). This was accompanied by M1-like metabolic reprogramming such as the buildup of itaconate and activated pentose phosphate pathway (PPP) (Fan et al. 2016b). In contrast, CA lung OTCs from another patient (UK049) with no COPD and much less macrophage

infiltration was unresponsive to WGPs in terms of immune/metabolic activation and tissue damages. The matched NC lung OTCs were insensitive to WGP treatment. Thus, this example not only demonstrates the value of ex vivo OTC models in probing reprogrammed metabolism in individual patients' TME in response to immunomodulation but also enables estimation of therapeutic index on target tissues without interferences from varying genetic, physiological, and nutritional backgrounds.

3. *Assessment of drug resistance in individual patient's TME and efficacy of combination therapy.* Here, we used [U-^{13}C]-glucose or [U-^{13}C,^{15}N]-Gln to track reprogrammed metabolism elicited by an FDA-approved immune checkpoint inhibitor Pembrolizumab (Pembro) in a matched pair of CA and NC lung OTCs derived from an NSCLC patient with primary lesion (Fan et al. 2021). We found that Pembro activated PPP and glycogen synthesis but attenuated glutamine oxidation via the Krebs cycle, which were accompanied by enhanced release of proinflammatory effectors in CA OTCs. These changes were akin to those in human Mφ in response to M1-type polarization and were associated with overall tissue damages. It is interesting to note that the response of glutamine oxidation in human M1-Mφ is opposite to that in mouse M1-Mφ described above. We also used digital spatial profiling (DSP) to compare 58 protein markers of cancer/immune cells' functional states and mitotic index across 12 different TMEs in Pembro-treated versus control CA OTCs. We found that two of the 12 TMEs had low HER2/3 expression relative to other TMEs and maintained high proliferative states despite displaying boosted effector functions of M1-type Mφ or CD8$^+$ T cells. Thus, the OTC study revealed the overall efficacy of Pembro against this PD1-positive NSCLC tissue but there appeared to be two TMEs that displayed resistance to Pembro-induced immune activation. We further showed by using brain-metastasized CA OTCs from another NSCLC patient that Pembro alone was ineffective, but Pembro and WGPs combined caused massive CA tissue damage and attenuated anabolic metabolism, which was accompanied by enhanced release of M1-type proinflammatory effectors (Fan et al. 2021). Thus, in addition to gaining molecular insights into drug resistance, the OTC model enables highly versatile treatment options and the use of costly tracers to be readily implemented on patients' target tissues without time-consuming development of the PDX model or approval for clinical trials. These merits can greatly facilitate rational choices of therapeutic options on an individual patient basis.

4. *Enhanced capacity of NSCLC OTCs in leucine uptake and metabolism into glycine.* Leucine is known to activate the mTOR signaling pathway, thereby enhancing protein synthesis (Han et al. 2012). This mechanism can account for the ability of leucine-rich diet in attenuating the symptoms of cancer cachexia in preclinical models by stimulating protein synthesis and suppressing protein degradation (Beaudry and Law 2022). Leucine-rich diets also reprogram tumor metabolism causing a shift from glycolysis to oxidative phosphorylation, which attenuates tumor aggressiveness and number of metastatic sites in tumor-bearing rats (Viana et al. 2019). On the other hand, leucine supplementation promotes the survival and growth of human PDAC cells (Wei et al. 2020). The latter can be related to the capacity of leucine catabolism to acetyl CoA for fueling lipid synthesis required for proliferation (Lee et al. 2019). In comparison, much less is known for leucine metabolism and tumor developmental consequences in human cancer tissues. The leucine transporter *SLC7A5* and catabolic enzyme genes (*BCAT* and *BCKDH*) were found to be overexpressed in human NSCLC but downregulated in human PDAC (Mayers et al. 2016) tissues. *SLC7A5* overexpression was related to immune suppressive TME and poor prognosis for NSCLC patients (Liu et al. 2022). A better understanding of leucine metabolism will help delineate its role in promoting or blocking tumor development in human cancer tissues.

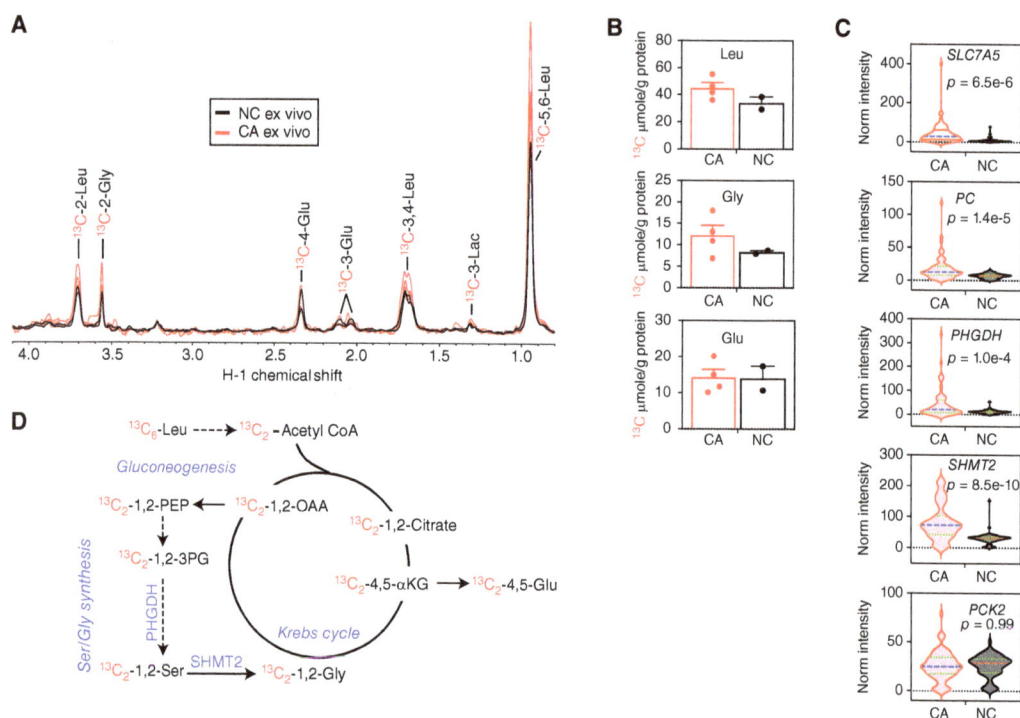

Figure 3. Ex vivo organotypic tissue cultures (OTCs) of human non-small-cell lung cancer (NSCLC) show enhanced [U-^{13}C]-Leu uptake. Matched pairs of cancerous (CA) (red dash) and noncancerous (NC) (black dash) OTCs from an NSCLC patient (UK121) were treated with ^{13}C$_6$-Leu for 24 hours as in Figure 2. At harvest, tissues were processed and extracted for polar metabolites as in Figure 2. Polar extracts were analyzed by 1D ^{1}H{^{13}C} HSQC for ^{13}C-labeled metabolites in A and B (CA $n = 4$; NC $n = 2$). The P-values for Leu and Gly data in B were 0.197 and 0.066, respectively. (C) Gene expression pattern for the BCAA transporter *SLC7A5*, gluconeogenic/ anaplerotic enzyme *PC*, and Ser/Gly synthesis enzymes *PHGDH/SHMT2* in bulk CA versus matched NC lung tissues resected from 63 NSCLC patients. (D) An example ^{13}C atom-resolved transformation pathway from [U-^{13}C]-Leu to the ^{13}C-labeled products Glu at 4,5 position (^{13}C$_2$-4,5-Glu) and Gly at 1,2 position (^{3}C$_2$-1,2-Gly).

As a proof-of-concept, we used the OTC model and [U-^{13}C]-Leu tracer to explore how leucine is metabolized in human CA versus NC lung tissues. Figure 3A shows ^{1}H{^{13}C}HSQC NMR analysis of the parent tracer and its ^{13}C-labeled products in CA versus NC lung OTCs of an NSCLC patient (UK121). Although nonstatistically significant due to a sizable variation in the CA OTC data, there appeared to be an enhanced buildup of ^{13}C-Leu and ^{13}C-Gly in CA versus NC OTCs (Fig. 3B). Such large variation in the metabolism of CA lung OTCs was evident for other NSCLC patients (Fan et al. 2021) and most likely reflects the tissue heterogeneity from slice to slice. We also saw a significant and comparable buildup of ^{13}C-glutamate in both CA and NC

OTCs, which presumably results from the oxidation of [U-^{13}C]-Leu to ^{13}C-acetyl CoA (Kohlmeier 2015) and subsequent conversion to ^{13}C-glutamate via the Krebs cycle and αKG transamination (cf. Fig. 3D). Consistent with the previous report (Mayers et al. 2016; Liu et al. 2022), we saw robustly enhanced gene expression of the leucine transporter *SLC7A5* in bulk CA versus matched NC lung tissues resected from 63 NSCLC patients. This was also the case for the anaplerotic/gluconeogenic enzyme *PC*, serine/glycine biosynthetic enzymes phosphoglycerate dehydrogenase (*PHGDH*)/serine hydroxymethyl transferase 2 (*SHMT2*) (Fig. 3C). These gene expression changes, together with the enhanced buildup of ^{13}C-Leu and ^{13}C-Gly, point to activa-

Cite this article as *Cold Spring Harb Perspect Med* doi: 10.1101/cshperspect.a041552

tion of leucine uptake and metabolism to glycine via the Krebs cycle, gluconeogenesis, and de novo serine–glycine synthesis pathway (Fig. 3D) in CA lung tissues.

De novo synthesis of glycine from leucine was also evident from a whole-body study of diabetic patients with [^{13}C-1]-leucine as tracer (Robert et al. 1985). In this whole-body study, hepatic gluconeogenesis presumably contributed dominantly to the synthesis of 3-phosphoglycerate (3PG), which is the precursor to serine/glycine synthesis (Fig. 3D). However, as there was no hepatic contribution in the lung OTC study, in-lung gluconeogenesis, at least as far as 3PG, constitutes a major pathway for leucine utilization to support glycine synthesis, which requires the expression of PCK. The *PCK2* gene is expressed in 63 NSCLC patients' CA and NC lung tissues (CA/NC ratio 1.31 ± 0.25), although with no statistically significant difference between them. However, *PC* (another key gluconeogenic enzyme gene) is consistently overexpressed in CA versus NC lung tissues (Fig. 3C), which could reflect a higher capacity for gluconeogenesis.

This example shows the ability of ex vivo OTC models in delineating target tissue metabolism without systemic influence. Enhanced leucine conversion to glycine to fuel purine nucleotide synthesis in CA lung tissues could offer growth/survival advantages in case of glucose deficiency in the TME. Metabolic insights gained from such human patient tissue studies should help guide future research on the role of leucine metabolism in human cancer development and progression.

PATIENT-DERIVED ORGANOIDS ARE EXCELLENT MODELS FOR PROBING CELL–CELL AND CELL–MATRIX INTERACTIONS IN THE TME

3D cell cultures including spheroids of established cell lines and patient-derived organoids (PDOs) are emerging to be much-preferred models than their 2D counterparts for mimicking the architecture and cell–cell/cell–matrix interactions intrinsic to the TME (Tomás-Bort et al. 2020; Barbosa et al. 2021). 3D cell models display protein/gene expression levels closer to in vivo models than the 2D counterparts and better recapitulate drug resistance (Barbosa et al. 2021). Mouse lung tumor–derived organoids were shown to retain more of the molecular features of the original tissues than their 2D cell counterparts, including tissue lineage gene expression patterns (Chen et al. 2023). PDOs in particular can emulate individual patient's TME via reconstitution with other TME cell types, thereby providing a powerful tool for resolving the metabolic interactions in the corresponding ex vivo OTC models and in-patient. In collaboration with Dr. Christine F. Brainson, we have isolated PDOs from the squamous cell carcinoma (SqCC) tissue of an NSCLC patient (UK022) (cf. Fig. 4C) and carried out an SIRM study for comparison with the corresponding CA OTCs. Figure 4 shows the transformations of [U-^{13}C]-glucose into various ^{13}C-labeled metabolites in CA PDOs (B) and CA OTCs along with NC OTCs (A). As seen in Figure 2, relative to NC OTCs (black dash), CA OTCs (red dash) exhibited an enhanced buildup of ^{13}C-labeled glycolytic products (lactate, Ala), Krebs cycle products (Glu), glycogen, and purine/pyrimidine nucleotides (AXP/UXP) but depletion of ^{13}C-glucose and/or G6P. These differences again recapitulate those observed in in-patient tracer studies (Sellers et al. 2015).

We also noted that relative to ^{13}C-lactate (^{13}C-Lac) in CA PDOs versus CA OTCs, there was a greater buildup of the ^{13}C-labeled Krebs cycle metabolites (succinate, glutamate, glutamine, glutathiones, and aspartate) and various nucleotides/nucleotide derivatives (*N*-acetylglucosamine-UDP, UDP-glucose, guanine/uracil/adenine nucleotides, and NAD$^+$) but a lower buildup of ^{13}C-glycogen. These data could reflect enhanced activities of the Krebs cycle and synthesis of glutathione and purine/pyrimidine nucleotides but an attenuated synthesis of glycogen in CA PDOs versus CA OTCs. Except for the glycogen synthesis, this was also the case for CA OTCs in comparison with matched NC OTCs (Fig. 4A). Thus, CA PDOs qualitatively recapitulate the reprogrammed metabolism of the parent CA tissue. The quantitative differences in metabolic activities between CA PDOs and OTCs could be attributed to the influence of other cell types on cancer cell metabolism in the TME of CA OTCs and/or the

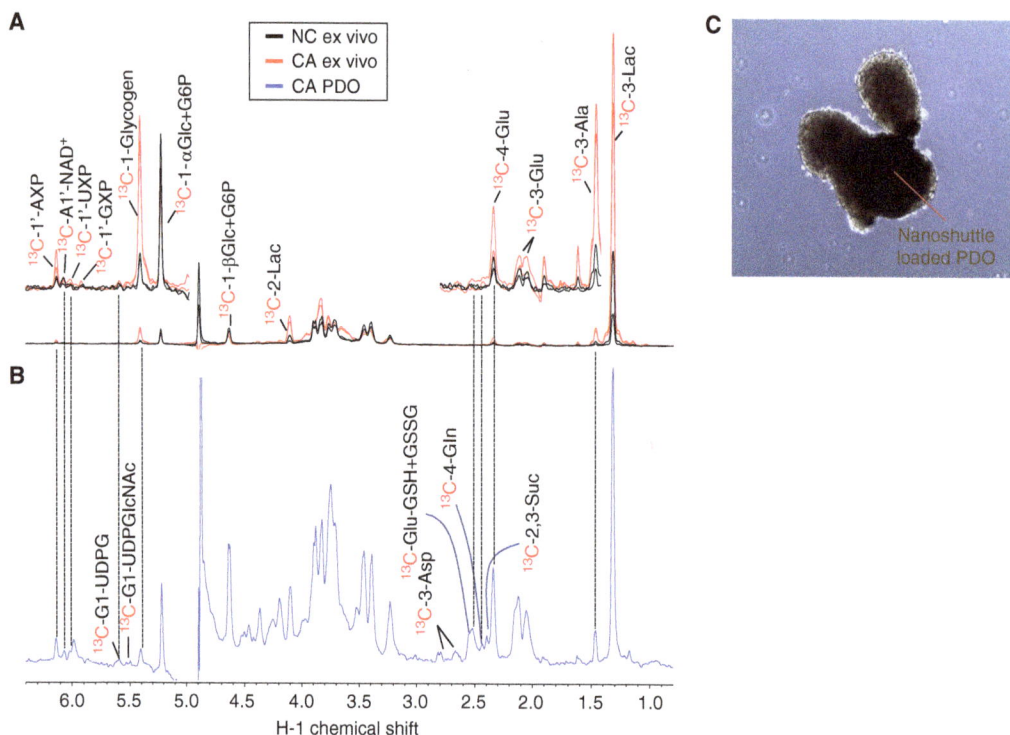

Figure 4. Comparison of metabolic activity in cancerous (CA) organotypic tissue cultures (OTCs) versus the corresponding patient-derived organoids (PDOs). Matched pairs of CA and noncancerous (NC) OTCs ($n = 2$) from a non-small-cell lung cancer (NSCLC) patient UK022 (A) was treated with $^{13}C_6$-glucose for 24 hours as in Figure 2. PDOs were isolated by Dr. Christine Brainson from the squamous cell carcinoma tissue of an NSCLC patient UK022. They were cultured as spheroids using Nanoshuttle as described previously (Fan et al. 2018) in full DMEM medium containing 0.2% [U-^{13}C]-Glc and 2 mM unlabeled Gln for 72 hours (B). (C) An example UK022 PDO loaded with Nanoshuttle; the image was taken with 10× objective. At harvest, OTCs were processed for polar metabolites as in Figure 2 and PDOs were rinsed of medium components, quenched in cold CH_3CN before extraction for polar metabolites as described in Fan et al. (2018). Polar extracts were analyzed by 1D $^1H\{^{13}C\}$ HSQC. (Lac) Lactate, (GSH/GSSG) reduced and oxidized glutathione, (Suc) succinate, (Glc) glucose, (G6P), glucose-6-phosphate, (UDPGlcNAc) N-acetylglucosamine-UDP, (UDPG) UDP-glucose, (GXP/UXP/AXP) guanine/uracil/adenine nucleotides.

contribution of other cell types to the metabolic activities of CA OTCs as CA PDOs should be more enriched in cancer cells (including cancer stem cells) than their tissue counterpart.

In another [U-^{13}C]-Glc-based SIRM study of PDOs isolated from the SqCC of NSCLC patient UK057, we compared the metabolic activities of CA PDOs with the corresponding CA OTCs and tumor xenograft in mice (PDTX). As shown in Figure 5, the ^{13}C fractional enrichment of various metabolites in PDOs (red square) largely tracked that of CA OTCs (black square) but deviated significantly from that of the PDTX (blue square).

The metabolites shown are those derived from glycolysis (a,c), the Krebs cycle (d–k,m), PPP (l), and purine/pyrimidine synthesis (n,o), including those resulting from the activity of anaplerotic PC (3,5 in d) and ME (1 in h) (Fig. 5). These data point to PDOs as a more accurate model than PDTX for recapitulating the metabolic activities of CA patient tissues.

To determine how CA PDOs metabolically interact with human macrophages (Mφ), we cocultured UK057 CA PDOs with a healthy volunteer's (UK096) Mφ differentiated from peripheral blood monocytes (PBMCs). Figure 6A shows

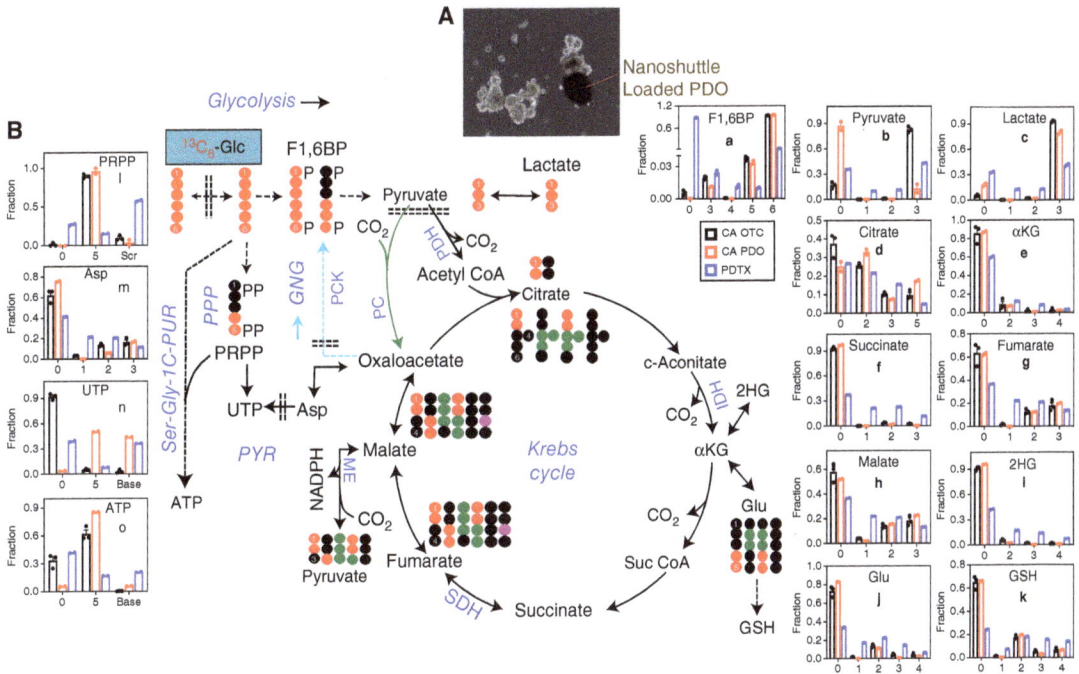

Figure 5. UK057 patient-derived organoids (PDOs) recapitulates cancerous (CA) organotypic tissue cultures (OTCs) in metabolic activity better than the patient-derived tumor xenograft (PDTX) model. $^{13}C_6$-glucose ($^{13}C_6$-Glc)-based stable isotope-resolved metabolomics (SIRM) studies were performed for 24 hours on CA lung OTCs ex vivo derived from a non-small-cell lung cancer (NSCLC) patient UK057 bearing squamous cell carcinoma, as described previously (Fan et al. 2021). A similar SIRM experiment was done on matched patient-derived CA organoids (A; image taken with a 20× objective) isolated by Dr. Christine Brainson, as described in Fan et al. (2018). (B) $^{13}C_6$-Glc was administered via liquid diet feeding for 18 hours on F0 mice bearing PDTX of UK057, as described in Sun et al. (2017). The analysis of polar extracts by ion chromatography, ultra high-resolution mass spectrometry (IC-UHRMS) is shown for PDOs (red square; $n = 2$), OTCs (black square; $n = 3$), and PDTX (blue square; $n = 2$) as fractional enrichment in selected isotopologues of metabolites in glycolysis, the Krebs cycle, the pentose phosphate pathway (PPP), glutathione (GSH) synthesis, gluconeogenesis (GNG), and serine–glycine, one-carbon purine (Ser-Gly-1C-PUR)/pyrimidine (PYR) synthesis pathways. Values on the x-axis represent the number of ^{13}C atoms in each isotopolog. ^{12}C (black dot), ^{13}C (red dot/green dot/pink dot) derived from PDH/PC/ME reactions in the Krebs cycle. (F1,6BP) Fructose-1,6-bisphosphate, (αKG) α-ketoglutarate, (2HG) 2-hydroxyglutarate, (PDH/PCB) pyruvate dehydrogenase/carboxylase, (IDH/SDH) isocitrate/succinate dehydrogenase, (ME) malic enzyme, (PCK) phosphoenolpyruvate carboxykinase.

the staining patterns of HLA-DR and CD206 in single or cocultures of PDOs and Mφ in response to M1 (LPS + IFN-γ), M2 (IL-4 + IL-13), or M2 + β-glucan (formulated as WGP) polarization treatments. The mannose receptor CD206 is known to be highly expressed in anti-inflammatory or M2-type and down-regulated in proinflammatory M1-type human Mφ (Buchacher et al. 2015; Raggi et al. 2017; Fan et al. 2022) while HLA-DR has been shown to be highly expressed in M2-like Mφ but down-regulated in fully po-

larized M2-Mφ, relative to the M1-Mφ counterpart (Buchacher et al. 2015). The expression patterns of these two markers in Mφ single cultures confirmed the M1- and M2-type polarization by LPS + IFN-γ and IL-4 + IL-13 treatments, respectively, but also showed that the M2-type Mφ was not fully polarized as HLA-DR was still expressed. WGP treatment of M2-type Mφ reduced the expression of both CD206 and HLA-DR, which points to repolarization toward the M1-type but with retention of some M2-type

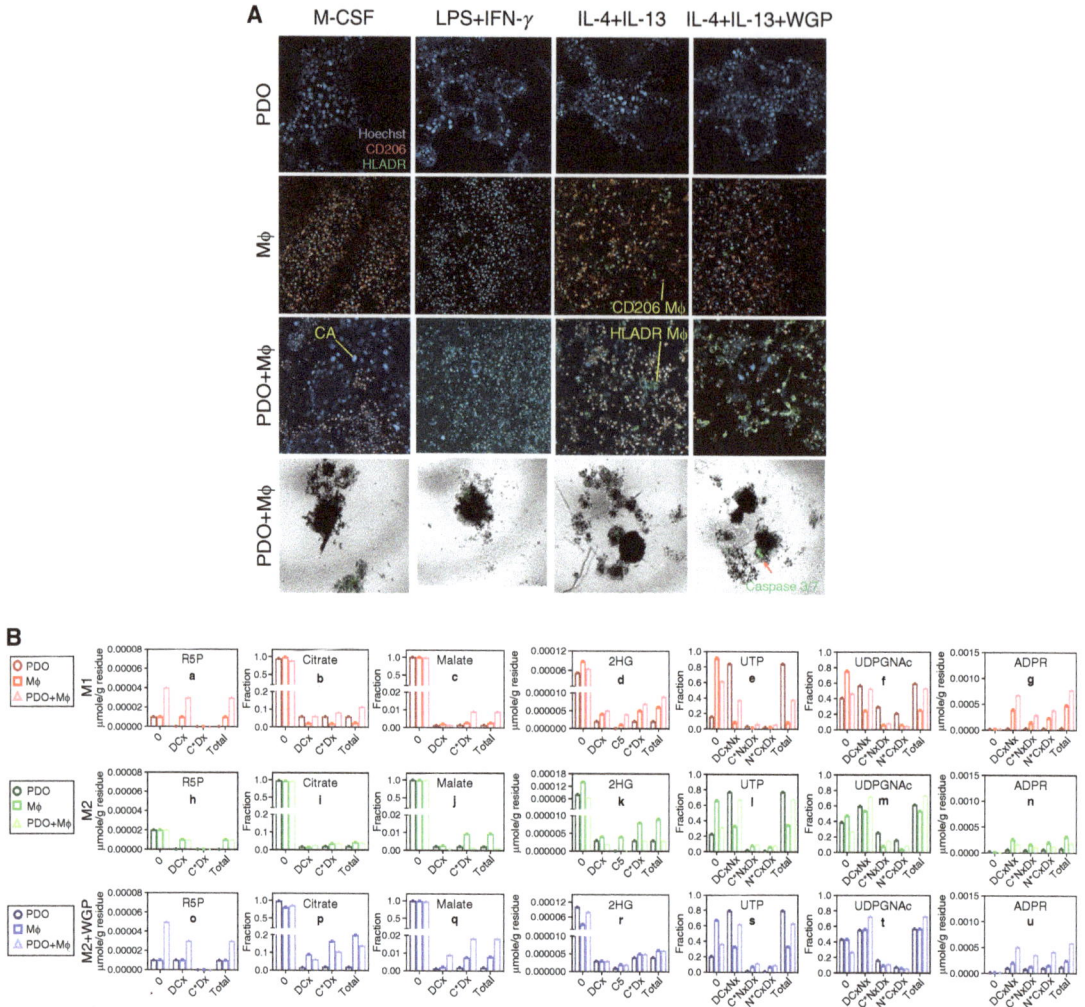

Figure 6. Distinct response of patient-derived organoids (PDOs), Mφ, and cocultures to differential polarization and whole glucan particulates (WGPs) treatment. PDOs (UK057's) (*A*) were grown in a 96-well plate using Nano-shuttles as described in Fan et al. (2018) as single and 1:1 cocultures with macrophages (Mφ) differentiated with m-CSF from a healthy volunteer's (UK096) peripheral blood monocytes (cf. Fan et al. 2022 for protocol) (each 200,000 cells total). The culture media contained DMEM/F12 base media supplemented with 10% FBS, 0.2% glucose, 2 mM Gln, and 78 µM L-Trp. For the m-CSF, LPS + IFN-γ (M1), IL-4 + IL-13 (M2), and IL-4 + IL-13 + WGP (M2 + WGP) polarization treatments, cells were incubated in the culture medium for 3 days with the respective addition of 100 ng/mL m-CSF (M0), 100 ng/mL LPS + 20 ng/mL IFN-γ (M1), 20 ng/mL each IL-4/IL-13 (M2), and 20 ng/mL each IL-4/IL-13, followed by supplementing an additional IL-4/IL-13 treatment with 100 µg/mL β-glucan (M2 + WGP) formulated as WGPs. All cells were incubated for a further 24 hours before staining for CD206 (M2 marker), HLA-DR (M1 marker), Hoechst (nuclear marker), and caspase 3/7 as live cells. Images (CD206, HLA-DR, and Hoechst) were acquired with a 20× objective on an Olympus confocal microscope (FV1200) or with a 4× objective on an EVOS M7000 microscope (caspase 3/7). In *B*, UK057's PDOs and UK096's Mφ were similarly grown as single and cocultures except for replacing unlabeled glucose, Gln, and Trp with 0.2% D_7-glucose, 2 mM $^{13}C_5$-Gln, and 78 µM $^{15}N_2$-Trp. Cells were quenched and extracted with cold 70% methanol for polar metabolites as described in Fan et al. (2018). Polar extracts (*n* = 2) were pooled before analysis for labeling patterns of metabolites with IC-UHRMS as in Figure 5. The *x*-axis denotes selected mass isotopologs as follows: 0: unlabeled; C5: $^{13}C_5$; DCx/DCxNx: ^{2}H with 0 − *x* number of $^{13}C/^{13}C$ and ^{15}N; C*NxDx: ^{13}C with 0 − *x* number of ^{15}N and ^{2}H; N*CxDx: ^{15}N with 0 − *x* number of ^{13}C and ^{2}H; total: total labeled; C1-xDx: $^{13}C_{1-x}$ with 0 − *x* number of ^{2}H.

properties, as we have observed previously (Fan et al. 2022). When Mφ was cocultured with PDOs, they did not change shape significantly under m-CSF or LPS + IFN-γ treatment but became enlarged with IL-4 + IL-13 or IL-4 + IL-13 + WGP treatments. These enlarged cells were high in HLA-DR but low in CD206 expression, which is akin to the property of fully polarized M1-Mφ (Buchacher et al. 2015). Enhanced HLA-DR expression was accompanied by an increase in the caspase 3/7 level (red arrow) in WGP-treated coculture of PDOs and M2-Mφ, which points to enhanced cell death in the cancer spheroid.

We also carried out a parallel SIRM study of the same set of UK057's PDO and UK096's Mφ cultures using a triple tracer cocktail of D_7-glucose, $^{13}C_5$-Gln, and $^{15}N_2$-Trp. This multiplexed tracer approach enabled simultaneous tracing of glucose, glutamine, and tryptophan metabolism while reducing sample requirements and avoiding sample batch artifacts compared with the single tracer approach. For example, in Figure 6B, significant ^{13}C labeling (C*NxDx) of ADP-ribose (ADPR; g,n,u) indicates active gluconeogenesis from $^{13}C_5$-Gln while sizable ^{15}N labeling (N*CxNx) of ADPR reflects $^{15}N_2$-Trp catabolism via the action of indoleamine 2,3-dioxygenase (IDO) in Mφ and Mφ-PDO cocultures. The higher ^{15}N enrichment in M1-Mφ (red square, g) than in M2-Mφ (green square, n) is consistent with the induction of IDO in M1-Mφ versus M2-Mφ, as observed previously (Fan et al. 2022). Also shown in Figure 6B were representative labeling patterns of metabolites in PDO-Mφ cocultures (red, green, and purple triangles) that could reflect mixed M1- (light, medium, and dark red bars) and M2-type (light, medium, and dark green bars) polarization. M1-type responses included enhanced enrichment or buildup of D-labeled (DCx) ribose-5-phosphate (R5P; a,o), D-labeled (DCxNx) ADP-ribose (ADPR; g,u)/UDP N-acetylglucosamine (UDP-GNAc; f,m,t), D-/^{13}C-labeled (C*Dx) 2-hydroxyglutarate (2HG; d,r), and ^{15}N-labeled ADPR (g,u). M2-type responses included increased enrichment of D-labeled citrate (b,p)/UTP (l,s) and ^{13}C-labeled UTP (e), as reported previously for UK096 Mφ (Fan et al. 2022). These changes could reflect, respectively, activation of PPP, ADP-ri-

bosylation, and 2HG-regulated processes such as prolyl hydroxylation or attenuated Krebs cycle activity and protein glycosylation in M1-Mφ versus M2-Mφ, as reasoned previously (Fan et al. 2022). Also noted was reduced enrichment of ^{13}C-labeled citrate/malate in the single M1-Mφ culture (red square, b,c) but increased enrichment in their PDO cocultures (red triangle, b,c) relative to the M2 counterparts (green square, green triangle, i,j), which could reflect, respectively, attenuated (M1-type) and boosted (M2-type) Krebs cycle activity in the single and cocultures. Moreover, WGP treatment repolarized M2-Mφ toward M1-type metabolic responses (purple triangle, o,r,u) while retaining some of the M2-type metabolic responses (purple triangle, p,q,t) in the coculture. The former can be related to the enhanced expression of HLA-DR and cell death while the latter to the persistent expression of CD206 in the coculture (Fig. 6A). We have previously associated metabolic responsiveness to WGPs to reduced mitotic index and cell death in NSCLC patient-derived CA OTCs (Fan et al. 2016b, 2022). Such pilot study of PDOs in culture with human Mφ demonstrates the utility of PDOs in modeling metabolic interactions in the patient's TME and associated tissue damages.

CONCLUDING REMARKS

The development of metabolomic technologies that support stable isotope tracer experimentation has made it practical to broadly and accurately resolve intersecting metabolic networks reprogrammed in human cancers, be they in vivo, ex vivo (OTCs), or in vitro (PDOs). Knowledge gained from in vivo patient studies provides the "benchmark" for numerous cancer models (from isolated cells and resected tissues to in vivo animal models) to recapitulate. It is a particularly difficult challenge to reproduce patient TMEs in models, as they lack the complete complexity of the patient's native state that is shaped by many variable physicochemical factors leading to highly heterogeneous and complex interactions of cancer cells with other cell types.

These interactions dictate metabolic reprogramming, a hallmark of cancer impacting all stages of cancer development and drug resistance. The ex vivo patient-derived OTCs represent a unique metabolic model for individual patients, as this model retains each patient's tissue architecture and TME while enabling a wide range of treatments, including the use of costly metabolic tracers or any desirable therapeutics for determining target tissue responses and manipulation of the TME. Using NSCLC patient-derived lung OTCs, we have shown that these models recapitulate the metabolic reprogramming of the patient tumors better than the corresponding PDX model. We have also shown that the PD-OTC model enables metabolic interrogation of immune cell response to immune modulators in an individual patient's TME context while revealing TME-dependent resistance of cancer cell proliferation to immune activation.

The importance of TME context on cancer metabolism is shown by the closer metabolic resemblance of the PD-OTC (with patient TME) to the PDO model than to the PDTX model (with mouse TME) of the same patient. The value of the PDO model in reconstituting patient tissue metabolism is also exemplified by the ability of the PDO immune cell coculture to recapitulate the metabolic responses of the PD-OTC model to immune modulators. Future research on PD-OTC and PDO models using 'omics technologies, particularly at single-cell/organelle resolution in situ will afford an unprecedented basic understanding of the TME dependence of cancer metabolic reprogramming on an individual patient basis. This should, in turn, translate into the identification of novel metabolic targets that block tumor-promoting TME interactions and drug resistance development.

ACKNOWLEDGMENTS

This research was funded by the National Institutes of Health, grant numbers 1P01CA163223-01A1 (to A.N.L. and T.W.-M.F.), 1U24DK0972 15-01A1 (to R.M.H., T.W.-M.F., and A.N.L.), 5R01 CA101199-02 (to T.W.-M.F.), 5R21ES025 669-02 (to T.W.-M.F.), and Edith D. Gardner (T.W.-M.F.) and Carmen L. Buck (A.N.L.) endowment funds. NMR and MS were recorded using the Metabolism Shared Resources supported in part by P30CA177558 (to BM Evers). We thank Drs. Yelena Chernyavskaya and James Sledziona for assisting in the PDO-Mφ coculture study, Dr. Christine Brainson for providing PDOs, and Drs. Salim El-Amouri and Jessica Macedo for assisting in the SIRM studies of PDOs. We also thank Dr. Angela Mahan for resecting the NSCLC patients' lung tissues.

REFERENCES

Baghban R, Roshangar L, Jahanban-Esfahlan R, Seidi K, Ebrahimi-Kalan A, Jaymand M, Kolahian S, Javaheri T, Zare P. 2020. Tumor microenvironment complexity and therapeutic implications at a glance. *Cell Commun Signal* **18:** 59. doi:10.1186/s12964-020-0530-4

Barbosa MAG, Xavier CPR, Pereira RF, Petrikaitė V, Vasconcelos MH. 2021. 3D cell culture models as recapitulators of the tumor microenvironment for the screening of anticancer drugs. *Cancers (Basel)* **14:** 190. doi:10.3390/cancers14010190

Beaudry AG, Law ML. 2022. Leucine supplementation in cancer cachexia: mechanisms and a review of the preclinical literature. *Nutrients* **14:** 2824. doi:10.3390/nu14142824

Boroughs LK, DeBerardinis RJ. 2015. Metabolic pathways promoting cancer cell survival and growth. *Nat Cell Biol* **17:** 351–359. doi:10.1038/ncb3124

Buchacher T, Ohradanova-Repic A, Stockinger H, Fischer MB, Weber V. 2015. M2 polarization of human macrophages favors survival of the intracellular pathogen chlamydia pneumoniae. *PLoS ONE* **10:** e0143593. doi:10.1371/journal.pone.0143593

Chastagnier L, Marquette C, Petiot E. 2023. In situ transient transfection of 3D cell cultures and tissues, a promising tool for tissue engineering and gene therapy. *Biotechnol Adv* **68:** 108211. doi:10.1016/j.biotechadv.2023.108211

Chen F, Byrd AL, Liu J, Flight RM, DuCote TJ, Naughton KJ, Song X, Edgin AR, Lukyanchuk A, Dixon DT, et al. 2023. Polycomb deficiency drives a FOXP2-high aggressive state targetable by epigenetic inhibitors. *Nat Commun* **14:** 336. doi:10.1038/s41467-023-35784-x

Commisso C, Davidson SM, Soydaner-Azeloglu RG, Parker SJ, Kamphorst JJ, Hackett S, Grabocka E, Nofal M, Drebin JA, Thompson CB, et al. 2013. Macropinocytosis of protein is an amino acid supply route in Ras-transformed cells. *Nature* **497:** 633–637. doi:10.1038/nature12138

Davies PSW. 2020. Stable isotopes: their use and safety in human nutrition studies. *Eur J Clin Nutr* **74:** 362–365. doi:10.1038/s41430-020-0580-0

Dhillon S. 2018. Ivosidenib: first global approval. *Drugs* **78:** 1509–1516. doi:10.1007/s40265-018-0978-3

Fan TW, Lane AN. 2016. Applications of NMR spectroscopy to systems biochemistry. *Prog Nucl Magn Reson Spectrosc* **92–93:** 18–53. doi:10.1016/j.pnmrs.2016.01.005

Fan T, Bandura L, Higashi R, Lane A. 2005. Metabolomics-edited transcriptomics analysis of Se anticancer action in human lung cancer cells. *Metabolomics* **1:** 325–339. doi:10.1007/s11306-005-0012-0

Fan TW, Lane AN, Higashi RM, Farag MA, Gao H, Bousamra M, Miller DM. 2009. Altered regulation of metabolic pathways in human lung cancer discerned by ^{13}C stable isotope-resolved metabolomics (SIRM). *Mol Cancer* **8:** 41. doi:10.1186/1476-4598-8-41

Fan TW, Lane AN, Higashi RM, Yan J. 2011. Stable isotope resolved metabolomics of lung cancer in a SCID mouse model. *Metabolomics* **7:** 257–269. doi:10.1007/s11306-010-0249-0

Fan TW, Lane AN, Higashi RM. 2016a. Stable isotope resolved metabolomics studies in ex vivo tissue slices. *Bio Protoc* **6:** e1730.

Fan TW, Warmoes MO, Sun Q, Song H, Turchan-Cholewo J, Martin JT, Mahan A, Higashi RM, Lane AN. 2016b. Distinctly perturbed metabolic networks underlie differential tumor tissue damages induced by immune modulator β-glucan in a two-case ex vivo non-small-cell lung cancer study. *Cold Spring Harb Mol Case Stud* **2:** a000893. doi:10.1101/mcs.a000893

Fan TW, El-Amouri SS, Macedo JKA, Wang QJ, Song H, Cassel T, Lane AN. 2018. Stable isotope-resolved metabolomics shows metabolic resistance to anti-cancer selenite in 3D spheroids versus 2D cell cultures. *Metabolites* **8:** 40. doi:10.3390/metabo8030040

Fan TWM, Bruntz RC, Yang Y, Song H, Chernyavskaya Y, Deng P, Zhang Y, Shah PP, Beverly LJ, Qi Z, et al. 2019. De novo synthesis of serine and glycine fuels purine nucleotide biosynthesis in human lung cancer tissues. *J Biol Chem* **294:** 13464–13477. doi:10.1074/jbc.RA119.008743

Fan TWM, Higashi RM, Chernayavskaya Y, Lane AN. 2020. Resolving metabolic heterogeneity in experimental models of the tumor microenvironment from a stable isotope resolved metabolomics perspective. *Metabolites* **10:** 249. doi:10.3390/metabo10060249

Fan TW, Higashi RM, Song H, Daneshmandi S, Mahan AL, Purdom MS, Bocklage TJ, Pittman TA, He D, Wang C, et al. 2021. Innate immune activation by checkpoint inhibition in human patient-derived lung cancer tissues. *eLife* **10:** e69578. doi:10.7554/eLife.69578

Fan TW, Daneshmandi S, Cassel TA, Uddin MB, Sledziona J, Thompson PT, Lin P, Higashi RM, Lane AN. 2022. Polarization and β-glucan reprogram immunomodulatory metabolism in human macrophages and ex vivo in human lung cancer tissues. *J Immunol* **209:** 1674–1690. doi:10.4049/jimmunol.2200178

Fu X, Deja S, Fletcher JA, Anderson NN, Mizerska M, Vale G, Browning JD, Horton JD, McDonald JG, Mitsche MA, et al. 2021. Measurement of lipogenic flux by deuterium resolved mass spectrometry. *Nat Commun* **12:** 3756. doi:10.1038/s41467-021-23958-4

Hanahan D, Weinberg RA. 2011. Hallmarks of cancer: the next generation. *Cell* **144:** 646–674. doi:10.1016/j.cell.2011.02.013

Han JM, Jeong Seung J, Park Min C, Kim G, Kwon Nam H, Kim Hoi K, Ha Sang H, Ryu Sung H, Kim S. 2012. Leucyl-tRNA synthetase is an intracellular leucine sensor for the mTORC1-signaling pathway. *Cell* **149:** 410–424. doi:10.1016/j.cell.2012.02.044

Hattori A, Tsunoda M, Konuma T, Kobayashi M, Nagy T, Glushka J, Tayyari F, McSkimming D, Kannan N, Tojo A, et al. 2017. Cancer progression by reprogrammed BCAA metabolism in myeloid leukaemia. *Nature* **545:** 500–504. doi:10.1038/nature22314

Hensley CT, Faubert B, Yuan Q, Lev-Cohain N, Jin E, Kim J, Jiang L, Ko B, Skelton R, Loudat L, et al. 2016. Metabolic heterogeneity in human lung tumors. *Cell* **164:** 681–694. doi:10.1016/j.cell.2015.12.034

Hou X, Zaks T, Langer R, Dong Y. 2021. Lipid nanoparticles for mRNA delivery. *Nat Rev Mater* **6:** 1078–1094. doi:10.1038/s41578-021-00358-0

Humpel C. 2015. Organotypic brain slice cultures: a review. *Neuroscience* **305:** 86–98. doi:10.1016/j.neuroscience.2015.07.086

Jones JG, Solomon MA, Cole SM, Sherry AD, Malloy CR. 2001. An integrated ^{2}H and ^{13}C NMR study of gluconeogenesis and TCA cycle flux in humans. *Am J Physiol Endocrinol Metab* **281:** E848–E856. doi:10.1152/ajpendo.2001.281.4.E848

King A, Selak MA, Gottlieb E. 2006. Succinate dehydrogenase and fumarate hydratase: linking mitochondrial dysfunction and cancer. *Oncogene* **25:** 4675–4682. doi:10.1038/sj.onc.1209594

Kodama M, Oshikawa K, Shimizu H, Yoshioka S, Takahashi M, Izumi Y, Bamba T, Tateishi C, Tomonaga T, Matsumoto M, et al. 2020. A shift in glutamine nitrogen metabolism contributes to the malignant progression of cancer. *Nat Commun* **11:** 1320. doi:10.1038/s41467-020-15136-9

Kohlmeier M. 2015. *Leucine.* Academic, Cambridge, MA.

Landau BR. 1999. Quantifying the contribution of gluconeogenesis to glucose production in fasted human subjects using stable isotopes. *Proc Nutr Soc* **58:** 963–972. doi:10.1017/S0029665199001275

Lane AN, Fan TW, Bousamra M II, Higashi RM, Yan J, Miller DM. 2011. Stable isotope-resolved metabolomics (SIRM) in cancer research with clinical application to nonsmall cell lung cancer. *OMICS* **15:** 173–182. doi:10.1089/omi.2010.0088

Lane AN, Higashi RM, Fan TW. 2020. Metabolic reprogramming in tumors: contributions of the tumor microenvironment. *Genes Dis* **7:** 185–198. doi:10.1016/j.gendis.2019.10.007

Lee JH, Cho YR, Kim JH, Kim J, Nam HY, Kim SW, Son J. 2019. Branched-chain amino acids sustain pancreatic cancer growth by regulating lipid metabolism. *Exp Mol Med* **51:** 1–11.

Leitch CA, Jones PJ. 1993. Measurement of human lipogenesis using deuterium incorporation. *J Lipid Res* **34:** 157–163. doi:10.1016/S0022-2275(20)41329-X

Le Page LM, Guglielmetti C, Taglang C, Chaumeil MM. 2020. Imaging brain metabolism using hyperpolarized ^{13}C magnetic resonance spectroscopy. *Trends Neurosci* **43:** 343–354. doi:10.1016/j.tins.2020.03.006

Liu M, Luo F, Ding C, Albeituni S, Hu X, Ma Y, Cai Y, McNally L, Sanders MA, Jain D, et al. 2015. Dectin-1 activation by a natural product β-glucan converts immunosuppressive macrophages into an M1-like phenotype. *J Immunol* **195:** 5055–5065. doi:10.4049/jimmunol.1501158

Liu Y, Ma G, Liu J, Zheng H, Huang G, Song Q, Pang Z, Du J. 2022. SLC7A5 is a lung adenocarcinoma-specific prognostic biomarker and participates in forming immunosuppressive tumor microenvironment. *Heliyon* **8:** e10866. doi:10.1016/j.heliyon.2022.e10866

Luengo A, Gui DY, Vander Heiden MG. 2017. Targeting metabolism for cancer therapy. *Cell Chem Biol* **24:** 1161–1180. doi:10.1016/j.chembiol.2017.08.028

Maher EA, Marin-Valencia I, Bachoo RM, Mashimo T, Raisanen J, Hatanpaa KJ, Jindal A, Jeffrey FM, Choi C, Madden C, et al. 2012. Metabolism of [U-^{13}C]glucose in human brain tumors in vivo. *NMR Biomed* **25:** 1234–1244. doi:10.1002/nbm.2794

Martínez-Reyes I, Chandel NS. 2021. Cancer metabolism: looking forward. *Nat Rev Cancer* **21:** 669–680. doi:10.1038/s41568-021-00378-6

Mayers JR, Torrence ME, Danai LV, Papagiannakopoulos T, Davidson SM, Bauer MR, Lau AN, Ji BW, Dixit PD, Hosios AM, et al. 2016. Tissue of origin dictates branched-chain amino acid metabolism in mutant *Kras*-driven cancers. *Science* **353:** 1161–1165. doi:10.1126/science.aaf5171

Mellor AL, Munn DH. 2008. Creating immune privilege: active local suppression that benefits friends, but protects foes. *Nat Rev Immunol* **8:** 74–80. doi:10.1038/nri2233

Merritt ME, Harrison C, Sherry AD, Malloy CR, Burgess SC. 2011. Flux through hepatic pyruvate carboxylase and phosphoenolpyruvate carboxykinase detected by hyperpolarized ^{13}C magnetic resonance. *Proc Natl Acad Sci* **108:** 19084–19089. doi:10.1073/pnas.1111247108

Nelson SJ, Kurhanewicz J, Vigneron DB, Larson PE, Harzstark AL, Ferrone M, van Criekinge M, Chang JW, Bok R, Park I, et al. 2013. Metabolic imaging of patients with prostate cancer using hyperpolarized [1-^{13}C]pyruvate. *Sci Transl Med* **5:** 198ra108. doi:10.1126/scitranslmed.3006070

Oba M, Tanaka M. 2012. Intracellular internalization mechanism of protein transfection reagents. *Biol Pharm Bull* **35:** 1064–1068. doi:10.1248/bpb.b12-00001

Pavlova NN, Thompson CB. 2016. The emerging hallmarks of cancer metabolism. *Cell Metab* **23:** 27–47. doi:10.1016/j.cmet.2015.12.006

Raggi F, Pelassa S, Pierobon D, Penco F, Gattorno M, Novelli F, Eva A, Varesio L, Giovarelli M, Bosco MC. 2017. Regulation of human macrophage M1-M2 polarization balance by hypoxia and the triggering receptor expressed on myeloid cells-1. *Front Immunol* **8:** 1097. doi:10.3389/fimmu.2017.01097

Robert JJ, Beaufrere B, Koziet J, Desjeux JF, Bier DM, Young VR, Lestradet H. 1985. Whole body de novo amino acid synthesis in type I (insulin-dependent) diabetes studied with stable isotope-labeled leucine, alanine, and glycine. *Diabetes* **34:** 67–73. doi:10.2337/diab.34.1.67

Ruigrok MJR, Maggan N, Willaert D, Frijlink HW, Melgert BN, Olinga P, Hinrichs WLJ. 2017. siRNA-mediated RNA interference in precision-cut tissue slices prepared from mouse lung and kidney. *AAPS J* **19:** 1855–1863. doi:10.1208/s12248-017-0136-y

Sellers K, Fox MP, Bousamra M, Slone SP, Higashi RM, Miller DM, Wang Y, Yan J, Yuneva MO, Deshpande R, et al. 2015. Pyruvate carboxylase is critical for non-small-cell lung cancer proliferation. *J Clin Invest* **125:** 687–698. doi:10.1172/JCI72873

Strohecker AM, Guo JY, Karsli-Uzunbas G, Price SM, Chen GJ, Mathew R, McMahon M, White E. 2013. Autophagy sustains mitochondrial glutamine metabolism and growth of *Braf*^{V600E}-driven lung tumors. *Cancer Discov* **3:** 1272–1285. doi:10.1158/2159-8290.CD-13-0397

Sun RC, Fan TWM, Deng P, Higashi RM, Lane AN, Le AT, Scott TL, Sun Q, Warmoes MO, Yang Y. 2017. Noninvasive liquid diet delivery of stable isotopes into mouse models for deep metabolic network tracing. *Nat Commun* **8:** 1646. doi:10.1038/s41467-017-01518-z

Sushentsev N, McLean MA, Warren AY, Benjamin AJV, Brodie C, Frary A, Gill AB, Jones J, Kaggie JD, Lamb BW, et al. 2022. Hyperpolarised ^{13}C-MRI identifies the emergence of a glycolytic cell population within intermediate-risk human prostate cancer. *Nat Commun* **13:** 466. doi:10.1038/s41467-022-28069-2

Thompson CB. 2009. Metabolic enzymes as oncogenes or tumor suppressors. *N Engl J Med* **360:** 813–815. doi:10.1056/NEJMe0810213

Tomás-Bort E, Kieler M, Sharma S, Candido JB, Loessner D. 2020. 3D approaches to model the tumor microenvironment of pancreatic cancer. *Theranostics* **10:** 5074–5089. doi:10.7150/thno.42441

Toro JR, Nickerson ML, Wei MH, Warren MB, Glenn GM, Turner ML, Stewart L, Duray P, Tourre O, Sharma N, et al. 2003. Mutations in the fumarate hydratase gene cause hereditary leiomyomatosis and renal cell cancer in families in North America. *Am J Hum Genet* **73:** 95–106. doi:10.1086/376435

Tredan O, Galmarini CM, Patel K, Tannock IF. 2007. Drug resistance and the solid tumor microenvironment. *J Natl Cancer Inst* **99:** 1441–1454. doi:10.1093/jnci/djm135

Viana LR, Tobar N, Busanello ENB, Marques AC, de Oliveira AG, Lima TI, Machado G, Castelucci BG, Ramos CD, Brunetto SQ, et al. 2019. Leucine-rich diet induces a shift in tumour metabolism from glycolytic towards oxidative phosphorylation, reducing glucose consumption and metastasis in Walker-256 tumour-bearing rats. *Sci Rep* **9:** 15529. doi:10.1038/s41598-019-52112-w

Wagenmakers AJ. 1999. Tracers to investigate protein and amino acid metabolism in human subjects. *Proc Nutr Soc* **58:** 987–1000. doi:10.1017/S0029665199001305

Warburg O. 1924. Über den Stoffwechsel der Carcinomzelle. *Naturwissenschaften* **12:** 1131–1137. doi:10.1007/BF01504608

Warburg O. 1956. On the origin of cancer cells. *Science* **123:** 309–314. doi:10.1126/science.123.3191.309

Wei Z, Liu X, Cheng C, Yu W, Yi P. 2020. Metabolism of amino acids in cancer. *Front Cell Dev Biol* **8:** 603837. doi:10.3389/fcell.2020.603837

White E, Lattime EC, Guo JY. 2021. Autophagy regulates stress responses, metabolism, and anticancer immunity. *Trends Cancer* **7:** 778–789. doi:10.1016/j.trecan.2021.05.003

Yan J, Lima Goncalves CF, Korfhage MO, Hasan MZ, Fan TWM, Wang X, Zhu C. 2023. Portable optical spectroscopic assay for non-destructive measurement of key metabolic parameters on in vitro cancer cells and organotypic fresh tumor slices. *Biomed Opt Express* **14:** 4065–4079. doi:10.1364/BOE.497127

Yuneva M. 2008. Finding an "Achilles' heel" of cancer: the role of glucose and glutamine metabolism in the survival of transformed cells. *Cell Cycle* **7:** 2083–2089. doi:10.4161/cc.7.14.6256

Zhong H, De Marzo AM, Laughner E, Lim M, Hilton DA, Zagzag D, Buechler P, Isaacs WB, Semenza GL, Simons JW. 1999. Overexpression of hypoxia-inducible factor 1α in common human cancers and their metastases. *Cancer Res* **59:** 5830–5835.

Cite this article as *Cold Spring Harb Perspect Med* doi: 10.1101/cshperspect.a041552

Cancer Metabolism: Aspirations for the Coming Decade

Ralph J. DeBerardinis,[1] Karen H. Vousden,[2] and Navdeep S. Chandel[3]

[1]Howard Hughes Medical Institute and Children's Research Institute, University of Texas Southwestern Medical Center, Dallas, Texas 75390, USA

[2]The Francis Crick Institute, London NW1 1AT, United Kingdom

[3]Department of Medicine, Biochemistry and Molecular Genetics, Northwestern University Feinberg School of Medicine, Chicago, Illinois 60611, USA

Correspondence: Ralph.Deberardinis@UTSouthwestern.edu

Fueled by technological and conceptual advancements over the past two decades, research in cancer metabolism has begun to answer questions dating back to the time of Otto Warburg. But, as with most fields, new discoveries lead to new questions. This review outlines the emerging challenges that we predict will drive the next few decades of cancer metabolism research. These include developing a more realistic understanding of how metabolic activities are compartmentalized within cells, tissues, and organs; how metabolic preferences in tumors evolve during cancer progression from nascent, premalignant lesions to advanced, metastatic disease; and, most importantly, how we can best translate basic observations from preclinical models into novel therapies that benefit patients with cancer. With modern tools and an incredible amount of talent focusing on these problems, the upcoming decades should bring transformative discoveries.

Who knows how Otto Warburg would react to learning that his work on glycolysis and respiration launched an entire field of cancer biology, still accelerating after a century of discoveries. Warburg died in 1970. That was a pivotal time in cancer research, 11 years after Hungerford and Nowell described the Philadelphia chromosome, and a few short years before Varmus and Bishop reported the cellular origin of oncogenes that caused cancer. These discoveries in cancer genetics sidelined the "metabolic theory of cancer," but only temporarily. Over the past few decades, advances in genetics, cell biology, molecular biology, and biochemistry have become integrated into cancer metabolism research. This produced a sea change in how we think about metabolic reprogramming and how we study it.

So what will the next few decades bring? Where are the current knowledge gaps, and how can we close them? Below, we propose a few areas where progress has been bottlenecked by a lack of knowledge, technological capabilities, or both. Discovery in these areas could change the trajectory of the entire field.

METABOLIC COMPARTMENTATION IN CANCER

Posters of metabolic pathways show the sequence of biochemical events connecting nutrients to end products, but they undersell the immense complexity of how these pathways operate in intact cells and tissues. In reality, metabolism is compartmentalized in various ways to enhance rapid flow from beginning to end, or to optimize flow by physically separating segments of the pathway from each other. Despite advances in the breadth and sensitivity of metabolic analysis, most assays still rely on bulk analysis of single tissues, making it difficult to probe spatial dimensions of metabolism. This is an important gap, because compartmentation contributes to flux regulation in many ways, including in cancer.

Metabolic Compartmentation within Cells

The sequestration of enzymes and pathways into different membrane-bound organelles is the most basic and widely studied aspect of metabolic compartmentation. Although enzyme localization within organelles has been known for decades, it has been difficult to obtain reliable assessments of the metabolic makeup of these compartments. New techniques enabling rapid harvest of mitochondria, lysosomes, peroxisomes, etc. (Chen et al. 2024) have helped in this regard. Assessing metabolism in more porous organelles like the nucleus is still a challenge. This is relevant to cancer research because of the reliance of epigenetic enzymes on metabolites, such as acetyl-CoA, S-adenosylmethionine, and α-ketoglutarate, within the nucleus.

Some pathways are compartmentalized without the help of membrane-bound organelles, instead using the physical clustering of enzymes to facilitate substrate channeling and prevent intermediates from diffusing into the aqueous milieu (Pareek et al. 2021). The term "metabolon" refers to a form of pathway compartmentation defined by physical clustering of sequential enzymes in the same pathway to promote channeling and perhaps to enable metabolites arising from different sources (e.g., inside the cell vs. taken up

from outside) to be processed differently (Srere 1987). The purinosome, composed of enzymes in de novo inosine monophosphate synthesis, is a classic metabolon that enables cluster channeling. This complex is assembled and disassembled during the cell cycle, presumably linking purine synthesis to genome replication (Chan et al. 2015). The mechanisms allowing enzymes to participate in metabolon-like clusters are undefined, but it would be reasonable to explore whether growth-factor signaling cascades contribute to this process. This could open up new insights into the nature of metabolic flux regulation in both healthy tissues and cancer.

Metabolic Compartmentation among Different Cell Types

The tumor microenvironment (TME) includes immune cells, stromal cells, endothelial cells, and others in addition to the malignant cells. Current metabolomic technologies generally miss this complexity by using homogenized tissue samples that lump together all cell types. Research over the next decade needs to get past this kind of bulk averaging analysis. Ultimately, we need to know the metabolic contributions of each cell type, how the metabolic properties of each cell type affect all the others, and how these metabolic interactions contribute to cancer progression. This will require significant technological advancements but should be worth the effort, because reductionist approaches have already identified examples of productive metabolic interactions among cell types in the TME. Coculture experiments revealed that pancreatic stellate cells produce and secrete alanine, which is taken up and metabolized by pancreatic cancer cells (Sousa et al. 2016). In vivo, preventing stellate cells from releasing alanine reduced their ability to promote tumor growth. Axons from peripheral nerves can also release nutrients for consumption by malignant cells (Banh et al. 2020). There are likely many more such examples, and we need better ways to directly probe the intact TME to systematically identify new aspects of metabolic cross talk. Although further technical advances are needed, it is possible that mass spectrometry imaging (MSI) will eventually allow us to assess metabolic interactions between cell types, with resolution at the level of individual cells. There are also opportunities to use genetically encoded metabolite sensors to study metabolic interactions in intact tissues.

Metabolic Compartmentation between Tumor and Distant Organs

Tumor metabolism influences and is influenced by metabolism in the rest of the body. We are only in the early stages of understanding how these interactions affect cancer progression and health of the patient. Recent discoveries emphasize the potential for this area of research. Autophagy provides cell-autonomous metabolic advantages to cancer cells, but inactivating autophagy in the host reduces growth of transplanted tumors in mice. This indicates that some benefits of autophagy are extrinsic to the tumor (Yang et al. 2018). One such benefit involves making nutrients systemically available to the tumor. Lack of hepatic autophagy causes the liver to release arginase-1. This depletes arginine from the bloodstream, inducing arginine starvation in tumors and reducing their growth (Poillet-Perez et al. 2018). Another example of organ-level metabolic compartmentation is the observation that glucose oxidation to CO_2 flows in part through lactate. In this pathway, glucose is taken up and converted to lactate in one tissue, then lactate is secreted into the bloodstream, taken up elsewhere, and oxidized to CO_2 in the tricarboxylic acid (TCA) cycle. This is relevant to cancer because the pyruvate oxidized in tumors is partially fed by circulating lactate, and this activity promotes metastasis in mice (Faubert et al. 2017; Hui et al. 2017; Tasdogan et al. 2020). Advances in isotope tracing and computational flux analysis should permit the discovery of other mechanisms by which the contributions of multiple organs determine metabolism in tumors. There is also a pressing need to understand the biology of cachexia, which contributes to morbidity and mortality in many forms of cancer. This systemic phenotype likely involves compartmentalized metabolic activities in the tumor, liver, adipose tissue, and muscle.

THE METABOLIC BASIS OF CANCER PROGRESSION

Tumor metabolism is thought to evolve during progression from pre-neoplastic lesions to locally invasive tumors to lethal metastatic dissemination. We should seek to identify metabolic liabilities at every stage. An area where we currently know very little is in the nascent aspects of cancer progression; specifically, tumor initiation and growth into lesions large enough to come to clinical attention. We need to explore these processes, which may involve a combination of metabolic effects of somatic mutation, altered epigenetics, and interactions with the microenvironment. Understanding these metabolic influences could help explain how common comorbidities such as obesity and diabetes increase the incidence of some kinds of cancer, and uncover interventions that could be used in at-risk individuals to reduce the number of patients who develop cancer. Mouse models will help, but the links between cancer and multifactorial metabolic conditions such as obesity and diabetes surely differ between humans and mice. We suggest that actionable discoveries will require intense clinical research specifically designed to uncover new aspects of pathophysiology in humans, followed by mechanistic work in mice and other experimental systems that recapitulate the most relevant components of the pathophysiology.

An orthogonal approach to studying the metabolic basis of cancer initiation is to focus on inborn errors of metabolism (IEMs) that cause cancer. These are rare monogenic diseases caused by germline mutations in genes encoding enzymes and other proteins involved in the metabolism. Because these are monogenic diseases, all aspects of the pathophysiology arise from a single defective node of the metabolic network. Some of these diseases enhance cancer risk, implying that certain metabolic perturbations are sufficient for cancer initiation in sensitive tissues (Erez and DeBerardinis 2015). This greatly simplifies how to think about the relationship between metabolism and cancer initiation. IEMs have already proven valuable in understanding the role of metabolic perturbation at the earliest stages of cancer. The seminal discovery that mutant isoforms of IDH1 and IDH2 produce *R*-2-hydroxyglutarate (*R*-2HG) in gliomas (Dang et al. 2009) is an example of this. Among over 1400 known IEMs, the only one associated with brain tumors is L-2-hydroxyglutaric aciduria, an autosomal-recessive disease caused by defects in the enzyme that converts *S*-2HG into α-ketoglutarate. The fact that enantiomers of the same metabolite accumulate in both L-2-hydroxyglutaric aciduria and in tumors with IDH1/2 mutations strongly implied that elevation of *R*-2HG directly contributes to malignancy, as opposed to any other putative effects of mutant IDH1/2. This insight informed the development of drugs targeting mutant IDH1/2 and stimulated basic research into mechanisms of transformation.

Other IEMs promote cancer in different organs, particularly the liver. In glycogen storage disease type 1A, loss of glucose-6-phosphatase (encoded by *G6PC*) causes excessive glycogen accumulation, hypoglycemia, and hepatic tumors. A fraction of sporadic, adult-onset hepatocellular carcinomas also contain mutations in *G6PC*, raising the possibility that glycogen accumulation and/or associated metabolic disturbances are sufficient to cause cancer. Indeed, work from genetically modified mice showed that glycogen induces liquid–liquid phase separation in hepatocytes in a manner that activates Yap and drives hepatocyte growth and tumorigenesis (Liu et al. 2021).

Most cancer-related deaths result from tumors with acquired therapy resistance and/or metastasis to distant organs. Metabolic evolution in these later stages of progression is an active area of study and has been reviewed elsewhere (Faubert et al. 2020). We certainly need better ways to prevent tumors from reaching these late stages and to treat the ones that do. Several challenges cells must surmount along the metastatic cascade impose metabolic liabilities, and some are targetable in mice. These include the need to resist oxidative stress after escape from the primary tumor and the need to maintain metabolic flexibility during dormancy to use whatever nutrients are available at the metastatic site (Piskounova et al. 2015;

Ubellacker et al. 2020; Parida et al. 2023). In both mice and patients, metastatic tumors activate the TCA cycle relative to tumors at the primary site (Bartman et al. 2023; Bezwada et al. 2024); the mechanistic basis for this shift is unclear but it occurs in multiple kinds of cancer, suggesting that it reflects a common metabolic demand during dissemination. Metabolic changes also accompany acquired therapy resistance because the cells emerging from cytotoxic therapy often share molecular properties with convergent metabolic preferences. For example, small-cell lung cancers that relapse after platinum-etoposide therapy are enriched for *MYC* overexpression, and this induces metabolic liabilities that can be exploited to kill these otherwise highly resistant tumors (Chalishazar et al. 2019; Huang et al. 2021). The principle that relapsed and metastatic tumors are selected from preexisting clones within heterogeneous primary tumors should make it possible to use lineage-tracing techniques to identify the metabolic properties of cells destined to drive cancer progression.

NEXT-GENERATION APPROACHES TO METABOLIC THERAPY

Many attempts have been made over the past 20 years to target tumor metabolism in patients, so far with limited success. Mutant-selective IDH1/2 inhibitors have been effective in patients whose tumors contain the relevant mutations. But most other metabolic inhibitors have failed to produce clinical benefits beyond standard therapies, and some have caused dose-limiting, on-target toxicities. This has led to calls for more basic research before proceeding with additional interventional trials (Zhang and Dang 2023).

There is no doubt that further exploration of fundamental mechanisms will help identify new pathways worth targeting and better explain how these activities support cancer progression. But regardless of how much preclinical work is carried out, we also need to rethink how we capitalize on information from model systems and how we deploy new investigational agents into clinical trials. The following are a few thoughts about approaches that could help increase the likelihood of success in clinical trials and reduce risks to patients unlikely to benefit from experimental agents.

First, there are untapped opportunities to incorporate metabolic analysis into patient stratification. Human tumor metabolism is incredibly heterogeneous, even among tumors from the same site. But most clinical trials studying metabolic inhibitors do not consider interpatient metabolic heterogeneity. They choose tumor types that seem to share metabolic properties as a group rather than developing ways to assess metabolic properties within individual tumors. Surrogate biomarkers like gene expression are too often used to infer metabolic activity, rather than assessing metabolism directly, and proof-of-concept preclinical studies too often use models of questionable metabolic fidelity to tumors in patients. These uncertainties add up to a recipe for failure. Think of the experience with mutant IDH1/2 inhibitors as a counterexample, where mutations in IDH1/2 were used as enrollment biomarkers, and levels of *R*-2HG could be used to assess pharmacodynamics. Other trials using metabolic inhibitors have nowhere near this level of clarity. Very few make a serious attempt to document which pathways are active in which tumors. Therefore, we cannot tell whether a therapeutic failure means that the drug failed to inhibit the target, the tumor compensated by activating an alternative pathway, or simply that too many of the wrong patients got the drug. Yes, we need more basic science around metabolic targets. But in parallel, we should be developing techniques to reliably assess metabolic activity in tumors on a patient-by-patient basis, then learning how to integrate these approaches into clinical trials. Magnetic resonance spectroscopy, positron emission tomography, metabolomics, and stable isotope tracing can all be used to assess tumor metabolism in individual patients. Perhaps better use of these techniques would improve the success rate of clinical trials.

Second, we can do more to develop rational combinations that include metabolic inhibitors. This is becoming essential because newer classes of therapies like targeted therapies and immunotherapies pervade modern clinical oncology. Demonstrating improvement over standard of care for a metabolic agent now often requires that it be tested in combination with other agents. Targeted therapies that inhibit growth factor signaling pathways block nutrient uptake and central carbon metabolism. Tumor cell metabolism is thought to contribute to immunosuppression within the TME. These considerations suggest ample opportunities to find contexts where metabolic blockade could synergize with existing drugs. Recent work with DRP-104 and similar molecules demonstrates this point (Leone et al. 2019; Pillai et al. 2024). These drugs are broadly acting antagonists of enzymes that use glutamine as a substrate. Blockade of these enzymes suppresses tumor cell growth directly, but the drugs also enhance antitumor immunity by making the TME more hospitable to cytotoxic T cells. This results in potent combinatorial effects between DRP-104 and checkpoint inhibitors, a remarkable finding given that many metabolic pathways are thought to be shared between tumor cells and cytotoxic T cells.

Finally, we believe the time is right to thoroughly examine the preventative and therapeutic effects of dietary modification, and to define contexts where particular diets could be useful in patients. Given the immense capacity of the human body to tolerate dietary modification, this approach could lead to many different applications in many kinds of cancer. Recent work in mice has demonstrated the extent to which the diet impacts tumor dependence on metabolic pathways and modulates therapeutic responses (Hopkins et al. 2018; Lien et al. 2021). Elimination of specific nutrients from the diet can be used in rational combination with metabolic inhibitors to suppress tumor growth in mice (Tajan et al. 2021). In addition to hypothesis testing about dietary therapies in experimental models, we suggest that all clinical trials involving metabolic therapies should incorporate rigorous dietary records of all participants. This may uncover unexpected combinations that modify responses to the drug.

CLOSING THOUGHTS

The history of cancer metabolism research mirrors the progression of cancer itself. Initiated by

Warburg, the field flourished for several decades before lying dormant, only to resurge together with new technologies and ideas, returning it to the leading edge of research. Discoveries from cancer metabolism have disseminated into many other areas of research, including stem cell biology, development, and immunity. The future of metabolism in cancer research is poised for significant advancements driven by an evolving understanding of metabolic reprogramming and its implications for tumor progression and therapy. Sophisticated animal models, advanced metabolic imaging techniques, and cooperative, multidisciplinary efforts will be crucial in translating findings from experimental models to clinical practice. This nuanced approach promises to reveal actionable metabolic vulnerabilities, leading to more effective and personalized cancer treatments.

REFERENCES

*Reference is also in this subject collection.

Banh RS, Biancur DE, Yamamoto K, Sohn ASW, Walters B, Kuljanin M, Gikandi A, Wang H, Mancias JD, Schneider RJ, et al. 2020. Neurons release serine to support mRNA translation in pancreatic cancer. *Cell* 183: 1202–1218.e25. doi:10.1016/j.cell.2020.10.016

Bartman CR, Weilandt DR, Shen Y, Lee WD, Han Y, TeSlaa T, Jankowski CSR, Samarah L, Park NR, da Silva-Diz V, et al. 2023. Slow TCA flux and ATP production in primary solid tumours but not metastases. *Nature* 614: 349–357. doi:10.1038/s41586-022-05661-6

Bezwada D, Perelli L, Lesner NP, Cai L, Brooks B, Wu Z, Vu HS, Sondhi V, Cassidy DL, Kasitinon S, et al. 2024. Mitochondrial complex I promotes kidney cancer metastasis. *Nature* doi:10.1038/s41586-024-07812-3

Chalishazar MD, Wait SJ, Huang F, Ireland AS, Mukhopadhyay A, Lee Y, Schuman SS, Guthrie MR, Berrett KC, Vahrenkamp JM, et al. 2019. MYC-driven small-cell lung cancer is metabolically distinct and vulnerable to arginine depletion. *Clin Cancer Res* 25: 5107–5121. doi:10.1158/1078-0432.CCR-18-4140

Chan CY, Zhao H, Pugh RJ, Pedley AM, French J, Jones SA, Zhuang X, Jinnah H, Huang TJ, Benkovic SJ. 2015. Purinosome formation as a function of the cell cycle. *Proc Natl Acad Sci* 112: 1368–1373. doi:10.1073/pnas.1423009112

* Chen WW, Pacold ME, Sabatini DM, Kanarek N. 2024. Technologies for decoding cancer metabolism with spatial resolution. *Cold Spring Harb Perspect Med* doi:10.1101/cshperspect.a041553

Dang L, White DW, Gross S, Bennett BD, Bittinger MA, Driggers EM, Fantin VR, Jang HG, Jin S, Keenan MC, et al. 2009. Cancer-associated IDH1 mutations produce 2-hydroxyglutarate. *Nature* 462: 739–744. doi:10.1038/nature08617

Erez A, DeBerardinis RJ. 2015. Metabolic dysregulation in monogenic disorders and cancer—finding method in madness. *Nat Rev Cancer* 15: 440–448. doi:10.1038/nrc3949

Faubert B, Li KY, Cai L, Hensley CT, Kim J, Zacharias LG, Yang C, Do QN, Doucette S, Burguete D, et al. 2017. Lactate metabolism in human lung tumors. *Cell* 171: 358–371.e9. doi:10.1016/j.cell.2017.09.019

Faubert B, Solmonson A, DeBerardinis RJ. 2020. Metabolic reprogramming and cancer progression. *Science* 368: eaaw5473. doi:10.1126/science.aaw5473

Hopkins BD, Pauli C, Du X, Wang DG, Li X, Wu D, Amadiume SC, Goncalves MD, Hodakoski C, Lundquist MR, et al. 2018. Suppression of insulin feedback enhances the efficacy of PI3K inhibitors. *Nature* 560: 499–503. doi:10.1038/s41586-018-0343-4

Huang F, Huffman KE, Wang Z, Wang X, Li K, Cai F, Yang C, Cai L, Shih TS, Zacharias LG, et al. 2021. Guanosine triphosphate links MYC-dependent metabolic and ribosome programs in small-cell lung cancer. *J Clin Invest* 131: e139929. doi:10.1172/JCI139929

Hui S, Ghergurovich JM, Morscher RJ, Jang C, Teng X, Lu W, Esparza LA, Reya T, Le Z, Yanxiang Guo J, et al. 2017. Glucose feeds the TCA cycle via circulating lactate. *Nature* 551: 115–118. doi:10.1038/nature24057

Leone RD, Zhao L, Englert JM, Sun IM, Oh MH, Sun IH, Arwood ML, Bettencourt IA, Patel CH, Wen J, et al. 2019. Glutamine blockade induces divergent metabolic programs to overcome tumor immune evasion. *Science* 366: 1013–1021. doi:10.1126/science.aav2588

Lien EC, Westermark AM, Zhang Y, Yuan C, Li Z, Lau AN, Sapp KM, Wolpin BM, Vander Heiden MG. 2021. Low glycaemic diets alter lipid metabolism to influence tumour growth. *Nature* 599: 302–307. doi:10.1038/s41586-021-04049-2

Liu Q, Li J, Zhang W, Xiao C, Zhang S, Nian C, Li J, Su D, Chen L, Zhao Q, et al. 2021. Glycogen accumulation and phase separation drives liver tumor initiation. *Cell* 184: 5559–5576.e19. doi:10.1016/j.cell.2021.10.001

Pareek V, Sha Z, He J, Wingreen NS, Benkovic SJ. 2021. Metabolic channeling: predictions, deductions, and evidence. *Mol Cell* 81: 3775–3785. doi:10.1016/j.molcel.2021.08.030

Parida PK, Marquez-Palencia M, Ghosh S, Khandelwal N, Kim K, Nair V, Liu XZ, Vu HS, Zacharias LG, Gonzalez-Ericsson PI, et al. 2023. Limiting mitochondrial plasticity by targeting DRP1 induces metabolic reprogramming and reduces breast cancer brain metastases. *Nat Cancer* 4: 893–907. doi:10.1038/s43018-023-00563-6

Pillai R, LeBoeuf SE, Hao Y, New C, Blum JLE, Rashidfarrokhi A, Huang SM, Bahamon C, Wu WL, Karadal-Ferrena B, et al. 2024. Glutamine antagonist DRP-104 suppresses tumor growth and enhances response to checkpoint blockade in *KEAP1* mutant lung cancer. *Sci Adv* 10: eadm9859. doi:10.1126/sciadv.adm9859

Piskounova E, Agathocleous M, Murphy MM, Hu Z, Huddlestun SE, Zhao Z, Leitch AM, Johnson TM, DeBerardinis RJ, Morrison SJ. 2015. Oxidative stress inhibits distant metastasis by human melanoma cells. *Nature* 527: 186–191. doi:10.1038/nature15726

Poillet-Perez L, Xie X, Zhan L, Yang Y, Sharp DW, Hu ZS, Su X, Maganti A, Jiang C, Lu W, et al. 2018. Autophagy maintains tumour growth through circulating arginine. *Nature* **563:** 569–573. doi:10.1038/s41586-018-0697-7

Sousa CM, Biancur DE, Wang X, Halbrook CJ, Sherman MH, Zhang L, Kremer D, Hwang RF, Witkiewicz AK, Ying H, et al. 2016. Pancreatic stellate cells support tumour metabolism through autophagic alanine secretion. *Nature* **536:** 479–483. doi:10.1038/nature19084

Srere PA. 1987. Complexes of sequential metabolic enzymes. *Annu Rev Biochem* **56:** 89–124. doi:10.1146/annurev.bi.56.070187.000513

Tajan M, Hennequart M, Cheung EC, Zani F, Hock AK, Legrave N, Maddocks ODK, Ridgway RA, Athineos D, Suárez-Bonnet A, et al. 2021. Serine synthesis pathway inhibition cooperates with dietary serine and glycine limitation for cancer therapy. *Nat Commun* **12:** 366. doi:10.1038/s41467-020-20223-y

Tasdogan A, Faubert B, Ramesh V, Ubellacker JM, Shen B, Solmonson A, Murphy MM, Gu Z, Gu W, Martin M, et al. 2020. Metabolic heterogeneity confers differences in melanoma metastatic potential. *Nature* **577:** 115–120. doi:10.1038/s41586-019-1847-2

Ubellacker JM, Tasdogan A, Ramesh V, Shen B, Mitchell EC, Martin-Sandoval MS, Gu Z, McCormick ML, Durham AB, Spitz DR, et al. 2020. Lymph protects metastasizing melanoma cells from ferroptosis. *Nature* **585:** 113–118. doi:10.1038/s41586-020-2623-z

Yang A, Herter-Sprie G, Zhang H, Lin EY, Biancur D, Wang X, Deng J, Hai J, Yang S, Wong KK, et al. 2018. Autophagy sustains pancreatic cancer growth through both cell-autonomous and nonautonomous mechanisms. *Cancer Discov* **8:** 276–287. doi:10.1158/2159-8290.CD-17-0952

Zhang X, Dang CV. 2023. Time to hit pause on mitochondria-targeting cancer therapies. *Nat Med* **29:** 29–30. doi:10.1038/s41591-022-02129-y

Index